Handbook of Nonprescription *Drugs*

ELEVENTH EDITION

Notices

The listing of selected brand names is intended only for ease of reference. The listed brand names are a representative sampling of drug products, not a comprehensive listing. The inclusion of a brand name does not mean the editors or publisher has any particular knowledge that the brand listed has properties different from other brands of the same drug, nor should its inclusion be interpreted as an endorsement by the editors or publisher. Similarly, the fact that a particular brand has not been included does not indicate the product has been judged to be in any way unsatisfactory or unacceptable.

The convention followed in this book to identify brand names of drugs and other products is to use initial capital letters (when appropriate). Nonproprietary, generic, or common names of such products are cited without initial capitalization.

The nature of drug information is that it is constantly evolving because of ongoing research and clinical experience and is often subject to interpretation. Although great care has been taken to ensure the accuracy of the information presented herein, the reader is advised that the authors, editors, reviewers, contributors, and publisher cannot be held responsible for the continued currency of the information or for any errors or omissions in this book or for any consequences arising therefrom. Readers are advised that decisions regarding drug therapy must be based on the independent judgment of the clinician, changing information about a drug (eg, as reflected in the literature and manufacturer's most current product information), and changing medical practices.

The editors, authors, and contributors have written this book in their private capacities. No official support or endorsement by any federal or state agency or pharmaceutical company is intended or inferred.

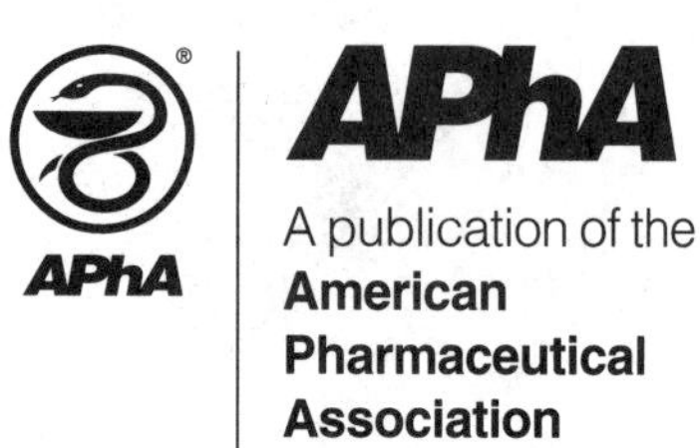

APhA

A publication of the
American Pharmaceutical Association

Handbook of Nonprescription *Drugs*

Published by

American Pharmaceutical Association

The National Professional Society of Pharmacists

2215 Constitution Avenue, NW

Washington, DC 20037

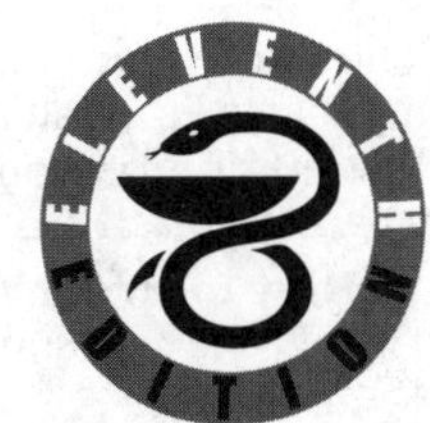

Dedicated
to William L. Blockstein
9th Edition Pharmaceutical Editor
and staunch APhA supporter

Tim R. Covington, PharmD
Pharmaceutical Editor

Rosemary R. Berardi, PharmD
Section Editor, Gastrointestinal Products

Linda L. Young
Managing Editor

Susan C. Kendall
Editorial Coordinator

Mary Jane Hickey
Director, Art and Production

Editorial Services: Publications Professionals, Inc

Anatomic Drawings: Walter Hilmers, Jr, Judith M. Guenther, Alexa L. Chun, Marie A. Dauenheimer

Color Illustration Contributors: Jean A. Borger, Richard C. Childers, Stanley Cullen, Alfred C. Griffin (deceased), Harold L. Hammond, R. Gary Sibbald

Printing: United Book Press, Inc

Library of Congress Catalog Card Number: 86-71446
ISSN 0889-7816
ISBN 0-917330-77-3

How to Order This Book
By phone: 800-878-0729—VISA, MasterCard, and American Express cards accepted.

Contents

Contributors

Advisory Panel

Manju T. Beier, PharmD
President, Geriatric Consultant Resources, Ann Arbor, Michigan

William L. Blockstein, PhD†
Professor Emeritus, School of Pharmacy, University of Wisconsin-Madison, Madison, Wisconsin

Carol A. Bugdalski, BS Pharmacy
Vice-President, Pharmacy, Arbor Drugs, Inc, Troy, Michigan

Brian Bullock, BS Pharmacy, MBA
Director, Benefit Management Services, Health Care Pharmacy Providers, Inc, Carrollton, Texas

Tom Dammer
National Accounts Manager, SmithKline Beecham Consumer Healthcare, Pittsburgh, Pennsylvania

Janet P. Engle, PharmD
Associate Dean for Academic Affairs, Clinical Associate Professor of Pharmacy Practice, College of Pharmacy, University of Illinois at Chicago, Chicago, Illinois

Edward G. Feldmann, PhD
President, Pharmaceutical Consultant Services, Falls Church, Virginia

Jack E. Fincham, PhD
Dean and Professor of Pharmacy Practice, School of Pharmacy, The University of Kansas, Lawrence, Kansas

Daniel A. Hussar, PhD
Remington Professor of Pharmacy, Philadelphia College of Pharmacy and Science, Philadelphia, Pennsylvania

Jerry D. Karbeling, BS Pharmacy
Community Pharmacist, Big Creek Pharmacy, Polk City, Iowa

Howard Maibach, MD
Dermatology Department, University of California Hospital, San Francisco, California

Milap C. Nahata, PharmD
Professor of Pharmacy and Pediatrics, College of Pharmacy, The Ohio State University, Columbus, Ohio

Chapter 1

Author

Tim R. Covington, MS, PharmD
Bruno Professor of Pharmacy, Director of Managed Care Institute, School of Pharmacy, Samford University, Birmingham, Alabama

Reviewers

Robert J. Anderson, PharmD
Professor, Southern School of Pharmacy, Mercer University, Atlanta, Georgia

Metta Lou Henderson, PhD
Professor of Pharmacy, Raabe College of Pharmacy, Ohio Northern University, Ada, Ohio

Dennis M. Williams, PharmD
Assistant Professor, School of Pharmacy, University of North Carolina, Chapel Hill, North Carolina

Chapter 2

Authors

Wendy Klein-Schwartz, PharmD
Associate Professor, School of Pharmacy, University of Maryland, Baltimore, Maryland

Brian J. Isetts, RPh, PhD, FASCP
Director of Pharmacy Operations, Red Wing Corner Drug and Clinic Pharmacy, Red Wing, Minnesota

Reviewers

Danial E. Baker, PharmD, FASCP, FASHP
Director, Drug Information Center and Clinical Pharmacy Programs, College of Pharmacy, Washington State University at Spokane, Spokane, Washington

Amy Broeseker, RN, PharmD
Assistant Professor, School of Pharmacy, Samford University, Birmingham, Alabama

Virginia J. Galizia, PhD
Associate Clinical Professor and Acting Dean, College of Pharmacy and Allied Health Professions, St. John's University, Jamaica, New York

William C. Gong, PharmD, FASHP
Director, Residency and Fellowship Programs, School of Pharmacy, University of Southern California, Los Angeles, California

Daniel A. Hussar, PhD
Remington Professor of Pharmacy, Philadelphia College of Pharmacy and Science, Philadelphia, Pennsylvania

† Deceased

Chapter 3

Authors
Wendy P. Munroe, PharmD
President, MedOutcomes, Inc, Richmond, Virginia
Marcus D. Wilson, PharmD
Assistant Professor of Clinical Pharmacy, Philadelphia College of Pharmacy and Science, Philadelphia, Pennsylvania

Reviewers
Stephen M. Caiola, MS
Associate Professor and Vice Chairman of Pharmacy Practice, School of Pharmacy, University of North Carolina, Chapel Hill, North Carolina
Diane Nykamp McCarter, PharmD
Professor of Pharmacy, Southern School of Pharmacy, Mercer University, Atlanta, Georgia
Susan M. Meyer, PhD
Director of Academic Affairs, American Association of Colleges of Pharmacy, Alexandria, Virginia

Chapter 4

Author
Arthur G. Lipman, PharmD
Professor of Clinical Pharmacy, College of Pharmacy and Pain Management Center, University Hospitals and Clinics, University of Utah Health Sciences Center, Salt Lake City, Utah

Case Studies Author
Micheline Goldwire, MS
Clinical Coordinator of Drug Information, Pharmacy Department, Texas Children's Hospital, Houston, Texas

Reviewers
Ann B. Amerson, PharmD
Professor, College of Pharmacy, University of Kentucky, Lexington, Kentucky
Richard D. Leff, PharmD, FCCP
Professor of Pediatrics and Pharmacy, University of Kansas, Kansas City, Kansas
James K. Marttila, PharmD
Pharmaceutical Manager, Mayo Foundation/Mayo Clinic, Rochester, Minnesota
J. Edwin Underwood, Jr, PharmD
Assistant Professor, School of Pharmacy, Samford University, Birmingham, Alabama

Chapter 5

Author
Arthur I. Jacknowitz, PharmD
Professor and Chair, Department of Clinical Pharmacy, School of Pharmacy, West Virginia University Health Sciences Center, Morgantown, West Virginia

Reviewers
Martin D. Higbee, PharmD
Associate Professor, College of Pharmacy, The University of Arizona, Tucson, Arizona
Phillip Oppenheimer, PharmD
Associate Dean, School of Pharmacy, University of Southern California, Los Angeles, California
Martha M. Rumore, PharmD, JD, FAPPM
Associate Professor, Arnold & Marie Schwartz College of Pharmacy, Brooklyn, New York
Craig S. Stern, PharmD, MBA, FASCP, FASHP
President, ProPharma Pharmaceutical Consultants, Inc, Northridge, California

Chapter 6

Authors
Leslie A. Shimp, MS, PharmD
Associate Professor of Pharmacy, College of Pharmacy, University of Michigan, Ann Arbor, Michigan
Constance M. Fleming, PharmD
Director of Experiential Programs, School of Pharmacy, Campbell University, Buies Creek, North Carolina

Reviewers
Connie Lee Barnes, PharmD
Assistant Professor, School of Pharmacy, Campbell University, Buies Creek, North Carolina
Charma A. Konnor, PharmD
Director, Division of Drug Quality Education, Food and Drug Administration, Rockville, Maryland
Geralynn B. Smith, MS
Assistant Professor, College of Pharmacy and Allied Health, Wayne State University, Detroit, Michigan
Linda Gore Sutherland, MBA, RPh
Coordinator, Drug Information Center, School of Pharmacy, University of Wyoming, Laramie, Wyoming

Chapter 7

Authors
Louise Parent-Stevens, PharmD
Clinical Assistant Professor, College of Pharmacy, University of Illinois at Chicago, Chicago, Illinois
David L. Lourwood, PharmD, BCPS
Clinical Assistant Professor of Pharmacy Practice, College of Pharmacy; Clinical Assistant Professor of Obstetrics and Gynecology, College of Medicine; University of Illinois at Chicago, Chicago, Illinois

Reviewers
Kim Coccodrilli Coley, PharmD
Assistant Professor, School of Pharmacy, University of Pittsburgh, Pittsburgh, Pennsylvania
Sandra Hardee Lilley, PharmD, BCPS
Assistant Professor, School of Medicine, East Carolina University, Greenville, North Carolina

Timothy D. Moore, MS, RPh
Administrative Director and Clinical Professor, The Ohio State University Hospitals, Columbus, Ohio
Ronald J. Ruggiero, PharmD
Clinical Professor, School of Pharmacy, University of California, San Francisco, California

Chapter 8

Author

Karen J. Tietze, PharmD
Associate Professor of Clinical Pharmacy, Philadelphia College of Pharmacy and Science, Philadelphia, Pennsylvania

Reviewers

Bruce C. Carlstedt, PhD
Associate Professor of Clinical Pharmacy, Purdue University, West Lafayette, Indiana
Jeffrey C. Delafuente, MS
Professor and Associate Chairman, Department of Pharmacy Practice, College of Pharmacy, University of Florida, Gainesville, Florida
H. Won Jun, PhD
Professor of Pharmaceutics, College of Pharmacy, The University of Georgia, Athens, Georgia
Jeff Taylor, MSc
Assistant Professor of Pharmacy Practice, College of Pharmacy, University of Saskatchewan, Saskatoon, Saskatchewan, Canada

Chapter 9

Authors

Dennis M. Williams, PharmD
Assistant Professor, School of Pharmacy, University of North Carolina, Chapel Hill, North Carolina
Timothy H. Self, PharmD
Professor of Clinical Pharmacy, College of Pharmacy, University of Tennessee, Memphis, Tennessee

Case Studies Coauthor

Cynthia Toso, PharmD
Drug Information Associate, Glaxo Wellcome Inc, Research Triangle Park, North Carolina

Reviewers

Carol E. Howard, MS, PharmD
Assistant Professor, School of Pharmacy, Samford University, Birmingham, Alabama
H. William Kelly, PharmD
Professor and Area Head of Pharmacy Practice, College of Pharmacy, University of New Mexico Health Sciences Center, Albuquerque, New Mexico
Craig S. Stern, RPh, PharmD, MBA, FASCP, FASHP
President, ProPharma Pharmaceutical Consultants, Inc, Northridge, California
Mark Stiling, BS Pharmacy, PharmD, RPh
Medical Services Manager, Bristol-Myers Squibb, Louisville, Kentucky

Chapter 10

Authors

M. Lynn Crismon, PharmD, FCCP
Professor of Clinical Pharmacy, Head of Clinical Pharmacy Division, College of Pharmacy, University of Texas at Austin, Austin, Texas
Donna M. Jermain, PharmD
Clinical Specialist, Scott & White Hospital, Temple, Texas

Case Studies Author

Micheline Goldwire, MS
Clinical Coordinator of Drug Information, Pharmacy Department, Texas Children's Hospital, Houston, Texas

Reviewers

Kenneth A. Bachmann, PhD, FCP
Distinguished University Professor and Chair, Department of Pharmacology, College of Pharmacy, The University of Toledo, Toledo, Ohio
Alice L. Paysinger, PharmD
Ambulatory Care Pharmacotherapy Specialist, Department of Veterans Affairs Medical Center, Jackson, Mississippi
Michael Z. Wincor, PharmD
Assistant Professor of Clinical Pharmacy, School of Pharmacy; Assistant Professor of Psychiatry and the Behavioral Sciences, School of Medicine; University of Southern California, Los Angeles, California

Chapter 11

Authors

Julianne B. Pinson, PharmD
Assistant Professor of Pharmacy Practice, School of Pharmacy, Campbell University, Buies Creek, North Carolina
C. Wayne Weart, PharmD
Professor of Community Pharmacy Practice and Administration, Associate Professor of Family Medicine, College of Pharmacy, Medical University of South Carolina, Charleston, South Carolina

Case Studies Author

Micheline Goldwire, MS
Clinical Coordinator of Drug Information, Pharmacy Department, Texas Children's Hospital, Houston, Texas

Reviewers

Stephen M. Caiola, MS
Associate Professor and Vice Chairman of Pharmacy Practice, School of Pharmacy, University of North Carolina, Chapel Hill, North Carolina
Bruce D. Clayton, BS, PharmD
Professor of Pharmacy Practice, College of Pharmacy and Health Sciences, Butler University, Indianapolis, Indiana
Rex W. Force, PharmD
Assistant Professor, Department of Family Medicine, College of Pharmacy, Idaho State University, Pocatello, Idaho

Robert P. Henderson, PharmD, FASHP, FCCP, BCPS
Professor of Pharmacy Practice, School of Pharmacy, Samford University; Clinical Pharmacy Specialist, Birmingham Baptist Medical Center Princeton; Birmingham, Alabama

Chapter 12

Authors

Clarence E. Curry, Jr, PharmD
Associate Professor of Pharmacy Practice, College of Pharmacy and Pharmaceutical Sciences, Howard University, Washington, DC

Demetris Tatum-Butler, PharmD
Clinical Pharmacy Supervisor, Laurel Regional Hospital, Laurel, Maryland

Reviewers

R. Randolph Beckner, PharmD, MHA
Pharmacy Coordinator, Barnes-Jewish Hospitals, St. Louis, Missouri

Eddie L. Boyd, MS, PharmD
Associate Professor, College of Pharmacy, University of Michigan, Ann Arbor, Michigan

Anthony T. Buatti, MBA
Adjunct Assistant Professor, College of Pharmacy and Allied Health Professions, St. John's University, Jamaica, New York

Janice A. Gaska, PharmD
Adjunct Associate Professor of Clinical Pharmacy, Philadelphia College of Pharmacy and Science, Philadelphia, Pennsylvania

Katheryn W. Russi, BS, MPA
Clinical Pharmacy Manager, Clinical Services Division, PCS Health Systems, Novi, Michigan

Chapter 13

Author

R. Leon Longe, PharmD
Professor, College of Pharmacy, The University of Georgia, Athens, Georgia

Case Studies Author

Micheline Goldwire, MS
Clinical Coordinator of Drug Information, Pharmacy Department, Texas Children's Hospital, Houston, Texas

Reviewers

Mark L. Britton, PharmD, CDE
Clinical Coordinator, Veterans Affairs Medical Center; Clinical Assistant Professor, College of Pharmacy, University of Oklahoma; Oklahoma City, Oklahoma

Joseph T. DiPiro, PharmD
Professor, Medical College of Georgia, University of Georgia, Augusta, Georgia

Herbert L. DuPont, MD
Chief, Internal Medicine Service, St. Luke's Episcopal Hospital, Houston, Texas

Wayne A. Kradjan, PharmD
Professor and Associate Dean, School of Pharmacy, University of Washington, Seattle, Washington

John J. Piecoro, Jr, MS, PharmD
Professor, Division of Pharmacy Practice and Science, College of Pharmacy, University of Kentucky, Lexington, Kentucky

Chapter 14

Author

Benjamin Hodes, PhD
Dean of Continuing Education, Professor of Pharmaceutics, School of Pharmacy, Duquesne University, Pittsburgh, Pennsylvania

Case Studies Author

Micheline Goldwire, MS
Clinical Coordinator of Drug Information, Pharmacy Department, Texas Children's Hospital, Houston, Texas

Reviewers

Thomas D. DeCillis
Captain, US Public Health Service (Retired); Panel Administrator, FDA OTC Review (Emeritus), Food and Drug Administration, Rockville, Maryland

Anthony Palmieri III, PhD
Director of Intellectual Property, The Upjohn Company, Kalamazoo, Michigan

Larry N. Swanson, PharmD
Professor and Chairman, Department of Pharmacy Practice, School of Pharmacy, Campbell University, Buies Creek, North Carolina

Chapter 15

Author

Kathryn K. Bucci, PharmD, BCPS
Associate Professor of Family Medicine and Clinical Associate Professor of Pharmacy Practice, Self Memorial Family Medicine Residency Program, Greenwood, South Carolina, and Medical University of South Carolina, Charleston, South Carolina

Reviewers

J. Fred Bennes, BS
School of Pharmacy, State University of New York at Buffalo, Buffalo, New York

Donald O. Fedder, DrPH, MPH
Professor of Pharmacy Practice, Director of Community Pharmacy Program, School of Pharmacy; Professor of Epidemiology and Preventative Medicine, School of Medicine; University of Maryland at Baltimore, Baltimore, Maryland

Robert A. Mangione, MS
Assistant Dean and Clinical Professor, College of Pharmacy and Allied Health Professions, St. John's University, Jamaica, New York

David E. Stewart, PharmD
Director of Pharmacy, Stones River Hospital, Woodbury, Tennessee

Chapter 16

Authors

Gary M. Oderda, PharmD, MPH
Professor and Chair, Department of Pharmacy Practice, College of Pharmacy, University of Utah, Salt Lake City, Utah

Jenifer C. Jennings, PharmD
Assistant Professor of Clinical Pharmacy, Department of Pharmacy Practice, College of Pharmacy, University of Utah, Salt Lake City, Utah

Reviewers
William D. King, RPh, MPH, DrPH
Associate Professor, Department of Pediatrics, GR Children's Hospital, School of Medicine, University of Alabama at Birmingham, Birmingham, Alabama
Alan H. Lau, PharmD
Associate Professor of Pharmacy Practice, College of Pharmacy, University of Illinois at Chicago, Chicago, Illinois
Anthony J. Silvagni, PharmD, DO, FACOFP
Vice President for Academic Affairs, Dean and Professor of Family Medicine and Clinical Pharmacology, University of Health Sciences, Kansas City, Missouri
Anthony R. Temple, MD
Executive Director, Medical Affairs, McNeil Consumer Products Company, Fort Washington, Pennsylvania

Chapter 17

Author
Michael L. Kleinberg, MS, FASHP
Vice President, Professional Services, Immunex Corporation, Seattle, Washington

Case Studies Author
Micheline Goldwire, MS
Clinical Coordinator of Drug Information, Pharmacy Department, Texas Children's Hospital, Houston, Texas

Reviewers
George B. Browning, BS
President, Medical Arts Pharmacy Inc, Melbourne, Florida
Mary M. Losey, MS
Director, Office of Student Services, School of Pharmacy, Purdue University, West Lafayette, Indiana
Gary Schmidt, RPh
Clinical Pharmacist, Veterans Administration Hospital, Madison, Wisconsin
Joan Lerner Selekof, RN, BSN, CETN
Enterostomal Therapy Nurse, University of Maryland Medical System, Baltimore, Maryland

Chapter 18

Authors
Condit F. Steil, PharmD, CDE
Associate Professor and Director, Center for Pharmaceutical Care Development in Community Practice, School of Pharmacy, Samford University, Birmingham, Alabama
R. Keith Campbell, RPh, FASHP, FAPP
Associate Dean and Professor of Pharmacy Practice, College of Pharmacy, Washington State University, Pullman, Washington
John R. White, Jr, PharmD
Assistant Professor, Washington State University, Spokane, Washington

Reviewers
Danial E. Baker, PharmD, FASCP FASHP
Director, Drug Information Center and Clinical Pharmacy Programs, College of Pharmacy, Washington State University at Spokane, Spokane, Washington
Charles Y. McCall, PharmD, FASHP
Associate Professor, College of Pharmacy, University of Georgia, Athens, Georgia
David A. Sclar, BS Pharmacy, PhD
Boehringer Ingelheim Scholar in Pharmaceutical Economics, Associate Professor of Health Policy and Administration, College of Pharmacy, Washington State University, Pullman, Washington
Kenneth A. Skau, PhD
Associate Professor of Pharmacology, College of Pharmacy, University of Cincinnati, Cincinnati, Ohio
Michael S. Torre, MS, RPh
Clinical Professor of Pharmacy, Department of Clinical Pharmacy Practice, College of Pharmacy and Allied Health Professions, St. John's University, Jamaica, New York

Case Studies Reviewer
Mike Soiland, RPh
Clinical Pharmacist, MedOutcomes, Inc, Richmond, Virginia

Chapter 19

Author
Loyd V. Allen, Jr, PhD
Professor and Chair, Department of Medicinal Chemistry and Pharmaceutics, College of Pharmacy, University of Oklahoma, Oklahoma City, Oklahoma

Reviewers
Carl J. Malanga, PhD
Associate Dean for Academic Affairs and Administration, School of Pharmacy, West Virginia University Health Sciences Center, Morgantown, West Virginia
Merlin V. Nelson, PharmD, MD
Department of Neurology, Henry Ford Hospital, Detroit, Michigan
Gail H. Rosen, PharmD, BCNSP
Nutrition Support Specialist, University of Maryland Medical System, Baltimore, Maryland
J. Ken Walters, PharmD
Director of Pharmacy Services, Sheppard & Enoch Pratt Hospital, Baltimore, Maryland

Chapter 20

Authors
Rosalie Sagraves, PharmD
Dean and Professor, College of Pharmacy, University of Illinois at Chicago, Chicago, Illinois

Claudia Kamper, PharmD
Assistant Professor, College of Pharmacy, University of Oklahoma, Oklahoma City, Oklahoma
Judi Doerr, RD/LD, CNSD, CDE
Nutrition Consultant, Addison Option Care Home IV and Nutritional Services, Oklahoma City, Oklahoma

Reviewers
Cynthia S. Kirman, PharmD
Director, Clinical Information Services, Value Rx Pharmacy Program, Bloomfield Hills, Michigan
Martha A. Ralls, PharmD
Assistant Professor of Pharmacy Practice, School of Pharmacy, Samford University, Birmingham, Alabama
Paul C. Walker, PharmD
Manager, Department of Pharmaceutical Services, Children's Hospital of Michigan, Detroit, Michigan

Chapter 21

Author
Paul L. Doering, MS
Distinguished Service Professor of Pharmacy Practice, College of Pharmacy, University of Florida, Gainesville, Florida

Reviewers
Robert L. Beamer, PhD
Professor of Medicinal Chemistry, Chairman of Department of Basic Pharmaceutical Sciences, College of Pharmacy, University of South Carolina, Columbia, South Carolina
Patricia A. Camazzola, PharmD
Director, Department of Pharmacy, Huron Valley Hospital, Commerce Township, Michigan
William Sanford Lackey, BS, FACA
Wil-Sant Inc, Tucson, Arizona
Nancy A. Letassy, PharmD
Ambulatory Care Clinical Specialist, Veterans Affairs Medical Center, Oklahoma City, Oklahoma
Larry N. Swanson, PharmD
Professor and Chairman, Department of Pharmacy Practice, School of Pharmacy, Campbell University, Buies Creek, North Carolina

Chapter 22

Authors
Mark W. Swanson, OD
Assistant Professor, Department of Optometry, School of Optometry, University of Alabama at Birmingham, Birmingham, Alabama
Jimmy D. Bartlett, OD
Professor of Optometry and Pharmacology, School of Optometry, University of Alabama at Birmingham, Birmingham, Alabama

Reviewers
Chris Bapatla, PhD
Director, Pharmaceutical Technical Affairs, Alcon Laboratories, Inc, Fort Worth, Texas
Alexander F. Demetro, PharmD
Pharmacist, Westwood Prescriptionists, San Jose, California
Richard G. Fiscella, RPh, MS
Assistant Professor, College of Pharmacy, University of Illinois at Chicago, Chicago, Illinois
John R. Yuen, PharmD
Pharmacist Specialist, Kaiser Permanente, Los Angeles, California

Chapter 23

Author
Janet P. Engle, PharmD
Associate Dean for Academic Affairs, Clinical Associate Professor of Pharmacy Practice, School of Pharmacy, University of Illinois at Chicago, Chicago, Illinois

Reviewers
William J. Benjamin, OD, PhD
Professor and Director of Clinical Research, School of Optometry, University of Alabama at Birmingham, Birmingham, Alabama
Timothy S. Lesar, PharmD
Assistant Director of Pharmacy, Albany Medical Center, Albany, New York
Thomas F. Patton, PhD
President, St. Louis College of Pharmacy, St. Louis, Missouri
John R. Yuen, PharmD
Pharmacist Specialist, Kaiser Permanente, Los Angeles, California

Chapter 24

Author
Keith O. Miller, PharmD
Assistant Director of Clinical Pharmacy, Wadley Regional Medical Center, Texarkana, Texas

Reviewers
Carl F. Emswiller, Jr, BS Pharmacy, FACA
Pharmacist, Emswiller Pharmacy, Leesburg, Virginia
E. Paul Larrat, PhD
Assistant Professor of Epidemiology, College of Pharmacy, University of Rhode Island, Kingston, Rhode Island
Michael S. Maddux, PharmD
Assistant Dean for Clinical Development, St. Louis College of Pharmacy, St. Louis, Missouri
Dennis Richmond, MD
Private Practitioner, Family Physician, Lafayette, Indiana

Chapter 25

Author
Arlene A. Flynn, RPh, MEd
Assistant Dean, College of Pharmacy, University of Illinois at Chicago, Chicago, Illinois

Reviewers
Paul L. Doering, MS
Distinguished Service Professor of Pharmacy Practice, College of Pharmacy, University of Florida, Gainesville, Florida
Lowell S. Lakritz, DDS
Private Practitioner, Lakritz & Salzmann, Madison, Wisconsin
Kevin M. Sims, DMD, BS Pharmacy
Department of Periodontics, School of Dentistry, University of Alabama at Birmingham, Birmingham, Alabama
Carl Stone, DDS, MA
Associate Professor, Mercy School of Dentistry, University of Detroit, Detroit, Michigan
Kenneth W. Witte, PharmD
Director of Pharmacy, Michael Reese Hospital, Chicago, Illinois

Chapter 26

Authors
Dennis P. West, PhD, FCCP
Professor of Dermatology, Northwestern University Medical School, Chicago, Illinois
Phillip A. Nowakowski, PharmD
Associate Director of Medical Affairs, GenDerm Corporation, Lincolnshire, Illinois

Reviewers
J. Fred Bennes, BS
School of Pharmacy, State University of New York at Buffalo, Buffalo, New York
Darrell F. Bennett, RPh
Student Health Services, California Polytechnic State University, San Luis Obispo, California
Emery W. Brunett, PhD
School of Pharmacy, University of Wyoming, Laramie, Wyoming
Anthony J. LaMonica, BS
President and Owner, Prescription Shoppe, Inc, Everett, Massachussetts

Chapter 27

Author
Joye Ann Billow, PhD
Professor of Pharmaceutical Sciences, College of Pharmacy, South Dakota State University, Brookings, South Dakota

Reviewers
Robert W. Bennett, MS
Associate Professor of Clinical Pharmacy, School of Pharmacy, Purdue University, West Lafayette, Indiana
Mary Beth Gross, PharmD, FASCP
Manager, Pharmacy Department, Mercy Hospital Medical Center, Des Moines, Iowa
Timothy J. Ives, PharmD, MPH
Associate Professor of Pharmacy, Clinical Associate Professor of Family Medicine, School of Pharmacy, University of North Carolina, Chapel Hill, North Carolina
Henry A. Palmer, PhD
Clinical Professor and Associate Dean, School of Pharmacy, University of Connecticut, Storrs, Connecticut
Charles D. Ponte, PharmD, RPh, CDE, FASHP
Professor of Clinical Pharmacy and Family Medicine, School of Pharmacy, West Virginia University Health Sciences Center, Morgantown, West Virginia

Chapter 28

Authors
Edwina Chan, PharmD
Assistant Professor, School of Pharmacy, Samford University, Birmingham, Alabama
Raymond Benza, MD
Associate in Cardiology and Internal Medicine, University of Alabama at Birmingham, Birmingham, Alabama

Case Studies Author
Micheline Goldwire, MS
Clinical Coordinator of Drug Information, Pharmacy Department, Texas Children's Hospital, Houston, Texas

Reviewers
Miriam P. Calhoun, BS
President, Miriam P. Calhoun, Inc, Potomac, Maryland
Karen Plaisance, PharmD
Associate Professor, School of Pharmacy, University of Maryland, Baltimore, Maryland
John G. Sowell, PhD
Professor of Pharmacology, School of Pharmacy, Samford University, Birmingham, Alabama

Chapter 29

Authors
Gary H. Smith, PharmD
Professor of Pharmacy Practice, College of Pharmacy, The University of Arizona, Tucson, Arizona
Victor A. Elsberry, PharmD
Assistant Professor of Pharmacy Practice, College of Pharmacy, The University of Arizona, Tucson, Arizona
Martin D. Higbee, PharmD
Associate Professor, College of Pharmacy, The University of Arizona, Tucson, Arizona

Reviewers
Miriam P. Calhoun, BS
President, Miriam P. Calhoun, Inc, Potomac, Maryland
Somnath Pal, MBA, PhD
Associate Professor of Pharmacy, College of Pharmacy and Allied Health Professions, St. John's University, Jamaica, New York
Debra Ricciatti-Sibbald, MS
Coordinator of Nonprescription Drugs, University of Toronto, Toronto, Ontario, Canada
Paul C. Walker, PharmD
Manager, Department of Pharmaceutical Services, Children's Hospital of Michigan, Detroit, Michigan

Chapter 30

Author

Edward M. DeSimone II, PhD
Associate Professor of Pharmaceutical and Administrative Sciences, School of Pharmacy and Allied Health Professions, Creighton University, Omaha, Nebraska

Case Studies Author

Micheline Goldwire, MS
Clinical Coordinator of Drug Information, Pharmacy Department, Texas Children's Hospital, Houston, Texas

Reviewers

Julie Rivkin Berman, PharmD
Clinical Specialist–Burn Center, Detroit Receiving Hospital and University Health Center, Detroit, Michigan
Martin J. Jinks, PharmD
Professor and Chair, Department of Pharmacy Practice, College of Pharmacy, Washington State University, Pullman, Washington
Katheryn W. Russi, BS, MPA
Clinical Pharmacy Manager, Clinical Services Division, PCS Health Systems, Novi, Michigan
Stewart B. Siskin, PharmD
Director, Clinical Research–Dermatology, Bristol-Myers Squibb Pharmaceutical Research Institute, Buffalo, New York

Chapter 31

Authors

Robert H. Moore III, PhD
Professor, School of Pharmacy, Samford University, Birmingham, Alabama
John D. Bowman, MS
Assistant Professor of Pharmacy Practice, School of Pharmacy, Samford University, Birmingham, Alabama

Reviewers

Robert W. Bennett, MS
Associate Professor of Clinical Pharmacy, School of Pharmacy, Purdue University, West Lafayette, Indiana
Julie Rivkin Berman, PharmD
Clinical Specialist–Burn Center, Detroit Receiving Hospital and University Health Center, Detroit, Michigan
Miriam P. Calhoun, BS
President, Miriam P. Calhoun, Inc, Potomac, Maryland
Walter T. Gloor, PhD
Consultant in Pharmaceutical Manufacturing, Hiwasse, Arkansas
Katheryn W. Russi, BS, MPA
Clinical Pharmacy Manager, Clinical Services Division, PCS Health Systems, Novi, Michigan

Chapter 32

Author

Henry Wormser, PhD
Professor of Medicinal Chemistry, College of Pharmacy and Allied Health Professions, Wayne State University, Detroit, Michigan

Reviewers

David C. Beck, MD
Clinical Assistant Professor of Dermatology, School of Medicine, Indiana University, West Lafayette, Indiana
Jerry D. Karbeling, BS Pharmacy
Community Pharmacist, Big Creek Pharmacy, Polk City, Iowa
Kenneth R. Keefner, RPh, PhD
Associate Professor, School of Pharmacy and Allied Health Professions, Creighton University, Omaha, Nebraska
Michael Kendrach, PharmD
Associate Director and Assistant Professor, School of Pharmacy, Samford University, Birmingham, Alabama
Robert B. Sause, PhD
Associate Professor, College of Pharmacy and Allied Health Professions, St. John's University, Jamaica, New York
Joel L. Zatz, PhD
Professor of Pharmaceutics, College of Pharmacy, Rutgers University–Busch Campus, Piscataway, New Jersey

Chapter 33

Author

Farid Sadik, PhD
Professor and Associate Dean, College of Pharmacy, University of South Carolina, Columbia, South Carolina

Reviewers

Richard N. Herrier, PharmD
Assistant Professor, College of Pharmacy, University of Arizona, Tucson, Arizona
Howard Maibach, MD
Dermatology Department, University of California Hospital, San Francisco, California
Victor A. Padrón, RPh, PhD
Associate Professor of Pharmaceutical and Administrative Sciences, School of Pharmacy and Allied Health Professions, Creighton University, Omaha, Nebraska
Robert B. Sause, PhD
Associate Professor, College of Pharmacy and Allied Health Professions, St. John's University, Jamaica, New York

Chapter 34

Authors

Nicholas G. Popovich, PhD
Professor of Pharmacy Practice, School of Pharmacy, Purdue University, West Lafayette, Indiana

Gail D. Newton, PhD
Assistant Professor of Pharmacy Practice and Administration, School of Pharmacy, Dusquesne University, Pittsburgh, Pennsylvania

Reviewers

Donald O. Fedder, DrPH, MPH
Professor of Pharmacy Practice, Director of Community Pharmacy Program, School of Pharmacy; Professor of Epidemiology and Preventative Medicine, School of Medicine; University of Maryland at Baltimore, Baltimore, Maryland

Thomas J. Holmes, Jr, PhD
Associate Dean for Student Affairs, School of Pharmacy, Campbell University, Buies Creek, North Carolina

Edward R. Hommel, DPM
Clinical Assistant Professor, Department of Family Medicine, School of Medicine, University of Wisconsin–Madison, Madison, Wisconsin

Damien Howell, MS, PT
Private Practitioner, Damien Howell Physical Therapy, Richmond, Virginia

Chapter 35

Authors

Varro E. Tyler, PhD, ScD
Lilly Distinguished Professor of Pharmacognosy, School of Pharmacy and Pharmacal Sciences, Purdue University, West Lafayette, Indiana

Steven Foster, BS
Associate Editor, American Botanical Council, Fayettville, Arkansas

Reviewers

R. Frank Chandler, PhD
Director and Professor, College of Pharmacy, Dalhousie University, Halifax, Nova Scotia, Canada

June H. McDermott, MS Pharmacy, MBA
Clinical Associate Professor, School of Pharmacy, University of North Carolina, Chapel Hill, North Carolina

E. John Staba, PhD
Professor Emeritus of Pharmacognosy and Medicinal Chemistry, College of Pharmacy, University of Minnesota, Minneapolis, Minnesota

Chapter 36

Author

Jack E. Fincham, PhD
Dean and Professor of Pharmacy Practice, School of Pharmacy, University of Kansas, Lawrence, Kansas

Reviewers

Donald J. Brideau, Jr, MD
Assistant Clinical Professor, School of Medicine, George Washington University, Mount Vernon Medical Group, Alexandria, Virginia

Cheryl Nunn-Thompson, PharmD, BCPS
Clinical Assistant Professor, Pharmacy Practice, Drug Information Specialist, College of Pharmacy, University of Illinois at Chicago, Chicago, Illinois

Jeff Shapiro, RPh
Chief Executive Officer, Shapiro's Drug Store, Inc, Hibbing, Minnesota

Holly Whitcomb, RPh
Community Pharmacist and Co-Owner, View Ridge United Drug, Seattle, Washington

William McGhan, PharmD
Professor of Pharmacy Administration, Philadelphia College of Pharmacy and Science, Philadelphia, Pennsylvania

Preface

Health care in the United States has undergone dramatic changes in the 1990s. Key trends that will continue to shape delivery of health care in the late 1990s include increased reliance on managed care to control costs, a growing interest in the quality of health care, and consumers' greater involvement in and assumption of responsibility for their own care. For health care providers, these trends create a practice environment that can be both extremely rewarding—as more attention is focused on helping patients become effective self-care and disease managers—and challenging—as fewer resources are available to provide this service.

The American Pharmaceutical Association believes that pharmaceutical care is an important component in the delivery of patient care and that it fills critical gaps in the health care environment just described. When pharmacists collaborate with other health care providers and with patients to outline a therapeutic plan and a system of patient follow-up and monitoring, the likelihood that patients can achieve the intended outcomes of therapy is greatly improved. With their knowledge of drug products and therapeutics, pharmacists are well positioned to deliver pharmaceutical care regardless of whether they practice in the community, hospital, managed care, or other pharmacy setting.

Nonprescription drug therapy is an essential component of pharmaceutical care, and the *Handbook of Nonprescription Drugs* seeks to provide a reference to support delivery of the related services. The 11th Edition has been expanded to include discussions of emerging self-care issues, such as herbs and phytomedicinal products, as well as clinical evaluation of nonprescription products that have become available since the last edition. Case studies have been incorporated in the chapters to aid readers in developing the problem-solving and interrogative skills required in nonprescription drug pharmacotherapy. Further, to provide quicker access to information, more subheads have been added and the chapter sections have been reformatted to present a straight-line discussion of conditions and their treatment.

Nonprescription drugs are used extensively to treat a range of self-limiting as well as chronic conditions. Annual purchases of nonprescription medications presently exceed $20 billion dollars. Sales of these medications are likely to grow to more than $30 billion by the year 2000. In addition, more than 600 products formerly available only by prescription have been made available as nonprescription drugs just in the last 20 years. This accelerating trend of reclassifying prescription drugs coupled with the emergence of new classes of nonprescription products will unleash a blizzard of powerful direct-to-consumer advertising to promote product use. Never before have consumers had a greater need for an accessible, learned intermediary to assist them in making the right decisions about product selection and use.

Pharmacists are strategically positioned in health care to assess patients needs, recognize conditions that are self-treatable with nonprescription drugs, and advise and counsel patients. If self-care with nonprescription drug therapy is appropriate, pharmacists can:

- Assess patient risk factors;
- Help in product selection;
- Counsel patients regarding proper use;
- Screen for allergies, adverse drug reactions and side effects, and drug-drug or drug-disease interactions;
- Monitor response to therapy;
- Discourage use of fraudulent or quack remedies;
- Assess the need for referral for medical services.

The 11th Edition of the *Handbook of Nonprescription Drugs* is a vital reference for clinicians providing these services to their patients. The patient assessment techniques and product information are presented as resources to enhance the delivery of pharmaceutical care and to facilitate the provider's role as a self-care adviser to consumers. The American Pharmaceutical Association is pleased to offer this valued resource and pledges an ongoing commitment to continuous expansion and refinement of this important publication.

John A. Gans, PharmD
Executive Vice-President
American Pharmaceutical Association

Introduction

The *Handbook of Nonprescription Drugs* is recognized as the worldwide standard on nonprescription pharmacotherapy. Since its inception in 1967, the *Handbook* has been the primary resource for accomplishing APhA's vision of providing pharmacists and pharmacy students with definitive, current information about patient self-care. The 11th Edition continues this tradition while also broadening its scope to encompass the role of pharmaceutical care in the late 1990s and to provide objective analysis of emerging self-care trends and products.

About the 11th Edition

Each new edition of the *Handbook* builds on the basis and innovations of prior editions and the numerous editors, authors, and reviewers who dedicated themselves to providing high-quality information and analyses. The 11th Edition has retained the following features of past editions that have become the gold standards of self-care and nonprescription pharmacotherapy:

- Assessment criteria;
- Pharmacoepidemiology of the condition;
- Anatomy and physiology of the affected area;
- Pathophysiology of the affected system;
- Signs and symptoms of the condition;
- Drugs indicated to treat the condition;
- Contraindications to drug use;
- Warnings and precautions relative to drug use;
- Adverse effect profile of drugs;
- Drug-drug interactions and potential clinical consequences;
- Special considerations regarding use of a particular drug in pediatric, geriatric, pregnant, or breast-feeding patients;
- Product selection guidelines;
- Administration and dosage guidelines;
- Guidelines for patient education and counseling.

In response to evolving health care trends and consumers' desire to play a greater role in their physical well-being, this edition features discussion of several new topics. To present the information in a readily accessible format, the 11th Edition has also undergone extensive reorganization, including the presentation of chapters and product tables in separate volumes.

New Features and Topics

Consumers' assertiveness in their own health care and interest in alternatives to manufactured drugs, along with the FDA's commitment to streamlining its approval process, provided the impetus for inclusion of three new chapters as well as new topics within several existing chapters. The three new chapters are:

- Herbs and Phytomedicinal Products;
- Smoking Cessation Products;
- First-Aid Products and Minor Wound Care.

New topics added to existing chapters include:

- In-home cholesterol tests;
- Melatonin;
- H_2-receptor antagonists;
- Commercial weight loss products and programs;
- Hair loss and hair regrowth products;
- Adult urinary incontinence.

In response to results from readership surveys, each 11th Edition chapter that discusses specific medical disorders features two case studies based on realistic interactions between patients and pharmacists. The case studies provide an alternative format for readers to use in developing the patient assessment, problem-solving, and interrogative skills needed in delivering pharmaceutical care to self-treating patients.

Reorganization and Formatting

The reordering of chapters in this edition provides a smooth transition from discussion of the continuing evolution of self-care and pharmacists' and the FDA's role in this movement to analyses of medical disorders for which nonprescription pharmacotherapy is appropriate. The majority of chapters that discuss disorders are now grouped by body systems. Any chapter that was added near the end of the production cycle as a result of FDA approval of new nonprescription drugs will be grouped with the appropriate body system in the next edition.

Based on the advisory panel's in-depth review of chapter contents and format, the 11th Edition editors and editorial staff made a concerted effort to streamline discussions of medical conditions and their treatments—

pharmacologic and nonpharmacologic—within a chapter. Input from the advisory panel and *Handbook* users prompted the standardization of subheads among chapters and the addition of numerous subheads within chapters to serve as guideposts for unearthing the *Handbook*'s plethora of "pearls of wisdom" about nonprescription pharmacotherapy. Presenting information in a readily accessible format will continue to be a priority in successive editions.

Cross-References to *Nonprescription Products: Formulations & Features*

APhA has determined that its commitment to providing annual updates of the product tables is best served by splitting the chapters and product tables into separate publications. Each *Handbook* chapter, however, contains cross-references that give the full titles of the appropriate product tables in the new publication *Nonprescription Products: Formulations & Features*. Other cross-references within a chapter will steer readers to in-depth discussions of topics presented either in other sections of that chapter or to separate chapters. When applicable, cross-references to the color photographs are also given.

Purchasers of the 11th Edition of the *Handbook* will receive both publications as part of the purchase price. Those individuals whose main interest is product information may purchase the *Nonprescription Products: Formulations & Features* only.

Acknowledgements

Scores of individuals with demonstrated expertise in nonprescription pharmacotherapy participated in this revamping of the *Handbook*. Although each participant is acknowledged in the list of contributors, the editors and editorial staff wish to express their deep gratitude to the authors and coauthors whose commitment to advancing the standards of self-care continued up to the time this edition went to press. These highly committed health care professionals diligently monitored FDA activities and, when necessary, moved quickly to supply discussion and analyses of newly approved nonprescription drugs.

The 155 peer reviewers, who were selected from many pharmacy practice settings and allied health professions, also merit special recognition and thanks. These individuals ensured that the chapter discussions of self-care and nonprescription pharmacotherapy included the perspectives of their respective practice settings or professions and that the information was of the highest quality.

The 12-member advisory panel undertook the massive task of evaluating the 10th Edition chapters and suggesting improvements for content and organization. The 11th Edition bears the imprint of this undertaking. These individuals, some of whom are also chapter authors, provided the foundation for this and successive editions.

Two APhA staff members undertook the Herculean task of launching the 11th Edition and shepherding it through the editorial and production stages. Linda L. Young, who served as Editorial Coordinator for the 9th Edition and Assistant Managing Editor for the 10th Edition, assumed the responsibilities of Managing Editor for the 11th Edition. As in past editions, she coordinated all facets of the *Handbook's* content and design, ensuring that final copy was accurate, current, and readily accessible. Ms Young also proved to be highly adept at anticipating problems with work flow and taking the necessary steps to keep the project on track.

Susan Kendall resumed the position of Editorial Coordinator for the 11th Edition and is responsible for updating the product tables for the *Nonprescription Products: Formulations & Features*. Ms Kendall kept abreast of the rapid growth of nonprescription product brands and categories by monitoring publications and the shelves of local pharmacies, and by continuing to update and refine her list of contacts at national manufacturers/distributors of nonprescription products. At the appointed time, she drew on all these resources and collaborated with editorial staff to provide the most comprehensive resource available on trade-name nonprescription products.

During the course of producing the 11th Edition, APhA lost one of its staunch supporters, and pharmacy educators lost one of their highly regarded peers. Dr William L. Blockstein served as pharmaceutical editor for the 9th Edition and as an advisory panel member for the 10th and 11th editions. APhA, the editors, and the editorial staff dedicate this edition to Dr Blockstein. His guidance and dedication will be sorely missed in future editions.

Tim R. Covington, PharmD
Pharmaceutical Editor

Rosemary R. Berardi, PharmD
Section Editor, Gastrointestinal Products

Symbols & Abbreviations

The 11th Edition marks a transition in style for technical content in the *Handbook of Nonprescription Drugs*. Past editions have used the American Chemical Society's style for abbreviated units of measurement and time, as well as for other technical material. This edition completes the shift from basic pharmaceutical science to pharmaceutical care by using the American Medical Association's style for most technical content.

Unless designated otherwise, the following selected abbreviations for units of measurement are used in running text, tables, and figures. The abbreviations for medical orders appear primarily in the case studies. Abbreviations of drug names, body systems, diseases, etc, are expanded at first mention in the chapters.

Units of Measurement

'	foot
"	inch
/	per
<	less than
>	greater than
≤	less than or equal to
≥	greater than or equal to
≈	approximately equal to
±	plus or minus
α-TE	alpha-tocopherol equivalent
bpm	beats per minute
c	cup
C	Celsius
Cal	large calorie
cc	cubic centimeter
cm	centimeter
cm^2	square centimeter
dL	deciliter
Eq	equivalent
F	Fahrenheit
fl oz	fluid ounce
ft	foot
g	gram
in.	inch
IU	international unit
kcal	kilocalorie
kg	kilogram
L	liter
lb	pound
m	meter
m^2	square meter
mcg	microgram
mcL	microliter
mcmol	micromole
mcU	microunit
mEq	milliequivalent
mg	milligram
mIU	milli-international unit
mL	milliliter
mm	millimeter
mm Hg	millimeters of mercury
mmol	millimole
mOsm	milliosmole

Units of Measurement *(continued)*

NE	niacin equivalent (tables only)
ng	nanogram (equals a millimicrogram)
nm	nanometer (equals a millimicron)
oz	ounce
pg	picogram (equals a micromicrogram)
ppm	parts per million
psi	pounds per square inch
RE	retinol equivalent
tbsp	tablespoon
tsp	teaspoon
U	unit
Vd	volume of distribution
vol/vol	volume per volume
wt/vol	weight per volume
wt/wt	weight per weight

Units of Time

AM	before noon
PM	after noon

Note: The following abbreviated units of time are used only in tables or figures.

h	hour
min	minute
mo	month
wk	week
y	year

Medical Orders

ac	before meals
bid	two times a day
hs	at bedtime
pc	after meals
po	by mouth
prn	as needed
q4h, q6h, etc	every 4 hours, every 6 hours, etc
qAM	every morning
qid	four times a day
qPM	every evening
tid	three times a day

CHAPTER 1

Self-Care and Nonprescription Pharmacotherapy

Tim R. Covington

The place of nonprescription drug therapy should not be undervalued in a contemporary system of health care delivery and financing. The sales volume of nonprescription drugs currently exceeds $20 billion annually and should reach well over $30 billion by the year 2000. A host of professional, economic, and public interest issues and opportunities are converging to enhance the position of nonprescription drug therapy in the disease management process.

Regrettably, until recently the nonprescription drug therapy domain has been neglected, undervalued, and/or underappreciated by many pharmacy practitioners. This has resulted in a substantial loss of market share by the pharmacy profession. It was not too long ago when America's pharmacies sold approximately 70% of all nonprescription drugs. Today, America's 60,000-plus pharmacies sell 45–50% of nonprescription drugs, with the majority of sales occurring in the nation's other 1 million-plus retail outlets. This situation is less than optimal if public interest is going to be served, therapeutic outcomes are to be maximized, and therapeutic misadventures are to be minimized.

Nonprescription drugs are powerful chemical entities that should be viewed just like prescription drugs relative to their pharmacology, toxicology, contraindications (absolute and relative), precautions for use, adverse effect profile, drug interaction potential, and special considerations in dosage and administration. Indeed, scores of nonprescription drugs were formerly prescription drugs. Moreover, all the expertise that is focused on the safe, appropriate, and effective use of prescription drugs should also be applied to nonprescription drug pharmacotherapy.

With a variety of clinical and economic factors fostering growth of nonprescription drug therapy, the pharmacy profession needs to seriously rethink its professional and business role in this regard. The following market forces and factors should be considered if pharmacy's professional and economic opportunities with nonprescription drug therapy are to be expanded:

- The public's value systems, attitudes, priorities, and levels of sophistication are changing with regard to health matters. The public is becoming increasingly health conscious and wants a better understanding of disease and disease management. Individuals want more control over their personal health care and want to self-medicate when appropriate.
- The reclassification of prescription drugs to nonprescription status has accelerated markedly and is expected to continue at a significant pace. At any point in time, there are approximately 50 prescription drugs in various stages of consideration for reclassification to nonprescription status by the Food and Drug Administration (FDA).
- Managed care and cost containment initiatives by managed care organizations continue to erode profit margins on legend drug dispensing. In more and more instances, profit margins on a $15–25 sale of nonprescription drugs exceed the profit margin on a $30–50 prescription dispensed at the average wholesale price minus a fixed percentage plus a dispensing fee. Further, nonprescription drug sales are typically cash and carry with no third-party constraints (eg, claim submission, 3- to 6-week wait for payment).
- America is aging. It should be noted that the elderly consume a disproportionately large share of both prescription and nonprescription drugs. The US population 65 years of age and older comprise approximately 13% of the total population, yet these 35 million Americans consume 25% of all prescription drugs and 33% of all nonprescription drugs sold.
- Approximately 60% of all dosage units consumed (prescription and nonprescription) are nonprescription drugs.
- Of approximately 3.5 billion health problems treated annually, some 2 billion (57%) are treated with a nonprescription drug.
- Well over 400 medical conditions are treatable with one or more nonprescription drugs as primary or major adjunctive therapy, and many of these conditions occur millions of times each year (Table 1).
- The per capita expenditure for nonprescription drugs is approximately $80 per year and growing.
- The cost-benefit ratio of appropriately used nonprescription drugs is very high. Nonprescription drugs account for less than two cents of every dollar spent on health care in the United States, yet the benefit derived is vast.
- The pharmacist is the most accessible health professional, is the only health professional that receives formal university-based education and training in nonprescription drug pharmacotherapy, and is perceived very favorably by the public. Thus, the pharmacist can and should differentiate him- or herself from other providers of the commodity by offering value-added informational services. Several of these factors will be discussed in more detail further on in this chapter.

Editor's Note: This chapter is based, in part, on the 10th edition chapters "The Self-Care Movement," written by Gary A. Holt and Edwin L. Hall, and "FDA's Review of OTC Drugs," written by William E. Gilbertson.

TABLE 1 Selected medical conditions amenable to nonprescription drug therapy[a]

Abrasions	Colds (viral upper respiratory infections)	Fever	Pharyngitis
Aches and pains (general, mild to moderate)	Congestion (chest, nasal)	Flatulence	Pinworm infestation
Acne	Conjunctivitis	Gastritis	Premenstrual syndrome
Allergic rhinitis	Constipation	Gingivitis	Prickly heat
Anemia	Contact lens care	Hair loss	Psoriasis
Arthralgia	Contraception	Halitosis	Ringworm
Asthma	Corns	Head lice	Seborrhea
Athlete's foot	Cough	Headache	Sinusitis
Bacterial infection (topical, superficial, uncomplicated)	Cuts (superficial)	Heartburn	Smoking cessation
Blisters	Dandruff	Hemorrhoids	Sprains
Blood pressure monitoring	Deficiency disorders (mineral, vitamin, enteral food supplements)	Impetigo	Strains
Boils	Dental care	Indigestion	Stye (hordeolum)
Burns (minor, thermal)	Dermatitis (contact)	Ingrown toenails	Sunburn
Calluses	Diabetes mellitus	Insect bites and stings	Swimmer's ear
Candidal vaginitis	Diaper rash	Insomnia	Teething
Canker sores	Diarrhea	Jet lag	Thrush
Carbuncles	Dry skin	Jock itch	Toothache
Chapped skin	Dysmenorrhea	Motion sickness	Vomiting
Cold sores	Dyspepsia	Myalgia	Warts (common and plantar)
	Feminine hygiene	Nausea	Xerostomia
		Nutrition (infant)	Wound care
		Obesity	
		Ostomy care	
		Otitis (external)	
		Periodontal disease	

[a]The pertinent nonprescription drug(s) for a particular condition may serve as primary or major adjunctive therapy.

The Self-Care Revolution

Many consumers desire and are taking a much more informed and active role in managing their own health care. The term "lifestyle medicine" has been coined to describe the partnership between informed health care consumers and health care providers. Documentation of the self-care revolution lies in the hundreds of self-help books, health-related newspaper features, television and radio programs, instructional audio and videotapes, and articles that proliferate in various magazines for the mass market. A host of factors may influence individual attitudes, values, and practices relative to self-care (Table 2). These attitudes, values, and practices vary from individual to individual. This stratification of the population at large should be taken into account by health care providers, and patients should be viewed as individuals with unique backgrounds and needs.

Surveys consistently demonstrate that consumers are increasingly self-medicating with nonprescription drugs. The following points reveal selected attitudes of nonprescription drug consumers about this practice[1]:

- Almost 7 in 10 consumers prefer to fight symptoms without taking medication, if possible.
- Approximately 9 out of 10 consumers realize they should take medication only when absolutely necessary.
- Eighty-five percent of consumers believe it is important to have access to nonprescription medications to help relieve minor medical problems.
- Of consumers who discontinued their nonprescription medication, 90% did so because their medical problem/symptoms were resolved.
- For problems treated with nonprescription medications, 94% of consumers report they would use the same product again for the same condition.
- Even though a medication may be available without a prescription, 94% of consumers agreed that care should be taken when using it.
- Nearly all consumers (93%) report that they read instructions before taking a nonprescription medication for the first time.
- Eighty-one percent of consumers believe that the pharmacist is a good source of nonprescription drug information.
- Fifty-four percent of consumers believe that the availability of products reclassified from prescription to nonprescription status has made it possible to save the time and expense of going to a physician for management of some conditions.
- Two out of every three consumers favor the reclassification process.

Over the past decade, the health problems most likely to be treated with a nonprescription drug have not changed substantially. Headache leads the list, fol-

TABLE 2 Selected attitudes, values, and practices likely to influence self-care behavior

Attitudes/Beliefs

Appreciation of the value of wellness and prevention initiatives in managing illness

Willingness to accept a significant degree of personal responsibility for one's own health

Motivation and commitment to become a learner relative to the disease in question and its proper treatment

Perception of the degree of seriousness of the medical condition one wishes to prevent or treat

Acceptance of traditional health care providers

Acceptance of the traditional health care delivery process

Willingness to communicate with legitimate, informed, mainstream health care providers

Tendency to be influenced by friends, relatives, alternative caregivers, and printed health information that is not mainstream

Demographics

Age

Family size

Gender differences

Socioeconomic position

Economics

Economic status (individual)

Cost of care (products and/or services)

Convenience/access to health care products and/or services

Availability of health care products and/or services

Education/Knowledge

Educational level of individual (public education, college/university education)

Baseline knowledge about the relevant medical condition(s)

Baseline knowledge about the relevant treatment regimen

Ability to comprehend/interpret consumer health information (verbal and written), package labeling, and package insert information

Access to quality consumer health information through the lay press, media, and so forth

Access to mentors and/or learned intermediaries who can assist in interpreting consumer health information as well as offer additional advice and counsel

Susceptibility to vague and/or misleading advertising or claims regarding alternative health care (eg, acupuncture, chelation therapy, megavitamin therapy, naturalism)

lowed by the common cold, muscle aches and pains (including sprains and strains), dermatologic conditions (eg, acne, cold sores, dandruff, dry skin, athlete's foot, jock itch), minor wounds (eg, cuts, scratches), premenstrual and menstrual symptoms, upset stomach, and sleeping problems.

Reports indicate that the average American experiences one potentially self-treatable health problem every 3–4 days and that approximately 90% of the US population consider themselves "a bit under the weather" one or more times each month. Individuals are more likely to self-treat or treat their children when they perceive their illness to be not serious enough to require medical intervention. In one survey, more than 50% of mothers had given their 3-year-olds one or more nonprescription medications within the prior 30 days.[2] An anecdotal report documented the fact that 16 nonprescription medications were on hand in the home for treatment of a child's various conditions. From an economics perspective, a patient was overheard extolling the virtues of nonprescription drugs, saying, "I can treat my headache for a dime. When I go to my doctor, my copayment for the office visit is $15.00 and my copayment on prescription drugs is $5.00 for generics and $15.00 for brand-name drugs. I try to take care of myself when I can."

Self-medication with nonprescription drugs is often the initial level of care in a tiered system of health care. To say that patients have choices in self-care therapy is an understatement. It is estimated that more than 300,000 nonprescription drug formulations are available to consumers. Many products are sold on a local or regional basis only. However, thousands of products have national distribution, and the many choices consumers have can be bewildering.

The self-care revolution involves and should encourage development of knowledge and skill in the promotion of wellness as well as in the treatment of medical conditions. Informed, appropriate, and responsible use of nonprescription drugs is a large part of self-care. Data suggest that the large majority of patients respect these drugs, recognize their limitations, and read labeling information carefully. Yet other consumers are uninformed or misinformed. Casual and inappropriate use of nonprescription drugs can lead to serious adverse consequences of both a direct (eg, adverse drug reaction, drug-drug interaction) and indirect (eg, delays in seeking appropriate medical attention) nature. Such practices should be discouraged and addressed through (1) adequate package labeling, (2) direct-to-consumer advertising that has a strong educational emphasis about the condition(s) being treated and the proper use of the nonprescription drug to ensure an optimal health outcome, and (3) patient education and counseling by pharmacists and other qualified health professionals regarding proper drug selection and use.

The Pharmacist's Responsibility in Pharmaceutical Care

In an era of health care reform and cost containment, numerous issues concerning the quality and cost of health care present practice opportunities to pharmacists. One significant practice opportunity is to serve and assist patients in the management of numerous self-limiting conditions and some chronic conditions with nonprescription drugs.

Self-care with nonprescription drugs should not be a random, uninformed process in which the patient acts alone by default. Consumers want and need more information on the appropriate use of such drugs. In addition to highly readable, understandable, and usable package labeling, patients need access to a qualified, learned intermediary to assist in nonprescription drug selection, use, and monitoring. That person is most logically the community-based pharmacist.

The pharmacist is uniquely qualified to serve the public interest in nonprescription pharmacotherapy because he or she receives university-level education and training in this area that is undergirded by in-depth instruction in pathophysiology, pharmacology, medicinal chemistry, pharmaceutics, and pharmacokinetics. The pharmacist's knowledge and ability are often enhanced by electronic and print databases. Further, the pharmacist is accessible to the public and strategically positioned in the community to serve as a provider of not only the drug but also information on how to maximize the value of drug therapy while minimizing any potential adverse consequences.

In the initial encounter with a patient seeking assistance with nonprescription drug use, the pharmacist should:

- Assess, by interview and observation, the patient's physical complaint/symptoms and medical condition;
- Differentiate self-treatable conditions from those requiring medical intervention;
- Advise and counsel the patient on the proper course of action (ie, no treatment with drug therapy, self-treatment with nonprescription products, or referral to a physician or other caregiver).

If self-treatment with one or more nonprescription drugs is appropriate, the pharmacist is positioned and intellectually equipped to perform the following patient care services:

- Assist in product selection;
- Assess patient risk factors (eg, contraindications, warnings, precautions, comorbidity, age, organ function);
- Counsel the patient regarding proper drug use (eg, dosage, administration technique, monitoring parameters);
- Maintain a patient drug profile that includes nonprescription as well as prescription drugs;
- Monitor drug therapy for:
  - Drug allergies or hypersensitivities;
  - Adverse drug reactions;
  - Drug-drug interactions;
  - An appropriate response to therapy;
  - Signs and symptoms of drug overuse and/or dependency;
- Discourage the use of fraudulent and "quack" remedies;
- Assess the potential of nonprescription drugs to mask symptoms of a more serious condition;
- Prevent delays in seeking appropriate medical attention.

The public's ability to discern appropriately information about the condition being treated and about the clinical significance of the product is highly variable. The array of product choices, line extensions, and overstated or vague and misleading marketing messages create confusion at the very least. Package labeling is generally limited in the breadth and depth of the message it communicates; it can never address the informational needs of patients for all clinical circumstances, and it can be difficult to read. Beyond this, comorbidity and polypharmacy create infinite special considerations in ensuring the safe, appropriate, and effective use of nonprescription drugs. Thus, the pharmacy-patient interaction is vital to optimal nonprescription pharmacotherapy. Further, the pharmacist and other health care providers should recognize the great difference between providing information to and educating patients. Validation of understanding is critical. Patients should be strongly encouraged to comment and ask questions.

The Self-Care/Pharmaceutical Care Synergy

In counseling medical students regarding the potential conflict associated with physicians treating themselves or their own family members, the famous British physician and philosopher, William Osler, warned that subjectivity and emotionalism may enter into treatment decisions. Objectivity in health care decision making is indeed important. Otherwise, caregivers may be tempted to let their emotions interfere with logical, analytical thought. Dr Osler concluded his presentation with his famous quote, "He who treats himself has a fool for a physician."

Such a statement seems to be in conflict with the self-care revolution in the United States. Today, however, many patients are highly literate, knowledgeable about their medical condition and drug therapy, and aware of available informational resources (eg, trade books, magazines, journals, Internet services) that can add objectivity to their decision-making process. Package labeling of nonprescription drugs, despite its many limitations, also fosters appropriate drug use. Nevertheless, most consumers could benefit substantially from consultation with a pharmacist committed to providing patient-focused, health outcome–oriented pharmaceutical care. The availability of a learned intermediary with access to an extraordinary drug information network is vital to optimal self-care practices. Pharmaceutical care and self-care are totally compatible, and the potential for synergy between the self-medicating patient and the committed pharmacist is vast.

Pharmaceutical care in its simplest form is defined as "the patient-focused provision of drug therapy and cognitive services for the purposes of achieving positive health outcomes and improved quality of life." If properly delivered, pharmaceutical care:

- Produces safe, appropriate, effective, and economical drug use;
- Maximizes the benefit of drug therapy;
- Prevents, identifies, and/or resolves drug-related problems and therapeutic misadventures;
- Assists in promoting optimal therapeutic outcomes;
- Delivers highly intellectual/informational, problem-based, outcome-oriented pharmacy services.

System failures in the health care delivery process dramatically validate the pharmaceutical care process and the need for a meaningful patient-pharmacist interaction. For example, approximately 30–50% of prescribed medication is taken incorrectly.[3] Hospital admissions and physician office visits to manage resultant drug-induced problems and therapeutic misadventures cost billions of dollars annually. The direct cost of therapeutic noncompliance and drug-induced morbidity and mortality is estimated to be $50–80 billion annually, which thus exceeds the annual cost of all diabetes care (approximately $50 billion). The indirect costs add another $50 billion per year to management costs.

In a managed care/managed cost environment, the focus on quality of care and improved health outcomes by payers of the nation's health care bills is accelerating rapidly. In an era of health care assessment and accountability, pharmaceutical interventions that produce value (ie, equal or better care at less overall cost) are viewed very favorably.

The basic tenets of pharmaceutical care are:

- Intellectual preparation and competence of the pharmacist;
- Proper attitude, motivation, and interpersonal skills of the pharmacist;
- A patient focus;
- A health outcome focus (therapeutic goal);
- A system for collecting and storing patient information;
- A system for identifying actual and potential drug-related problems;
- The ability of the pharmacist and the infrastructure of pharmacy practice to develop and execute an action plan, document intervention, and measure ultimate clinical and economic value;
- Effective participation of the pharmacist in a patient-monitoring process.

Pharmaceutical care principles and practices are not and should not be limited to legend drug pharmacotherapy. Higher levels of pharmaceutical care are needed in the nonprescription pharmacotherapy domain as well. More initiatives by pharmacists in the delivery of pharmaceutical care services to self-medicating patients is strongly encouraged.

FDA Regulation of Drugs

The first major federal legislation enacted to regulate drugs was the Pure Food and Drugs Act of 1906. "Unsafe" and "nonefficacious" drug products were not actually prohibited by the statute; drugs were required to meet only the standards of strength and purity claimed by manufacturers. Drug safety was not mandated by law until the passage of the 1938 Federal Food, Drug, and Cosmetic Act (1938 Act). Legislation for this new law had been under consideration since 1933, but final passage was compelled by the deaths of more than 100 individuals, many of them children, who used the newly marketed elixir of sulfanilamide, which contained the toxic solvent ethylene glycol (antifreeze) as the vehicle.

The 1962 amendments to the 1938 Act require that all new drugs be shown to be effective for their intended uses. This legislation thus required the FDA to review the effectiveness of the 4,500 new drug products, including 512 nonprescription drugs that had been approved for safety since 1938. In the mid-1960s, the FDA contracted for a review of these drugs through the National Academy of Sciences/National Research Council (NAS/NRC). The agency took the information from the NAS/NRC and, by a procedure called the Drug Efficacy Study Implementation (DESI), determined the effectiveness of all prescription drugs. As the DESI was nearing completion, it became clear that it was time for an extensive examination of the nonprescription drug marketplace. In 1972, the FDA initiated a massive scientific review of the active ingredients in nonprescription drug products to ensure that they were safe and effective and bore fully informative labeling. This review process is often referred to as the over-the-counter (OTC) drug review.

The FDA is also responsible for the reclassification of drugs from prescription to nonprescription status and the establishment of regulations for package labeling.

Quality Assurance of Nonprescription Drugs

Strict manufacturing and distribution standards exist for nonprescription as well as prescription drugs. A detailed presentation of those standards and processes is beyond the scope and purpose of this book. The FDA drug approval process and the OTC drug review process are presented briefly, however, because of their historical significance and professional relevance.

The Drug Approval Process

The 1938 Act required that all new drugs—that is, new drug products introduced after 1938—be proven safe for human use before being marketed and be cleared in advance through a new drug application (NDA). Products marketed prior to 1938 were exempted from the NDA provision under what is commonly referred to as the grandfather clause. Some currently marketed nonprescription drugs, such as aspirin, still fall under this clause. However, the FDA's OTC drug review has evaluated all nonprescription drugs for safety, effectiveness, and labeling, regardless of the date of marketing entry.

Even today, the 1938 Act, as amended, defines a market divided into "new" drugs, which are defined by law as being recognized as safe and effective (RASE), and those that are generally recognized as safe and effective (GRASE); often these latter drugs are referred to as "old" drugs, but such a legal definition does not exist. A new chemical entity never before marketed in the United States would be classified as a new drug and, in most cases, initially approved for prescription use only.

Through NDA procedures, a prescription drug may be reclassified to nonprescription status but remain a new drug. An NDA for a nonprescription drug product can also be approved directly (without reclassification), such as occurred with ibuprofen 200 mg (a dose that was never available by prescription). When a new drug is used for many years by many patients (referred to in the law as "used for a material time and material extent"), it can be considered GRASE. Another mechanism to gain general recognition status for nonprescription drugs has been provided by the FDA's OTC drug review (see the section The OTC Drug Review Process).

New Drug Application An NDA is necessary for a drug that is defined by law as not being recognized as safe and effective (NRASE) until it has been precleared and approved by the agency. Under existing public procedures, some data related to the approval and contained in the NDA (eg, a summary of the safety data and clinical studies) are publicly available. However, trade information (eg, final formulation ingredients and quantities) is held confidential.

The approved NDA is manufacturer specific and allows only the sponsor to market the product. Any other manufacturer interested in marketing a similar product would also first need to seek FDA approval through an appropriate NDA. In some cases, a full NDA is not necessary for the second manufacturer; an abbreviated application may be submitted instead, eliminating the need for duplicative testing.

All NDAs must contain complete (exact) labeling information, with final printed labeling usually being the last step prior to approval (see the section Nonprescription Drug Labeling). Most subsequent revisions in labeling require preapproval through a supplement to the application. Therefore, labeling is highly restricted and often takes considerable time to change. Similarly, except for some minor changes, the final product formulation cannot be changed without an applicable approved supplement to the application. Finally, periodic submissions—for example, a brief summary of significant new information from the previous year that might affect the safety, effectiveness, or labeling, including any actions taken by the sponsor as a result of these findings—are required in order to report postmarketing information. Distribution data, minor labeling revisions, chemistry, and manufacturing and control changes must also be reported.

Monographs An OTC monograph is developed for a drug that is defined by law as GRASE. A manufacturer desiring to market a monographed drug need not seek prior clearance from the FDA. In this case, marketing is not exclusive; any manufacturer may market a similar product without specific approval. Under the monograph approach, all data and information supporting GRASE status are publicly available. The OTC drug review has established the monographs through a complex, public process. Each individual rulemaking has resulted in an extensive, administrative, public record.

For the final monograph, the manufacturer has considerable flexibility in labeling. All the required monograph labeling must be included; for example, antacids must include terms such as *heartburn, acid indigestion,* and *sour stomach*. In addition, language not included in the monograph may be used in the label without prior approval. For example, *hospital tested* or *pleasant-tasting antacid* are terms considered outside the scope of the monograph but permissible in antacid labeling. However, even though these permissible terms are not precleared, they are subject to the general labeling provision of the 1938 Act and may not be false or misleading.

Monographs primarily address active ingredient(s) in the product, and in most cases, final formulations are not subject to monograph specifications. Manufacturers are free to include any inactive ingredients that serve a pharmaceutical purpose, provided those ingredients are safe and do not interfere with either product effectiveness or any required final product testing. In a few instances, even though the product contains GRASE ingredients, it may need to meet a monograph testing procedure; for example, antacids must pass an acid-neutralizing test.

Because the drugs in the monograph system are GRASE, there has not yet been any requirement to report adverse events. Historically, any changes in ingredient status and labeling for these drugs have occurred as a result of adverse drug findings reported in the literature or through similar public mechanisms. With the ever-increasing use of nonprescription drugs, however, the FDA believes it is important to develop a new and more effective formal mechanism to monitor and screen reports of adverse drug effects and unexpected events associated with their use.

New Drug Approval Of all drugs approved since the laws were established to require evidence of safety and efficacy, nearly 90% are considered new in both a medical and legal sense. Most have been approved for prescription use only.

The new drug approval process requires that all new drugs be proven effective as well as safe before they can be marketed. No drug is absolutely safe; there is always some risk of an adverse reaction. When the benefits outweigh the risks, however, the FDA considers a drug safe enough to approve. This risk-to-benefit assessment is critical for drug approval.

Most approved nonprescription NDAs were approved prior to the OTC drug review. When the program began, most potential applications with ingredients or claims that were also within the purview of the review were deferred. Until the review is completed, interim marketing of products is permissible; however, these products are subject to the appropriate final monograph, at which time, products with any marketing factors outside the monograph (eg, ingredient, dosage, or claim) will require new drug approvals.

NDAs are also necessary for unique delivery systems to ensure the bioavailability of the active component. For example, whereas an ingredient in the monograph could be marketed in an immediate-release form, the same ingredient in a sustained-release product would require an NDA.

More recently, NDAs have been the route of approval for many ingredients (not considered in the review) that have been reclassified from prescription to nonprescription status. These include ibuprofen, loperamide, miconazole, clotrimazole, clemastine, and permethrin.

The OTC Drug Review Process

Although an estimated 300,000 individual nonprescription drug products are currently being marketed, these products contain only about 700 distinct active ingredients. The number of individual products may seem high; however, each manufacturer's or distributor's labeled product is considered a separate drug product. Thus, in determining the logistics of the review, the FDA decided that a DESI-type, product-by-product determination, as described previously, would not be feasible because of the sheer volume of nonprescription pharmaceuticals. Pragmatism dictated a review that focused on the ingredients used in these products, subdivided by therapeutic category. For example, instead of examining individual antacid products, of which there are estimated to be more than 8,000, the FDA evaluated only the active ingredients, such as aluminum hydroxide, magnesium carbonate, and sodium bicarbonate. Because the process focuses on active ingredients, the FDA's OTC drug review is vastly different from that applied to a new nonprescription ingredient as part of an NDA, which evaluates final dosage forms.

The Rulemaking Process The OTC drug review is a three-phase rulemaking process. The process culminates in the promulgation of regulations establishing standards for both the active ingredients and labeling in each nonprescription therapeutic drug category.

Phase I of the OTC drug review was carried out by FDA-appointed advisory review panels; the panels have completed Phase I activities. Panel members were scientifically qualified individuals and nonvoting technical liaison members representing consumer and industry interests. The panels were charged with reviewing the ingredients and labeling of marketed nonprescription drug products to determine whether they could be classified as GRASE for use in self-treatment.

The panels classified ingredients of nonprescription drug products into three categories:

- *Category I*: generally recognized as safe and effective (GRASE) for the claimed therapeutic indication;
- *Category II*: not generally recognized as safe and effective (NRASE) or having unacceptable indications;
- *Category III*: insufficient data available to permit final classification.

The panels also recommended labeling (including therapeutic indications), dosage instructions, and warnings about side effects and the potential for misuse and abuse.

The panel phase of the review lasted a decade, with more than 300 individuals participating in this project. Findings were based largely on a review of 14,000 volumes of data.

Throughout the OTC drug review, the FDA encouraged manufacturers of drugs under consideration to reformulate and relabel their products to comply with panel recommendations before completion of the rulemaking proceeding. Consequently, the public usually received the benefits of the review before the final regulations were issued.

Phase II of the OTC drug review is the FDA's evaluation of the panels' findings, consideration of public comments, and study of any new data that may have become available. The agency then publishes its tentative conclusions as a proposed rule (tentative final monograph). This document offers the first clear signal of the agency's ultimate intentions. After the tentative final monograph is published, a period of time is allotted for objections or requests for a public hearing; new data may also be submitted during this period.

Phase III begins after objections and new data have been considered, and requests for a hearing have been processed. The FDA then issues a final rule, usually in the form of a final monograph. Other final regulations, sometimes referred to as nonmonographs (in which data are insufficient to establish any ingredients or even a monograph), are also developed. These nonmonograph regulations describe ingredients that cannot lawfully be marketed or claims that are unacceptable in labeling.

Preclearance by the FDA (ie, submission of an NDA for a nonprescription drug product) is not required if the regulatory standards described in the monographs are met. In essence, the FDA has already precleared the active ingredient(s) and labeling, and the final formulation is consigned to the manufacturer. Monographs usually become effective 1 year after publication in the *Federal Register*, after which date all affected nonprescription drug products must meet all regulatory specifications.

After an OTC drug monograph is finalized, new conditions that are not specified in the final regulations (ie, ingredients, combination of ingredients, indications, and labeling) will still need to be approved. Manufacturers have two separate approaches to gain marketing clearance: submit supportive data in the form of a petition to amend a final monograph to include the new marketing conditions, or submit an NDA for nonprescription drug use.

Impact of the Review The OTC drug review has generated substantial amounts of new data on nonprescription drugs, and additional data have been developed on many of the ingredients to demonstrate their safety and effectiveness. However, ingredients that could not be shown to be both safe and effective for their intended uses have been (and continue to be) dropped from formulations. A few ingredients were found to be so unsafe that they were removed from the market before the full rulemaking process was completed.

Collectively, the review panels examined 722 active ingredients for different uses. Some ingredients have more than one use, resulting in 1,454 ingredients for specific uses with the following results:

- About one third of the ingredients were judged to be safe and effective for their intended use.
- One third of the ingredients were found to be largely ineffective, and a few were found to be potentially unsafe.
- One third of the ingredients needed additional data to establish safety and effectiveness. Many have already been upgraded based on new information or additional studies.

Through a separate rulemaking (commonly referred to as the OTC wrap-up regulation—phase I), the agency proposed to remove 259 ingredients (142 in Category II and 117 in Category III) covering 22 classes of nonprescription drug products. The FDA gave interested parties 60 days to object but stated that no new scientific data could be submitted. In all instances, it had provided manufacturers with numerous opportunities to prove that the ingredients were effective and had received no significant comments or data. As a result of comments that were received, some minor changes were made, and the final rule, which was published in 1990, removed 223 ingredients.

A second similar rulemaking in 1993 (OTC wrap-up regulation—phase II) removed 415 ingredients (323 in Category II and 92 in Category III) covering seven classes of nonprescription drug products. In almost every case, the drug manufacturers had already reformulated their products.

Nonprescription Drug Labeling

Labels on nonprescription drug containers and packaging material should provide detailed information, so consumers can properly select and use the drugs. The message should not be constrained by the size of the container or package. Significant concerns about labeling comprehensibility, readability, and comprehensiveness continue to be expressed.

Comprehensibility

FDA regulations require that nonprescription drug labeling contain terms that are likely to be read and understood by the average consumer, including the person of low comprehension, under customary conditions of purchase and use. This is indeed challenging because in standardizing labeling information for the average consumer, there will always be a significant percentage of the population that is "below average" in its ability to read, comprehend, discern, and act properly on label information. An estimated 20% of the US adult population is functionally illiterate (eg, reading below a fifth-grade level, experiencing difficulty in reading and accurately comprehending a food package label or restaurant menu). In population subsets, the rate of functional illiteracy may exceed 40%. Approximately 35% of the US population reads and comprehends at a sixth- to tenth-grade level.

Labeling information that exceeds an individual's ability to interpret, comprehend, and apply that information produces major obstacles to the safe, appropriate, and effective use of nonprescription drugs. It is estimated that at least one half of all consumers of nonprescription drugs would benefit from counseling on how to interpret product labels properly.[3]

Readability

The FDA and manufacturers of nonprescription drugs have been actively engaged in initiatives to increase drug label readability over the last several years. Label standardization that is being considered addresses text, format, and the provision of essential information in the same order and in the same area of every drug label. Uniformity in print size, pictograms, icons, color, color contrast, type face, type size, type spacing, columns, margins, paragraphs, upper- versus lower-case lettering, bulleting, numbering, and language simplification are also being considered. One option being evaluated is the use of a "drug facts" box similar to the "nutrition facts" box on food labeling.

Label format should continue to focus on special populations with impaired vision. For example, a 45-year-old needs 50% more light than a 20-year-old and a 70-year-old needs approximately three times as much light as a 20-year-old to read well. Nonprescription drug manufacturers cannot control light, but they can compensate for low light and poor visual acuity by using larger print for the most critical messages. A threshold print size—4.5 points, while not optimal, has been suggested as a minimum—should be considered for use in nonprescription drug package labeling.

Essential Information

Essential information that should be displayed prominently on all nonprescription drug labeling consists of the following elements.

Product Name/Ingredients Large print on the package label should enable the reader to accurately identify the product trade name, generic name, classification, and strength of all therapeutic ingredients. Inactive ingredients (eg, formulation factors, adjuvants) should also be listed by name and amount present.

Product Indications/Claims Labels should include only the FDA-approved indication (use) for the active ingredient(s). It would be useful if package labeling linked the ingredient with its specific indication (eg, dextromethorphan for cough, pseudoephedrine for upper respiratory congestion).

Package Contents In addition to strength, concentration, and net quantity, package labeling should include the dosage form used (eg, tablet, chewable tablet, capsule, syrup, suspension, elixir, suppository, ophthalmic preparation), the dosage units or volume contained in the package, an indication that a tamper-resistant seal has been applied, and the course of action to take if the seal or band is broken or missing.

Directions for Use Labels must clearly instruct the patient on the proper way to take the product (eg, orally, topically), the proper dosage and the frequency of administration (given the patient's age, pregnancy, and other special considerations), and, in some cases, the length of time to take the medication. Special storage procedures (eg, refrigerate, avoid heat or cold extremes, avoid overexposure to sunlight) must be included.

Contraindications/Warnings/Precautions/Adverse Effects If a drug is contraindicated, all appropriate circumstances requiring the contraindication (eg, pregnancy, glaucoma, hypersensitivity) should be included on the label. Label information should caution women who are pregnant or breast-feeding to check with a health professional before taking the medication. Pediatric and geriatric populations may also have special informational needs that should be included on the label, particularly with regard to dosing and safety closures. Precautionary statements such as time limits on use, removal from the reach of children, and action to take in case of an accidental overdose should be included on the label. Potential side effects (eg, drowsiness, dizziness, nausea, diarrhea, blurred vision, elevation of blood pressure, tachycardia) that might debilitate or endanger the user to any degree should also be listed, as should drug-drug interactions of greatest potential clinical significance.

Indications for Seeking Medical Attention Package labeling that recognizes the limitations of nonprescription drugs and advises consultation with a health professional if symptoms persist or worsen over a relatively short period of time is strongly encouraged.

Manufacturer's Information The manufacturer's and/or distributor's name, address, and toll-free telephone number are useful information in matters related to recalls, unexpected adverse effects, and other unanticipated issues.

Expiration Date and Batch Code The expiration date is required and should remain distinguishable over time. The batch code is necessary for recall purposes.

Label Flags Flags or side panels in prominent type should be readily apparent on package labels when significant changes are made in a product (eg, its formulation) or its label information (eg, indications, contraindications, warnings, precautions, adverse effects, drug interactions, and/or dosage or administration guidelines).

Limitations

Overreliance on package labeling as the primary patient education process is fraught with potential patient risk. A package label can never address the infinite management issues associated with drug use, particularly in the presence of multiple disease states (comorbidity) and a complex regimen of prescription and/or nonprescription drugs (polypharmacy). Thus, package labeling should acknowledge and encourage dialogue with the pharmacist as well as the physician when patients have questions or concerns about nonprescription drug use.

Package Inserts

Finally, the FDA, nonprescription pharmaceutical manufacturers, and manufacturer trade associations may ultimately acknowledge that the breadth and depth of patient information needed to ensure the maximization of positive health outcomes and the minimization of adverse consequences from drug use may not be achievable with total reliance on a package label or container. Accordingly, patient package inserts for nonprescription drugs may be necessary to communicate the appropriate depth and breadth of information to patients in a readable and user-friendly format.

Drug Reclassification: Prescription to Nonprescription

The FDA OTC drug review is responsible for the reclassification of many drugs from prescription to nonprescription status. In 1991 the FDA announced the establishment of the Nonprescription Drug Advisory Committee to review and evaluate the safety and effectiveness of nonprescription drug products while serving as a forum for the exchange of views regarding the prescription and nonprescription status of various drugs. This process has produced more than 50 reclassifications from prescription-only to nonprescription status over the past 20 years.

Recognizing the vital and emerging role of nonprescription drug therapy in the health care process, a version of the 1996 FDA reform bill titled The Drugs and Biological Product Reform Act would establish, within the FDA Center for Drug Evaluation and Research, an office with sole responsibility for reviewing and acting upon "all applications or petitions to switch a drug from prescription to over-the-counter status" and "all other matters related to nonprescription drugs."[4] A scientific advisory panel would provide the majority of recommendations. Whether such legislation will pass and be promulgated was not known at press time. The fact that such legislation is being proposed, however, reflects a higher priority for nonprescription drugs in the US Congress and the FDA than was previously in evidence.

Criteria for Reclassification

Until 1951, federal law did not contain criteria for determining whether a drug should be limited to prescription use. This decision was left to the manufacturer, and different manufacturers made different decisions about the same drug formulations, leading to confusion among manufacturers, regulators, health professionals, and the general public. There were questions related to the FDA's authority to permit refill authorizations or to limit drug prescribing to physicians. To end the confusion, in 1951 Congress enacted an amendment to the 1938 Act, specifying three classes of drugs that were limited to prescription use:

- Certain habit-forming drugs listed by name;
- Drugs not safe for use except under the supervision of a licensed practitioner because of toxicity or other potential for harmful effect, the method of use, or the collateral measures necessary for use;
- Drugs limited to prescription under an NDA.

These statutory definitions, along with the basic statutory language requiring adequate directions for use, are still the principal criteria for determining prescription versus nonprescription drug classification.

In considering reclassification, the second criterion is probably the most essential and is worthy of close examination. The assessment of the overall margin of safety includes not only those considerations described in the statute (toxicity, potential for harmful effects, method of use, and collateral measures necessary to use), but also the potential for abuse and misuse and the benefit-to-risk ratio.

Many drugs administered to treat serious disease conditions may cause adverse effects. These drugs must be used carefully to achieve the appropriate level of effectiveness without endangering patient safety. They are therefore too toxic to be used for self-treatment and will continue to be classified as prescription drugs. However, because any drug can be misused with some toxic result, the possibility that a drug can be misused is not the sole basis for prescription classification. Because all drugs have both benefits and risks—for example, most antihistamines may cause drowsiness—some degree of risk must be tolerated for patients to receive the benefits. However, consumers can be informed of the risks through adequate directions for use in product labeling.

It is very difficult to set exact standards or reclassification criteria because so many factors must be carefully considered. The classification process is judgmental and based on a variety of factors related to an individual drug's use, risks, and benefits. The information that must be gathered from the expert opinions of advisors and consultants regarding a drug's nonprescription status includes but is not limited to the following:

- Is the condition self-diagnosable?
- Is the condition self-treatable?
- What is the product's toxicity?
- Does the product possess misuse and/or abuse potential?
- Is the product habit-forming?
- Do methods of use preclude nonprescription availability?
- Do the benefits of availability outweigh the risks?
- Can adequate directions for use be written?
- Can warnings against inappropriate and/or unsafe use be written?
- Can labeling be read and understood by the ordinary individual?

Further scientific scrutiny typically addresses the following questions as well:

- Does the reclassification candidate have special or unique toxicity within its pharmacologic class?
- Does the reclassification candidate have an adequate margin of safety?
- Does the reclassification candidate's frequency of dosing affect its safe use?
- Has the reclassification candidate been used for a sufficiently long time (eg, 3–5 years) on the prescription market to yield a full characterization of its safety profile?
- Has the reclassification candidate's safety profile been defined at high doses?
- Has a vigorous risk analysis been performed? If so, what are the results?
- Is there a full understanding of the pharmacodynamics of the reclassification candidate?
- Is the minimally effective dose of the proposed nonprescription indication known?
- Has the efficacy literature been reviewed in a way that supports the expected use and labeling of the reclassification candidate?
- Have potential drug interactions for the reclassification candidate been characterized?
- What is the worldwide clinical and marketing experience of the reclassification candidate?

Many FDA personnel and external experts are consulted in an effort to form a consensus on each reclassification candidate. The process is lengthy and thorough.

Mechanisms for Reclassification

Four basic mechanisms exist for the reclassification of a prescription drug to nonprescription status.

Mechanism 1 A full NDA may be submitted for a currently marketed prescription drug. The application might contain new clinical studies to support a specific nonprescription indication using a lower prescription strength. For example, a prescription drug may be available at 25 mg, 50 mg, and 100 mg, and the studies supporting nonprescription use are conducted using the 25-mg dosage. In this case, because new studies have been conducted, the sponsor of the approved NDA will have marketing exclusivity for several years. Other manufacturers would need to duplicate the studies during that period.

Mechanism 2 The "switch regulation" provides that drugs limited to prescription use under an NDA can be exempted from that limitation if the FDA determines the prescription requirements to be unnecessary for the protection of the public health. The regulation allows a petition for such an exemption to be initiated by the FDA or by any interested person. Before the nonprescription drug review began in 1972, the FDA used this mechanism to reclassify 25 ingredients to nonprescription status, the last one being the antifungal tolnaftate in 1971.

Mechanism 3 A prescription drug that already has an approved NDA can be reclassified to nonprescription status through the filing and agency approval of a supplement to the NDA. This alternative has in most respects replaced the reclassification regulation procedure. The FDA determines whether the drug, which was previously limited under the terms of its NDA, has now been shown to be safe for nonprescription use. In some cases, the same prescription dosage is considered for nonprescription status. Heavy reliance is placed on the extent of marketing experience and the degree of adverse findings. Under either the reclassification regulation or the supplement to the NDA, the reclassified drug product remains a "new drug" requiring premarket approval and periodic reports to the FDA.

Mechanism 4 Finally, using a completely different process, nearly 40 ingredients have been reclassified through the OTC drug review. Asked to make recommendations on any drugs that could be safely converted to nonpre-

Christine Forand

TABLE 3 Selected list of reclassified drug ingredients

Ingredient	Use/Indication	Ingredient	Use/Indication
Acidulated phosphate fluoride	Dental rinse	Ketoprofen	Analgesic
Brompheniramine maleate	Antihistamine	Loperamide	Antidiarrheal
Butoconazole	Antifungal	Miconazole	Antifungal
Chlorpheniramine maleate	Antihistamine	Minoxidil	Baldness
Cimetidine	Heartburn	Naproxen	Analgesic
Clemastine fumarate	Antihistamine	Nicotine polacrilex	Smoking cessation
Clotrimazole	Antifungal	Oxymetazoline	Decongestant
Dexbrompheniramine	Antihistamine	Permethrin	Pediculicide
Diphenhydramine	Antihistamine	Phenylephrine	Decongestant
Doxylamine	Sleep aid	Phenylpropanolamine	Decongestant
Dyclonine	Oral anesthetic	Pseudoephedrine	Decongestant
Ephedrine sulfate	Bronchodilator, vasoconstrictor	Pyrantel pamoate	Pinworm treatment
Famotidine	Heartburn	Ranitidine	Heartburn
Haloprogin	Antifungal	Sodium fluoride	Dental rinse
Hydrocortisone	Antipruritic, anti-inflammatory	Stannous fluoride	Dental rinse/gel
Ibuprofen	Analgesic	Tolnaftate	Antifungal
		Triprolidine	Antihistamine
		Xylometazoline	Decongestant

scription status, the advisory panels recommended changing many ingredients—including hydrocortisone, diphenhydramine, nystatin, and oxymetazoline—from prescription use to nonprescription drug availability. In some cases, the dosage was increased for marketed nonprescription ingredients (eg, 2 mg of chlorpheniramine was elevated to 4 mg). Comments and petitions by manufacturers as part of the nonprescription drug review have also contributed to enlarging the number of available nonprescription ingredients.

A selected list of former prescription drugs that are now available over the counter is included in Table 3.

A Third Class of Drugs?

It is becoming more and more apparent that optimal drug therapy is the single most critical process in the management of most medical conditions. Drug therapy represents 7–10% of the nation's total health care cost and, by reliable estimates, is solely or primarily responsible for the management of 85–90% of all acute and chronic illness. Drug therapy (prescription and nonprescription) is the "best buy" in American health care; its return on investment being unrivaled in the health care process.

Drug therapy should not, however, be viewed as a benign panacea for the management of acute and chronic illness. Rather, every drug should be viewed as a "two-edged sword," with the potential to do great good, but also to do harm if not used properly. Package labeling addresses the potential risks associated with drug use under categories of information familiar to all pharmacists and physicians. These categories include contraindications, warnings, precautions, adverse reactions, drug interactions, and administration and dosage guidelines.

Even with all the attention directed toward the safe, appropriate, and effective use of prescription drugs, there is abundant evidence of therapeutic mismanagement with both prescription and nonprescription drugs. For example, the annual direct cost of therapeutic noncompliance and drug-induced morbidity and mortality is estimated to be \$50–80 billion; the indirect cost (eg, lost productivity, lost wages) is estimated to be an additional \$50 billion per year.[5] Moreover, drug-related morbidity and mortality appear to be responsible for as many as 28% of hospital admissions (>8 million per year) at a cost in excess of \$47 billion annually, as well as an estimated 17% of all physician office visits (115 million per year) at an annual cost of approximately \$7.5 billion. Ultimately, approximately 140,000 Americans die annually from failure to consume drugs properly.

These figures should compel society to do a better job of managing drug therapy. Even if they are overstated by a factor of as much as 10–15%, the results are still staggering. Close to 15% of the nation's total health care expenditure—at least twice as much as the nation's total expenditure on drug therapy—appears to be directed toward managing the complications of drug therapy.

If system failures exist in managing prescription drug therapy, one can be assured that similar failures exist in nonprescription pharmacotherapy where even more patient management factors are left to chance or to the patients' own devices. Complications and adverse consequences related to nonprescription drug use are more anecdotal than those associated with prescription drug use, but they do exist. Ironically, drugs that were previously limited to prescription use because of statutory language (eg, [1] habit forming; [2] not safe for use except under the supervision of a licensed practitioner because of toxicity or other potential for harmful effect, method of use, or collateral measures necessary for use; [3] limited to prescription use under an NDA; or [4] requiring adequate directions for use) can suddenly be sold uncontrolled in virtually any retail outlet in America when nonprescription status is conferred.

The "black or white," "all or none" classification system of prescription-only or nonprescription-general access leaves no room for "shades of gray"—drugs in a transitional category—and no consistent opportunity for a pharmacist to confer with a patient on nonprescription drug selection and use issues. In the nonprescription drug domain, there is no regulation or legislation that differentiates the pharmacist from any employee in any retail sales outlet that sells nonprescription drugs (eg, department store, gas station, "quick-shop," grocery store, hardware store). Drugs that were formerly in prescription-only status are even sold in vending machines as soon as they are reclassified. This practice raises serious public interest questions.

The National Consumers League notes that most developed and industrialized nations of the world have at least three classes of drugs. Many groups favor moving prescription drugs to nonprescription status, when it is safe to do so, but most acknowledge that some drugs fall somewhere in between. Great Britain enjoys a three-class system (ie, prescription only, general sales nonprescription, and restricted sales by pharmacists). This last category is often referred to as a "third class of drugs." In supporting a third class of drugs that fosters patient-pharmacist interaction, John Ferguson, secretary-registrar of the Royal Pharmaceutical Society of Great Britain, suggests that general availability of nonprescription drugs makes potent pharmaceuticals a mere commodity to be distributed like soap, cornflakes and panty hose, and he notes that Great Britain's three-class system has withstood the test of time.[6]

Since 1964, the American Pharmaceutical Association has supported a third class of drugs that would require pharmacist consultation before consumer purchase. Since 1987, it has specifically proposed that all drugs being considered for reclassification from prescription to nonprescription status be placed in a third class for a period of 2 or more years as a way to increase surveillance. Many currently available nonprescription drugs, as well as many prescription drugs currently being considered for reclassification, would qualify for transitional status because of their side effect profile, drug interaction potential, and/or potential for misuse or abuse. For drugs in this transitional third class, the pharmacist could assist patients in selection and use, counsel patients, identify potential problems, resolve actual problems, and monitor the patient's progress. This active clinical involvement and surveillance, which is not possible in the approximately 1 million nonpharmacy retail outlets in the United States that currently sell nonprescription drugs, could help to determine whether a drug is too toxic or is subject to misuse and/or abuse to the extent that it should not be moved from the transitional class to general use. Advocates of a third class of drugs have confidence in the pharmacist's unique ability to operate in the best interest of the public relative to the use of a few drugs of particularly noteworthy risk.

In 1995, the General Accounting Office (GAO) of the US Congress completed a 3-year study requested by Representative John Dingell (D, Mich) to determine whether there were significant benefits or costs associated with a third class of drugs based on experience in 10 countries. The GAO report concluded that, at this time, no major improvements in nonprescription drug use are likely to result from restricting the sale of some nonprescription drugs to pharmacies or by pharmacists.[7] This conclusion disappointed many consumer groups and organized pharmacy as it contradicts the reality of the marketplace and problems such as ephedrine misuse and abuse, laxative dependency, rebound congestion from overuse of topical nasal decongestants, and hypervitaminosis, to name a few. Some would argue that the GAO report did not research public interest issues in adequate depth. Arguments that a transitional third class of drugs is anticompetitive and/or anticonsumer and would create a pharmacist's monopoly, increase consumer costs, and restrain trade are arguably superficial, flawed, and diminished by public interest issues.

More and more groups are declaring that a third class of drugs is an idea whose time has come. The current health care reform environment, which emphasizes disease management initiatives, optimal drug therapy outcomes, and quality health care at a reasonable cost, creates a positive environment for further initiatives to create a real or de facto third class of drugs.

Marketing Issues

Product Line Extensions

The matter of line extensions (eg, new doses, new formulations), while not a pure labeling issue, must be addressed more vigorously by the FDA and nonprescription drug manufacturers. From a marketing perspective, it is understandable that a manufacturer would see a potential benefit in trading on the name recognition of a previously successful brand-name product. However, if product line extensions create redundancy, distortion, misinterpretation, consumer confusion, and inappropriate patient drug selection and use decisions, marketing considerations must not override the safety and efficacy issues, which should be paramount.

Some companies capitalize on consumer recognition, trust, and loyalty to a brand name that originally applied to a single ingredient at a specific dose to treat a specific symptom (eg, fever) or symptom complex (eg, headache, fever, joint and muscle pain). When brand names are used as the prefix with a variety of suffixes (eg, PM, EX, DM, AF, Cold and Flu, Non-Drowsy, Extra, Allergy-Sinus-Headache, Advanced Formula, PH, Day/Night, and Plus), many consumers can and do become confused, if not bewildered.

Some product line extensions that carry the innovator brand name as the prefix retain the active ingredient of the innovator product, but strengths may vary. A few manufacturers with six or more product line extensions continue to use the innovator brand name as the prefix, but use none of the active ingredient of the innovator products and attach a vague suffix that provides little indication of the active therapeutic ingredient(s) in the extension product. Such practices are contrary to the public health interest and fly in the face of labeling initiatives designed to assist patients in better understanding nonprescription drug products and their proper selection, use, and monitoring.

Manufacturers of nonprescription drugs should be encouraged to consider the following guidelines in addressing some of the inherent problems of line extensions.[8]

- Product line extensions should be discouraged unless they meet a significant consumer need. In such cases, packaging and labeling should clearly distinguish the new product from existing products also marketed under the same brand name.
- Brand names should be restricted to products that contain the same active ingredient(s). A change in the product ingredient profile should warrant a new brand name.
- Application of truly descriptive suffixes to existing brand-name products should be allowed only when one or more active ingredients have been added to an existing formulation (eg, Robitussin DM).
- Standard nomenclature of abbreviations for individual active ingredients commonly added to existing nonprescription formulations should be used.
- A product reclassified from prescription-only to nonprescription status should be allowed to retain its brand name only if the nonprescription product contains the same active ingredient(s).

Nonprescription Drug Advertising

Although it can prohibit the sale of falsely advertised products, the FDA does not regulate or have authority over nonprescription drug advertising. Such authority rests with the Federal Trade Commission. As defined in the Federal Trade Commission Act, *advertisement* shall mean[9]:

> Any written or verbal statement, illustration or depiction, other than a label or in the labeling, which is designed to promote the sale of a product, whether the same appears in television or radio broadcast, newspaper, magazine, leaflet, circular, book insert, catalog, sales promotional material, billboard, or in any display intended for use at the point of sale of the product.

In the 1970s, the Federal Trade Commission Act was amended to prohibit advertisers, when describing the therapeutic benefits of nonprescription products, from using language not approved by the FDA for labeling. In 1973, the National Association of Broadcasters and the Nonprescription Drug Manufacturers Association developed a code of guidelines for manufacturers to follow in creating television advertisements for nonprescription drugs. According to these guidelines, which set standards for truthfulness and honesty, an advertisement should[10]:

- Urge the consumer to read and follow label directions;
- Emphasize uses, results, and advantages of the product advertised;
- If it references scientific or consumer studies, present actual research performed and interpret results honestly and accurately;
- Not contain claims of product effectiveness that are unsupported by clinical or other scientific evidence;
- Not reference doctors, hospitals, or nurses unless such representations can be supported by independently conducted research;
- Not be presented in a manner that suggests prevention or cure of a serious condition that must be treated by a licensed practitioner;
- Not dramatize the ingestion of a medication unless it is informing the consumer of proper medication administration;
- Not present negative or unfair reflections upon competing nonprescription products unless those reflections can be scientifically supported and presented in a manner such that consumers can perceive differences in the uses.

Print advertising should be held to the same integrity standards as the electronic media. Vigilance is warranted in monitoring advertising, however, to ensure that advertisements do not contain false or misleading claims.

Both consumers and health professionals should become "students" of advertising messages. Our society needs to become more analytical as we receive marketing messages, particularly those that are subjective, superficial, vague, or potentially misleading. Health professionals, particularly the pharmacist and physician, need to assist patients in separating fact from ambiguity with regard to nonprescription drug use. Public health educators-at-large (eg, the pharmacist and physician) are well qualified and positioned to protect and serve the public interest as an objective, informed source of nonprescription drug information. This counterbalance to marginal advertising is necessary and appropriate.

Summary

Self-care is expected to play an increasingly important role in health care. Nonprescription pharmacotherapy represents a significant element of the self-care process. Consumers, manufacturers, governmental agencies, and professional groups, particularly pharmacists, should become even more intent on recognizing that each group fulfills essential functions in ensuring the safe, appropriate, effective, and economical use of nonprescription drugs.

References

1. *Self-Medication in the '90s: Practices and Perceptions.* Washington, DC: Nonprescription Drug Manufacturers Association; 1992 May: 9–13.
2. Gadomski A. Rational use of over-the-counter medications in young children. *JAMA.* 1994 Oct 5; 272: 1063–4.
3. Johnson JA, Bootman JL. Drug-related morbidity and mortality: a cost of illness model. *Arch Intern Med.* 1995 Oct 9; 155: 1949–56.
4. FDA office would be established under House FDA reform bill. *FDC Reports—The Tan Sheet.* 1996 Apr 1; 3–4.
5. Silvestri M. The 1990s: establishment of a pharmacist legend class of drugs? Paper presented at Indianapolis, Ind: 87th NABP Annual Meeting; May 1991.
6. Martin S. Exploring the benefits of a third class of drugs. *Am Pharm.* 1991; NS31: 29–32.
7. GAO finds third class of drugs not supported by available evidence. *FDC Reports—The Tan Sheet.* 1995 Aug 28; 3: 1–6.
8. Rupp MT, Parker JM. Drug names: when marketing and safety collide. *Am Pharm.* 1993 May; 39–42.
9. Hewitt NM, Lausier JM, Rosenbaum S. Labeling and advertising of OTC medicines: special emphasis on Rx to OTC switch products. *Clin Res Reg Affairs.* 1994; 11: 207–23.
10. *Voluntary Codes and Guidelines for the OTC Medicines Industry.* Washington, DC: Nonprescription Drug Manufacturers Association; 1991.

CHAPTER 2

Patient Assessment and Consultation

Wendy Klein-Schwartz and Brian J. Isetts

Self-care, self-diagnosis, and self-medication are important components of the health care system in the United States. Rather than seek the attention of a physician, many people self-diagnose and treat their symptoms with nonprescription drugs and home remedies. Several factors increase the extent of self-treatment, including age (over 75 years), sex (female), socioeconomic status, and symptomatology (the number of distinct and separate symptoms).[1] Another factor is the trend of reclassifying prescription drugs to nonprescription status.

In 1994, more than $13 billion was spent on nonprescription drugs. Of the total sales, 45.9% of these expenditures were made in pharmacies[2]; the rest were made in food stores and mass merchandising outlets.

An additional, and somewhat onerous, statistic that is prompting pharmacists to assess and consult with all patients relates to the magnitude of "drug misadventures."[3] The fact that society spends more than $75 billion annually on managing such misadventures[4] suggests that pharmacists are being presented with a mandate to change the way pharmacy is being practiced.

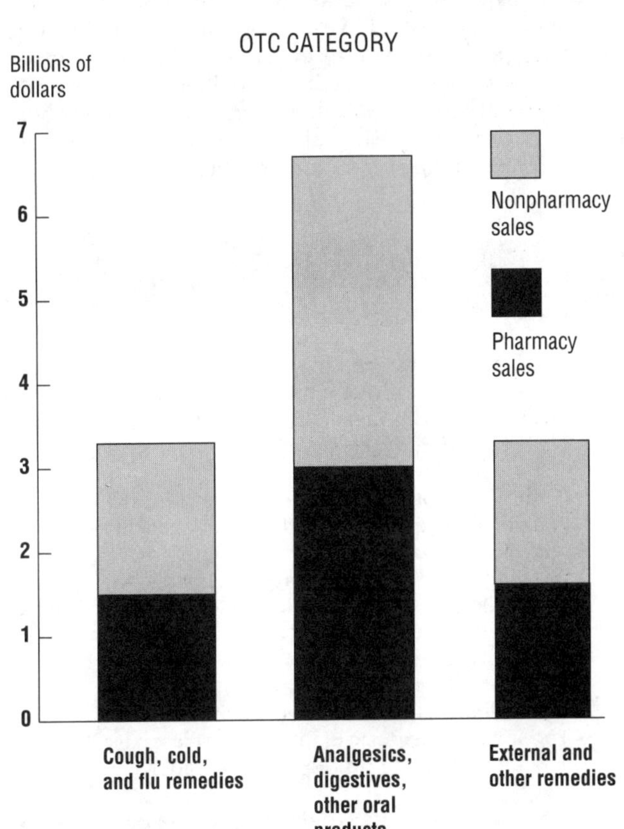

FIGURE 1 Expenditures for nonprescription drugs in 1990 (sales in billions of dollars). Data extracted from *Drug Topics*. 1995 May; 139: 52–61.

The Professional Mandate

Nonprescription drugs allow individuals to manage many medical problems rapidly, economically, and conveniently without unnecessary visits to a physician. However, appropriate use of a nonprescription product, like that of any other drug, requires certain restrictions and limitations. Although warnings are required on the labels of these products, labeling alone may be inadequate; the patient may often need assistance in selecting and properly using nonprescription drugs. Because inappropriate use and misuse of nonprescription drugs can increase the risk of drug misadventures, resulting in increased cost and a more seriously ill patient, the pharmacist's role in counseling and assessment can be crucial.

Patient Use/Evaluation of Pharmacy Services

Many patients do not appreciate or are not aware of the need for professional assistance in selecting nonprescription drugs. This attitude has recently become more evident from the large number of nonprescription products purchased in nonpharmacy outlets, such as supermarkets and local convenience stores, where such assistance is not available.[2] Figure 1 gives a general indication of the percentage of nonprescription products purchased in nonpharmacy outlets.

The pharmacist is what differentiates the nonprescription drug department in a pharmacy from a similar department in a food store. To serve patients better, pharmacies need to maximize the personal service of the pharmacist. Patient inquiries should always be referred to the pharmacist, who must actively promote the value of a pharmacist's guidance in selecting and monitoring treatment with a nonprescription drug. It is essential to increase the patient's awareness of the importance of consulting the pharmacist, not only when

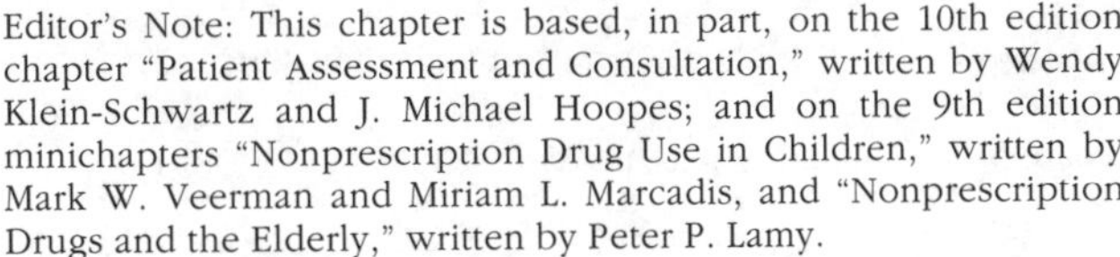
Editor's Note: This chapter is based, in part, on the 10th edition chapter "Patient Assessment and Consultation," written by Wendy Klein-Schwartz and J. Michael Hoopes; and on the 9th edition minichapters "Nonprescription Drug Use in Children," written by Mark W. Veerman and Miriam L. Marcadis, and "Nonprescription Drugs and the Elderly," written by Peter P. Lamy.

considering a drug for the first time but also when making subsequent purchases.

A number of factors influence the patient's choice of a pharmacy. Service, convenience, and price are important considerations.[5] An analysis of patient use of nondispensing pharmacy services found that, although they had not used most of the services available, most patients had obtained advice on nonprescription medications and minor health problems. Patients rank providing nonprescription drug information as a very important pharmacy service.[6]

The majority of patients considered pharmacists to be competent and to have a professional relationship with their patients.[7] Not all evaluations of pharmacists' counseling, however, have been positive. Patients have indicated that community pharmacists make themselves available to answer drug-related questions but generally do not voluntarily provide counseling.

Pharmaceutical Care

The pharmacist's changing societal responsibility to participate in the patient's drug therapy has led to the development of the concept of pharmaceutical care. Pharmaceutical care entails designing, implementing, and monitoring a therapeutic plan, in cooperation with the patient and other health professionals, to produce specific therapeutic outcomes.[8] Under this concept, each time a patient presents a therapeutic request (ie, a question about self-care or drug therapy, a request for a new prescription), the pharmacist systematically works with the patient and other health care providers to identify any actual or potential drug therapy problems and to review and determine the best response to *all* the patient's drug-related needs. This system is referred to as the "comprehensive pharmaceutical care process."[9] Within this process, the pharmacist reviews all the medications

TABLE 1 Pharmacist's assessment questions

1. Does the patient need this drug regimen?
   Does the patient have a medical condition? (Misusing drug unintentionally? Addicted? Using for recreation?)
   Does this condition call for this drug regimen? (Avoidable adverse drug reaction? Nondrug therapy indicated? Duplicate therapy?)
2. Is this drug/form the most effective and safe?
   For the medical condition? (Consider condition onset time, potency, acute/chronic use, oral/topical use, potential adverse reactions)
   For the patient? (Consider age, sex, pregnancy/lactation, race)
   With other diseases? (Consider patient's other disease states)
   With the patient's history? (Refractory condition? Allergic/intolerant?)
   Considering cost?
3. Is this dosage the most effective and safe?
   Too low? (Consider weight, patient class, disease states)
   Too high or changing too fast? (Consider weight, patient class, disease states)
4. If side effects are unavoidable, does the patient need additional drug therapy for side effects?
5. Will drug storage/administration impair efficacy or safety?
   (Consider lost potency, timing of doses, incorrect dosing technique)
6. Will any drug interactions impair efficacy or safety?
   Drug-drug interactions? (Consider prescription and nonprescription drugs, samples, social drugs)
   Drug-food interactions? (Consider food affecting drug, drug affecting nutrition)
   Drug-laboratory interactions?
7. Will the patient follow this drug regimen?
   Is the regimen available to the patient? (Drug unavailable? Unaffordable?)
   Is the patient physically able to follow the regimen? (Cannot swallow/administer drug?)
   Is the patient mentally able/willing to follow the regimen? (Cannot remember? Does not know how? Not motivated? Dislikes form/dosing?)
8. Does the patient need any additional drug regimen?
   For untreated condition? Synergism? Prophylaxis?
9. Does the patient need any nondrug therapy or information?
   (Consider other products, referral to health professional or support group, information about disease state)

Reprinted from Tomechko MA et al. Q and A from the pharmaceutical care project in Minnesota. *Am Pharm.* 1995; NS35(4): 34.

that a patient is taking as a prerequisite of assessment and consultation. Table 1 presents an overview of the pharmacist's assessment questions.

Assessing Drug Therapy Problems

Every profession has a clinical decision-making process dictated by the needs of society. The identification of drug therapy problems represents a primary clinical decision-making process for the pharmacist. As depicted in Table 1, the goal of each patient encounter is to prevent, detect, and resolve drug therapy problems. To do this, the pharmacist must establish an efficient method of gathering pertinent information so that any such problems can be assessed. Since the single most important piece of information is an accurate accounting of all medications that the patient is currently using, the pharmacist must obtain these data first. One way to do this efficiently is to print out the patient's medication profile for the previous 6–12 months and go through this list of medications with the patient. The list is then supplemented by a discussion of the patient's use of physician samples, medications obtained from other pharmacies, and self-care remedies that the patient has on hand in the home. The next step is to tie the use of each of these medications to the patient's specific medical conditions. Throughout the encounter, the pharmacist is working to identify any possible drug therapy problems. Table 2 presents a general outline of the categories of drug therapy problems and their causes.

In practice, it may seem quite innocuous to respond to a request such as "What is the best vitamin?" by simply directing the patient to the least expensive multivitamin with minerals. Unfortunately, the pharmacist cannot truly know what the best vitamin is for the patient unless the patient's drug therapy problems have been assessed. For the young patient currently taking no active medications and occasionally skipping meals, the least expensive multivitamin with minerals may be appropriate. However, that same multivitamin with minerals given to a patient with kidney disease could be fatal.

Improving Patient Compliance

Noncompliance is a drug therapy problem that causes significantly increased morbidity, hospitalizations, and health care expenditures.[10] Factors affecting compliant behavior include patient satisfaction and motivation.[11] Because pharmacists can help patients make medication decisions based on an understanding of the patient's own choices (eg, lifestyle, environment, values, and attitudes) as well as of associated risks, they can have a strong influence on patient compliance.[12]

TABLE 2 Categories of drug therapy problems and their causes

Assessment	Drug therapy problems	Causes
Indication	Unnecessary drug therapy	No medical indication; addiction or recreational drug use; nondrug therapy more appropriate; duplicate therapy; treatment for avoidable adverse reaction.
Effectiveness	Wrong drug	Dosage form inappropriate; contraindications present; condition refractory to drug; drug not indicated for condition; more effective medication available; drug interaction.
	Dosage too low	Dose incorrect; frequency inappropriate; duration inappropriate; storage incorrect; administration incorrect; drug interaction.
Safety	Adverse drug reaction	Unsafe drug for patient; allergic reaction; incorrect administration; drug interaction; dosage increase or decrease too fast; undesirable effect.
	Dosage too high	Dose incorrect; frequency inappropriate, duration inappropriate; drug interaction.
Compliance	Inappropriate compliance	Drug product not available; patient cannot afford drug product; patient cannot swallow/administer drug; patient does not understand instructions; patient prefers not to take medication.
Untreated indication	Needs additional drug therapy	Untreated condition; synergistic therapy; prophylactic therapy.
	None known	—

Reprinted from Tomechko MA et al. Q and A from the pharmaceutical care project in Minnesota. *Am Pharm*. 1995; NS35(4): 35.

Counseling Patients

Advising patients on self-treatment is an important part of pharmacy practice and provides the pharmacist with an opportunity to act in a primary care role. Often the patient's first contact with the health care system, the pharmacist can assess the situation and recommend a course of action. This may include recommending a nonprescription drug, dissuading the patient from buying medication when drug therapy is not indicated, recommending nondrug treatment, or referring the patient to another health care practitioner. If the pharmacist deters healthy people from using more costly health care services or products and refers more seriously ill patients to physicians, health care delivery in the United States should be improved.

Communication

Interventions by pharmacists through consultation and effective educational strategies can enhance patient compliance. For this to happen, however, good communication between the pharmacist and patient is necessary.[11,13] Thus, the pharmacist must have effective communication skills.

When a pharmacist responds to a patient's therapeutic request, the ensuing interaction can be referred to as a therapeutic dialogue. The goal of this patient–pharmacist interaction is to establish a therapeutic relationship. A therapeutic relationship is a partnership between the patient and the pharmacist characterized by trust and a reciprocal agreement to work together to prevent drug therapy problems and to identify and solve such problems when they occur.[9] This relationship allows the pharmacist to gather detailed, and sometimes intimate, information from the patient. In return, the patient expects the pharmacist to share knowledge and expertise to ensure safe and effective drug therapy. Because the pharmacist is not expected to gather every possible piece of information in a single patient encounter, scheduled follow-up and reassessment are vital components of this therapeutic relationship.

Establishing a viable patient–pharmacist relationship is a dynamic process affected by numerous variables. A positive interaction one day could be followed by a negative interaction a few days later for reasons unrelated to the care provided by the pharmacist (eg, loss of work, marital turmoil, a cloudy day, etc). The pharmacist must become adept at searching for and interpreting nonverbal cues (eg, facial expression, body position), as well as at responding to voice tones, inflection, and mood. When a patient is experiencing a drug therapy problem but does not have the time or inclination to deal with it when meeting with the pharmacist, the pharmacist must seek to schedule an alternative time to gather additional information.

General Principles of Communication

An effective patient–pharmacist relationship will be established if the pharmacist is a capable, empathetic source of information. Because the pharmacist's underlying attitude toward the patient will influence the quality of communication, the effective pharmacist must eliminate barriers by avoiding biases toward a patient's level of education, socioeconomic or cultural background, interests, or attitude. In addition, the patient must be assured that any information discussed with the pharmacist will be strictly confidential.

Because people may resent being told what they already know, the pharmacist should first determine the patient's level of knowledge. When interacting with patients, the pharmacist should use words that a layperson can understand and avoid using complex medical terms.

Effective communication occurs when a receiver of a message hears and understands exactly what the sender wishes to communicate. One way to ensure this is known as "active listening," a process in which the receiver repeats the information back to the sender. As information is exchanged, the participants change roles as receivers and senders of information. The message received is influenced by its content and context, as well as by how it is sent. Pharmacists can improve communication by paying attention to the interaction between sender and receiver.

Effective Questioning

Skillful questioning is a mark of a good communicator. The patient should feel that the pharmacist's questions convey a genuine desire to be of help. Because a patient may be uncooperative if the questions suggest only superficial curiosity, the pharmacist should explain the reason for asking personal questions: for example, "For me to select a product for your specific problem, I need some additional information."

Generally, two types of questions are used. Open-ended questions—for example, "Would you please tell me more about the symptoms you have?"—are valuable for gathering various kinds of information. Such questions allow more flexibility and provide more information than questions that can be answered with only yes or no. They also enable a good interviewer to collect more information faster and establish better communication. If the patient's response wanders, however, the pharmacist must keep the conversation focused. To be sure that a patient understands dosage instructions, the pharmacist could ask, "So that I know that I haven't forgotten to tell you anything, would you please tell me how you're supposed to take this medicine?"

Summarizing the important points or redirecting the conversation with a specific, closed-ended question may also be useful. Closed-ended questions—for example, "How long have you had this pain?"—help the pharmacist to gather specific information or to clarify information obtained through open-ended questions. It is important to ask one question at a time; the use of two questions in rapid succession or of multiple-choice questions will only cause confusion and restrict communication.

Effective Listening

Listening is an important component of communication. It means that the patient is free to state the problem completely and is assured of receiving the pharmacist's undivided attention. The pharmacist must focus on the patient and exclude distracting elements such as the telephone and the computer screen. The pharmacist often must clarify the details of the patient's problem and should be receptive to the patient's response to questions. In addition, the pharmacist should respond with empathy, perhaps by paraphrasing the patient's words or by reflecting on what was said in terms of the patient's own experience. For instance, after listening to a complaint of pain, the pharmacist might say, "You have a sharp, stabbing pain in your wrist, is that right?" and end with a statement such as "That must be very uncomfortable." Interrupting or demonstrating disinterest or disapproval may inhibit the patient's discussion of problems and concerns. Alternatively, encouraging the patient to talk, exploring the patient's comments, and expressing understanding facilitate communication. The pharmacist should reinforce correct decisions the patient has made while reserving judgment, and should communicate warmth, feeling, and interest in the patient's concerns.

Nonverbal Communication

Nonverbal communication skills are also important in counseling patients. Body language, such as posture and facial expression, communicates strong, direct messages. The pharmacist should be very aware both of his or her own nonverbal behavior as well as of the patient's. An open body posture—facing the patient with arms and legs uncrossed—indicates openness, honesty, and a willingness to communicate and listen. It is important to maintain an appropriate distance from the patient; the pharmacist should be close enough for confidential communication to occur without making the patient uncomfortable. If the patient backs away or moves closer, the pharmacist should maintain the new distance that the patient has established. It is also important for the pharmacist to maintain eye contact with the patient and to control his or her facial expressions to avoid showing negative emotions such as disapproval or shock.

The patient's nonverbal communication is equally important. If a patient has a closed body posture—arms crossed, legs crossed, body turned away from the pharmacist—the pharmacist may need to find out why the patient is uncomfortable and try to allay those concerns. The pharmacist should also watch the patient's facial expressions for signs of anxiety, nervousness, and even physical symptoms such as pain.

Physical Barriers to Communication

For good communication to occur, physical barriers should be removed or minimized. High counters, glass separators, and elevated platforms inhibit communication; the pharmacist should try to be at the same eye level as the patient. Discussions between the patient and the pharmacist should be as private and uninterrupted as possible. If the pharmacist expects or perceives that a patient is uncomfortable discussing the problem, a quiet or private counseling area should be used. Ideally, a specific private area of the pharmacy should be designated for patient consultation.

Communication Techniques for Special Populations

Special techniques may be required with some patients.[14,15] Writing down the information, using legible handwriting or a word processor with a printer that provides quality copy, may be necessary if the patient is deaf or hearing impaired. However, pharmacists should also remember that up to 20% of Americans are functionally illiterate.[16] If a hearing-impaired patient reads lips, the pharmacist should be physically close to and directly in front of the patient, and should maintain eye contact while speaking. In addition, the pharmacist should speak slowly and distinctly in a low-pitched, moderately toned voice since yelling only serves to distort the sound further. A quiet, well-lit environment is essential because background noise and dimness can markedly diminish a hearing-impaired individual's ability to communicate. The pharmacist should also use visual reinforcement, such as pointing to the part of the body that hurts or to the directions on the container.

When counseling a blind patient, a pharmacist should first identify him- or herself as a pharmacist. Because a blind patient cannot perceive most nonverbal communication, the pharmacist should depend on tone of voice and verbal feedback to convey empathy and interest in the patient's problem. If touching seems appropriate, the pharmacist should first ask the blind person if it would be acceptable.

The Patient Interview

Counseling patients about self-treatment is a primary care activity that carries with it a great professional responsibility. The initial interaction between the patient and the pharmacist is often initiated by the patient (Figure 2). The patient may approach the pharmacist with a symptom, often in the form of a question such as "What do you recommend for. . . ?" Or the patient may ask a product-related question such as "Which of these two products do you recommend?" The pharmacist should also intervene when a patient selects a product that seems contraindicated or has significant potential for causing problems.

Information-Gathering Process

Before formulating a plan for self-treatment or physician referral, the pharmacist must obtain enough information to identify and assess the problem. The most important piece of information the pharmacist must obtain is an accurate accounting of each active medication the patient is using to treat all of his or her medical conditions. On the surface it may seem like a formidable task to gather this information efficiently in the 3- to 5-minute time frame of a typical patient interview. As previously noted, one way to obtain this information is to print out the patient's medication profile every time the patient presents with a new prescription, nonprescription drug, or general medication question. An alternative method is to have a computer screen placed in the counseling area to review the patient's current medications.

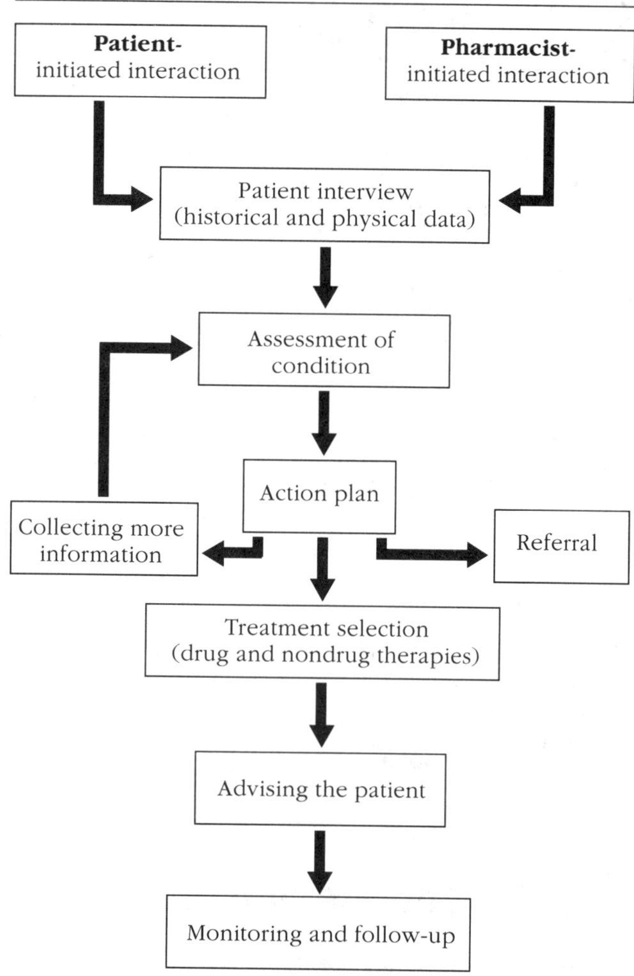

FIGURE 2 Patient-pharmacist consultation process.

Once the pharmacist has this patient prompt in place, the interview process can begin with the pharmacist saying, "I would like to review each of the medications you are currently taking so that the medication that we select (or is prescribed) for you fits together with your current regimen. Here is a list of the medications you have received at our pharmacy. Let's take a minute to see which ones you are currently taking as well as what other medications you may be using." Sometimes it is helpful for the pharmacist to have the patient close his or her eyes and relate what is in the medicine cabinet at home or describe his or her daily medication schedule.

When an accurate picture of the patient's active medication list has been attained, the pharmacist should tie all active medications to each of the patient's medical conditions. It is at this point that the patient's drug allergies and relative medical history may be taken. Here the interview process is dictated by the patient's knowledge level as well as by the amount of time available to continue the interaction. Thus, to obtain the needed information quickly and efficiently, the pharmacist should approach the problem logically and keep the questioning direct and to the point. With experience, the pharmacist will be able to gather the necessary information to assess a particular condition within a few minutes.

Fortunately, within the context of providing comprehensive pharmaceutical care, the pharmacist need not try to obtain all relevant information in one encounter. The follow-up step of care continues the initial assessment process and allows the pharmacist the luxury of obtaining additional information. The weight of a 10-month-old child, the smoking history of a patient with emphysema, the allergy history of a patient with a sinus infection, and the calcium intake of a postmenopausal woman are examples of information that may be essential during the course of one patient encounter and less essential during the course of another. With continual practice, the pharmacist learns to use every patient encounter to gather whatever additional information is needed. The pharmacist also develops a sense for when to bring the interview to a close and how to establish appropriate follow-up.

Historical Data

A broad overview of the entire patient enables the pharmacist to identify the condition that the patient seeks to treat and to make the most appropriate recommendation, which may or may not include a drug. Patients may initially present incomplete and vague information. To determine what the specific symptoms are and whether they are amenable to self-treatment, the pharmacist can ask the following questions:

- Can you describe the problem?
- When did the problem start?
- How long does it last? Does it come and go, or is it continuous?
- Does the problem limit your daily activities (sleeping, eating, working, walking, etc)?
- Is this a new problem, or is it the recurrence or worsening of an old one?
- Are there other problems that occur concurrently?
- Does any food, drug, or physical activity make the problem worse?
- Does anything relieve the problem? What has relieved it in the past?
- What has been done so far to treat the problem?

The next step in the process is to gather patient-specific data. The pharmacist should selectively elicit the following information:

- Who is the patient? Is the patient the person in the pharmacy or someone else?
- How old is the patient?
- Is the patient male or female? If the patient is female, is she pregnant or breast-feeding?
- Does the patient have any other medical problems that may alter the expected effects of a given nonprescription drug or be aggravated by the drug's effects? Is the complaint related to a chronic disease?
- Does the patient have any allergies?
- Is the patient on a special diet? Does the patient have any special nutritional requirements?
- Is the patient using any prescription, nonprescription, or social drugs (eg, vitamins or food supplements, caffeine, nicotine, alcohol, or marijuana)? How long has the patient been taking these drugs?
- Has the patient experienced adverse drug reactions in the past?

Throughout the encounter, the pharmacist is formulating a hypothesis based on the identification of actual or potential drug therapy problems. The pharmacist should determine whether the patient has misinterpreted the condition, done any harm by waiting to seek advice, or worsened the condition by previous self-treatment.

Observed Physical Data

Besides the historical data, physical data are extremely helpful in assessing the medical problem. Physical data include pulse rate, heart sounds, respiration rate, age, and weight. Pharmacists have been routinely collecting physical data for years, and some have acquired additional skills that have greatly expanded their ability to assess and monitor patients' medical conditions. Depending on the pharmacist's training and skills, physical data are collected by all or some of the following techniques: observation or inspection, palpation or manipulations, percussion, and auscultation. The importance of each technique in the process of data collection depends on the body system involved. For example, the skin is easily assessed by inspection and palpation, the lungs require percussion and auscultation, and all four skills are essential in examining the abdomen. However, most pharmacists obtain physical data exclusively through observation.

Good observational skills are very valuable. Many clues to a patient's general health and to the seriousness of a condition can come from simple observation. The degree of discomfort caused by pain may be judged from a patient's facial expressions or lack of use of a particular limb. Toxicity from an infection may be manifested by lethargy and pallor. The pharmacist would need to inspect the patient's skin before offering advice about a skin rash, which may result from a simple contact phenomenon or may suggest systemic disease.

Assessment of Condition

Assessment is the evaluation of all the data—historical and physical—collected from the patient to determine the etiology and severity of the medical condition. Determining etiology and severity is essential for reaching appropriate conclusions about treatment and the need for referral. Assessment of severity will vary depending on the problem. Some conditions, such as diabetes with hyperglycemia or polyuria, may be considered severe only when they reach certain levels. Other conditions may be considered severe only when patients become symptomatic or when the symptoms begin to impair the activity of the patient. For instance, the pharmacist may elect not to recommend a cough suppressant for a patient with an intermittent cough unless the cough is nonproductive and is keeping the patient awake at night.

Many times, however, the etiology and severity of a condition cannot be determined conclusively because certain data may not be accessible. In such situations, and especially when the available information suggests that a certain etiology is responsible or that the condition may be particularly severe, referral may be required. For example, an acutely inflamed joint that is swollen, warm to the touch, tender, and painful may be caused by trauma, bacterial infection, gout, or rheumatoid arthritis. Because a final assessment may require examination of the joint fluid, the patient should be referred to a physician. In general, the more severe the problem, the greater the potential for referral.

Finally, certain groups of patients are at greater risk for complications and require more careful evaluation. These groups include elderly patients, infants and children, patients with certain chronic diseases such as diabetes or renal or heart disease, patients with multiple medical conditions and those who are taking multiple medications, recently hospitalized patients, and patients treated by several physicians.

Action Plan

After collecting all the available information and assessing the patient's condition, the pharmacist must quickly formulate an action plan. Often the pharmacist must do this without having all the desired information. Areas of uncertainty will always exist, but a well-considered plan can help ensure proper management of the patient. A sound action plan requires paying careful attention to five specific areas:

- Collecting more information;
- Selecting physician referral;
- Selecting self-treatment;
- Advising the patient on self-treatment;
- Maintaining follow-up contact.

Collecting More Information

The pharmacist may need more information to assess the patient's condition. This may require specific action, such as talking to a parent or another adult, or calling a physician. Communication between the pharmacist and the physician is often desirable to avoid conflict in the management of the patient and to overcome the problem of overlapping responsibilities. In some situations, such communication may even be necessary. This occurs when the pharmacist must:

- Obtain data on preexisting medical conditions to determine whether self-treatment is appropriate;
- Determine if the physician wants to deal with the problem over the phone with the patient;
- Determine if the physician wants to see the patient, or if the patient should be referred to an urgent care center or a hospital emergency department;
- Provide information on the reason for referral.

Selecting Physician Referral

When enough information is available to assess the condition, the pharmacist must decide whether to refer the patient to a physician or advise self-treatment. If the plan involves physician referral, the pharmacist must consider both the type of treatment center to which the patient will be referred (physician's office or emergency care facility) and the urgency for treatment. Some conditions do not require the immediate attention or extensive evaluation of emergency care treatment.

When advising a patient to see a physician, the pharmacist should discuss with the patient why the referral should be made, using tact and firmness so that the patient is not frightened unnecessarily but is convinced of the need for concern. Physician referral is indicated in any of the following situations:

- The symptoms are too severe to be endured by the patient without definitive diagnosis and treatment.
- The symptoms are minor but have persisted and do not appear to be due to some easily identifiable cause.
- The symptoms have returned repeatedly for no readily recognizable cause.
- The pharmacist is in doubt about the patient's medical condition.

Selecting Self-Treatment

Advising self-treatment requires the pharmacist to consider several factors. First, a measurable and achievable therapeutic objective must be identified, based on the condition and the patient. Then, with this determined, a therapeutic modality—either drug or nondrug—may be recommended. For example, the objective in a patient who has a productive cough but is having difficulty producing sputum would be to increase sputum production. Thus, an expectorant would be the agent of choice. However, in a patient with a dry, nonproductive cough, the therapeutic objective would be to suppress the cough, in which case a cough suppressant would be selected. Selecting a specific treatment requires reviewing drug variables (dosage forms, ingredients, side effects, adverse reactions, relative effectiveness, and price) and matching them with patient variables (age, sex, drug history, other physiologic problems, and ability to pay).

Should self-treatment without drugs be indicated, selection of the nondrug modality would similarly be modified based on patient variables. For example, the pharmacist may recommend that a patient with vomiting and diarrhea only drink fluids for a 24-hour period to provide bowel rest. However, if the patient is an insulin-dependent diabetic, the pharmacist must modify this recommendation because diabetic patients must maintain a specific caloric intake. Communicating with the physician is a must in this situation.

To measure the success of treatment, the pharmacist should set indices based on the therapeutic objective, the toxic or adverse effects of the treatment, the nature and severity of the condition, and the ability of the patient to understand the condition and its treatment. The objectives in treating sinusitis with decongestants, for example, are to facilitate drainage and relieve symptoms such as headache. Achievement of the first objective can be determined by observing or asking about the nature of nasal discharge (quantity, color, and viscosity); achievement of the second, by simply asking about the headache. Indices of toxicity are those symptoms indicative of an excessive dose or an untoward reaction. Indices that suggest the problem may be worsening and may require special attention should be identified. Finally, indices relating to patient understanding of the condition and its treatment can include determination of the appropriateness of the patient's questions to the pharmacist as well as his or her response to the pharmacist's queries. The patient's compliance with the agreed-upon treatment plan can also be considered.

Advising the Patient on Self-Treatment

The fourth step in the action plan is to advise the patient on self-treatment. The primary purposes here are to educate the patient and to obtain the consent necessary to enact the plan. Specifically, the pharmacist should give advice in the following areas:

- Reasons for self-treatment;
- Description of the drug and/or treatment;
- Administration of the drug and/or treatment;
- Side effects and precautions;
- General treatment guidelines.

In advising the patient about the suggested treatment plan, the pharmacist should summarize the patient's condition, explaining the significance of the symptoms and outlining the reasons for treatment. The therapeutic objective(s) should be clearly explained. Should the patient desire information on alternative treatments, the pharmacist should be prepared to present alternative treatments, with their relative merits, without biasing the information and jeopardizing the patient–physician relationship. The pharmacist should then discuss the nonprescription drug(s) selected, describing both the therapeutic action of the ingredients (eg, decongestants, antihistamines, or laxatives) in lay terms and the effect the product(s) will have on the patient's symptoms and condition. Finally, the patient should be told about the available dosage forms and the availability of any generic product.

Administration guidelines should be explained clearly and concisely. Because many patients may remember only part of the information, some thought should be given to deciding what is most important for the patient to remember. Covering a few of the most important points is better than overwhelming a patient with a lot of information. Additionally, patients will remember dosage instructions better if administration is linked to specific times of the day rather than just assigned "three times daily." Having patients review their normal daily activities will help them establish the best times to take their medication. It is also important to include information about length of treatment.

The patient should be told about the most common side effects or adverse reactions associated with a drug and instructed on how to manage them. Special warnings about activities, other drugs, foods, or beverages that should be avoided, as well as about medical conditions that may be complicated by use of the drug, should also be discussed. Information should be written down if it is extensive or complex.

Finally, the pharmacist should offer the patient general treatment guidelines that may be helpful in managing the condition. These guidelines might include lifestyle changes, additional products or services, and informational sources, as well as a list of signs and symptoms that indicate whether the drug is working or causing adverse effects and when a physician's advice is needed. In addition, the patient should be told of the normal response time to the treatment, the time required to resolve the condition, and what to do if response is delayed.

Maintaining Follow-up Contact

Follow-up allows the pharmacist to determine whether self-treatment has resulted in an appropriate therapeutic response and whether the patient has complied inappropriately or experienced any drug therapy problems, including drug-related toxicity. The pharmacist should decide whether active monitoring and follow-up are necessary and, if they are, should arrange a follow-up plan with the patient. The pharmacist may tell the patient to call at an appropriate interval or may inform the patient that the pharmacist will make a follow-up contact.

Many problems encountered by the pharmacist do not need follow-up. However, the patient should be encouraged to check back if the condition does not improve within a specific period of time or if problems with the medication develop. To this end, the pharmacist might state: "Please let me know whether you feel better in a couple of days," or "If your cough is not better in a few days, you should see your physician. Be sure to tell your physician that you have been taking this medicine."

Follow-up serves several additional functions. It provides feedback that allows a pharmacist to assess whether his or her communication skills require modification and whether useful information has been provided. At the same time, the patient will sense that the pharmacist cares. The pharmacist's concern for the correct use of the nonprescription drugs will also reinforce that these products are drugs and must be used carefully.

Pharmaceutical Care for High-Risk and Special Groups

Four groups of patients—the very young, elderly persons, pregnant patients, and nursing mothers—often experience a higher incidence of drug therapy problems than other patients. Because these problems could have dire consequences, these high-risk patients require special attention. Awareness of their physiologic state, possible pathologic conditions, and special social context is necessary for the proper assessment of their medical conditions and recommendation of treatment.

In many respects, geriatric and pediatric patients require surprisingly similar considerations. Both groups share a need for drug dosages that are different from those for other age groups because of:

- Their altered pharmacokinetic parameters;
- Their decreased ability to cope with illness or drug side effects because of physiologic changes associated with either normal aging or child development;
- Their patterns of impaired judgment because of either altered sensory function or immaturity;
- The different drug effects unique to their age groups;
- The adverse drug effects unique to their age groups;
- A need for special consideration in administering medications.

Yet because each of these four groups is heterogeneous, it is also important to consider these features for each individual patient.

Pediatric Patients

In considering nonprescription drugs for the pediatric age group, it should be noted that the pediatric population may vary substantially among age groups. It is often appropriate to differentiate relatively distinctive pediatric age periods, as follows:

- *Preterm neonate (premature)*: gestational age of less than 38 weeks;
- *Full-term neonate*: gestational age of 38–42 weeks;
- *Newborn*: first postnatal month of life;
- *Infant (baby)*: 1–12 months of age;
- *Toddler (young child)*: 1–5 years of age;
- *Older child*: 6–12 years of age;
- *Adolescent*: 13–18 years of age;

Package labeling will often encourage medical evaluation in children under the age of 1 or 2 years. Also, some package labeling will provide dosage guidelines specific to age groups.

Physiologic Differences

Pediatric patients are at risk for drug therapy problems as their body and organ functions are in a continuous state of development. While both hepatic metabolism and renal elimination of drugs are usually slower in neonates and young infants, they improve rapidly over the first year of life. Additionally, children metabolize some drugs more rapidly than adults do. Illness in children is potentially more serious because their physiologic state is less tolerant of changes. Children are also very susceptible to fluid loss, so fever, vomiting, or diarrhea represent greater potential risks to them.

Effects of Altered Drug Pharmacokinetics

The pharmacokinetic properties of drugs (eg, absorption, distribution, metabolism, elimination) in pediatric patients may be quite different from those seen in adults, and may vary significantly in pediatric age periods.

Absorption The gastrointestinal (GI) absorption of drugs is influenced by many factors, including gastric pH, gastric emptying time, motility of the GI tract, enzymatic activity, blood flow/perfusion of the GI mucosa, permeability and maturation of the mucosal membrane, and concurrent disease process.[17–19] Significant changes in these factors occur during the first few years of life.

The pH of the stomach changes significantly during the first few months of life. At birth, the pH is basic, ranging from 6 to 8.[20] The pH decreases rapidly to 1–3 within a few days but then slowly increases during the next few weeks to reach about 5.[20] The gastric acidity then falls slowly until adult values are reached at about 2 or 3 years of age.[18] Changes in pH affect the absorption of drugs that are weak acids and weak bases. Because drugs are more completely absorbed as unionized compounds, weak acids have a decreased absorption in neonates and infants because of the higher pH in those populations.[21]

Gastric emptying in both the neonate and the infant is prolonged and reaches adult values after 6–8 months.[22] Intestinal transit time is initially prolonged in the neonate, but intestinal motility increases within several months, leading to variable and unpredictable drug absorption. Delayed intestinal motility can lead to increased drug bioavailability because the drug remains available for a long time for absorption in the intestinal tract.[23]

Both bile acids and pancreatic enzymes are reduced in the newborn infant. The effect is most noticeable in the absorption of lipid-soluble drugs such as vitamins D and E.[24]

Disease states can also have a pronounced effect on drug absorption. Pediatric patients with previous GI surgery may have a shortened intestinal length, which results in decreased bioavailability of a drug. Infantile diarrhea and gastroenteritis also decrease transit time, leading to lower absorption of drugs.[25]

Distribution The distribution of a drug in the body is most often expressed in terms of its volume of distribution (Vd). A higher Vd means more drug is concentrated in other areas of the body (eg, fat, muscle, body water) relative to the concentration in the blood. Several differences in pediatric age groups affect the distribution of drugs when compared with that in adults.[26]

One major factor in determining the distribution of water-soluble drugs is total body water (TBW). TBW represents the relationship of body water to total body weight. In adults, water comprises about 55% of total body weight. However, neonates have a much higher Vd because their TBW is about 75%. This decreases rapidly in the first year of life; adult values are reached by about 12 years of age.[27] A water-soluble drug has a lower serum concentration for a given milligram-per-kilogram dose in a neonate or infant than it has for the same milligram-per-kilogram dose in an adult.[28]

The changes in body fat with age are just the opposite. A full-term infant will have an average of 12% body fat. This percentage increases with age to about 21% and 33%, respectively, in adult males and females.[26]

Plasma protein binding is also an important parameter in the Vd of a drug. The higher the amount of drug bound to plasma proteins, the lower the amount of "free" drug available to exert a pharmacologic action. Drugs administered to neonates and infants have lower protein binding than those administered to adults; adult values occur at about 1 year of age.[17,20] Lowered protein binding is a result of decreased serum proteins and a decreased drug affinity for binding to proteins.[29] Drugs that have a high degree of protein binding exert a greater effect in the younger age group because of the relatively low quantities of binding proteins.

Metabolism The metabolism of drugs is primarily the responsibility of the liver. The liver handles drugs in one of two ways: (1) by changing the structure of the drug through oxidation, reduction, demethylation, or hydrolysis or (2) by conjugating the drug molecule to make it more water soluble.[18,22] Nonconjugating reactions are primarily the function of mixed-function oxidase systems (cytochrome P-450). The activity of these reactions remains low in the neonate, and each hepatic metabolic process matures at a different rate. This delayed maturation of metabolic processes makes it difficult to characterize the elimination of drugs undergoing biotransformations, but the metabolic processes begin in the neonate at 20–40% of the adult activity level.[30] Conjugating reactions are even more variable and probably slower to mature in the developing neonate and infant. Glucuronidation does not approach adult values until about 70 days of life.[31,32]

Once the metabolic function of the liver matures, it may actually exceed the adult capacity to metabolize drugs on a milligram-per-kilogram-per-day basis. This increased capacity probably occurs because the liver weighs proportionately more in children than in adults, creating a higher relative metabolic surface area.[33]

Excretion/Elimination Excretion or elimination is primarily the function of the kidneys; this process also undergoes significant age-related changes. At birth, the glomerular filtration rate (GFR) is approximately 30% or less than that of adults.[34] The GFR increases significantly in the first 2 weeks of life and reaches adult values by 1 year of age.[34] Therefore, drugs eliminated primarily by glomerular filtration require special dosage considerations during this period. Renal tubular secretion and reabsorption also mature with age but at a rate slightly slower than the GFR.[22,35]

Other Potential Drug Therapy Problems

The pharmacist should be sensitive to the potential for drug therapy problems among children. For some illnesses such as diarrhea, nondrug therapy is often more appropriate than therapy with nonprescription antidiarrheal drugs. In some situations, specific drugs are contraindicated; for example, aspirin should not be administered to young children with certain viral illnesses because of its association with Reye's syndrome (see Chapter 4, "Internal Analgesic and Antipyretic Products"). For younger children, solid dosage forms are inappropriate, and the pharmacist will need to guide parents to liquid medications or chewable tablets.

Inaccurate Dosing Inaccurate dosing is another potential problem. Labeling on nonprescription drugs generally uses age-based guidelines for determining dosages; however, many products do not provide dosage information for children under 6 years of age. Following the nonprescription drug's label instructions for dosing an older child can result in too high a dose and potential toxicity for a younger child. For some drugs, children

TABLE 3 Average pediatric weight by age grouping

Age	Average weight	
	Pounds	**Kilograms**[a]
Birth	7.3	3.3
6 mo	17.0	7.7
1 y	21.6	9.8
15 mo	23.0	10.5
2 y	27.0	12.3
3 y	32.0	14.5
4 y	36.4	16.5
5 y	41.0	18.6
6 y	46.0	20.9
7 y	52.0	23.6
8 y	57.2	26.0
9 y	62.0	28.2
10 y	68.0	30.9

[a]1 kg equals 2.2 lb.

Reprinted from Nykamp D. Nonprescription medications in the pediatric population. *Am Pharm*. 1995 Apr; 35: 10–29.

require a larger milligram-per-kilogram dose than adults do because they metabolize the drugs more rapidly. Body surface area may be the best measure because it correlates well with all the body parameters, but body surface area is not easily determined. Because nonprescription medications have a wide therapeutic index (the ratio of the toxic dose to the therapeutic dose), safe doses may generally be determined by weight. Average weight at different ages is included in Table 3.

Improper Administration Selecting the proper drug and dosage is of no benefit unless the medication is administered. Proper administration of medications to pediatric patients requires an appreciation of dosage forms, delivery methodology, routes of administration, palatability, and many other factors. This chapter segment focuses on oral medications.

Liquids are relatively easy to administer, and the dose can be titrated to the patient's weight; therefore, liquid medications are often used in pediatrics. Because elixirs and syrups can have a high alcohol and sugar content, respectively, these liquid forms may be less desirable than suspensions and solutions. A suspension may also mask the disagreeable taste of a drug.

Problems with drug administration can result in the child receiving the wrong dose. The volume delivered by household teaspoons ranges from 2.5 to 7.8 mL and may also vary greatly when the same spoon is used by different individuals.[36,37] The American Academy of Pediatrics Committee on Drugs highly recommends the use of appropriate liquid administration devices, which include a medication cup, cylindrical dosing spoon, oral dropper, and oral syringe. Ease of administration and accuracy should be considered when choosing one of the dosing devices. Plastic medication cups are fairly accurate for volumes of exact multiples of 5 mL (ie, 5 mL, 10 mL, 15 mL). With higher-viscosity liquids, the oral syringe is preferable to the other oral dosing devices because the syringe completely expels the total measured dose. Potent liquid medications should be administered with an oral syringe to ensure that the correct dose is given; the pharmacist should briefly explain to parents how to use and read an oral syringe. However, drawing up the dose in the syringe requires dexterity.

The use of precision oral dosing devices helps ensure adequate therapeutic response by reducing the incidence of underdoses and eliminating adverse drug effects from potential overdoses. These devices may also enhance acceptance of medication by infants and children.[38] Parents may need instructions on using these devices to measure doses accurately, as well as advice on giving medications to reluctant or struggling children. The pharmacist may need to demonstrate to parents and older children how to take the medication.

Tablets or capsules can usually be swallowed by a child over 4 years of age. Tablets that are not sustained-release or enteric-coated formulations may be crushed; most capsules may be opened and the contents sprinkled on small amounts of food (applesauce, jelly, or pudding) to ensure that all the drug is taken. If the child does not eat the full portion, underdosing can occur. The child may be more cooperative if allowed to choose what flavored drink to use and, if multiple drugs are prescribed, which medication to take first. Table 4 presents selected guidelines for administering oral medications to pediatric patients.

Adverse Effects Adverse reactions are another potential drug therapy problem in children. Side effects may be different in children than in adults. For example, as in the elderly population, antihistamines and central nervous system (CNS) depressants may cause excitation in children.

Noncompliance Noncompliance may occur when children refuse to take the medication or parents give up before the child receives the entire dose. Noncompliance can also occur when parents do not understand instructions or do not pass them on to day care providers, who, along with other individuals, may need written directions.[39]

Assessment and Counseling

Assessment and counseling for pediatric patients usually involve the parents. For younger children, the pharmacist works with the parents to recommend treatment and assess drug therapy problems. For older children, the pharmacist can involve the child in effective counseling.[39] Some tips for pediatric counseling include explaining what the medication is; using the word *medicine*, not *drug*; discussing different dosage forms and the importance of medication timing; preparing special vials for school; preparing the child for the medicine's taste; and demonstrating how to take the medicine.

TABLE 4 Selected medication administration guidelines for oral medications

Infants

- Use a calibrated dropper or oral syringe.
- Support the infant's head while holding the infant in the lap.
- Give small amounts of medication to prevent choking.
- If desired, crush nonenteric-coated or slow-release tablets to a powder and sprinkle them on small amounts of food.
- Provide physical comforting while administering medications to help calm the infant.

Toddlers

- Allow the child to choose a position in which to take the medication.
- If necessary, disguise the taste of the medication with a small volume of flavored drink or small amounts of food. A rinse with a flavored drink or water will help remove an unpleasant aftertaste.
- Use simple commands in the toddler's jargon to obtain cooperation.
- Allow the toddler to choose which medications (if multiple) to take first.
- Provide verbal and tactile responses to promote cooperative taking of medication.
- Allow the toddler to become familiar with the oral dosing device.

Preschool children

- If possible, place a tablet or capsule near the back of the tongue and provide water or a flavored liquid to aid the swallowing of the medication.
- If the child's teeth are loose, do not use chewable tablets.
- Use a straw to administer medications that could stain teeth.
- Use a follow-up rinse with a flavored drink to help minimize any unpleasant medication aftertaste.
- Allow the child to help make decisions about dosage formulation, place of administration, which medication to take first, and the type of flavored drink to use.

Geriatric Patients

Social, economic, physiologic, and age-related health factors place elderly patients at high risk for medical problems and prompt them to be large consumers of nonprescription drugs. Indeed, the elderly as a group consume more drugs than any other age segment of our society. A 10-year study of more than 4,509 elderly individuals found that nonprescription drug use in this population increased significantly from 1978 through 1988.[40] Close to two thirds of ambulatory elderly patients use nonprescription drugs.[41] Furthermore, 40% of all drugs used in nursing homes and 80% of all drugs used in assisted living facilities are nonprescription drugs. The elderly's response to drug therapy is more scattered and unpredictable than that of other populations. Pharmacokinetic, pharmacodynamic, and various nonpharmacologic factors predispose the elderly to potential problems with nonprescription drugs.[41] To deliver comprehensive pharmaceutical care to ambulatory elderly patients, pharmacists must recognize the special needs and risks of this group.

Effects of Physiologic Aging

Normal aging is associated with physiologic changes that predispose patients to disease. The elderly often suffer from impaired vision (eg, difficulty reading and differentiating colors) and hearing loss. The pharmacist should be aware of patient behaviors that indicate visual or hearing loss and should take these impairments into consideration when communicating with the elderly patient.[42] Additional instructions for nonprescription drugs may need to be provided in larger, high-contrast, dark print.

Subtle changes in mental status, such as confusion, may be anticipated in elderly patients in whom illness has caused anxiety over their state of health. Fifteen to twenty percent of community-living elderly are thought to be cognitively impaired to varying degrees, making comprehension of directions even more difficult.[43] Patients may not remember the names of all their medications or may not be able to remember instructions later as the result of memory impairment. Because of memory lapses, some elderly patients may require unique drug delivery systems (eg, transdermal patches, sustained-release preparations, etc) to help them adhere to their dosage regimen. Elderly patients with cognitive impairment are less likely to read and interpret labels correctly,[44] which further emphasizes their need for special dosage form considerations.

The elderly are believed to confuse at least one third of their problems with age-associated problems and therefore to misreport their symptoms.[45] Accurate perception (and reporting) of symptoms is vital to the successful use of any drug. In addition, elderly patients are often reluctant to share health information with others.

Aging alters the absorption, distribution, metabolism, and elimination of certain drugs, increasing the susceptibility of the elderly patient to drug therapy problems (Table 2). Such pharmacokinetic changes can result in an unexpected accumulation of these drugs to toxic levels.[42,46]

The aging process, as well as many chronic diseases, can alter a patient's nutritional status. The elderly most at risk for undernourishment or malnutrition are homebound patients and nursing home residents; poverty, multiple chronic diseases, multiple drug therapy, or a combination of these factors may cause malnutrition in these patients. The patient's nutritional status and weight are important because they can also alter the pharmacokinetics and pharmacodynamics of drugs.

Effects of Altered Drug Pharmacokinetics

Absorption Pharmacokinetic changes, which have been well described in literature, are caused not only by advancing age but also by the effects of disease states and often by multiple drug use. For example, coexisting diseases may alter the absorption of some drugs, so too may antacids, either by chelation or by pH changes. These factors may alter the rate of absorption, the extent of absorption, or both.

Distribution Similarly, drug distribution is age and disease dependent, and changes can lead to altered drug action. As the ratio of lean body weight to lipid tissue changes with age—lean body weight decreases while lipid tissue increases—the Vd of water-soluble drugs decreases, possibly promoting more intense action of these drugs. Extracellular and other body fluids also decrease with age, thereby decreasing the Vd of water-soluble drugs. $Alpha_1$-acid glycoprotein, a plasma protein, increases with age in healthy elderly patients, whereas albumin levels decrease by 4% per decade of life.[47,48] The effect is greater in those 70 years of age and older, and there is a high prevalence of abnormally low serum albumin in the very old. Therefore, drugs that are highly protein bound should show altered distribution patterns in elderly patients.

Metabolism Theoretically, elderly patients should have reduced rates of hepatic drug metabolism because of age-related changes. The weight of the liver is correlated with body weight; both decrease beginning in the fifth or sixth decade of life. Both hepatic function and blood flow decrease with age, but changes are effected by many other factors, such as smoking and alcohol intake. Nevertheless, it is generally agreed that elderly patients probably have diminished capacity to metabolize drugs and that it is primarily the oxidative drug-metabolizing mechanism that changes with age.

Excretion/Elimination Age-related changes in renal function and drug elimination must also be considered. Renal function declines with age but to a variable degree and at a variable rate. Little decline is observed in about one third of the elderly; in the rest, normal renal function at age 70 may be 40% less than at age 30.[49] The GFR declines with age, even in the absence of cardiovascular, renal, or acute illnesses. The decline is more rapid in men than in women. Altered physiologic processes, such as reduced cardiac output, cardiac contractility, total vascular resistance, and hypotension, may also reduce the GFR. Furthermore, the renal function of older people is more vulnerable to insults imposed by drug therapy and overall stress.

Effects of Altered Drug Pharmacodynamics

Pharmacodynamics (eg, the hypoglycemic effect, the extent and duration of pain relief, and the effect of a drug on heart rate) represent the physiologic and psychologic responses to a drug or a combination of drugs and are of major interest in the pharmacologic management of chronic diseases of the elderly. The pharmacodynamics of a drug govern the type, intensity, and duration of drug action or, more precisely, the duration of a given concentration of a drug at its site of action. As is the case with pharmacokinetics, pharmacodynamics change with age (and disease), but it is still difficult to differentiate between normal aging effects and pathophysiologic effects and their influence on pharmacodynamics. Advancing age heightens the interplay between the aging processes and chronic diseases, which has made it difficult to clearly identify those pharmacodynamic changes that are only age associated.

Few studies have simultaneously investigated both pharmacokinetics and pharmacodynamics. In general, drug action altered with age has been ascribed to the elderly's reduced reserve capacity and changes in the autonomic nervous system, CNS, cardiovascular system, endocrine system, and drug receptors.

Reduced Physiologic Reserve The elderly are more susceptible to decompensation under stress because of the loss of physiologic reserve. For example, the perfusion of vital organs is often diminished in the elderly, and small changes in blood flow (perhaps induced by drugs) can endanger organ function because the organ's functional reserve capacity is reduced. Older people are less able to regulate blood glucose levels, blood pH, pulse rate, blood pressure, and oxygen consumption. Therefore, it is not unreasonable to assume that drugs can bring about unanticipated (although not unpredictable) adverse effects on the elderly's functional reserve.

Altered Hemostatic and Thermoregulatory Mechanisms There is evidence that the efficiency of postural stability is reduced with advancing age.[50] Any drugs that affect this homeostatic mechanism (eg, antihistamines that affect the CNS) can decrease the body's ability to maintain balance, possibly leading to a greater incidence of falls and fractures.

The efficiency of the thermoregulatory mechanism, which controls body temperature, decreases with advancing age.[51] Impaired shivering, defective vasoconstriction, and poor appreciation of low temperatures are more prevalent in the elderly.

Altered Drug-Receptor Interactions A drug has affinity and intrinsic activity in relation to each of its receptors. Affinity is the efficiency with which a drug binds to its receptors; intrinsic activity is the drug's power to generate a stimulus. Drugs with both affinity and intrinsic activity are defined as agonists. Drugs that have affinity but lack intrinsic activity are defined as antagonists.

Most drugs bind to receptors and thus initiate their action. Age-related altered drug action may also be related to altered drug-receptor interactions. It has been postulated that a given receptor site or drug concentration produces a greater pharmacodynamic effect in the elderly than in younger persons. However, generalizations cannot be drawn because the number of receptors is not fixed but is regulated by a number of factors, including certain diseases states (ischemia, hypertension, heart failure, cardiac hypertrophy), drugs (glucocorticoids, hormones, adrenergic agonists and antagonists), and the aging process itself. There may be receptor changes with age in certain parts of the body but not in others. The CNS cholinergic receptors decline in the basal ganglia but probably not in other brain regions. Receptors, in adapting to drug therapy, may also become supersensitive or desensitized. For example, alterations in insulin receptors account for some forms of insulin resistance. Age-related changes have been documented for brain benzodiazepine receptors and for several hormone receptors.[52,53] Most studies, however, have concentrated on the cholinergic, the dopamine, and the beta-adrenergic receptors.

Drug-receptor response, defined as the pharmacologic response after a drug-end organ interaction, may be increased or decreased in the elderly. It has been suggested for some time that the elderly appear to be more "sensitive" to some drugs. Drugs whose pharmacodynamic effects in the elderly have been most intensively studied include the barbiturates, the benzodiazepines, warfarin, heparin, and morphine.

Altered Neurologic Functions Between 20 and 80 years of age, brain weight is reduced by 20%, and there may be neuronal dropout of up to 25% in some areas of the brain.[54,55] Neuronal loss in the superior frontal and temporal regions and the striatum has been reported.[56] There is also an age-related decline in dopamine receptors.[57]

Evidence indicates that, with advanced age, there is increased conduction time, decreased cerebral blood flow, and possibly increased permeability of the blood-brain barrier.[58] Both subjective and objective evidence indicates that the elderly have an enhanced CNS sensitivity to drugs, prompting a reduced dose requirement (perhaps by as much as 50%) for some drugs.[59]

Increased brain sensitivity and other changes, such as decreased coordination, prolongation of reaction time, and impairment of short-term memory, manifest as increased frequency of confusion, frequency of urinary incontinence, and number of falls (particularly among elderly women). Drug therapy may exaggerate all these changes, particularly if drugs are used in the "usual" dose or if multiple drugs are used.

The most clear-cut evidence of enhanced brain sensitivity to the action of some drugs and thus of altered and age-associated pharmacodynamic drug actions exists for the benzodiazepines.[60] Confusion, ataxia, immobility, and incontinence have been demonstrated when some of these drugs are given in the normal adult dose to elderly patients.[61] Impairment of neurologic function in elderly patients prescribed these drugs appears to be the rule rather than the exception.

Control of bowel and bladder function is lessened with advancing age. A further decrease in efficiency is likely with laxative use. Drugs with anticholinergic action and other CNS drugs may lessen neurologic control. Antihistamines have sedative properties that may reduce bladder control in the elderly.[62] The impact of nonprescription drugs is often increased when such drugs are added to an already existing therapeutic regimen.

Altered Cardiovascular Functions The action of cardiac drugs in the elderly is assumed to differ from that in younger people because measurements start from a different point. For example, the cardiac index changes with age; the elderly have a higher peripheral resistance and intrinsic heart rate and a lower vagal restraint. Sinus node and atrioventricular node dysfunction increase with age; maximum heart rate decreases. Peak cardiac output at exercise also declines with age. The lower maximum exercise heart rate is largely the result of changes in response to beta-adrenergic stimulation.[63] Total left ventricular mass increases, decreasing maximum coronary blood flow. Adaptation of the aging heart to stress is diminished because of a delayed and reduced reaction of the sympathetic nervous system.[64] Reduced work performance and oxygen consumption at maximal workload are associated with a lesser capacity to increase heart rate, cardiac output, and ejection fraction.

The maximal response of the myocardium to catecholamines is reduced with aging.[65] The heart manifests an increased sensitivity to the toxic effects of some drugs (eg, digoxin), which is heightened in the presence of hypokalemia but manifests a lessened increase in contractility to cardiac glycosides.[66]

Changes in the cardiovascular system also involve changes in blood vessels. Between 20 and 80 years of age, vessel elasticity and distensibility are reduced by 90%, leading to increased arterial blood pressure.[67] An increase in peripheral resistance is mainly responsible for essential hypertension. In both normotensive and hypertensive elderly patients, plasma renin and aldosterone concentrations decline. Increases in plasma renin activity in response to sodium depletion or diuretics may also be reduced. The elderly generally present with a relatively reduced fluid volume; extracellular volume is decreased to the greatest degree. Therefore, these hemodynamic and fluid volume changes are expected to change the response of the elderly to drugs.

Additionally, the elderly are more likely than younger people to become symptomatically orthostatic, even without drugs. As many as 5% of elderly patients show a drop in systolic hypertension upon standing; one contributing factor is the reduced sensitivity of the baroreceptor system, which does not allow the elderly to compensate as efficiently for either elevated or reduced blood pressure. Therefore, all drugs that could cause orthostatic hypotension, particularly if used in combination, should be used cautiously in the elderly.[68,69] The risk of orthostatic hypotension is further increased in elderly patients with volume depletion, caused by salt and/or water depletion, or with circulatory changes, caused by infections or fever.[69,70]

Altered Endocrine Functions Age-related changes in the endocrine system have been documented. The reduced availability of hormones results in diminished endocrine regulatory mechanisms with age, as well as with deficiencies in hormonal feedback mechanisms.[70]

Alterations in pancreatic and adrenal hormone levels result in decreased glucose tolerance with age and an increased susceptibility to drug-induced hypoglycemia. Some elderly suffer from a decreased release of insulin while others have a decreased number of insulin receptors and/or postreceptor abnormalities.[71] Production of sex hormones also decreases with age.[58] In women, reduced estrogen levels have been correlated with a greater incidence of osteoporosis. Because of hormonal changes, women are also more susceptible to orthostatic hypotension. Decreased thyroid levels make the elderly more sensitive to the action of digitalis and increase the risk of drug-induced hypothermia.[72]

Altered Immunologic Functions Some, but not all, immunologic functions show a gradual decline with age. The thymus probably has less power than the central immunologic organs and the bone marrow to maintain functional levels of peripheral T-lymphoid population.

The immune function is under complex regulatory control, and immunologic changes are probably caused by disturbances in that regulatory process. Indeed, age-related changes in immune function reflect several different alterations. Overall, T cells are diminished in function; the deficiency includes most T-cell effector and regulatory functions, with the possible exception of T suppression. All these factors combine to decrease cellular immune competence.[73,74] Infections are more prevalent in the elderly; however, the infections common in older people (influenza, pneumococcal pneumonia) are not usually associated with immune deficiency as are infections caused by opportunistic organisms.

Apparently, elderly patients who are prescribed nonsteroidal anti-inflammatory drugs (NSAIDs) (and who may also take self-prescribed nonprescription NSAIDs) are at heightened risk of gastric and duodenal ulceration. Elderly women, especially those receiving diuretics, appear to be at particular risk.

Altered GI Functions Aging is associated with secretory and morphologic changes in the stomach. Muscular atrophy, thinning of gastric mucosa, and infiltration of the submucosa with elastic fibers are evident in the stomachs of 80% of patients over 50 years of age.[75,76] Intestinal blood flow may be reduced by as much as 50% by age 65, being further diminished by stress, congestive heart failure, hypoxia, and hypovolemia. Tension, fear of disease and death, depressive illness, anxiety, and worry influence stomach motility and secretory function. Chronic gastritis, irritable colon, heartburn, ulcerlike distress, and nausea can result.

Gastric secretion declines with age. Gastric cell function decreases and gastric pH is generally elevated. Furthermore, gastric secretion is diminished in diabetes.

Gastric emptying is about 2.5 times faster in younger than in older persons because it is under the control of the CNS, which may lose efficiency with advancing age. Slowing of gastric emptying follows a reduction in gastric acid secretion; gastric emptying is also negatively affected by stress, lack of ambulation, gastric ulcer, intestinal obstruction, myocardial infarct, and diabetes mellitus. Some drugs (eg, antacids, anticholinergics, isoniazid, lithium, narcotic analgesics) delay gastric emptying. Fatty meals delay gastric emptying more in the elderly than in younger people. A delay in gastric emptying permits gastrotoxic agents a longer residence time, and, therefore, more opportunity to exert their toxic effect.

NSAID-Induced Adverse Effects As people age, their use of NSAIDs increases, and the adverse effects of these drugs also increase disproportionally. One reason may be that NSAIDs are overprescribed. Of course, many NSAIDs may also be obtained without a prescription. The potential gastrotoxicity of these drugs may be enhanced by their simultaneous administration with other gastrotoxic drugs, coffee, or alcohol.[77,78] Through inhibition of the protective effects of GI prostaglandins and via local noxious effects, salicylates and other NSAIDs can cause superficial gastric and duodenal erosions and ulcer formation, which could then result in GI bleeding and perforations. Decreased platelet aggregation can enhance the potential for bleeding. All NSAIDs can interfere with platelet function and prolong bleeding time. Mucosal lesions of the stomach and duodenum are often reported in patients taking NSAIDs. Elderly patients may be especially susceptible to NSAID-associated peptic ulcer disease.

With advancing age, renal blood and plasma flow decrease, and the kidney's ability to concentrate urine decreases, as does its maximum diluting ability and its ability to compensate for abnormalities of the acid-base balance and electrolytes. The elderly do not conserve sodium efficiently. Therefore, the two broad excretory functions of the kidneys—preservation of body fluid volume and maintenance of their composition—are adversely affected by aging. NSAIDs can exacerbate the severity of renal disease by blocking interrenal cyclo-oxygenase (reduction of renal prostaglandin secretion). This risk is increased in volume-depleted elderly.

Other Potential Drug Therapy Problems

Duplicate Therapy Elderly patients can receive unnecessary drug therapy when drugs are added to their therapeutic regimen without a reevaluation of the entire regimen to determine whether drugs should also be deleted. Duplicate therapy may occur because elderly patients may be seeing multiple providers for their various medical problems. Many elderly people have serious and multiple diseases such as coronary artery disease, chronic renal failure, or congestive heart failure, which can be aggravated by concurrent therapy for other acute problems. Concomitant illness or certain drugs may contraindicate the use of other drugs. It is also important to consider whether the elderly person is requesting a nonprescription drug to treat an adverse reaction from another medication.

Appropriate Dosing/Dosage Forms Normal drug doses may be too high in the elderly because of impaired hepatic and renal function. This would necessitate either lowering the dose or increasing the dosing interval. Further, elderly patients may experience difficulty with some dosage forms (eg, swallowing large tablets, using inhalers) because of physical impairment.

Poor Compliance Poor compliance in the elderly may result from difficulty swallowing or administering the drug. It may also result from an inability to afford the drug because of a limited or fixed income.[19] The elderly may also lack the social supports to supply the aid required by an illness.

The Pregnant Patient

Pregnancy introduces a very important variable in drug therapy. Drug therapy during pregnancy may be necessary to treat medical conditions or may be considered to manage common complaints of pregnancy such as vomiting or constipation. However, because most drugs cross the placenta to some extent, a mother who takes a drug might expose her fetus to it. Thus, the desire to ease the mother's discomfort must be balanced with concern for the developing fetus.

A study among 4,186 women during the first trimester found that 66% used at least 1 drug, with a mean

TABLE 5 FDA categories for evaluating the safety of drugs during pregnancy

A: Adequate studies in pregnant women have not demonstrated a risk to the fetus in the first trimester of pregnancy, and there is no evidence of risk in later trimesters.

B: Animal studies have not demonstrated a risk to the fetus, but there are no adequate studies in pregnant women . . . or . . . Animal studies have shown an adverse effect, but adequate studies in pregnant women have not demonstrated a risk to the fetus during the first trimester of pregnancy, and there is no evidence of risk in later trimesters.

C: Animal studies have shown an adverse effect on the fetus, but there are no adequate studies in humans; the benefits from the use of the drug in pregnant women may be acceptable despite its potential risks . . . or . . . There are no animal reproduction studies and no adequate studies in humans.

D: There is evidence of human fetal risk, but the potential benefits from the use of the drug in pregnant women may be acceptable despite its potential risks.

X: Studies in animals or humans demonstrate fetal abnormalities, or adverse reaction reports indicate evidence of fetal risk. The risk of use in a pregnant woman clearly outweighs any possible benefit.

number of drugs for all subjects and for drug users being 1.3 and 2.9, respectively.[79] Nonprescription drugs accounted for 68% of the drugs used; the nonprescription drugs used most often were oral analgesics (acetaminophen and aspirin), antacids, and cold and allergy products.

Potential Problems

Teratogenic Effects Several factors are important in determining whether a drug taken by a pregnant woman will adversely affect the fetus. Two such factors are the stage of pregnancy and the ability of the drug to pass from maternal circulation to fetal circulation via the placenta. The first trimester, when organogenesis occurs, is the period of greatest teratogenic susceptibility for the embryo and is the critical period for inducing major anatomical malformations. However, exposure at other periods of gestation may be no less important because the exact critical period depends on the specific drug in question.

Drug therapy problems are also important considerations in the pregnant patient. Although dosage guidelines for some prescription drugs are different in the pregnant patient from those in other patients, there is no information on dosage adjustments for nonprescription drugs. Unnecessary drug therapy should be avoided. Nondrug therapy is often more appropriate than drug therapy in the pregnant patient. Use of cigarettes and alcohol should also be limited since they have been associated with increased risk to the fetus.[80–83]

In the pregnant patient, the primary concern is related to the safety of the drug. All practitioners should be familiar with the A-B-C-D-X system for evaluating the safety of drugs in pregnancy (Table 5).[84] Often the issue is not whether there is a more effective drug available but whether there is a safer drug available. For example, there is evidence regarding the association of aspirin with congenital defects, the incidence of stillbirths, neonatal deaths, or reduced birth weight.[79,84] Use of aspirin late in pregnancy has been associated with increases in the length of gestation and the duration of labor. These effects are related to aspirin's inhibition of prostaglandin synthesis. In addition, because aspirin affects platelet function, perinatal aspirin ingestion has been found to increase the incidence of hemorrhage in both the pregnant woman and the newborn during and following delivery. Therefore, aspirin use during pregnancy should be avoided, especially during the last trimester. Instead, because acetaminophen is generally considered safe for use in pregnancy, it is the nonprescription drug of choice for antipyresis and analgesia when taken in standard therapeutic doses.[79] Naproxen, a nonsteroidal anti-inflammatory drug, can be taken early in pregnancy.[84] However, naproxen should not be used late in pregnancy since it is a potent prostaglandin synthetase inhibitor and can not only cause problems in the newborn but also affect the duration of gestation and labor.

Noncompliance Nausea and vomiting associated with the pregnancy may make it difficult for the pregnant patient to comply with taking oral medications.

Management of the Pregnant Patient

The pharmacist can aid the self-treating pregnant woman in deciding which drug or nondrug treatments she should consider and when self-treatment may be harmful to her or her unborn child. The decision to suggest a drug must be based on both an up-to-date knowledge of the literature and a very critical risk-to-benefit evaluation of the mother and the fetus. The assessment and management of the pregnant patient require observation of the following principles.

First, the pharmacist must be alert to the possibility of pregnancy in any woman of childbearing age who has certain key symptoms of early pregnancy, such as nausea, vomiting, and frequent urination. Any woman who fits this description should be warned not to take a drug that might be of questionable safety if she is pregnant.

Second, the pharmacist should similarly advise the pregnant patient to avoid using drugs, in general, at any stage of pregnancy unless it is deemed essential by the patient's physician. Similarly, the safety and effectiveness of homeopathic and herbal remedies in pregnancy have not been established.

Third, the pharmacist should advise the pregnant patient to increase her reliance on nondrug modalities as treatment alternatives. For example, the first approach to nausea and vomiting should be eating small, frequent meals and avoiding foods, smells, or situations that cause vomiting. Next, taking an effervescent glucose or buffered carbohydrate solution may be effective. Only if these measures are ineffective should an antihistamine or antiemetic be considered. Physician consultation may be indicated at this point.

Last, the pharmacist should refer the patient to a physician for certain problems that carry increased risk of poor outcomes in pregnancy (eg, high blood pressure, vaginal bleeding, urinary tract infections, rapid weight gain, or edema).

The Nursing Mother

Drug use while breast-feeding can cause an adverse effect in the infant. The concentration of a drug in the mother's milk depends on a number of factors, including the concentration of the drug in the mother's blood; the drug's molecular weight, lipid solubility, degree of ionization, and degree of binding to plasma and milk proteins; and the active secretion of the drug into the milk. Other important considerations include the relationship between the time of taking a drug and the time of a breast-feeding, as well as the drug's potential for causing toxicity in infants. Additionally, some drugs (eg, decongestants) may decrease milk supply.

When advising a nursing mother on self-treatment, the pharmacist should decide if a drug is really necessary, recommend the safest drug (eg, acetaminophen instead of aspirin) if one is necessary, and advise the mother to take the medication just after a breast-feeding or just before the infant's lengthy sleep periods.[85]

When taken in therapeutic dosages, most drugs are not present in breast milk in sufficient amounts to cause significant harm to the infant. However, several drugs are contraindicated for use while breast-feeding, and several others should be used cautiously by nursing mothers. The amount of caffeine in caffeine-containing beverages is not harmful, but higher doses could cause irritability and poor sleep patterns in infants. There are also many nonprescription drugs for which data on their transfer into breast milk and their possible clinical effects are not available.

The American Academy of Pediatrics Committee on Drugs published a statement on drugs in human milk.[85] Of the nonprescription drugs included in the statement, aspirin and other salicylates are the only ones that were considered to have had significant effects on some nursing infants and that nursing mothers should therefore take with caution. Nonprescription drugs that are usually considered compatible with breast-feeding include[84,85]:

- *Analgesics*: acetaminophen, ibuprofen, naproxen, and ketoprofen;
- *Antacids*;
- *Antidiarrheals*: kaolin-pectin and attapulgite;
- *Antihistamines*: brompheniramine, chlorpheniramine, diphenhydramine, and triprolidine;
- *Antisecretory agents*: cimetidine, famotidine, ranitidine, and nizatidine;
- *Cough preparations*: dextromethorphan;
- *Decongestants*: phenylephrine, phenylpropanolamine, and pseudoephedrine;
- *Fluoride*;
- *Laxatives*: bran type, bulk-forming type, docusate, glycerin suppositories, magnesium hydroxide, and senna;
- *Vitamins*.

Summary

The use of nonprescription drugs represents an important component of the health care system. Many people diagnose their own symptoms, select a nonprescription drug product, and monitor their own therapeutic response. Properly used, nonprescription drugs can relieve the minor physical complaints of patients and permit physicians to concentrate on more serious illnesses. If used improperly, however, these products can create a multitude of problems.

To be of greatest service to patients, pharmacists must continually update their therapeutic knowledge and improve their interpersonal communication skills. As pharmacists continue to expand their patient-counseling services, people will learn of these services and will seek their pharmacist's assistance whenever they are in doubt about self-treatment. The result will be better-informed patients who will not only use the professional services of pharmacists but also recognize the contributions of pharmacists to health care.

References

1. Montagne M, Bleidt B. How to help the elderly self-medicate. *US Pharm*. 1989 Jun; 14: 53–60.
2. Scanning OTC/HBC sales. *Drug Topics*. 1995 May; 139: 52–61.
3. Manasse HR Jr. Medication use in an imperfect world: drug misadventuring as an issue of public policy: parts 1 and 2. *Am J Hosp Pharm*. 1989 Jun; 46: 929–44, 1141–52.
4. Johnson JA, Bootman JL. Drug-related morbidity and mortality. A cost-of-illness model. *Arch Intern Med*. 1995 Oct; 155: 1949–56.
5. Meade V. Patients satisfied with pharmacy services, survey shows. *Am Pharm*. 1994 Jul; NS34: 26–8.
6. Hirsch JD, Gagnon JP, Camp R. Value of pharmacy services: perceptions of consumers, physicians, and third party prescription plan administrators. *Am Pharm*. 1990 Mar; NS30: 20–5.
7. Monsanto HA, Mason HL. Consumer use of nondispensing professional pharmacy services. *Drug Intell Clin Pharm*. 1989 Mar; 23: 218–23.
8. Hepler CD, Strand LM. Opportunities and responsibilities in pharmaceutical care. *Am J Hosp Pharm*. 1990 Mar; 47: 533–43.
9. Tomechko MA et al. Q & A from the Pharmaceutical Care Project in Minnesota. *Am Pharm*. 1995 Apr; NS35: 30–9.
10. Sullivan SD, Kreling DH, Hazlet TK. Noncompliance with medication regimens and subsequent hospitalizations: a literature analysis and cost of hospitalization estimate. *J Res Pharm Econ*. 1990; 2: 19–23.
11. Fisher RC. Patient education and compliance: a pharmacist's perspective. *Patient Educ Counselor*. 1992 Jun; 19: 261–71.
12. Schulz RM, Brushwood DB. The pharmacist's role in patient care. *Am Pharm*. 1991 Dec; NS31: 882–8.
13. McNally DL, Wertheimer D. Strategies to reduce the high cost of patient noncompliance. *Md Med J*. 1992 Mar; 41: 223–5.
14. Chermak G, Jinks M. Counseling the hearing-impaired older adult. *Drug Intell Clin Pharm*. 1981 May; 15: 377–82.

15. Smith DL. The patient and his medications. In: *Medication Guide for Patient Counseling*. 2nd ed. Philadelphia: Lea and Febiger; 1981: 3–46.
16. Epstein D. More counseling called for in medicating the illiterate. *Drug Topics*. 1988 Nov; 132: 15.
17. Boreus LO. *Principles of Pediatric Clinical Pharmacology*. New York: Churchill, Livingstone; 1982.
18. Young SL. *J Pharm Practice*. 1989; 2: 13–20.
19. Balistreri WF. In: *Nutrition During Infancy*. Tsang RS, Nichols BL, eds. Philadelphia: CV Mosby. 1988; 35–57.
20. Morselli PL. *Clin Pharmacokinet*. 1976; 1: 81–98.
21. Mirkin BL. *Pediatr Ann*. 1976 Sep: 542–57.
22. Morselli PL et al. *Clin Pharmacokinet*. 1980; 5: 485–527.
23. Silverio J, Poole JW. *Pediatrics*. 1973; 51: 578–80.
24. Matthews LW, Drotar D. *Pediatr Clin N Am*. 1984; 31: 133–52.
25. Greene HL et al. *J Pediatr*. 1975; 87: 695–704.
26. Friss-Hansen B. *Pediatrics*. 1971; 47: 264–74.
27. Friss-Hansen B. *Pediatrics*. 1961; 28: 169–81.
28. Siber GR et al. *J Infect Dis*. 1975; 78(suppl): 959–82.
29. Kurz H et al. *Eur J Clin Pharmacol*. 1977; 11: 463–7.
30. Neims AH et al. *Ann Rev Pharmacol Toxicol*. 1976; 16: 426–45.
31. Odell GB et al. In: *Care of the High-Risk Neonate*. Klaus MH, Fanaroff AA, eds. Philadelphia: WB Saunders; 1973: 183–204.
32. Datton GJ. *Ann Dev Pharmacol Ther*. 1978; 18: 17–36.
33. Haley TJ. *Drug Metabol Rev*. 1983; 14: 295–335.
34. Loggie JMH et al. *J Pediatr*. 1975; 86: 485–96.
35. Arant BS. *J Pediatr*. 1978; 92: 705–12.
36. Arny HV. *Am Pharm Assoc J*. 1917; 6: 1056.
37. Wilbert WI. *Am J Pharm*. 1902; 74: 120.
38. McKenzie M. *US Pharm*. 1981; 55: 66.
39. Martin S. Catering to pediatric patients. *Am Pharm*. 1992 Jan; NS32: 47–50.
40. Steward RB et al. Changing patterns of therapeutic agents in the elderly: a ten-year overview. *Age Ageing*. 1991 May; 20: 182–8.
41. Lamy PP. Nonprescription drugs and the elderly. *Am Fam Physician*. 1989 Jun; 39: 175–9.
42. Mallet L. Counseling in special populations: the elderly patient. *Am Pharm*. 1992 Oct; NS32: 71–81.
43. Lamy PP. *Pharm Internat*. 1986; 7: 46.
44. Meyer ME, Schuna HH. Assessment of geriatric patients' functional ability to take medication. *Drug Intell Clin Pharm*. 1989 Feb; 23: 171–4.
45. Levkoff SE et al. *J Am Geriatr Soc*. 1988; 36: 622.
46. Montamat SC, Cusack BJ, Vestal RE. Management of drug therapy in the elderly. *N Engl J Med*. 1989 Aug; 321: 303–9.
47. Cooper J, Gardner C. *J Am Geriatr Soc*. 1988; 36: 660.
48. Brown EM, Winograd CH. *J Am Geriatr Soc*. 1988; 36: 653.
49. Schmucker DL, Lonergan ET. *Rev Biol Res Aging*. 1987; 3: 509.
50. Swift GC. *Br Med J*. 1988; 296: 913.
51. Collins KJ et al. *Br Med J*. 1977; 1: 353.
52. Severson JA. *J Am Geriatr Soc*. 1984; 32: 24.
53. Bar SR, Roth J. *Arch Intern Med*. 1977; 137: 474.
54. Tomlinson BE, Henderson G. In: *Neurobiology of Aging*. Terry RD, Gershon S, eds. New York: Raven Press; 1976.
55. Anderson JM et al. *J Neurol Sci*. 1983; 58: 235.
56. Bell MJ. *Acta Neuropathologia*. 1977; 37: 111.
57. Wagner HN et al. *Science*. 1983; 221: 2164.
58. Lamy PP. *Prescribing for the Elderly*. Littleton, Mass: PSG Publishing; 1980.
59. Scott JC, Stanski DR. *J Pharmacol Exper Ther*. 1987; 240: 59.
60. Schmucker DL. *Pharmacol Rev*. 1985; 37: 133.
61. Evans JG, Jarvis EH. *Br Med J*. 1972; 4: 133.
62. Willington FL. Urinary incontinence: a practical approach. *Geriatrics*. 1980 Jun; 35: 41–8.
63. Schwartz JB, Abernethy DR. *Geriatrics*. 1987; 21: 349.
64. Bend F. *Ztg Kardiol*. 1985; 74(suppl 1): 49.
65. Guarnieri T et al. *Am J Physiol*. 1980; 239: H501.
66. Lakatta EG et al. *Circ Res*. 1975; 36: 262.
67. Fleisch JH. *Pharmacol Ther*. 1980; 8: 477.
68. Gribbin B et al. *Circ Res*. 1971; 29: 424.
69. Caird FI et al. *Br Heart J*. 1973; 35: 527.
70. Snyder SH. *N Engl J Med*. 1970; 300: 465.
71. Davidson MB. *Metabolism*. 1979; 28: 688.
72. Orlander P, Johnson DG. *Otolaryngol Clin North Am*. 1982; 15: 439.
73. Makinodan T, Kay MMB. *Adv Immunol*. 1980; 29: 287.
74. Price GB, Makinodan T. *J Immunol*. 1972; 108: 302.
75. Lamy PP. *Geriatr Med Today*. 1988; 7(4): 30.
76. Lamy PP. In: *Side Effects of Anti-inflammatory Drugs*. Rainsford KD, Velo GP, eds. Lancaster, England: MTP Press; 1986.
77. Goulson K, Cooke AR. *Br Med J*. 1968; 14: 664.
78. Lamy PP. *Generations*. 1988; 12(4): 9.
79. Buitendijk S, Bracken MB. Medication in early pregnancy: prevalence of use and relationship to maternal characteristics. *Am J Obstet Gynecol*. 1991 Jul; 165: 33–40.
80. American Academy of Pediatrics Committee on Environmental Hazards. Effects of cigarette smoking on the fetus and child. *Pediatrics*. 1976 Mar; 57: 411–3.
81. Fielding JE. Smoking and pregnancy. *N Engl J Med*. 1978 Feb; 298: 337–9.
82. Clarren SK, Smith DW. The fetal alcohol syndrome. *N Engl J Med*. 1978 May; 298: 1063–7.
83. Shaywitz SE, Cohen DJ, Shaywitz BA. Behavior and learning difficulties in children of normal intelligence born to alcoholic mothers. *J Pediatr*. 1980 Jun; 96: 978–82.
84. Briggs GG, Freeman RK, Yaffe SJ. *Drugs in Pregnancy and Lactation: A Reference Guide to Fetal and Neonatal Risk*. 4th ed. Baltimore: Williams and Wilkins; 1994: 65a–73a, 176c–9c, 363f–4f, 613n–4n.
85. American Academy of Pediatrics Committee on Drugs. Transfer of drugs and other chemicals into human milk. *Pediatrics*. 1994; 93: 137–50.

CHAPTER 3

In-Home Testing and Monitoring Products

Wendy P. Munroe and Marcus D. Wilson

Questions to ask in patient assessment and counseling

Fecal Occult Blood Test Kits

- *Have you ever suffered from any bowel disorder? Have you or anyone in your family had colorectal cancer? Have any family members suffered from stomach or colon problems (eg, ulcers or hemorrhoids)?*
- *Are you currently experiencing known bleeding such as hemorrhoidal or menstrual bleeding?*
- *What nonprescription or prescription medications are you currently taking?*
- *Do you have any visual limitations?*

Ovulation Prediction Test Kits

- *Do you have any chronic medical conditions?*
- *Are you consulting or have you consulted a doctor who specializes in fertility problems?*
- *How "regular" are your periods?*
- *Have you ever used a product like this? If so, which one?*
- *Do you have any visual limitations?*

Pregnancy Test Kits

- *How late is your period?*
- *Do you have any chronic medical conditions?*
- *What nonprescription or prescription medications are you currently taking?*
- *Have you ever used a pregnancy test before? If so, which one?*
- *Do you have any visual limitations?*

Cholesterol Test Kit

- *Do you have any conditions that cause excessive bleeding from a finger prick?*
- *Do you have any chronic medical conditions?*
- *What nonprescription or prescription medications are you currently taking?*
- *Have you ever used this product before?*

Home Blood Pressure Monitoring Devices

- *Do you or any family members have a history of high blood pressure?*
- *Are you taking any medications to control high blood pressure?*
- *Have you been instructed on the use of a blood pressure monitor?*
- *Have you monitored your own blood pressure in the past? If so, what type of device did you use?*
- *Do you have difficulty with your hearing or sight?*

In 1977 the home diagnostics market made a quantum leap when Warner-Lambert introduced the first home pregnancy test kit. Since then, the market has continued to grow, with the development of an expanded array of products and more user-friendly versions of established ones. In the 12 months ending November 30, 1994, the sale of home test kits grew 17%, reaching total sales of $647.3 million.[1]

Several forces are driving this growth. One is the increasing public interest in health, fitness, and preventive medicine. Home testing and monitoring kits allow patients to test themselves at their convenience in their homes, which encourages their active participation in their own health care. A second impetus for growth is that these kits can help patients reduce health care costs by avoiding unnecessary physician visits and seeking earlier treatment.

Important advances in technology have led to simplified tests that can be accurately and easily performed at home. A major advance has been the use of an enzyme-linked immunoassay (ELISA) with monoclonal antibodies. These immunoglobulin molecules, which are structurally similar to the antibodies that B lymphocytes normally produce in response to an antigen stimulus,[2] are purified antibodies that are engineered to recognize and bind to a specific antigen. Thus, they make home test kits highly sensitive, accurate, and easy to use.

This chapter discusses several home test kits: fecal occult blood detection tests, ovulation prediction tests, pregnancy tests, cholesterol tests, and blood pressure measurement devices. (The products used in the self-monitoring of asthma and diabetes are presented in Chapter 9, "Asthma Products," and Chapter 18, "Diabetes Care Products and Monitoring Devices.")

Editor's Note: This chapter is based, in part, on a chapter with the same title that appeared in the 10th edition but was written by Susan M. Meyer.

Use/Selection of Home Diagnostic Kits

Home testing and monitoring kits are designed to serve two basic purposes: early disease detection and disease therapy monitoring. Pharmacists can play an important role in helping patients to select and use the kits appropriately and to understand their limitations.

General Principles of Use

The Food and Drug Administration (FDA) requires home tests to be 95–99% accurate.[3] To achieve these accuracy rates, the products must be used as intended. A 1989 study that evaluated the reliability of selected home pregnancy tests demonstrated a 93.5% accuracy rate in home use.[4] The authors concluded that inaccurate test results occurred because patients did not follow directions correctly and used improper techniques.

Although testing procedures and kit contents vary among manufacturers, the mechanism of action for each category of tests is basically the same. Patients should follow these general guidelines for using home test kits:

- Because these products use monoclonal antibodies and various chemicals, reagent stability is a concern. Patients should always check the test kit expiration date and follow the manufacturer's instructions for storage.
- Patients should read the instructions entirely before attempting to perform a test. They should note the time of day the test is to be conducted, the length of time that is required, and any necessary equipment. This will allow the patient to schedule the best time and place to conduct the test.
- Many kits require that the user wait a specified length of time between steps. In these cases, the timing must be precise. Patients should use an accurate timing device that measures seconds.
- Many kits require the user to observe a color change to read the test results; therefore, someone must be present who does not have color-defective vision or other visual impairment.
- The instructions must be followed exactly and in sequence. Patients who have questions about the testing procedure or interpretation of the results should consult a pharmacist or other health professional. Most kits offer a toll-free number to call for assistance.
- It is important that patients understand they are self-*testing*, not self-*diagnosing*. Positive test results should be reported to a physician immediately for definitive diagnosis and management. Negative test results should be questioned if the patient is experiencing definite symptoms of a suspected condition. If there is any question about the results, the patient should seek the advice of a health professional.

Product Selection Guidelines

With the variety of diagnostic products available, deciding which test to recommend to patients is quite challenging. The major variables to consider include the test's complexity, ease of reading results, presence of a control, and cost.

Complexity of the Test Procedure

Since human error plays such an important part in the ultimate value of these products, simplicity of use deserves major consideration. Each step and manipulation required is a potential source of error. Some of the tests are more user-friendly than others; simple tests are generally more desirable.

Ease of Reading Results

In most home test kits, the result is indicated by a change in color. With some products this color change is easily discernible (eg, the appearance of a plus sign or a check mark) whereas other products require that the user recognize subtle variations in shade. The latter results are more open to misinterpretation.

Presence of a Control

When possible, patients should select a test that includes a control to ensure that the test has been performed correctly.

Cost

Many products provide more than one test per kit. Thus, when considering cost, patients should determine the cost per test *unit*.

Fecal Occult Blood Kits

Fecal occult blood testing products can be used as an adjunct to more invasive tests to detect any gastrointestinal bleeding. The best-known use of these tests is for colorectal cancer screening; one early and common symptom of colorectal cancer is rectal bleeding.

How They Work

The in-home tests are designed to detect occult blood in feces with a colorimetric assay for hemoglobin. The heme portion of hemoglobin acts as an oxidizing agent, catalyzing the oxidation of the test reagent, tetramethylbenzidine, which produces a blue-green color. The appearance of this color indicates that the test is positive.

Occult blood may be present on the surface or in the matrix of the stool.[5] In general, matrix blood originates in the upper gastrointestinal tract while surface blood comes from the lower tract. The kits are more likely to detect blood from lower gastrointestinal abnormalities such as colorectal cancer.

The reagent is sandwiched between two layers of biodegradable paper and is placed in the toilet bowl following a bowel movement. These kits are based on the premise that a significant amount of fecal blood will remain on the surface of the toilet bowl water after a bowel movement.

Choosing a Test

Two nonprescription products, ColoCARE and EZ Detect, are available (see product table "Fecal Occult Blood Test Kits"). The differences between the two are minor. The main advantage of EZ Detect is that it imposes no dietary restrictions because the results are not affected by red meat or vitamin C.

ColoCARE contains three pads for testing three consecutive bowel movements. Immediately after a bowel movement, the ColoCARE pad is floated in the toilet bowl, printed side up. The pad is observed for 30 seconds for the appearance of a blue or green tint in the test area. This color change should be considered a positive sign of the presence of hemoglobin. Two control areas on the bottom of each pad indicate if the test is functioning properly. The left area should always turn blue or green and the right area should not change color. If this does not occur, the pad should be discarded and the test repeated after the next bowel movement.[6]

The EZ Detect kit contains five test pads and a positive control chemical package. Before using EZ Detect, the patient should use one test pad to perform a water quality check. If any trace of blue appears in the cross-shaped area when the pad is floated in the toilet water, another toilet bowl should be used. The same testing procedure is then used with the EZ Detect test pad as with the ColoCARE. Three consecutive bowel movements are tested. A positive result is indicated after 2 minutes by the appearance of a blue cross on the test pad. If no positive results are obtained in the three tests, a test pad quality check may be performed with the remaining pad. The patient should flush the toilet and empty the contents of the positive control chemical package into the bowl as it refills. The remaining test pad should then be floated in the water, printed side up. A blue cross should appear within 2 minutes, indicating that the test pads were working properly. If the blue cross does not appear, the test results are invalid and the patient should call the assistance line provided with the product.[7]

Factors That Affect Results

Medications that may cause gastritis may also cause sufficient bleeding to produce false-positive results; thus, they should be avoided for at least 2–3 days before and during the test period.[8] These medications include aspirin, nonsteroidal anti-inflammatory drugs, steroids, and reserpine. Rectally administered medications should also be avoided. However, patients should be advised to consult their physicians before discontinuing any prescribed medications.

Toilet bowl cleaners also may produce false-positive results.[8] Before using these tests, patients should flush the toilet twice to remove any chemicals and cleansers from the bowl. With ColoCARE, vitamin C in excess of 250 mg per day may interfere with the peroxidase action of hemoglobin, causing false-negative results.[8] Another restriction with this product is that red meat should be avoided for 2–3 days before and during the test period. This is because the test is *not* specific for human blood and may produce positive results if red meat is consumed.

Patient Counseling

The pharmacist should advise patients to follow the package instructions carefully. The following points about fecal occult blood tests should also be stressed:

- These tests should not be performed during times of known bleeding, such as hemorrhoidal or menstrual bleeding.
- Dietary fiber intake should be increased for several days before testing. Roughage increases the accuracy of the test by stimulating bleeding from lesions that might not otherwise bleed.[5]
- Because bleeding from cancerous lesions may be intermittent, the tests should be performed on three consecutive bowel movements to increase the chance of detecting a possible lesion. Patients should be instructed to complete all three stool tests even if the first two produce negative results.
- Those evaluating the results of fecal occult blood tests must remember that this is a screening method and is not specific to a particular disease.

A positive test result may indicate any medical condition that causes a loss of blood through the gastrointestinal system, such as hemorrhoids, peptic ulcers, colitis, diverticulitis, polyps, and esophageal varices. The primary value of these tests is to alert patients and physicians that a thorough workup may be needed. The kits are *not* intended to replace other diagnostic procedures.

Ovulation Prediction and Pregnancy Test Kits

The Female Reproductive Cycle

The female reproductive cycle, which is approximately 28 days in length, is under hormonal control. At the beginning of the cycle (day 1 through approximately day 13), low levels of circulating estrogen and progesterone cause the hypothalamus to secrete gonadotropin-releasing hormone (GnRH), which in turn stimulates the release of follicle-stimulating hormone (FSH) and low levels of luteinizing hormone (LH) from the anterior pituitary. This combination of hormones is responsible for promoting the development of several follicles within an ovary during each cycle. At one point in the development, one follicle is singled out and continues to mature while the others regress. At midcycle (approximately day 14 or 15), circulating LH levels significantly increase and cause final maturation of the follicle. Ovulation (rupturing of the follicle and release of the ovum) occurs approximately 20–48 hours after this LH surge. Cells in the ruptured follicle then luteinize and form the corpus luteum, which begins to secrete progesterone and estrogen. For approximately 7–8 days after ovulation, the corpus luteum continues to develop and to secrete estrogen and progesterone, which inhibit further secretion of FSH and LH.

If fertilization occurs, trophoblastic cells produce the hormone human chorionic gonadotropin (HCG). HCG causes the corpus luteum to continue to produce progesterone and estrogen, which forestall the onset of menses while the placenta develops and becomes functional. As early as day 7 after conception, the placenta produces HCG, the concentration of which continues to increase during early pregnancy. Some HCG is excreted in the urine, and maximum levels of HCG are reached 6 weeks after conception. HCG levels decline over the following 4–6 weeks and then stabilize for the remainder of the pregnancy.

If fertilization does not occur during a cycle, the corpus luteum degenerates, circulating levels of progesterone and estrogen diminish, and menstruation occurs (days 1–5). Resulting low levels of progesterone and estrogen cause the release of GnRH from the hypothalamus, and the hormonal cycle begins again.[9,10]

Basal Thermometry

For many years, women have measured basal body temperature to predict the time of ovulation. This is because resting basal body temperature is usually below normal during the first part of the female reproductive cycle. After ovulation, basal body temperature rises to a level closer to normal (ie, 98.6°F [37°C]).

Women who use this method of ovulation prediction take their temperature (orally, rectally, or vaginally) with a basal thermometer each morning before arising. These temperature measurements are then plotted graphically. A rise in temperature is a signal that ovulation has occurred. When the increase occurs, women seeking to become pregnant should have intercourse as soon as possible to maximize their chances of conception.

Choosing a Test

The only equipment necessary for basal body temperature monitoring is a basal thermometer. Although basal thermometry is a relatively simple method of ovulation prediction, recording and interpreting temperature data can be confusing. In addition, some women may have difficulty reading mercury thermometers accurately. Because the temperature increase that follows ovulation is small (0.4°–1.0°F [0.2°–0.6°C]), women who have trouble reading a thermometer may miss it altogether.[11]

The Bioself Fertility Indicator uses computer technology to avoid these potential problems, providing a digital temperature reading in just 2 minutes. The device can also store temperature readings in its memory for 120 consecutive days. The user must input the date of the first day of menses each month. The device then processes temperature measurements and cycle information to calculate the user's average cycle length and predict the user's most fertile days. The device's indicator lights, activated each morning when the temperature is taken, display the predictions. Specifically, a green light means that the woman is in the most infertile period of her cycle, a red light indicates that a woman's fertility is low but that conception is possible, and a flashing red light signals that a woman is in her most fertile period and that her likelihood of conception is highest.

Two clinical studies have demonstrated that the Bioself Fertility Indicator is 90% effective in indicating a time window that includes a woman's highly fertile period.[12,13] However, knowing this time window does not guarantee that a woman will conceive, even when the device is used properly.

Factors That Affect Results

Several factors, such as emotions, movements, and infections, can influence the basal metabolic temperature. Eating, drinking, talking, and smoking should be postponed until after each measurement is obtained.

Patient Counseling

Patients who use basal thermometry as a method of predicting ovulation should be advised of the following:

- The Bioself Fertility Indicator device may be used to record oral, rectal, or vaginal temperature. However, it is critical that users choose one method for temperature measurement and use it consistently, and that temperature readings be taken at approximately the same time each morning. An alarm is built into the device to remind users when it is time to obtain a measurement.
- The temperatures should be taken just before arising each morning after at least 5 hours of sleep.
- Women who do not conceive after using this device for three consecutive cycles may wish to use another unique feature of it. Specifically, the device includes a modem that enables the user to transmit data stored in the device to the manufacturer by telephone. The company then mails a printout to the user that indicates the number of days the device was used, the lengths of the last six menstrual cycles, a graphic plot of daily temperature measurements for the last 120 days, and fertility-level estimates for the same period. The woman may then provide this information to her fertility specialist as a starting point for consultation.

Ovulation Prediction Kits

Ovulation prediction kits, which estimate the time of ovulation, are marketed to women who are having trouble conceiving and need to pinpoint ovulation.

How They Work

These tests indicate the increase and decrease of LH. LH is normally present throughout the menstrual cycle but increases sharply just prior to ovulation. The LH surge appears in the serum approximately 20–48 hours before ovulation. Approximately 8–12 hours after it appears, the LH surge is detectable in the urine.

Ovulation prediction kits use monoclonal antibodies specific to LH and use an ELISA to elicit a color change indicative of the amount of LH in the urine.[14] The LH surge is revealed by a difference in color or color intensity from that noted on the previous day of testing. The intensity of the color on the test stick or in the test solution is directly proportional to the amount of LH in the urine sample.

Choosing a Test

The kits available vary in the complexity of the procedure, the length of time needed to complete the test, and the number of individual tests provided (see product table "Ovulation Prediction Test Kits"). With the simplest kits, a woman urinates onto a test stick and reads the result in 3 minutes. The more complicated products require a series of precisely timed manipulations involving test tubes and droppers. The more steps that are involved, the greater is the potential for human error.

Factors That Affect Results

Medications that are used to promote ovulation (eg, menotropins) may cause a false-positive result each time the tests are used because LH levels are artificially elevated. The true LH surge can be detected in patients receiving clomiphene so long as testing does not begin until the second day after drug therapy ends. Medical conditions associated with high levels of LH, such as menopause and polycystic ovary syndrome, may also cause false-positive results. A false-positive result may also be obtained if the user is already pregnant.[14] If the patient has recently discontinued using oral contraceptives, the start of ovulation may be delayed for one to two cycles. Thus, it would not be appropriate for this individual to use an in-home ovulation prediction test kit until fertilization has been attempted unsuccessfully for several months following discontinuation of the oral contraceptives.

Patient Counseling

The pharmacist should advise patients to follow the package instructions carefully and should stress the following points about ovulation prediction tests:

- The first day of testing should be 2–3 days before ovulation is expected. The kit contains directions to help the woman determine when to begin testing, based on the average length of her past three menstrual cycles. If her cycle varies by more than 3–4 days each month, she should use the length of the shortest cycle to determine the starting date.
- It is important to follow the manufacturer's specific directions regarding the timing of urine collection. Generally, the early morning is recommended because the LH surge usually begins early in the day and the urine concentration is relatively consistent at this time. Some products do not specify a time of day, requiring only that a consistent time be used. In this case, the woman should not have urinated for at least 4 hours before testing and should restrict her fluid intake before testing so that her urine will not be diluted.
- The urine sample should be tested immediately after collection. If this is not feasible, the urine may be stored under refrigeration for the length of time specified in the directions for each product. The sample must reach room temperature by standing 20–30 minutes before the testing procedure is begun. The woman should not redisperse any sediment that may be present in the sample.
- The woman is looking for the test's first significant increase in color intensity, which indicates that the LH surge has occurred and that ovulation will occur within a day or two. Once ovulation occurs, the ovum remains viable for fertilization for a period of 12–24 hours.[15] Because sperm may live up to 72 hours, the optimal days for fertilization are the 2 days before ovulation, the day of ovulation, and the day after ovulation. For the greatest chance of achieving pregnancy, intercourse should take place within the 24 hours after the LH surge.
- Once the LH surge is detected, the woman should discontinue testing. Remaining tests can be used at a later date, if necessary.
- If the LH surge is not detected, one of the following possibilities may have occurred: (1) the test may not have been performed properly, (2) the woman may not have ovulated, or (3) the test may have been used too late in the cycle. The woman should carefully review the testing procedure and consider testing for a longer period in the next cycle to increase her chances of detecting the LH surge.
- It is generally recommended that these products not be used for longer than 3 months. If a woman has not conceived within this time, she should consult her physician.

Home Pregnancy Tests

The fastest-growing segment of the home diagnostic market is the home pregnancy test. One third of women who think they may be pregnant have reportedly used these products.[16] Early detection of pregnancy is desirable because it allows the woman to make decisions regarding prenatal care and lifestyle changes to avoid potential harm to the fetus.

How They Work

The pregnancy tests available for home use are designed to detect the presence of HCG in the urine.[17] HCG, a hormone produced by the trophoblast of the fertilized ovum, is detectable in the urine within 1–2 weeks after conception and is considered a diagnostic indicator of pregnancy. The original in-home pregnancy test kits used the hemagglutination inhibition reaction method to detect HCG in the urine. However, there were numerous limitations associated with this method for detecting pregnancy.

Most of the kits on the market today use monoclonal or polyclonal antibodies in an enzyme immunoassay.[17] These antibodies, which act against HCG, are bound to a solid surface such as a stick, bead, or filter. If urinary HCG is present, it will complex with the antibodies. Another antibody, one that is linked to an enzyme that will react with a chromogen to produce a distinctive color, is added. The HCG is then "sandwiched" between the antibody linked to the enzyme and the antibodies bound to the solid surface. Washing or filtering the testing device removes unbound substances; a chromogen that will react with the enzyme is then added. These antibody-based tests are very sensitive and specific; if correctly used, they have a reported accuracy of more than 95%.[18]

Choosing a Test

The available products vary in the complexity of the testing procedure and the length of time needed to complete the test (see product table "Pregnancy Test Kits"). With the simplest kits, a woman urinates onto a test stick and can read the result in 3 minutes. The more steps that are involved, the greater is the potential for human error.

Factors That Affect Results

The antibody pregnancy tests are less susceptible to interference from other substances than were the original hemagglutination inhibition tests. However, false-negative results may occur with these tests if they are performed too soon after conception or if the urine sample was refrigerated and not allowed to return to room temperature.

Patient Counseling

The pharmacist should advise patients to follow the package instructions carefully, especially with regard to the following points:

- The instructions will specify the number of days the woman must wait after menses is due before performing the test. Performing the test too early may produce false-negative results. Most tests on the market may be used as early as the day of a missed menstrual period.
- Generally, the first morning urine should be used because the levels of HCG, if present, will be concentrated at that time. Some tests allow the use of a sample collected at any time, as long as the woman restricts her fluid intake 4–6 hours prior to urine collection.
- The woman should use the urine collection device provided in the kit rather than use some other container. Waxed cups may cause erroneous results in antibody-based tests because wax particles can clog the test matrix. Soap residue in household containers can also interfere with the test reaction.
- The urine sample should be tested immediately after collection. If this is not possible, the urine may be stored in the refrigerator, but it must be allowed to reach room temperature before testing. Chilled urine may produce false-negative results. Also, the woman should be careful not to redisperse any sediment that may be present in the sample.
- If the test result is positive, the woman should assume she is pregnant and see her family physician or an obstetrician as soon as possible.
- If the test result is negative, the woman should review the procedure and make sure she performed the test correctly. If she did not wait the number of days recommended by the manufacturer, she should wait the prescribed time and test again if menses has not begun. If the results of the second test are negative and menses still has not begun, the woman should seek the advice of a physician.

Home Cholesterol Test Kit

A 1988 FDA survey found that only 30% of people with high cholesterol were aware of their condition. The US Department of Health and Human Services recommends efforts to increase to 60% the proportion of adults with high blood cholesterol who are not only aware of their condition but also taking action to alleviate the problem.[19] Consistent with this goal, the National Cholesterol Education Program recommends that all adults aged 20 and older have their total cholesterol measured at least every 5 years.[20] One means to achieve this first critical step in minimizing the risk for cardiovascular heart disease is the use of home cholesterol testing.

The Advanced Care Cholesterol Test is the only marketed nonprescription test kit that enables patients to measure their total blood cholesterol at home (see product table "Cholesterol Test Kits"). The test kit includes one test cassette, a single-use lancet, one gauze pad, one adhesive bandage, an instruction booklet, a question-and-answer booklet, and a chart for interpreting the test results.

How It Works

The Advanced Care test device is a palm-sized, single-use, noninstrumented, plastic cassette that is read like a thermometer. Cholesterol obtained from a blood sample of one to two drops is converted into hydrogen peroxide through two chemical reactions involving cholesterol esterase and cholesterol oxidase. The peroxide then reacts with horseradish peroxidase and a dye to produce the color that rises along the test's measurement scale. Two separate indicator spots change color to show that the test is functioning properly. One spot also indicates that the test has been completed and it is time to read the scale.

The first step in completing the test is to wash the hands thoroughly with soap and warm water. After drying the hands, the patient should select the outside of one fingertip for the test. The patient should then lance the fingertip, wipe away the first sign of blood with the gauze pad, lower the hand below the heart, and milk the finger from base to tip to obtain a large, hanging drop of blood. This drop should be touched to the bottom of the sample well of the test cassette. Additional drops should then be added until the black fill line is covered completely.

After at least 2 but no more than 4 minutes, the patient should pull the clear plastic tab on the right side of the cassette until it clicks into place and a red line appears. After another 10–12 minutes, when the "END" indicator turns green, the patient should measure the height of the purple column against the scale printed on the cassette. This number should then be interpreted using the paper result chart included in the kit. Patients must use only the result chart that comes with the kit because a chart from another test kit may give an inaccurate result.

Factors That Affect Results

Good finger-pricking technique is necessary to avoid erroneous results. Two or three hanging drops of blood are needed; excessive squeezing and milking of the finger will affect the quality of the blood sample. If sufficient blood cannot be obtained from the first finger prick, a second finger should be used. A low cholesterol value may result if the blood sample is too small or if it takes longer than 5 minutes to collect the necessary amount of blood.

Doses of 500 mg or more of vitamin C or standard doses (eg, 325–1,000 mg) of acetaminophen should be avoided for 4 hours before the test because these may interfere with test results.

A number of studies have demonstrated that the test's accuracy (on average, 97% when performed according to package directions) is comparable to that of instrumented laboratory methods.[21–23]

Patient Counseling

The pharmacist should advise patients to follow the package instructions carefully and to pay special attention to the following points:

- The cassettes are stable at room temperature.
- Used cassettes are considered potentially biohazardous and should be disposed of appropriately.
- Because of the risk of excessive bleeding from the finger prick, the test should *not* be used by patients with hemophilia or by those who take anticoagulants. These people should have their cholesterol tested by physicians only.
- This product only measures total cholesterol. Any consumer who obtains a result of 200 mg/dL or greater should see a physician for a repeat measurement, lipid profile, and appropriate medical workup.

Home Blood Pressure Monitoring Devices

The consequences of untreated hypertension are well documented. Long-standing elevations in blood pressure can lead to damage to the heart, kidney, lungs, eyes, and vessels and to an increase in morbidity and mortality.[24–27] In the United States, cardiovascular disease, to which hypertension is a major contributor, takes the life of one of every two persons. With more than 50 million people with high blood pressure,[24] fewer than 25% are well controlled. The remaining patients are either not identified, identified but not treated, or treated and not controlled. The reasons for this are multiple, but a significant factor seems to be the lack of patient motivation, which leads to noncompliance. Hypertension is an asymptomatic disease. Its treatment often involves significant lifestyle changes and the institution of drug therapies. These measures inevitably produce side effects, so that the patient who was without symptoms of disease is suddenly symptomatic. Patient education and empowerment play a large role in improving patient compliance with antihypertensive efforts. This, in turn, helps reduce morbidity and mortality, maintains or improves the patient's quality of life, and improves the patient's use of health care resources.[28]

Teaching patients to take their own blood pressure at home is an excellent means of achieving these goals. Home blood pressure monitoring (HBPM) gives patients a sense of control over their health. Patients can measure their progress toward a goal blood pressure level. In addition, HBPM provides valuable data on blood pressure values, which can be obtained away from the physician's office. Thus, although the office measurement of blood pressure is still the mainstay of monitoring, hypertension experts strongly encourage the use of HBPM in the routine care of most patients with hypertension or suspected hypertension.[24,29] This sentiment was most recently expressed by a committee of national hypertensive experts at the 1995 annual meeting of the American Society of Hypertension.

Of note in this regard is the fact that the market for HBPM devices has grown steadily over the last decade. Sales in 1993 reached 2.75 million units, representing a 17% increase over 1992. With the increased emphasis on home monitoring, the market will continue to expand.

How They Work

There are two types of indirect measurement of blood pressure: auscultatory (measurement of sound) and oscillometric (measurement of vibration) (see product table "Electronic Oscillometric Blood Pressure Monitor Products"). Currently, there are three categories of monitors for home use: mercury column, aneroid, and digital. Mercury and aneroid meters involve auscultation with the use of a stethoscope to detect Korotkoff's sounds, which are produced by the motion of the arterial wall in response to changes in arterial pressure. Oscillometric sensors, which are often used with digital meters, measure blood pressure by detecting blood surges underneath the cuff as it is deflated. The detection device, which is usually indicated on the cuff with a tab or other marking, is placed directly over the brachial artery. The brachial artery can be found by palpating 1–2 inches above and just to the inside of the antecubital space. As cuff pressure increases during the measurement procedure, the brachial artery is compressed and blood flow is obstructed. As cuff pressure is gradually released, blood flow is reestablished and Korotkoff's sounds can be heard in different phases. Phase I, which corresponds to systolic pressure, can be identified when at least two consecutive "beats" are heard as cuff pressure is decreased. The nature of the sounds changes over the next three phases. Diastolic pressure is identified as phase V, the disappearance of sound.

Using the appropriate size cuff is essential for accurate measurement of a patient's blood pressure (Table 1). If the cuff is too small, blood pressure readings can be significantly overestimated. Several monitors are supplied with a large cuff; many others allow for the purchase of a large cuff separately. A thigh cuff for home monitoring is currently not available. For those patients requiring a thigh cuff, a wrist monitor may be a useful alternative. For wrist cuffs, instructions on cuff placement should be followed closely: careful attention must be paid to the level of the wrist in relation to the heart. Because these devices are also highly sensitive to changes in

TABLE 1 Arm circumferences for determining appropriate cuff size

Arm circumference (adult)[a]	Cuff size
<31 cm	Regular adult cuff
31–40 cm	Large adult cuff
>40 cm	Thigh cuff[b]

[a]Arm circumference should be calculated by measuring around the midpoint of the upper arm. Remeasure the patient's arm periodically, especially if he or she has recently gained or lost significant weight.

[b]For those patients needing a thigh cuff, a wrist monitor should be considered.

Source:

Soghikian K et al. Home blood pressure monitoring. Effect on use of medical services and medical care costs. *Med Care.* 1992; 30: 855–65.

Egmond J et al. Accuracy and reproducibility of 30 devices for self-measurement of arterial blood pressure. *Am J Hypertens.* 1993; 6: 873–9.

wrist level, it is best to support the arm on a table with a pillow to raise the wrist to the appropriate level. Many clinicians feel that the finger cuffs currently on the market lack sufficient accuracy and reliability to warrant their routine use.

Choosing a Device

No single device is best for every patient. The choice of device is individualized, based on characteristics such as the patient's ability and willingness to learn, physical handicaps, economic status, and preference.

Mercury Column Devices

The reference standard in blood pressure measurement remains the mercury column blood pressure (BP) meter (Figure 1). These devices typically come with a cuff and an inflation bulb. The tubing from the cuff is attached to a column of mercury encased in a glass gauge. The stethoscope is usually sold separately.

Although mercury BP meters are the most accurate and reliable of the devices, their routine use for home measurement is discouraged because they are cumbersome and pose the risk of mercury toxicity should the glass tubing break. However, the devices are often used in the professional environment, especially for the calibration of aneroid devices. Good eyesight and hearing are required to use them effectively. Should it happen that the mercury does not rest at zero when the cuff is removed, lying flat, and completely deflated, the device will need to be recalibrated.

Aneroid Devices

Next to the mercury column BP meters, the aneroid devices are the most accurate and reliable monitors. They are light, portable, and very affordable, and they pose no risk from mercury toxicity. They also include several features that make patient teaching much easier. First, many devices now come with a stethoscope attached to the cuff (Figure 2); this keeps the patient from having to hold the bell of the stethoscope in place. Second, a D-ring on the cuff allows a single user to place the cuff on the arm easily. Third, a few manufacturers offer a gauge that is attached to the inflation bulb; again, this makes it easier to manipulate the equipment since there are fewer pieces to control. While these monitors are considered the option of choice for home use, they do require more careful patient instruction and follow-up. Good eyesight and hearing are necessary for accurate results. For patients with reduced visual capacity, however, there are gauges available with large-type print on the face of the gauge.

At the bottom of the face of each aneroid device, there is a small box. When the cuff is completely deflated and lying on the table, the needle of the gauge should rest in the box. If the needle is outside the box, the gauge should be recalibrated. Many manufacturers sell recalibration tools to allow health care professionals to adjust the devices themselves.

Digital Devices

With advancing technology, digital devices have become more accurate, reliable, and easy to use and have thus skyrocketed in popularity. These devices include semiautomatic (manually inflating), fully automatic (auto-inflating), wrist, and finger blood pressure monitors (Figure 3). Such features as printouts, a pulse monitor, a digital clock, automated inflation and deflation, memory, a large display, a D-ring for the cuff, a preformed cuff, and fuzzy logic differentiate many of the devices. These features also add significantly to the price.

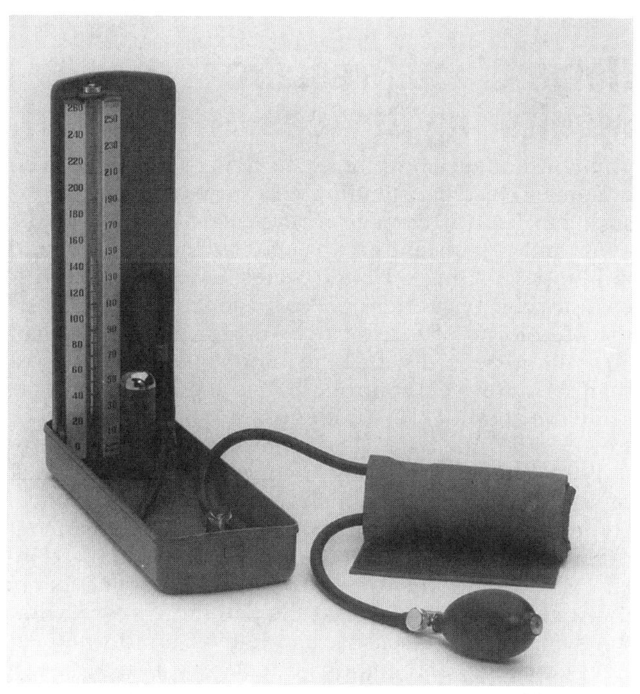

FIGURE 1 Mercury blood pressure meter. Reprinted from *Am Pharm.* 1989; NS29: 578.

A major drawback to the digital monitors is the inability of the user to determine if the device is out of calibration. In addition, many of the devices currently on the market lack extensive accuracy and reliability data and are often found to be inadequate for routine use.[30–33] This leads many clinicians to recommend the use of the aneroid devices over the easier-to-use digital products.

Proper Technique

While the actual measurement of blood pressure is a relatively simple procedure, many people consistently do it incorrectly. Blood pressure is naturally variable and can change in seconds. Thus, proper technique is essential to reduce measurement variability and improve the quality of results. It should be remembered that the normal range for blood pressures was established with patients in the resting state, so any variation from this setting can produce artificial results.

For the person who is doing the actual monitoring, following the steps outlined below will help improve the accuracy of blood pressure readings whether they are taken by the physician in his or her office, by the pharmacist in the pharmacy, or by the patient at home.

- Make sure the room is at a comfortable temperature.
- Seat the patient in a comfortable chair, with the back supported and the feet straight ahead and flat on the floor.
- Make sure the patient's arm is supported with the midpoint of the upper arm at heart level. The patient who is taking his or her own blood pressure should place the arm on a table.
- Remove restrictive clothing from the arm.
- Place the cuff on the arm to be measured. The cuff should be snug but not tight enough to restrict blood flow.
- Have the patient rest for at least 5 minutes in this position.
- Measure the blood pressure.
- Take two to three measurements separated by at least 2 minutes using the same arm.
- Record the results and include the time and date of the measurement, as well as any medications, including antihypertensive medications, currently being taken and the time of the last dose of each.
- Supply these results to the patient's primary care provider.

Factors That Affect Results

The results of a 1991 study examining the blood pressure monitoring technique of physicians demonstrated that not one of 114 physicians performed this procedure accurately.[34] The most common error was failure to use the correct size cuff. Using a cuff that is too small can significantly overestimate a patient's blood pressure, sometimes by as much as 20–30 mm Hg. Table 1 provides guidelines for choosing the correct size cuff. Holding the arm higher or lower than heart level can also significantly alter readings.

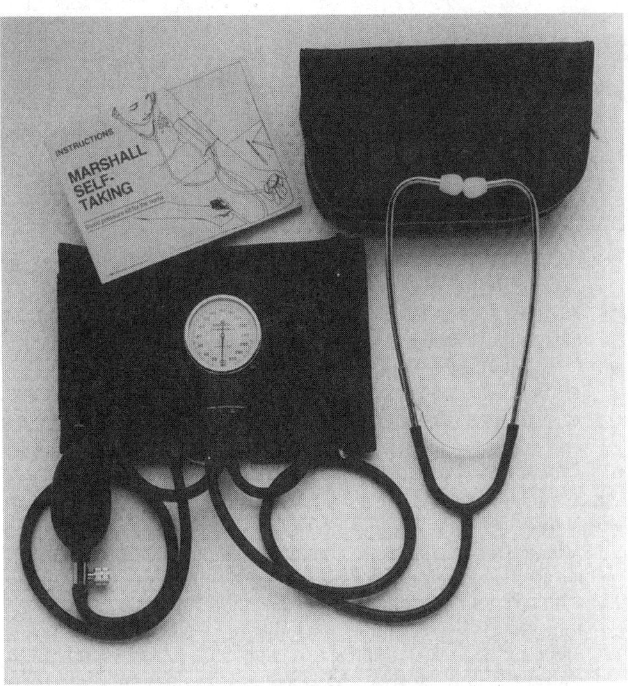

FIGURE 2 Aneroid blood pressure meter. Photograph provided by Omron Healthcare, Inc, Vernon Hills, Illinois.

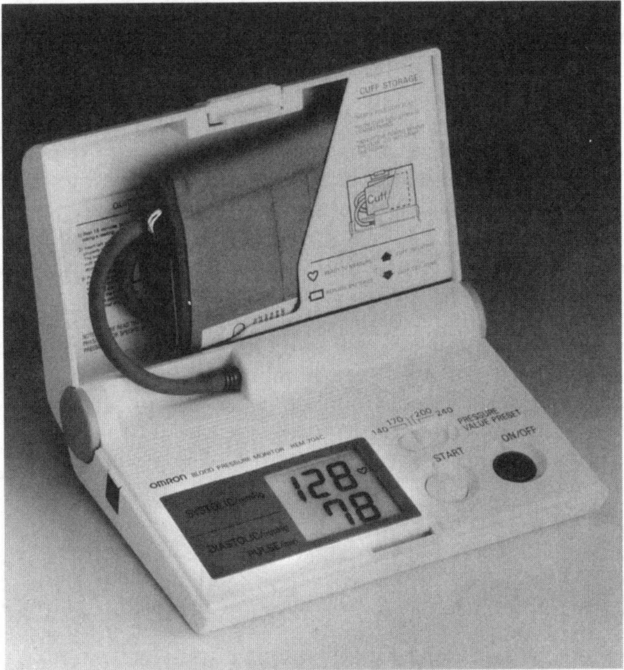

FIGURE 3 Digital blood pressure meter. Photograph provided by Omron Healthcare, Inc, Vernon Hills, Illinois.

Patient Counseling

To obtain maximal results with HBPM, it is essential that patients choose the correct device and be adequately trained in its usage. The pharmacist can play a major role in this regard by motivating the patient to perform HBPM; guiding the patient in product selection; training the patient to use the device appropriately; and facilitating communication between the patient, the patient's family, and the patient's primary care provider regarding any antihypertensive therapy.

In addition, pharmacists should instruct patients who are measuring blood pressure at home to avoid smoking and the ingestion of caffeine-containing beverages for at least 30 minutes prior to taking measurement. Since eating or taking a hot bath can lower blood pressure, patients should also be told to wait 10–15 minutes after a bath and 30 minutes after eating before taking measurement. They should also know to allow plenty of time to relax first; if they are pressured by time, their results can be elevated. Finally, pharmacists should caution patients not to self–adjust blood pressure medications on the basis of home measurements unless specifically instructed to do so by their physicians.

Future Home Diagnostic Kits

As the products of biotechnology become more sophisticated, easier to use, and less costly, more tests will become available on a nonprescription basis for in-home use. In addition, manufacturers will continue to strive to make their products more accurate and reliable.

One product that may be on the market in the near future is a home test kit for human immunodeficiency virus (HIV). The FDA has indicated a willingness to approve a nonprescription home specimen collection kit system for HIV testing. Previously, the agency believed that such testing should be restricted to professional use in a health care environment. Public health experts hope a home kit will expand access to HIV testing.[35]

It is expected that these tests will require the user to prick a finger with a lancet, allow two drops of blood to be absorbed by a special paper with a unique identification number, and mail the specimen to the company, where it will be tested using standard laboratory screening. About a week after mailing the specimen, the user will call a toll-free number and, after providing the test identification number, receive counseling, the test result, and referral to local care should the test result be positive. In this way, users can maintain their anonymity.

Summary

To advise patients properly on product selection, pharmacists must be familiar with the testing procedures for each available product. Manufacturers are continually introducing new products and modifying current ones to provide more user-friendly versions. To keep up-to-date, pharmacists should request product information from the manufacturers by calling the toll-free numbers or contacting the sales representatives.

References

1. Home diagnostic kits. *Drug Topics.* 1995 Jan 9; 139: 46.
2. Tami JA et al. Monoclonal antibody technology. *Am J Hosp Pharm.* 1986; 43: 2816–25.
3. Miller SW. Update on self-monitoring products. *NARD J.* June 1992; 114: 51–4.
4. Hick J, Josefsohn M. Reliability of home pregnancy test kits in the hand of lay persons. *N Engl J Med.* 1989; 320: 320–1. Letter.
5. Gray SL. Fecal occult blood testing for colorectal cancer. *Am Pharm.* 1992; NS32: 814–5.
6. ColoCARE product information. Beaumont, Tex: Helena Laboratories; Sep 1991.
7. EZ-Detect product information. Newport Beach, Calif: NMS Pharmaceuticals, Inc; October 1994.
8. Fecal occult blood test kits. *USP DI Drug Information for the Health Care Professional.* 13th ed. Rockville, Md: United States Pharmacopeial Convention, Inc; 1993: 1387–9; 1995: 1306–8.
9. Reiders TP, Ruggiero RJ, Steadman S. *Methods of Birth Control: Assessment Skills for Pharmacists.* Palo Alto, Calif: Syntex Laboratories; 1985: 2–5.
10. Inglis JK. *A Textbook of Human Biology.* 3rd ed. New York: Pergamon Press; 1986: 252–3.
11. *Instructions and Use.* Bioself Fertility Indicator instruction booklet. Self-care: 4.
12. Labrecque M, Drevin J, Rioux JE. Validity of the Bioself 110 fertility indicator. *Fertil Steril.* 1989; 63(4): 604–8.
13. Ismail M et al. An evaluation of the Bioself 110 fertility indicator. *Contraception.* 1989; 30: 53.
14. Ovulation prediction test kit for home use. *USP DI Drug Information for the Health Care Professional.* 13th ed. Rockville, Md: United States Pharmacopeial Convention, Inc; 1993: 2118–9; 1995: 2101–2.
15. Engle JP. Ovulation predictors. *Am Druggist.* Mar 1993; 207: 55–6.
16. Gannon K. Who is most apt to turn to a home pregnancy test? *Drug Topics.* 1992; 136: 46.
17. Pregnancy test kits for home use. *USP DI Drug Information for the Health Care Professional.* 13th ed. Rockville, Md: United States Pharmacopeial Convention, Inc; 1995: 2298–300.
18. Caiola SM. The pharmacist and home-use pregnancy tests. *Am Pharm.* 1992; NS32: 57–60.
19. *Healthy People 2000.* Washington, DC: US Department of Health and Human Services; 1990: 402.
20. National Cholesterol Education Program. 1993 panel report. *JAMA.* 1993; 269(23): 3015.
21. Warnick GR. Compact analysis systems for cholesterol, triglycerides and high density lipoprotein cholesterol. *Curr Opin Lipidol.* 1991; 2: 343–8.
22. Schuman AJ. A guide to office cholesterol testing. *Contemp Pediatr.* 1991; 8: 17–42.
23. Allen MP et al. A noninstrumented quantitative test system and its application for determining cholesterol concentration in whole blood. *Clin Chem.* 1990; 36: 1591–6.
24. Joint National Committee on Detection, Evaluation, and Treatment of High Blood Pressure. The fifth report of the Joint National Committee on the Detection, Evaluation, and Treatment of High Blood Pressure (JNC V). *Arch Intern Med.* 1993; 153: 154–83.
25. Stamler J, Neaton JD. Blood pressure, systolic and diastolic, and cardiovascular risk. US population data. *Arch Intern Med.* 1993; 153: 598–615.

26. Pyorala K et al. Prevention of coronary heart disease in clinical practice. Recommendations of the task force of the European Society of Cardiology, European Atherosclerosis Society and European Society of Hypertension. *Eur Heart J.* 1994; 15: 1300–31.
27. Luepker RV. Patient adherence: a "risk factor" for cardiovascular disease. *Heart Dis Stroke.* 1993; 2: 418–21.
28. Soghikian K et al. Home blood pressure monitoring. Effect on use of medical services and medical care costs. *Med Care.* 1992; 30: 855–65.
29. Kaplan NM. Measurement of blood pressure. In: Kaplan NM, ed. *Clinical Hypertension.* Baltimore: Williams and Wilkins; 1994: 23–45.
30. Harrison DW, Kelly PL. Home health-care: accuracy, calibration, exhaust, and failure rate comparisons of digital blood pressure monitors. *Med Instrum.* 1987; 21: 323–8.
31. O'Brien E et al. Inaccuracy of seven popular sphygmomanometers for home measurement of blood pressure. *J Hypertens.* 1990; 8: 621–34.
32. Evans CE et al. Home blood pressure–measuring devices: a comparative study of accuracy. *J Hypertens.* 1989; 7: 133–42.
33. Egmond J et al. Accuracy and reproducibility of 30 devices for self-measurement of arterial blood pressure. *Am J Hypertens.* 1993; 6: 873–9.
34. McKay DW et al. Clinical assessment of blood pressure. *J Hum Hypertens.* 1990; 4: 639–45.
35. Conlan MF. FDA open to home test kits for detecting HIV virus. *Drug Topics.* 1995; 139: 60.

CHAPTER 4

Internal Analgesic and Antipyretic Products

Arthur G. Lipman

Questions to ask in patient assessment and counseling

Pain Characteristics

- *Where is the pain? Is it in one place, such as a particular muscle or area of skin, or does it spread to other parts of the body?*
- *On a scale of zero to 10, with zero being no pain and 10 being pain as bad as you can imagine, what is your level of pain now?*
- *Have you ever had pain like this before? If so, what caused it and what helped it?*
- *Is any part of your body red and swollen? Have you recently sustained a physical injury?*
- *How long have you had this pain? Has it changed or remained constant in character and intensity?*
- *What words best describe your pain (eg, sharp, dull, aching, burning, electrical, stabbing)? Is it constant or does it come and go? Did it develop suddenly or gradually?*
- *Does the pain occur at any particular time of the day? What makes it worse or better? Is it relieved by changing your body position?*
- *Do you have any other symptoms that you feel might be associated with the pain (eg, visual disturbances, numbness, weakness, a tingling sensation, dizziness, unusual drowsiness, nausea, vomiting, fever, mental confusion, unusual sensitivity to light or sounds)?*

Drug Therapy for Pain

- *Have you had this pain before? If so, what medications did you take to relieve or manage the pain?*
- *What medications have you already taken? How much and for how long? How effective were they?*
- *Do aspirin or other pain relievers upset your stomach?*
- *Have you ever had an allergic reaction to aspirin or any other medication for pain, swelling, or fever?*
- *What allergies or reactions have you ever had to foods, dyes, or food additives?*
- *Have you ever had hives or a recurrent skin rash?*
- *Have you ever had an ulcer or stomach problem?*
- *Have you ever had asthma, nasal polyps, or a breathing problem?*
- *Do you now have or have you ever had asthma, allergies, ulcers, gout, high blood pressure, heart failure, kidney disease, or a blood-clotting disorder?*
- *Are you now taking medication for gout, arthritis, asthma, high blood pressure, or diabetes?*
- *Are you currently taking any drug that may thin your blood? Have you taken any such drug within the last week?*
- *What other prescription or nonprescription drugs are you now taking?*
- *(If the patient is under 15 years of age) Has your child had recent symptoms of influenza or chickenpox?*
- *(If the patient is a woman of child-bearing age) Are you pregnant? Are you breast-feeding? If you are pregnant, do you plan to breast-feed?*

Fever

- *How long have you been ill? (If the patient is a child) How long has your child been ill?*
- *How high is your [your child's] fever? How long has the fever been present?*
- *How did you measure the temperature (ie, by the oral, axillary, rectal, or ear canal method)?*
- *What activities preceded this fever?*
- *What other symptoms do you have?*
- *What medication or other treatment have you used to treat the fever?*
- *Have you ever had a convulsion, seizure, or brain disorder?*

Pain is the most common reason that patients seek medical care, and patients come to pharmacies for analgesics more often than they do for any other type of nonprescription medication. Yet pain is perhaps the most misunderstood of the common ailments, perhaps because of the limited coverage that pain management receives in most health professional curricula. Much of what we now know about the pathophysiology of pain and the appropriate use of analgesics has only recently been discovered.

Fever is among the most common symptoms for which parents seek nonprescription drugs to treat their children. One of five emergency room visits for children is related to fever, and more than 10% of children between the ages of 1 to 24 months have fevers when they are seen in pediatricians' offices.

Because nonprescription analgesics available in the United States are also antipyretic agents, it is logical to consider these two categories of medications together. Nonprescription analgesic/antipyretic use has increased 50% in the United States during the past 5 years because of increased consumer demand, changes from prescription to nonprescription status for several dosage forms, and increased advertising.

Providing accurate information on pain and fever and their management is both a real need and an excellent opportunity for pharmaceutical care.

Pain

Mechanism of Pain Perception

Many traditional dictionary definitions of pain describe it as a physical phenomenon (eg, localized physical suffering associated with a bodily disorder). This is very different from the currently accepted definition of the International Association for the Study of Pain, which describes pain as an unpleasant sensory and emotional experience associated with actual or potential tissue damage or described in terms of such damage.[1] The latter definition recognizes that pain can have physical, affective, and learned components; it is not necessarily a result of physical injury.

As defined above, pain is a "sensory and emotional experience." The sensory component derives from transmission of peripheral pain impulses to the central nervous system (CNS). Nociceptors are peripheral pain receptors that are activated by noxious stimuli in the periphery and send the pain stimulus to the spinal cord via afferent, nociceptive nerve fibers (Figure 1). The afferent nerve impulses pass through the dorsal route ganglion where neurotransmitters are synthesized. From there, the impulses go into the dorsal horn of the spinal cord, where they synapse with both ascending fibers that send the pain message to the brain and efferent fibers that return to the periphery to complete the nerve circuit. It is important to note that the efferent fibers pass through the sympathetic chain ganglia; this helps to explain the chronic pain syndromes that are maintained by sympathetic nervous stimulation. Such pain is called sympathetically maintained pain.

Within the dorsal horn of the spinal cord, many substances, including substance P, are involved in the transmission and modulation of pain. Much research now focuses on the role of the amino acid glutamate, which acts on *N*-methyl-D-aspartate (NMDA) receptors found on postsynaptic membranes. NMDA antagonists will most probably become important drugs for the management of neuropathic pain in the foreseeable future; however, it is doubtful whether clinically useful NMDA antagonists will be available without a prescription.

The dorsal horn of the spinal cord contains large numbers of nociceptive nerve endings. High concentrations of opioid receptors, endorphins (endogenous opioid substances), alpha$_2$ sympathetic receptors, and serotonin-containing neurons are also found here. When activated by endorphins or opioid drugs, opioid receptors impede the release of excitatory neurotransmitters. Alpha$_2$ sympathetic receptors also decrease pain when activated by norepinephrine. Increased serotonin levels within the nerves may also have an antinociceptive effect. The mechanism of action has been assumed to be related to the fact that these drugs increase levels of norepinephrine and serotonin in the nerves through inhibition of the reuptake of these neurotransmitters. Recent evidence suggests that action of these drugs at sodium channels leading to nerve membrane stabilization may be the major mechanism. Nonprescription analgesics have minimal effect within the dorsal horn.

Pain due to noxious stimuli such as mechanical or thermal insults is immediate (acute). Pain due to ongoing tissue damage and many diseases normally is caused by numerous chemical substances including prostaglandins, bradykinin, and histamine. These pain-facilitating chemicals are present in normal tissue, but their production and release are enhanced by tissue damage. Pain itself enhances the production and release of these chemical mediators. That helps explain why untreated (or undertreated) acute pain may progress to a chronic pain syndrome.

When acute pain is not adequately managed, the sympathetic "fight or flight" phenomenon may be maintained, causing ongoing adrenaline release. This, in turn, results in increased, ongoing pain and anxiety. That helps to explain why antianxiety medications sometimes are useful adjuncts in the management of pain.

Somatic pain occurs when pain impulses are transmitted from peripheral nociceptors to the CNS via nociceptive nerve fibers. Common sites of origin of somatic pain are muscles, fascia, bones, and nerves. Somatic pain is most commonly myofascial (ie, arising from muscles or the fascia that surround them). Myofascial pain arises from localized tender areas in muscle or the surrounding fascia, which are known as trigger points. Trigger points, which can occur following injury or immobility of the affected tissues, cause a reproducible, referred pain pattern when pressed.

Myofascial pain is amenable to treatment with nonprescription drugs, whereas osteopathic and neuropathic pain are usually treated with prescription drugs or other forms of treatment. Tricyclic antidepressants are often

---

Editor's Note: This chapter is based, in part, on two chapters in the 10th edition "Internal Analgesic Products" and "Antipyretic Drug Products," which were written by W. Kent Van Tyle and Thomas E. Lackner, respectively.

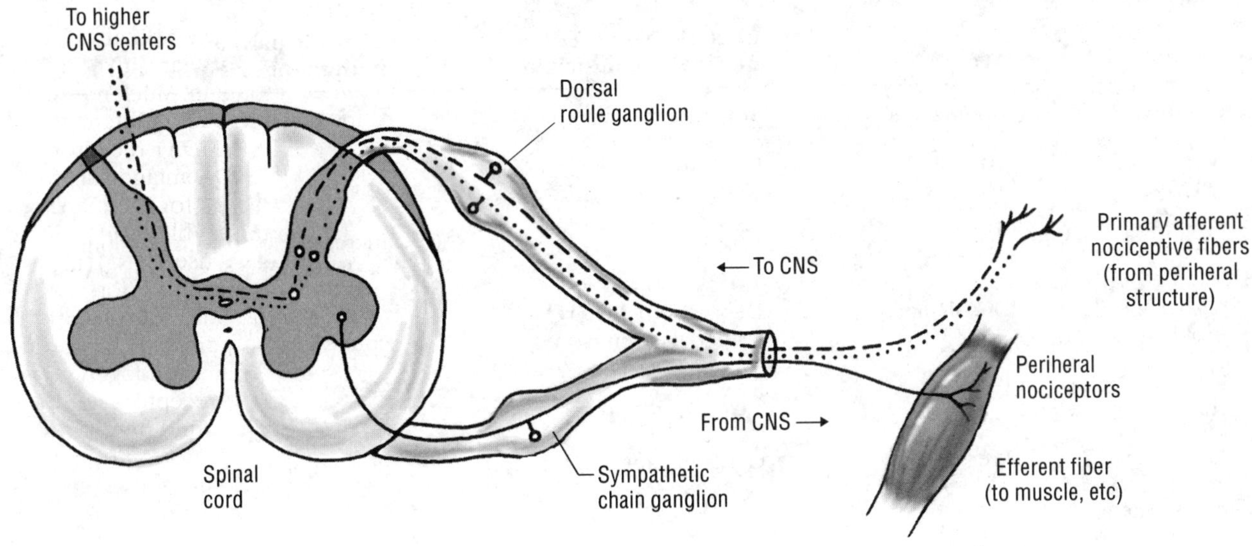

FIGURE 1 Pain pathways from the periphery to the central nervous system.

used as hypnotics in various types of chronic pain and are agents of choice in the management of neuropathic pain.

Classification and Management of Pain

Studies of patient satisfaction with pain control consistently document that only one half to three quarters of patients receive acceptable relief of both postoperative and cancer pain, although these types of pain can be well managed more than 90% of the time with modalities that are readily available. This dissatisfaction has led to several federal initiatives on pain management. The 1979 report to the White House of the Federal Interagency Committee on New Therapies for Pain and Discomfort documented the need for dramatically improved pain management.[2] In 1985, the US Public Health Service's Interagency Committee on Pain and Analgesia identified the need for better education of both health professionals and the public on pain and pain management, the need for improved pain research, and the importance of implementing a new public policy related to pain and analgesia.[3] *The Integrated Approach to the Management of Pain,*[4] the 1986 report of the National Institutes of Health, concluded that pain should be considered as three distinct entities: acute pain, chronic pain associated with malignant disease, and chronic pain not associated with malignant disease. Nonprescription analgesics may be useful in all three types of pain, but they are only adjunctive for most chronic, nonmalignant pain syndromes. Table 1 illustrates how these three types of pain differ.

Types of Pain

Acute Pain Acute pain is an immediate reaction to noxious stimuli such as mechanical (eg, fracture, muscle sprain) or thermal injuries. Analgesics often prevent acute pain from progressing to more serious disorders.

Chronic Malignant Pain Chronic pain associated with malignant disease includes the pain of any advanced, progressive disorder, not just cancer. Examples of such disorders are multiple sclerosis, amyotrophic lateral sclerosis (Lou Gehrig's disease), acquired immunodeficiency syndrome (AIDS), end-stage renal or hepatic failure with pain, and painful end-stage respiratory disease. The principles of managing chronic malignant pain are also appropriate for diseases causing intermittent pain (eg, sickle-cell disease). Important guidelines for the management of acute and cancer pain have been published by the American Pain Society[5] and for the management of cancer pain by the World Health Organization.[6]

Chronic Nonmalignant Pain Chronic pain not associated with malignant disease is the most complex, most misunderstood, and least well managed of the three major categories of pain. This type of pain is related to a progressive, debilitating process; arthritides may or may not be classified as chronic nonmalignant pain, depending on whether the disease is truly progressive or is manifested as periodic exacerbations and remissions. Chronic nonmalignant pain patients often take excessive doses of acetaminophen and salicylates, which can lead to toxicities. The management of chronic nonmalignant pain often requires an interdisciplinary approach.

Nonprescription analgesics may be useful adjuncts

TABLE 1 Categories of pain[a]

	Acute	Chronic pain of nonmalignant origin	Chronic pain of malignant origin
Duration	Hours to days	Months to years	Unpredictable
Associated pathology	Present	Often none	Usually present
Prognosis	Predictable	Unpredictable	Increasing pain with possibility of disfigurement and fear of dying
Associated problems	Uncommon	Depression, anxiety, secondary gain issues	Many, especially fear of loss of control
Nerve conduction	Rapid	Slow	Slow
Autonomic nervous system involvement	Present	Generally absent	Present or absent
Biological value	High	Low or absent	Low
Social effects	Minimal	Profound	Variable—usually marked
Treatment	Primarily analgesics	Multimodal: often largely behavioral, drugs usually play a minor role	Multimodal: drugs usually play a major role

[a]Most people's definition of pain would describe acute pain. The characteristics and management principles of acute pain differ from those of the two types of chronic pain. It is important to determine the type of pain involved before recommending a therapy or making referrals for evaluation and management of pain.

for some chronic nonmalignant pain, but these drugs are of limited value in most such syndromes. Not all pain—and relatively little chronic, nonmalignant pain—responds to analgesics alone. Therefore, practitioners should learn about resources in their communities to which they can refer patients whose pain is not effectively managed with analgesic medications.

Pain Management

Acute pain and chronic malignant pain are often indications for aggressive drug therapy. These types of pain are often undertreated, leading to unnecessary and avoidable suffering. Therefore, whenever there is pain due to ongoing tissue damage, it is preferable for patients to take analgesic medications on a regular schedule to help prevent the recurrence of pain. Patients with this type of pain should be advised not to take analgesics "as needed" (ie, after pain recurs).

However, additional mechanisms are probably involved. Inflammation is characterized by erythema or redness, edema, and tenderness or hyperalgesia at the site. Multiple mediators, including histamine, bradykinin, 5-hydroxytryptamine, leukotrienes, and prostaglandins of the E series, participate in the inflammatory response. Because pain and inflammation increase prostaglandin production, drugs that inhibit peripheral prostaglandin production (eg, nonsteroidal anti-inflammatory drugs [NSAIDs]) reduce the transmission of pain impulses from the periphery to the CNS.

Conversely, chronic nonmalignant pain management is often inappropriately treated with analgesic and other CNS depressant drugs that are not effective as primary treatment modalities. This can produce adverse effects, dependence, psychologic complications, and worsening pain. Although analgesics and adjunctive medications can be important in the management of many chronic nonmalignant pain syndromes, rehabilitation and behavioral treatments are the principal treatment modalities for these types of pain more often than analgesics.

As in all clinical care, the underlying disorder should be treated, not just the presenting symptom. Simply masking symptoms with analgesics or other medications may allow the underlying disease to progress to the detriment of the patient. Nonprescription or prescription medications should not be used in lieu of appropriate referral of these patients for evaluation by an appropriate interdisciplinary pain treatment team. Such teams should include, at a minimum, a physician with pain expertise (most commonly an anesthesiologist or neurologist), a rehabilitation specialist (most commonly a physical therapist), and a mental health professional (most commonly a psychologist with behavioral medicine expertise). Such teams increasingly include pharmacists who assess, monitor, and consult on drug therapy.[7]

The federal initiative that has the greatest potential for improving pain management is the publication of clinical practice guidelines on the management of acute pain in 1992[8] and cancer pain in 1994[9] by the Public Health Service's Agency for Health Care Policy and Research (AHCPR). These two publications and their accompanying Quick Reference Guides for Clinicians (abbreviated forms) as well as Patient Guides (published in both English and Spanish) are available (currently at no charge) from the AHCPR Publications Clearinghouse, PO Box 8547, Silver Spring MD 20907 (800–358–9295). The clinical practice guideline on cancer pain management is also distributed by the National Cancer Institute Cancer Information Service (800–4CANCER [422–6237]). Both documents provide important, scientifically based information in a well-referenced and easy-to-read format.

Selected Pain-Associated Conditions Responsive to Nonprescription Analgesics

Headache

Headaches are the most common pain complaint. More than 75% of the population experience muscle contraction headaches at some time, and 20–25% of the population experience migraine headaches. Many headaches—including some severe vascular headaches—respond well to nonprescription analgesics. Headaches result from dysfunction, injury, or displacement of pain-sensitive cranial structures.

Muscle Contraction Headache Muscle contraction or tension headaches are a type of myofascial pain. These headaches result from tight muscles in the upper back, neck or scalp, or from myofascial trigger points in the muscles of the cervical area, occiput or scalp. They commonly present as bilateral, diffuse pain, often over the top of the head and extending to the rear and base of the skull. Patients often describe the pain as "tight" or "pressing," as if the head were constricted by a band. The pain is usually more gradual in onset than the pain of vascular headaches and produces more of an aching than a throbbing sensation. Tension headaches may be associated with emotional stress or anxiety and may continue for several days.[10] Acute muscle contraction headaches usually respond well to nonprescription analgesics. However, chronic muscle contraction headaches often require physical therapy and relaxation exercises for management. Generally, physical therapy emphasizing stretching and strengthening of the affected muscles is safer and more effective than prescription medications for muscle contraction headaches.

Vascular/Migraine Headache Vascular headaches may be due to distention or dilation of intracranial arteries or traction or displacement of large intracranial veins or their meningeal covering. Most vascular headaches are migraine headaches. Many patients use the term migraine to denote any bad headache. Therefore, clinicians should ensure that purported migraine headaches are truly that before suggesting treatment that is appropriate for migraine, but not muscle contraction, headaches.

Migraine headaches are recurrent, hemicranial, and throbbing. They are classified as either classic or common. Classic migraines start with an aura (ie, neurologic symptoms including shimmering or flashing areas or blind spots in the visual field, difficulty speaking, and [usually] one-sided muscle weakness). These symptoms may last for up to half an hour, and the throbbing headache pain that follows may last from several hours to 1–2 days. Common migraine does not have an aura; it begins immediately with the throbbing headache pain. Both forms of migraine are often associated with nausea, vomiting, photophobia, phonophobia, light headedness, and vertigo. Women have a five times higher incidence of migraine headaches than do men, and for some women, migraine headaches recur at specific times during the menstrual cycle.[10] For some patients, NSAIDs or acetaminophen effectively controls migraine headache pain if dosed properly; these nonprescription analgesics may actually abort a migraine headache if taken soon after onset.

Vascular-Muscle Contraction Headache Mixed vascular-muscle contraction headaches may occur. Most commonly one type causes the other. Treatment of the underlying type of headache often suffices. It is not always necessary to treat both types.

Sinus Headache Sinus headache occurs when infection or blockage of the paranasal sinuses causes inflammation or distention of the sensitive sinus walls. Sinus headache is usually localized to the periorbital area or forehead. Pain tends to occur upon awakening and may subside gradually after the patient has been upright for a while. Stooping or blowing the nose often intensifies the pain. In addition to nonprescription analgesics, decongestants are often useful in facilitating drainage of the sinuses and thus in relieving pain.[10] (See Chapter 8, "Cold, Cough, and Allergy Products.") Persistent sinus pain and/or discharge suggests possible bacterial infection and requires referral for medical evaluation.

Other Types of Headaches Other headaches amenable to nonprescription drug treatment may be caused by fever or "hangover." A hangover caused by an accumulation of acetaldehyde, a toxic metabolite of ethyl alcohol, often responds to acetaminophen or NSAIDs; however, the condition does not fully resolve for several hours until the acetaldehyde is eliminated from the body by normal metabolic and excretory processes. Nonprescription stimulants such as caffeine may provide some relief in headaches related to fatigue, but making up any sleep deficit is important in reducing the incidence and severity of this type of headache. Headaches can also be caused by eye strain or infection, or be a manifestation of anxiety or depression. Nonprescription medications are usually not effective in treating these types of headaches.

Myalgia

Diffuse muscle pain, which tends to be a dull, constant aching, is common and can result from systemic infections (eg, influenza, Coxsackievirus, measles, other illnesses) and from strenuous exertion. Prolonged tonic contraction produced by exercise, tension, or poor posture and body mechanics can also produce muscle pain. Diffuse muscle soreness and aching may be the initial symptom of rheumatoid arthritis (RA), preceding joint involvement by weeks or months.[11]

Muscle pain usually responds well to nonprescription analgesics and adjunctive treatment with heat or massage. The nonprescription analgesics should be started soon after the injury, taken on a regular schedule while the noxious stimulus is present, and taken in sufficient doses. However, remobilization of the affected area soon after the injury is the appropriate treatment. Although it may be appropriate to rest an injured muscle for a few days, failure to mobilize the area once the acute injury is healing often results in the muscle becoming tight, weak, and overly contracted (guarded). Trigger points then commonly arise. They can arise in any muscle, but are most commonly seen in major muscle groups. If muscle pain becomes chronic, the painful area may require application of ice or vapo-coolant sprays, or injections—typically using local anesthetics (trigger point injections)—to facilitate remobilization. Chronic muscle pain often requires structured physical therapy. Analgesics and trigger point injections facilitate physical therapy for chronic muscle pain syndromes; however, the drugs are not curative.

Periarticular Pain

Joints consist of cartilage covering the articulating surfaces of bone; surrounding synovial membrane; and periarticular supporting structures, including ligaments and tendons. Bursae resemble synovial membranes and provide the surface and lubrication on which these supporting structures move. Injury or inflammation of the tissues surrounding a joint (ie, the joint capsule, tendons, ligaments, and bursae) can cause pain. Localized tenderness is often present, and the pain can be elicited by maneuvers that stress the structure but not the associated joint. Periarticular pain tends to be nocturnal and often involves the shoulder, elbow, or knee. It responds well to nonprescription analgesics and limitation of motion in the affected joint.[12]

Arthralgia

Joint pain often involves inflammation of the synovial membrane (synovitis). Cartilage loss with associated synovitis can be the result of mechanical stress and wear, such as in degenerative joint disease (DJD, or osteoarthritis), or of erosive processes, such as in RA.

Degenerative Joint Disease DJD affects 85% of persons over the age of 70, and symptoms usually begin in the fifth or sixth decade of life. The primary complaint is joint stiffness and aching in weight-bearing joints. Joint stiffness lasts only a few minutes following initiation of joint motion. Degenerative changes of the upper extremities usually affect the joints of the fingers but rarely involve wrists, elbows, or shoulders. DJD of the hip, knee, and spine does occur and can be disabling. Earlier stages of DJD respond well to nonprescription analgesics. Weight loss is indicated to relieve stress on the affected joints of obese patients with DJD. Acetaminophen is an analgesic of choice for most DJD pain. For acute flares when inflammation exacerbates the problem, NSAIDs and local heat are often beneficial. Progressive disease, especially of weight-bearing joints, requires orthopedic management beyond the scope of nonprescription analgesics.[13]

Rheumatoid Arthritis RA symptoms commonly appear between the third and seventh decade of life, and the disease occurs more often in women than in men. This is a systemic disease that may begin with a prodrome of fatigue, weakness, joint stiffness, arthralgia, and myalgia appearing several weeks before joint swelling. Multiple joints of the hands, wrists, and feet show symmetrical involvement. Involved joints become warm, red, and swollen, and range of motion is limited. RA is a progressive disease that persists in affected joints and leads to joint deformity. Duration of morning stiffness can be used to assess severity and progression. Because the onset and progression of RA are slow and often subtle, many patients attempt self-medication in its initial stages. The therapeutic goal of managing RA—to control inflammation and induce remission—normally requires more than just nonprescription analgesics although NSAIDs are a mainstay of therapy. Education, exercise, and good nutrition are important in the control of RA. Because many RA patients have progressive, disabling disease that is best managed with a multimodal approach that includes education, physical therapy, nutritional counseling and medications, pharmacists should ensure that patients receive referral for appropriate care by clinicians with expertise in managing this disease.[14]

Assessment of Pain

Pharmacists can perform a brief assessment of pain with a few well-chosen questions. Assessment should include inquiry about the etiology, duration, location, and severity of pain as well as factors that relieve and exacerbate it. Nonprescription analgesics are often appropriate for managing acute pain if it is not too severe and the complaints are not suggestive of a serious underlying disorder. Patients with pain that has lasted longer than is normally expected from the underlying cause, or pain of more than 2 weeks duration, should usually be referred for medical evaluation. Asking whether the pain is mild, moderate, or severe often leads to inconsistent reports. Simple, validated rating scales should be used. The two most common methods are the verbal numerical rating scale and the visual analog scale (VAS). If using the verbal scale, the pharmacist should ask patients to rank the present pain on a scale of zero to 10, with zero being no pain and 10 being pain as bad as the patient can imagine. The VAS allows patients to graphically quantify their pain by marking on a 10-cm line the distance along the line that indicates the level of the present pain. To quantify the pain, the pharmacist measures the line with a metric ruler and records the pain level using a scale of 1 to 100.

Other scales are available for pain rating in children, adolescents, non-English speakers and other special populations.[8] It is important to use validated scales, not empirical ratings such as mild, moderate, or severe.

Fever

Fever is one of the most common reasons that parents seek medications for their children. Most fevers are self-limited and nonthreatening; however, fever can cause a great deal of discomfort and, in some cases, may indicate serious underlying pathology (eg, an acute, infectious process) for which prompt medical evaluation is indicated. The principal reason for treating fever is to alleviate discomfort. Treatment should target the underlying cause whenever possible. Serious complications of fever are uncommon and overly aggressive fever management may be more dangerous than the fever itself.

Fever is defined as a body temperature that is higher than the normal core temperature of 98.6°F (37°C). It is a sign of an upward displacement of the body's thermoregulatory set-point.[15] A rectal temperature above 101.8°F (38.8°C), an oral temperature above 100°F (37.8°C), or an axillary (armpit) temperature above 99°F (37.2°C) is considered abnormal.[16] Axillary temperatures range from 0.7°F (0.4°C) higher to 3.6°F (2°C) lower than rectal temperature. This discrepancy is normal, it should not be ascribed to improper measurement technique. Axillary temperatures are considered meaningful when they exceed 100.4°F (38°C), whereas the rectal temperature will usually exceed 100.4°F. Normal body temperature may range 2–2.5°F (1–1.5°C) from these norms and diurnal rhythm causes variances in body temperature during the day. The average rectal temperature for an 18-month-old baby is 100°F (37.8°C); therefore, 50% of infants have normal rectal temperatures above 100°F. Rectal temperatures of healthy children may approach 101°F (38.3°C) in the late afternoon or after physical activity.[17]

Although fever is a common symptom, it is often misunderstood and poorly treated. One study revealed that 20% of the population apparently does not know how to measure body temperature properly; many more persons do not know how to interpret the results.[18] Pharmacists and other health professionals can improve drug therapy outcomes by teaching patients self-assessment skills and the proper ways to measure and manage fever appropriately.

Mechanisms of Normal Thermoregulation and Fever

Body temperature is regulated by the thermoregulatory center located in the anterior hypothalamus.[17] Temperature-sensitive neurons in both the hypothalamus and the skin continuously transmit information about body temperature to the hypothalamic "thermostat." Physiologic and behavioral homeostatic mechanisms can then be invoked to maintain body temperature within the normal range. Examples of behavioral adaptations to temperature changes or extremes include putting on additional clothing, adjusting air conditioning, rubbing the hands together, and seeking shade for relief from the hot sun. Compensatory physiologic mechanisms include heat dissipation (eg, sweating, vasodilation, hyperventilation) in response to heat, and heat production or conservation (eg, shivering, vasoconstriction) in response to cold. Compensatory effects are mediated by alterations in the secretory rates of thyroid-stimulating hormone and catecholamines. Normal thermoregulation prevents wide fluctuations in body temperature so that the average body temperature is usually maintained at 97.7°–99.5°F (36.5°–37.5°C).

Normal body temperature varies throughout the day, peaking daily between 5 and 7 PM, and reaching its lowest point between 3 and 5 AM.[15,19] This consistent rhythm occurs at all ages above 2 years and is more pronounced in children than in adults. Body temperature can vary by as much as 1.8°F (1°C) in adults and as much as 2.5°F (1.4°C) in children each day. Because circadian variation continues during febrile illness, patients may be incorrectly described as febrile when they have a relatively normal temperature in the early morning and a moderately high evening temperature, which is misinterpreted as fever.

Pyrogens are fever-producing substances that activate the body's host defenses, resulting in an increase in the hypothalamic heat regulatory set-point. Pyrogens can be exogenous (originating outside the body) or endogenous (originating within the body).

Prostaglandins of the E series are produced in response to circulating pyrogens and act on the anterior hypothalamus to elevate the thermoregulatory set-point.[15] In response to these prostaglandins and to changes in monoamine concentration, the hypothalamus appears to direct the reestablishment of body temperature to correspond to the elevated set-point. Within hours, body temperature reaches this new set-point and fever occurs. During the period of upward temperature readjustment, the patient experiences chills due to peripheral vasoconstriction and skeletal muscle tone increases to maintain homeostasis. Because the new set-point is regulated by negative feedback, body temperature rarely exceeds 106°F (41.1°C). NSAIDs and acetaminophen, which inhibit the synthesis of E series prostaglandins in the CNS in response to endogenous pyrogens, possess antipyretic activity.

Patients' ability to perceive fever varies. Some individuals quite accurately perceive elevations in their body temperature. Others (eg, those with tuberculosis) are unaware of temperatures as high as 102.9°F (39.4°C).[20] Furthermore, fever may be ignored because of more unpleasant concomitant symptoms.

Etiology of Fever

Fever is usually caused by a microbiological agent, often a virus for which specific anti-infective therapy is not available. Fever may also be induced by certain drugs or physiologic processes, or be of unknown origin.

Microbe-Induced Fever

Most febrile episodes are due to infection by exogenous pyrogens, including viruses, bacteria, fungi, yeasts, and protozoa. Elevated temperatures associated with bacterial infections are generally higher than those associated with viral infections, but there is no absolute temperature at which these infections can be differentiated. Nor is there any basis for differentiating viral from bacterial infections according to the magnitude of temperature reduction from antipyretic drug therapy.[21] Fever

TABLE 2 Selected agents responsible for episodes of drug-induced fever

Cardiovascular
Methyldopa
Quinidine
Procainamide
Hydralazine
Nifedipine

Antimicrobial
Penicillin G
Ampicillin
Methicillin
Cloxacillin
Cephalothin
Cephapirin
Cefamandole
Tetracycline
Lincomycin
Sulfonamide
Sulfamethoxazole–trimethoprim
Streptomycin[a]
Vancomycin
Colistin
Isoniazid
Para-aminosalicylic acid
Nitrofurantoin
Mebendazole

Antineoplastic
Bleomycin
Daunorubicin
Procarbazine
Cytarabine
Streptozocin
6-Mercaptopurine
L-Asparaginase
Chlorambucil
Hydroxyurea

Central nervous system
Phenytoin
Carbamazepine
Chlorpromazine
Nomifensine
Haloperidol
Triamterene
Benztropine[a]
Thioridazine
Trifluoperazine[a]
Amphetamine

Anti-Inflammatory
Ibuprofen
Tolmetin
Aspirin

Other
Iodide
Cimetidine
Levamisole
Metroclopramide
Clofibrate
Allopurinol
Folate
Prostaglandin E_2
Ritodrine
Interferon
Propylthiouracil

[a]Fever seen during drug overdose.
Adapted with permission from Mackowiak PA, LeMaistre CF. *Ann Intern Med.* 1987; 106: 729.

from exogenous pyrogens, such as infectious organisms, is often less marked in elderly patients than in younger individuals.[22] Consequently, infection may not be easily recognized in older patients if fever is the primary assessment criterion.

Pathology-Induced Fever

Noninfectious pathologic causes of fever include malignancies, tissue damage (eg, myocardial infarct [MI], surgery), metabolic disorders (eg, hyperthyroidism, gout), antigen-antibody reactions, and dehydration. Each of these etiologies can trigger the production and release of endogenous pyrogens from liver and spleen cells, monocytes, eosinophils, and neutrophils.

Signs and symptoms that help distinguish among fever-inducing disorders include headache, sweating, generalized malaise, tachycardia, arthralgia, myalgia, back pain, irritability, and anorexia.[23] However, fever caused by the release of endogenous pyrogens from malignant cells is difficult to distinguish from fever due to infections in cancer patients. High body temperature dulls intellectual functioning and causes disorientation and delirium, especially in individuals with preexisting dementia, cerebral arteriosclerosis, or alcoholism. Reducing high temperature may alleviate CNS symptoms in some individuals.

Drug-Induced Fever

Many drugs may induce fever. Table 2 lists drugs that have been associated with this iatrogenic condition. The incidence of drug-induced fever is unknown, but the condition may account for more than 3% of all adverse drug reactions. Failure to discontinue the offending agent can result in substantial morbidity and even mortality. However, drug-induced fever often goes unrecognized because consistent signs and symptoms are lacking.[24]

Drug-induced fever probably is not related to atopy, sex, age, or systemic lupus erythematosus, as was previously believed. It is now believed to be a hypersensitivity reaction or idiosyncrasy in most cases.[25] However, drugs may cause fever by interfering with peripheral heat dissipation, increasing basal metabolic rate, invoking cellular immune response, structurally mimicking endogenous pyrogens, and inflicting direct tissue damage. The method of drug administration can also cause fever (eg, thrombophlebitis and septicemia from intravenous catheterization; phlebitis from caustic agents; the excessively rapid infusion of vancomycin; and release of endogenous pyrogens from sterile abscesses formed after multiple intramuscular injections).

Some drugs elevate body temperature by altering normal thermoregulatory mechanisms. Large doses of phenothiazines or anticholinergic agents decrease sweating and thus reduce heat dissipation. Thyroid hormones may increase the metabolic rate and thus increase heat generation. Other drugs may modify the behavioral response to the climatic temperature. For example, obtundation from sedatives may impair the normal behavioral withdrawal response from high environmental temperature.

Occasionally, fever may be a direct result of the pharmacologic effect of a drug. For example, the release of endotoxin from bacteria following the initiation of antibiotic therapy (eg, penicillin for syphilis) can result in high fever, chills, hypotension, myalgia, and leukocytosis.[25] This phenomenon (the Jarisch-Herxheimer reaction) may occur within hours after parenteral antibiotic therapy is begun. Fever may also result from the release of endogenous pyrogens associated with cellular injury or death following cancer chemotherapy. Similarly, the administration of drugs that possess oxidizing activity to individuals who have a glucose-6-phosphate dehydrogenase deficiency may cause fever secondary to the release of endogenous pyrogens from damaged erythrocytes.[25]

Some drugs or their metabolites and some biologic preparations have antigenic properties that can produce a hypersensitivity reaction. Although drug fever usually develops after 7-10 days of treatment, fever and other symptoms may occur shortly after initiation of therapy when previous exposure and sensitization have occurred.[25] The onset of drug fever caused by antineoplastic agents often comes within 7 days of initiation of therapy. Fever caused by cardiac drugs may not occur until more than 10 days have passed.[24]

Drug fever is distinguished by (1) fever occurring during or shortly after treatment with a drug previously reported to cause fever or other allergic symptoms, (2) fever accompanied by other manifestations of allergy, and (3) temperature elevation despite patient improvement.[26] One study of drug-induced fevers identified skin rash in only 18% of patients, and fewer than half of those individuals experienced urticaria. Furthermore, a generally mild eosinophilia was present in only 22% of the patients. The presence of high fever and shaking chills may make it hard to differentiate drug fever from infection. Bradycardia is uncommon with drug fever.[24] Drug fever should not be excluded on the basis of a shift to the left in the white blood cell differential count because this occasionally accompanies drug-induced fever.[27] Diurnal temperature variation in drug fever is often minimal.

The management of drug-induced fever involves discontinuation of the suspected drug whenever possible. If feasible, all medications should be temporarily discontinued. If the fever is drug induced, the patient's temperature will generally decrease within 24–48 hours after the offending drug is withdrawn. After patient safety and the need to definitively identify the offending drug have been considered, each medication may be restarted, one at a time, while monitoring for fever recurrence. If an implicated drug cannot be discontinued, systemic corticosteroids may be given to suppress fever and minimize other allergic symptoms. Risk of fever associated with parenteral drug administration is decreased with (1) proper catheter placement and care, (2) avoidance of frequent intramuscular injections, and (3) use of recommended infusion rates. Dosage reduction of phenothiazines, anticholinergic agents, and thyroid hormone may decrease temperature and should be considered if these drugs are suspected of causing fever, particularly in elderly patients.

Fever in persons taking neuroleptic medications (eg, phenothiazines, butyrophenones, thioxanthenes) could be secondary to neuroleptic malignant syndrome, a potentially life-threatening condition.[28] The high fever of neuroleptic malignant syndrome is often accompanied by muscle rigidity, abnormal body movements, sweating, tachycardia, high or low blood pressure, incontinence, and altered consciousness including delirium, stupor, or coma. Although neuroleptic malignant syndrome may occur in anyone taking these medications, it is most common in young males and possibly individuals who are dehydrated. When this syndrome is suspected, the neuroleptic medication should be discontinued and a physician contacted immediately.

Complications of Fever

Serious complications of fever are rare. Harmful effects (eg, dehydration, delirium, seizures, coma, irreversible neurologic or muscle damage) are most likely to occur at temperatures above 106°F (41.1°C). However, even lower body temperature elevations may be life-threatening in patients with heart disease because of an increased demand for oxygen in conjunction with increased cardiac output and heart rate.[15] Increased risk and lower tolerance to elevated body temperature exist in infants and in patients with brain tumors or hemorrhage, CNS infections, preexisting neurologic damage, and decreased ability to dissipate heat.[29,30]

Febrile seizures are seizures associated with fever in the absence of another cause, such as acute metabolic disorder or CNS inflammation. These occur in about 2–4% of all children between 6 months and 5 years of age.[31,32] Simple febrile seizures generally last no longer than 15 minutes, have no features characteristic of focal origin, and do not recur during a single febrile episode.[33] Significant neurologic sequelae (eg, impaired intellectual development) are unlikely following a single pediatric febrile seizure that is not complicated by status epilepticus.[34] However, the prevalence of epilepsy may be somewhat higher following a febrile seizure, particularly after a complex seizure or when severe electroencephalogram abnormalities exist.[34]

Unlike simple febrile seizures, complex febrile seizures in children are repetitive during the course of a single febrile episode, generally last longer than 15 minutes, and exhibit signs characteristic of a focal origin. Complex seizures are believed to be precipitated by fever in children with preexisting or latent epilepsy.[31]

Although both the magnitude and rate of temperature increase appear to be critical determinants in precipitating febrile seizures, the temperature at which a particular child will seize is unpredictable. Most initial febrile seizures occur in children under 3 years of age. Seizures occurring after that age are usually unrelated to fever. The risk for a febrile seizure is increased in children who have experienced a previous febrile seizure (especially if it occurred before 1 year of age or was a complex febrile seizure), who have a documented seizure or other CNS disorder, or whose family history includes febrile seizures.[32,34]

Prophylaxis against febrile seizures with antiepileptic drugs should be reserved for individuals at high risk of subsequent epilepsy. Antipyretics rarely will prevent febrile seizures in children predisposed to them. For such therapy, valproate or diazepam is now considered the drug of choice.[35] Phenobarbital is no longer considered optimal therapy; two reports failed to find a decrease in the seizure recurrence rate with the barbiturate, and cognitive performance may be impaired even after the drug is discontinued.[35,36]

Status epilepticus, which is characterized by recurrent or repetitive seizures without intervening periods of normal consciousness, occurs in only about 1–2% of children who experience a febrile seizure. Unlike simple febrile seizures, status epilepticus can result in permanent brain damage, renal failure, cardiorespiratory arrest, and death if not controlled. Any person experiencing such seizures requires immediate medical attention.

Measurement of Body Temperature

Normal body temperature varies according to the individual's age and level of physical and emotional stress, the environmental temperature, the time of day, and the anatomical site at which the temperature is measured.[15,17,19] Body temperature may be measured at rectal, axillary, oral, or tympanic (ear canal) sites. The rectal method is more consistently accurate than the oral or axillary readings. However, most individuals, especially children, prefer the other, more comfortable methods of temperature measurement.

Body temperature may be measured using various types of thermometers. During the course of an illness, the same thermometer should be used because the readings from different thermometers may vary. Regardless of the site or method used, thorough hand washing should precede and follow all temperature measurements.

Types of Thermometers

Mercury-in-glass and electronic thermometers are commonly used for temperature measurement. Both are accurate when used appropriately. The advantages of mercury-in-glass thermometers over electronic thermometers are (1) patient familiarity, (2) low cost, (3) light weight, and (4) compact size. However, mercury-in-glass thermometers can break, rendering them useless and potentially dangerous. Although the elemental mercury contained in the thermometers manufactured today is nonabsorbable through the gastrointestinal (GI) tract and is nontoxic, many patients still fear mercury poisoning from a broken thermometer. The real danger is from glass fragments; patients should discard chipped thermometers. In addition, mercury-in-glass thermometers register slowly and must be disinfected before each use. Such thermometers should be stored in a cool location and out of direct sunlight because they may be damaged by excessive heat.[37]

Electronic thermometers are available for oral, rectal, and axillary temperature measurement. These instruments may require about 30 seconds for equilibration. They register quickly and are not subject to glass breakage and the attendant risk of cuts. The use of disposable covers with these thermometers eliminates the need for disinfection following their use. In addition, the electronic digital temperature display makes these thermometers easier to read than the traditional glass thermometers.

Glass thermometers intended for oral use have a long, thin bulb designed to reach well under the tongue. In contrast, the bulb of the rectal thermometer is short and thick, permitting insertion in the rectum with little risk of breakage. Although a rectal thermometer can be used for oral temperature measurement, an oral thermometer should never be inserted into the rectum because oral thermometers are more fragile; they may break and injure rectal tissue. The same thermometer should never be used both rectally and orally because effective disinfection is difficult. To ensure reliable measurement, the patient should neither engage in vigorous physical activity nor heat or cool the oral cavity artificially by smoking or by drinking hot or cold beverages for at least 5 minutes (preferably 20 minutes) before temperature is measured.

Body temperature can also be determined by tympanic membrane blood temperature measurement with instruments developed for that use only. The tip of the instrument, which is placed in the ear canal, measures body temperature by sensing infrared radiation from the blood vessels in the eardrum. The tympanic membrane is close to the hypothalamus, and the blood supply to these two anatomical areas is at the same temperature. This measurement therefore provides an accurate reading of the body core temperature.[38] The instructions that come with the instrument on inserting the thermometer into the ear canal and properly positioning it should be followed carefully to ensure that the infrared radiation that is measured is from the tympanic membrane, not adjacent areas. The technique varies somewhat for young infants and older patients. The instrument provides an error message if the measurement is not performed correctly. The measurement takes only 1 second, is simple and accurate, and can be performed on a sleeping child. Inexpensive, disposable lens covers (sheaths) for the filter probe eliminate the need to disinfect the instrument between uses. The instruments are still relatively expensive, but the cost has decreased in recent years, and many families with young children now find the convenience of one of these thermometers sufficient to offset the cost.

Skin thermometers—adhesive temperature strips that are applied to the skin and change color over a particular temperature range—are not sufficiently accurate or reliable.[39] In one study, temperature strips failed to detect 66% of fevers of 100°F (37.8°C) or higher.[40] This method of temperature measurement is less reliable than either glass or electronic thermometers.

Subjective assessment of fever typically involves feeling a part of the body, such as the forehead. However, fever was unrecognized by this method in up to 26% of children with documented fever, whereas 6% of children who were thought to have a fever did not.[41]

Types of Temperature Measurement

Oral Measurement Before a patient's oral temperature is measured using a mercury-in-glass thermometer, the thermometer should be inspected for cracks or imperfections. It should then be disinfected by drawing it through a swab moistened with an antiseptic (eg, alcohol, povidone iodine solution). Next it should be rinsed with cool water; hot water should never be used as it may break the thermometer. After disinfection, the thermometer should be rotated at or slightly below eye level to confirm that the displayed temperature is below 96°F (35.6°C). If the reading is higher, the thermometer should be shaken in a rapid, downward, snapping motion until the mercury column falls below the 96°F level. When counseling patients about mercury-in-glass thermometers, pharmacists should demonstrate the correct shaking motion. The user should be advised to shake the thermometer over a bed, carpet, or other soft surface to reduce the likelihood of breakage if the thermometer slips from the hand.

The thermometer should then be placed under the tongue, positioned slightly to one side of the mouth, and left in place until the temperature reading is consistent. Although the literature recommends insertion for

6–10 minutes, 3–4 minutes is usually sufficient.[42] The patient's lips should be kept closed around the thermometer to hold it in place and to prevent air from flowing over the thermometer. Saliva should be removed from the thermometer by wiping from the stem toward the bulb. After the recorded temperature is noted, the mercury should be shaken down to less than the 96°F (35.6°C) level and the thermometer disinfected as described previously.

To measure oral temperature with an electronic thermometer, the probe should be removed from the thermometer base in which it is stored. The temperature set-point should be verified as specified by the manufacturer. The thermometer probe should then be inserted into a probe sheath following the same instructions for placement in the mouth as for a glass thermometer. After the electronic thermometer indicates that the temperature has been measured, the probe should be removed from the mouth, the contaminated sheath discarded, and the temperature display read. The probe should be returned to the base to reset the thermometer. Electronic thermometers can be used for children as young as 3 years of age because these instruments are not breakable if bitten and pose no risk of accidental cuts.

Oral temperature should not be taken when an individual is mouth breathing or hyperventilating; has recently had oral surgery; is not fully alert; or is uncooperative, lethargic, or confused. Oral thermometers are not appropriate for use in most children under 3 years because young children usually find it difficult to maintain a tight seal around the oral thermometer.[37,43]

Rectal Measurement To measure rectal temperature using a mercury-in-glass thermometer, a rectal (security bulb) thermometer should be disinfected and calibrated in the same manner as an oral thermometer. The thermometer bulb should then be lubricated with a water-soluble lubricant to allow easy passage through the anal sphincter and reduce the risk of trauma.

Rectal body temperature measurement in infants and young children is best accomplished by placing the child face down over the parent's lap, separating the buttocks with the thumb and forefinger of one hand, and inserting the thermometer gently and calmly in a direction pointing toward the child's umbilicus with the other hand. In infants, the thermometer should be inserted to the length of the bulb; in young children, it should be inserted about 1 inch into the rectum.[17] The thermometer should be held in place (in a straight line along its angle of insertion) for at least 3 minutes and cleaned by wiping from the stem toward the bulb. The temperature should be read at or slightly below eye level. The thermometer should be disinfected as previously described for the oral method, and any remaining lubricant should be wiped from the anus.

In the relatively uncommon situation when rectal temperature is measured in an adult, the patient should to lie on one side with the legs flexed to about a 45-degree angle from the abdomen, and the bulb should be inserted ½–2 inches into the rectum. This is done by holding the thermometer ½–2 inches from the bulb and inserting it until the finger touches the anus. To facilitate passage of the thermometer through the anal sphincter, the patient should be told to take a deep breath; this helps to divert the patient's attention to another activity. If the patient has hemorrhoids, insertion of a thermometer into the rectum should be particularly gentle to avoid causing pain and injury.

TABLE 3 Equations to convert temperatures °Celsius ↔ °Fahrenheit and selected temperature conversions

Celsius = 5/9 (°F–32)

Fahrenheit = (9/5 × °C) + 32

Sample conversions

Celsius	Fahrenheit
36°	96.8°
37°	98.6°
38°	100.4°
39°	102.2°
40°	104.0°
41°	105.8°
42°	107.6°

Risks associated with taking rectal temperature include injury from broken glass, retention of the thermometer, rectal or intestinal perforation, and peritonitis.[44] The patient should never be left unattended while the rectal thermometer remains in place because a positional change may cause the thermometer to be expelled or broken. Rectal temperature measurement is relatively contraindicated in patients who are neutropenic, have had recent rectal surgery or injury, or have rectal pathology (eg, obstructive hemorrhoids), as well as in newborns who are more susceptible to mucosal perforation.[44] Many parents cannot use a rectal thermometer correctly or read it accurately.[18] Confusion also often results from the difference between the Celsius and Fahrenheit scales and from normal variations in temperature among rectal, oral, and axillary sites of measurement. These differences should be emphasized when instructing individuals on the proper use of fever thermometers. Fahrenheit and Celsius temperatures are compared in Table 3.

Axillary Measurement Axillary temperature measurement is recommended for adults who are not candidates for oral or rectal temperature measurement (eg, somnolent individuals recovering from rectal surgery or severe diarrhea). Axillary temperature measurement may also be preferred in children 3 months to 5 years of age because intrusive rectal procedures can be very frightening to preschool children, children with diarrhea, or infants with severe diaper rash. However, because axillary temperature measurement is generally considered unreliable for detecting fever in infants and young children, rectal temperature measurement is preferred for infants under 3 months of age.[45–47]

Most oral thermometers can also be used to measure axillary temperature. This is accomplished by placing the thermometer in the armpit and holding the arm pressed against the body for at least 10 minutes or as long as the thermometer instructions indicate.

Ear Canal Measurement Tympanic thermometers provide digital readouts, and many can be set to provide either a rectal or an oral temperature equivalent. A clean disposable lens cover should be placed over the insertion end of the instrument before it is inserted into the ear canal. The instrument should not be inserted until the digital instruction panel indicates that it is ready for use. The tip should be aimed into the canal by pointing the lens of the instrument toward the patient's eye. The button should be pressed for the amount of time indicated in the instructions, typically 1 second. The digital panel can be read immediately.

Treatment of Fever

The decision to treat fever is based on several considerations. Patient discomfort associated with fever is an indication for antipyretic therapy, but arguments against such treatment include (1) the generally benign and self-limited course of fever, (2) the possible elimination of a diagnostic or prognostic sign, (3) the attenuation of enhanced host defenses (ie, possible therapeutic effect of fever), and (4) the untoward effects of antipyretic drugs.

There is no correlation between the magnitude or pattern of temperature elevation (ie, persistent, intermittent, recurrent, or prolonged) and the underlying etiology or severity of the disease.[48] Furthermore, when associated with an infectious disease, effective antibiotic therapy is generally guided by microbiologic cultures and sensitivity, epidemiologic, and other diagnostic data. In the febrile neutropenic patient with negative cultures, antipyretic therapy should be periodically interrupted to determine the need for continued anti-infective therapy.[49] An agent lacking anti-inflammatory activity, such as acetaminophen, should be used when anti-inflammatory effects may mask the clinical signs of a particular disease (eg, septic joint, rheumatic fever).[50]

The argument that fever is an adaptive response and that elevated body temperature may be beneficial is often overstated. Although the growth of some pathogenic microorganisms is impaired by higher than normal temperatures, the benefits of fever appear to be limited to regional cutaneous infections.[51] Fever itself is rarely beneficial to the host response to infection. Fever increases oxygen consumption, production of carbon dioxide, and cardiac output. The minimal benefits of low-grade fever on host defense mechanisms (eg, antigen recognition, T helper lymphocyte function, leukocyte motility) do not appear to favorably alter the course of infectious diseases.[52] Data from animal studies suggest that the abolition of fever may enhance and prolong viral shedding.[53] Aspirin has been associated with increased shedding of rhinovirus in adults.[54]

Treatment of fever with oral antipyretic agents is indicated if the oral temperature exceeds 102°F (38.9°C).[15] When a lower temperature and its associated discomfort are present, nonpharmacologic or pharmacologic intervention may be used. All nonprescription antipyretic agents are also analgesics, and the discomfort associated with a fever of less than 102°F may be the primary indication for any of the nonprescription analgesic/antipyretic medications (ie, acetaminophen, aspirin, ibuprofen, naproxen sodium, ketoprofen).

A physician should be contacted at the first sign of fever in a child predisposed to seizures. In such individuals, antipyretic medication should be administered every 4 hours with one dose given during the night, and therapy should be continued for at least 24 hours. The need for additional therapy, such as anticonvulsant medication, should be determined by the physician.

If a fever-induced seizure occurs, sponging with tepid (lukewarm) water should be initiated and the physician notified immediately. Nonpharmacologic treatment should consist of providing light clothing, removing blankets, maintaining room temperature at 78°F (25.6°C), and supplying sufficient fluid intake to replenish insensible losses.

When the body temperature exceeds 104°F (40°C), body sponging with tepid water can be started to facilitate heat dissipation. However, body sponging is not routinely recommended for children with a temperature under 104°F because this procedure is usually uncomfortable and often causes the child to shiver, which could raise the temperature even higher. Ideally, sponging should follow oral antipyretic therapy by 1 hour to permit the therapeutic reduction of the hypothalamic set-point and thereby permit a more sustained temperature-lowering response. Unlike acetaminophen and NSAIDs, topical sponging does not reduce the hypothalamic set-point. Sponging can be useful, however, because only a small temperature gradient between the body and the sponging medium is necessary to achieve an effective antipyretic response. Ice water baths or spongings with hydroalcoholic solutions (eg, isopropyl or ethyl alcohol) are uncomfortable, unnecessary, and not recommended. Alcohol poisoning can result from cutaneous absorption or inhalation of topically applied alcohol solutions.[55]

In addition to the above-mentioned measures to lower body temperature, fluid intake in febrile children should be increased by at least 1 oz of fluids per hour (eg, soft drinks, fruit juice, water, or other fluids), unless oral fluids are contraindicated.

Because infants younger than 3 months are at greater risk of serious outcomes from fever than are older children, they should be evaluated by a physician when their temperature rises above 100°F. For infants older than 3 months, a rectal temperature that is above 104°F is cause for contacting a physician immediately and withholding antipyretic medication pending the physician's directive.

Nonprescription Analgesic/ Antipyretic Agents

The nonprescription analgesic/antipyretic agents available in the United States are the salicylates (ie, aspirin, choline salicylate, magnesium salicylate, and sodium salicylate), acetaminophen, ibuprofen, naproxen sodium, and ketoprofen (see product table "Internal Analgesic and Antipyretic Products"). The strengths of nonprescription products containing ibuprofen, naproxen sodium, or ketoprofen are lower than those of prescription-strength products containing these agents.

The selection of an analgesic/antipyretic medication should be based on the agent's clinical effective-

TABLE 4 Dosages of nonprescription analgesic/antipyretic agents commonly used for pain or inflammation

	Dosage (maximum)	
Agent	**Analgesic**	**Anti-inflammatory**
Acetaminophen	650–1,000 mg, 3–4 times/day (4,000 mg/day)	—
Aspirin	650–1,000 mg every 4 h (4,000 mg/day)	2,400–3,900 mg/day for 5–7 days
Ibuprofen	200–400 mg every 4–6 h (1,200 mg/day)	400–800 mg, 3–4 times/day[a] (3,200 mg in 2 wk)
Naproxen sodium	220 mg every 6–8 h (660 mg/day)	275–550 mg, 2 times/day[a] (1,650 mg/day for 2 wk)
Ketoprofen	12.5–25 mg every 6–8 h (75 mg/day)	50–75 mg, 3–4 times/day[a,b] (300 mg/day)

[a]Dosage exceeds that recommended in nonprescription product labeling.

[b]Dosage should be reduced in elderly and renally impaired patients.

Information extracted from Whelton A. Renal effects of over-the-counter analgesics. *J Clin Pharmacol.* 1995; 35: 453–63.

ness, the incidence and severity of adverse effects associated with its use, its absolute and relative contraindications, the convenience of its administration, and the cost of therapy. Acetaminophen, aspirin, ibuprofen, and naproxen sodium are the most popular and effective antipyretic agents available without a prescription. Ketoprofen, which was approved for nonprescription use more recently, is pharmacodynamically and pharmacokinetically very similar to ibuprofen. Many patients may find its efficacy comparable to that of ibuprofen. Under most circumstances, these drugs are equally effective and have similar times to onset of effect and similar times to peak antipyretic activity. Their antipyretic durations of action are also similar, but naproxen sodium may have a slightly longer analgesic duration.

Both acetaminophen and the NSAIDs are effective analgesics and contribute to the relief of numerous discomforting symptoms that often accompany fever. The onset of antipyretic activity after an oral dose of one of these agents occurs within about 30 minutes to 1 hour. Maximum temperature reduction is evident between 2 and 3 hours after the dose, and antipyretic effects are generally sustained for 4–6 hours. Because the average maximum reduction in temperature is usually only 2–3°F (1.1°–1.7°C), "normalization" of temperature may not occur and should not necessarily be a goal of therapy. The most important objective of fever management is to relieve patient discomfort. Because of the causal relationship between salicylates and Reye's syndrome in children under 15 years of age who have influenza or herpes zoster-varicella virus infections (see the section Reye's Syndrome), aspirin is rarely used as a pediatric antipyretic in the United States today.

The dosages of nonprescription analgesics/antipyretics commonly used for pain or inflammation are listed in Table 4.[56] Dosages recommended by the FDA are given in the following discussions of these agents.[57]

Salicylates

The active moiety of all salicylates is salicylic acid, but that compound is too irritating to be used systemically. Therefore, esters of salicylic acid and salicylate esters of organic acids that can be administered orally and rectally have been formulated. Table 5 lists adult dosages of commercially available nonprescription salicylates. FDA recommended dosages are given in text discussions of the individual salicylates.

The more water soluble choline salicylate offers the advantage of being stable in an oral solution. Sodium salicylate and magnesium salicylate offer no advantages over aspirin except that patients allergic to aspirin may be able to tolerate these forms.

Indications

Salicylates are effective in treating mild to moderate pain and fever from a variety of etiologies. These agents are most commonly used for musculoskeletal indications. They are usually ineffective in pain of visceral origin.

Dosage

The adult oral aspirin dosage recommened by the FDA for mild to moderate pain and fever is 325–650 mg every 4 hours, or 325–500 mg every 3 hours, or 650–1,000 mg every 6 hours while symptoms persist, not to exceed 4 g in 24 hours.[57] The recommended pediatric antipyretic doses are listed in Table 6. Aspirin dosages in the range of 4–6 g per day are often needed to produce anti-inflammatory effects. Because the maximum analgesic dosage for self-medication with aspirin is 4 g per day in divided doses, anti-inflammatory efficacy often will not occur unless the drug is used at the high end of the acceptable dosage range. Therefore, many clinicians now recommend NSAIDs as drugs of choice in inflammatory disorders such as rheumatoid arthritis.

TABLE 5 Adult dosages of nonprescription salicylates

Agent	Dosage forms	Usual adult dosage
Aspirin	Tablets, effervescent, enteric coated, buffered; suppositories; chewing gum	650–975 mg (three 325-mg doses) or 1,000 mg (two 500-mg doses) every 4–6 h, not to exceed 4,000 mg/day
Choline salicylate	Oral solution (870 mg/5 mL)	870 mg every 3–4 h, not to exceed 6 daily doses
Magnesium salicylate	Tablets (325 and 500 mg)	650 mg every 4 h or 1000 mg, 3 times/day
Sodium salicylate	Tablets, enteric coated (325 and 650 mg)	650 mg every 4 h

Overdose

Mild salicylate intoxication (salicylism) occurs with chronic therapy that produces toxic salicylate plasma concentrations. Chronic intoxication in adults generally requires taking salicylate doses of approximately 90–100 mg/kg within 24 hours for at least 2 days. Symptoms include headache, dizziness, ringing in the ears, difficulty in hearing, dimness of vision, mental confusion, lassitude, drowsiness, sweating, thirst, hyperventilation, nausea, vomiting, and occasional diarrhea. These symptoms, which may mimic the signs and symptoms of the disease being treated, are all reversible upon lowering the plasma concentration to a therapeutic range.

Acute salicylate intoxication is categorized as mild (<150 mg/kg), moderate (150–300 mg/kg), or severe (>300 mg/kg). Symptoms depend on serum salicylate levels and include lethargy, tinnitus, tachypnea and pulmonary edema, convulsions, coma, nausea, vomiting, hemorrhage, and dehydration. Acid-base disturbances are prominent and range from respiratory alkalosis to metabolic acidosis. Initially, salicylate affects the respiratory center in the medulla, producing hyperventilation and respiratory alkalosis. In severely intoxicated adults and in most salicylate-poisoned children under 5 years of age, respiratory alkalosis rapidly progresses to metabolic acidosis.[58] Children are more prone to develop high fever in salicylate poisoning. Hypoglycemia resulting from increased tissue glucose use may be especially serious in children. Bleeding may occur from the GI tract or mucosal surfaces, and petechiae are a prominent feature at autopsy.

Emergency management of acute salicylate intoxication is directed toward preventing the absorption of salicylate from the GI tract. Emergency medical personnel and poison control centers commonly advocate using ipecac syrup at home to empty the stomach for mild to moderate unintentional ingestions by children under 6 years of age. When the patient is to be seen in an emergency department, the emetic, gastric lavage, or activated charcoal may be used depending upon the attending physician's preference and the clinical situation. Therefore, in such cases, ipecac syrup or activated charcoal should be used only if recommended by emergency department personnel. Vomiting should be induced even if the patient has vomited spontaneously. Adults and children over 12 years of age should be given 30 mL of ipecac syrup followed by 8 oz of water, clear liquids, or carbonated beverages, and should be ambulated to stimulate emesis. If emesis does not occur in 20–30 minutes, the process should be repeated with the same ipecac dose.

For children 1–12 years of age, the recommended dose of ipecac syrup is 15 mL (1 tbsp or 3 tsp) followed by 8 oz of water, clear liquids, or carbonated beverages. The same 15-mL dose of ipecac syrup should be repeated if vomiting does not occur within 20–30 minutes. In children under 1 year of age, vomiting should be induced only under medical supervision.

Administering ipecac syrup or other oral liquids to a person who is convulsing or not completely conscious is absolutely contraindicated because of the potential for aspiration.[59,60] Further guidelines on the use of ipecac syrup or activated charcoal in preventing absorption of salicylate are included in Chapter 16, "Emetic and Antiemetic Products."

TABLE 6 Recommended pediatric antipyretic doses: acetaminophen and aspirin

Body weight	Age (y)	Single dose (mg)[a]
Acetaminophen		
(10–15 mg/kg)	<2	Physician directed
	2–3	160
	4–5	240
	6–8	320
	9–10	400
	11–12	480
	Adult	650
Aspirin		
(10–15 mg/kg)	<2	Physician directed
	2–3	162
	4–5	243
	6–8	324
	9–10	405
	11–12	486
	Adult	650

[a]Individual doses may be repeated every 4–6 hours as needed, up to four to five daily doses. Do not exceed five doses in 24 hours.

Pharmacokinetics of Aspirin and Other Salicylates

Salicylates inhibit prostaglandin synthesis from arachidonic acid by inhibiting cyclo-oxygenase, an enzyme essential for prostaglandin synthesis. Prostaglandins sensitize nociceptors to the chemical or mechanical initiation of pain impulses. The resulting decrease in prostaglandins reduces the sensitivity of pain receptors to the initiation of pain impulses at sites of inflammation and trauma. Although some evidence suggests that aspirin might also produce analgesia through a central mechanism, its site of action is primarily peripheral.[61]

Salicylates are absorbed by passive diffusion of the nonionized drug in the stomach and small intestine. Factors affecting absorption include dosage form, gastric pH, gastric emptying time, dissolution rate, and the presence of antacids or food. Because enteric-coated aspirin is absorbed only from the small intestine, its absorption is markedly slowed by food, which increases the gastric emptying time. Buffered aspirin products are absorbed more rapidly than nonbuffered products, but this has little therapeutic significance in terms of onset of drug effect.[62] Rectal absorption of salicylate is slow and unreliable. By the rectal route, aspirin is only 60–75% bioavailable and produces peak salicylate levels of about half those achieved with an equivalent oral dose.[63]

Endoscopic evaluation comparing the gastric damage produced by buffered and nonbuffered aspirin products suggests that there is no difference in the amount of gastric damage produced by either product.[64] However, enteric coating eliminates the local gastric irritation produced by aspirin.[65,66] Equivalent doses of plain, buffered, or enteric-coated aspirin produce essentially the same plasma levels of salicylate; however, the time to peak is delayed with the enteric-coated product.[67] Thus, for patients requiring rapid pain relief, enteric-coated aspirin is inappropriate because of the delay in absorption and time to analgesic effect. However, for patients requiring prolonged aspirin therapy, such as that required for the management of RA, enteric-coated aspirin may be preferred because it produces less gastric mucosal injury than either plain or buffered aspirin.

Timed-release aspirin is formulated to prolong the product's duration of action by slowing dissolution and absorption. Because of this delayed absorption, such products are not useful for rapid pain relief but may be useful as bedtime medication. Bioavailability comparison of a single 1.3-g dose of plain aspirin versus 1.3 g of a timed-release formulation (Measurin) revealed plasma salicylate concentrations to be higher for the first 4 hours following administration with the plain aspirin product and higher during the 4- to 8-hour interval with the timed-release product.[68] But although comparisons of three timed-release aspirin products (Measurin, Verin, and Zorprin) demonstrated all three to be equally bioavailable, they were not bioequivalent. Fifty percent of the administered dose was recovered in the urine approximately 9 hours following administration of Measurin compared with 18–19 hours for both Verin and Zorprin.[69] These data suggest that the pharmacokinetics profiles are not identical for the various sustained-release aspirin products and that the duration of therapeutic efficacy is, therefore, product dependent.

Sustained-release aspirin products may produce less GI irritation than regular aspirin.[70] However, aspirin-induced reversible deafness has been reported to occur to a much greater extent with high-dose sustained-release aspirin than with equivalent daily doses of plain aspirin.[71]

Effervescent aspirin solutions (eg, Alka-Seltzer) are rapidly absorbed because disintegration does not have to occur. However, there is no evidence that such products produce more rapid or effective analgesia than oral solid dosage forms of salicylates. Moreover, effervescent aspirin solutions contain large amounts of sodium and must be avoided by patients requiring restricted sodium intake (eg, those with hypertension, heart failure, or renal failure).

Therapeutic Considerations for Use

Impaired Platelet Aggregation and Hematologic Effects Aspirin is the prototype NSAID. Chemically, aspirin is acetylsalicylic acid. The acetyl moiety makes aspirin a more effective anti-inflammatory agent than other salicylates, and aspirin is the salicylate of choice for most patients. However, that moiety also acetylates platelets causing irreversible inhibition of platelet aggregation. This effect provides a unique advantage in preventing blood clots, but it can also be a unique disadvantage due to the increased risks of bleeding.

Platelet aggregation is an important, secondary hemostatic mechanism. Aspirin can potentiate bleeding from capillary sites such as those found in the GI tract (with ulcers), tonsillar beds (following tonsillectomy), and tooth sockets (following dental extractions). A single 650-mg dose of aspirin can double the bleeding time. Aspirin therapy should be discontinued at least 48 hours before surgery and should not be used to relieve the pain of tonsillectomy, dental extraction, or other surgical procedures except under the close supervision of a physician or dentist. Some surgeons and dentists routinely recommend cessation of aspirin a week before surgery. That probably is not necessary for patients with normal hematopoietic systems. These patients will produce sufficient new platelets within 48 hours to provide efficient platelet aggregation–induced blood clotting.

Because of this effect on hemostasis, aspirin is contraindicated in patients with hypoprothrombinemia, vitamin K deficiency, hemophilia, history of any bleeding disorder, or history of peptic ulcer disease (PUD). By contrast, acetaminophen does not affect platelet aggregation or bleeding time. A daily dose of 1,950 mg of acetaminophen for 6 weeks was found to have no effect on bleeding time in hemophiliacs.[72] When peripheral anti-inflammatory activity is not needed and aspirin's effect on hemostasis is a concern, acetaminophen is an appropriate analgesic for self-medication. Most other NSAIDs impair platelet aggregation while the drugs are at analgesic serum levels, but these effects resolve as the drug is cleared from the serum. The prescription salicylate compounds salsalate[73] and choline magnesium trisalicylate[74] do not have appreciable effects on platelet aggregation and are reasonable alternatives when a peripheral anti-inflammatory agent is indicated. Sodium salicylate does not affect platelets, but it does increase prothrombin time.

Salicylates do not normally affect leukocyte, platelet, or erythrocyte count; hematocrit; or hemoglobin.

However, chronic blood loss from the GI tract resulting from continued use of aspirin-containing products can cause iron-deficiency anemia and alter hematologic indices.

Effect on Uric Acid Elimination Salicylates can affect uric acid secretion and reabsorption by the renal tubules. The resulting effect on plasma uric acid is dose related. Doses of 1–2 g per day inhibit tubular uric acid secretion without affecting reabsorption and may increase plasma uric acid levels, which can precipitate or worsen an attack of gout. Moderate doses of 2–3 g per day have little effect on uric acid secretion. High doses of more than 5 g per day may decrease plasma uric acid by increasing its renal excretion, but because these are toxic salicylate doses, they should not be used in the clinical management of gout or hyperuricemia. All salicylates should be avoided in patients with a history of gout or hyperuricemia.

Gastrointestinal Irritation and Bleeding Aspirin produces local GI damage by penetrating the protective mucous and bicarbonate layers of the gastric mucosa and permitting the back diffusion of acid, causing cellular and vascular erosion. There are two distinct mechanisms by which this occurs: a local irritant effect from the drug contacting the gastric mucosa and a systemic effect from prostaglandin inhibition. Gastritis is a local effect that can occur without risk of ulceration. Conversely, ulceration is due to systemic activity and it can be asymptomatic until it is advanced. Contributing mechanisms include inhibition of mucosal prostaglandin synthesis, reduction and alteration of mucus secretion, and reduction of bicarbonate secretion. Endoscopic evaluation of healthy volunteers showed that 650 mg of aspirin produced multiple gastric petechiae and erythema within 1 hour in all subjects. A second group taking 650 mg aspirin every 6 hours for 24 hours showed multiple antral erosions in all subjects and duodenal erosions and petechiae in half the volunteers.[75] In a prospective endoscopic analysis of patients taking 2.5 g of aspirin per day for at least 3 months, 20% had gastric ulcers, 40% had gastric erosions, 75% had gastric erythema, and 4% had duodenal ulceration.

GI blood loss with aspirin is dose dependent. Normal subjects with no aspirin exposure lose approximately 0.5 mL of blood per day in the stool. Moderate aspirin intake increases this amount to 2–6 mL per day, and up to 15% of patients will lose in excess of 10 mL per day. Chronic GI bleeding of this magnitude can deplete total body iron and produce iron deficiency anemia. Patients experiencing aspirin-induced blood loss may or may not be positive for fecal occult blood, depending on the dose and duration of aspirin therapy. Aspirin use should be discontinued for at least 3 days prior to a test for fecal occult blood.

In a small percentage of patients, aspirin use can produce massive GI bleeding (acute hemorrhagic gastritis), resulting in the vomiting of blood (hematemesis) or the presence of large amounts of digested blood in the stools (melena). Recent aspirin ingestion has been associated with about half of all cases of acute hemorrhagic gastritis, and the incidence of hospital admissions for major upper GI bleeding attributable to regular aspirin use is estimated to be about 15 cases per 100,000 admissions per year.[76] Elderly patients, patients with a history of gastric ulceration or bleeding, and those with alcoholic liver disease are at increased risk for acute hemorrhagic gastritis with aspirin use and therefore should avoid aspirin. In addition, patients who take aspirin should be advised that ingesting aspirin with alcohol appears to increase the incidence of GI bleeding.[77]

Aspirin Allergy Many patients report that they are allergic to aspirin because they have experienced gastritis or heartburn following its use. These are common side effects, not allergy or hypersensitivity, and they are not contraindications to future trials of aspirin. True aspirin allergy is uncommon, occurring in less than 1% of patients. Manifestations of aspirin allergy include hives (urticaria), edema, difficulty in breathing, bronchospasm, rhinitis, or shock; these adverse effects usually occur within 3 hours of aspirin ingestion. Aspirin allergy is usually allergy to acetylated salicylates, not to all salicylates; therefore, nonacetylated salicylates may be used by many patients who are allergic to aspirin. Aspirin is the only acetylated salicylate available in the United States. Aspirin allergy occurs most commonly in patients with urticaria, asthma, and nasal polyps. In patients with only one of these conditions, the incidence of aspirin allergy has been reported to range from 10 to 30%.[78] Patients with chronic urticaria often develop an urticarial reaction to aspirin, and those with asthma or nasal polyps normally develop bronchospasm and/or rhinorrhea. However, the level of these adverse effects may not be clinically problematic.

Patients intolerant to aspirin may also cross-react with other chemicals or drugs. Up to 15% of patients who are allergic to aspirin may cross-react when exposed to tartrazine (Food Drug and Cosmetic yellow dye #5), which can be found in many drugs, in foods such as soft drinks and colored candy, and in colored desserts such as puddings and frostings. The cross-reaction rates for acetaminophen and ibuprofen in documented aspirin-intolerant patients are 6% and 97%, respectively. High cross-reaction rates in aspirin-intolerant patients are also reported with some prescription NSAIDs. Thus, patients with a history of aspirin intolerance should be advised to avoid all aspirin- and NSAID-containing products and to use acetaminophen for analgesic self-medication.

However, even though the cross-reaction rate for acetaminophen is low, aspirin-intolerant patients may exhibit urticarial or bronchospastic symptoms with this drug.[79] Other nonprescription analgesics that have a low risk of cross-reactivity include sodium salicylate and choline salicylate.[80] In 182 documented aspirin-intolerant patients given either sodium or choline salicylate, no symptoms of intolerance were observed.[81]

Pregnancy/Lactation Aspirin consumption during pregnancy may produce adverse maternal effects including anemia, antepartum or postpartum hemorrhage, and prolonged gestation and labor. The increased duration of gestation and labor results from the inhibition of prostaglandin synthesis. Aspirin ingestion on a regular basis during pregnancy may increase the risk for complicated deliveries, including cesarean sections and breech and forceps deliveries. However, controlled study data supporting this concern are lacking. In 1990, FDA required oral and rectal nonprescription drug products that contain aspirin to carry labels that warned against using the drugs during the last 3 months of pregnancy unless the patient is directed to do so by a physician.

Aspirin readily crosses the placenta and can be found in higher concentrations in the neonate than in the mother. Salicylate elimination is slow in the neonate because of the immature and underdeveloped capacity to form glycine and glucuronic acid conjugates in the liver and reduced urinary excretion resulting from low glomerular filtration rates.[82,83]

Fetal effects of in utero aspirin exposure include intrauterine growth retardation, congenital salicylate intoxication, decreased albumin-binding capacity, and increased perinatal mortality. In utero mortality results, in part, from antepartum hemorrhage or premature closure of the ductus arteriosus. In utero aspirin exposure within 1 week of delivery can produce hemorrhagic episodes and/or pruritic rash in the neonate. Reported neonatal bleeding complications include petechiae, hematuria, cephalhematoma, subconjunctival hemorrhage, and bleeding from circumcision. An increased incidence of intracranial hemorrhage in premature or low-birth weight infants has also been reported after maternal aspirin use near birth.[84] The relationship between maternal aspirin ingestion and congenital malformation is unresolved. An association between maternal aspirin ingestion, oral clefts, and congenital heart disease has been reported. However, other studies have failed to demonstrate any increased risk for fetal malformation resulting from maternal aspirin exposure.[83]

Aspirin and other salicylates are excreted into breast milk in low concentrations. Following single-dose oral salicylate ingestion, peak milk levels occur at about 3 hours, producing a milk to maternal plasma ratio of 0.03:0.08. Adverse effects on platelet function in the nursing infant exposed to aspirin via the mother's milk have not been reported but still must be considered a potential risk.[85]

In summary, both increased maternal morbidity and fetal morbidity and mortality have been reported with perinatal aspirin exposure. The role of salicylates in producing fetal malformation during first-trimester exposure is unresolved. Women should be advised to avoid aspirin during pregnancy, especially during the last trimester, and when breast-feeding. At these times, acetaminophen is the preferred analgesic for self-medication.

Reye's Syndrome Reye's syndrome is an acute, potentially fatal illness occurring almost exclusively in children under 15 years of age. The syndrome produces fatty liver with encephalopathy. It is characterized by vomiting, progressive CNS damage, signs of hepatic injury, and hypoglycemia. The onset usually follows a viral infection with influenza (type A or B) or varicella-zoster (ie, chickenpox). Within 1–7 days, persistent vomiting generally occurs along with stupor, possibly progressing to generalized convulsions and coma. Other neurologic symptoms include listlessness, lethargy, disorientation, hostility, combativeness, inability to recognize family members, incessant moaning or screaming, twitching, and jerking. The mortality rate may be as high as 50%.[86]

Although the cause of Reye's syndrome is unknown, viral and toxic agents, especially salicylates, have been associated with it. The Centers for Disease Control and Prevention (CDC) has been consistently monitoring for an association between Reye's syndrome and ibuprofen since 1977, and none has been identified.[87] The data suggest that nonsalicylate NSAIDs are not associated with this syndrome.

Three case-controlled retrospective studies reported in the early 1980s by the state health departments of Arizona, Michigan, and Ohio suggested an association between the development of Reye's syndrome and the ingestion of aspirin during the antecedent viral illness. After reviewing the available data, the CDC, the American Academy of Pediatrics, the FDA, and the US surgeon general issued a warning that aspirin and other salicylates should be avoided in children and young adults who have influenza or chickenpox. Since 1988 the FDA has required that the following Reye's syndrome warning be added to the labels of nonprescription aspirin and aspirin-containing products:

> Children and teenagers should not use this medicine for chickenpox or flu symptoms before a doctor is consulted about Reye's syndrome, a rare but serious illness associated with aspirin use.

In 1993, the FDA proposed that the warning be revised slightly and extended to all nonprescription products containing bismuth subsalicylate (which is not an analgesic/antipyretic, per se) except those marketed solely for diarrhea.[88] The Aspirin Foundation of America and manufacturers of nonaspirin salicylate drugs objected to the proposed change, and a final rule had not been published by mid-1996.

The PHS's Reye's Syndrome Task Force conducted its study in the peak influenza season between January 1985 and May 1986 in 70 pediatric tertiary care centers throughout the United States and reported its findings in 1987.[89] More than 90% of the subjects who developed Reye's syndrome had taken salicylates. The independent risk of nonaspirin salicylate use could not be assessed. The study also found that risk of developing Reye's syndrome correlated with the salicylate dose, with those subjects who received higher doses being at greater risk.

The dose dependency of Reye's syndrome risk was further evaluated using data from the PHS's Main Study of Reye's Syndrome and Medications.[90] Aspirin doses as low as 15 mg/kg per day were associated with a sevenfold increase in the risk for developing Reye's syndrome. Based on these data, there is no safe minimum dose of aspirin for children and teenagers with influenza or chickenpox, and the drug should be completely avoided.

Because of concerns of potential bias in the previously cited PHS study, an epidemiologic investigation was conducted to assess whether the findings of that study were flawed. After controlling for five potential sources of bias in the study, a strong association was confirmed between the use of salicylate during an antecedent viral infection and the subsequent development of Reye's syndrome.[91] Thus, it is imperative that pharmacists warn against giving products containing aspirin or nonaspirin salicylates to children and teenagers who have influenza or chickenpox. In such cases, acetaminophen is the preferred nonprescription analgesic/antipyretic. A simple viral upper respiratory infection (eg, a common cold) is not a contraindication to aspirin use; however, symptoms of this type of infection may mimic some of those seen in influenza and chickenpox. Therefore, many clinicians recommend a conservative approach of aspirin avoidance when symptoms resembling influenza are present. The use of aspirin as a pediatric antipyretic has all but ceased in the United States, as have reports of Reye's syndrome.

Drug Interactions

Aspirin, the other nonprescription salicylates, acetaminophen, ibuprofen, naproxen sodium, and ketoprofen interact with several other important drugs and drug classes. Adverse effects of the drugs are additive with other agents or diseases that cause similar disorders. Patients at increased risk of toxicity from NSAIDs include individuals with marked renal or hepatic impairment (ie, uremia, cirrhosis, hepatitis); patients with metabolic disorders (ie, hypoxia, hypothyroidism); patients with unstable disease (ie, cardiac arrhythmias, intractable epilepsy, brittle diabetes); patients with status asthmaticus; and elderly patients in general because of the increased incidence of multiple system disorders. Clinically important drug interactions that have been reported with aspirin and other nonprescription analgesic/antipyretic drugs are listed in Table 7.[92]

Valproic Acid Analgesic doses of aspirin may increase the free fraction of valproic acid in plasma, markedly causing enhanced neurologic toxicity such as drowsiness and behavioral disturbances. The mechanism appears to be a combination of protein-binding displacement and decreased clearance of valproic acid. Patients taking valproic acid should avoid salicylates; naproxen and acetaminophen are safe nonprescription analgesic alternatives.[93]

Sulfonylureas Hypoglycemic effect of sulfonylurea oral antidiabetic agents may be enhanced by the concurrent administration of any salicylate that increases insulin secretion at doses greater than 2 g per day. The decreased protein binding of the sulfonylurea may also play a role. Patients taking sulfonylurea oral hypoglycemic drugs to control diabetes should avoid all salicylate-containing products and consider acetaminophen as an appropriate alternative.[92]

Uricosuric Drugs The uricosuric effect of both probenecid and sulfinpyrazone may be antagonized by the concurrent administration of salicylate, resulting in the worsening of hyperuricemia and the possible exacerbation of gout. The effect and magnitude of this interaction are salicylate dose dependent. Doses of aspirin greater than 5 g per day are uricosuric but are also toxic. An occasional dose of aspirin or other salicylate is unlikely to cause serious problems in patients taking uricosuric drugs, but all salicylates should be avoided in such patients to minimize risk. Acetaminophen is the best nonprescription alternative.[92]

Ethanol Ethanol can interact with both acetaminophen and NSAIDs, increasing the risk of hepatic toxicity with acetaminophen and gastropathy with the NSAIDs. Ethanol also increases fecal blood loss resulting from aspirin ingestion, possibly doubling daily GI blood loss when compared with that induced by aspirin in the absence of ethanol. This effect results both from the GI erosive effects of ethanol and aspirin and from an enhanced prolongation of bleeding time due to ethanol's potentiation of the antiplatelet effect of aspirin. The ingestion of ethanol plus 1 g of aspirin 1 hour after a standard breakfast significantly elevated the blood alcohol concentration compared with that of subjects who did not receive aspirin. In such patients, ethanol bioavailability is increased because gastric alcohol dehydrogenase is inhibited, thus allowing greater GI absorption of ethanol.[94] Pharmacists should advise patients not to consume ethanol and aspirin together because of the potential for enhanced irritation or GI bleeding, or enhanced neurologic impairment from the ethanol. If ethanol is to be consumed during analgesic use, acetaminophen should be recommended for self-medication as a "safer" alternative to NSAIDs.

Methotrexate Salicylates may increase the toxicity of methotrexate by displacing the drug from protein-binding sites and decreasing its renal excretion. Serious sequelae, including pancytopenia, have been reported with this drug combination. Patients receiving methotrexate must be warned against self-medication with any nonprescription analgesic containing any form of salicylate. Acetaminophen has been used concurrently with methotrexate without producing an increase in methotrexate toxicity.[92]

Oral Anticoagulants Aspirin in doses greater than 3 g per day can have a hypoprothrombinemic effect that can be additive to that produced by oral anticoagulants such as warfarin. In addition, the GI erosion and the inhibition of platelet aggregation produced by aspirin may further increase the bleeding risk if aspirin is used concurrently with an oral anticoagulant. An increased incidence of GI bleeding has been reported in patients receiving warfarin and as little as 500 mg per day of aspirin. Thus, patients receiving oral anticoagulants should be cautioned to avoid all nonprescription analgesic products containing aspirin or other salicylates and to consider acetaminophen as an appropriate nonprescription analgesic alternative.[58]

Other Salicylate-Drug Interactions A large number of additional drug–drug interactions have been documented, many of which are not as clinically significant as those mentioned previously. Pharmacists should review current drug interaction references for newly identified interactions when monitoring the therapy of patients taking high-dose salicylates.

Aspirin and Myocardial Infarct Prophylaxis

As noted previously, aspirin is known to inhibit prostaglandin synthesis within the platelet irreversibly and to retard platelet aggregation for the life span of the aspirin-exposed platelet. Because platelet aggregation has a role in thrombin clot formation, aspirin's antithrombotic

TABLE 7 Clinically important drug interactions with nonprescription analgesic/antipyretic agents

OTC analgesic/ antipyretic	Drug	Potential interaction	Management/Preventive measures
Ibuprofen, high-dose salicylates	Phenytoin	Phenytoin displaced from serum protein–binding sites if phenytoin metabolism is saturated or folate levels are low	Monitor unbound phenytoin levels; adjust dose, if indicated; ensure that patient has sufficient folate
Aspirin	Valproic acid	Oxidation of valproate inhibited; up to 30% reduction in clearance	Avoid concurrent use; use naproxen instead of aspirin (no interaction)
NSAIDs (several)	Digoxin	Renal clearance inhibited	Monitor digoxin levels; adjust doses as indicated
NSAIDs (several)	Aminoglycosides	Renal clearance inhibited	Monitor antibiotic levels; adjust doses as indicated
NSAIDS (several)	Antihypertensive agents; beta-blockers, ACE inhibitors, vasodilators, diuretics	Antihypertensive effect antagonized; hyperkalemia may occur with potassium-sparing diuretics and ACE inhibitors	Monitor blood pressure and cardiac function; monitor potassium levels
NSAIDs	Oral anticoagulants	Risk of bleeding, especially GI bleeding, increased	Avoid concurrent use, if possible; risk is lowest with salsalate and choline magnesium trisalicylate
NSAIDs (some)	Lithium	Renal clearance inhibited	Monitor lithium levels; adjust doses as indicated; interaction less likely with aspirin than with ibuprofen or naproxen
NSAIDs	Alcohol	Increased risk of GI bleeding	Avoid concurrent use, if possible; minimize alcohol intake when using NSAID
NSAIDs (several)	Methotrexate	Methotrexate clearance decreased	Avoid NSAIDs with high-dose methotrexate therapy; monitor levels with concurrent treatment
Naproxen	Probenecid	Naproxen clearance inhibited	Monitor for adverse effects
Naproxen	Aluminum hydroxide	Naproxen absorption decreased	Increase naproxen dose as needed
Salicylates	Antacids in high doses	Salicylate levels possibly reduced 25%	Determine if salicylate doses should be increased
Salicylates (moderate to high doses)	Sulfonylureas	Hypoglycemic activity increased	Avoid concurrent use, if possible; monitor blood glucose levels when changing salicylate dose
Salicylates	Corticosteroids	Salicylate clearance possibly increased with long-term, high-dose salicylate therapy	Monitor salicylate levels when changing steroid dose; adjust salicylate dose, if indicated

Note: NSAIDs include the salicylates.

activity has been used clinically under medical supervision to prevent transient ischemic attack, thrombotic stroke, MI in unstable angina patients, and vascular reocclusion following both percutaneous transluminal coronary angioplasty and coronary artery bypass grafts. Aspirin has also been used clinically in post-MI patients to prevent the risk of future thromboembolic events.

In 1993, the FDA proposed that all nonprescription drug products containing aspirin, buffered aspirin, and aspirin in combination with an antacid contain the following notice[95]:

> **IMPORTANT:** See your doctor before taking this product for your heart or other new uses of aspirin, because serious side effects could occur with self-treatment.

No final rule on that proposal had been published as of mid-1996.

Nonacetylated Salicylates

Choline Salicylate Choline salicylate (Arthropan) is an oral liquid salicylate preparation. It is absorbed from the stomach more rapidly than aspirin tablets, but this may not be clinically important.[57] A 5-mL dose of choline salicylate (174 mg/mL, or 870 mg) is equivalent to 650 mg of aspirin in salicylate content. The FDA recommended adult dosage is 435–870 mg every 4 hours, or 435–670 mg every 3 hours, or 870–1,340 mg every 6 hours, not to exceed 5,325 mg in 24 hours. For patients who find the fishy odor of the liquid product unacceptable, choline salicylate oral solution may be mixed with fruit juice, a carbonated beverage, or water just before administration. However, it should not be mixed with any alkaline solution, including antacids, because the liberation of choline exaggerates the fishy odor of the product. Comparative analgesic/anti-inflammatory efficacy studies are not available for choline salicylate. However, the product was found to be less effective than either aspirin or acetaminophen as an antipyretic in children.[96]

Magnesium Salicylate A study comparing the analgesic efficacy of 500 mg of aspirin taken four times daily with 500 mg of magnesium salicylate taken four times daily in patients with chronic degenerative arthritis found similar reductions in objective pain scores for the two drugs at the end of 12 weeks.[97] Magnesium salicylate is available as the tetrahydrate (Arthriten, Backache); as a consequence, the salicylate content of 377 mg of magnesium salicylate tetrahydrate is equivalent to that of 325 mg of sodium salicylate. The FDA recommended adult dosage of magnesium salicylate for nonprescription use is 377–754 mg every 4 hours, or 377–580 mg every 3 hours, or 754–1,160 mg every 6 hours, not to exceed 4,640 mg in 24 hours. The maximum 24-hour dose of magnesium salicylate contains 264 mg (11 mEq) of magnesium. Thus, patients with compromised renal function must avoid using magnesium salicylate because of the potential for decreased renal excretion of magnesium with its subsequent accumulation and the production of systemic magnesium toxicity.

Sodium Salicylate Divided oral doses of enteric-coated aspirin and enteric-coated sodium salicylate, 4.8 g per day, have been shown to be equally effective in the treatment of rheumatoid arthritis. Both drugs have produced similar degrees of pain relief, increased grip strength, reduced joint tenderness, and decreased digital joint circumference.[98] Patients allergic to aspirin may be able to tolerate sodium salicylate. However, sodium salicylate is less effective than an equal dose of aspirin in reducing pain or fever. The FDA recommended adult nonprescription anti-inflammatory dosage of sodium salicylate is 325–650 mg every 4 hours, or 325–500 mg every 3 hours, or 650 mg to 1 g every 6 hours, not to exceed 4 g in 24 hours. The maximum 4-g dose of sodium salicylate contains 560 mg (25 mEq) of sodium; consequently, patients on strict sodium restriction should avoid using sodium salicylate.

Comparison of Aspirin and Nonacetylated Salicylates

When doses containing equivalent amounts of salicylate are given, it appears that aspirin and the nonacetylated salicylates are equally well absorbed and produce similar plasma salicylate levels. However, choline salicylate oral solution produces peak plasma salicylate levels sooner than the oral solid dosage forms.[99]

Because aspirin's effect on platelet aggregation with a prolongation of bleeding time requires the participation of the acetyl moiety, nonacetylated salicylates do not affect platelet aggregation or bleeding time significantly.[73,100–102] With the exception of this difference, the nonacetylated salicylates have the same contraindications and interactions as aspirin because all other salicylate effects result from the production of salicylic acid. However, nonacetylated salicylates are weaker prostaglandin synthesis inhibitors than aspirin and, as such, appear to cause less GI erosion and bleeding, fewer renal complications, and a low level of cross-reactivity in aspirin-intolerant patients.[80,103]

Acetaminophen

Indications

Acetaminophen is an effective analgesic and antipyretic. Animal studies of acetaminophen at high doses have demonstrated weak anti-inflammatory activity that is not useful clinically. Unlike salicylates, acetaminophen produces analgesia through a central rather than a peripheral effect on the nervous system.[61] Acetaminophen is effective in relieving mild to moderate pain of nonvisceral origin.

Dosage

The FDA recommended adult dosage of acetaminophen is 325–650 mg every 4 hours, or 325–500 mg every 3 hours, or 650–1,000 mg every 6 hours, not to exceed a total of 4 g in 24 hours. Table 6 lists recommended oral pediatric doses. Rectal bioavailability of acetaminophen is approximately 50–60% of that achieved with oral administration. Equal doses of acetaminophen and aspirin administered by the same route produce equivalent degrees of analgesia.[104]

Acetaminophen is available for oral administration

in various liquid and solid dosage forms, including rectal suppositories and capsules. The capsules contain tasteless granules that can be emptied onto a teaspoon containing a small amount of drink or soft food. Patients and parents should not add the contents of the capsules to a glass of liquid because large numbers of granules may adhere to the side of the glass. Mixing with a hot beverage can result in a bitter taste.

Overdose

The American Association of Poison Control Centers reports that acetaminophen accounted for 66% of overdoses with nonprescription analgesics; ibuprofen accounted for 19% of reports and aspirin 15%.[105] Fifty-eight percent of analgesic overdoses were in children under 6 years of age, and 38% of these ingestions resulted in treatment in a health care facility. Less than 1% of the poisonings resulted in major morbidity.

Of 4,801 nonprescription analgesic overdoses in children, only 0.3–0.4% resulted in severe or life-threatening effects, and there were no deaths in this group. In 5,333 adult exposures, severe or life-threatening results occurred in 5.4% taking aspirin, 5.2% taking acetaminophen, and 1.6% taking ibuprofen; 11 deaths occurred with aspirin, 10 with acetaminophen, and none with ibuprofen.[106]

Symptoms are often absent for hours following an acute overdose of acetaminophen. During the first 2 days after an acute overdose, symptoms may not reflect the potential seriousness of the exposure. Early symptoms of acetaminophen intoxication include nausea, vomiting, drowsiness, confusion, and abdominal pain. Clinical manifestations of hepatotoxicity begin 2–4 days after the acute ingestion of acetaminophen and include increased plasma transaminases (both aspartate and alanine aminotransferase), increased plasma bilirubin with jaundice, and prolonged prothrombin time. In nonfatal cases, the hepatic damage is reversible over a period of weeks or months. The most serious adverse effect of acute overdose with acetaminophen is a dose-dependent, potentially fatal hepatic necrosis.[107] Renal tubular necrosis and hypoglycemic coma may also occur. In adults, hepatotoxicity may occur after ingestion of a single dose of 10–15 g (150–250 mg/kg) of acetaminophen; doses of 20–25 g or more are potentially fatal.

Because of the potential seriousness of acetaminophen overdose, all cases should be referred to a poison control center or other medical personnel experienced in managing such cases. Approximately 65% of acetaminophen overdoses in children are effectively managed in the home, compared with only about 18% for adult acetaminophen overdose.[106] Immediate first-aid management of acute acetaminophen poisoning includes the induction of vomiting with ipecac syrup. Activated charcoal may also be effective in reducing the absorption of acetaminophen; however, it can also adsorb the specific antidote for acetaminophen hepatotoxicity, *N*-acetylcysteine, and presumably reduce its efficacy. If activated charcoal is administered on an in-home, first-aid basis for acetaminophen overdose, this information must be made known to emergency medical personnel administering *N*-acetylcysteine so that appropriate dose adjustments can be made.[108] Dosing recommendations for both ipecac syrup and activated charcoal are included in Chapter 16, "Emetic and Antiemetic Products." Pharmacists and other caregivers are strongly encouraged to coordinate with a poison center any non–hospital-based management of poisoning or drug overdose.

Therapeutic Considerations for Use

Acetaminophen sometimes is underdosed, especially in young patients. This occurs when parents reuse the 0.8-mL dropper provided with infant drops (80 mg/0.8 mL) to measure a dose of an equivalent volume of acetaminophen elixir in a concentration of 160 mg/5 mL, incorrectly assuming the same strength. In addition, rapidly growing infants quickly outgrow previous dose requirements. Therefore, recalculation of the pediatric dose according to present age and body weight is appropriate at the time of each treatment course.[109]

Acetaminophen crosses the placenta but is considered safe for use during pregnancy. It appears in breast milk, producing a milk to maternal plasma ratio of 0.50:1.0. Based on a 1,000 mg maternal dose, the estimated maximum infant dose is 1.85% of the maternal dose. The only adverse effect reported in nursing infants exposed to acetaminophen through breast milk is a rarely occurring maculopapular rash, which subsides when drug exposure is discontinued. The American Academy of Pediatrics considers acetaminophen use to be compatible with breast-feeding.[85]

Acetaminophen has no effect on the urinary excretion of uric acid, on prothrombin synthesis, or on platelet aggregation and bleeding time.[110] In addition, it produces less GI irritation, erosion, and bleeding than aspirin or other salicylates. Acetaminophen also has a very low incidence of cross-reactivity in aspirin-intolerant patients. Thus, for patients who cannot take aspirin or another salicylate because of contraindications due to adverse effects on bleeding time, uric acid excretion, GI bleeding, aspirin intolerance, or concurrent drug therapy, acetaminophen is an appropriate nonprescription analgesic alternative.

Acetaminophen is potentially hepatotoxic in doses exceeding 4 g per day. Patients with preexisting liver disease who are taking other potentially hepatotoxic drugs, who do not eat regularly, and who ingest alcohol more than occasionally are at increased risk for acetaminophen-induced hepatotoxicity. A retrospective case series study of the association between acetaminophen-induced hepatotoxicity with fasting and alcohol use demonstrated that hepatotoxicity was associated with fasting and, less commonly, with alcohol use when the drug was taken at doses of 4–10 g per day.[111] Patients should be advised to avoid alcohol and fasting, if possible, when taking acetaminophen.

Drug Interactions

Clinically important drug interactions of acetaminophen are listed in Table 7. Acetaminophen produces no therapeutically significant drug interactions with the possible exception of zidovudine (azidothymidine, or AZT). It has been reported that patients with AIDS and AIDS-related complex who were taking zidovudine experienced an increased incidence of bone marrow suppression if they concurrently received acetaminophen.[112] Both acetaminophen and zidovudine are metabolized by hepatic glucuronidation; competition for the same metabolizing system may produce increased levels of zidovudine, resulting in increased bone marrow suppression. In a subsequent attempt to clarify this interaction, four patients receiving 200 mg of zidovudine were administered 650 mg of acetaminophen every 6 hours for 48 hours. Acetaminophen had no significant effect on peak times of zidovudine plasma levels or on the plasma half-life of zidovudine. However, the total availability of zidovudine to plasma with concurrent acetaminophen decreased by 19%.[113] In a study to ascertain whether concurrent treatment with acetaminophen impairs the clearance of zidovudine, 27 patients with clinical manifestations of human immunodeficiency disease who received 200 mg of zidovudine were concurrently treated with one of three acetaminophen regimens: 325 mg for 3 days, 650 mg for 3 days, or 650 mg for 7 days. Neither zidovudine clearance nor the production of the zidovudine glucuronide conjugate was impaired by the concurrent acetaminophen treatment. Zidovudine clearance was increased by 5%, 11%, and 33%, respectively, with the three acetaminophen regimens. The increased total clearance of zidovudine probably resulted from increased nonhepatic or renal clearance of zidovudine. From baseline until 2 weeks after the last dose of acetaminophen was administered, there were no statistically significant changes in hemoglobin concentration, leukocyte count, absolute neutrophil count, or platelet count in the three acetaminophen treatment groups.[114]

These studies suggest that concurrent administration of acetaminophen with zidovudine does not produce increased plasma levels of zidovudine and that the short-term use of acetaminophen (less than 7 days) does not increase the risk of myelosuppression and neutropenia in AIDS patients receiving zidovudine. Aspirin should probably be avoided by AIDS patients receiving zidovudine because the prolonged antiplatelet effect of aspirin could increase their bleeding risk. For these patients, the short-term or intermittent use of acetaminophen is the recommended nonprescription analgesic for self-medication.

Ibuprofen

Indications

Ibuprofen has analgesic, antipyretic, and anti-inflammatory activity; it is also useful in managing mild to moderate pain of nonvisceral origin and dysmenorrhea. Its analgesia apparently results from the peripheral inhibition of cyclo-oxygenase and the subsequent inhibition of prostaglandin synthesis.

Dosage

The analgesic dosage of nonprescription ibuprofen for patients over 12 years of age is 200–400 mg every 4–6 hours, not to exceed 1,200 mg in 24 hours. A dose-effect relationship has been demonstrated for ibuprofen analgesia in the range of 100–400 mg. On a milligram-to-milligram basis, ibuprofen is approximately 3.5 times more potent than aspirin as an analgesic, and the analgesic effect may last up to 6 hours.[115] The anti-inflammatory dose of ibuprofen is 300–600 mg every 4–6 hours, exceeding the maximum daily dose of ibuprofen recommended for nonprescription use. However, anti-inflammatory efficacy can be achieved within the recommended maximum daily dose range.

TABLE 8 Recommended analgesic/antipyretic dosages for ibuprofen, naproxen sodium, and ketoprofen

Agent	Age	Dosage (maximum)
Ibuprofen	6 mo–12 y	7.5 mg/kg (30 mg/kg/day)
	>12 y	200–400 mg every 4–6 h (1,200 mg/day)
Naproxen sodium	<12 y	Not recommended
	12–65 y	220–440 mg every 8–12 h (660 mg/day)
	>65 y	220 mg every 12 h (440 mg/day)
Ketoprofen	<16 y	Not recommended
	>16 y	12.5 mg every 6–8 h; may take second dose after 1 h, if needed (75 mg/day)

The FDA approved the oral pediatric suspension of ibuprofen as a nonprescription drug in 1995. This 100 mg/5 mL suspension (Children's Motrin) is indicated for children aged 2–11 years as an antipyretic and for relief of minor aches and pains due to colds, influenza, sore throat, headaches, and toothaches. The duration of action may be as long as 8 hours. Dosage information is listed in Table 8.

Primary dysmenorrhea is estimated to occur in up to 50% of women during their reproductive years. It is characterized by uterine cramps, backache, vomiting, diarrhea, headache, mild fever, and malaise. The symptoms occur shortly before and during the onset of menses and result from increased endometrial production of prostaglandins during this period.[116] In numerous clinical trials, ibuprofen has been shown to be superior to aspirin, nonacetylated salicylates, and acetaminophen for the symptomatic relief of primary dysmenorrhea.[116] Symptomatic relief appears to result from the inhibition of prostaglandin production in the uterus. The recommended dose of ibuprofen for primary dysmenorrhea is 400 mg every 4–6 hours as needed for the 2–3 days that symptoms persist.[9]

Overdose

Overdose of ibuprofen usually produces minimal symptoms of toxicity and is rarely fatal. In an analysis of more than 1,500 reports of overdose with ibuprofen, only 0.4% of children and 1.6% of adults exhibited major or life-threatening effects; there were no fatalities. Eighty-six percent of children and 41% of adults evidenced no symptoms from the drug exposure.[106] In a prospective study of 329 cases of ibuprofen overdose, it was found that GI and CNS symptoms (in 42% and 30% of patients, respectively) were most common and included nausea, vomiting, abdominal pain, lethargy, stupor, coma, nystagmus, dizziness, and lightheadedness. Hypotension, bradycardia, tachycardia, dyspnea, and painful breathing were also reported. In this study, 43% of ibuprofen-overdose patients were asymptomatic.[117] Unless contraindicated by convulsions or unconsciousness, appropriate first-aid treatment of ibuprofen overdose includes the induction of vomiting with ipecac syrup or the administration of activated charcoal. (See Chapter 16, "Emetic and Antiemetic Products.")

Therapeutic Considerations for Use

The most frequent adverse effects of ibuprofen involve the GI tract and include dyspepsia, heartburn, nausea, anorexia, and epigastric pain. Ibuprofen produces less GI bleeding than aspirin. In patients receiving one of these two medications for at least 1 year, aspirin produced a 15-mL blood loss over 4 days in contrast to only a 3-mL loss with ibuprofen.[118] A gastroscopic evaluation of patients on either ibuprofen or aspirin for 3–12 months revealed that 50% of those receiving aspirin evidenced gastric lesions compared with only 18% of those receiving ibuprofen.[119]

In dosages of 600–1,800 mg per day, ibuprofen increased bleeding time by inhibiting platelet aggregation. However, ibuprofen's effect on platelet aggregation, unlike that of aspirin, is reversible within 24 hours after medication is discontinued.[120] Ibuprofen does not significantly affect whole blood clotting time or prothrombin time. Because alcohol ingestion has been shown to increase by 3.5–fold the prolongation of bleeding time produced by ibuprofen, patients self-medicating with ibuprofen should be cautioned against the concurrent use of alcohol.[121] In dosages of 1,200–2,400 mg per day, ibuprofen does not appear to affect the hypoprothrombinemia produced by warfarin.[122] However, because plasma protein–binding displacement of warfarin by ibuprofen can occur and because of the drug's antiplatelet activity and its potential for increased GI bleeding, ibuprofen should not be recommended for self-medication to patients who are concurrently taking anticoagulants.

Ibuprofen may decrease renal blood flow and glomerular filtration rate as a result of inhibition of renal prostaglandin synthesis. This may increase blood urea nitrogen and serum creatinine values, often with concomitant sodium and water retention. This effect is of greatest clinical importance in patients with preexisting renal impairment or congestive heart failure. Advanced age, hypertension, use of diuretics, diabetes, and atherosclerotic cardiovascular disease appear to increase the risk of renal toxicity with ibuprofen.[123–125] As a result, patients with a history of impaired renal function, congestive heart failure, or diseases that compromise renal hemodynamics should not self-medicate with ibuprofen.

Ibuprofen is contraindicated in patients with a history of intolerance to aspirin or to any other NSAID. Cross-reactivity with ibuprofen is reported to be 97% in documented aspirin-intolerant patients. Patients with a history of asthma may experience a worsening of their bronchospastic symptoms with ibuprofen.

There is no evidence that ibuprofen is teratogenic in either humans or animals. However, because all potent prostaglandin synthesis inhibitors can cause delayed parturition, increased postpartum bleeding, prolonged labor, and adverse fetal cardiovascular effects (closure of the ductus arteriosus), ibuprofen use is contraindicated during the third trimester of pregnancy. In lactating women taking up to 2.4 g of ibuprofen per day, there is no measurable excretion of ibuprofen into breast milk. The American Academy of Pediatrics considers ibuprofen compatible with breast-feeding.[85]

The safety of ibuprofen in children was demonstrated by a practitioner-based, randomized clinical trial of ibuprofen at doses of 5 mg/kg or 10 mg/kg and acetaminophen at a dose of 12 mg/kg. This study, which involved a total of 84,192 children, demonstrated that the risk of hospitalization for GI bleeding, renal failure, or anaphylaxis was not increased following short-term use of ibuprofen as compared with acetaminophen in children.[126]

Drug Interactions

Clinically important drug interactions of ibuprofen are listed in Table 7.

Digoxin Ibuprofen has been reported to increase plasma digoxin concentrations when taken by patients receiving digoxin. The clinical significance of this interaction is uncertain. Worsening heart failure with fluid overload and blunting of furosemide responsiveness may occur with the administration of ibuprofen to patients with congestive heart failure. Because of the uncertainty of a possible ibuprofen-digoxin interaction and the potential for ibuprofen-induced furosemide refractoriness with symptomatic deterioration, pharmacists should advise patients with a history of congestive heart failure to avoid self-medicating with any ibuprofen-containing products.[92]

Antihypertensive Drugs Ibuprofen antagonizes the blood pressure-lowering effects of certain antihypertensive drugs, including diuretics, angiotensin-converting enzyme inhibitors, beta blockers, and centrally acting antihypertensives. Forty-five patients with essential hypertension controlled with at least two antihypertensive drugs were given ibuprofen (400 mg every 8 hours), acetaminophen (1 g every 8 hours), or placebo (2 capsules every 8 hours) for 3 weeks. At the end of 3 weeks, the ibuprofen-treated group experienced a 5.8-mm Hg increase in sitting mean arterial pressure and a 6.6-mm Hg increase in supine mean arterial pressure, both of which were statistically significant when compared with placebo treatment. By contrast, the acetaminophen-treated group showed no change in blood pressure during the 3-week test interval.[127] Thus, pharmacists should advise hypertensive patients selecting a nonprescription analgesic that ibuprofen may antagonize their blood pressure medication and that acetaminophen is a better choice.

Lithium The concurrent use of ibuprofen in lithium-stabilized patients is reported to produce increased plasma lithium levels and enhanced lithium toxicity. In a study of nine psychiatric patients on chronic lithium therapy (600–900 mg per day), the administration of ibuprofen, 1,800 mg per day for 6 days, decreased lithium clearance by 34% and increased serum lithium by 34% (range 12–66%). Three patients showed increased tremor, a dose-dependent adverse reaction to lithium.[128] Similar results have been obtained in healthy subjects concurrently given lithium (900 mg per day) and ibuprofen (1,200 mg per day) for 7 days.[129] Based on limited controlled studies, it appears that aspirin does not adversely affect lithium clearance.[130] Consequently, it is imperative that pharmacists advise patients taking lithium to avoid all ibuprofen-containing nonprescription analgesics. For such patients, acetaminophen is considered the best alternative analgesic because it has little, if any, effect on renal prostaglandin synthesis. Lithium-treated patients may also safely self-medicate with aspirin.

Methotrexate There is a potentially serious interaction between methotrexate and ibuprofen as well as the other NSAIDs. An anecdotal report of an 18-year-old male undergoing intravenous methotrexate therapy for osteogenic sarcoma supports the potential severity of the methotrexate-ibuprofen interaction. Unknown to the oncology team, this patient was self-medicating with ibuprofen (400 mg every 4 hours) for his leg pain. Twenty hours into his methotrexate infusion, his serum creatinine, which was 0.9 mg/dL before he began infusion, was found to be 2.3 mg/dL, and folinic acid rescue was begun immediately. It is postulated that ibuprofen competes with methotrexate for renal proximal tubular secretion, causing decreased renal clearance of methotrexate and resulting in nephrotoxicity.[131] Based on limited reports, it is imperative that patients receiving methotrexate as outpatient therapy be warned not to self-medicate with nonprescription analgesic products containing either ibuprofen or aspirin. For such patients, acetaminophen is the only nonprescription analgesic considered safe.

Naproxen Sodium

Naproxen sodium was approved for use as a nonprescription analgesic, anti-inflammatory agent, and antipyretic in 1994 (Aleve). This NSAID is very similar to nonprescription ibuprofen. Naproxen sodium has a similar onset of activity but its duration of action may be somewhat longer. The American Academy of Pediatrics considers naproxen compatible with breast-feeding.[85]

Indications

The labeled indications for the nonprescription form of the drug are relief of minor pain associated with headache, the common cold, toothache, muscle ache, backache, arthritis, and muscle cramps as well as the reduction of fever.

Dosage

The maximum daily dosage listed on the labeling for patients aged 12–65 years is three 220-mg tablets; doses should be taken 8–12 hours apart (Table 8). Patients over 65 years of age should not take more than one tablet every 12 hours unless directed to do so by a physician. The labeling stipulates that children under 12 years of age should use the drug only under a physician's supervision.

Overdose

The presentation and management of a naproxen sodium overdose should be similar to an ibuprofen overdose. Severe metabolic acidosis has been reported following naproxen sodium overdose.[132] Movement disorder has also been associated with naproxen sodium poisoning.

Drug Interactions

Clinically important drug interactions of naproxen are listed in Table 7. Naproxen sodium has a similar drug interaction profile to that of ibuprofen. Similar to the other nonprescription NSAIDs, naproxen may increase the risk of bleeding when administered concurrently with oral anticoagulants; therefore, such concurrent use should be avoided. Some studies suggest that naproxen may decrease the antihypertensive activity of some beta-blockers.[133] Other reports, however, suggest that this interaction may not be clinically important.[134] If this interaction were to occur, it might be obviated by adjusting the dose of the antihypertensive agent. Again, similar to the other NSAIDs, naproxen may reduce the antihypertensive and diuretic activity of furosemide.[135] In addition, serum lithium levels may be increased by concurrent use of naproxen. If the two drugs were used concurrently, careful monitoring of lithium levels and careful attention to dosage compliance would be needed. Finally, concurrent use of naproxen and methotrexate may cause major toxicity because of methotrexate's prolonged half-life and decreased methotrexate elimination.[136] Obviously, concurrent use of these two drugs should also be avoided.

Ketoprofen

Ketoprofen was approved for nonprescription use as an analgesic and antipyretic in 1995 (Orudis KT, Actron).

Indications

Like ibuprofen and naproxen sodium, ketoprofen is a propionic acid derivative NSAID; therefore, its indications (analgesia, anti-inflammatory activity, and antipyresis) and pharmacologic activity are the same as these two agents. Ketoprofen has also been used effectively in juvenile rheumatoid arthritis in children aged 2–16 years; however, labeling of the nonprescription products recommends that the drug be used only in patients over 16 years of age.

Dosage

One 12.5-mg tablet of ketoprofen appears to be equivalent to one 200-mg tablet of ibuprofen. The recommended dosage for patients over 16 years of age is 12.5 mg every 6–8 hours, not to exceed 75 mg in 24 hours (Table 8). If needed, a second dose may be taken after 1 hour.

Adverse Effects

Adverse effects related to ketoprofen are also similar to those of the other propionic acid derivative NSAIDs; these effects include gastric mucosal damage, inhibition of platelet aggregation, and renal effects. When administered at doses higher than nonprescription doses, ketoprofen has produced headache in more than 3% of the patients. Other dose-related side effects include visual disturbance in 1–3% of patients, peripheral edema in 2% of patients, and hepatic dysfunction in less than 1% of patients. At normal nonprescription doses, these effects are rare.

No evidence of teratogenicity or toxicity to embryos has been uncovered in studies of pregnant animals given high doses of ketoprofen. There is also no evidence of adverse effects on fertility. The product labeling, however, recommends that this drug not be used by nursing mothers.

Drug Interactions

A life-threatening interaction of ketoprofen and methotrexate has been reported. Of four patients who experienced severe methotrexate toxicity resulting from concurrent ketoprofen administration, three ultimately died from methotrexate toxicity.[137]

Comparative Efficacy of Nonprescription Analgesics/Antipyretics

Aspirin versus Acetaminophen

Numerous controlled studies have demonstrated the equivalent analgesic efficacy of aspirin and acetaminophen on a milligram-for-milligram basis in various pain models, including postoperative pain, cancer pain, episiotomy pain, and oral surgery pain. Aspirin and acetaminophen have similar dose-response and time-effect curves and are equipotent and equianalgesic for the relief of most pain.[104,138] In a controlled study involving 269 patients, acetaminophen (1 g) and aspirin (650 mg) produced similar efficacy in the treatment of moderate to severe headache. The apparent superiority of aspirin on a milligram-for-milligram basis may be the result of an inflammatory component to the headache pain that would be unresponsive to acetaminophen.[139] However, acetaminophen (1 g) has been shown to be superior to aspirin (650 mg) in the control of pain secondary to dental surgery or episiotomy.[140,141] This difference is most probably due to the inequivalent doses, not superiority of acetaminophen as an analgesic.

Aspirin versus Ibuprofen

Ibuprofen has been shown to be at least as effective as aspirin in treating various types of pain, including dental extraction pain, dysmenorrhea, and episiotomy pain. A double-blind, single-dose study of postepisiotomy pain found ibuprofen (400 mg) to be more effective than aspirin (600mg).[142] Another double-blind, single-dose study that compared the efficacy of oral ibuprofen (100, 200, or 400 mg) with that of aspirin (650 mg) in treating moderate to severe pain after the extraction of impacted teeth estimated 100 mg of ibuprofen to be as effective as 650 mg of aspirin.[143] Single-dose analgesic studies often provide different outcomes than those of multiple dose studies, which characterize more accurately how the drugs are used clinically.

Controlled clinical trials have shown that ibuprofen is as effective as, but not superior to, aspirin in the treatment of rheumatoid arthritis. A double-blind, crossover, randomized study with 18 rheumatoid arthritic patients compared aspirin (3.6 g per day), ibuprofen (1.2 g per day), and placebo. Both aspirin and ibuprofen were superior to placebo for symptomatic control but were not different from each other. Both drugs reduced morning stiffness and improved grip strength to an equivalent degree. However, aspirin appeared superior to ibuprofen in the reduction of joint size.[144] It is noteworthy that the daily aspirin dose approached the maximum for safe use while the ibuprofen dose was relatively low.

Ibuprofen versus Acetaminophen

In postpartum patients with moderate to severe episiotomy pain, a single ibuprofen dose (400 mg) was found to be superior to acetaminophen (1 g) in producing analgesia. This superior analgesic effect was manifested by a more rapid onset and prolonged effect and by a greater area under the analgesic time-effect curve.[145] In reducing the severity and duration of migraine headache, ibuprofen 400 mg taken every 4 hours was significantly superior to acetaminophen 900 mg taken every 4 hours.[146] And in a multicenter study involving 706 patients, a single 400-mg oral dose of ibuprofen provided superior analgesia following oral surgery compared with 1 g of acetaminophen.[147] Numerous comparisons of oral ibuprofen and acetaminophen in various pain models suggest that 100–200 mg of ibuprofen is approximately equianalgesic to 650 mg of acetaminophen. Ibuprofen has a clear superiority, however, in pain conditions associated with inflammation.

A double-blind, randomized, parallel group study of 7.5 mg/kg ibuprofen syrup and 10 mg/kg acetaminophen syrup demonstrated no significant difference in temperature reduction over time among 154 children with infectious diseases that produced fever. However, the ibuprofen produced significantly greater temperature reductions during the first 4 hours of treatment.[149]

Naproxen versus Ibuprofen

One 200-mg nonprescription naproxen sodium tablet appears to be very similar in indications and efficacy to one 200-mg ibuprofen tablet. The onset of activity is similar between the two NSAIDs. Naproxen sodium's duration of action is somewhat longer than that of ibuprofen, but the clinical significance of that difference is not clear.[148] Naproxen sodium and ibuprofen are very similar pharmacologically and similar effects should be expected. Both are propionic acid derivative NSAIDs, and extensive clinical experience with these agents has demonstrated great similarity. Nonetheless, some RA patients do report better response to one NSAID than to another for reasons that are unclear. It is less probable, but still possible, that such differences will occur at the maximum nonprescription doses of an NSAID; these higher doses are often required by arthritic patients.

Combination Products Containing Caffeine or Antihistamines

Many nonprescription analgesics are available as combination products containing aspirin, ibuprofen, or acetaminophen as primary ingredients plus caffeine or an antihistamine. The adjuvant ingredients are claimed to enhance the analgesic efficacy of the product. There is some evidence to support the enhanced efficacy of such combination product. Other studies have failed to demonstrate a benefit from the adjuvants.

Thirty clinical studies involving more than 10,000 patients have been analyzed to assess the value of caffeine as an analgesic adjuvant. These studies were based on various pain models, including postpartum uterine cramping, episiotomy pain, oral surgery pain, and headache. Caffeine was combined with aspirin or acetaminophen alone and with aspirin-acetaminophen combinations. In 21 of 26 studies reviewed, the relative potency of the analgesic with caffeine was greater than that of the analgesic in the absence of caffeine. The pooled relative potency estimate for caffeine-containing analgesics is 1.41 (with a 95% confidence interval of 1.23–1.63), as compared with an analgesic potency of 1.0 for the analgesic in the absence of caffeine. This analysis suggests that to obtain the same amount of response from an analgesic without caffeine would require a dose approximately 40% greater than that required in the presence of caffeine.[150]

The adjuvant effect of caffeine has also been reported for ibuprofen analgesia. In a double-blind study, a single oral dose of ibuprofen (100 or 200 mg) with and without caffeine (100 mg) was evaluated for pain relief in 298 patients with postoperative pain after the surgical removal of impacted third molars (wisdom teeth). Subjects self-rated their pain relief hourly for 8 hours. Relative potency estimates indicated that the caffeine-ibuprofen combination was 2.4–2.8 times as potent as ibuprofen alone. The combination also had a more rapid onset and a longer duration of analgesic action than ibuprofen alone.[151]

In addition, enhanced analgesia has been reported for various antihistamine-analgesia combinations, including orphenadrine-acetaminophen and phenyltoloxamine-acetaminophen. The adjuvant effect of phenyltoloxamine citrate (60 mg) in combination with acetaminophen (650 mg) was evaluated in 200 female inpatients experiencing episiotomy pain using a self-rating pain relief scale. Compared with acetaminophen alone, the phenyltoloxamine-acetaminophen combination produced significantly greater pain relief at all points from 30 minutes through 6 hours after administering acetaminophen alone.[152] A growing body of clinical literature supports the enhancement of analgesia by the inclusion of either caffeine or an antihistamine with a nonprescription analgesic.

Finally, combination dosage forms containing a decongestant and either acetaminophen or an NSAID are also available. Such combinations appear logical for use in sinus headaches or other indications in which both analgesia and decongestion are needed.

Case Studies

Case 4–1

Patient Complaint/History

A mother presents to your pharmacy with her 5-year-old son BH, who has had a fever of 100°F (37.8°C) for the past 12 hours. She apparently used a rectal thermometer to take the infant's oral temperature; she described the thermometer bulb as being short and thick. Thinking BH may have the flu, the mother has selected Children's Motrin and Children's Tylenol to treat the fever. When questioned about treatment of previous fevers, the mother reveals that she has successfully treated BH's fevers with Tylenol. She now wonders whether the new product Children's Motrin would be better for treating the present fever and asks which product she should purchase. She also asks about the appropriate method to administer the medication.

BH has no history of drug allergies and is not presently receiving any medications; further, he has no symptoms other than fever.

Clinical Considerations/Strategies

The following considerations/strategies are provided to aid the reader in (1) determining whether treatment of the patient's condition with nonprescription medications is warranted, (2) selecting the appropriate nonprescription medication, and (3) developing a patient counseling strategy to ensure optimal therapeutic outcomes:

- Suggest a response to the mother's question about which product—Children's Tylenol versus Children's Motrin—is best for treating the infant's fever.
- Consider the appropriateness of a variety of nonprescription medications (acetaminophen, aspirin, ibuprofen, naproxen, ketoprofen) for treatment of fever in children.
- Identify precautions, adverse effects, and drug interactions, if any, associated with the use of the recommended nonprescription medication regimen.
- Assess the complications that could result from a high fever in children.
- Assess the appropriateness of using a rectal thermometer to take an oral temperature.
- Discuss the appropriate use of oral and rectal thermometers.
- Develop a patient education/counseling strategy that will:
  - Ensure that the mother understands the appropriate use of the recommended nonprescription medication regimen;
  - Ensure that the mother understands when to contact the physician about the infant's symptoms.

Case 4–2

Patient Complaint/History

JO, a 25-year-old female college student, presents to the pharmacist with complaints of a headache that she is unsure of how to treat. She has used ibuprofen, acetaminophen, or aspirin to relieve previous headaches; none of these medications caused adverse effects. When questioned about her symptoms, the patient describes a headache that may be related to sinus congestion; she feels pain in her forehead that intensifies in the morning. She has no other symptoms.

JO has been taking a decongestant/antihistamine (pseudoephedrine/chlorpheniramine) combination product, which has not relieved the sinus pain. To treat heartburn, she is also currently taking Pepcid AC 40 mg hs and antacids prn.

Clinical Considerations/Strategies

The following considerations/strategies are provided to aid the reader in (1) determining whether treatment of the patient's condition with nonprescription medications is warranted, (2) selecting the appropriate nonprescription medication, and (3) developing a patient counseling strategy to ensure optimal therapeutic outcomes:

- Suggest an appropriate treatment regimen for the patient's headache.
- Identify the precautions and adverse effects associated with the recommended nonprescription medication regimen.
- Identify and assess medications you would not recommend to manage this patient's symptoms because of the presence of an ulcer.
- Develop a patient education/counseling strategy that will:
  - Ensure that the patient understands the appropriate use of the recommended nonprescription medication regimen;
  - Ensure that the patient understands when to contact a physician about her symptoms.

Summary

In determining which medication to recommend, pharmacists should consider the condition being treated; the nature and origin of the complaint; the accompanying symptoms; concomitant history of asthma, urticaria, aspirin or NSAID intolerance, PUD, gout or hyperuricemia, clotting disorders, and concomitant hypertension, or diabetes. It is also important to review concurrent prescription and nonprescription medications. In addition to efficacy, factors to be considered in recommending a medication include formulation factors that may give the patient more prompt relief or fewer side effects, and the potential for adverse effects and drug interactions. Because of its minimal anti-inflammatory activity, acetaminophen may not be as effective as aspirin, ibuprofen, naproxen sodium, or ketoprofen for pain associated with inflammation. Because of decreased rectal bioavailability, larger acetaminophen and aspirin doses may be needed if the medication is administered rectally.

Acetaminophen, aspirin, ibuprofen, and naproxen sodium are the most commonly used nonprescription antipyretic agents available today. The recent introduction of ketoprofen offers an alternative NSAID that should be comparable. Under most circumstances, these drugs are equally effective and have similar times to onset of effect, similar times to peak antipyretic activity, and similar duration of action. These agents exert antipyretic activity by lowering the elevated hypothalamic set-point primarily through inhibiting prostaglandin synthesis and release at the thermoregulatory center. When concurrent anti-inflammatory effects are desired, an NSAID should be used because acetaminophen lacks significant anti-inflammatory activity. All of these antipyretic agents are also effective analgesics and contribute to the relief of numerous discomforting symptoms (eg, myalgia, arthralgia, headache) that often accompany fever.

Ongoing studies of new indications for, and toxicity from, nonprescription analgesic/antipyretic agents have suggested new potential uses and the need for some caution in self-medication with these drugs. Ongoing studies continue to suggest the usefulness of aspirin in prevention and treatment of primary vascular events (ie, for acute MIs and unstable angina).[153] Daily low-dose aspirin ingestion provided significant protection against MI, stroke, and death among high risk patients (ie, those with unstable angina, suspected MI, transient ischemic attacks). Daily or alternate day low-dose aspirin may also be beneficial for other at-risk patients, including those with stable angina or peripheral vascular disease or those undergoing vascular procedures. The effectiveness of antiplatelet therapy in patients at low risk has not yet been demonstrated. Aspirin has been associated with decreased risk of colorectal cancer in men.[154] Epidemiologic evidence has suggested that regular aspirin use may also reduce the risk of lung, colon, and breast cancers.[155] These associations are not definitive and do not apply equally to both sexes and across all ages. Additional studies are needed to confirm or refute these preliminary findings.

Adverse reactions to nonprescription analgesics continue to be a concern.[156] NSAID-induced GI bleeding and nephropathy, and acetaminophen-induced hepatic damage are real phenomena that mandate that patients use these medications wisely. Pharmacists can markedly improve the outcomes of nonprescription analgesic/antipyretic use by discussing risk factors with patients and recommending drugs with the best risk-to-benefit ratios for specific patients.

Nonprescription analgesic/antipyretic agents are effective medications that can greatly increase patient comfort when used correctly. Correct use of these drugs is more apt to occur if pharmacists educate patients on how to manage pain and fever, counsel patients on drug selection and use when these symptoms occur, and refer patients to physicians for more comprehensive evaluation and treatment when indicated. By monitoring patients who take these medications for therapeutic and toxic outcomes, pharmacists can make meaningful contributions to their patients' comfort and well-being and provide good pharmaceutical care.

References

1. Mersky H. Pain terms: a list with definitions and notes on usage, IASP Subcommittee on Taxonomy. *Pain*. 1979; 6: 249–53.
2. National Institutes of Health. *The Interagency Committee on New Therapies for Pain and Discomfort: Report to the White House*. US Department of Health Education and Welfare, Public Health Service; May 1979.
3. Pinkert TM. Report from the Interagency Committee on Pain and Analgesia: a Public Health Service initiative. *J Pain Symptom Manag*. 1986; 1: 174–7.
4. National Institutes of Health Consensus Development Conference. The integrated approach to the management of pain. *J Pain Symptom Manag*. 1987; 2: 35–44.
5. American Pain Society. *Principles of Analgesic Use in the Treatment of Acute Pain and Chronic Cancer Pain*. 3rd ed. Skokie, Ill: American Pain Society; 1992.

6. World Health Organization. *Cancer Pain Relief and Palliative Care.* Technical Report Series 804. Geneva: World Health Organization; 1990.
7. Russell SW. Interdisciplinary versus multidisciplinary pain management. *J Pharm Care Pain Symptom Control.* 1993; 1(2): 89–94.
8. Acute Pain Management Guideline Panel. *Acute Pain Management: Operative or Medical Procedures and Trauma; Clinical Practice Guideline.* AHCPR Pub No 92–0032. Rockville, Md: US Department of Health and Human Services, Agency for Health Care Policy and Research; 1992.
9. Jacox A et al. *Management of Cancer Pain. Clinical Practice Guideline.* AHCPR Pub No. 94–0592. Rockville, Md: Public Health Service, Agency for Health Care Policy and Research; 1994.
10. Martin JB. Headache. In: Wilson JD, Braunwald E, Isselbacher KJ, et al, eds. *Harrison's Principles of Internal Medicine.* 12th ed. New York: McGraw-Hill; 1991: 108–15.
11. Griggs RC. Pain, spasm, and cramps of muscle. In: Wilson JD, Braunwald E, Isselbacher KJ, et al, eds. *Harrison's Principles of Internal Medicine.* 12th ed. New York: McGraw-Hill; 1991: 173–6.
12. Gilliland BC. Relapsing polychondritis and miscellaneous arthritides. In: Wilson JD, Braunwald E, Isselbacher KJ, et al, eds. *Harrison's Principles of Internal Medicine.* 12th ed. New York: McGraw-Hill; 1991: 1484–90.
13. Brandt KD, Kovalov-St. John K. Osteoarthritis. In: Wilson JD, Braunwald E, Isselbacher KJ, et al, eds. *Harrison's Principles of Internal Medicine.* 12th ed. New York: McGraw-Hill; 1991: 1475–9.
14. Lipsky PE. Rheumatoid arthritis. In: Wilson JD, Braunwald E, Isselbacher KJ, et al, eds. *Harrison's Principles of Internal Medicine.* 12th ed. New York: McGraw-Hill; 1991: 1437–43.
15. Mackowiak PA, ed. *Fever: Basic Mechanisms and Management.* New York: Raven Press; 1991.
16. Adam D, Stankov G. Treatment of fever in childhood. *Eur J Pediatr.* 1994; 153: 394–402.
17. Hoekelman RA. The physical examination of infants and children. In: Bates B, ed. *A Guide to Physical Examination and History Taking.* 5th ed. Philadelphia: JB Lippincott; 1991: 136–7, 577.
18. Eskerud JR, Hoftvedt BO, Laerum E. Fever: management and self-medication. Results from a Norwegian population study. *Fam Pract.* 1991; 8: 148–53.
19. Stephenson LA, Kolka MA. Effect of gender, circadian period, and sleep loss on thermal responses during exercise. In: Pandolf KB, Sawka MN, Gonzalez RR, eds. *Human Performance Physiology and Environmental Medicine at Terrestrial Extremes.* Indianapolis: Benchmark Press; 1988: 267–304.
20. MacGregor RR. A year's experience with tuberculosis in a private urban teaching hospital in the postsanatorium era. *Am J Med.* 1975 Feb; 58: 221–8.
21. Wasserman M et al. Utility of fever, white blood cells, and differential count in predicting bacterial infections in the elderly. *J Am Geriatr Soc.* 1989 Jun; 37: 537–43.
22. Jones PC et al. Fever in the elderly: production of leukocyte pyrogen by monocytes from elderly persons. *Gerontology.* 1984 May/Jun; 30: 182–7.
23. Dale DC. The febrile patient. In: Wyngaarden JB, Smith LH, Bennett JC, eds. *Cecil Textbook of Medicine.* 19th ed. Philadelphia: WB Saunders; 1992: 1567–8.
24. Mackowiak PA, LeMaistre CF. Drug fever: a critical appraisal of conventional concepts. *Ann Intern Med.* 1987 May; 106: 728–33.
25. Patterson R, Anderson J. Allergic reactions to drugs and biologic agents. *JAMA.* 1982 Nov; 248: 2637–45.
26. Murray HW, Mann JJ. *Ann Intern Med.* 1975 Jul; 83: 84–5.
27. Lysy J, Oren R. Drug fever with a shift to the left. *DICP Ann Pharmacother.* 1990 Jul/Aug; 24: 782.
28. Guze BM, Baxter LR Jr. Neuroleptic malignant syndrome. *N Engl J Med.* 1985 Jul; 313: 163–6.
29. McCarthy PL, Dolan TF. Hyperpyrexia in children. *Am J Dis Child.* 1976 Aug; 130: 849–51.
30. Akerren Y. On hyperpyretic conditions during infancy and children: a clinical study of fever. *Acta Pediatr.* 1943; 31: 1–72.
31. Fishman MA. Febrile seizures: the treatment controversy. *J Pediatr.* 1979 Feb; 94: 177–84.
32. Verity CM, Butler NR, Golding J. Febrile convulsions in a national cohort followed up from birth: I. prevalence and recurrence in the first five years of life. *Br Med J.* 1985 May; 290: 1307–10.
33. Ellenberg JH, Nelson KB. Febrile seizures and later intellectual performance. *Arch Neurol.* 1978 Jan; 35: 71–2.
34. Verity CM, Butler NR, Golding J. Febrile convulsions in a national cohort followed up from birth: II. medical history and intellectual ability at 5 years of age. *Br Med J.* 1985 May; 290: 1311–5.
35. Farwell JR et al. Phenobarbital for febrile seizures—effects on intelligence and on seizure recurrence. *N Engl J Med.* 1990 Feb; 322: 364–9.
36. Newton RW. Randomized controlled trial of phenobarbital and valproate in febrile convulsions. *Arch Dis Child.* 1988 Oct; 63: 1189–91.
37. Erickson R. Oral temperature differences in relation to thermometer and technique. *Nurs Res.* 1980 May/Jun; 29: 157–64.
38. Shinozaki T et al. *Crit Care Med.* 1988; 16: 148.
39. Reisinger KS, Kao J, Grant DM. Inaccuracy of the Clinitemp skin thermometer. *Pediatrics.* 1979 Jul; 64: 4–6.
40. Lewit EM, Marshall CL, Salzer JE. An evaluation of a plastic strip thermometer. *JAMA.* 1982 Jan; 247: 321–5.
41. Siebenaler ME. Taking a baby's temperature: is it common knowledge? *Am J Maternal Child Nurs.* 1985 Jan/Feb; 10: 71.
42. Baker NC et al. The effect of type of thermometer and length of time inserted on oral temperature measurements of afebrile subjects. *Nurs Res.* 1984 Mar/Apr; 33: 109–11.
43. Tandberg D, Sklar D. Effect of tachypnea on the estimation of body temperature by an oral thermometer. *N Engl J Med.* 1983 Apr; 308: 945–6.
44. Greenbaum EI et al. Rectal thermometer–induced pneumoperitoneum in the newborn. *Pediatrics.* 1969 Oct; 44: 539–42.
45. Eoff MJ, Joyce B. Temperature measurements in children. *Am J Nurs.* 1981 May; 81: 1010–1.
46. Weisse ME et al. Axillary vs rectal temperatures in ambulatory and hospitalized children. *Pediatr Infect Dis J.* 1991 Jul; 10: 541–2.
47. Ogren JM. The inaccuracy of axillary temperatures measured with an electronic thermometer. *Am J Dis Child.* 1990 Jan; 144: 109–11.
48. Musher DM et al. Fever patterns: their lack of clinical significance. *Arch Intern Med.* 1979 Nov; 139: 1225–8.
49. Done AK. Treatment of fever in 1982: a review. *Am J Med.* 1983 Jun; 74(6A): 27–35.
50. Done AK. Uses and abuses of antipyretic therapy. *Pediatrics.* 1959 Apr; 23: 774–80.
51. Rodbard D. The role of regional body temperature in the pathogenesis of disease. *N Engl J Med.* 1981 Oct; 305: 808–14.
52. Roberts NJ Jr. Impact of temperature elevation on immunologic defenses. *Rev Infect Dis.* 1991 May/Jun; 13: 462–71.
53. Brunell PA. Contagion and varicella-zoster virus. *Pediatr Infect Dis.* 1982 Sep/Oct; 1: 304–7.
54. Stanley ED et al. Increased virus shedding with aspirin treatment of rhinovirus infection. *JAMA.* 1975 Mar; 231: 1248–51.
55. Steele RW et al. Evaluation of sponging and of oral antipyretic therapy to reduce fever. *J Pediatr.* 1970 Nov; 77: 824–9.
56. Whelton A. Renal effects of over-the-counter analgesics. *J Clin Pharmacol.* 1995; 35: 453–63.

57. Internal analgesic, antipyretic, and antirheumatic drug products for over-the-counter human use: tentative final monograph. *Federal Register.* 1988 Nov; 53: 46255–7.
58. Temple AR. Pathophysiology of aspirin overdosage toxicity, with implications for management. *Pediatrics.* 1978 Nov; 62(5 pt, suppl 2): 873–6.
59. Danel V, Henry JA, Glucksman E. Activated charcoal, emesis, and gastric lavage in aspirin overdose. *Br Med J.* 1988 May; 1: 1507.
60. Curtis RA, Barone J, Giacona N. Efficacy of ipecac and activated charcoal/cathartic: prevention of salicylate absorption in simulated overdose. *Arch Intern Med.* 1984 Jan; 144: 48–52.
61. Piletta P, Porchet HC, Dayer P. Central analgesic effect of acetaminophen but not of aspirin. *Clin Pharmacol Ther.* 1991 Apr; 49: 350–4.
62. Mason WD. Kinetics of aspirin absorption following oral administration of six aqueous solutions with different buffer capacities. *J Pharm Sci.* 1984 Sep; 73: 1258–61.
63. Kanto J et al. Bioavailability of rectal aspirin in neurosurgical patients. *Acta Anaesthesiol Scand.* 1981 Feb; 25: 25–6.
64. Lanza FL. Endoscopic studies of gastric and duodenal injury after the use of ibuprofen, aspirin, and other nonsteroidal anti-inflammatory agents. *Am J Med.* 1984 Jul; 77(suppl 1A): 19–24.
65. Hoftiezer JW et al. Comparison of the effects of regular and enteric-coated aspirin on the gastroduodenal mucosa of man. *Lancet.* 1980 Sep; 2(8195, pt 1): 609–12.
66. Hawthorne AB et al. Aspirin-induced gastric mucosal damage: prevention by enteric-coating and relation to prostaglandin synthesis. *Br J Clin Pharmacol.* 1991 Jul; 32: 77–83.
67. Lanza FL, Royer GL, Nelson RS. Endoscopic evaluation of the effects of aspirin and enteric-coated aspirin on gastric and duodenal mucosa. *N Engl J Med.* 1980 Jul; 303: 136–8.
68. Hollister LE. Measuring Measurin: problems of oral prolonged-action medications. *Clin Pharmacol Ther.* 1972 Jan–Feb; 13: 1–5.
69. Lobeck F, Spigiel RW. Bioavailability of sustained-release aspirin preparations. *Clin Pharm.* 1986 Mar; 5: 236–8.
70. Brandslund I, Rask H, Klitgaard NA. Gastrointestinal blood loss caused by controlled-release and conventional acetylsalicylic acid tablets. *Scand J Rheumatol.* 1979; 8: 209–13.
71. Miller RR. Deafness due to plain and long-acting aspirin tablets. *J Clin Pharmacol.* 1978 Oct; 18: 468–71.
72. Mielke CH et al. Hemostasis, antipyretics, and mild analgesics: acetaminophen vs aspirin. *JAMA.* 1976 Feb; 235: 613–6.
73. Estes D, Kaplan K. Lack of platelet effect with the aspirin analog, salsalate. *Arthritis Rheum.* 1980; 23: 1301–7.
74. Danesh BJ et al. Therapeutic potential of choline magnesium trisalicylate as an alternative to aspirin for patients with bleeding tendency. *Scottish Med J.* 1987; 32: 167–8.
75. Ivey KJ. Mechanisms of nonsteroidal anti-inflammatory drug-induced gastric damage. *Am J Med.* 1988 Feb; 84(suppl 2A): 41–8.
76. Levy M. Aspirin use in patients with major upper gastrointestinal bleeding and peptic ulcer disease: a report from the Boston Collaborative Drug Surveillance Program, Boston University Medical Center. *N Engl J Med.* 1974 May; 290: 1158–62.
77. Needham CD et al. Aspirin and alcohol in gastrointestinal haemorrhage. *Gut.* 1971 Oct; 12: 819–21.
78. Lee TH. Mechanism of aspirin sensitivity. *Am Rev Resp Dis.* 1992; 1456(suppl): S34–S36.
79. Settipane GA. Aspirin and allergic diseases: a review. *Am J Med.* 1983 Jun; 74(6A): 102–9.
80. Savitsky ME, Wiens JA. Cross-reactivity in aspirin-sensitive patients. *Drug Intell Clin Pharm.* 1987 Apr; 21: 338–9.
81. Samter M, Beers RF Jr. Intolerance to aspirin: clinical studies and consideration of its pathogenesis. *Ann Intern Med.* 1968 May; 68: 975–83.
82. Levy G, Procknal JA, Garrettson LK. Distribution of salicylate between neonatal and maternal serum at diffusion equilibrium. *Clin Pharmacol Ther.* 1975 Aug; 18: 210–4.
83. Levy G, Garrettson LK. Kinetics of salicylate elimination by newborn infants of mothers who ingested aspirin before delivery. *Pediatrics.* 1974 Feb; 53: 201–10.
84. Briggs GG, Freeman RK, Yaffe SJ. *Drugs in Pregnancy and Lactation.* 3rd ed. Baltimore: Williams and Wilkins: 1990.
85. Committee on Drugs, American Academy of Pediatrics. The transfer of drugs and chemicals into human breast milk. *Pediatr.* 1994; 93: 137–50.
86. Isselbacher KJ, Podolsky DK. Infiltrative and metabolic diseases affecting the liver. In: Wilson JD, Braunwald E, Isselbacher KJ, et al, eds. *Harrison's Principles of Internal Medicine.* 12th ed. New York: McGraw-Hill; 1991: 1352–5.
87. Rosefsky JB. Ibuprofen safety. *Pediatrics.* 1992; 89: 166–7. Letter.
88. *Federal Register.* 1993; 58(201): 14228
89. Hurwitz ES et al. Public Health Service study of Reye's syndrome and medications: report of the main study. *JAMA.* 1987 Apr; 257: 1905–11.
90. Pinsky PF et al. Reye's syndrome and aspirin: evidence for a dose-response effect. *JAMA.* 1988 Aug; 260: 657–61.
91. Forsyth BW et al. New epidemiologic evidence confirming that bias does not explain the aspirin/Reye's syndrome association. *JAMA.* 1989 May; 261: 2517–24.
92. Johnson AF, Siedemann P, Day RV. NSAID-related adverse drug interactions with clinical relevance. *Int J Clin Pharmacol* Ther. 1994; 32: 509–32.
93. Goulden KJ et al. Clinical valproate toxicity induced by acetylsalicylic acid. *Neurology.* 1987 Aug; 37: 1392–4.
94. Roine R et al. Aspirin increases blood alcohol concentrations in humans after ingestion of ethanol. *JAMA.* 1990 Nov; 264: 2406–8.
95. *Federal Register.* 1993; 58(201): 14224.
96. Wilson JT et al. Efficacy, disposition and pharmacodynamics of aspirin, acetaminophen and choline salicylate in young febrile children. *Ther Drug Monit.* 1982; 4: 147–80.
97. Stern SB. Clinical evaluation of the analgesic effect of magnesium salicylate. *Med Times.* 1967 Oct; 95: 1072–6.
98. Preston SJ et al. Comparative analgesic and anti-inflammatory properties of sodium salicylate and acetylsalicylic acid (aspirin) in rheumatoid arthritis. *Br J Clin Pharmacol.* 1989 May; 27: 607–11.
99. McEvoy GK, ed. *AHFS Drug Information.* 1995 ed. Bethesda, Md: American Society of Hospital Pharmacists, Inc; 1995.
100. Sutor A, Bowie EJ, Owen CA. Effect of aspirin, sodium salicylate, and acetaminophen on bleeding. *Mayo Clin Proc.* 1971 Mar; 46: 178–81.
101. Binder R, Durocher J, Mielke H. Treatment of pain in hemophilia: effect of drugs on bleeding time. *Am J Dis Child.* 1974 Mar; 127: 371–3.
102. Stuart JJ, Pisko EJ. Choline magnesium trisalicylate does not impair platelet aggregation. *Pharmatherapeutica.* 1981; 2: 547–51.
103. Roth SH. Salicylates revisited: are they still the hallmark of anti-inflammatory therapy? *Drugs.* 1988 Jul; 36: 1–6.
104. Mehlisch DR. Review of the comparative analgesic efficacy of salicylates, acetaminophen, and pyrazolones. *Am J Med.* 1983 Nov; 75(suppl 5A): 47–52.
105. Litowitz TL, Clark LR, Soloway RA. 1993 Annual Report of the American Association of Poison Control Centers Toxic Exposure Surveillance System. *Am J Emerg Med.* 1994; 12: 546–8.
106. Veltri JC, Rollins DE. A comparison of the frequency and severity of poisoning cases for ingestion of acetaminophen, aspirin, and ibuprofen. *Am J Emerg Med.* 1988 Mar; 6: 104–7.
107. Ellenhorn MJ, Barceloux DG. *Medical Toxicology.* New York: Elsevier; 1988.

108. Ekins BR et al. The effect of activated charcoal on *N*-acetylcysteine absorption in normal subjects. *Am J Emerg Med.* 1987 Nov; 5: 483–7.
109. Gribetz B, Conley SA. Underdosing of acetaminophen by parents. *Pediatr.* 1987; 80: 630–3.
110. Clissold SP. Paracetamol and phenacetin. *Drugs.* 1986; 32(suppl 4): 46–59.
111. Whitcomb DC, Block GD. Association of acetaminophen hepatotoxicity with fasting and alcohol use. *JAMA.* 1994; 272: 1845–50.
112. Richman DD et al. The toxicity of azidothymidine (AZT) in the treatment of patients with AIDS and AIDS-related complex: a double-blind, placebo-controlled trial. *N Engl J Med.* 1987 Jul; 317: 192–7.
113. Steffe EM et al. The effect of acetaminophen on zidovudine metabolism in HIV-infected patients. *J Acquir Immune Defic Syn.* 1990; 3(7): 691–4.
114. Sattler FR et al. Acetaminophen does not impair clearance of zidovudine. *Ann Intern Med.* 1991 Jun; 114: 937–40.
115. Miller RR. Evaluation of the analgesic efficacy of ibuprofen. *Pharmacotherapy.* 1981 Jul–Aug; 1: 21–7.
116. Chan WY. Prostaglandins and nonsteroidal antiinflammatory drugs in dysmenorrhea. *Ann Rev Pharmacol Toxicol.* 1983; 23: 131–49.
117. McElwee NE et al. A prospective, population-based study of acute ibuprofen overdose: complications are rare and routine serum levels not warranted. *Ann Emerg Med.* 1990 Jun; 19: 657–62.
118. Schmid FR, Culic DD. Antiinflammatory drugs and gastrointestinal bleeding: a comparison of aspirin and ibuprofen. *J Clin Pharmacol.* 1976 Aug–Sep; 16: 418–25.
119. Caruso I, Bianchi, Porro G. Gastroscopic evaluation of anti-inflammatory agents. *Br Med J.* 1980 Jan; 280: 75–8.
120. Royer GL, Seckman CE, Welshman IR. Safety profile: fifteen years of clinical experience with ibuprofen. *Am J Med.* 1984 Jul; 77(1A): 25–34.
121. Deykin D, Janson P, McMahon L. Ethanol potentation of aspirin-induced prolongation of the bleeding time. *N Engl J Med.* 1982 Apr; 306: 852–4.
122. Penner JA, Albrecht PH. Lack of interaction between ibuprofen and warfarin. *Curr Ther Res Clin Exp.* 1975 Dec; 18: 862–71.
123. Schooley RT, Wagley PF, Lietman PS. Edema associated with ibuprofen therapy. *JAMA.* 1977 Apr; 237: 1716–7.
124. Ciabattoni G et al. Effects of sulindac and ibuprofen in patients with chronic glomerular disease. *N Engl J Med.* 1984 Feb; 310: 279–83.
125. Blackshear JL, Davidman M, Stillman MT. Identification of risk for renal insufficiency from nonsteroidal anti-inflammatory drugs. *Arch Intern Med.* 1983 Jun; 143: 1130-4.
126. Lesko SM, Mitchell AM. An assessment of the safety of pediatric ibuprofen. *JAMA.* 1995; 273: 929–33.
127. Radack KL, Deck CC, Bloomfield SS. Ibuprofen interferes with the efficacy of antihypertensive drugs: a randomized, double-blind, placebo-controlled trial of ibuprofen compared with acetaminophen. *Ann Intern Med.* 1987 Nov; 107: 628–35.
128. Ragheb M. Ibuprofen can increase serum lithium level in lithium-treated patients. *J Clin Psychiatry.* 1987 Apr; 48: 161–3.
129. Kristoff CA et al. Effect of ibuprofen on lithium plasma and red blood cell concentrations. *Clin Pharm.* 1986 Jan; 5: 51–5.
130. Ragheb M. The clinical significance of lithium–nonsteroidal anti-inflammatory drug interactions. *J Clin Psychopharmacol.* 1990 Oct; 10: 350–4.
131. Cassano WF. Serious methotrexate toxicity caused by interaction with ibuprofen. *Am J Pediatr Hematol Oncol.* 1989 Winter; 11: 481–2.
132. Martinez R, Smith D, Frankel L. Sever metabolic acidoses after acute naproxen sodium ingestion. *Ann Emerg Med.* 1989; 18: 129–31.
133. Wong DG et al. Effect of nonsteroidal antiinflammatory drugs on control of hypertension by beta-blockers and diuretics. *Lancet.* 1986; 1: 997.
134. Schuna AA et al. Lack of interaction between sulindac or naproxen and propranolol in hypertensive patients. *J Clin Pharmacol.* 1989; 29: 524.
135. Davis A et al. Interactions between non-steroidal antiinflammatory drugs and antihypertensives and diuretics. *Aust N Z J Med.* 1986; 16: 537–46.
136. Dupuis LL et al. *J Rheumatol.* 1990; 17: 1469.
137. Thyss A et al. Clinical and pharmacokinetic evidence of a life-threatening interaction between methotrexate and ketoprofen. *Lancet.* 1986 Feb; 1: 256–8.
138. Cooper SA. Comparative analgesic efficacies of aspirin and acetaminophen. *Arch Intern Med.* 1981 Feb; 141: 282–5.
139. Peters BH, Fraim CJ, Masel BE. Comparison of 650 mg aspirin and 1,000 mg acetaminophen with each other, and with placebo in moderately severe headache. *Am J Med.* 1983 Jun; 74(6A): 36–42.
140. Mehlisch DR, Frakes LA. A controlled comparative evaluation of acetaminophen and aspirin in the treatment of postoperative pain. *Clin Ther.* 1984; 7: 89–97.
141. Hopkinson JH III et al. Acetaminophen (500 mg) versus acetaminophen (325 mg) for the relief of pain in episiotomy patients. *Curr Ther Res.* 1974 Mar; 16: 194–200.
142. Sunshine A et al. Ibuprofen, zomepirac, aspirin, and placebo in the relief of postepisiotomy pain. *Clin Pharmacol Ther.* 1983 Aug; 34: 254–8.
143. Jain AK et al. Analgesic efficacy of low-dose ibuprofen in dental extraction pain. *Pharmacotherapy.* 1986 Nov-Dec; 6: 318–22.
144. Huskisson EC et al. A new look at ibuprofen. *Rheumatol Phys Med.* 1970; 10(suppl 10): 88–98.
145. Schachtel BP, Thoden WR, Baybutt RI. Ibuprofen and acetaminophen in the relief of postpartum episiotomy pain. *J Clin Pharmacol.* 1989 Jun; 29: 550–3.
146. Pearce I, Frank GJ, Pearce JM. Ibuprofen compared with paracetamol in migraine. *Practitioner.* 1983 Mar; 227: 465–7.
147. Mehlisch DR et al. Multicenter clinical trial of ibuprofen and acetaminophen in the treatment of postoperative dental pain. *J Am Dent Assoc.* 1990 Aug; 121: 257–63.
148. Anonymous. *Am J Hosp Pharm.* 1994; 51: 588.
149. Autret L et al. Comparative efficacy and tolerance of ibuprofen syrup and acetaminophen syrup in children with pyrexia associated with infectious diseases and treated with antibiotics. *Eur J Clin Pharmacol.* 1994; 46: 197–201.
150. Laska EM et al. Caffeine as an analgesic adjuvant. *JAMA.* 1984 Apr; 251: 1711–8.
151. Forbes JA et al. Effect of caffeine on ibuprofen analgesia in postoperative oral surgery pain. *Clin Pharmacol Ther.* 1991 Jun; 49: 674–84.
152. Sunshine A et al. Augmentation of acetaminophen analgesia by the antihistamine phenyltoloxamine. *JClin Pharmacol.* 1989 Jul; 29: 660–4.
153. Antiplatelet trialists collaboration. Collaborative overview of randomized trials of antiplatelet therapy: I. prevention of death, myocardial infarction, and stroke by prolonged antiplatelet therapy in various categories of patients. *Br Med J.* 1994; 308: 81–106.
154. Giovannucci E et al. Aspirin use and the risk of colorectal cancer and adenoma in male health professionals. *Ann Intern Med.* 1994; 121: 241–6.
155. Schreinemachers DM, Everson RB. Aspirin use and lung, colon, and breast cancer incidence in a prospective study. *Epidemiology.* 1994; 5(2): 138–46.
156. Strom BL. Adverse reactions to over-the-counter analgesics taken for therapeutic purposes. *JAMA.* 1994; 272: 1866–7.

CHAPTER 5

External Analgesic Products

Arthur I. Jacknowitz

Questions to ask in patient assessment and counseling

- *How long has the pain been present? How did it first appear? How often does it occur? Have you experienced it before?*
- *Can you relate the pain to any specific event, such as an accident, overwork, or a sports-related activity?*
- *Is the pain in a joint or in the muscle? If the pain is in a joint, is the joint red, swollen, or warm to the touch?*
- *Is the pain worse when you get up in the morning, and does it tend to subside as the day goes on?*
- *Does the pain move to other areas of the body?*
- *Has any specific treatment been helpful in alleviating the pain?*
- *Do you have a fever or any flu symptoms?*

Painful injuries as a result of our active lifestyles and the prevalence of arthritis have led to the increased use of external analgesics. In 1990, external analgesics were the undisputed nonprescription drug growth leader, with sales increasing by more than 25% over the previous year. No other category came close.[1] In 1994, sales continued to increase, albeit not so dramatically, jumping by more than 8% over sales in the previous year. In fact, this category of nonprescription drugs is expected to account for estimated increases of 11% annually from 1995 to 1998, resulting in total sales of almost $400 million by that latter year.[2]

Approximately 40 million Americans currently suffer from all forms of arthritis, and the Centers for Disease Control and Prevention (CDC) expects that number to increase by 50% by the year 2020. In fact, 40% of adults over the age of 50 are regular users of external pain relievers, and arthritis patients account for more than 75% of total usage. External analgesics are also popular among younger, more active people. However, the marketing focus of these agents has shifted from sports-induced to arthritis pain since 30% of all nonprescription analgesics are used to alleviate pain and inflammation accompanying the latter disorder.[3]

Mechanism of Muscular Pain Perception

Pain is one of the most common ailments for which people seek advice and help from health care providers. But although everyone is familiar with the sensation of pain, people experience it differently. Nevertheless, the International Association for the Study of Pain developed a definition of it nearly 20 years ago that is accepted by pain clinicians and researchers today; according to this definition, pain is an "unpleasant sensory and emotional experience associated with actual or potential tissue damage or described in terms of such damage."[4] It is a multidimensional experience that involves both a discriminative capacity and an interpretation of a stimulus in terms of present and past encounters.

More than thirty years ago, the gate-control theory of pain was proposed to integrate physiologic components of pain.[5] It postulated that a neural mechanism in the spinal cord acts like a gate that can control the transmission of pain impulses to the brain. According to this theory, pain signals are carried from specialized pain receptors to the spinal cord via two types of nerve fibers: small, unmyelinated fibers (type C fibers) and large, myelin-containing nerve cells (type A delta fibers) (Figure 1). The small fibers conduct impulses slowly and are associated with dull, aching, and lingering pain. The large fibers are linked with immediate pain, characterized as sharp and precise with a pricking sensation.

Small and large nerve fiber impulses can oppose each other. In fact, mild stimulation of large fibers can attenuate pain felt from the activation of small fibers, a finding that helps to explain the efficacy of topical counterirritants. An example is the effect of applying an external analgesic (stimulating large fibers) to diminish the pain caused by a sports-related knee injury (activating small fibers).

Pain receptors are present in most areas of the body, including skeletal muscles. Stimuli activating these receptors cause sensory impulses to be transmitted via the nerve fibers to the brain, which may integrate and evaluate the signals as a perception of pain.[6]

Because of its pendulous structure, the shoulder area is subject to continuous gravitational pull and therefore endures more stress and strain than any other articulation of the body. The prehensile grasp, which raised humans above our ancestors, has resulted in the development of a shoulder girdle that sacrifices stability for mobility and is a major cause of muscular pain.[7] Although painful conditions affecting the shoulder are more prevalent in elderly persons, they often occur in ath-

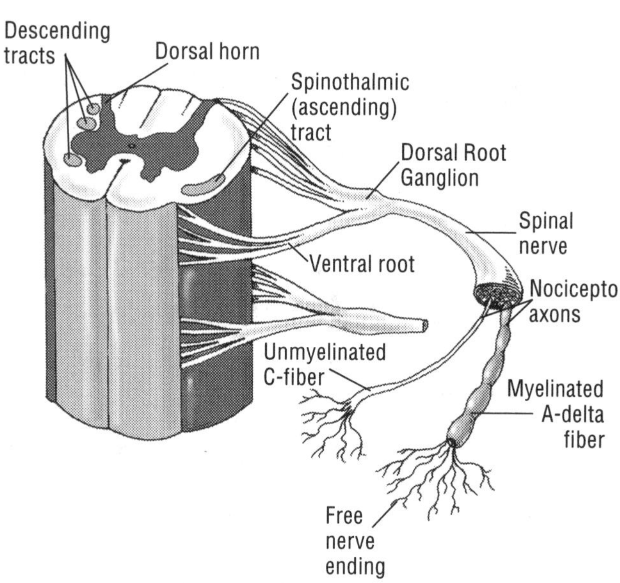

FIGURE 1 Afferent "pain" fiber input into the spinal cord. These specialized sets of afferent units carry pain signals to the spinal cord via either small, unmyelinated fibers (type C fibers) or large, myelin-containing nerve cells (type A delta fibers). Adapted with permission from *Hosp Formul.* 1985 Sep; 20: 973.

letes[8] and in those engaged in certain occupations in which the arms are used vigorously and repetitively.[9]

Types of Muscular Pain

Overuse Injuries

Skeletal muscle pain is quite common, especially among persons who are not accustomed to strenuous exercise. Motivated by a heightened awareness of the beneficial effects of exercise, more Americans than ever are exercising regularly, making exercise-induced injuries more common. Such injuries are caused by equal and opposite reactions, which result either in macrotrauma or microtrauma.[10] Macrotrauma, a sudden catastrophic injury, occurs when an equal and opposite force exceeds the inherent tensile strength of a body structure such as a bone, ligament, muscle, or tendon, causing the structure to collapse. In contrast, microtrauma is a microscopic subclinical injury that results from repeated activity that, over a period of time, overwhelms the tissue's ability to repair itself. By definition, this pain and dysfunction is described as "overuse syndrome" and is most often encountered in the form of tendinitis.[11] Repetitive microtrauma from exercise-related activities can also break down bursae, cartilage, bone, and nerve.

Tendinitis

Tendinitis, resulting from a strain or injury of tendons, is often seen at times of maximum physical effort, such as during athletic competition (Figure 2). There are three distinct pathologic phases.[12] The first phase includes the development of the acute inflammatory response. As inflammation continues and remains untreated, excessive proliferation of connective tissue occurs. Microscopically, the tissue changes in this second phase are characterized by the development of young, vascular elements with fibroblastic growth. In the third phase, persistent and chronic inflammation results in further overgrowth of connective tissue plus tendon degeneration, which may lead to rupture. The pathologic changes occurring in each of the three phases appear to be related primarily to repetitive intrinsic tension overload in the muscle–tendon unit.

Although tendinitis in the shoulder area is a major cause of pain, athletes often suffer injury of tendons in other areas of the body. In fact, it has been said that Achilles tendinitis is the most common injury in sports.[11] (See Chapter 34, "Foot Care Products.") Other examples of this common injury include biceps tendinitis, which occurs in the throwing athlete such as a football quarterback or baseball pitcher; patellar tendinitis, which occurs in the volleyball and basketball player; and iliotibial-band tendinitis, which occurs in the runner. In a recent prospective study of sports injuries in elderly athletes (those over 60 years of age),[13] the investigators found that shoulder as well as Achilles tendon and calf complaints were significantly more common in elderly athletes than in younger ones. In addition, although both groups sustained injuries primarily to the knee joint, young athletes suffered this injury more often than elderly ones. Most of the injuries in the elderly (70%) were overuse injuries, but these accounted for less than half of the injuries (41%) in the young.[13]

Many factors contribute to producing an overuse injury such as tendinitis. In industry, these factors include poorly designed equipment, awkward working positions, lack of job variation, long work hours, inadequate rest breaks, and bonuses for high work rates and

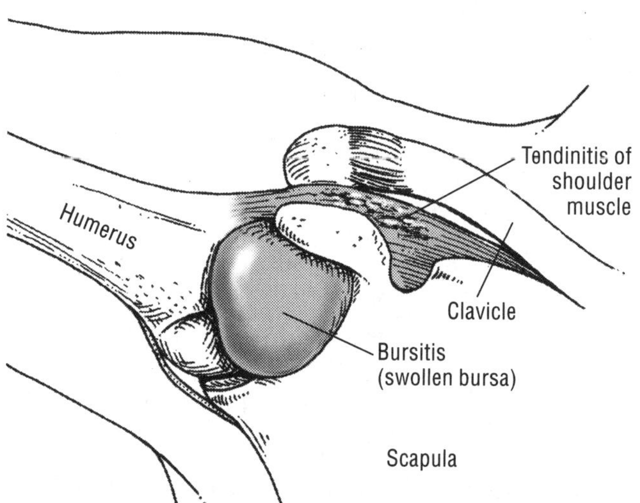

FIGURE 2 Bursitis and tendinitis. These two painful injuries, which often result from overuse of a joint or tendon, can cause inflammation, swelling, and tenderness in the injured area. Adapted with permission from *US Pharm.* 1995 Jan; 20 (1).

overtime.[14] In athletics, contributing factors can include the athlete's age, poor technique, and improper conditioning; exercise of prolonged intensity or duration; and poorly designed equipment for specific activities (such as poor cushioning of athletic shoes).[10]

As of October 1994, the Food and Drug Administration (FDA) had received reports of 25 cases of tendon rupture (22 of them occurring outside the United States) associated with fluoroquinolone antibiotics.[15] The ruptures occurred 2 days to 6 weeks after the initiation of therapy. Of the 25 patients, 16 had relevant risk factors, including concomitant corticosteroid therapy, advanced age, and chronic renal dialysis. On the basis of these reports, the FDA updated the labeling for all commercially available fluoroquinolones to incorporate a warning about the possibility of tendon rupture. This includes a recommendation to discontinue treatment with these antibiotics at the first sign of tendon pain or inflammation and to refrain from exercise until the diagnosis of tendinitis can be excluded.

Bursitis

Bursae are sacs formed by two layers of synovial tissue that are located at sites of friction between tendon and bone or skin and bone. The bursae enable the tendons and muscles to move over bony prominences. With overuse, repetitive trauma from either friction of the overlying tendon or external pressure may cause the bursa to become inflamed, with resultant fluid buildup in the bursal wall. This condition, termed *bursitis*, is a common cause of localized pain, tenderness, and swelling, which is worsened by any movement of the structure adjacent to the bursa (Figure 2). It may be an acute pain due to either macro- or microtrauma, or it may be chronic pain, in which case an infectious cause should be suspected. Infection or trauma can be documented by appropriate studies of aspirated fluid. It should be noted, however, that most cases of bursitis are due to overuse. This is particularly true in sports that involve repetitive overhead throwing motions, such as baseball, swimming, gymnastics, skiing, and weight lifting. Runners commonly are afflicted with bursitis of the knees, hips, ankles, and feet.[16]

Bursitis is a common cause of joint pain and often results in limited motion of adjacent joints, especially when the inflamed bursa is superficial and obvious redness and swelling are present. Symptoms of bursitis that mimic arthritic pain can be distinguished by a physical examination. For instance, direct pressure over the joint capsule of the shoulder does not cause pain in bursitis although it does in arthritis. (See Chapter 4, "Internal Analgesic and Antipyretic Products.")

Occupational Repetition Strain

Another overuse injury, described as the new industrial epidemic,[17] involves occupational repetition strain injuries. These muscle and tendon injuries of the upper limbs, shoulder girdle, and neck are caused by an overload on particular muscles due to awkward working postures or repeated use; the overload causes pain, fatigue, and a decline in work performance. Assembly line workers and typists are likely candidates for this type of strain injury, which has become a major cause of injury and disability in industry with considerable social and economic consequences.[18]

While such injuries are traditionally linked to blue-collar workers, a recent warning indicated that filling 100 prescriptions a day qualifies as repetitive motion and that pharmacists and others who work at computer keyboards are at risk for developing muscle and tendon injuries.[19] It is of interest that in 1993, a British court ruled that repetitive strain injury does not exist as a separate medical condition. Rather than referring to this disorder as an injury, the court described it as a pain syndrome occurring in the workplace. However, the association of that pain with a specific type of work has yet to be clearly defined and has led to a strongly worded editorial advising employers and employees to pay attention to workplace factors, such as stress and appropriate work breaks, to reduce the incidence of this syndrome.[20] In the United States, although repetitive strain injury claims have been touted as the "asbestos of the 90's," litigation against major corporations such as IBM has been stalled by a vigorous defense involving the work ethic of both employer and employee rather than the equipment.[21]

Soft Tissue Injury

Sprain, *bruise*, and *strain*—terms used to characterize injury to soft tissue—are defined as follows[22]:

- A sprain is a partial or complete rupture of a ligament.
- A bruise is a rupture of tissue resulting in a hematoma.
- A strain is a partial tear of muscles.

Sprains occur as a result of a joint being forced beyond its normal range of motion (eg, a hyperextended knee) or forced in a plane through which little or no motion actually exists (eg, a lateral ankle sprain). The abnormal forces producing the sprain can be rapid, as exemplified by a clipping injury in football, or slow, as observed with a slow, twisting fall in skiing. Although ligaments behave differently, depending on how quickly or slowly they are stretched, either mechanism can induce injury. Most strains, on the other hand, occur during forceful muscle action. The injury might occur soon after an activity has begun, such as coming out of the blocks when a race has just started, or with an interruption of some motion, such as momentarily losing one's footing on a slippery surface.[23] When these injuries occur, the muscles become sore and painful, and movement becomes difficult.

Arthritis

Arthritic pain may be caused by rheumatoid arthritis, which may involve almost all peripheral joints, tendons, bursae, and the cervical spine; or by osteoarthritis, which involves degeneration of cartilage with secondary changes in joints. Endogenous neuropeptides have been implicated in the pathogenesis of both rheumatoid arthritis and osteoarthritis and can enhance cartilage destruction.[24] In experimental studies in animals, a direct correlation has been found between the release of the neurotransmitter substance P by specific joints and the degree of inflammation in those joints. In addition, substance P activates rheumatoid synovial cells to produce prostaglandins and metalloproteinases.[25] Although both types of rheumatic disorders are chronic systemic diseases, local treatment of painful joints coupled with rest may give temporary symptomatic relief.

Lower Back Pain

Just as the prehensile grasp has imposed a stress upon the shoulder girdles of humans, so has erect posture predisposed the lower spine to the painful twinge of an aching back. At least 70% of the population experiences lower back pain at some time in their lives. Lower back pain rivals the common cold as the leading cause of absenteeism from work.[26] However, unlike the overuse injuries described previously, this regional musculoskeletal disorder is due primarily to a sedentary lifestyle (particularly one disrupted by bursts of activity), as well as to poor posture, improper shoes, excess body weight, poor mattresses and sleeping posture, and improper technique in lifting heavy objects. Thus, back pain is primarily a disease of living. Although most victims recover within a few days to a few weeks with conservative treatment, lower back pain is significantly likely to recur if the initial episode of pain is severe; advancing age also increases the risk of recurrence.

In addition to injuries, the causes of backache include:

- Congenital anomalies;
- Osteoarthritis;
- Spinal tuberculosis;
- Referred pain from diseased kidneys, pancreas, liver, or prostate.

Emotional factors, including tension, anxiety, repressed anger, and other manifestations of "psychosocial prestress," have also been postulated to correlate with the occurrence of lower back pain, but a comprehensive review of the literature could not confirm a relationship between lower back pain and temperament.[27]

Other Types of Muscular Pain

Acute, temporary stiffness and muscle pain can also result from cold, dampness, rapid temperature changes, and air currents. In some cases, visceral stimuli resulting from cardiovascular disease (such as angina pectoris) or gastrointestinal complaints (such as disorders of the gallbladder and esophagus) are felt as referred pain in the skeletal muscles of the shoulder. These episodes tend to be sudden in onset but are self-limiting (ie, the condition will resolve with or without treatment in a short time). Elimination of the cause and/or symptomatic treatment generally provides relief.[6]

Patient Assessment

To assess the patient's condition accurately before recommending a nonprescription counterirritant preparation, the pharmacist should ask the patient the following questions:

- How long has the pain been apparent? What kind of pain is it? Is it debilitating? Is it recurrent? Conditions amenable to nonprescription treatment are self-limiting. Pain that has been apparent for longer than 7 days may indicate a more serious underlying condition. Furthermore, prolonged use of external analgesics can increase the sensitivity to and decrease the effectiveness of these products.[28] Patients experiencing prolonged pain should be evaluated by a physician.
- Is there any apparent cause for the pain? Often, muscular or joint pain can be brought on by simple overexertion, such as unaccustomed exercise or other physical activity; such pain is a valid indication for nonprescription external analgesics.
- Can the patient locate and describe the pain? If so, and if the pain is mild, it may be appropriate to recommend a nonprescription product. However, if the patient has difficulty locating the origin of the pain, it may be referred pain. For example, pain in the lumbar area may be referred from pelvic viscera and may be an early manifestation of disease in these organs. Nor should nonprescription treatment be recommended if the pain is severe.
- If the pain is in a joint, is the joint red, swollen, warm, and tender to the touch? If so, there may be a fracture or rupture of ligaments or tendons, and/or arthritic involvement. Nonprescription products used in this condition would delay an accurate diagnosis.
- Has the patient been diagnosed by a physician as having any type of arthritic condition? If so, and if the patient is under medical supervision for such a condition, it may be appropriate to recommend only a counterirritant preparation as adjunctive treatment. The rationale for this therapy is that the topical analgesic helps the patient over intermittent painful episodes, thus reducing his or her intake of oral analgesics, which may pose a greater risk of adverse reactions.
- Is the patient taking any other prescription or nonprescription medication? Knowledge of the patient's medication history enables the pharmacist to recommend an appropriate external analgesic while minimizing the risk of both duplication of therapy and drug-drug interactions.

Topical analgesics are very inexpensive when compared with many oral antiarthritic agents. Therefore, a positive economic factor may also exist.

Arthritic conditions should not be self-diagnosed or self-treated. (See Chapter 4, "Internal Analgesic and Antipyretic Products.") If the pharmacist determines that the condition is minor and that there are no serious underlying conditions, it may be appropriate to recommend a nonprescription preparation. However, the pharmacist should advise the patient that if the symptoms persist or are not relieved by the preparation within 7 days, or if the symptoms clear up and occur again within a few days,[28] the medication should be discontinued and a physician should be consulted. The pharmacist should also arrange a follow-up consultation to review the patient's condition. This may prevent prolonged ineffective self-treatment that allows a more serious underlying disease to progress.

Treatment

External analgesics are topically applied substances that may have either local analgesic, local anesthetic, local antipruritic, or counterirritant effects. It is important to differentiate these four groups. The topical analgesic, anesthetic, and antipruritic agents depress cutaneous sensory receptors for pain, burning, and itching, and they act directly on the skin to diminish or obliterate these symptoms caused by burns, cuts, abrasions, insect bites, and other cutaneous lesions. (See Chapter 31, "Burn and Sunburn Products," and Chapter 33, "Insect Sting and Bite Products.") Topical counterirritants are included among the external analgesics because they are applied to the intact skin to relieve pain (see product table "External Analgesic Products"). They differ from the other three types of agents, however, in that they relieve pain indirectly by stimulating cutaneous receptors to induce sensations such as cold, warmth, and sometimes itching.[28] These induced sensations distract from the deep-seated pain in muscles, joints, and tendons, which are distant from the skin surface where the counterirritant is applied. Some counterirritant agents, when present in low concentrations, actually depress cutaneous receptors in a manner similar to local anesthetics, analgesics, and antipruritics. For example, menthol in concentrations below 1.0% depresses cutaneous receptors while it stimulates them in concentrations above 1.25%. Because percutaneous absorption of active ingredients is not desired with counterirritant external analgesic products, they are considered a distinct class of analgesic products.

Mechanism of Action

Counterirritants

Counterirritation, the paradoxical pain-relieving effect achieved by producing less severe pain to counter a more intense one, has been known for centuries. The Greeks and probably the Egyptians knew about these effects and referred to them in numerous manuscripts.[29] Today, to counter pain of pathologic origin, pain sufferers produce bearable pain by biting their lips, clenching their fists, digging their nails into the palms of their hands,[30] or using counterirritant preparations.

Counterirritants are medications applied to the skin at pain sites to produce a mild, local, inflammatory reaction. The objective is to provide relief at another site that is usually adjacent to, or underlying, the skin surface being treated. Pain is only as intense as it is perceived to be, and the perception of other sensations caused by the counterirritant or its application, such as massage, warmth, or redness, causes the sufferer to disregard the sensation of pain. The intensity of response depends on the irritant used, its concentration, the solvent in which it is dissolved, and the duration of its contact with the skin.[30]

Several theories have been proposed to explain the action of irritant drugs:

- Stimulation of sensory nerve endings in the skin causes reflexive stimulation of vasomotor fibers to the viscera. These reflexes are mediated through the cerebrospinal axis and dilate the visceral vasculature.[31]
- Stimulation of sensory nerve endings in the skin may have a reflex effect on axons, resulting in peripheral vasodilation. The vasodilation produces an increase in the blood flow to the muscles by changing the thermal gradient that extends from the skin to the deeper structures.[32]
- Summation of pain stimuli produces intense stimulation of the areas of pain interpretation of the brain, partly abating visceral pain stimuli.

According to this last theory, stimuli originating in the viscera or muscles are transmitted, along with sensations from the skin, over fibers in a common pathway and are referred to the same area of the spinal cord as the stimuli from the skin (Figure 1). If the intensity of the stimulation from the skin is increased by a drug's irritant action, the character of the visceral or muscle pain is modified. With intense skin stimulation, the referred pain stimuli may be partly or completely obliterated insofar as the sensorium is concerned. The patient's attention is diverted from the muscular or visceral structure by the application of the counterirritant drug.[33]

Some counterirritants also cause vasodilation of cutaneous vasculature. These drugs, known as rubefacients, produce reactive hyperemia; it is hypothesized that this increase in blood pooling and/or flow is accompanied by an increase in localized skin temperature, which then may exercise a counterirritant effect. This positive thermal response for some agents has been documented by thermography.[34] Although not considered a rubefacient, a topical analgesic containing menthol and methyl salicylate has reportedly produced a three- to fourfold increase in blood flow to the skin in five subjects.[35] Unpublished data reported subsequently from the same study indicated that the warming effect may go deeper than the skin.[36] Indeed, a temperature-sensitive needle inserted into the lateral thigh muscle of three of the subjects recorded a 3.6°C (6.6°F) rise in temperature after the counterirritant was applied. However, the author cautioned that the massage alone may have caused the muscle temperature to rise. An increase in skin temperature and underlying muscle temperature has also been observed after topical applications of a commercially available preparation containing menthol and eucalyptus oil.[37] But however it is produced, the degree of irritation must be controlled because strong irritation may cause erythema and blistering.

There is no evidence that the risk of adverse reactions to counterirritants increases when the application site is lightly bandaged. However, there is an increased risk of irritation, redness, or blistering with tight bandaging or occlusive dressing.[28]

Undoubtedly, the action of counterirritants in relieving pain has a strong psychologic component. Indeed, these agents may exert a placebo effect through pleasant aromatic odors or the sensation of warmth or coolness they produce on the skin.

Analgesics, Anesthetics, and Antipruritics

Topical analgesics other than counterirritants act by overcoming the stimulus that causes the pain. To do this, they must first be percutaneously absorbed. The effects following this absorption are then systemic in nature, resulting in the relief of any deep-seated pain provided

TABLE 1 Classification of nonprescription counterirritant external analgesics

Group	Characteristics	Ingredients	Concentration (%)
A	Induce redness and irritation; are more potent than other commonly used counterirritants	Allyl isothiocyanate	0.5–5.0
		Ammonia water	1.0–2.5
		Methyl salicylate	10–60
		Turpentine oil	6–50
B	Produce cooling sensation; have strong organoleptic properties	Camphor	3–11
		Menthol	1.25–16
C	Cause vasodilation	Histamine dihydrochloride	0.025–0.1
		Methyl nicotinate	0.25–1.0
D	Incite irritation without rubefaction; are equal in potency to Group A ingredients	Capsicum	0.025–0.25
		Capsicum oleoresin	0.025–0.25
		Capsaicin	0.025–0.25

Adapted from *Federal Register*. 1979; 44: 69874.

that the interstitial fluid drug concentration obtained is sufficiently high.[38] The action is the same as that produced by an internal analgesic. (See Chapter 4, "Internal Analgesic and Antipyretic Products.")

Pharmacologic Agents

Ingredients of Proven Safety and Effectiveness

The following ingredients have been recognized as safe and effective (Category I) counterirritants for use in adults and children over the age of 2 years by the FDA Advisory Review Panel on Over-the-Counter (OTC) Topical Analgesic, Antirheumatic, Otic, Burn, and Sunburn Prevention and Treatment Drug Products. According to the FDA's proposed ruling on external analgesic products, issued in February 1983, "although it is true that by 6 months of age a child's skin is similar to an adult's with regard to any absorption, there are enough other differences between adults and children under 2 years of age to require different standards of practice in the use of drugs."[28] Table 1 classifics the counterirritants by their relative potencies.

Allyl Isothiocyanate Allyl isothiocyanate, also known as volatile oil of mustard and essence of mustard, is derived from powdered seeds of the black mustard plant and other species of mustard. It can also be prepared synthetically or by distillation after expression of the fixed oil. Depending or the variety of mustard, the yield of allyl isothiocyanate is approximately 1%.

In high concentrations, allyl isothiocyanate is absorbed rapidly from intact skin as well as from all mucous membranes. Because penetration into the skin is rapid, ulceration may occur if the agent is not removed soon after application. A poultice, erroneously termed a *mustard plaster*, has often been used as a home remedy. It is prepared by mixing equal parts of powdered mustard and flour and moistening with water to form a paste. The paste is then spread on a towel or piece of material and placed on the affected area. The person who is preparing a mustard plaster should take care to avoid inhaling this powerful irritant; allyl isothiocyanate is one of the most toxic essential oils and should never be tasted or inhaled undiluted.[39] The continuous release of allyl isothiocyanate by the presence of water and body heat may cause the inflammatory action to go beyond redness to blistering; therefore, the poultice should not remain on the skin for more than a few minutes.

Allyl isothiocyanate is considered to be safe and effective for topical nonprescription use in concentrations of 0.5–5.0%. It should be applied to the affected areas no more than three or four times a day; this dosage is for adults and children over 2 years of age.[28]

Stronger Ammonia Water Stronger ammonia water, also known as strong ammonia solution, stronger ammonium hydroxide solution, and Spirit of Hartshorn, is an aqueous solution of ammonia containing 27–30% by weight of ammonia. Because it is caustic and the vapors are irritating, this product should be handled with care and the vapors should not be inhaled. Inhalation of ammonia vapor causes sneezing and coughing and, in high concentrations, can cause pulmonary edema. Asphyxia has been reported following edema or spasm of the glottis. In addition, ammonia vapor is an eye irritant and can cause weeping, conjunctival swelling, and temporary blindness.[40] Thus, to be safe and effective for topical use by adults and children over 2 years of age, the product must be diluted. The concentration used is a 1.0–2.5% solution of available ammonia, which should be applied to the affected area no more than three or four times a day.[38]

Methyl Salicylate Methyl salicylate occurs naturally as wintergreen oil or sweet birch oil; gaultheria oil and teaberry oil are other names for the natural compound. Synthetic methyl salicylate is prepared by the esterification of salicylic acid with methyl alcohol. In either form, methyl salicylate is the most widely used counterirritant and has been categorized as safe and effective for use as a nonprescription analgesic when used in the appropriate dosage.[38] At very low concentrations (0.04%), methyl salicylate is used in oral preparations for its pleasant flavor and aroma. Indeed, it has been used as a flavoring agent in candies, cough drops, lozenges, chewing gum, toothpastes, and mouthwashes. However, ingestion of more than small amounts of the substance is hazardous because of its high salicylate content. Although the average lethal dose of methyl salicylate is estimated to be 10 mL for children and 30 mL for adults,[41] as little as 4 mL has caused death in infants and 5 mL has caused death in children.[42] Thus, while a survey by the FDA advisory review panel considering methyl salicylate found that oral ingestion of this ingredient from products formulated as ointments caused no deaths and that few cases manifested severe symptoms,[38] regulations require the use of child-resistant containers for liquid preparations containing more than 5% methyl salicylate.[43]

Even though the agent possesses a high degree of safety for topical use and has had a long marketing history, a single case report emphasizes the importance of avoiding the use of a heating pad in conjunction with counterirritants containing methyl salicylate.[44] The heating pad produced the elevated temperature, vasodilation, and occlusion necessary to greatly enhance percutaneous absorption of menthol and methyl salicylate, which caused full-thickness skin and muscle necrosis as well as persistent interstitial nephritis.

In addition, a clinical study was undertaken to determine the effects of exercise and heat exposure on the percutaneous absorption of methyl salicylate in six healthy volunteers.[45] The results indicated that a threefold increase in systematic availability of salicylate occurred under heat exposure and exercise as judged by plasma and urine data. The authors cautioned that if individuals were subjected to extreme heat or strenuous physical activity, the resultant increase in absorption of topically applied preparations could lead to adverse systemic reactions. Therefore, patients should be told not to use heating pads or other heating devices in conjunction with all topically applied external analgesics and not to apply these products after strenuous exercise, especially during hot and humid weather. Rather, these products should be applied after the body has cooled down.

The rate and extent of percutaneous absorption of various commercially available methyl salicylate preparations were studied after the agents were left in place for 10 hours under occlusive dressing.[46] It was found that only about 12–20% of the amount of salicylate applied to the skin was absorbed into the systemic circulation during this period. Furthermore, both the skin permeability coefficient for methyl salicylate and the percentage of salicylate absorbed decreased when the agents were applied to different areas of the body in this order: abdomen > forearm > instep > heel > plantar. The slower absorption from the foot regions was primarily attributed to fewer hair follicles and a thicker stratum corneum. The authors concluded that topical application of products containing methyl salicylate results in low plasma salicylate concentrations and that the usefulness of these preparations is limited to their local effects.

The recommended topical dosage of methyl salicylate for adults and children over 2 years of age is a 10–60% concentration applied to the affected area no more than three or four times a day.[38] Because percutaneous absorption can occur, this product should be used with caution in individuals who are sensitive to aspirin or who suffer from severe asthma or nasal polyps, conditions associated with aspirin sensitivity. In an isolated case report,[47] a patient sensitive to aspirin experienced allergic symptoms when exposed to various products containing methyl salicylate, including candy, toothpaste, and liniment. The patient reacted to all products, experiencing throat discomfort and soreness with the oral products and a marked swelling and itching with the topical preparation. However, because the patient did not previously report allergic reactions when methyl salicylate and aspirin were used together, the author concluded that the case was a coincidence rather than the result of cross-reactivity. Nevertheless, patients who report an allergy to aspirin should be cautioned to avoid products containing methyl salicylate.

Turpentine Oil Turpentine oil is commonly misnamed "turpentine." The oil used for medicinal purposes must be of higher quality than that used commercially. Medicinal turpentine oil, known as spirits of turpentine or rectified turpentine oil, is prepared by steam distillation of turpentine oleoresin collected from various species of pine trees.

Turpentine oil is both a primary irritant and a sensitizer. As an irritant, it usually acts by defatting the skin, causing dryness and fissuring. It is often used as a cleanser for removing paints and waxes, and it can cause hand eczema by irritating sensitive skin.

Turpentine oil has been used as an ingredient in counterirritant preparations with a long history of safety and efficacy. The recommended dosage for adults and children over 2 years of age is a 6–50% concentration applied to the affected area no more than three or four times a day.[38] Application of turpentine liniments to the skin in greater amounts may cause local burning and irritation, gastrointestinal upset, and respiratory symptoms in susceptible individuals.[48] A case report has been published of a man known to be sensitive to turpentine who applied a liniment containing turpentine oil to a bruised neck and trunk and who subsequently developed erythema multiforme.[49] The authors of the original case report concluded that immune complexes were formed with the antigen terpene, resulting in a severe dermatologic reaction.

In a recent communication, the CDC noted that cutaneous application of large enough amounts of turpentine has been associated with vesicular eruptions, urticaria, and vomiting. The article describes a 56-year-old man who developed skin blistering after applying turpentine to relieve himself of "seed ticks." Citing the results of a survey regarding the use of this remedy among adults in rural Mississippi, the CDC recommended that "health-care providers should be aware of potential drug interactions, toxicity and adverse reactions as well as possible treatment benefits that may be associated with plant-derived therapies."[50]

Several human fatalities from the ingestion of turpentine oil have been reported. An oral dose of 140 mL in adults (15 mL in children) may be fatal.

Menthol Menthol is either extracted from peppermint oil (which contains 30–50% concentration of menthol) or prepared synthetically. It may be used safely in small quantities as a flavoring agent and has found wide acceptance in candy, chewing gum, cigarettes, cough drops, toothpaste, nasal sprays, and liqueurs. Menthol has also been used extensively in inhalant preparations for the relief of nasal congestion. Menthol is usually combined with other ingredients with antipruritic or analgesic properties, such as camphor.[28]

When menthol is used in topical preparations in concentrations of 0.1–1.0%, it depresses sensory cutaneous receptors and acts as an antipruritic. However, there are no controlled studies to attest to the efficacy of menthol as a topical treatment for this condition.[51] When used in higher concentrations of 1.25–16.0%, it acts as a counterirritant: applied to the skin, menthol stimulates the nerves that perceive cold while depressing the nerves that perceive pain. The initial feeling of coolness is soon followed by a sensation of warmth. An experimental study demonstrated that exposure to 2.0% menthol solution caused the threshold for warmth to rise significantly whereas the threshold for heat pain remained unchanged.[52] Although menthol-induced sensations of cold masking sensations of warmth may explain these results, the author considered a direct effect of the menthol molecule on warmth receptors (ie, inhibition or desensitization) to be a more likely explanation. It has also been postulated that menthol exerts its action on the perception of cold and warmth by influencing the movement of calcium in thermoreceptors.[53] A recent review summarizes the pharmacology, mechanism of action, therapeutic use, and toxicology of this naturally occurring compound.[54]

A review of reactions to menthol has been published.[55] Menthol causes sensitization in certain individuals although the sensitization index is low.[56] Symptoms include urticaria, erythema, and other cutaneous lesions, such as contact dermatitis. More recently, peppermint-flavored toothpaste has been implicated in exacerbating wheezing and dyspnea in a young woman with a history of asthma.[57] Despite menthol's widespread record of safety, two patients were recently identified who experienced allergic contact dermatitis owing to the menthol content of peppermint oil: one experienced cheilitis; the other, eczema affecting the upper lip. Of interest was the 18- to 24-month history of these conditions prior to their diagnosis.[58] The fatal dose of menthol in humans is approximately 2 g.[59] However, this may be an underestimate since in acute studies, menthol appears to be a substance of very low toxicity.[54]

The recommended dosage for menthol when used as a counterirritant for adults and children over 2 years of age is 1.25–16.0% applied to the affected area no more than three or four times a day.[38] To facilitate application, a soft, flexible pad containing a layer of menthol in a gel formulation was introduced in 1994.

Camphor Although camphor occurs naturally and is obtained from the camphor tree, approximately three fourths of the camphor used is prepared synthetically. The natural product is dextrorotatory; the synthetic product is optically active.

In concentrations of 0.1–3.0%, camphor depresses cutaneous receptors and is used as a topical analgesic, anesthetic, and antipruritic. In concentrations exceeding 3%, particularly when combined with other counterirritant ingredients, camphor stimulates the nerve endings in the skin and induces relief of pain and discomfort by masking moderate to severe deeper visceral pain with a milder pain arising from the skin at the same level of innervation.[60] When applied vigorously, it produces a rubefacient reaction.

Application of topical camphor products should be made no more than three or four times a day. The recommended concentration for external use as a counterirritant for adults and children over 2 years of age is 3–11%. Higher concentrations are not more effective and can cause more serious adverse reactions if accidentally ingested.[28] (The risk of toxicity relates to both the concentration of camphor in the ingested product and the rate of absorption of camphor into the body.) Accordingly, preparations with camphor concentrations exceeding 11%, such as camphorated oil (camphor liniment), which is a solution of 20% camphor in cottonseed oil, are not considered safe for nonprescription use and have been removed from the market.[61] In children, 5 mL of a 20% camphor liniment is a potentially lethal dose, and death resulting from respiratory depression or complications of status epilepticus can occur.[62] In 1994, the American Academy of Pediatrics' Committee on Drugs noted that although nonprescription camphor–containing preparations cannot exceed 11%, its toxicity continues. They advised parents to be aware of these products and their potential danger, and they recommended that because other therapies exist for all indications for camphor use, modalities that do not contain camphor should be used.[63]

It is of interest that in 1980, the FDA review panel charged with evaluating external analgesics recommended that camphor products for external use be limited to a concentration of 2.5% because of concerns regarding camphor toxicity and the agent's low benefit-to-risk ratio.[64] However, the FDA has yet to take final action on the panel's recommendation.

Histamine Dihydrochloride As a Category I external analgesic agent, histamine dihydrochloride in a 0.025–0.10% concentration is considered to be a safe and effective counterirritant when applied no more than three or four times a day. Application of products containing histamine dihydrochloride results in vasodilation and causes percutaneous absorption of histamine from an ointment vehicle containing other medicinal agents. Aqueous vehicles seem to be superior to ointments for percutaneous absorption.[38]

Methyl Nicotinate Methyl nicotinate, used in a 0.25–1.0% concentration, is a safe and effective counterirritant when applied no more than three or four times a day. As noted with other counterirritants, methyl nicotinate is not indicated in children under the age of 2 years.

Although nicotinic acid is inactive topically, this ester possesses a marked power of diffusion and readily penetrates the cutaneous barrier. A recent comparative study on the release kinetics of methyl nicotinate from topical formulations found that the highest penetration rate occurred when methyl nicotinate was incorporated into hydrophilic gels.[65] Vasodilation and elevation of skin temperature result from very low concentrations. It has been shown that indomethacin, ibuprofen, and aspirin significantly depress the skin's vascular response to methyl nicotinate. Because these three drugs suppress prostaglandin biosynthesis, it was concluded that the vasodilator response to methyl nicotinate is mediated at least in part by prostaglandin biosynthesis.[66] Susceptible persons who apply methyl nicotinate over large areas may experience a drop in blood pressure and pulse rate and syncope due to generalized vascular dilation.[38]

In this regard, a study was undertaken to explore the possibility of age and racial differences in methyl nicotinate–induced vasodilation of human skin.[67] The results indicated an equivalent response among young Caucasian and African-American subjects (26–30 years of age) and elderly Caucasian subjects (63–80 years of age) when calculating time-to-peak response, the area under the time-response curve, and the time for the response to decline to 75% of its maximum value. These results were unexpected because differences in percutaneous absorption between black and white human skin have been described in several studies.[68]

Capsicum Preparations Capsicum preparations (capsaicin, capsicum, and capsicum oleoresin) are derived from the fruit of various species of plants of the nightshade family. Capsicum contains about 1.5% of an irritating oleoresin, the major component of which is capsaicin (0.02%). Capsaicin is the major pungent ingredient of hot (chile) pepper. When applied to normal skin, capsaicin elicits a transient feeling of warmth. More concentrated solutions produce a sensation of burning pain. However, as a result of tachyphylaxis, this local effect diminishes with repeated applications. Capsicum preparations do not cause blistering or reddening of the skin, even in high concentrations, because they do not act on capillaries or other blood vessels.

To determine the reason for this feeling of warmth, investigators applied a solution of capsaicin to the skin, followed by an intradermal injection of histamine to test for chemical responsiveness.[69] Although the capsaicin-treated sites responded by developing a wheal and itch, the flare response did not occur. This latter response, also known as axon reflex vasodilation (Figure 3), is postulated to be under the control of substance P, a neurotransmitter that is thought to function in the passage of painful stimuli from the periphery to the spinal cord and higher structures.[70] High concentrations of substance P are also present in sensory nerves supplying sites of chronic inflammation.[71]

Substance P is found in slow-conducting, unmyelinated type C neurons that innervate the dermis and epidermis. It is released in the skin in response to endogenous (stress) and exogenous (trauma, injury) factors. It appears that pruritic stimuli along with pain impulses are conveyed to central processing centers via type C fibers in the skin for which capsaicin has selective activity. Local application of capsaicin to the peripheral axon appears to affect substance P primarily by depleting it from sensory neurons that have been implicated in mediating cutaneous pain. The depletion occurs both peripherally and centrally—presumably, the result of impulse initiation. When substance P is released, burning pain and redness occur initially but abate with repeated applications. The net effect may be analogous to cutting a nerve or ligating it, which also depletes the substance P content of the neuron.[72] There is no evidence to date, however, that topical application of low concentrations of capsaicin causes any permanent neurologic injury.[73]

Substance P is one of the many neuropeptides that have been isolated from peripheral nerve cells; its depletion by capsaicin has assumed an increasing role in the treatment of certain cutaneous disorders, including:

- Postherpetic neuralgia[74,75];
- Psoriasis[76];
- Postmastectomy pain[77];
- Reflex sympathetic dystrophy;
- Diabetic neuropathy.[70,78]

Several recently published reviews have discussed the use of topical capsaicin in the treatment of cutaneous disorders.[79–81] Capsaicin has also been used to relieve post-traumatic amputation stump pain[82,83] and intractable itching associated with hemodialysis,[84] and its use in the treatment of notalgia (dorsalgia) paresthetica (characterized by localized episodic itch or skin pain usually close to the medial border of the shoulder blade) has recently been reported.[85] The symptoms of erythromelalgia, a syndrome that is characterized by burning, discomfort, warmth, and dermal erythema of one or more extremities; exacerbated by dependency or heat exposure; and relieved by elevation or cooling of the affected limb,[86] can also be alleviated by this agent. Idiopathic trigeminal neuralgia[87] and the syndrome of fibromyalgia[88] have also been reported to be amenable to capsaicin therapy.

Although capsaicin in concentrations of 0.025% and 0.075% share the same indications, the more concentrated formula has been recently studied in diabetic neuropathy[89–91] and has also been reported in a single case study to alleviate the constant aching and burning foot pain accompanying Guillain-Barré syndrome[92]; studies using the 0.025% concentration have primarily focused on its use in the relief of arthritis pain[93,94] and postherpetic neuralgia.[74,75] The role of neuropeptides and capsaicin in the treatment of musculoskeletal pain due to osteoarthritis and rheumatoid arthritis was discussed in a seminar sponsored by the manufacturer and reported in a journal supplement.[95] In evaluating the response to capsaicin in the treatment of chronic postherpetic neuralgia, investigators found that the effect was not dependent on age of the patient, duration or localization of the neuralgia, sensory disturbances, or character of the pain, nor was it associated with the incidence, time course, or severity of capsaicin-induced burning. In this study, almost half the patients "substantially" improved after the 8-week trial, about 40% reported no benefit, and 12.5% discontinued therapy because of side effects. Of those who responded initially, three quarters were still improved a year after the onset of the study.[96]

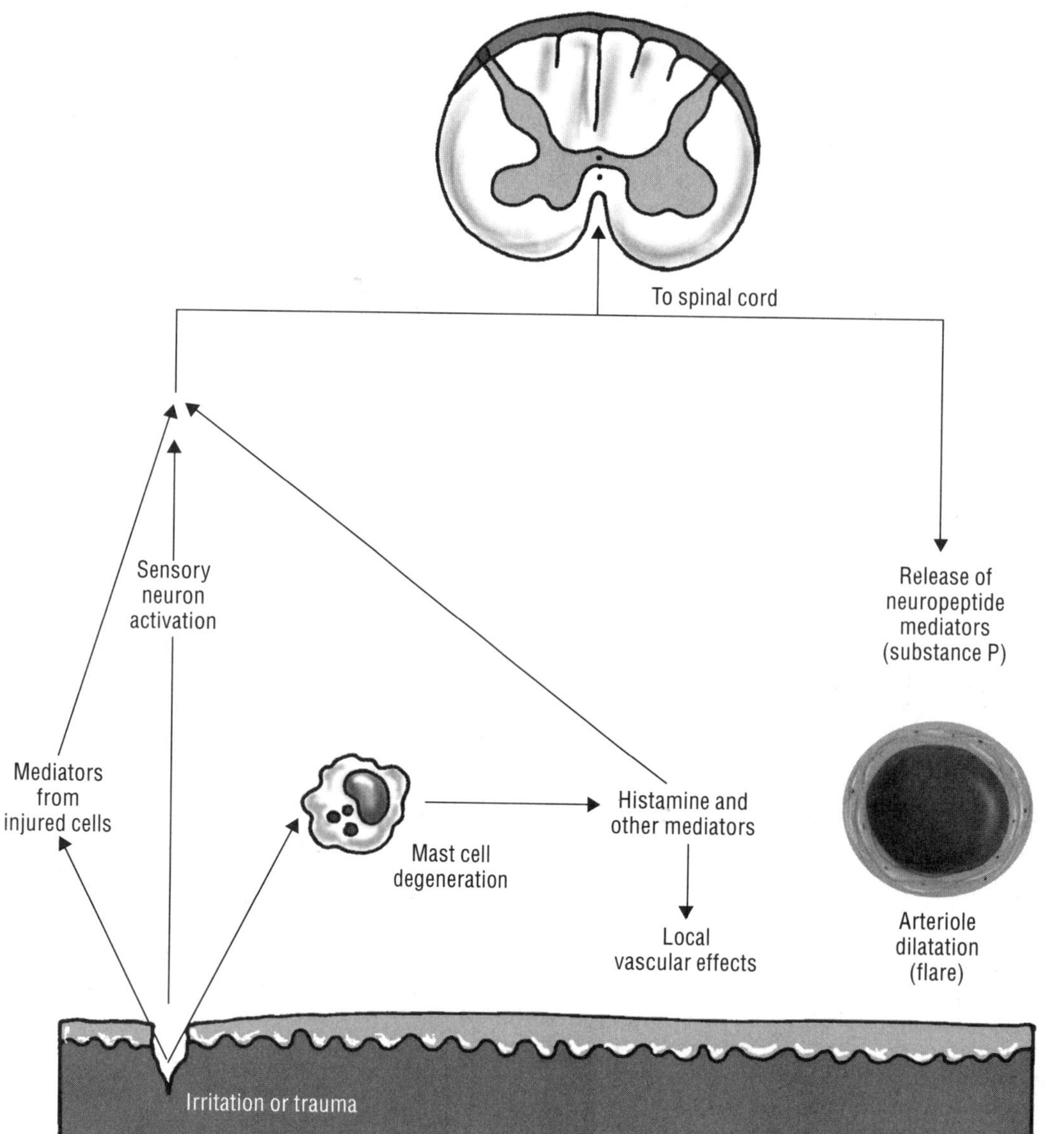

FIGURE 3 The axon reflex concept. Impulses created by the noxious stimulus of a peripheral branch of a sensory neuron are conducted not only in the usual direction to the spinal cord, but also into neuron branches located near blood vessels. (Arrowheads show the direction of impulse propagation.) The axon flex enables the spread of vasodilation (flare) beyond the site of the original stimulus. Histamines and other mediators contribute to activation of axon reflexes and to local vascular effects. Adapted with permission from *Neuroscience*. 1988; 24: 748.

The use of capsaicin as an adjuvant analgesic has also been recently reviewed.[73] Unfortunately, it has been difficult to prove the suggested positive results of open label trials because the initial burning sensation produced by capsaicin has made it impossible to maintain blinding in placebo-controlled studies. In any event, even though a number of case reports and clinical trials appear to demonstrate a statistically significant change in rating scales of pain severity and relief, this does not necessarily indicate clinical effectiveness. Yet there is an apparent persistent benefit in those patients who respond, remain improved, and do not continue to need capsaicin. A meta-analysis undertaken to help clarify the results of the studies published on the many uses of capsaicin reported that, "given the intractable nature of the conditions being treated and the poor performance of other treatments, many clinicians will feel justified in using topical capsaicin on the strength of the available evidence."[97]

The recommended dosage for adults and children over 2 years of age is a concentration of capsicum preparation that yields 0.025–0.25% capsaicin, applied to the affected area no more than three or four times a day.[38] It appears that efficacy decreases and local discomfort increases when capsaicin is applied less often because the drug's duration of action is 4–6 hours. Pain relief is usually noted within 14 days after therapy has begun, but will occasionally be delayed by as much as 4–6 weeks. It should also be noted that, because of variations between lots of capsicum, the concentration range for this drug cannot be expressed as a percentage and must be calculated for each lot.

Combination Products Two or more safe and effective active ingredients may be combined when each active ingredient contributes to the claimed effect and the combination does not decrease the safety or effectiveness of any individual active ingredient. There are four separate chemical and/or pharmacologic groups of counterirritants, which provide four qualitatively different types of irritation. Many marketed preparations aim for at least two such effects when greater potency is desired. Table 1 lists the individual ingredients and classifies them according to their relative potency and acceptable concentration ranges. Many products combine active ingredients from one group of counterirritants with one, two, or three other active ingredients, provided that each active ingredient is from a different group. General guidelines for nonprescription drug combination products state that Category I active ingredients from the same therapeutic category should not ordinarily be combined unless there is some benefit over the single ingredient in terms of enhancing effectiveness, safety, patient acceptance, or quality of formulation.[28] In this case, combination products containing only camphor and menthol as active ingredients have been identified.[28]

It is irrational to combine counterirritants with local anesthetics, topical antipruritics, or topical analgesics. Because these agents depress sensory cutaneous receptors, their effects would be opposed by the counterirritants, which stimulate cutaneous sensory receptors. It is also irrational to combine counterirritants with skin protectants because the protectants act in opposition to the counterirritants and may nullify their effects.[38]

Ingredients of Unproven Effectiveness and/or Safety

Eucalyptus Oil Eucalyptus oil is a naturally occurring volatile oil with a characteristic, aromatic, camphoraceous odor. One of the chief constituents of eucalyptus oil is eucalyptol. Both have been categorized as flavors and have mild irritant and rubefacient actions causing a sensation of warmth. Marketing experience of a topical analgesic product containing small amounts of eucalyptus oil revealed no evidence of toxicity. Nevertheless, a case report emphasized the profound central nervous system depression experienced after accidental ingestion.[98] In a recent status report of certain Category II and III active ingredients in external analgesic products, the FDA advised that eucalyptus oil "had not been shown to be generally recognized as safe and effective" for its intended use and that it should be eliminated from nonprescription counterirritant products.[99] However, a product has been recently introduced containing natural eucalyptus oil as an "inactive" ingredient (Eucalyptamint). The recommended topical dosage for adults and children over 2 years of age is a 0.5–3.0% concentration applied to the affected area not more than three or four times a day.

Trolamine Salicylate Trolamine salicylate (formerly known as triethanolamine salicylate), although a salicylate salt, is not a counterirritant analgesic. The exact mechanism by which salicylates produce their analgesic effect is not known, but it is generally accepted that they act in part centrally and in part peripherally as anti-inflammatory agents that inhibit prostaglandins, bringing subsequent relief of pain. Data exist to show that trolamine salicylate is absorbed from the skin[100]; 10 g of a 10% cream, applied topically, may result in a concentration of salicylate in synovial fluid of approximately 60% of that obtained from a 500-mg oral dose of aspirin. However, the FDA concluded in 1983 after a comprehensive review of submitted documents that the data were still insufficient to support a general recognition of the effectiveness of trolamine salicylate as a nonprescription external analgesic.[28]

Although the FDA's review of the data indicated that trolamine salicylate studies did not show any significant differences between active drug and placebo, several reports published after the review suggest that trolamine may be effective in alleviating neuralgia caused by unaccustomed strenuous exercise[101] and muscle soreness induced by a reproducible program of weight training.[102] A study documenting a unique use of trolamine was designed to evaluate the degree of pain relief and the increase in playing time among musicians with moderate or severe localized pain in the arms, wrists, hands, and fingers. After 750 mg of trolamine given over a 6-hour period was compared with placebo in a double-blind crossover trial, the investigators concluded that topical use of trolamine was associated with a diminution of pain and an increase in playing time.[103] Additional studies should help clarify the use of this agent as an external analgesic.

In 1994, a major manufacturer of external analgesics containing trolamine salicylate asked the FDA to reopen the administrative record for this category of nonprescription drugs; the purpose was to include an additional double-blind, placebo-controlled clinical trial intended to support the efficacy of this ingredient in relieving the stiffness and pain associated with arthritis. The results submitted by the manufacturer indicated that trolamine salicylate provided significant improvement over placebo in arthritis relief.[104] The FDA has yet to act on this request.

Topical NSAIDs Current clinical investigations are ongoing with topical nonsteroidal anti-inflammatory drugs (NSAIDs) that have been marketed for a number of years in Europe.[105] Objective data showing minimal systemic absorption of these agents and consequent low plasma concentrations along with high tissue penetration provide support for their promotion as a convenient and safe alternative for treating painful and inflammatory musculoskeletal conditions.[106] However, a recent report has provided evidence that even when they are applied topically, NSAIDs can cause renal disease and should be used with caution in those patients at risk.[107] Yet another case-control study of more than 1000 patients treated for upper gastrointestinal bleeding or perforation showed that topical NSAIDs are not significantly associated with these adverse reactions.[108]

These preparations presumably act locally in a manner analogous to their systemic mechanism of action. Therefore, their application on acute soft tissue strains and sprains, where the target tissue is situated closer to the skin surface, may prove to be their optimal use as therapeutic agents.[109]

More than a decade ago, the FDA Arthritis Advisory Committee discussed problems associated with the evaluation of these products and offered recommendations for enhancing the ability to discriminate between the topical NSAID and the comparison topical placebo. No additional information has been forthcoming.[110]

Dosage Forms

Because percutaneous absorption of counterirritant drugs is generally undesirable, the finished product should consist of ingredients and vehicles that keep skin penetration to a minimum. The ideal topical drug vehicle should be[111]:

- Easy to apply and remove;
- Nontoxic, nonirritating, and nonallergenic;
- Cosmetically acceptable, nongreasy, and nondehydrating;
- Homogeneous;
- Bacteriostatic;
- Chemically stable;
- Pharmacologically inert.

The FDA urged manufacturers to list all inactive ingredients voluntarily,[28] and this listing has been for the most part implemented. The nonprescription counterirritant preparations are usually available as liniments, gels, lotions, sprays, creams, and ointments.

Liniments Solutions or mixtures of various substances in oil, alcoholic solutions of soap, or emulsions are called liniments. They are intended for external application and should be so labeled. They are applied to the affected area of the skin with friction and rubbing; the oil or soap base facilitates application and massage. The vehicle for a liniment is selected on the basis of the kind of action of the desired components.[112] Liniments with an alcoholic or hydroalcoholic vehicle are useful when rubefacient or counterirritant action is desired; oleaginous liniments are used primarily when massage is desired. By their nature, oleaginous liniments are less irritating to the skin than alcoholic liniments.[112] Liniments should not be applied to skin that is broken or bruised.

Gels Gels used for the delivery of counterirritants are more appropriately classified as jellies because they are generally clear, composed of water-soluble ingredients, and of a more uniform and semisolid consistency. A greater sensation of warmth is experienced with a gel than with equal quantities of the same product as a lotion or ointment. Products formulated as gels promote a more rapid and extensive penetration of the medication into the skin and hair follicles. Patients should be advised against using excessive amounts of gels or rubbing them vigorously into the skin because increased penetration may cause an unpleasant burning sensation.[112]

Lotions Lotions—suspensions of solids in an aqueous medium—are applied to the skin, usually without friction, for the protective or therapeutic value of their constituents. Depending on the ingredients, lotions may be alcoholic or aqueous and are often emulsions. Their fluidity allows for rapid and uniform application over a wide surface area and makes them especially suited for application to hairy body areas. Lotions are intended to dry on the skin soon after application, leaving a thin layer of their active ingredients on the skin's surface. In many instances, the cosmetic aspects of the lotion are of great significance. Because lotions tend to separate while standing, the label should include the instruction to shake the product before each use.[112]

Ointments Ointments are semisolid preparations intended for external application to the skin. Ointments are applied to the skin to elicit one of three general effects: a surface activity, an effect within the stratum corneum, or a more deep-seated activity requiring penetration into the epidermis and dermis. These semisolid dosage forms are particularly desirable for counterirritation because the agents are applied with massage.[113]

Clinical Considerations Dosage forms referred to as "greaseless" are oil-in-water formulations, are therefore "water washable," and are usually preferred for daytime use. In the past, many formulations contained lanolin or anhydrous lanolin as a vehicle. However, because both of these vehicles are obtained from wool fat (to which many people are allergic), these animal waxes are no longer used in contemporary formulations.

The longer any active ingredient remains in contact with the skin, the longer its duration of action. There seems to be little agreement on how long the preparations should be left in contact with the skin for optimal results; however, a practical guideline is that preparations should be used no more than three or four times a day. Although it is desirable to protect clothing from stains by covering the application site, the covering should not be tightly applied. Tight bandages increase the risks of irritation, redness, and blistering. Therefore, proper application techniques are essential.

Labeling of Preparations

Labeling approved by the FDA advisory review panel on topical analgesics identifies the product as an "external analgesic," a "topical analgesic," or a "pain-relieving" cream, lotion, or ointment. However, these terms may not necessarily be similar to manufacturer's advertising claims.[38]

Labeling of preparations must list the active ingredients, including their concentrations, and identify them by their officially recognized, "established" names. Recently, manufacturers have voluntarily listed inactive ingredients on the label. The manner of usage and the frequency of applications should also be indicated.[38]

The labeling for indications states that these preparations should be used "for the temporary relief of minor aches and pains of muscles and joints." In addition, the labeling recommended by most of the panel includes claims for "simple backache, arthritis pain, strains, bruises, and sprains."[38] These terms were selected because they would be readily and easily understood by the general population.

It is acceptable to use terms describing certain physical or chemical qualities of the counterirritant preparations as long as these terms do not imply that any therapeutic effects occur. Terms such as *nongreasy, soothing, cooling action, penetrating relief, warming relief,* and *cool comforting relief* are considered acceptable in labeling.

As with all nonprescription drug products, external analgesics are intended to achieve a beneficial effect within a reasonable period of time. However, claims related to product performance are unacceptable unless they can be substantiated by scientific data. Claims such as "fast," "quick," "prompt," "swift," "immediate," and "remarkable" are misleading and would not signal any property that is important to the safe and effective use of these products.[28]

Nondrug Measures

Although the nonprescription preparations described in this chapter have their own merit as therapeutic agents, there are simple physical methods of inducing counterirritation. Perhaps the most frequently used method is heat applied by means of a heat lamp, hot water bottle, heating pad, or moist steam pack. Under normal conditions, collagen recoils like a spring once the load is released. After a stretching injury, however, the collagen tissue does not return to its resting length. Heat helps to restore the elastic property of collagen by increasing the viscous flow. Heat also acts selectively on free nerve endings in the tissue and on peripheral nerve fibers to increase the pain threshold. This results in an analgesic effect.[114] However as noted previously,[44] heat should be applied with extreme caution, if at all, in conjunction with a counterirritant preparation. Severe burning or blistering of skin, muscle and skin necrosis, and interstitial nephritis have resulted from the simultaneous use of a counterirritant preparation and heat.

Massaging the painful area is another method of producing counterirritation. The therapeutic benefits of massage have been known for centuries. It is possible that the beneficial effects of some counterirritants used in treating musculoskeletal disorders may be largely due to the rubbing and massage involved in the application of the medication. Massage increases the flow of blood and lymph in the skin and underlying structures. Studies comparing massage with other modalities are nonexistent because it is difficult to prepare protocols for the conduct of controlled objective clinical studies documenting the therapeutic effectiveness of massage techniques. Many clinicians have found that massage is therapeutically beneficial in select situations and use it extensively.

Patient Counseling

Precautions

Pharmacists should provide the following important information to patients using counterirritant preparations[115]:

- This product is for external use only. Do not use it near the eyes or apply it to mucous membranes. If some of the product is accidentally swallowed, contact a poison information center or physician immediately.
- Discontinue use of this product if your condition worsens or if there is only a transient improvement. If symptoms persist for more than 7 days or if the pain is constant and felt in any position, consult a physician.
- Do not apply this product to open wounds or to broken, damaged, or sunburned skin.
- Do not apply this product more than three or four times a day, except on the advice and under the supervision of a physician.
- Avoid excessive exposure to sunlight or sunlamps after using this product. Do not use a hot water bottle or electric heating pad concurrently with this product. Do not apply this product before a sauna or professional massage.
- If you apply a covering over this product, do not bandage it tightly.
- Wash your hands thoroughly after applying this product. If arthritic hand joints are the site, wait 30 minutes after application before washing them.
- Do not handle or insert contact lenses following application without washing your hands.
- Massage only a small amount into the affected area of your skin.
- Do not apply this product on children under 2 years of age, except on the advice and under the supervision of a physician.
- Keep this and all other medications out of the reach of children.
- Preparations in this therapeutic class are not interchangeable even though product names are often similar. It is important to read the listing of ingredients or to seek the advice of a pharmacist prior to selecting a product.

Adverse Effects

Self-treatment with nonprescription counterirritant preparations may result in harm if directions are not followed exactly. Some individuals overreact to the irritant properties of counterirritants and develop rashes and blisters. In addition to irritation, counterirritants also may produce sensitization, in which case immune complexes are involved. It may be difficult to distinguish between direct topical irritation and topical sensitization. Therefore, the labeling of preparations must indicate prompt discontinuation if excessive skin irritation develops. Skin in sensitive areas (ie, behind the knees) may be particularly susceptible to irritation. It is of interest that the FDA is considering extending the Reye's syndrome warning that is currently required for aspirin-containing medications to those products that contain nonaspirin salicylates. Although intended to provide information to consumers about salicylate excipients (ie, flavors), this warning, if extended, can also clarify whether methyl salicylate or trolamine salicylate plays a role in the etiology of this syndrome.[116]

Drug Interactions

A letter to the editor in a 1990 issue of *JAMA* describes two patients who were receiving maintenance warfarin therapy and whose prothrombin time was markedly prolonged by their concomitant use of salicylate-containing external analgesics (both methyl salicylate and trolamine salicylate were implicated).[117] The authors comment that the external analgesics' exacerbation of the anticoagulant response underscores the need to make patients aware of the wide range of drug interactions that can occur when warfarin is prescribed. A more detailed description of 11 patients who had an abnormally elevated international normalized ratio after significant usage of topical methyl salicylate ointment later that year confirmed this initial report.[118] It is useful to remember that the risk of adverse clinical effects of drug interactions with warfarin can be minimized by:

- Knowing all the drugs the patient is taking;
- Restricting drugs to those that are genuinely indicated and keeping therapy as simple as possible;
- Educating the patient as to the importance of not changing or adding to the medication, whether prescription or nonprescription, without first consulting a physician or pharmacist;
- Avoiding occasional use of those drugs known to cause clinically important interactions;
- Keeping changes in drug therapy to a minimum, and monitoring coagulation status closely for a number of weeks after any changes.

Case Studies

Case 5–1

Patient Complaint/History

PB, a 75-year-old female with a previous history of congestive heart failure, was admitted to the hospital with a chief complaint of difficulty in breathing. She was subsequently found to have an acute pulmonary embolism. While in the hospital, she developed atrial fibrillation and received anticoagulation therapy with heparin followed by warfarin. After a 10-day hospitalization, she was discharged with an international normalized ratio (INR) level of 2.4.

One month later, PB presented to the hospital emergency room with vaginal bleeding, irregular heartbeat, and orthostatic hypotension. Ecchymoses were seen on the extremities; gross bleeding from the vagina was also evident. The hemoglobin level, which had been 110 g/L during her previous hospitalization, was now 80 g/L. Her INR level was 5.5; her platelet count was 2.85×10^9 g/L; and her blood salicylate levels were 0.80 mmol/L.

After fluid replacement, blood transfusions, and parenteral vitamin K were administered, the patient had an uncomplicated recovery. Her INR level returned to 2.6. Prior to her discharge from the hospital, PB revealed that she had frequently applied large quantities of topical methyl salicylate and menthol to the skin over her foot, knee, elbow, shoulder, and finger joints to treat joint pain.

Clinical Considerations/Strategies

The following considerations/strategies are provided to aid the reader in (1) determining whether treatment of the patient's condition with nonprescription medications is warranted, (2) selecting the appropriate nonprescription medication, and (3) developing a patient counseling strategy to ensure optimal therapeutic outcomes:

- Describe the probable etiology of the bleeding.
- Determine which ingredients in external analgesic formulations should not be used by patients receiving warfarin therapy.
- Propose an alternative nonprescription external analgesic for this patient.
- Develop a patient education/counseling strategy that will:
  - Explain the risk of using nonprescription salicylates concurrently with warfarin;
  - Explain the indications for which use of external analgesics is appropriate as well as what precautions should be observed during therapy;
  - Discuss the overt signs and symptoms of complications related to excessive levels of unbound warfarin in the blood.

Case 5–2

Patient Complaint/History

Five days ago, SR, an 18-year-old male high school athlete, complained of swelling and pain in his left ankle immediately following a track meet. The pain continued for several days. The physician's examination of the ankle revealed tenderness and warmth over the ankle area; however, no indication of bone, joint, or ligament damage was noted on the X-rays or computerized axial tomography (CAT) scan. The physician instructed SR to wrap the injured ankle and refrain from adding any stress to it.

Except for the ankle injury and a seasonal allergy for which he takes terfenadine 60 mg bid, SR is in good general health. His parents came to the pharmacy today seeking advice on a pain reliever that can be applied directly to the ankle.

Clinical Considerations/Strategies

The following considerations/strategies are provided to aid the reader in (1) determining whether treatment of the patient's condition with nonprescription medications is warranted, (2) selecting the appropriate nonprescription medication, and (3) developing a patient counseling strategy to ensure optimal therapeutic outcomes:

- Assess the need for nonpharmacologic therapy, including resting the ankle, applying ice, and elevating the ankle.
- Determine whether the patient has other allergies that would contraindicate the use of certain formulations of external analgesics.
- Select the most appropriate analgesic (ie, external vs internal) and provide instructions for appropriate use.
- Develop a patient education/counseling strategy that will:

- Explain the selection and proper use of external analgesics (eg, indications, warnings/precautions, adverse effects, interaction potential, and administration and dosage guidelines);
- Discuss the concomitant use of bandages when applying external analgesics;
- Identify appropriate nonpharmacologic therapy for the management of sprains and strains.

Summary

Counterirritant external analgesic agents contribute to decreasing the pain and discomfort associated with many minor aches and pains of muscles and joints. However, they must be used correctly to be safe and effective.

Patients should be advised that the oral toxicity of counterirritant preparations is variable; some agents, such as capsicum preparations, have a low oral toxicity whereas other agents, such as methyl salicylate and camphor, are highly toxic when ingested orally. Although some percutaneous absorption occurs when counterirritants are topically applied, the amount absorbed is insignificant if the ingredients do not exceed the maximum recommended effective concentrations and the environmental conditions are normal (ie, the counterirritant is not applied during or after strenuous exercise in high outdoor heat).

Pharmacists can play an important role in patient education by instructing patients on the proper use of these agents. Because external analgesic drug products temporarily relieve only minor pain, patients should understand the degree of relief that can reasonably be expected and the amount of time that it takes for relief to occur. Patients should also be advised when self-treatment is not indicated and when a physician should be consulted.

References

1. Hammacher DP and Associates. *NARD J.* 1991; 133(12): 47–48.
2. Gannon K. *Drug Topics.* 1994; 138(7): 35.
3. Hammacher DP and Associates. *NARD J.* 1995; 137(1): 71–2.
4. Merskey H. *Pain.* 1979; 6: 249–52.
5. Melzack R, Wall PD. *Science.* 1965; 150: 971–9.
6. Reisner-Keller LA. In: Herfindal ET et al, eds. *Clinical Pharmacy and Therapeutics.* 5th ed. Baltimore, Md: Williams and Wilkins; 1992: 880–4.
7. Booth RE Jr, Marvel JP Jr. *Orthop Clin North Am.* 1975; 353–79.
8. Jobe FW, Jobe CM. *Clin Orthop.* 1983; 173: 117–24.
9. Halder NM. *Arthritis Rheum.* 1977; 20: 1019–25.
10. Puffer JC, Zachazewski MS. *Am Fam Phys.* 1988; 38: 225–32.
11. Herring SA, Nilson KC. *Clin Sports Med.* 1987; 6: 225–39.
12. Nirschi RP. In: Petron PA, ed. *Symposium on Upper Extremity Injuries in Athletes.* St Louis, Mo: CV Mosby; 1986: 322–36.
13. Kannus P et al. *Age Ageing.* 1989; 18: 263–70.
14. Evans G. *Br Med J.* 1987; 294: 1569–70.
15. Szarfman A, Chin M, Blum MD. *N Engl J Med.* 1995; 332: 193. Letter.
16. McCarthy P. *Physician Sports Med.* 1989; 17(11): 115–25.
17. Ferguson D. *Med J Aust.* 1984; 140: 318–9.
18. Brown CD et al. *Med J Aust.* 1984; 140: 329–32.
19. *NARD J.* 1994: 136(4): 11.
20. Brooks P. *Br Med J.* 1993; 307: 1298.
21. *New York Times.* May 29, 1995: 19.
22. *Drug Ther Bull.* 1976; 14: 66–7.
23. Garrick JG, Webb DR. *Sports Injuries—Diagnosis and Management.* Philadelphia, Pa: WB Saunders Co; 1990: 14–22.
24. Altman RD, Aven A, Holmberg CE. *Semin Arthritis Rheum.* 1994; 6(suppl 3): 25–33.
25. Harris ED Jr. *N Engl J Med.* 1990; 322: 1277–89.
26. Quinet RJ, Hadler NM. *Semin Arthritis Rheum.* 1979; 8: 261–87.
27. Crown S. *Rheumatol Rehabil.* 1978; 17: 114–24.
28. *Federal Register.* 1983; 48: 5854–67.
29. Kane K, Taub A. *Pain.* 1975; 1: 125–38.
30. Gossel TA. *US Pharm.* 1987; 12(8): 26.
31. Swinyard EA, Pathak MA. In: Goodman AG et al, eds. *The Pharmacological Basis of Therapeutics.* New York: Macmillan; 1980: 950.
32. Post BS. *Arch Phys Med Rehabil.* 1961; 42: 791.
33. Aviado DM, ed. *Krantz and Carr's Pharmacological Principles of Medical Practice.* 8th ed. Baltimore, Md: William and Wilkins; 1972: 801.
34. Lewis DW, Verhonick PJ. *Appl Radiol.* 1977; 6: 114.
35. Shellock FG. *Med Sci Sports Exerc.* 1987; 19: S49.
36. Barone J. *Physician Sports Med.* 1989; 17(2): 162–8.
37. Hong C-Z, Shellock FG. *Am J Phys Med Rehabil.* 1991; 70: 29–33.
38. *Federal Register.* 1979; 44: 68831–9841.
39. Olin BR, ed. *The Lawrence Review of Natural Products.* Facts and Comparisons Division, JP Lippincott: St. Louis, Mo; Feb 1992.
40. Reynolds JEF, ed. *Martindale: The Extra Pharmacopoeia.* 30th ed. London: Pharmaceutical Press; 1993: 1336.
41. Budavari S, ed. *The Merck Index.* 11th ed. Rahway, NJ: Merck and Co; 1989: 6038.
42. Reynolds JEF, ed. *Martindale: The Extra Pharmacopoeia.* 30th ed. London: Pharmaceutical Press; 1993: 24.
43. Trapnell K. *J Am Pharm Assoc.* 1976; NS16: 147.
44. Heng MCY. *Cutis.* 1987; 39: 442–4.
45. Danon A et al. *Eur J Clin Pharmacol.* 1986; 31: 49–52.
46. Roberts MS et al. *Aust N Z J Med.* 1982; 12: 303–5.
47. Speer F. *Ann Allergy.* 1979; 43: 36–7.
48. Reynolds, JEF, ed. *Martindale: The Extra Pharmacopoeia.* 30th ed. London: Pharmaceutical Press; 1993: 1424–5.
49. Fisher AA. *Cutis.* 1986; 37: 101–102,104.
50. Centers for Disease Control and Prevention. *MMWR.* 1995 Mar; 44: 204–7.
51. Greco PJ, Ende J. *J Gen Intern Med.* 1992; 7: 340–9.
52. Green BG. *Physiol Behav.* 1986; 38: 833–8.
53. Schafer K, Braun HA, Renipe L. *Experientia.* 1991; 47: 47–50.
54. Eccles R. *J Pharm Pharmacol.* 1994; 46: 618–30.
55. Fisher AA. *Cutis.* 1986; 38: 17–8.
56. Blondeel A et al. *Contact Dermatitis.* 1978; 4: 270–6.
57. Sporlock BW, Dailey TM. *N Engl J Med.* 1990; 323: 1845–6.
58. Wilkinson SM, Beck MH. *Contact Derm.* 1994; 30: 42–3.
59. Reynolds JEF, ed. *Martindale: The Extra Pharmacopoeia.* 29th ed. London: Pharmaceutical Press; 1989: 1586.
60. Phelam WJ III. *Pediatrics.* 1976; 57: 428–31.
61. Gossel TA. *US Pharm.* 1983; 8(4): 12, 14, 16.
62. *Pediatr Clin North Am.* 1986; 33: 375–9.
63. Committee on Drugs. *Pediatrics.* 1994; 94: 127–8.
64. *Federal Register.* 1980; 45: 63878.
65. Nastruzzi C et al. *Int J Pharm.* 1993; 90: 43–50.

66. Wilkin JK et al. *Clin Pharmacol Ther.* 1985: 38: 273–7.
67. Guy RH et al. *J Am Acad Dermatol.* 1985; 12: 1001–6.
68. Anderson KE, Maibach HI. *J Am Acad Dermatol.* 1979; 1: 276–82.
69. Bernstein JE et al. *J Invest Dermatol.* 1981; 76: 394–5.
70. Bernstein JE. *Semin Dermatol.* 1988; 7: 304–9.
71. Lembeck F et al. *Neuropeptides.* 1981; 1: 175–80.
72. Fitzgerald M. *Pain.* 1983; 15: 109–30.
73. Watson CPN. *J Pain Symptom Manage.* 1994; 9: 425–33.
74. Bernstein JE et al. *J Am Acad Dermatol.* 1987; 17: 93–6.
75. Watson CPN et al. *Pain.* 1988; 33: 333–40.
76. Bernstein JE et al. *J Am Acad Dermatol.* 1986; 15: 504–7.
77. Watson CPN et al. *Pain.* 1989; 38: 177–86.
78. Todd FT, Varipapa RJ. *N Engl J Med.* 1989; 321: 474–5.
79. Carter RB. *Drug Devel Res.* 1991; 22: 109–23.
80. Gossell TA. *US Pharm.* 1990; 15(12): 27, 28, 30, 32.
81. Rumsfield JR, West DP. *DICP: Ann Pharmacother.* 1991; 25: 381–7.
82. Weintraub M et al. *Lancet.* 1990 Oct; 336: 1003–4.
83. Rayner HC et al. *Lancet.* 1990 Nov; 336: 1276–7.
84. Breneman DL et al. *J Am Acad Dermatol.* 1992; 26: 91–4.
85. Wallengren J, Klinker M. *J Am Acad Dermatol.* 1995; 32: 287–9.
86. Muhiddin KA et al. *Postgrad Med J.* 1994; 70: 841–3.
87. Fusco DM, Alessandri M. *Anesth Anal.* 1992; 74: 375–7.
88. McCarty DJ et al. *Semin Arthritis Rheum.* 1994; 23(suppl 3): 41–7.
89. Donofrio PD et al. *Arch Intern Med.* 1991; 151: 2225–9.
90. Dailey GE et al. *Diabetes Care.* 1992; 15: 159–65.
91. Tandan R et al. *Diabetes Care.* 1992; 15: 8–18.
92. Morgenlander JC et al. *Ann Neurol.* 1990; 28: 199.
93. Deal CL et al. *Clin Ther.* 1991; 13: 383–95.
94. McCarthy GM, McCarthy DJ. *J Rheumatol.* 1992; 19: 604–7.
95. Altman RD, Gottlieb NL, Howell DS, eds. *Semin Rheum Arthritis.* 1994; 23(suppl 3): 1–51.
96. Peikert A, Hentrich M, Ochs G. *J Neurol.* 1991; 238: 452–6.
97. Zhang WY, Po, ALW. *Eur J Clin Pharmacol.* 1994; 46: 517–22.
98. Patel S, Wiggins J. *Arch Dis Child.* 1980; 55: 405–6.
99. *Federal Register.* 1990; 55: 46918.
100. Rabinowitz JI et al. *J Clin Pharmacol.* 1982; 22: 42–8.
101. Politino V et al. *Curr Ther Res.* 1985; 38: 321–7.
102. Hill DW, Richardson JD. *J Orthop Sports Phys Training.* 1989; 11: 19–23.
103. Hochberg FH et al. In: *Medical Problems of Performing Artists.* Philadelphia, Pa: Hanley and Belfus; 1988: 9–14.
104. *The Tan Sheet.* May 9, 1994: 25.
105. Heyneman CA. *Ann Pharmacother.* 1995; 29: 780–2.
106. Fourtillan JB, Girault J. *Drug Invest.* 1992; 4: 435–40.
107. O'Callaghan CA, Andrews PA, Ogg CS. *Br Med J.* 1994; 308: 110–1.
108. Evans JMM et al. *Br Med J.* 1995; 311: 22–6.
109. Memeo A, Garofoli F, Peretti G. *Drug Invest.* 1992; 4: 441–9.
110. Weisman MN et al. *Arthritis Rheum.* 1995; 34: 931.
111. Carr DS, Bennett TA. *Pharm Times.* 1991; 57(3): 112–9.
112. Nairn JG. In: *Remington's Pharmaceutical Sciences.* 19th ed. Easton, Pa: Mack; 1995: 1508–23.
113. Block LH. In: *Remington's Pharmaceutical Sciences.* 19th ed. Easton, Pa: Mack; 1995: 1585.
114. Sherman M. *J Am Pharm Assoc.* 1980; NS20: 46.
115. Gossell TA. *US Pharm.* 1992; 17(9): 22–24, 26.
116. *The Tan Sheet.* Jan 9, 1995: 11.
117. Littleton F Jr. *JAMA.* 1990 Jun; 263: 2888.
118. Yip ASB et al. *Postgrad Med J.* 1990; 60: 367–9.

CHAPTER 6

Vaginal and Menstrual Products

Leslie A. Shimp and Constance M. Fleming

Questions to ask in patient assessment and counseling

- *What symptoms are you currently experiencing?*
- *Describe the severity of your symptoms.*
- *At what time in the menstrual cycle do your symptoms occur?*
- *Are these symptoms the same as or different from symptoms you have experienced in previous menstrual cycles?*
- *Are your menses heavier or lighter than usual?*
- *Have you experienced unusual menstrual bleeding? Has this occurred at midcycle or at the usual time of menses?*
- *Is your menstrual cycle shorter or longer than usual?*
- *Have you missed a period?*
- *Have you experienced an abnormal vaginal discharge? Has it been discolored or accompanied by itching and burning or by an abnormal odor?*
- *Have you experienced vaginal dryness and/or difficult or painful sexual intercourse?*
- *Have you experienced any abdominal cramping, lower abdominal pain, or lower back pain?*
- *Have you experienced one or more of the following symptoms just prior to your period: mood swings, low self-esteem, depression, anger, hostility, anxiety, tension, jumpiness, lack of energy, difficulty concentrating, food craving, overeating, insomnia, weight gain, fluid retention, breast tenderness and/or bloating?*
- *Are you now experiencing a high fever, dizziness, nausea, vomiting, diarrhea, sunburnlike rash, muscle aches, and/or mental confusion? What is the relationship between the onset of these symptoms and your menstrual period?*
- *Do you use menstrual pads or tampons? Which contraceptive method do you use?*
- *What medication(s) are you currently taking?*
- *What medication(s) have you taken previously to control your symptoms?*
- *Are you allergic or hypersensitive to any drugs? If yes, which one(s)?*

Vaginal Disorders and Feminine Hygiene

Vaginal Physiology

The vagina, often referred to as the female genital tract or birth canal, extends 7–9 cm in length from the vestibule to the cervix of the uterus. The anatomical position of the vagina is dorsal to the urinary bladder and ventral to the rectum. A thin fold of mucous membrane, the hymen, is found at the lower end of the vagina. Following intercourse, trauma, or medical procedures, this membrane is torn, leaving a fragmented membrane or "tabs" (hymenal caruncles).

The wall of the vagina consists of three layers: the mucosa, the muscular coat, and the adventitial connective tissue. The mucosal surface consists primarily of typical stratified squamous epithelium 150–200 mcm in thickness while the submucosal tissue comprises a network of large veins and smooth muscle fiber. The muscular coat consists of two layers, an external longitudinal layer and an internal circular layer, which are not totally separate; the longitudinal layer is the thicker and stronger of the two. The adventitial coat is a thin layer of dense connective tissue, which contains nerve bundles and nerve cells and which blends with other tissue and joins the vagina to the surrounding structures. The lower end of the vagina is encompassed by paired masses of erectile tissue on either side of the vaginal opening. The vagina itself is void of glands; most lubrication comes from glands found in the cervix.[1–4]

The mature vagina is colonized by a variety of organisms, including certain species of *Lactobacillus*, *Streptococcus*, *Staphylococcus*, and *Gardnerella vaginalis*. Other organisms, including *Candida albicans* and anaerobic bacteria, may also be isolated in the absence of active infection. Various factors determine the number and type of endogenous organisms. These factors include vaginal pH, glycogen concentration, and glucose content. The normal vagina has an acidic pH (usually between 3.8 and 4.2). This relatively acid environment is maintained by lactic acid production from bacteria and vaginal epithelial cells that use glycogen and glucose as

---

Editor's Note: This chapter, which is based, in part, on the 10th edition chapter "Menstrual Products," has been updated and expanded to include discussions of vaginal infections and douching. The core material of these discussions appeared in the 10th edition chapters "Topical Anti-Infective Products," written by Dennis P. West and Susan V. Maddux, and "Personal Care Products," written by Donald R. Miller and Mary Kuzel.

substrates. Growth of *Lactobacillus* species aids in both maintaining a low pH and preventing overgrowth by potential vaginal pathogens. Pregnant women have a higher vaginal pH and may therefore be more prone to candidal infection. Vaginal pH also increases during menstruation, and this increase may predispose menstruating women to cyclic fungal vaginal infections. Estrogens are thought to maintain the glycogen content and thickness of vaginal epithelial cells and hence to ensure the integrity of the protective lining of the vaginal tract.[5,6]

The healthy vagina is cleansed daily by secretions that lubricate the vaginal tract. Such discharges, which consist of endocervical mucus, endogenous vaginal flora, and epithelial cells,[6,7] are a normal physiologic response to vaginal irritants such as feminine hygiene deodorant products, vaginal douches and other cleansing products, contraceptive products and devices, or tampons. In addition, an increase in mucus production is normal during ovulation, sexual excitement, or emotional flares. These normal vaginal discharges, referred to as leukorrhea, are odorless and clear or white.

In summary, normal vaginal physiologic mechanisms maintain an environment that discourages the overgrowth of pathogenic organisms. When this environment is altered, the potential for infection is increased.

Vaginal Infections

It has been estimated that more than 25% of women's visits to sexually transmitted disease clinics are owing to infectious vaginitis or vulvovaginitis.[8] In addition, approximately 10% of office visits to primary care physicians are in response to vaginal symptoms.[9] About 40% of women who experience vaginal symptoms have some type of vaginal infection.[8]

Common symptoms of vaginitis may include vaginal discharge, pruritus, irritation, soreness, dysuria (pain on urination), and dyspareunia (pain during sexual intercourse).[8] Unfortunately, although each of the most common vaginal infections has its own characteristic signs and symptoms, distinguishing one infection from another is often difficult for clinicians. Symptoms may be similar for different infections, and characteristic symptoms may be absent in some patients.[10,11] Nevertheless, in view of the large number of women seeking diagnosis and treatment for vaginal infections and the recent Food and Drug Administration (FDA) approval of nonprescription antifungal compounds for vaginal use, it is imperative that the pharmacist be able to help patients decide about the appropriateness of self-treatment and understand the therapeutic management of the three most common vaginal infections.

Types of Vaginal Infections

Three types of infections account for most vaginal symptoms: bacterial vaginosis, candidal vulvovaginitis, and trichomoniasis.[10,12] Bacterial vaginosis (the commonly accepted term for noninflammatory vaginal infections) is the most common type, accounting for 30–50% of vaginal infections; candidal vulvovaginitis accounts for about 20–25% of infections, and trichomoniasis accounts for about 15–20%. Infections may also be mixed, with more than one causative organism, and vaginal symptoms may be noninfectious (eg, atrophic vaginitis, allergic or chemical dermatologic reaction).[8]

Bacterial Vaginosis Bacterial vaginosis is the most common type of vaginal infection in women of childbearing age. Historically, bacterial vaginosis has been referred to by several names, including "nonspecific vaginitis," *Haemophilis* vaginitis, and *Gardnerella* vaginitis. The organisms responsible for this infection are not well defined. However, bacterial vaginosis is the result of a change in normal vaginal flora with an increase in anaerobes (eg, *Peptostreptococcus*, *Bacteroides*) and a decrease in *Lactobacillus*.[8,13,14]

Half of the women with bacterial vaginosis are thought to be asymptomatic; the other half report a vaginal discharge with a "fishy" odor. This hallmark symptom is most prominent following intercourse. Standard diagnostic criteria require that three of four conditions be present: (1) a vaginal pH of greater than 4.5, (2) the presence of clue cells, (3) a positive amine test producing a fishy odor, and (4) a homogeneous vaginal discharge.[8,10,13]

Predisposing factors are thought to include pregnancy; the use of an intrauterine device; lactation; and sexual activity, particularly at the onset of a new sexual relationship or involving intercourse with multiple sexual partners.[15] In general, bacterial vaginosis is benign, rarely resulting in adverse health outcomes. However, it may be associated with pelvic inflammatory disease (PID), preterm labor and premature rupture of the fetal membranes, and urinary tract infections.[10,16,17]

Trichomoniasis Trichomoniasis is caused by the protozoa *Trichomonas vaginalis* and is classified as a sexually transmitted disease (STD). Repeated occurrences of the infection are common. The prevalence of trichomoniasis varies by practice sites: "5% of women in family-planning clinics, 13% to 25% of women attending gynecology clinics, 50% to 75% of prostitutes, and 7% to 35% of women in STD clinics."[8] However, physician visits in the United States for trichomoniasis have declined by 40% over the last two decades, and this decline follows a similar trend worldwide.[14]

Trichomoniasis is primarily a disease of young women; two thirds of cases occur in women less than 30 years of age.[14] Other predisposing factors are sexual activity, multiple sex partners, pregnancy, and menopause.[15] Between 50% and 75% of women complain of a profuse, frothy, or foamy vaginal discharge. This discharge may be white, yellow, gray, or green and may be malodorous. Less frequently, women report lower abdominal pain, pruritus, and/or "strawberry" spots.[8,10,15] These symptoms most commonly occur during or immediately following menstruation; however, between 10% and 50% of women are asymptomatic.[8]

Candidal Vulvovaginitis About 75% of women experience at least one candidal vaginal infection during their childbearing years, and up to 40% experience a subsequent infection. However, only a small percentage of women, less than 5%, experience recurrent candidal vulvovaginitis.[8,18] *Candida* fungi are the causative organisms of this vaginal infection; about 85% of cases are caused by *Candida albicans*. The incidence of non-*albicans* candidal infections has increased in the last two decades, and *Candida tropicalis* and *Candida glabrata* now account for a significant minority of candidal vaginal infections.[14] Candidal vulvovaginitis has also been referred to as "yeast infection" and "moniliasis."

The characteristic symptoms of candidal vulvovaginitis are intense pruritus (itching); a thick, whitish vaginal discharge (often referred to as "curdlike" or "cottage cheese–like") with no offensive odor, and vulvar or vaginal erythema.[8,10] Urinary tract symptoms (eg, frequency, dysuria) are infrequent symptoms of candidal infections.[8,11] Most symptomatic women experience vaginal or vulvar pruritus and/or irritation, but fewer than one half report a vaginal discharge and few report an odor to the discharge. The symptom most apt to differentiate a candidal vaginal infection from that of bacterial vaginosis and trichomoniasis is the absence of an offensive odor of the vaginal discharge.[11]

A number of physiologic and behavioral factors have been studied as possible risk factors for candidal vulvovaginitis. These factors include pregnancy, the use of estrogen-containing oral contraceptives, diabetes mellitus, diet, treatment with broad-spectrum antibiotics or immunosuppressant drugs, human immunodeficiency virus (HIV) infection, tight-fitting clothing (eg, panty hose), gastrointestinal (GI) colonization, and sexual activity.[8,18,19]

During pregnancy or during the use of estrogen-containing oral contraceptives, the vagina may be more susceptible to candidal infections. This may be because estrogen increases the glycogen content of the vagina or alters immune function, decreasing the ability of cells to resist infection. In addition, candida cells contain estrogen and progesterone receptors which, when stimulated, result in candida proliferation. However, recent studies do not support an increased risk of candidal infections with low-dose oral contraceptives, and studies on risk during pregnancy are inconsistent. Patients with diabetes mellitus are known to be at greater risk for skin and vaginal candidal infections, particularly if glycemic control is poor. Studies associating higher urinary sugar levels with greater risk for candidal vaginal infections have suggested that diet is an important factor. Foods shown to produce elevated urinary sugar are milk (>1 qt per day), yogurt, cottage cheese, and artificial sweeteners. More studies are needed to determine the importance of diet as a risk factor for candidal vaginal infections. Paradoxically, it has been suggested that consumption of yogurt may have a potential prophylactic benefit against candidal vulvovaginitis.[20]

A number of patients report developing candidal vaginal infections during or just after treatment with broad-spectrum antibiotics such as tetracycline, ampicillin/amoxicillin, and cephalosporins. The proposed mechanism is a decrease in normal vaginal flora, especially *Lactobacillus*, allowing an overgrowth of candida. However, neither an increase in vaginal candida nor a decrease in *Lactobacillus* occurs in all women who have taken antibiotics, and most women who demonstrate an increase in candida in the vagina are asymptomatic. Nonetheless, there may be a subgroup of patients who are susceptible to candidal vulvovaginitis following exposure to systemic antibiotics. Patients who are taking systemic corticosteroid, antineoplastic, or immunosuppressant drugs may be at increased risk of developing candidal infections. This risk is well known for certain patient populations such as organ transplant recipients and acquired immunodeficiency syndrome (AIDS) patients.

Studies do not demonstrate a consistent association between tight-fitting, nonabsorbent clothing or panty hose and vaginal candidal infections. Clothing of this type may increase risk by creating a warm and moist environment. A GI reservoir of candida with the transfer of the candida organism from the rectum to the vagina was thought to explain recurrent vaginal candidal infections in some patients. However, further studies found that vaginal infections recurred even though rectal cultures for candida were decreased or negative following oral antifungal therapy. It has been suggested that simultaneous oral and vaginal antifungal therapy may provide better cure rates; however, long-term studies are needed. One study found that the frequency of sexual intercourse was related to the likelihood of candidal vaginal infections; the author suggests that sexual intercourse may facilitate movement of candida into the vagina and cause minor vaginal trauma that results in an increased risk for vaginitis. It is also possible that greater exposure to semen may increase the risk for candidal vulvovaginitis as seminal fluid promotes mycelial formation and increases the virulence of candida.[19] The treatment of candidal vaginal infections does not include treatment of the male partner, however. No controlled studies have shown that treatment of male partners prevents recurrence of candidal vaginal infections in women.

Assessment of Vaginal Infections

The only vaginal infection for which effective nonprescription treatment is available is candidal vulvovaginitis. As noted previously, differentiating vaginal infections on the basis of reported signs and symptoms is difficult. However, given the availability of nonprescription topical vaginal antifungal preparations and the cost and inconvenience of physician evaluation, many patients prefer to self-treat empirically for presumed vulvovaginal candidiasis. Pharmacists can advise patients when it is appropriate to self-treat for vaginal symptoms and when physician evaluation, including pelvic examination and laboratory examination of vaginal secretions, is indicated.

Self-treatment is most appropriate when the woman (1) has infrequent vaginal symptoms (no more than three vaginal infections per year and no vaginal infection within the last 2 months); (2) has previously had physician-diagnosed candidal vulvovaginitis; and (3) has current symptoms consistent with the characteristic signs and mild to moderate symptoms of candidal vulvovaginitis—in particular, a nonmalodorous discharge and no urinary tract symptoms. In one study examining physician attitude toward the availability of nonprescription antifungals, more than 40% of physicians stated they would encourage patients who had previously experienced a diagnosed candidal vaginal infection to self-assess and self-treat similar subsequent vaginal symptoms.[12]

Self-treatment is inappropriate for women who are pregnant and for girls under 12 years of age. Similarly, patients with concurrent symptoms such as fever or pain in the lower abdomen, back, or shoulder should be referred for evaluation by a physician, as should patients who are taking certain medications (eg, systemic corticosteroids, antineoplastic agents) or who have medical conditions (eg, diabetes mellitus, HIV infection) that may predispose them to candidal infections.

By definition, recurrent candidal vulvovaginitis occurs when a woman experiences at least four (documented) infections within a 12-month period.[21] Self-treatment is not appropriate for recurrent vaginal symptoms. Patients with such symptoms should be evaluated for the possibility of a mixed infection or a non-*albicans* strain of candida that may be resistant to standard therapy. Recurrent candidal infections often require long-term suppressive prophylactic therapy. Repeated use of the nonprescription antifungal vaginal preparations for chronic vaginal symptoms may delay the diagnosis of important medical conditions or the institution of effective drug therapy. About two thirds of physicians who were surveyed reported seeing patients who had delayed treatment because of inappropriate use of nonprescription products.[12] In addition, frequent or recurrent episodes of vulvovaginal candidal may be an early sign of HIV infection. The FDA now requires that the labeling of nonprescription products for the treatment of vulvovaginal candidal infection include a statement that indicates the possible association between recurrent candidal infections and HIV. The "warnings" section of these medications now includes statements similar to the ones that follow:

> If your symptoms return within 2 months, or if you have infections that do not clear up easily with proper treatment, consult your doctor. You could be pregnant or there could be a serious underlying medical cause for your infections, including diabetes or a damaged immune system (including damage from infection with HIV, the virus that causes AIDS).

An algorithm for an appropriate approach to the patient with vaginal symptoms is presented in Figure 1.

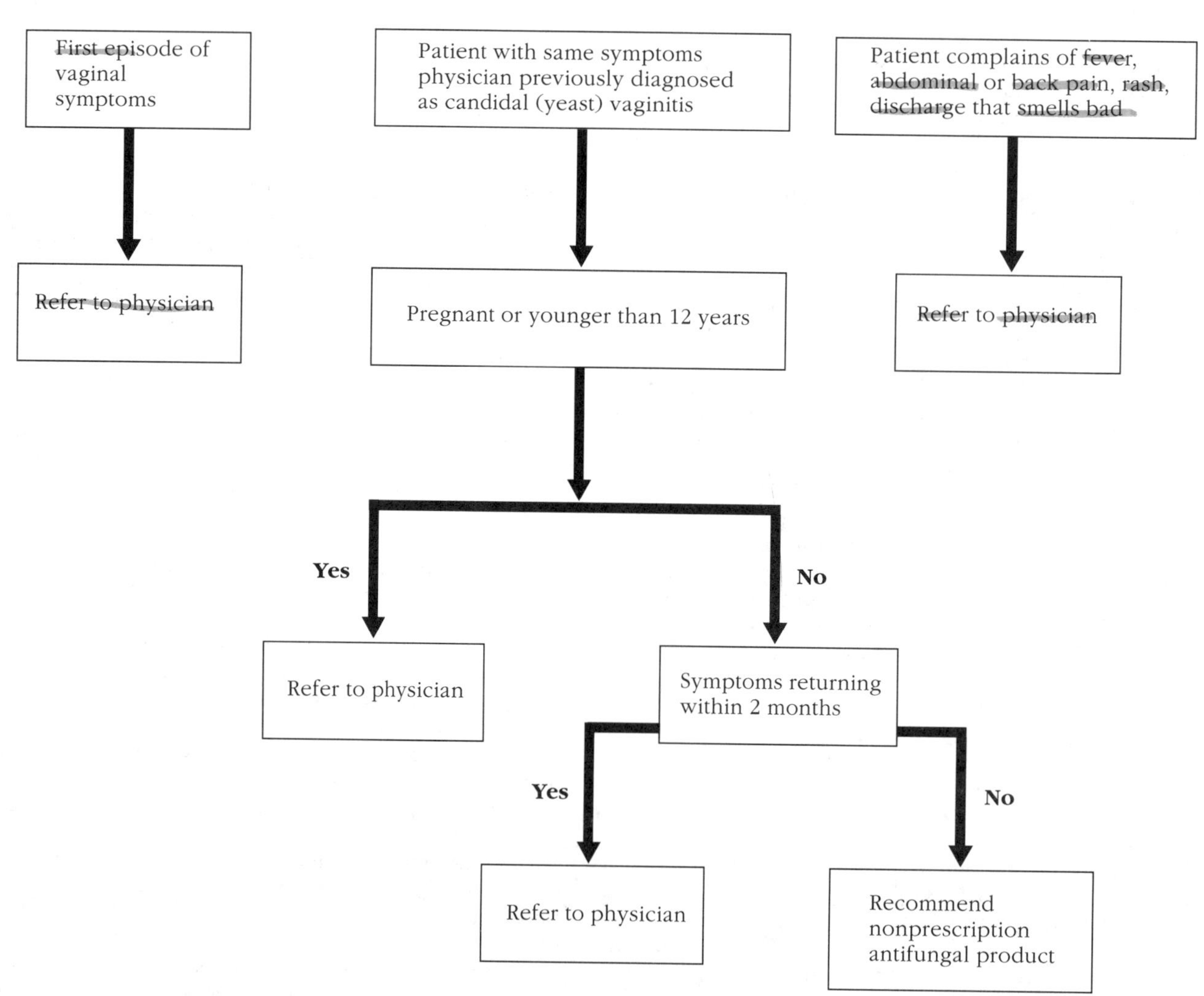

FIGURE 1 Management of patients with symptoms of a vaginal infection.

Drug Treatment of Vaginal Infections

Vaginal Antibacterial/Antiprotozoal Agents The treatment of bacterial vaginosis and trichomoniasis usually requires prescription medications. Metronidazole vaginal gel in a 0.75% concentration (MetroGel-Vaginal) and clindamycin vaginal cream in a 2% concentration (Cleocin) are approved for the treatment of bacterial vaginosis. Clindamycin cream is the treatment of choice for women during their first trimester of pregnancy.[8,10,15] The standard therapy for trichomoniasis is currently oral metronidazole (Prostat, Flagyl) as a single 2-g dose, as a 1-g dose taken twice a day for 1 day, or as a 250-mg or 500-mg dose taken three times a day for 7 days. For optimal efficacy, sexual partners must be treated concurrently with similar dosing. The routine treatment of sexual partners is not warranted for bacterial vaginosis. Because of the risk for congenital defects, metronidazole should be avoided during the first trimester of pregnancy, and its use in the second or third trimester is controversial. Patients treated with metronidazole should be instructed to avoid ethanol consumption because of the possibility of a "disulfiram-like" reaction (nausea, flushing, headache) noted when the two are taken together.[15] As alternatives, oral ampicillin, amoxicillin, and ampicillin/clavulanic acid have been used to treat bacterial vaginosis, and clotrimazole vaginal tablets have been used to treat trichomoniasis, but unfortunately, these therapies are less successful.[5–7,22]

Vaginal Antifungal Agents Currently, recommended initial therapy for candidal vulvovaginitis is with an imidazole product. Before the discovery of imidazole compounds, a 14-day regimen of nystatin taken twice a day was the treatment of choice. Nystatin (available by prescription only) is a polyene antifungal available in cream and tablet form for topical use. Nystatin damages the cytoplasmic membrane of fungi and is effective in approximately 80% of all cases of candidal vulvovaginitis.[5]

There are currently four topical imidazole derivatives available in the United States for treating candidal vulvovaginitis: butoconazole, clotrimazole, miconazole, and tioconazole (see product table "Vaginal Antifungal Products"). These products are available as vaginal creams, suppositories, and tablets. Studies have shown the imidazoles to be equally effective and without major toxicities; effectiveness rates are approximately 85–90%.[5–7] Clinical studies have demonstrated that terconazole, which is often grouped with the imidazoles but is more appropriately classified as a triazole, possesses comparable efficacy to the imidazoles in the treatment of candidal vulvovaginitis.[23,24] At this time, butoconazole, miconazole, and clotrimazole are available as nonprescription medications.

The major antifungal effect of the imidazole and triazole compounds is accomplished by altering the membrane permeability of the fungi. These agents inhibit cytochrome P-450 enzymes in the fungal cell membrane, thereby decreasing synthesis of the essential fungal sterol ergosterol. The reduced membrane ergosterol content is accompanied by a corresponding increase in lanosterol-like methylated sterols. These lanosterol-like sterols cause structural damage to fungal membranes, resulting in the loss of normal membrane function.[25,26]

The topical vaginal preparations that contain imidazole are not appreciably absorbed. One pharmacokinetic study with vaginal application of clotrimazole found that between 3% and 10% of a dose was systemically absorbed. This study also revealed that fungicidal clotrimazole concentrations were detectable in the vaginal fluid for up to 3 days after a single 500-mg intravaginal dose.[27] A study of intravaginally administered radiolabeled miconazole demonstrated that approximately 1% of the dose was excreted in the urine and that the radioactivity of whole blood was too low for measurement.[28] In contrast, approximately 5–16% of terconazole is absorbed and may cause the patient to experience flulike symptoms.[10]

Side effects from topical therapy are minimal. Topical imidazoles and triazoles are associated with vulvovaginal burning, itching, and irritation in about 7% of patients.[29,30] These side effects are more likely to occur with the initial application of the vaginal preparation and are similar to symptoms of the vaginal infection. Abdominal cramps, headache, penile irritation, and allergic reactions are rare.

The success rates of the topical imidazoles and triazoles in the treatment of candidal vulvovaginitis are similar. Different treatment durations have been studied. Initially, antifungal treatment regimens of 14 days were used; this duration is still recommended for nystatin therapy. Recommended durations of treatment for other vaginal antifungals include 7 days (6 days for prescription-only butoconazole), 3 days, and a single-dose regimen (approved only for the 500-mg clotrimazole vaginal tablet or 6.5% tioconazole vaginal ointment). Currently, the 7-day regimens of clotrimazole and miconazole and the 3-day regimen of butoconazole are available without a prescription. A summary of recommended nonprescription regimens is presented in Table 1. Information on currently available prescription and nonprescription products and regimens for acute infections, recurrent infections, and prophylactic therapy is presented in the review by Reed and Eyler.[10]

Selection of cream, tablet, or suppository formulations can be left to patient preference. If vulvar symptoms are significant, a cream preparation or the combination of a cream and vaginal suppositories/tablets is preferable so that vulvar application can accompany intravaginal administration.

Appropriate directions for proper use are listed in Table 2. These directions should be discussed with the patient, preferably in a private counseling area. The pharmacist should also inform the patient of potential local reactions, including temporary burning, itching, and irritation. The patient must be instructed to stop using the antifungal product and call her physician if she develops abdominal cramping, headache, urticaria, hives, or skin rash. The vaginal antifungals can be used during menses, and women should be instructed to continue therapy if menses begin during the course of therapy. However, some patients object to using the vaginal antifungals during menses; postponement of treatment may be reasonable. The pharmacist should also emphasize the importance of continuing therapy despite early symptomatic relief. Relief of symptoms can occur as early as several hours after initiation of therapy, but relief of symptoms is not synonymous with cure.[29] The patient

TABLE 1 Nonprescription vaginal antifungal preparations

Antifungal agent (Brand name)	Dosage forms
Clotrimazole (Gyne-Lotrimin, Mycelex-7, generic)	1% cream (45 g)
	100-mg tablets (7)
	Combination pack (7 tablets and 7 g of cream)
Miconazole (Monistat-7, generic)	2% cream (45 g) Prefilled applicators
	100-mg suppository
	Combination pack (7 tablets and 7 g of cream)
Butoconazole (Femstat)	2% cream (20 g)
	Prefilled applicators (35 g)

Reprinted from *Drug Topics Redbook*. Montvale, NJ: Medical Economics; 1995: 526–607.

should also be instructed to obtain a physician evaluation if there has been no improvement or worsening of symptoms after 3 days of therapy, if symptoms are incompletely resolved after the full course of therapy, or if symptoms recur within 2 months of stopping therapy.

Other Drug Treatments for Candidiasis Other topical vaginal agents that have been used to treat candidiasis include povidone-iodine, gentian violet, boric acid, and *Lactobacillus* preparations. A number of nonspecific nonprescription preparations, including Vagisil and Yeast-Gard (benzocaine and resorcinol) and Vaginex (tripelennamine), are also being marketed; however, use of these agents is rarely appropriate, given the obvious advantages of the imidazole derivatives. These advantages include superior efficacy and improved patient compliance associated with ease of use, less frequent local reactions, and shorter treatment durations.

Nondrug Measures for Treating Candidiasis Consumption of yogurt has also been suggested as a measure to decrease candidal vulvovaginitis, particularly for women who experience recurrent infections. One study found a decrease in the incidence of this vaginal disorder in women ingesting 8 oz of yogurt (containing viable *Lactobacillus acidophilus* cultures) daily.[20] Home remedies such as vaginal douches of yogurt or vinegar have also been used to treat this condition but are generally not effective.[5,25]

Vaginal Douche Products

Studies confirm that douching remains a relatively common practice, given that more than half of all women douche regularly or intermittently.[31] The National Survey of Family Growth reported that douching rates in 1988 were similar in all age groups among women of reproductive age.[32] However, douching rates were influenced by race, geographic region, socioeconomic status, and education. In one study, race was the most important predictor of douching practices; two thirds of African-American women douched compared with one third of Caucasian women.[32] Geographic region was another strong predictor of douching, with women living in the South being more likely to douche than women in other regions of the United States. Both education and socioeconomic status were inversely related to the practice of douching.

The most frequent reason stated for douching is to achieve good vaginal hygiene. Because vaginal douches mechanically irrigate the vagina, thus clearing away mucus and other accumulated debris, they may be used as cosmetic cleansing agents. Women who commonly douche may do so after their menstrual period, after using various contraceptive jellies and creams, after sexual intercourse, to clear out accumulations of vaginal discharge, or simply to feel clean and refreshed. An alternative cleansing method for vaginal and perineal areas involves gently washing the vagina and the vulvar, perineal, and anal regions with the fingers using lukewarm water and mild soap.[33] How often women douche for nontherapeutic purposes is unknown. Some nonprescription douche products recommend douching no more than twice weekly.[34]

Douche products are available as liquids, liquid concentrates to be diluted with water, powders to be dissolved in water, and powders (insufflations) to be instilled as powders (see product table "Feminine Hygiene Products"). Premixed douche products in disposable applicators are widely available and convenient to use as they eliminate the care and cleansing requirements of nondisposable equipment.

Douche Ingredients

Antimicrobial Agents Most antimicrobial agents in douche products are present in concentrations that provide preservative properties but no therapeutic antimicrobial activity. These agents include benzethonium and benzalkonium chloride, chlorothymol, hexachlorophene, and parabens.[35] Other compounds, such as boric acid, cetylpyridinium chloride, oxyquinoline, and sodium perborate, may be included for their supposed antiseptic or germicidal activity; however, their value as antimicrobials is also highly questionable in the concentrations used. Because many manufacturers do not list concentrations of ingredients when the products are considered cosmetics, assessing the efficacy of those ingredients for their labeled purpose is impossible.

The possibility of local irritation, sensitization, and contact dermatitis exists with many antimicrobial agents found in douches. If these effects are encountered, the patient should discontinue using the product and consult a health care provider.

TABLE 2 Directions for vaginal antifungal products

1. It is advisable to start the treatment at night before going to bed. A supine position will reduce leakage of the product from the vagina.
2. Wash the entire vaginal area with mild soap and water and dry completely before applying the product.
3. To open the tube, unscrew the cap; place the cap upside down on the end of the tube. Push down firmly until the seal is broken. (For vaginal tablets/suppositories, remove the protective wrapper.)
4. Attach the applicator to the tube by turning the applicator clockwise. (For vaginal tablets/suppositories, place the product into the end of the applicator barrel.)
5. Squeeze the tube from the bottom to force the cream into the applicator. Do this until the inside piece of the applicator is pushed out as far as possible and the applicator is completely filled with cream. Remove the applicator from the tube.
6. While standing with your feet slightly apart and your knees bent or lying on your back with your knees bent, gently insert the applicator into the vagina as far as it will go comfortably. Push the inside piece of the applicator in and place the cream as far back in the vagina as possible. (For vaginal tablets/suppositories, insert the applicator into the vagina and press plunger until it stops to deposit the product.) Remove the applicator from the vagina. You may want to wear a sanitary napkin or pad during the time you are using the vaginal product, because some leakage will likely occur. Do not use a tampon to prevent leakage.
7. After use, recap the tube (if using cream) and clean the applicator. The applicator can be cleaned by pulling the two pieces apart and washing them with soap and warm water.
8. Continue using the product according to product instructions.
9. Complete the full course of therapy and use on consecutive days, even during menstrual flow.
10. Avoid sexual contact during treatment. If intercourse does occur, do not use condoms, diaphrams, or cervical caps; the antifungal may damage the contraceptive device and increase the risk of pregnancy.
11. If no improvement is noted after 3 days, if a worsening of symptoms is noted after 3 days, or if symptoms are still present after you have completed the course of therapy, contact your physician.

Counterirritants Counterirritant compounds such as eucalyptol, menthol, phenol, and thymol are included in douche products for their local anesthetic or antipruritic effects; however, the efficacy of these agents has not been substantiated. Aromatic agents may be added to mask odors and to produce a soothing and refreshing feeling.

Astringents Astringent substances such as ammonium and potassium alums and zinc sulfate are included in some douches to reduce local edema, inflammation, and exudation. The astringent concentration is important because many astringents are irritants in moderate or high concentrations but are ineffective if too dilute.

Proteolytics At least one proteolytic agent, papain, is included in a douche product to "break down" the excess vaginal discharge. Papain is an enzyme that attacks proteinaceous material; it may elicit inflammatory and allergic reactions.

Surfactants Docusate sodium, nonoxynol 4, and sodium lauryl sulfate are used to facilitate the douche's spread over vaginal mucosa and penetration of mucosal folds. This surfactant or detergent effect lowers surface tension and increases wettability; its cosmetic or clinical value, however, is not readily apparent. Cetylpyridinium chloride, benzalkonium chloride, and benzethonium chloride also have mild surfactant properties.

Substances Affecting pH Many vaginal douche products are buffered or contain substances that purposely render them either acidic or alkaline. For example, sodium perborate and sodium bicarbonate provide alkalinity whereas lactic, citric, and acetic acid provide acidity. A douche solution may actually wash out glycogen, lactic acid, and other acids and render the vaginal pH alkaline for a short time.

One of the most commonly used douches is a vinegar and water douche. This douche can be prepared by mixing ¼–⅓ cup of household white vinegar with 2 quarts of warm water.

Povidone-Iodine Povidone-iodine (eg, Betadine) has a greater potential than acetic acid douches to reduce total bacteria but may allow pathogenic species to proliferate, increasing the risk for vaginal infection.[36] Although few allergic reactions have been reported with intravaginal povidone-iodine, it may be systemically absorbed and should not be used by individuals allergic to iodine-containing products. Absorption poses a particular hazard to pregnant women, in whom repeated vaginal applications may result in iodine-induced goiter and hypothyroidism in the fetus.[37,38]

Douche Equipment

Two types of syringes are available for douching purposes: the douche bag and the bulb douche syringes. The douche bag (fountain syringe or folding feminine syringe) holds 1–2 quarts of fluid and comes with tubing and a shut-off valve. Two types of tips are supplied, one for enema use (the shorter rectal nozzle) and one for douching. The two tips are not interchangeable; vaginal infections may occur if the rectal tip is also used for douching.

Bulb douche syringes are available as both disposable and nondisposable products. The nondisposable units hold 8–16 oz of fluid while the disposable units contain 3–9 oz. The flow rate is regulated by the amount of hand pressure exerted when the bulb is squeezed.

Gentle pressure is recommended because excess pressure may force fluid through the cervix and cause inflammation. Instructions for the proper use of these devices are found in Table 3.

Potential Adverse Effects of Douches

Studies have not proven douching to be either safe or desirable. Contrarily, it is documented that frequent douching may lead to an increased risk for PID, sterility, and/or ectopic pregnancy.[32] Additional problems include irritation or sensitization from douche ingredients and disruption of normal vaginal flora and vaginal pH. Douching may alter the vaginal chemical environment, leading to an increased risk for acquiring a sexually transmitted disease or cervical cancer. Manufacturers recommend that women who suspect that they have PID or any sexually transmitted disease should stop douching and immediately consult a physician.

Douching Guidelines

To use douches safely, appropriately, and effectively, patients should be instructed as follows:

- Strictly follow the manufacturer's instructions.
- Keep all douche equipment clean.
- Use lukewarm water to dilute products.
- Never instill a douche with forceful pressure.
- Do not use these products for birth control.
- Do not douche until at least 8 hours after intercourse if a diaphragm, cervical cap, or contraceptive jelly, cream, or foam is used.
- Do not douche 24–48 hours before any gynecologic examination.

Specific manufacturer warnings are as follows:

- If vaginal dryness or irritation occurs, discontinue use.
- Do not use during pregnancy unless under the advice and supervision of your physician.
- Use this product only as directed for routine cleansing.
- Do not douche more often than twice a week except on the advice of your doctor.

TABLE 3 Douching instructions

Bulb douche syringe method

1. Choose a douching position that is comfortable for you. There are two recommended positions: (a) sitting on the toilet or (b) standing in the shower. Whichever you choose, remember that douching is easier when you are relaxed.
2. Gently insert the nozzle about 3 in. into your vagina. Avoid closing the lips of the vagina.
3. Squeeze bottle gently, letting the solution cleanse the vagina and then flow freely from the body.
4. After douching, throw away bottle and nozzle.

Douche bag method

1. Fill the douche bag with the prescribed solution or with a warm water/vinegar solution.
2. Lie back in the tub with knees bent. Place the douche bag about 1 ft above the height of your hips. Do not place it or hang it any higher as this will cause the pressure of fluid entering the vagina to be too high.
3. Insert the nozzle into the vagina about 1½ in. Aim the nozzle up and back toward the small of the back. While holding the labia closed around the nozzle, release the clamp slowly to allow fluid to enter the vagina. Rotate the tip and allow fluid to enter the vagina until the vagina feels full. Stop the flow of fluid and hold the fluid in the vagina for about 30–60 seconds. Release and allow the fluid to flow out; repeat until the douche bag is empty.

Menstruation and Menstrual Disorders

The menstrual cycle is a regular physiologic event for women beginning during adolescence and usually continuing through late middle age. During the menstrual cycle, some women experience unpleasant symptoms such as abdominal pain and cramping, headache, and fluid retention. Many women use nonprescription products and seek advice from a pharmacist on how best to manage their symptoms.

The pharmacist should be familiar with common menstrual symptoms and disorders, as well as with the risks associated with the misuse of menstrual products (eg, toxic shock syndrome). The pharmacist should be able to interview a woman, assess her symptoms, determine their severity, recommend a product or activity to produce symptomatic relief, or refer the patient to a physician when appropriate. The pharmacist should also be able to evaluate available nonprescription preparations and recommend safe and effective therapy, including nondrug adjunctive measures, for symptomatic relief.

The Menstrual Cycle

Menstruation results from the monthly cycling of female reproductive hormones. In contrast to male fertility, which is relatively constant, female fertility is cyclic, occurring once monthly around the midpoint of the menstrual cycle. A single menstrual cycle is the time between the onset of one menstrual flow (menstruation or menses) and the beginning of the next.

Onset and Cessation of Menstruation

The average age at which menarche (the initial menstrual cycle) occurs in US women is 12.5 years; however, menarche may occur as early as age 9 or as late as age 17. The onset of menstruation may be influenced by race, genetic factors, nutritional status, exercise intensity, and psychologic factors. The variability in the onset of menstruation parallels the variation in onset of puberty, which can begin as early as age 9 and as late as age 14. Two of the earliest signs of puberty among females are a growth spurt and the beginning of breast development. On average, there is a 2-year lag period between the beginning of breast development and the onset of menarche.[39]

Menopause is defined as the cessation of menstrual flow, or the last menstrual cycle. However, this term is also commonly used to refer to the perimenopausal or climacteric period, the years just before and after menopause. Menopause is associated with a depletion of ovarian follicles. The average age for onset of menopause in women is 51 years; however, menopause may occur as early as age 45 and as late as age 55. The age at which it occurs is not related to race, body size, age at menarche, number of pregnancies, lactation, or prior oral contraceptive use.[40] Alterations and irregularities in the menstrual cycle, which are often one of the earliest signs of the climacteric, typically begin when a woman is 40–45 years of age. These changes are related to changing hormone levels. The usual overt change is for the menses to become lighter and irregular; ovulation may occur less often. The anovulatory cycles are related to a decline in progesterone levels.[40] The decline in estrogen levels affects many tissues because estrogen receptors are located throughout the body. Some degree of estrogen-deprivation symptoms are experienced by almost all peri- and postmenopausal women. The most common of these symptoms are hot flashes, sleep disturbances, psychologic symptoms, and vaginal dryness.[41]

Menstrual Physiology

The menstrual cycle results from the hormonal activity of the hypothalamus, pituitary gland, and ovaries (hypothalamic–pituitary–ovarian axis). The hypothalamus is a cluster of nerve cell bodies located in the center of the brain. The arcuate nuclei of the hypothalamus play an important role in regulating the menstrual cycle via production of gonadotropin-releasing hormone (GnRH). Low levels of estradiol and progesterone, occurring at the end of the previous menstrual cycle, stimulate the hypothalamus to release GnRH, which is then immediately transported to the anterior pituitary. The pituitary gland is located adjacent to the hypothalamus in a bony depression called the sella turcica. GnRH stimulates pituitary gonadotroph cells to synthesize and secrete luteinizing hormone (LH) and follicle-stimulating hormone (FSH) into the general circulation. FSH released from the anterior pituitary gland stimulates a group of ovarian follicles to mature. These maturing follicles then begin to secrete the estrogen estradiol, which influences follicular development and promotes the growth of the uterine endometrium. In addition, the increasing estradiol levels promote the midcycle surge in LH from the pituitary gland. This LH surge then stimulates the cells of the graafian follicles to secrete progesterone, which helps to maintain the endometrial lining and to inhibit hormonal secretions of the hypothalamus and pituitary gland.

Two principal reproductive events, each hormonally controlled, occur during each menstrual cycle. The first is the maturation and release of an ovum (egg) from the ovaries; the second is the preparation of the endometrial lining of the uterus for the implantation of a fertilized ovum.[42,43] The first 12–18 months of the menstrual cycle may be irregular and anovulatory (not associated with ovum release) as the complex endocrine system involved in the reproductive cycle achieves synchronization and maturation.[43,44]

The average menstrual cycle lasts 28 days; the normal range for cycle length is 21–35 days.[45] The first day of the menstrual flow is called day 1 of the cycle. Menses usually last 4–6 days (± 2 days). Most of the blood loss occurs during days 1 and 2.[42,46] The major components of menstrual fluid are endometrial cellular debris and blood. Average blood loss is 30–35 mL (range 20–80 mL) per cycle. A loss of more than 80 mL per cycle is considered abnormal.

Phases of the Menstrual Cycle

The events of the menstrual cycle can be described in phases that reflect changes in the ovary (follicular, ovulatory, and luteal phases) or in the uterine endometrium (menstrual, proliferative, and secretory phases).

Follicular/Menstrual Phase Cycle day 1 (the first day of menstrual blood flow) is the beginning of the follicular phase in the ovary and of the menstrual phase in the uterus. The follicular phase, during which the final maturation of a single dominant follicle occurs, is quite variable in length; it lasts an average of 14 days but can range in length between 7 and 22 days.

Ovulatory/Proliferative Phase By about cycle day 7, a single ovarian follicle becomes dominant. This follicle continues to develop and secrete increasing amounts of estradiol while the other follicles regress and degenerate. Once it is mature and capable of ovulation, this follicle is known as the graafian follicle. The ovulatory phase of the cycle is approximately 3 days in length. During this phase, the LH surge occurs. This is a 36- to 48-hour period when several large waves or pulses of LH are released, thus increasing serum LH levels as much as 10-fold. The LH surge catalyzes the final steps in the maturation of the ovum and also stimulates the production of prostaglandins and proteolytic enzymes, which are necessary for the rupture of the follicle wall and ovulation (release of a mature ovum). Increasing levels of progesterone also play a role in stimulating the production of proteolytic enzymes. During the LH surge, levels of estradiol decrease, sometimes accompanied by midcycle endometrial bleeding. Ovulation typically occurs within 24 hours after the LH surge; however, this time has been reported to be as little as 16 hours and as many as 48 hours after the surge. Ovulation releases 5–10 mL of follicular fluid, which contains the oocyte mass; this event may cause abdominal pain (mittelschmerz) for some women.[39,42–45]

Luteal/Secretory Phase The luteal phase is the time between ovulation and the beginning of menstrual blood flow. In contrast to the follicular phase, the luteal phase is more constant in length, averaging 13–14 days (± 2 days). After the graafian follicle ruptures, its walls collapse and its cells take up lipid and lutein pigment, which gives it a yellow appearance. This transformed graafian follicle is now referred to as the corpus luteum. The duration of the luteal phase is consistent with the functional period (about 10–12 days) of the corpus luteum, during which time the corpus luteum secretes progesterone, estradiol, and androgens. The increased levels of estrogen and progesterone alter the character of the two outer layers of the uterine endometrial lining. The glands of the endometrium mature, proliferate, and become secretory in nature (secretory phase) as the uterus prepares for the implantation of a fertilized egg. Progesterone and estrogen levels reach their peaks in the middle of the luteal phase, and levels of LH and FSH decline in response to the increase in these two hormones. If pregnancy occurs, human chorionic gonadotropin (HCG) released by the developing embryo supports the function of the corpus luteum until the placenta develops enough to begin secreting estrogen and progesterone. If pregnancy does not occur (no production of HCG), the corpus luteum ceases to function and estrogen and progesterone levels decline, causing the endometrial lining of the uterus to become edematous and necrotic. The decrease in progesterone also allows prostaglandin synthesis. Following prostaglandin initiation of vasoconstriction and uterine contractions, the sloughing of the outer two endometrial layers occurs. The decline in estrogen and progesterone also results in an increase in GnRH and the renewed production of LH and FSH, which begins a new menstrual cycle.[39,42–45] Figure 2 presents a graphic display of the events of the normal menstrual cycle.

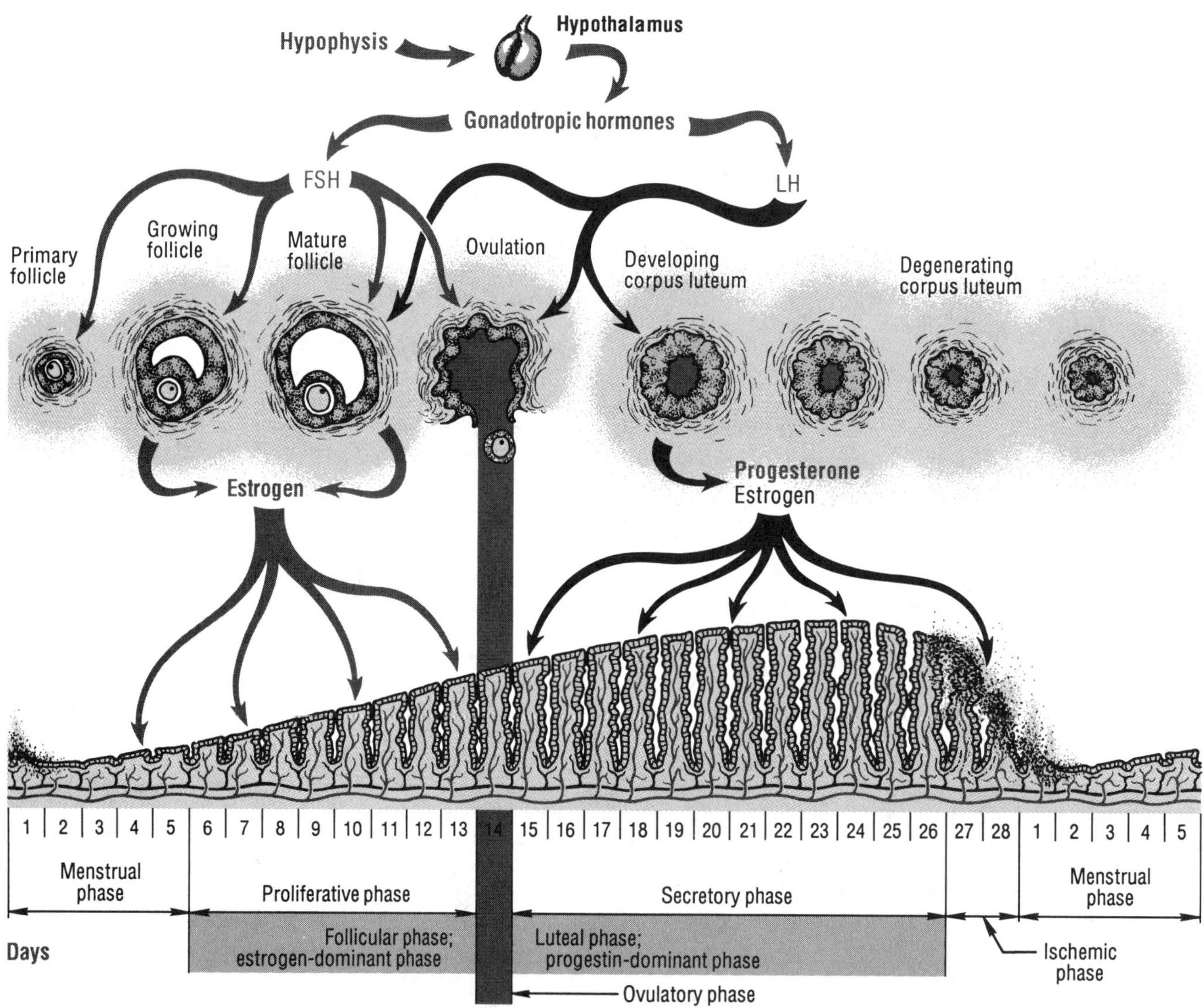

FIGURE 2 Schematic drawing illustrating the interrelations of the hypothalamus, hypophysis (pituitary gland), ovaries, and endometrium. One complete menstrual cycle and the beginning of another are shown. Changes in the ovaries, called the ovarian cycle, are promoted by the gonadotropic hormones, FSH and LH. Hormones from the ovaries (estrogens and progesterone) then promote changes in the structure and function of the endometrium. Thus, the cyclical activity of the ovary is intimately linked with changes in the uterus. From Moore KL. *The Developing Human*. 2nd ed. Philadelphia: WB Saunders; 1977.

Menstrual Disorders

Dysmenorrhea

Dysmenorrhea (ie, difficult or painful menstruation)[47] is one of the most common gynecologic problems in the United States. It occurs in approximately 50% of postpubescent women. Approximately 40% of adult women experience some degree of painful menstrual cramps and up to 10% may be functionally impaired for 1–3 days per month. This dysfunction translates into an estimated 650 million work hours lost per year at a cost in excess of $3 billion in lost productivity. Similarly, 10–18% of adolescent girls report missing school regularly because of dysmenorrhea.[39,47,48,50]

Types of Dysmenorrhea Dysmenorrhea is divided into primary and secondary disease. Primary dysmenorrhea is idiopathic and is associated with pain at the time of menstruation with no identifiable organic pelvic disease. Occurring most often in young women, it usually develops within 6–12 months of menarche and generally affects women during their teenage years and early 20s. Primary dysmenorrhea occurs only during ovulatory cycles; therefore, its prevalence increases between early adolescence, when about 39% of 12-year-olds ovulate, and older adolescence, when approximately 72% of 17-year-olds ovulate.[39] Its prevalence decreases after 30–35 years of age.[47,48] Primary dysmenorrhea pain lasts from a few hours up to 48–72 hours.[47,48] Although it is experienced as lower midabdominal or suprapubic pain, which is cramping in nature, the pain may radiate to the lower back and upper thighs and may be accompanied by symptoms such as nausea, vomiting, fatigue, nervousness, dizziness, diarrhea, and headache.[39]

Secondary dysmenorrhea is usually associated with pelvic pathology. Possible causes include endometriosis, PID, ovarian cysts, benign uterine tumors, endometrial cancer, adhesions, cervical stenosis, and congenital abnormalities. Secondary dysmenorrhea may also be caused by the presence of intrauterine devices.[39,47] Because symptoms of dysmenorrhea are similar to those of endometriosis, ectopic pregnancy, and PID, physician evaluation is necessary to rule out the presence of secondary causes of dysmenorrhea. Secondary dysmenorrhea is suggested if dysmenorrhea initially appears years after menarche (at 30 years of age or older); if dysmenorrhea occurs throughout the duration of menstrual flow (for more than 2–3 days); or if the patient experiences irregular menstrual cycles, menorrhagia, or a history of PID or infertility.[50]

Etiology of Dysmenorrhea Evidence suggests that dysmenorrhea is related to prostaglandin levels. Both the endometrium and the myometrium of the uterus have the capacity to synthesize prostaglandins. Prostaglandin levels in the endometrium and menstrual fluid of women with dysmenorrhea have been found to be elevated. Researchers have reported prostaglandin serum levels to be 5–13 times greater in women with dysmenorrhea than in women without dysmenorrhea. The symptoms of primary dysmenorrhea are very similar to those produced by the administration of a prostaglandin to induce labor. Finally, administration of prostaglandin synthesis inhibitors such as nonsteroidal anti-inflammatory drugs (NSAIDs) has been shown to reduce the symptoms of dysmenorrhea.[47,48,52]

Prostaglandin serum levels rise as progesterone levels decrease during the luteal phase of the menstrual cycle. Concurrently, the levels of prostacyclin (a smooth-muscle relaxant) decrease. This combination of biochemical events can lead to strong uterine contractions and significant vasoconstriction, resulting in uterine hypoxia and pain in some women.[48] Several physiologic changes have been identified that contribute to the development of this pain: an elevation of myometrial resting tone, an elevation of contractile myometrial pressure, and an increased frequency of uterine contractions. During normal menses, contraction pressure is 50–80 mm Hg, each contraction lasts about 15–30 seconds, and about one to four contractions occur every 10 minutes. These normal contractions help to expel menstrual fluids. With dysmenorrhea, however, contraction pressure can exceed 400 mm Hg, contractions may last longer than 90 seconds, and the time between contractions may be less than 15 seconds.[50] Both the intrauterine pressure and the number of uterine contractions have been shown to be directly related to the pain of dysmenorrhea because both of these conditions produce a decrease in blood flow and tissue hypoxia.[39,47,48]

In a subset of women with primary dysmenorrhea, prostaglandin levels were not found to be elevated and the administration of prostaglandin synthesis inhibitors did not alleviate their pain. One hypothesis suggests that leukotrienes, which, like prostaglandins, are formed from arachidonic acid, may cause the pain. Leukotrienes induce uterine contractions and vasoconstriction similar to the action of prostaglandins. In addition, some evidence exists that vasopressin (a substance that can produce dysrhythmic uterine contractions) may also be involved in the etiology of primary dysmenorrhea.[48]

A number of factors have been associated with the occurrence or severity of dysmenorrhea. As mentioned previously, dysmenorrhea is most common in young women and less so in women beyond the late 20s. This decrease in incidence and severity may be related to pregnancy because during late pregnancy, uterine adrenergic nerves virtually disappear and only a portion regenerate after childbirth.[52] Lifestyle alterations may also alleviate symptoms to varying degrees. Smoking tobacco or consuming excessive amounts of ethanol has been associated with more severe dysmenorrhea; the severity reportedly increases with the number of cigarettes smoked per day. The basis for this effect is unknown, but it has been hypothesized that nicotine-induced vasoconstriction is involved.[53,54] Evidence regarding the benefit of exercise is conflicting.[39,48,53]

Assessment of Dysmenorrhea Before recommending any product to a patient experiencing symptoms of dysmenorrhea, the pharmacist should establish the onset of pain in relation to the onset of menses. Primary dysmenorrhea produces abdominal and lower back pain that begins within 1–2 days before the onset of menses and ceases during the first several days of menstrual blood flow. Pain that does not follow this pattern and that is severe or different in character from pain occurring during previous menstrual cycles should be evaluated promptly by a physician. It is important that adolescents who experience symptoms be educated about dysmenorrhea and realize this condition can be treated with products that can provide symptomatic relief.

They should also be reassured about the "normality" of dysmenorrhea.

Treatment of Dysmenorrhea The treatment of dysmenorrhea varies with the severity of symptoms. For mild symptoms, an analgesic agent such as acetaminophen or aspirin and the application of local heat to the abdomen or lower back may be adequate (see product table "Internal Analgesic and Antipyretic Products").[42] However, aspirin has only a limited effect on prostaglandin synthesis and is therefore only moderately effective in treating women with more than minimal symptoms.[47] When used for menstrual discomfort, the adult dosing of aspirin or acetaminophen is 325–650 mg every 4 hours, 325–500 mg every 3 hours, or 650–1,000 mg every 6 hours as needed, not to exceed 4,000 mg per day. Aspirin is best taken with food or a full glass of water.

Before recommending aspirin, the pharmacist should question the patient about allergy or intolerance to aspirin, disease states that are relative contraindications to aspirin therapy (eg, peptic ulcer disease, gastritis, bleeding disorders, asthma, or renal insufficiency), and current medication usage. Clinically significant aspirin-drug interactions occur with anticoagulants, probenecid, phenytoin, oral hypoglycemics, and high doses of antacids (eg, 60–120 mL of an aluminum–magnesium hydroxide suspension).

The principal nonprescription agents for the treatment of moderate dysmenorrhea are NSAIDs, which inhibit the production and action of prostaglandins. Three NSAIDs are available as nonprescription products: ibuprofen 200 mg; naproxen sodium 220 mg; and ketoprofen 12.5 mg. In clinical trials, these NSAIDs were found to be effective in 66–90% of patients. However, clinical trial doses were higher (ibuprofen 400 mg qid; ketoprofen 50–100 mg qid; naproxen sodium 275 mg qid) than the labeled nonprescription doses.[48,49] Therapy should begin at the onset of pain after menstrual flow begins. It should be explained to patients that the NSAID is used as much to prevent cramps as to relieve pain.[42] Optimal pain relief is achieved when these agents are taken on a scheduled rather than an as-needed basis. Therefore, ibuprofen should be taken every 4–6 hours, ketoprofen every 4–8 hours, and naproxen sodium every 8–12 hours for the first 48–72 hours of menstrual flow because this is when prostaglandin release is maximal.[48] The recommended ibuprofen dosage is 400 mg taken initially and every 6 hours thereafter as needed. However, the nonprescription dosage of 200 mg taken every 4–6 hours may be used at first; if it is not effective, 400 mg taken every 6 hours should be recommended, not to exceed 1,200 mg per day. The prescription dosage of naproxen sodium recommended for dysmenorrhea is 550 mg followed by 275 mg every 6–8 hours. However, the labeled nonprescription dosage is 220–440 mg taken initially followed by 220 mg every 8–12 hours, not to exceed 660 mg per day. Similarly, the prescription dose of ketoprofen ranges from 25–100 mg every 6–8 hours, but the labeled nonprescription dose is 12.5–25 mg taken initially and then every 4–8 hours, not to exceed 75 mg per day or 25 mg within any 4- to 6-hour period. NSAID drug therapy should be undertaken for three to six menstrual cycles, with changes in the agent and/or dosage before a judgment is made as to the effectiveness of these agents.[47]

Each of these agents has a side effect profile: naproxen sodium is more likely to cause drowsiness, shortness of breath, and tinnitus than is either ibuprofen or ketoprofen; ketoprofen and naproxen are associated with a greater incidence of fluid retention, constipation, and headache than is ibuprofen; and ketoprofen is more likely to cause gas/bloating, diarrhea, or nervousness/irritability than is either ibuprofen or naproxen. Side effects from a few days of use are limited. Those most commonly associated with short-term NSAID therapy include GI symptoms (eg, upset stomach, vomiting, heartburn, abdominal pain, diarrhea, constipation, and anorexia) and central nervous system side effects (eg, headache and dizziness). The GI side effects of these agents may be decreased by taking the drugs with food.

Relative contraindications to the use of these NSAIDs include a history of allergy to aspirin (bronchospastic reaction) or to any other NSAID, active GI disease (eg, peptic ulcer disease, gastroesophageal reflux disease, or ulcerative colitis), and bleeding disorders.[42,48]

The patient with more severe dysmenorrhea or with dysmenorrhea that does not respond to nonprescription therapy should be referred to a physician. A trial with another prescription NSAID or therapy with an oral contraceptive may be prescribed. Approximately 80–90% of women with dysmenorrhea can be successfully treated with NSAIDs, oral contraceptives, or the combination. If these agents fail to relieve dysmenorrhea, a calcium channel blocker or transcutaneous electrical nerve stimulation may be prescribed. Unfortunately, despite the efficacy of drug therapy for dysmenorrhea, many women remain untreated and continue to experience the pain and activity limitations imposed by this condition.[52]

Amenorrhea

Amenorrhea is defined as the absence or abnormal cessation of menses.

Types of Amenorrhea *Primary amenorrhea* is the term used for the disorder when a female adolescent does not begin menstruation. Amenorrhea is diagnosed if menses has not occurred by age 14 in a female who has not had any secondary sexual development, or by age 16 in a female whose secondary sexual development has occurred. *Secondary amenorrhea* refers to a cessation of menses for 3 months or longer in a woman who was previously having menses. This disorder has many etiologies. In the general population, about 2–5% of women experience amenorrhea; among athletes, a prevalence of 3–66% has been reported.[55]

Etiology of Amenorrhea Possible causes include gonadal failure, reproductive tract anomalies, emotional stress, weight loss or gain, poor nutrition, anorexia nervosa, excessive exercise, hyperthyroidism, hypothyroidism, and previous exposure to radiation or chemotherapy used to treat childhood malignancies.[44,56]

Exercise-induced amenorrhea can be manifested as either primary or secondary amenorrhea, depending on the age at which intense athletic training occurs. If such training is begun before the onset of menarche, it can delay onset and increase the likelihood of menstrual cycle irregularity. More than 80% of competitive swimmers and runners who begin athletic training before menarche experience irregular menses or amenorrhea; this incidence is lower (approximately 40%) among athletes who experienced menarche before beginning strenuous training.[57] Although the exact cause of exercise-induced amenorrhea has not been established, this condition has been shown to correlate with exercise intensity, nutrition, emotional stress, and anxiety associated with competition. Changes in levels of hormones involved in the normal menstrual cycle have also been noted; estradiol, progesterone, and LH levels have all been found to be decreased during strenuous athletic training.[57,58] Fortunately, exercise-induced amenorrhea is readily reversed with a decrease in the intensity of training and/or a 2–3% increase in body weight.[58] The major risk associated with this type of amenorrhea is a possibly irreversible decrease in bone density and associated stress fractures of bones. According to one study, 49% of amenorrheic runners developed stress fractures while no fractures occurred among eumenorrheic runners.[55] It is unclear whether the decrease in bone density (peak bone mass) from exercise-induced amenorrhea will contribute to a greater risk for osteoporosis and bone fractures postmenopausally.[57,58]

Treatment of Amenorrhea The treatment of amenorrhea is based on its etiology. Treatment of primary amenorrhea caused by gonadal failure may be managed by hormone replacement therapy consisting of a combination oral contraceptive or a combination of conjugate estrogens (eg, Premarin) and medroxyprogesterone (eg, Provera). Chromosome disorders and reproductive tract anomalies often require a combination of hormone replacement (eg, cortisone, estrogens, or progesterone) and surgical therapy.[44]

Normogonadotropic amenorrhea can be caused by malnutrition, including anorexia, or excessive exercise as part of endurance training. To resume menses, these patients should modify their lifestyle; such modifications may include reduced exercise, reduced stress, and adequate intakes of calcium, caloric fat, and protein. Many athletes who have exercise-associated amenorrhea are reluctant to gain weight or decrease their intensity of physical training. In this case, treatment with combined oral contraceptives may be instituted to protect against the loss of bone mass caused by the low estrogen levels associated with exercise-associated amenorrhea.[44]

Amenorrhea caused by psychologic trauma or emotional stress often resolves with psychotherapeutic counseling.[44]

Menorrhagia

Menorrhagia is excessive menstrual blood loss occurring with either menses lasting for more than 7 days or a total blood loss of more than 60–80 mL of blood. Women who repeatedly experience a cyclic menstrual blood loss of more than 80 mL may develop low hematocrit, low hemoglobin, and low serum iron levels. About 15–20% of healthy women have experienced menorrhagia, which is one of the most common causes of iron deficiency in reproductive-age women.[46,59]

Etiology of Menorrhagia A number of systemic illnesses and endocrine disorders (eg, renal and hepatic disease, uterine tumors or polyps, thyroid dysfunction, and diabetes mellitus) may cause menorrhagia. In addition, a number of medications, including anticoagulants, oral contraceptives, postmenopausal hormone replacement therapy, oral or intramuscular progestins, neuroleptics, and chemotherapy, can cause abnormal vaginal bleeding. Intrauterine devices may also cause excessive menses.[59]

Treatment of Menorrhagia Estrogen-progestin combination oral contraceptives are effective in decreasing the thickness of the endometrial lining and thus reducing menstrual blood loss. NSAIDs are also effective in decreasing menorrhagia; these agents may achieve their effect by altering the balance between the vasoconstrictor thromboxane A_2 and the vasodilator prostacyclin. An increased production of leukotrienes, which are powerful vasoconstrictors, has also been suggested as a mechanism by which NSAIDs benefit the patient.[46] NSAIDs are most effective when given for several days premenstrually and then regularly during menses.[59]

Dysfunctional Uterine Bleeding

Dysfunctional uterine bleeding (DUB) is a syndrome of irregular menses with periods of prolonged, heavy menstrual flow alternating with amenorrhea for which there is no identifiable etiology.[46,60] DUB most commonly occurs during the first 2 years following menarche and during the perimenopausal period. It is usually the result of anovulatory cycles. In the first year following menarche, about 50% of menstrual cycles are anovulatory.[46]

Etiology of DUB The amount of bleeding during menses is a function of the number of days the endometrium has been exposed to estrogen stimulation. Normally, menses occurs about 13–14 days following ovulation. In anovulatory cycles, no midcycle surge in LH occurs, so the endometrium remains in the proliferative phase rather than switching to a secretory phase. Bleeding eventually occurs when the endometrium has grown to such a thickness that it can no longer be supported. Excessive fibrinolytic activity and changes in uterine prostaglandin production also appear to contribute to DUB.[46,60]

Treatment of DUB The management of DUB is directed toward regulating the menstrual cycle to avoid excessive bleeding and anemia. In mild cases, therapy is usually initiated with just iron supplementation. If the condition is more severe, an estrogen-progestin combination oral contraceptive may be prescribed to regulate the menstrual cycle. Hormone therapy is usually continued until the hemoglobin level and iron store are normalized. After hemoglobin is normalized, iron therapy is continued for at least 3 months to restore body iron stores.[60]

Midcycle Pain and Bleeding

Midcycle bleeding (spotting) is a relatively common phenomenon; microscopic bleeding is demonstrated in 60–94% of women at midcycle. This type of intermenstrual bleeding, which may be accompanied by short-lived abdominal pain, is typically due to the decrease in ovarian estrogen production, which occurs at midcycle. At the time of ovulation, estrogen levels may decrease by 25–33%. Bleeding of this type is self-limited and does not require therapy.[46] Intermenstrual bleeding, commonly referred to as spotting or breakthrough bleeding, is also associated with use of an oral contraceptive, particularly during the first 3 months of therapy. Forgetting to take pills or taking them at an inconsistent time every day can cause intermenstrual bleeding, as can drug interactions that may reduce the contraceptive efficacy of the oral contraceptive. Clinically significant drug interactions with estrogen-containing oral contraceptives occur with antibiotics, anticonvulsants, rifampin, and griseofulvin. A sudden discontinuation of high-dose vitamin C (≥1,000 mg per day) can also cause spotting.[42]

Premenstrual Syndrome

Premenstrual syndrome (PMS) is a condition surrounded by controversy owing to the lack of agreement regarding its definition, etiology, and treatment. PMS can be defined as a cyclic disorder composed of a combination of physical and emotional (mood) changes that occur during the luteal phase of the menstrual cycle and improve significantly or disappear within the first several days of menstrual flow. Attempts have been made to standardize the diagnosis and study of PMS, also known as late luteal phase dysphoric disorder, by specifying a strict set of criteria for diagnosis (Table 4).

Symptoms of PMS Approximately 70–90% of women experience some physical or mood changes prior to the onset of menses. These changes are regarded as part of the normal menstrual cycle and are referred to medically as molimina. Common symptoms include minor weight gain, abdominal bloating, mild fatigue, and irritability. Sixty-six percent of women report positive changes such as increased energy, creativity, and work productivity. Very few women who experience premenstrual symptoms experience a decline in their ability to function normally, and less than 1% report regularly missing work as a result of their symptoms.[61,62] Only a small percentage of women, probably less than 10%, experience symptoms severe enough to meet the criteria in Table 4.[61,63,64]

Etiology of PMS Many biophysiologic and endocrinologic theories have been developed to explain the etiology of PMS, but it remains unknown. Nonetheless, a variety of therapies paralleling these theories have been advocated. One of the more publicized theories has been the progesterone-deficiency theory. However, inadequate progesterone levels have not been clearly demonstrated as an etiologic factor in studies, and well-controlled clinical trials have not shown a benefit from progesterone therapy.[62–65] Similarly, neither aldosterone, endorphin, nor prolactin levels have been found to be different in control subjects versus symptomatic patients.[62,65,66]

Another popular theory hypothesizes that a deficiency of vitamin B_6 might occur secondary to depletion by estrogen and suggests that vitamin B_6 might be an effective treatment for PMS. However, no evidence exists for altered vitamin B_6 absorption or metabolism, and controlled trials have not found vitamin B_6 to be any more efficacious than placebo in treating PMS.[62–65] Still, one study reported a high percentage of physicians (60%) who prescribed vitamins for women with premenstrual symptoms and a significant number of patients (40%) who had taken vitamin B_6.[67] Vitamin B_6 supplementation is not without risk; high doses (2–6 g per day) have been associated with the development of peripheral neuropathy,[63,65] and one report suggests that even doses of about 50 mg per day might be associated with neuropathy.[64]

TABLE 4 Criteria for diagnosing premenstrual syndrome

1. Symptoms must occur in most menstrual cycles, beginning after ovulation and decreasing within several days after the onset of menses.

2. Symptoms must include at least five of the following (and at least one of the first four):

   Marked mood swings;

   Persistent and marked anger or irritability;

   Marked anxiety, tension, or feeling of being "keyed up" or "on edge";

   Markedly depressed mood, feeling of hopelessness, low self-esteem;

   Decreased interest in usual activities;

   Lack of energy; feeling of being easily fatigued;

   Difficulty concentrating;

   Marked change in appetite, overeating, food cravings;

   Hypersomnia or insomnia;

   Other physical symptoms, such as breast tenderness or swelling, headaches, joint or muscle pain, bloating, or weight gain.

3. The condition seriously interferes with work or usual activities, or with social relationships with others.

4. The condition is not merely a worsening of the symptoms of another disorder (eg, depression, panic disorder, or personality disorder).

5. The criteria specified above are confirmed by prospective daily self-ratings during at least two symptomatic menstrual cycles.

Information extracted from Robinson GE, Garfinkel PE. *Can J Psychiatry*. 1990; 35(3): 199–206.

Yet another theory holds that PMS is caused by a prostaglandin E_1 deficiency. Accordingly, evening primrose oil (efamol), which contains 72% gamma linoleic acid, a prostaglandin E_1 precursor, has been advocated for the treatment of PMS. Several placebo-controlled trials have shown an improvement in breast tenderness and depression when 4 g of efamol were given daily throughout the cycle for at least three to four cycles.[65] However, response to placebo was also high and more studies are needed.[65,66]

Psychologic theories for the etiology of PMS have also been suggested. There is some evidence that PMS severity may be affected by disturbed family relationships and negative attitudes toward menstruation.[66] In addition, women's expectations may affect their rating of symptoms such as fluid retention; in one study, women who were told they were premenstrual reported a greater degree of fluid retention than those who were told they were intermenstrual.[66] In two well-controlled, double-blind studies, the benzodiazepine alprazolam was rated by both patients and physicians as more effective than placebo in alleviating symptoms.[65]

Lastly, there have been nutritional theories for the etiology of PMS. While the benefit of nutritional therapy for PMS is unproven, many clinicians recommend a balanced diet combined with the avoidance of salty foods and simple sugars (which aggravate fluid retention) and caffeine (which increases irritability).[62,63,65]

Treatment of Premenstrual Syndrome The initial treatment of the symptoms of PMS is generally conservative, consisting of education and nondrug measures. Women with symptoms of PMS should be educated about the syndrome and encouraged to elicit family support and understanding. Other management recommendations include avoiding stress, developing effective coping mechanisms for managing stress, learning relaxation techniques, incorporating regular exercise into the lifestyle, and making appropriate dietary alterations (eg, lowering sodium intake and avoiding caffeine).[65] For symptoms that are not responsive to nondrug therapy, a number of medications have been prescribed with variable and limited success (Table 5).[68] Because PMS is a multisymptom disorder, however, a single therapeutic agent is unlikely to address all symptoms; thus, specific agents should be selected to address the major symptoms experienced by the patient.

One of the most common premenstrual complaints is fluid accumulation. The FDA has examined the usefulness and safety of nonprescription diuretics to relieve water retention, weight gain, bloating, swelling, and a full feeling. Three nonprescription diuretics—ammonium chloride, caffeine, and pamabrom—are contained in commercially available menstrual products (see product table "Menstrual Products"). Ammonium chloride is an acid-forming salt with a short duration of effect; it is taken in oral doses of up to 3 g per day (divided into three doses) for no more than 6 consecutive days. Larger doses of ammonium chloride (4–12 g per day) can produce significant GI and central nervous system adverse effects. Ammonium chloride is contraindicated in patients with renal or liver impairment because metabolic acidosis may result.[69]

Caffeine, a xanthine, promotes diuresis by inhibiting the renal tubular reabsorption of sodium and water. It is safe and effective as a diuretic in dosages of 100–200 mg every 3–4 hours. Tolerance to the diuretic effect may occur. Patients should be reminded that caffeine may cause anxiety, restlessness, or insomnia (if taken within several hours of bedtime), and that additive side effects (nervousness, irritability, nausea, or tachycardia) might occur if other caffeine-containing beverages, foods, or medications are consumed concurrently. Caffeine may also cause GI irritation, so patients with a history of peptic ulcer disease should avoid it.[69,70] Patients taking monoamine oxidase inhibitors or other xanthine medications (eg, theophylline, aminophylline, oxtriphylline, or dyphylline) should avoid diuretics that contain caffeine.

Pamabrom, a derivative of theophylline, is contained in combination products (along with analgesics and antihistamines) and is marketed for the treatment of PMS.

TABLE 5 Medications prescribed for treatment of PMS symptoms

Symptom	Drug therapy
Anxiety	Alprazolam; buspirone; transdermal estradiol
Depression/ mood swings	Vitamin B_6 (50 mg/day); antidepressants (TCA; SSRI); calcium (1,000 mg/day); magnesium (360 mg/day); transdermal estradiol; danazol
Fatigue	Vitamin B_6 (50 mg/day)
Fluid retention	Spironolactone
Bloating	Calcium (1,000 mg/day); magnesium (360 mg/day); transdermal estradiol; bromocriptine
Irritability	Vitamin B_6 (50 mg/day); calcium (1,000 mg/day); danazol
Mastalgia	Evening primrose oil; danazol; bromocriptine; tamoxifen
Suppression of ovulation	Oral contraceptive (combined/ progestin-only); progesterone; leuprolide

Information extracted from Parker PD. Premenstrual syndrome. *Am Fam Physician*. 1994; 50(6): 1309–17.

It is taken in doses of up to 200 mg per day (50 mg four times daily).[69]

The NSAIDs have shown some evidence of efficacy in managing symptoms of PMS. These agents may be most useful for women who experience both dysmenorrhea and PMS; reducing symptoms associated with dysmenorrhea may help improve a woman's ability to tolerate PMS-related symptoms.[62,63,65,66] Several smooth-muscle relaxants, antihistamines, sympathomimetic amines, and herbal preparations have also been evaluated for the treatment of dysmenorrhea and PMS, but none of these agents is classified as Category I (safe and effective).[69]

Atrophic Vaginitis and Vaginal Dryness

Etiology and Symptoms At menopause, vaginal lubrication declines secondary to the decrease in estrogen levels. Among the common complaints associated with menopause are atrophic vaginitis and associated dyspareunia.[71,72] Atrophic vaginitis is inflammation of the vagina related to atrophy of the vaginal mucosa secondary to decreased estrogen levels. Symptoms include vaginal irritation, burning, itching, and dyspareunia.[73] The most common cause of secondary superficial dyspareunia is also a lack of adequate vaginal lubrication.[71,72] This condition is most common in postmenopausal women and breast-feeding women. The pharmacist should inquire about the onset of these symptoms; self-treatment is most appropriate for those women who have previously been able to maintain adequate vaginal lubrication. Severe vaginal dryness or dyspareunia should be evaluated by a physician.

Treatment of Vaginal Dryness Vaginal dryness can often be treated with topical lubricants (see product table "Vaginal Lubricants"). One study found that about half the women with vaginal dryness had tried "something," including such substances as butter, baby oil, and petroleum jelly (Vaseline), before seeking medical attention.[72] The pharmacist should question patients about the use of any vaginal or feminine hygiene products because such products may cause or worsen vaginal irritation and dyspareunia.[74]

Water-soluble lubricants (eg, Gyne-Moistrin, KY Jelly, and Replens) and moisturizing skin lotions (eg, Lubriderm and Keri-lotion) are acceptable vaginal lubricants.[72] Vaseline should not be used because it is difficult to remove from the vagina. If the patient is using a condom or diaphragm, only water-soluble lubricants should be used because other products may impair the efficacy of these contraceptive methods. Water-soluble lubricant gels can be applied both externally and internally. Initially, the patient should be instructed to use a liberal quantity of lubricant (up to 2 tbsp) and then to tailor the quantity and frequency of use to her specific needs. If the patient is treating dyspareunia, the lubricant should be applied to both the vaginal opening and the penis. If the use of nonprescription lubricants does not produce adequate benefit or is aesthetically unappealing to the patient, oral or topical estrogen replacement therapy may be prescribed.[72]

The Pharmacist's Role in Assessment of Menstrual Disorders

Before recommending any product for a patient, the pharmacist should obtain a clear and complete description of the patient's current symptoms, including their severity, onset, similarity to symptoms experienced during other menstrual cycles, relationship to onset of menstrual bleeding, and the patient's explanation for their occurrence. The pharmacist should also gather pertinent information such as current medication therapy, treatment previously tried, outcome of prior therapy (efficacy, dose, duration, side effects), drug allergies, hypersensitivities, or intolerances, and whether symptoms were evaluated by a physician. All conditions of menstrual dysfunction (ie, amenorrhea, menorrhagia, DUB, and midcycle pain and bleeding), with the exception of minor midcycle pain and bleeding, should be evaluated by a physician. Because many possible etiologies exist for these conditions, appropriate therapy and prognosis depend on an accurate diagnosis. The pharmacist should instruct the patient to see a physician for any of the following problems:

- Abnormal vaginal bleeding or discharge;
- Atrophic vaginitis or vaginal dryness;
- Dyspareunia;
- Irregular menstrual cycles or amenorrhea or dysmenorrhea;
- Significant alterations in mood;
- Breast tenderness.

Although symptoms may not be bothersome, pharmacists should encourage patients to seek medical evaluation to avoid potential long-term adverse consequences (eg, osteoporosis or endometrial cancer associated with long-term amenorrhea) or the delayed diagnosis and treatment of a potentially serious medical condition.

Pharmacists discussing premenstrual symptoms with patients should emphasize that minor symptoms such as bloating and weight gain, fatigue, irritability, mood swings, changes in appetite, and breast tenderness are not uncommon. If these symptoms are more severe, evaluation by a physician is encouraged. In addition, pharmacists should inquire about prior self-treatment and discuss any potential dangers inherent in prior therapy (eg, neuropathy associated with vitamin B_6 therapy). Pharmacists should also dispel some common myths about the adverse effect of the menstrual cycle on the ability of women to function normally.

Most women who purchase nonprescription drugs for menstrual cycle–related symptoms are healthy. Recommendations for any nonprescription drug should be accompanied by adequate patient counseling regarding the appropriate use of the product and other adjunctive measures.

Menstrual Products and Toxic Shock Syndrome

Feminine Cleansing Products

The pharmacist should be familiar with feminine hygiene products and should know how to advise a patient regarding their appropriate use and which symptoms related to their use require referral to a physician (see product table "Feminine Hygiene Products").

Feminine Pads and Tampons

Feminine pads are used to absorb menstrual and other vaginal discharges. They are made of an absorbent cotton, synthetic, or cellulose (derived from wood pulp) material that is covered with a lightweight paper gauze to reduce irritation. A layer of cellulose or thin plastic is incorporated into the side of the pad worn away from the perineum to minimize leakage and the soiling of undergarments. Most styles are held in place with adhesive strips on the underside of the pad, which affix to the undergarment.

Feminine pads are available in a wide variety of sizes and absorbencies. Because most women experience their heaviest menstrual flow on day 2 of the menstrual cycle, "super" or "maxi" pads may be used at this time. During the days of heaviest flow, pads may need to be changed every 2–4 hours; changing them every 4–6 hours may be adequate for days of lesser menstrual flow. Frequent changing of sanitary pads minimizes the development of unpleasant odors arising from the breakdown of blood products and vaginal secretions; it also helps to minimize irritation and chafing of the perineum and upper inner thighs. Applying powder to the inner thighs may also alleviate chafing. "Mini" or "light" pads and "junior" or "teen" pads are designed to accommodate the smaller anatomy and lighter flow of the adolescent female. The narrower width of these pads may reduce chafing and irritation. Many women prefer the new, less cumbersome light pads for the first and last days of their cycles. These light pads or the thin shields may also be used to protect undergarments from being stained by vaginal creams, vaginal tablets, suppository leakage, or normal vaginal secretions.

Tampons are intravaginal inserts made of cellulose, cotton, or synthetic materials (viscose rayon or polyacrylate rayon) and designed to absorb menstrual and other vaginal discharges. They have the advantage over feminine pads of being worn internally, which lessens chafing, odor, bulkiness, and irritation. Some tampons are "scented," however, and some fragrances may cause local irritation and allergic reactions, such as allergic contact dermatitis. The FDA evaluated feminine pads and tampons and has classified unscented menstrual pads into performance Class I, which indicates that the device meets only the general controls applicable to all devices. Scented menstrual pads and both unscented and scented menstrual tampons have been classified into performance Class II, which requires the future development of standards to ensure the safety and efficacy of the products.[75]

Both the composition of tampons and their high absorbency have been associated with toxic shock syndrome (TSS).[76] In response to this association and in an effort to decrease the likelihood of TSS, tampon manufacturers have altered the composition and lowered the absorbency of tampons.[76] In addition, the FDA changed the requirement for the labeling of tampons so that terms such as *regular* and *super*, which are used to indicate the absorbency of tampons, have a uniform meaning and indicate a specific range of fluid absorbed per tampon.[77] Four descriptive terms are now used: *junior* (6 g or less of fluid absorbed), *regular* (6–9 g), *super* (9–12 g), and *super-plus* (12–15 g). Higher-absorbency products (>15 g) are not prohibited, but no products are currently marketed with these higher absorbencies.[77]

Toxic Shock Syndrome

Toxic shock syndrome was a term originally coined by Todd and coworkers in 1978 to describe a severe multisystem illness characterized by high fever, profound hypotension, severe diarrhea, mental confusion, renal failure, erythroderma, and skin desquamation.[78] In 1980, these symptoms were recognized as affecting a relatively large number of young, previously healthy, menstruating women, and the term *toxic shock syndrome* was applied to their illness. The Centers for Disease Control and Prevention case definition of TSS is shown in Table 6.[79]

TABLE 6 CDC[a] case definition of toxic shock syndrome

Fever: temperature ≥102°F (38.9°C)

Rash: diffuse macular erythroderma

Desquamation: 1–2 weeks after onset of illness, particularly on palms and soles

Hypotension: systolic blood pressure ≤90 mm Hg, orthostatic drop in diastolic ≥15 mm Hg; orthostatic syncope or dizziness

Involvement of three or more of the following organ systems:

- Gastrointestinal: vomiting or diarrhea at onset of illness
- Muscular: severe myalgia or twice-normal creatine phosphokinase
- Mucous membranes: vaginal, oropharyngeal, or conjunctival hyperemia
- Renal: twice-normal blood urea nitrogen or creatinine or pyuria (more than five white blood cells in a high-power field)
- Hepatic: twice-normal bilirubin or transaminases
- Hematologic: platelets <1,000,000/mm^3

Central nervous system: disorientation or alterations in consciousness without focal neurologic signs when fever and hypotension are absent

Negative results on the following tests, if obtained: blood, throat, or cerebrospinal fluid cultures (blood culture may be positive for *S aureus*)

Serologic tests for Rocky Mountain spotted fever, leptospirosis, or measles

[a]Centers for Disease Control and Prevention.

Incidence of TSS TSS is commonly divided into menstrual and nonmenstrual cases. Nonmenstrual TSS is much less common; only about one third of TSS cases are of this type. TSS can occur in both men and women; about one third of the nonmenstrual cases occur in men. The current incidence of TSS in the United States is unknown, but it has declined dramatically since 1980, when 812 cases of menstrual TSS were reported to the Centers for Disease Control; in 1988, only 53 cases were reported.[79]

Menstrual TSS has been found to affect primarily young women between the ages of 15–19 years. One reason for the greater incidence in young women is the absence of preexisting antibodies to the TSS toxin. By the age of 20–25, more than 90% of both men and women have detectable antibodies to this toxin.[78] However, in almost all cases of TSS, an absent or low titer of antibody to toxic shock syndrome toxin 1 (TSST-1), an exotoxin that causes TSS, has been found.[80] TSS is also more common in Caucasian women than in women of other racial groups. This is primarily owing to a difference in the usage of menstrual products (ie, tampons versus menstrual pads). Other explanations include a difference in the susceptibility to TSS and the inability to recognize the characteristic early rash in dark-skinned individuals.[79] The early data also indicated a possible difference in the geographic distribution of menstrual TSS; in 1981 and 1982, more cases occurred in the Mountain and North Central states than on either coast.[81] However, subsequent data do not reveal any geographic variation in incidence.[78]

Etiology/Manifestation of TSS Obviously, TSS is a severe, life-threatening disease. Known to result from infections (at any site) with toxin-producing strains of *Staphylococcus aureus*, TSS is essentially a consequence of the systemic effects of the toxin. The major cause of TSS is TSST-1, an exotoxin produced by 90–100% of the strains of *S aureus* associated with menstrual TSS and by 60–75% of the strains associated with nonmenstrual TSS.[79,82] The effects of TSST-1 are due to both the direct effects of the toxin and the toxin's ability to induce production of two cytokines. The biologic properties of TSST-1, either directly or via the other cytokines, include induction of fever, enhanced susceptibility to endotoxin shock, blockade of the reticuloendothelial system, lymphocyte mitogenicity, enhancement of delayed-type hypersensitivity skin reactions, inhibition of neutrophil chemotaxis, and suppression of immunoglobulins. Further study of *S aureus* has shown that the presence of *Escherichia coli* can facilitate its growth and the production of TSST-1. Other toxins are also associated with the production of TSS.[79]

The clinical manifestations of TSS characteristically evolve quite rapidly. Within 8–12 hours an individual can move from a state of good health to full-blown TSS, which includes high fever, myalgias, vomiting and diarrhea, erythroderma, decreased urine output, severe hypotension, and shock.[78,79] The hypotension is characteristically profound; even individuals with mild cases often experience syncope.[79] This hypotension is due to several factors, including a decrease in vasomotor tone, which allows for the pooling of blood in the periphery; a leaking of fluid from the intravascular space to the interstitial space ("second-spacing"); depressed heart function; and volume depletion caused by vomiting, diarrhea, and fever. Multisystem organ involvement typically occurs in TSS. Myalgias, muscle weakness, arthralgias, and GI symptoms (vomiting, diarrhea, and abdominal pain) typically occur early in the illness and affect almost all patients. Neurologic manifestations also occur in almost all cases. Encephalopathy from cerebral edema can be manifested as headache, confusion, agitation, lethargy, and seizures. Both acute renal failure and adult respiratory distress syndrome are also common in this condition.

Dermatologic manifestations are also characteristic of TSS; both the early rash and subsequent skin desquamation are required for a definite diagnosis. The early rash is often described as a sunburnlike, diffuse, macular erythroderma that is not pruritic. It usually appears on the lower abdomen and thighs but may involve the perineum, torso, or extremities. This rash is often most intense in the area of infection, perhaps reflecting a high local concentration of toxin or mediators. It usually disappears after 3 days, and about 1–3 weeks later, desquamation of the skin on the patient's soles and palms begins. A second rash (very erythematous, pruritic, and maculopapular) occurs in more than 50% of patients. Telogen effluvium, a late dermatologic manifestation that is a common, nonspecific reaction to severe sepsis and stress, may also be seen. Telogen effluvium describes the loss of hair and/or nails, which can occur after 4–16 weeks; growth is restored in 5–6 months.[79,80]

Risk Factors for TSS Risk factors for menstrual TSS have been identified. The strongest predictor of risk is the use of tampons. One study found that women who use tampons have a 33 times greater risk than those who do not.[79,81] A case-control study from 1986 to 1987 found that the use of all major tampon brands was associated with the increased risk although the risk varied by the brand of tampon.[76] The risk also varied with the absorbency of the tampon: two studies found that for every 1-g increase in absorbency, the risk for TSS increased 34–37%.[76,81] Additionally, the occurrence of TSS has been related to tampon composition, which can alter the presence of several factors (eg, oxygen, magnesium, and glucose) that can influence the production of toxin by *S aureus*.[78] Since the early 1980s, when the association between tampon usage and TSS was first noted, the absorbency and composition of tampons have changed dramatically. Nonetheless, the risk for TSS continues to be greater in tampon users than in other individuals, and the greatest risk is associated with the use of higher-absorbency tampons. Finally, patterns of tampon use may affect risk for TSS. Continuous use of tampons for at least 1 day of menses has been shown to correlate with an increased risk for menstrual TSS.[76] This association persisted even after the investigators controlled for the absorbency of the tampon product.

The question of whether tampons induce changes in vaginal microflora has received considerable attention. Both qualitative and quantitative changes in vaginal microflora (aerobic and anaerobic) occur during the menstrual cycle. Neither the type of menstrual product used nor the composition of tampons affected either of these parameters for women who had previously used tampons.[83] However, one study found a change in the number of staphylococci present when women who had previously used menstrual pads switched to tampons.[76] Tampons do not appear to act as a focus for microbial growth. Bacterial counts from vaginal swabs were consistently higher than those obtained from tampons; lower levels of bacterial counts were obtained from tampons after both 2 and 6 hours of use.

In addition to tampons, the risk for TSS has been associated with the use of all barrier contraceptives, including diaphragms, cervical caps, and cervical sponges. This risk has been calculated to be about 10–12 times greater for women who use these forms of contraception than for women who do not. Neither oral contraceptive use nor use of an intrauterine device has been related to the development of TSS.[84]

The Pharmacist's Role in TSS Counseling A pharmacist should be able to counsel a patient about the prevention of TSS, emphasizing that the risk for this condition is quite small; recent data suggest an incidence of 1–2.5 per 100,000 menstruating women.[76] Avoidance or reduction of risk can be accomplished if patients follow the guidelines listed below:

- To reduce the risk for TSS to almost zero, women should use sanitary pads instead of tampons.
- To lower the risk for TSS while using tampons, women should use the lowest-absorbency tampons compatible with their needs and should alternate the use of menstrual pads (eg, at night) with the use of tampons. Although frequent changing of tampons has not been found to reduce the risk for TSS, changing them at least four to six times per day is often suggested.
- Women should wash their hands with soap before inserting anything into the vagina (eg, a tampon, a diaphragm, a contraceptive sponge, or a vaginal medication).

- Women should follow instructions for vaginal contraceptive products carefully. A sponge or diaphragm or cervical cap should not be left in place in the vagina longer than recommended and should not be used during a menstrual period.
- During the first 12 weeks after childbirth, women should not use tampons, contraceptive sponges, or a cervical cap, and it may be best to avoid using a diaphragm as well.
- Every woman should be encouraged to read the insert on TSS enclosed in the tampon package and familiarize herself with the early symptoms of TSS. These include a high fever, muscle aches, a sunburnlike rash appearing after a day or two, weakness, fatigue, nausea, vomiting, and diarrhea.
- If the early symptoms of TSS occur, the tampon should be removed immediately and emergency medical treatment should be sought.[78] In severe cases, TSS can cause dizziness, faintness, shock, and even death.

Women who have had TSS are at higher risk for recurrent episodes, especially during the first year after the illness, because it takes at least that long for protective antibodies to reappear. Prevention of TSS for these patients includes avoidance of tampons; administration of oral antistaphylococcal antibiotics during menses until there is a rise in the TSST-1 titer[79,80]; and the use of nonbarrier forms of contraception, at least until the TSST-1 titers rise.[84]

Case Studies

Case 6–1

Patient Complaint/History

MP, a 34-year-old female, enters the pharmacy and requests advice on the use of a nonprescription vaginal antifungal product. Based on her symptoms, which include a clumpy white vaginal discharge and intense vulvar itching, the patient thinks that she has a "yeast" infection. She has selected Monistat 7 (100-mg) vaginal suppositories for purchase.

During further conversation with the pharmacist, MP explains that her physician prescribed the Monistat 7 suppositories for a couple of previous yeast infections that occurred about 2 years ago. Because she expects her "period" in the next several days, the patient asks about using suppositories during her menses.

MP is in good general health with no chronic medical problems. Her patient profile reveals seasonal allergic rhinitis and intermittent sinusitis but no drug allergies. She currently takes chlorpheniramine 4 mg hs or bid prn; Ortho-Novum 1/35 21 one tablet daily for 21 days, 7 days off; amoxicillin 500 mg tid; and Sudafed 30–60 mg qid prn.

Clinical Considerations/Strategies

The following considerations/strategies are provided to aid the reader in (1) determining whether treatment of the patient's condition with nonprescription medications is warranted, (2) selecting the appropriate nonprescription medication, and (3) developing a patient counseling strategy to ensure optimal therapeutic outcomes:

- Assess the appropriateness of self-treatment of the vaginal symptoms: Are the symptoms similar to those that the patient experienced previously? Are they consistent with candidal vulvovaginitis?
- Assess the appropriateness of the selected dosage form.
- Discuss with the patient her possible risk factors for candidal vulvovaginitis.
- Develop a patient education/counseling strategy that will:
  - Explain when self-treatment is appropriate for vaginal symptoms, what symptomatic relief to expect, when physician evaluation is necessary, and what risks are associated with uninformed self-treatment for recurrent vaginal symptoms;
  - Explain the optimal use of the vaginal antifungal and the potential side effects of this therapy.

Case 6–2

Patient Complaint/History

LB, a 27-year-old female, comes to the pharmacy counter and asks whether Advil or Aleve is better for dysmenorrhea. She reveals that in her late teens a physician diagnosed her as having primary dysmenorrhea.

The patient's symptoms, which include severe cramping, backache, and diarrhea, usually occur when her period begins and last about 2 days. After she married and began taking "the Pill," her symptoms improved a great deal. However, she recently stopped taking the oral contraceptive because she and her husband want to start a family. Since then she has experienced symptoms of dysmenorrhea every month. Further, because of menstrual cramps, she has missed 2 days of work in each of the last 2 months. LB recently saw her nurse clinician about the symptoms, who confirmed that they were consistent with dysmenorrhea and added that their intensity would most likely diminish following a pregnancy. Until she becomes pregnant, the patient wants to take something to relieve the symptoms and avoid missing work.

LB is in good general health. Her patient profile shows an allergy to sulfa drugs, which is manifested as hives. Minor medical problems include mild acne for which she applies erythromycin topical solution 2% once daily hs. The recently discontinued contraceptive is listed as Brevicon 21-Day.

Clinical Considerations/Strategies

The following considerations/strategies are provided to aid the reader in (1) determining whether treatment of the patient's condition with nonprescription medications is warranted, (2) selecting the appropriate nonprescription medication, and (3) developing a patient counseling strategy to ensure optimal therapeutic outcomes:

- Compare and contrast the patient-selected nonprescription NSAIDs (ie, indications, warnings/precautions, drug interactions, and adverse effects).
- Discuss dosage recommendations for the use of nonprescription NSAIDs (ie, dose, frequency of administration, and duration of therapy) to relieve symptoms of primary dysmenorrhea.

- Develop a protocol for the management of ambulatory patients with dysmenorrhea; include initial drug selection, initial dose selection, dose modifications, possible switch to another NSAID, and medical referral.
- Develop a nondrug therapy that could be recommended as an adjunct to the drug management of dysmenorrhea.
- Develop a patient education/counseling approach that will explain the optimal use of an NSAID for the treatment of dysmenorrhea.

Summary

Nonprescription topical imidazole therapy for vaginal infections requires that the pharmacist counsel the patient on the proper selection and use of these products (drugs and dosage forms). The pharmacist must also be able to identify symptomatic patients who should be referred to a physician. With advice and consultation from the pharmacist, many patients with uncomplicated candidal vulvovaginitis can be safely and appropriately managed.

Most women function normally and require minimal or no pharmacologic intervention for menstrual cycle–related symptoms. If necessary, the relief of many minor menstrual symptoms may be accomplished with nonprescription products. However, more severe symptoms and specific menstrual disorders, such as amenorrhea, dysmenorrhea, menstrual dysfunction, and significant PMS symptoms, may require referral to a physician for evaluation.

References

1. Fawcett DW. *A Textbook of Histology*. 11th ed. Philadelphia: WB Sanders; 1986: 896–8.
2. Gray H. *Anatomy of the Human Body*. 13th ed. Clemente CD, ed. Philadelphia: Lea and Febiger; 1985: 1578–81.
3. Moore KL. *Clinically Oriented Anatomy*. 2nd ed. Baltimore: Williams and Wilkins; 1985: 370–3.
4. Tortora GJ, Grabowski SR. *Principles of Anatomy and Physiology*. 7th ed. New York: Harper Collins College Publishers; 1993: 943–5.
5. Rein MF. Vulvovaginitis and cervicitis. In: Mandell GL, Douglas RG, Bennett JE, eds. *Principles and Practice of Infectious Diseases*. New York: Churchill Livingstone; 1990: 953–65.
6. McCue JD. Evaluation and management of vaginitis: an update for primary care practitioners. *Arch Intern Med*. 1989; 149: 565–68.
7. Eschenbach DA. Vaginal infection. *Clin Obstet Gynecol*. 1983; 26: 186–202.
8. Sobel JD. Vulvovaginitis. *Dermatol Clin*. 1992; 10(2): 339–59.
9. Paavonen J, Stamm WE. Lower genital tract infections in women. *Infect Dis Clin North Am*. 1987; 1: 179–98.
10. Reed BD, Eyler A. Vaginal infections: diagnosis and management. *Am Fam Physician*. 1993; 47(8): 1805–16.
11. Schaaf VM, Pérez-Stable EJ, Borchardt K. The limited value of symptoms and signs in the diagnosis of vaginal infections. *Arch Intern Med*. 1990; 150: 1929–33.
12. Taylor CA, Lipsky MS. Physicians' perceptions of the impact of the reclassification of vaginal antifungal agents. *J Fam Pract*. 1994; 38: 157–60.
13. MacDermott RI. Bacterial vaginosis. *Br J Obstet Gynaecol*. 1995; 102: 92–4.
14. Kent HL. Epidemiology of vaginitis. *Am J Obstet Gynecol*. 1991; 165: 1168–76.
15. Goode MA. Infectious vaginitis. Selecting therapy and preventing recurrence. *Postgrad Med*. 1994; 96: 85–8, 91–8.
16. McCutchan JA et al. Evaluation of new anti-infective drugs for the treatment of vaginal infections. *Clin Infect Dis*. 1992; 15(suppl 1): S115–22.
17. Schlitch JR. Treatment of bacterial vaginosis. *Ann Pharmacother*. 1994; 28: 483–7.
18. Reed BD. Risk factors for candida vulvovaginitis. *Obstet Gynecol Surv*. 1992; 47(8): 551–60.
19. Foxman B. The epidemiology of vulvovaginal candidiasis: risk factors. *Am J Public Health*. 1990; 80: 329–31.
20. Hilton E et al. Ingestion of yogurt containing *Lactobacillus acidophilus* as prophylaxis for candidal vaginitis. *Ann Intern Med*. 1992; 116: 353–7.
21. Sobel JD. Pathogenesis and treatment of recurrent vulvovaginal candidiasis. *Clin Infect Dis*. 1992; 14(suppl 1): S148–53.
22. Holmes KK, Handsfield HH. Sexually transmitted diseases. In: Wilson JD et al, eds. *Harrison's Principles of Internal Medicine*. New York: McGraw-Hill; 1991: 524–33.
23. Thomason JL. Clinical evaluation of terconazole: United States experience. *J Reprod Med*. 1989; 34(suppl): 597–601.
24. Kjaeldgaard A. Comparison of terconazole and clotrimazole vaginal tablets in the treatment of vulvovaginal candidosis. *Pharmatherapeutica*. 1986; 4: 525–31.
25. Koerign PL, Santiago TM. Drugs for treatment of vulvovaginal candidiasis: comparative efficacy of agents and regimens. *DICP Ann Pharmacother*. 1990; 24: 1078–83.
26. Cauwenbergh G, Bossche HV. Terconazole pharmacology of a new antimycotic agent. *J Reprod Med*. 1989; 34(suppl): 588–92.
27. Ritter W et al. Pharmacokinetic fundamentals of vaginal treatment with clotrimazole. *Chemotherapy*. 1982; 28(suppl 1): 37–42.
28. Abrams LS, Weintraub HS. Disposition of radioactivity following intravaginal administration of 3H-miconazole nitrate. *Am J Obstet Gynecol*. 1983; 147: 970–1.
29. Nixon SA. Vulvovaginitis: the role of patient compliance in treatment success. *Am J Obstet Gynecol*. 1991; 165: 1207–9.
30. Ernest JM. Topical antifungal agents. *Obstet Gynecol Clin North Am*. 1992; 19(3): 587–607.
31. Rosenberg MJ et al. Vaginal douching. *J Reprod Med*. 1991; 36(10): 753–8.
32. Aral SO, Mosher WD, Cates W Jr. Vaginal douching among women of reproductive age in the United States: 1988. *Am J Public Health*. 1992; 82: 210–4.
33. McGowan L. Peritonitis following the vaginal douche and a proposed alternative. *Am J Obstet Gynecol*. 1965; 90(4): 506–9.
34. Gossel TA. Feminine hygiene products. *US Pharm*. 1992; 17(5): 24–32.
35. Gossel TA. Feminine hygiene products: why your advice is needed. *US Pharm*. 1986; 11(5): 20–7.
36. Onderdonk AB et al. Quantitative and qualitative effects of douche preparations on vaginal microflora. *Obstet Gynecol*. 1992; 80(pt 1): 333–8.
37. Safran M, Braverman LE. Effect of chronic douching with polyvinylpyrrolidone-iodine on iodine absorption and thyroid function. *Obstet Gynecol*. 1982; 60: 35–40.
38. Mahillon I et al. Effect of vaginal douching with povidone-iodine during early pregnancy on the iodine supply to mother and fetus. *Biol Neonate*. 1989; 56: 210–7.
39. Neinstein LS. Menstrual problems in adolescents. *Med Clin North Am*. 1990; 74(5): 1181–203.
40. Willis J. Demystifying menopause. *FDA Consumer*. 1988 Jul/Aug; 22: 24–9.

41. Shimp LA. Hormone replacement therapy. *J Mich Pharm Assoc.* 1991; 29(6): 218–21.
42. Hatcher RA et al. The menstrual cycle. In: *Contraceptive Technology, 1990–1992.* 15th ed, rev. New York: Irvington Publishers; 1990: 39–46.
43. Espey LL, Halim IA. Characteristics and control of the normal menstrual cycle. *Obstet Gynecol Clin North Am.* 1990; 17(2): 275–98.
44. Kustin J, Rebar RW. Menstrual disorders in the adolescent age group. *Prim Care.* 1987; 14(1): 139–66.
45. Franz WB. Basic review: endocrinology of the normal menstrual cycle. *Prim Care.* 1988; 15(3): 607–16.
46. Field CS. Dysfunctional uterine bleeding. *Prim Care.* 1988; 15(3): 561–74.
47. Avant RF. Dysmenorrhea. *Prim Care.* 1988; 15(3): 549–59.
48. Dawood MY. Dysmenorrhea. *Clin Obstet Gynecol.* 1990; 33(1): 168–78.
49. Kauppila A, Puolakka J, Ylikorkala O. The relief of primary dysmenorrhea by ketoprofen and indomethacin. *Prostaglandins.* 1979; 18(4): 647–53.
50. Johnson J. Level of knowledge among adolescent girls regarding effective treatment for dysmenorrhea. *J Adolesc Health Care.* 1988; 9: 398–402.
51. Smith RP. Cyclic pelvic pain and dysmenorrhea. *Obstet Gynecol Clin North Am.* 1993; 20: 753–64.
52. Jensen DV, Andersen KB, Wagner G. Prostaglandins in the menstrual cycle of women. *Dan Med Bull.* 1987; 34(3): 178–81.
53. Sundell G, Milsom I, Andersch B. Factors influencing the prevalence and severity of dysmenorrhea in young women. *Br J Obstet Gynaecol.* 1990; 97: 588–94.
54. Barry JA. Dysmenorrhoea: periods can be a pain. *Aust Fam Physician.* 1988; 17(3): 174–5.
55. Putukian M. The female triad. Eating disorders, amenorrhea, and osteoporosis. *Med Clin North Am.* 1994; 78: 345–56.
56. Doody KM, Carr BR. Amenorrhea. *Obstet Gynecol Clin North Am.* 1990; 17(2): 361–87.
57. Henley K, Vaitukaitis JL. Exercise-induced menstrual dysfunction. *Ann Rev Med.* 1988; 39: 443–51.
58. Olson BR. Exercise-induced amenorrhea. *Am Fam Physician.* 1989; 39(2): 213–21.
59. Long CA, Gast MJ. Menorrhagia. *Obstet Gynecol Clin North Am.* 1990; 17(2): 343–59.
60. Coupey SM, Ahlstrom P. Common menstrual disorders. *Pediatr Clin North Am.* 1989; 36(3): 551–71.
61. Johnson SR. The epidemiology and social impact of premenstrual symptoms. *Clin Obstet Gynecol.* 1987; 30(2): 367–76.
62. Chihal HJ. Premenstrual syndrome: an update for the clinician. *Obstet Gynecol Clin North Am.* 1990; 17(2): 457–79.
63. Robinson GE. Premenstrual syndrome: current knowledge and management. *Can Med Assoc J.* 1989; 140: 605–10.
64. Wickes SL. Premenstrual syndrome. *Prim Care.* 1988; 15(3): 473–87.
65. Robinson GE, Garfinkel PE. Problems in the treatment of premenstrual syndrome. *Can J Psychiatry.* 1990; 35(3): 199–206.
66. Lurie S, Borenstein R. The premenstrual syndrome. *Obstet Gynecol Surv.* 1990; 45(4): 220–8.
67. Kendall KE, Schnurr PP. The effects of vitamin B_6 supplementation on premenstrual symptoms. *Obstet Gynecol.* 1987; 70(2): 145–9.
68. Parker PD. Premenstrual syndrome. *Am Fam Physician.* 1994; 50(6): 1309–17.
69. *Federal Register.* 1988; 53: 46194–202.
70. Leonard TK, Watson RR, Mohs ME. The effects of caffeine on various body systems: a review. *J Am Diet Assoc.* 1987; 87: 1048–53.
71. Gass ML, Rebar RW. Management of problems during menopause. *Compr Ther.* 1990; 16(2): 3–10.
72. Sarazin SK, Seymour SF. Causes and treatment options for women with dyspareunia. *Nurse Pract.* 1991; 16(10): 30–41.
73. Chantigian PDM. Vaginitis: a common malady. *Prim Care.* 1988; 15(3): 517–45.
74. Sandberg G, Quevillon RP. Dyspareunia: an integrated approach to assessment and diagnosis. *J Fam Pract.* 1987; 24(1): 66–9.
75. *Federal Register.* 1980; 45: 12713.
76. Reingold AL et al. Risk factors for menstrual toxic shock syndrome: results of a multistate case–control study. *Rev Infect Dis.* 1989; 2(suppl 1): S35–41.
77. Nightingale SL. New requirements for tampon labeling. *Am Fam Physician.* 1990; 41(3): 999–1000.
78. Reingold AL. Toxic shock syndrome: an update. *Am J Obstet Gynecol.* 1991; 165: 1236–9.
79. Freedman JD, Beer DJ. Expanding perspectives on the toxic shock syndrome. *Adv Intern Med.* 1991; 36: 363–97.
80. Chesney PJ. Clinical aspects and spectrum of illness of toxic shock syndrome: overview. *Rev Infect Dis.* 1989; 11(suppl 1): S1–7.
81. Broome CV. Epidemiology of toxic shock syndrome in the United States: overview. *Rev Infect Dis.* 1989; 11(suppl 1): S14–21.
82. Chow A. Microbiology of toxic shock syndrome: overview. *Rev Infect Dis.* 1989; 11(suppl 1): S55–60.
83. Onderdonk AB et al. Normal vaginal microflora during use of various forms of catamenial protection. *Rev Infect Dis.* 1989; 11(suppl 1): S61–7.
84. Schwartz B et al. Nonmenstrual toxic shock syndrome associated with barrier contraceptives: report of a case–control study. *Rev Infect Dis.* 1989; 11(suppl 1): S43–9.

CHAPTER 7

Contraceptive Methods and Products

Louise Parent-Stevens and David L. Lourwood

Questions to ask in patient assessment and counseling

- *What type of contraceptive method are you now using?*
- *What contraceptive products have you used before?*
- *What did you like or dislike about your current or previous contraceptive method?*
- *Are you in a monogamous relationship now?*
- *What does your partner like or dislike about your current or previous contraceptive method?*
- *Have you discussed contraception and sexual health matters with your physician or another health care provider?*
- *Do you belong to a religious faith that has specific guidelines concerning family planning?*
- *Do you have children already? Do you want additional children?*
- *Do you know what your risks are for being infected with the virus that causes acquired immunodeficiency syndrome (AIDS) or with other sexually transmitted diseases?*
- *How do you protect yourself from sexually transmitted diseases, including AIDS?*

Throughout history, people have sought ways to control their fertility in order to choose the number and timing of their pregnancies. The earliest recorded methods of contraception include coitus interruptus, mentioned in the Book of Genesis of the Bible; barrier methods, such as the vaginal pessaries made of crocodile dung used in ancient Egypt; and early cervical caps made from lemon halves, a method said to have been used by Casanova.[1] As knowledge of reproductive physiology has evolved, a wider variety of safe and reliable methods of contraception has been developed.

According to the 1992 Ortho Birth Control Study of 15- to 44-year-old US women at risk for unintended pregnancy, oral contraceptives are the most widely used method of conception control; 39% of all women aged 15 to 44 use the birth control pill as their primary method of contraception. The next most prevalent method is sterilization of either the male or the female. After that, 25% of the women surveyed relied on condoms, 5% used spermicides, 4% used the diaphragm, and 1% had received a hormonal implant. Some patients reported using multiple methods. Overall, 94% of women aged 15 to 44 years reported using some form of birth control.[2]

In the United States and worldwide, reliance on nonprescription methods of contraception is widespread. The fact that nonprescription contraceptive products are accessible and relatively inexpensive makes them very important for those who do not have access to family planning services, choose not to use physicians or clinics, or are unable or unwilling to use a prescription contraceptive method. Even if a prescription product is chosen as the primary contraceptive method, low-cost and low-risk nonprescription methods may be appropriate at different times during a person's sexually active life.

Uses for Contraceptive Products

Unwanted Pregnancies

Consistent and proper use of a contraceptive, whether prescription or nonprescription, will significantly reduce the incidence of unwanted pregnancies. Moreover, a recent survey of women undergoing counseling for unplanned pregnancies found that inconsistent or improper use of contraceptives was responsible for 74% of unwanted pregnancies.[3] Given that at least 40% of pregnancies in the United States are unplanned,[4,5] it is apparent that much more attention needs to be paid to family planning and contraceptive counseling.

Of particular concern is the high risk of pregnancy in the adolescent population. The 1988 National Survey of Family Growth found that 38% of 15- to 17-year-old women and 74% of 18- to 19-year-old women had experienced sexual intercourse. Of the teenagers who were sexually active, only 65% used a contraceptive method during their first sexual encounter. Among teenagers who used a contraceptive method during their first sexual encounter, the most popular choice of contraceptive was condoms (47%). Withdrawal was used by as many teenagers as birth control pills (8%). However, 35% of the sexually active adolescents used no contraceptive method.[4] The teenage pregnancy rate in the United States (11% of 15- to 19-year-olds), which is high compared with that in other developed countries, may have much to do with the fact that the average US teenager has unprotected intercourse for an average of 1 year before seeking contraceptive advice.[4,6]

Editor's Note: This chapter is based, in part, on the chapter with the same title that appeared in the 10th edition but was written by Louise Parent-Stevens and Roberta S. Carrier.

Reasons why adolescents delay seeking contraceptive advice include fear about the perceived dangers of contraceptives, fear of parental discovery, and belief that they cannot get pregnant because of their young age or low frequency of intercourse.[7] However, half of all adolescent pregnancies occur within the first 6 months after the initiation of sexual intercourse, with 20% occurring during the first month.[8] Eighty-five percent of teenage pregnancies are unintended.[5] Only one in three sexually active teenagers consistently uses contraception. Often contraceptives are not used until after the young woman becomes pregnant. Clearly, efforts to disseminate accurate reproductive information as well as to provide access to contraceptive products are vital to addressing this serious public health problem.

Sexually Transmitted Diseases

In addition to the risk of pregnancy, sexually active persons who do not use condoms place themselves at significant risk for acquiring a sexually transmitted disease (STD). Adolescents and young adults under the age of 25 years account for two thirds of all cases of STDs.[9] Among 13- to 19-year-old females, heterosexual intercourse with a partner infected with human immunodeficiency virus (HIV, the AIDS virus) is responsible for more than 50% of newly reported AIDS cases. Additionally, females constitute a greater portion of newly diagnosed AIDS cases in the teenage population than in older populations.[10] Often adolescents engage in risky behavior because they perceive themselves to be immune to contracting AIDS.[11] Education of this population must include the real probability that risky sexual behavior may lead to the acquisition of this deadly disease.

Types of Sexually Transmitted Diseases

There are more than 20 STDs, both bacterial and viral, that may have severe, long-standing consequences on the health and reproductive capabilities of those infected. The presence of some STDs may increase a person's susceptibility to and risk of acquiring the HIV infection.[12]

AIDS The incidence of AIDS is increasing almost exponentially. The first 100,000 cases of the full-blown disease were reported over a 99-month period (June 1981–August 1989); however, the next 100,000 cases were reported over a period of just 27 months (September 1989–November 1991).[13] The female portion of reported cases among adults and adolescents has increased from 3% in 1981 to 13% in 1992–1993. About a quarter of the women with AIDS are 20–29 years old, suggesting that many were infected in their teen years.[10,14]

The known routes of transmission of AIDS are (1) blood and blood products (via transfusions, the sharing of contaminated needles and syringes, and accidental contamination from needle sticks); (2) mucous membrane exposures (saliva, seminal fluid, and vaginal fluids, including menstrual blood); and (3) perinatal and peripartum transmission to infants. In the United States, at least 65% of HIV infections are transmitted via heterosexual or homosexual intercourse.[15] Table 1 provides a list of safer sex options as well as high-risk sexual activities.

Chlamydia Chlamydia is now the most commonly occurring STD in the United States. Chlamydia is an obligate intracellular parasite that often does not present with immediate symptoms for the female but may lead to pelvic inflammatory disease (PID), infertility, and chronic pelvic pain. As many as 3 million cases of chlamydia infection may occur in women annually.[16] Women infected with chlamydia most often present with a mucopurulent discharge from the cervix. Unfortunately, many women do not recognize this discharge as abnormal.

Men often present with nongonococcal urethritis (NGU). This infection is caused by chlamydia in up to 50% of cases, yet it may also be caused by other sexually transmittable organisms such as *Ureaplasma urealyticum*, *Trichomonas vaginalis*, and herpes simplex virus. NGU is believed to occur more often than gonorrhea in men, with more than 2 million cases estimated to occur annually.[16] Symptoms in men include dysuria, urinary frequency, and mucoid to purulent urethral discharge. It is important to realize that many men will have asymptomatic infections. Several complications, including urethral strictures and epididymitis, may occur in a male with untreated NGU.

NGU may be transmitted to female sexual partners with complications as listed above for chlamydia. Chlamydia may be transmitted by a pregnant woman to the fetus and result in neonatal infections such as ophthalmia or pneumonia.

Gonorrhea Gonorrhea remains a major STD in the United States. Approximately 700,000 cases of gonorrhea were reported in 1992. When unreported cases are added, an estimated 1.5 million cases of gonorrhea occur annually.[16] Males who are symptomatic will present with dysuria, increased urinary frequency, and a purulent urethral discharge. Women with gonorrhea may have an abnormal vaginal discharge, abnormal menses, or dysuria. Gonorrhea may also present in the pharynx and the anus. Pharyngeal involvement will most often present as acute pharyngitis. Anal disease will produce symptoms of diarrhea, tenesmus, or constipation. Up to one fourth of men infected with gonorrhea and as many as three fourths of women may be asymptomatic.

Up to 40% of untreated women with gonorrhea may develop PID with complications as previously described. Men, when untreated, are at increased risk for epididymitis, urethral stricture, and sterility.[16] In both sexes, gonorrhea may also disseminate to involve the skeletal, cardiovascular, and nervous systems. Finally, gonorrhea may be transmitted to newborns who may present with ophthalmia neonatorum, scalp abscesses (at the site of fetal monitors), rhinitis, and anorectal infections.

Herpes Infections Herpes genitalis is caused by herpes simplex virus types 1 or 2, both of which are DNA viruses that cannot be clinically distinguished. Type 2 infection is more common in genital infections. Symptomatic primary disease may affect as many as 200,000 persons each year.[16] Recurrent infections are much more common, with as many as 30 million Americans being infected.

Both sexes may present with single or multiple vesicles, which are usually quite pruritic. These vesicles, which may appear anywhere on the genitalia, spontaneously

TABLE 1 Safer sex options for physical intimacy

Safe

Massage
Hugging
Body rubbing
Dry kissing
Masturbation
Hand-to-genital touching (hand job) or mutual masturbation
Erotic books and movies
All sexual activities when both partners are monogamous, trustworthy, and known by testing to be free of HIV

Possibly safe

Wet kissing with no broken skin, cracked lips, or damaged mouth tissue
Vaginal or rectal intercourse using latex or synthetic condom correctly
Oral sex on a man using a latex or synthetic condom
Oral sex on a woman using a latex or synthetic barrier such as a female condom, dental dam, or modified male condom, especially if she does not have her period or a vaginal infection with discharge
All sexual activities when both partners are in a long-term monogamous relationship and trust each other

Unsafe in the absence of HIV testing and trust and monogamy

Any vaginal or rectal intercourse without a latex or synthetic condom
Oral sex on a man without a latex or synthetic condom
Oral sex on a woman without a latex or synthetic barrier such as a female condom, dental dam, or modified male condom, especially if she is having her period or has a vaginal infection with discharge
Semen in the mouth
Oral-anal contact
Sharing sex toys or douching equipment
Blood contact of any kind, including menstrual blood, or any sex that causes tissue damage or bleeding

Reprinted with permission from Hatcher RA et al. *Contraceptive Technology*. 16th rev ed. New York: Irvington Publishers; 1994: 55.

rupture to form a shallow ulcer that may be quite painful. Lesions then spontaneously resolve with minimal scarring. First, or primary, clinical infections often take longer to heal and are more often symptomatic. Subsequent, or recurrent, infections are usually milder and resolve quicker. Recurrent infections may be asymptomatic in some individuals. It is important to realize that drug therapy for herpes does not result in cure but only ameliorates the symptoms and hastens the healing of the ulcers. Thus, patients with herpetic genital infections remain infectious all their lives. Patients are most infectious at the time of active occurrences.

Genital herpes has been associated with an increased risk for contracting HIV infections. This risk is especially high when ulcers are present.

Syphilis Syphilis currently affects 40,000 persons each year in the United States, with a higher prevalence among persons in the lower socioeconomic strata.[16] Over the past decade, syphilis reached its highest level in the past 40 years. Recent syphilis outbreaks have been associated with the exchange of sex for drugs, particularly crack cocaine.

Symptoms of syphilis vary, based on the stage of the disease. Primary syphilis presents with a classic chancre. This chancre is a painless, indurated ulcer located at the site of exposure. Any genital lesions should be suspected of being indicative of syphilis. In men, this chancre may appear on the penis; in women, the chancre may be difficult to see because it is found on the internal structures of the genital tract. Chancres may also appear inside the anus, in the pharynx, on the lips, or on the fingers of infected individuals.

The secondary stage of syphilis may present as a highly variable skin rash. Mucous patches, condylomata lata, lymphadenopathy, and alopecia are also common. Latent syphilis will be asymptomatic. Patients who are untreated may present with sequelae of late disease, including neurosyphilis, cardiovascular disease, and localized gumma formation.

Hepatitis B Hepatitis B is not often thought of as a sexually transmittable disease, yet it can often be passed by sexual activity. It is estimated that 5–20% of segments of the US population may show evidence of past hepatitis and that about 150,000 new cases are transmitted sexually each year.[32] Heterosexual intercourse is now the predominant mode of hepatitis transmission.

Most hepatitis infections are asymptomatic. Symptoms, when noted, may include a serum sickness–like prodrome (skin eruptions, urticaria, arthralgia, and arthritis), lassitude, anorexia, nausea, vomiting, headache, fever, dark urine, jaundice, and moderate liver enlargement with tenderness. Long-term complications of hepatitis can include chronic, persistent, and active hepatitis; cirrhosis; hepatocellular carcinoma; hepatic failure; and death.

Trichomoniasis Trichomoniasis is predominantly noted as a vaginal infection. The infection usually presents with a frothy, excessive vaginal discharge; other symptoms include erythema, edema, and pruritus of the external genitalia. Also, dysuria and dyspareunia may be common. In some women, however, trichomoniasis may be asymptomatic. Men will rarely present with symptoms but may present with urethritis, balanitis, or cutaneous lesions on the penis. It is important to realize that symptomatology alone will not distinguish the etiology of the disease. Complications of trichomoniasis include common recurrent infections and infections secondary to excoriations. Increased risk of PID, low birth weight, and prematurity may occur.

Bacterial Vaginosis Bacterial vaginosis is a syndrome caused by several species of vaginal bacteria, including *Gardnerella vaginalis*, *Mycoplasma hominis*, and various anaerobes such as *Mobiluncus*. Common symptoms include an excessive or malodorous vaginal discharge; erythema, edema, and pruritus of the external genitalia may also be seen. Recurrent infections may be common in untreated patients, as may be secondary infections due to excoriations. An increased risk of PID and premature childbirth may be common in patients with bacterial vaginosis.

Prevention of STDs

Given the prevalence of these diseases and the fact that well over 1 million Americans are HIV-positive, the prevention of STDs must be a priority. As health care practitioners in a position to offer much-needed health information, pharmacists must keep current in their knowledge of all aspects of the prevention and treatment of STDs, especially with respect to AIDS.

The only sure way to guard against infection with the AIDS virus through sexual contact is to abstain from sex or to remain in a mutually monogamous relationship with an uninfected individual. If neither action is feasible, the next option is to use latex (not natural membrane) condoms for any oral, anal, or vaginal intercourse.[17] Most data indicate that the male condom can protect against HIV transmission, and some authorities believe the female condom may provide similar protection.[18] However, the high failure and pregnancy rates of 20–25% reported with the female condom strongly suggest a lack of adequate protection against STDs. In populations at risk, individuals who consistently use male condoms have demonstrated a significantly lower seroconversion rate (an indicator of infection with the AIDS virus) than those who do not use condoms or who use them inconsistently.[19–21]

It is very important to emphasize that condom use does not guarantee safety because condoms can break.[22,23] Laboratory data are being accumulated that suggest that the spermicide nonoxynol-9 in proper concentrations may be somewhat effective in killing the AIDS virus and might offer additional protection when used with condoms.[20,24,25] However, recent data have also indicated that spermicide-mediated vulvovaginal microabrasions could increase a woman's susceptibility to HIV. While the quality of the data to date is questionable, women with compromised vulvar and vaginal tissue may be at an increased risk for susceptibility to HIV.[26,27]

Timing is important in the proper use of the male condom. Patients must realize that seminal fluid can leak from the erect penis in some men. This preejaculatory fluid can contain HIV, other pathogens, and viable sperm.[28,29] Thus, for proper use in safer sex, the condom must be placed on the penis well before contact is made with the partner's mouth, vagina, anus, or any broken skin.

Other contraceptive methods have also been studied for their efficacy in preventing transmission of AIDS.[18,30,31] However, as indicated in Table 2, the use of other nonprescription barrier methods (eg, the diaphragm and cervical cap) has thus far shown limited protection against AIDS as well as against other STDs.[32] The same

TABLE 2 Effects of contraceptives on bacterial and viral STD

Contraceptive method	Bacterial STD	Viral STD
Latex male condoms	Protective	Protective
Polyurethane male condoms	Probably protective	Probably protective
Natural membrane condoms	Protective	Possibly not protective
Female condom	Possibly protective against recurrent vaginal trichomoniasis	Possibly protective
Spermicides	Protective against cervical gonorrhea and chlamydia	Undetermined in vivo
Diaphragms	Protective against cervical infection; associated with vaginal anaerobic overgrowth	Protective against cervical infection
Hormonal	Associated with increased cervical chlamydia, protective against symptomatic PID[a]	Not protective
Intrauterine device	Associated with PID in first month after insertion	Not protective
Natural family planning	Not protective	Not protective

[a]Pelvic inflammatory disease (PID).

Adapted with permission from Hatcher RA et al. *Contraceptive Technology*. 16th rev ed. New York: Irvington Publishers; 1994: 81.

is true for hormonal contraceptives, such as oral contraceptives and parenteral products (eg, depot medroxyprogesterone acetate and levonorgestrel implants). It is also important to keep in mind that some STDs, such as syphilis and herpes, may be spread via external skin lesions. Condoms and spermicides may not be effective in preventing these types of infection.

Because compliance with safer sex practices, especially with regard to condom use, is poor even among those at risk, other behavioral factors aimed at lowering risk should be stressed.[33] These changes include changes in lifestyle and sexual practices.

Choice of Contraceptive Method

There is no perfect method of birth control. Throughout life a woman's reproductive priorities change; her contraceptive choice may change as well. The method selected should be well thought out by the couple involved. The major points to be considered should include safety, effectiveness, accessibility, and acceptability of each method to each sexual partner.

Safety factors to consider in choosing a method of contraception include the risk of side effects as well as protection against infectious STDs, including HIV. It is important that sexually active individuals who are infertile, through either surgical or natural causes, be aware that they are still at risk for contracting and transmitting STDs. Other safety considerations are the potential for method-associated adverse effects on future fertility as well as on the fetus, should unintended conception occur.

The effectiveness of a contraceptive method is reported in two ways: the accidental pregnancy rate in the first year of *perfect* use (method-related failure rate) and the accidental pregnancy rate in the first year of *typical* use (use-related failure rate) (Table 3). The lowest expected rate—that of perfect use—is very difficult to measure and indicates the method's theoretical effectiveness, assuming accurate and consistent use of the method every time intercourse occurs. The more realistic rate of typical use includes pregnancies that may have occurred because of inconsistent or improper use of the method. Reported use-related failure rates may vary, depending on the population studied. Effectiveness increases with increasing length of use of a particular method. Declining fertility in an older user population may contribute to increased effectiveness rates. In addition, couples who use contraception to prevent pregnancy have fewer failures than those who use contraceptives to space the births of their children.[34]

The percentage of people who continue with a given contraceptive method after a year of use is an indication of the method's acceptability (Table 3). Important factors in determining a method's acceptability include user's religious beliefs and future reproductive plans, partner's supportiveness, complexity of method use, degree of interruption of spontaneity, "messiness," and cost. Pharmacists should be aware of the safety, effectiveness, accessibility, acceptability, and relative cost of the different contraceptive methods to help their patients make informed decisions.

Condoms

Male Condoms

Condoms—also known as rubbers, sheaths, prophylactics, safes, skins, or pros—are the most important barrier contraceptive device in an era of infectious STDs. The condom was originally described in the 16th century by Fallopius as a means of protecting the wearer from syphilis.[1] Apart from its role as a contraceptive, its importance in disease prevention is second only to that of abstinence.

Types of Condoms The sheath described by Fallopius was made of linen. Current-day materials, which include latex, polyurethane and lamb cecum (natural membrane, or skin), are much more comfortable for users and their partners.

Condom sales increased by 20% from 1986 to 1988, and the sale of latex condoms treated with spermicide increased by 116%. This increase was attributed to an extensive public health campaign following the release of the US surgeon general's report on AIDS, which recommended that persons at risk use condoms regularly to help prevent HIV transmission.[35] Latex condoms have also been shown to protect against various other STDs[16] (Table 2). Latex condoms come in a variety of colors, styles, shapes, and thicknesses (ranging from 0.03 mm to approximately 0.1 mm). Other available features include reservoir tips, ribs, studs, lubrication, and spermicidal lubrication.[36]

The polyurethane condom has been shown in vitro to be impermeable to HIV; clinical studies to confirm this effect in vivo are ongoing.[37] Additionally, the polyurethane condom is more expensive than latex condoms (Table 4). Until more information is available on the efficacy of the polyurethane condom, its use should be restricted to patients with latex allergies. Condoms made from lamb cecum provide less protection from STDs than do latex condoms because the presence of pores in the membrane may allow the passage of viral organisms, including HIV and the hepatitis B virus.[38] They are also more expensive. Skins should be recommended only for those who have a latex allergy[39] or are not at risk for STDs, such as those in a long-term, mutually monogamous relationship with an uninfected person. There are two brand names of natural membrane condoms on the market, and one polyurethane condom is currently available in the United States although others are under development (see product table "Condom Products").

Breakage Rate Since 1976, condom quality has been under the purview of the Food and Drug Administration (FDA). The Center for Devices and Radiological Health is responsible for monitoring the quality of domestically produced as well as imported condoms.[24,40] The testing program was expanded in 1987 because of concerns about protection from the AIDS virus. The United States uses a water-leak test as the standard. The failure rate per batch is not to exceed 4 condoms per 1,000. Of batches that met the quality guidelines, the average failure rate was 2.3 per 1,000 tested.[24] In 1994, the FDA also adopted the air burst test as one of the tools for testing condoms. In this test, a sample of condoms from a given lot is inflated to the bursting point while a meter measures

TABLE 3 First-year failure/continuation rates of various contraceptive methods[a,b]

Method (1)	% who experience accidental pregnancy in first year of use: Typical use[b] (2)	Perfect use[c] (3)	% who continue using contraceptive method for one year[a] (4)
Chance[d]	85	—	—
Spermicides[e]	21	6	43
Withdrawal	19	4	—
Natural family planning	20	—	67
Calendar (rhythm) method	—	9	—
Cervical mucus (ovulation) method	—	3	—
Symptothermal method[f]	—	2	—
Basal body temperature (postovulation) method	—	1	—
Cervical cap[g]			
Parous women	36	26	45
Nulliparous women	18	9	58
Diaphragm[g]	18	6	58
Condom[h]			
Male	12	3	63
Female	21–25[i]	5	56
Pill	3	—	72
Progestin only	—	0.5	—
Combined (estrogen/progestin)	—	0.1	—
Intrauterine device			
Progesterone T	2.0	1.5	81
Cu T 380A	0.8	0.6	78
Depo-Provera	0.3	0.3	70
Norplant (6 capsules)	0.09	0.09	85
Sterilization			
Female	0.4	0.4	100
Male	0.15	0.10	100

Note. Emergency contraceptive pills: Treatment initiated within 72 hours after unprotected intercourse reduces the risk of pregnancy by at least 75%. The treatment schedule is one dose as soon as possible (but no more than 72 hours) after unprotected intercourse and a second dose 12 hours after the first. The hormones that have been studied in the clinical trials of postcoital hormonal contraception are found in Nordette, Levlen, Lo/Ovral (one dose is four pills), Triphasil, Tri-Levlen (one dose is four yellow pills), and Ovral (one dose is two pills).
Lactational amenorrhea method: This is a highly effective, temporary method of contraception. However, to maintain effective protection against pregnancy, another method of contraception must be used as soon as menstruation resumes, the frequency or duration of breast-feeding is reduced, bottle feeding is introduced, or the baby reaches 6 months of age.

[a]Among couples attempting to avoid pregnancy, the percentage who continue to use a method for 1 year.

[b]Among typical couples who initiate use of a method (not necessarily for the first time), the percentage who experience an accidental pregnancy during the first year if they do not stop use for any other reason.

[c]Among couples who initiate use of a method (not necessarily for the first time) and who use it perfectly (both consistently and correctly), the percentage who experience an accidental pregnancy during the first year if they do not stop use for any other reason.

[d]The percentages failing in columns (2) and (3) are based on data from populations in which contraception is not used and from women who cease using contraception to become pregnant. Among such populations, about 89% become pregnant within 1 year. This estimate was lowered slightly (to 85%) to represent the percentage who would become pregnant within 1 year among women now relying on reversible methods of contraception if they abandoned contraception altogether.

[e]Foams, creams, gels, vaginal suppositories, and vaginal film.

[f]Cervical mucus (ovulation) method supplemented by calendar in the preovulatory phase and by BBT in the postovulatory phase.

[g]With spermicidal cream or jelly.

[h]Without spermicides.

[i]Extrapolated from 6 month failure rates.

Adapted with permission from Hatcher RA et al. *Contraceptive Technology*. 16th rev ed. New York: Irvington Publishers; 1994: 113–4.

TABLE 4 Cost of contraceptive methods, based on assumption of 100 acts of intercourse annually

Method	Unit cost	Annual cost	Comments
Cervical Cap	$45 + $50–150 for fitting	Cost of spermicide: $85	
Male condom			
Latex	$0.50	$50	Add cost of spermicide, if used
Synthetic	$1.50–2.00	$150–200	Add cost of spermicide, if used
Female condom	$2.50–3.00	$250–300	Add cost of spermicide, if used
Diaphragm	$20 + $50–150 for fitting	Cost of spermicide: $85	
Depo-Provera	$35/injection	$140	
Intrauterine Device			
Progestasert	$120 + $40–50 for insertion/tests	$160	
Cu T 380A	$235 + $40–50 for insertion/tests	$28, if retained 10 years[a]	
Norplant	$350/kit + $150–250 for insertion/removal	$130–170, if retained 5 years[a]	5-year cost: $650–850
Pill	$10–25/cycle	$130–300	
Spermicides	$0.85/application	$85	

[a]Norplant and Cu T 380A have considerably higher annual costs if the devices are removed prior to expiration; however, Wyeth Laboratories will refund the cost of implants if they are removed before 6 months.

Adapted with permission from Hatcher RA et al. *Contraceptive Technology*. 16th rev ed. New York: Irvington Publishers; 1994: 133.

the pressure withstood by the condoms before breaking. To meet FDA standards for this test, no more than 1.5% of condoms in a lot should break before inflating to a minimum of 16 L of air. This test, which may reflect the potential for breakage more accurately than the water-leak test, is felt to be a better measure of condom elasticity.[41] Alternative condom-testing methods under investigation are the use of a fluorescent microsphere that approximates the size of the AIDS virus to evaluate for leaks and an electrical process that tests for conduction of an electrical current through minute holes in the latex.[41,42]

The incidence of condom breakage is unknown. However, breakage rates from studies vary widely: one break per 164 acts of intercourse (a rate of 0.6%) was reported in a general population of health care workers[36]; rates of 0.5% for anal acts and 0.8% for vaginal acts were reported in a study conducted in brothels in Australia[43]; a rate of 5% was reported in a Danish study using both female prostitutes and hospital personnel[22]; and an 8% incidence of tearing or slippage during anal intercourse was reported in a study of Dutch homosexuals.[23] In one report of three study sites, breakage rates ranged from 6.7 to 12.9%.[44] In this and one other study, however, multiple incidences of breakage were reported by a limited group of study patients, indicating that breakage may be related as much to the individual user as it is to manufacturing defects.[44,45] Behaviors that have been associated with an increased risk of condom breakage are incorrect placement of the condom, use of an oil-based lubricant, reuse of condoms, and increased duration and intensity of coitus. Past use of condoms without breakage problems indicates a decreased likelihood of condom breaks.[45] One study found that the use of additional lubrication with lubricated condoms increased the likelihood of condom slippage, leading to the possible spillage of semen.[46] Initial studies with the polyurethane condom suggest that it has a breakage rate similar to that of the latex condom.[37]

Failure Rate The use-related failure rate for condoms is 10–13 pregnancies per 100 women during the first year of use.[36] Efficacy of condoms does appear to increase, however, with increasing duration of use; one study found a pregnancy rate of only 0.6% in experienced users.[16] The most common cause of use-related failure with condoms, as with all other contraceptive methods, is the lack of consistent, proper use. An important part of being able to use a product effectively is understanding the directions for use. A recent review of the reading level required to understand the printed instructions included in condom packaging found that although many Americans do not have the reading skills of a high school graduate, condom instructions are written at or above a high school reading level.[47] Because condoms are often purchased in drug stores, pharmacists are the obvious primary source of verbal information on the correct use of condoms. Unfortunately, in one recent survey of 31 pharmacies, only 31% of the pharmacists were able to appropriately educate a patient on the proper selection and use of a condom.[48] It is imperative that pharmacists maintain and continually update their contraceptive knowledge base.

Proper Use/Storage Condoms should be placed on the erect penis before any genital contact because precoital involuntary urethral secretions of the male may contain semen or viable sperm. Rather than interrupting foreplay, many couples find it very pleasurable to incorporate condom use into foreplay by having the woman put the condom on her partner.[36] If the condom does not have a reservoir tip, one should be improvised by

TABLE 5 Guidelines for proper condom use

1. Use only condoms that are fresh (not previously opened) and that have been stored in a dry, cool place (not a wallet or car glove compartment).
2. *Always* use latex condoms unless you are in a monogamous relationship with someone you *know* is not infected with HIV.
3. Do *not* attempt to test the condom for leaks before using; this only increases the risk of tearing.
4. Condoms occasionally break. You should always have a vaginal spermicidal product (foam, cream, or jelly) available and insert it as soon as possible if a condom break or spill occurs.
5. Be aware that long fingernails or jewelry may easily tear condoms.
6. Unroll the condom onto the erect penis before the penis comes into *any* contact with the vagina. *This is very important for preventing both pregnancy and disease.* If you start to put the condom on backward, discard that condom and use a fresh one.
7. If you are not using a reservoir-tipped condom, leave 1/2 inch of space between the end of the condom and the tip of the penis by pinching the top of the condom as you unroll it. This leaves space for the ejaculate and decreases the risk of breakage.
8. If your partner has vaginal dryness, you may want to use additional lubrication. This will help decrease the risk of tears and breakage. Only *water-based lubricants* such as K-Y Jelly and Lubrin are safe for use with condoms. Oil-based lubricants, such as Vaseline and Crisco, weaken condoms and increase the chance of breakage. Spermicidal agents may be used as lubricants with condoms and may increase the effectiveness of the condom as well.
9. After ejaculation, withdraw the penis immediately. Hold on to the rim of the condom as you withdraw to prevent the condom from slipping off, especially if you have used additional lubrication.
10. Check the condom for tears and then discard.
11. If a tear has occurred, *immediately* insert spermicidal foam, cream, or jelly containing a high concentration of spermicide into the vagina. *Do not* use *suppositories* or a vaginal *film* in these cases, as the delay time for dissolution may decrease the product's efficacy.

leaving a half-inch space at the tip. Air should be squeezed from this reservoir by pinching it as the condom is unrolled to its full length. Persons using the polyurethane condom should be advised that it is not as elastic as the latex condom and will not fit as snugly. Nor does it have a reservoir tip, so a space must be left at the tip as when using a non–reservoir-tipped latex condom.[37] To minimize tears, care should be taken with rings and fingernails, and adequate lubrication should be ensured before vaginal or anal entry. If the condom should break while it is being put on, it must be replaced immediately. If breakage or leakage occurs after ejaculation, a spermicidal product (cream, jelly, or foam) should be inserted immediately although the protective value of this procedure is uncertain. Once ejaculation has occurred, the man should withdraw his penis while it is still erect, holding on to the base of the condom to prevent it from slipping off and spilling semen. Spermicidal condoms or the combined use of a vaginal spermicide and a condom may minimize the risk of pregnancy should leakage occur. Specific guidelines for proper condom use are given in Table 5.

If the latex condom user wants a lubricant, the pharmacist must stress the importance of using lubricants that do not harm or weaken the strength and integrity of the condom. Latex condom users should definitely avoid any oil-based lubricants, including Vaseline, Vaseline Intensive Care lotion, baby oil, and corn oil.[49,50] These products cause rapid deterioration of the latex and may lead to breaks in the condom. (Ability to wash off a substance with water is not a good indicator of whether the substance contains an oil-based ingredient.) Appropriate water-based lubricants to use with latex condoms include products such as K-Y Jelly, Ortho Personal Lubricant, or any of the spermicidal creams or jellies. A list of lubricants that are safe or unsafe to use with latex condoms can be found in Table 6. The polyurethane condom, which comes prelubricated, is not subject to degradation by oil-based products.[37]

Excessive heat or overexposure to ozone at levels found in some metropolitan areas will significantly decrease the integrity of the latex within 6 hours; consequently, proper storage of condoms is very important. Pharmacists should emphasize that condoms must be protected from light and excessive heat.[51] The shelf life of condoms under optimal conditions, as packaged by the manufacturers, is 3–5 years; the user should always check for discoloration, brittleness, or stickiness, and condoms displaying any of these characteristics should be discarded.[24]

Advantages/Disadvantages For the vast majority of people, condoms are an effective, acceptable, inexpensive, safe, and nontoxic method of birth control. The most frequent complaint is decreased sensitivity of the glans penis and decreased sexual pleasure for the male. Strategies for countering this problem might include the use of very thin condoms, ridged condoms, or—in a monogamous relationship with an HIV-negative individual—natural membrane condoms.

It is estimated that 1–2% of the population may be sensitized to latex.[52] These patients may develop condom contact dermatitis from the use of latex condoms. This condition, which may occur in the male or female partner, may be characterized by immediate localized itching and swelling (urticarial reaction) or a delayed eczematous reaction. In patients with severe sensitivity, the reaction may spread beyond the area of physical contact with the latex.[53] Patients should be asked if they can wear rubber gloves or blow up a balloon without developing itching. The sensitizers are usually antioxidants or accelerators used in processing the rubber.[39] Because different manufacturers use different processes,

TABLE 6 Lubricants and products that are safe or unsafe to use with latex condoms

Safe	Unsafe
Aloe-9	Baby oils
Aqua-Lube	Burn ointments
Aqua-Lube Plus (spermicidal)	Coconut oil/butter
Astroglide	Edible oils
Carbowax	(eg, olive, peanut, corn, sunflower)
Contraceptive foams	Hemorrhoidal ointments
(eg, Emko, Delfen, Koromex)	Insect repellents
Contraceptive creams and gels	Margarine/dairy butter
(eg, Prepair, Contraceptrol)	Mineral oil
Duragel	Palm oil
Egg white	Petroleum jelly (eg, Vaseline)
ForPlay Lubricant	Rubbing alcohol
Glycerin (USP)	Suntan oil
H-R Lubricating Jelly	Vaginal creams
Intercept	(eg, Monistat, Estrace, Femstat, Vagisil, Premarin,
Koromex Gel	Rendell's Cone, Pharmatext Ovule)
Lubafax	(eg, Elbow Grease, Hot Elbow Grease, Shaft)
Lubrin Insert	Some sexual lubricants
Norform Insert	
Ortho-Gynol	
Personal Lubricant	
Prepair Lubricant	
Probe	
Saliva	
Semicid	
Silicones DC 360	
Transi-Lube	
Water	

Reprinted with permission from Hatcher RA et al. *Contraceptive Technology*. 16th rev ed. New York: Irvington Publishers; 1994: 158.

changing brands may alleviate the problem. In one study, reactions in patients allergic to latex ranged from 0% to 76%, depending on the brand used.[54] If switching brands does not eliminate the irritation, polyurethane or lamb cecum condoms may be used if their limitations are recognized. Also, some patients may be sensitized to components of the lubricant or spermicide. Changing brands or using a condom without spermicide may resolve the problem.

Female Condom

Because of concerns over the lack of means for women to protect themselves against pregnancy and STDs (especially HIV), a female condom was developed. The Reality condom is made of polyurethane rather than latex. It is thinner than the male condom and is resistant to degradation by oil-based lubricants. It is prelubricated and comes with additional lubricant. The condom is secured by a circular ring that fits like a diaphragm over the cervix. An outer ring, which dangles outside the vagina, is designed to protect the external genitalia. The female condom is designed for one-time use and may be inserted up to 8 hours before intercourse. It should then be removed immediately after intercourse and before the woman stands up.

Failure Rate The 6-month pregnancy failure rate among all users of the female condom is 12.4%, similar to that for users of diaphragms and cervical caps; among perfect users, however, the 6-month pregnancy failure rate has been documented to be as low as 2.6%. The extrapolated annual pregnancy failure rates for the female condom are 21–25% for all users and 5% for perfect users[55] (Table 3).

Advantages/Disadvantages Advantages of the female condom include a reduced chance of breakage, less mess than spermicides, no known significant adverse effects, and easy access without prescription. This product offers a means of control and protection by the woman. It has been shown to be impermeable to HIV in vitro,[56] and its use has been associated in one study with a decrease in the recurrence rate of vaginal trichomonas.[57] However, with an estimated annual pregnancy rate of up to 25%, it is questionable whether the female condom affords true protection against STDs.

Some disadvantages noted include the expense (female condoms cost significantly more than male condoms), a cumbersome and unattractive appearance, vaginal irritation, decreased sensation for some women, increased noise ("squeaking") if lubrication is inadequate, and some difficulty with insertion for those not experienced in using tampons. While most of these disadvantages should not significantly affect the proper use of the female condom, they may limit its acceptance.

Vaginal Contraceptives

Vaginal contraceptives (spermicides) use surface-active agents to immobilize (kill) sperm. The effective spermicides include nonoxynol-9, octoxynol-9, and menfegol. Nearly all currently available products use nonoxynol-9. No products containing menfegol are currently marketed in the United States; however, several are available in Asia.

Types of Spermicides

Spermicides come in a variety of dosage forms: jelly, cream, foam, suppository, and film (see product table "Spermicide Products").

Vaginal Creams and Jellies When using a vaginal cream or jelly without a diaphragm or cervical cap, the user should be careful to choose a product with a higher concentration of spermicide, not one with a lower concentration designed for use in conjunction with barrier methods. Products with a higher concentration of spermicide may be used alone or with a diaphragm or cervical cap. Creams have better lubricating and spreading qualities whereas gels may be less messy. A full applicator of spermicide should be deposited high in the vagina, near the cervix. These agents are effective immediately and may be inserted up to 30–60 minutes in advance of intercourse. The product should be reapplied if intercourse is repeated or occurs more than 60 minutes after the initial application. In addition, douching should be delayed until at least 8 hours after the last act of intercourse. Allergic reactions, although rare, may be experienced by either partner. Couples having oral-genital sex may find the taste of some of these products unpleasant.[36]

When a spermicide is used with a diaphragm or cervical cap, the barrier is filled one-third full with spermicide and positioned over the cervix, with placement checked as instructed by the health care practitioner. The spermicide-filled barrier may be inserted up to an hour before intercourse.

The diaphragm is to be left in place for at least 6 hours after intercourse; if coitus is repeated before 6 hours have elapsed, additional cream or jelly should be inserted intravaginally without removing the diaphragm. If 6 hours have elapsed since intercourse, the diaphragm should be removed and washed and new spermicide should be applied before it is used again.[36] A study by Leitch found that contraceptive jelly retained its spermicidal activity for up to 12 hours and that cream was effective for up to 24 hours after application.[58] If this finding is confirmed by other research, the time restrictions on insertion before intercourse and on reapplication of spermicide for repeated intercourse may be liberalized.

The cervical cap need not be removed if intercourse is repeated and may be left in place for up to 48 hours. To ensure full protection in the event of repeated intercourse, it is advisable to apply another dose of spermicide intravaginally without removing the cervical cap.[36]

Vaginal Foams When used alone, contraceptive foams appear to have better efficacy rates than do other vaginal contraceptives, possibly because they are more evenly distributed and adhere better to the cervical area and vaginal walls. Their availability and ease of use also make vaginal contraceptive foams an excellent product to use in combination with condoms, a good backup method for women who use oral contraceptives, and useful for women with newly inserted intrauterine devices (IUDs). However, women experiencing vaginal dryness may find vaginal contraceptive foams to provide inadequate lubrication compared with creams and jellies.

Strict attention must be paid to the directions for use for each product; some require two full applicators whereas others require only one for an effective dose. For convenience, applicators may be prefilled before use. Prefilled unit-dose applicators are also commercially available. Contraceptive foam, like creams and jellies, may be inserted up to an hour before coitus; it is effective immediately on insertion and, like the other vaginal preparations, should be applied as close to the cervix as possible. Douching should be delayed until at least 8 hours after the last act of intercourse to allow adequate time for the spermicide to act.

Vaginal Suppositories Vaginal suppositories are solid or semisolid dosage forms that are activated by the moisture in the woman's vaginal tract. They must be inserted high up in the vagina at least 10–15 minutes before intercourse. There may be some occasions when the suppository will not completely dissolve, resulting in an unpleasant, gritty sensation. As with other medicated suppositories, there is a risk that the woman may forget to unwrap the product or choose the wrong orifice for insertion, so the pharmacist should make certain the user understands the directions. Efficacy of vaginal suppositories is low. They are generally not recommended because more efficacious vaginal products are available. Vaginal suppositories do not require refrigeration.

Contraceptive Film Vaginal contraceptive film, available in the United States since 1987, is made in England and has been used in Europe for more than a decade. The film contains 28% nonoxynol-9 as its active ingredient and is available in packets of 3, 6, or 12 paper-thin 2-inch square sheets. The film is activated by vaginal secretions. It is inserted on the tip of a finger and placed at the cervix, where it should be allowed to dissolve for at least 5 minutes before intercourse. Patients should be advised not to place the film over the penis for insertion. This method does not ensure proper placement and does not allow adequate time for dissolution. The film is effective for 2 hours. It is unknown how widely marketed or used this product is, or how the film compares in effectiveness with other vaginal contraceptive products.[36]

Failure Rate

Spermicides used alone have a relatively high failure rate among typical first-year users (Table 3).[36] Of these products, vaginal foam appears to be most effective when it is used consistently. Efficacy improves greatly if spermicides are used in conjunction with barrier methods such as diaphragms, cervical caps, or condoms. If the woman wants to douche after using a vaginal spermicide, she should wait at least 8 hours after intercourse before doing so.

Advantages/Disadvantages

Spermicides are easy to use and readily available without prescription, and most forms are relatively inexpensive. Unit-dose containers of foam and suppositories can be carried in a purse quite discreetly. Spermicides are very useful as a backup method to other contraceptive products such as condoms, and they can also serve as a backup method if a birth control pill has been missed. If vaginal lubrication is desired, spermicidal creams or jellies are very good choices. There is also a growing body of literature suggesting that spermicides are possibly somewhat protective in vivo against many STDs, including chlamydia and gonorrhea.[59–61] Although studies have shown that nonoxynol-9 inactivates HIV in vitro and can apparently decrease transmission of simian immunodeficiency virus in monkeys,[62] a study of Rwandan women was unable to demonstrate a decreased risk of HIV infection in women who used vaginal spermicides.[16] Of concern is the increased incidence of vaginal ulceration in women using spermicides, which has been reported in some studies[26] and which may lead to enhanced transmission of the HIV virus.[16,36] Until more definitive data on the efficacy of spermicides in preventing HIV transmission between humans are available, protection against HIV infections must not be assumed.[62,63]

While studies suggest that the simultaneous use of condoms and spermicides can lead to pregnancy prevention rates that are similar to those of oral contraceptives and IUDs,[64] the relatively low use-effectiveness rate of spermicides used alone is their major disadvantage. Each product has very specific directions for use, dosage, and timing of administration with respect to coital activity. Therefore, users must be reminded to pay strict attention to the directions for use for each product. Some people are hypersensitive (allergic) to the components, and others find spermicidal products excessively messy. Very frequent use or use of high-concentration products may lead to irritation or damage of the vaginal and cervical epithelium.[16,65] There has been concern about a possible association between spermicide use and birth defects or miscarriage. After two very large population studies,[66,67] however, the FDA has concluded that no increased risk of birth defects can be attributed to spermicides.[68]

Natural Family Planning

Natural family planning methods, also called periodic abstinence, rhythm, or fertility awareness methods, use various techniques to determine a woman's period of fertility. The information provided by these techniques is helpful in pinpointing the time of ovulation and optimal time for conception. Natural family planning is the only method of contraception approved by the Roman Catholic Church and is widely used around the world.

Natural family planning can be divided into four methods: calendar, basal body temperature, cervical mucus, and symptothermal. Each of these methods requires the woman to keep detailed records of her menstrual cycles and other symptoms associated with cyclical hormonal levels. The data acquired, such as basal body temperature (BBT) or the character and quantity of cervical mucus (Figure 1), are recorded on detailed monthly charts. After a period of instruction and with the information provided by charts from several months, a woman is usually able to predict her most fertile time. With this information, a couple can choose to abstain from sexual intercourse during this period if they want to avoid pregnancy.[69] (See Chapter 6, "Vaginal and Menstrual Products," for a review of menstrual physiology and biochemistry.)

Methods of Natural Family Planning

Calendar Method The calendar method (also known as the rhythm method) is based on records of monthly menstrual cycle lengths. The estimated day of ovulation, considered to be 14±2 days before the onset of menstruation, is used to determine the woman's fertile period. The fertile period is calculated on the basis of estimates of the viable life of ova and sperm.[70] The fertilizable life of the ovum (egg) is estimated to be from 6 to 24 hours following ovulation, as measured by peaks in estrogen and luteinizing hormone (LH). Sperm is considered to be viable for 48–72 hours. The fertile period for a woman with records of her last 12 months of cycles is found by

TABLE 7 How to calculate the interval of fertility using the calendar or rhythm method

If the shortest cycle has been (no. of days)	The first fertile (unsafe) day is	If the longest cycle has been (no. of days)	The last fertile (unsafe) day is
21[a]	3rd day	21	10th day
22	4th	22	11th
23	5th	23	12th
24	6th	24	13th
25	7th	25	14th
26	8th	26	15th
27	9th	27	16th
28	10th	28	17th
29	11th	29	18th
30	12th	30	19th
31	13th	31	20th
32	14th	32	21st
33	15th	33	22nd
34	16th	34	23rd
35	17th	35	24th

[a]Day 1, first day of menstrual bleeding.

Reprinted with permission from Hatcher RA et al. *Contraceptive Technology 1990–1992.* 15th ed. New York: Irvington Publishers; 1990: 341.

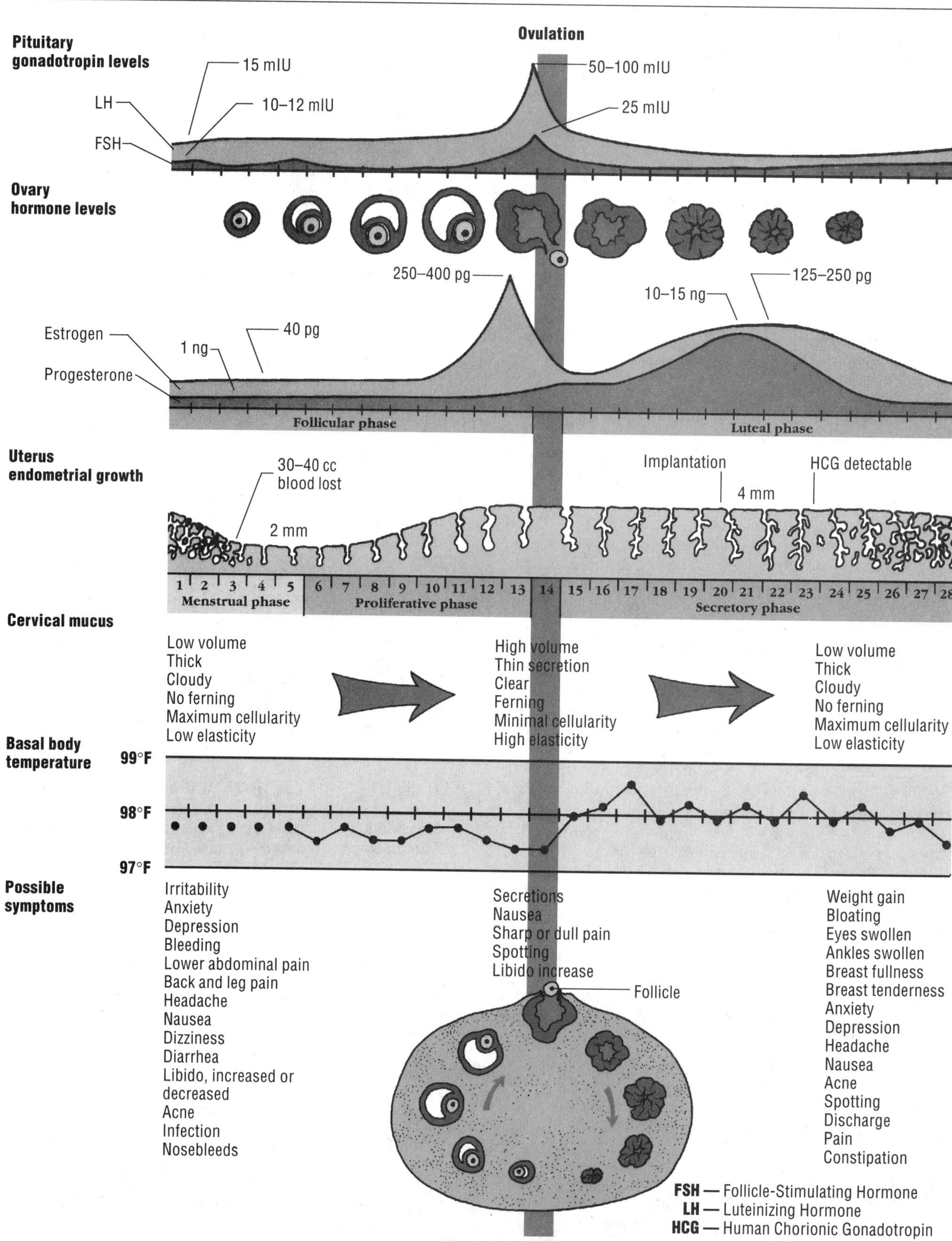

FIGURE 1 Primary menstrual cycle events: hormone levels, ovarian and endometrial patterns, cyclical temperature, and cervical mucus changes. Reprinted with permission from Hatcher RA et al. *Contraceptive Technology 1990–1992.* 15th ed. New York: Irvington Publishers; 1990: 42.

subtracting 18 days from the shortest cycle to determine the first fertile day and subtracting 11 days from the longest cycle to determine the last fertile day. For example, if a woman's shortest cycle in the last year was 25 days and her longest was 30 days, her fertile period would be from day 7 to day 19 of her cycle (Table 7).

The calendar method is considered the least effective of the natural family planning methods, primarily because of natural variations in the length of a woman's normal menstrual cycle. Although it is still widely used as the sole contraceptive method, such reliance results in many unintended pregnancies (Table 3).[69,70] Consequently, family planners do not currently recommend using it as the sole method of contraception but suggest instead that the calendar method be used in conjunction with other methods of natural family planning.

Basal Body Temperature Method In the BBT method, the woman measures her body temperature every day in the morning and charts this temperature. The temperature should be taken with a mercury or electronic digital thermometer that is calibrated in increments of 0.1°F (0.05°C). Such a thermometer allows the detection of small changes in body temperature. It is very important to obtain the temperature before embarking on *any* physical activity (ie, the temperature should be taken before getting out of bed) and to obtain it at the same time every day. Oral or rectal temperature may be used, but any given individual should use one method (site) consistently.

These charts can be used to estimate the time of ovulation because the BBT usually drops 12–24 hours before ovulation and then rises sharply over a 24- to 48-hour period to about 0.4–1.0°F (0.2–0.5°C) above the lowest point (the *nadir*) (Figure 2).[69–71] This sharp rise, called the *thermal shift*, is due to high progesterone levels. The *safe* (infertile) *period* is considered to begin after 3 days of postnadir temperature elevation and to last until the start of the next menstrual cycle. Because this method is not absolutely accurate in predicting when ovulation occurs, the postmenstrual or preovulatory safe period is difficult to determine, and those who engage in unprotected intercourse during this period have a higher pregnancy rate.

Electronic digital thermometers are more accurate than mercury thermometers and have a shorter recording time (45–90 seconds). Because the activity of shaking down a thermometer may cause the woman's body temperature to change, mercury thermometers must be shaken down each night rather than immediately before use in the morning.

For patients who feel that they may have difficulty interpreting shifts in their BBT, there is a computerized monitor, Bioself Fertility Indicator, which registers and stores the BBTs. The computer uses the collected data to indicate periods of infertility, fertility, and high fertility. It has a six-cycle memory, and printouts of stored temperatures are available from the manufacturer. However, this product is only as good as the information it records. A woman must still take her temperature at the same time every morning before any physical activity. Anything that affects her BBT will interfere with the ability of the computer to generate an accurate indicator of her fertility levels.

Poor correlation of the thermal shift with ovulation reduces the accuracy of the BBT method. Furthermore, some women have monophasic menstrual cycles and do not have a definite or significant temperature dip or

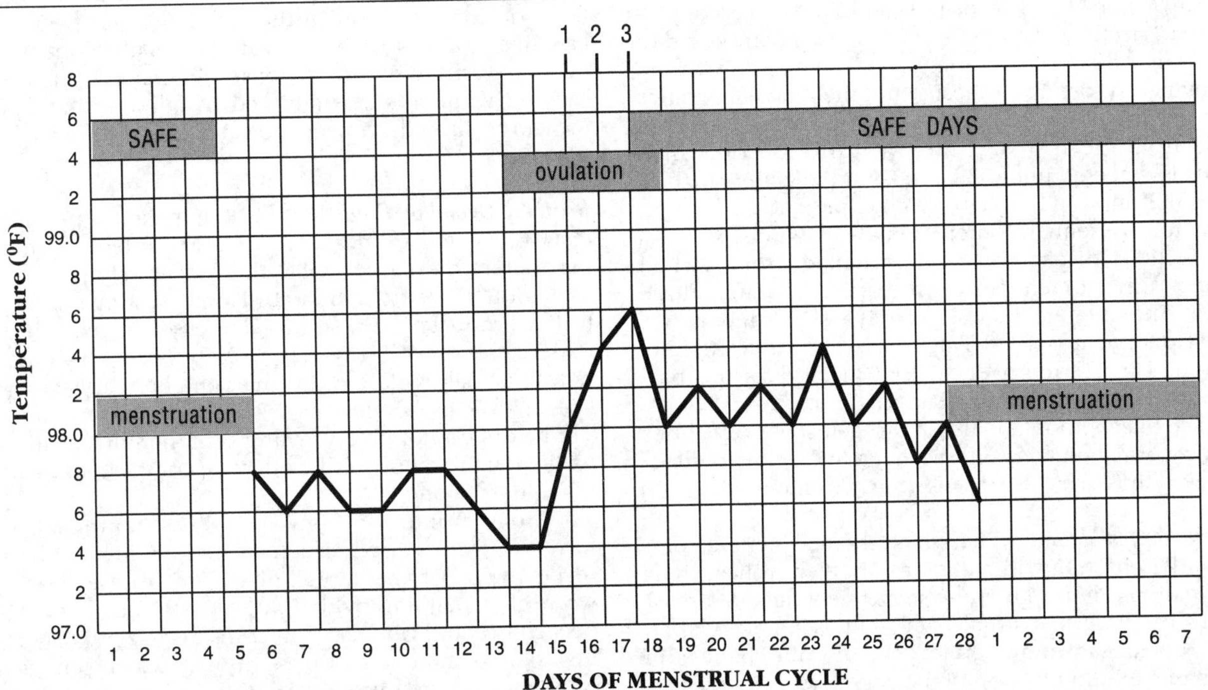

FIGURE 2 Basal body temperature variations during a model menstrual cycle. Reprinted with permission from Hatcher RA et al. *Contraceptive Technology 1990–1992*. 15th ed. New York: Irvington Publishers; 1990: 343.

TABLE 8 Summary of cervical mucus (ovulation) method of fertility regulation

Approximate cycle day: Phase	How identified	Intercourse allowed?
1–5: Menstruation[a]	Bleeding	No
6–9: Dry days	Absence of cervical mucus	On alternate nights only
10: Fecund period begins	Onset of sticky mucus secretion	No
16: Peak fecund day	Last day on which slippery mucus (resembling raw egg white) is observed	No
20: Fecund period ends	Evening of the 4th day after the peak day	After the fecund period ends
20–29: Safe period	From end of fecund period until onset of bleeding	Yes

[a]The cycle begins on the first day of menstruation.

Reprinted with permission from Hatcher RA et al. *Contraceptive Technology*. 16th rev ed. New York: Irvington Publishers; 1994: 337.

rise. Stress, fever, lactation, and use of an electric blanket may affect BBT, and temperature changes are difficult to interpret just before and during menopause.[71] At such times, it is best for the couple to use one or more alternative methods of contraception.

Cervical Mucus Method The cervical mucus method is based on the rather consistent changes in cervical mucus that take place during a normal menstrual cycle. Every day, the woman observes the mucus at the vulva (vaginal orifice) and charts its character and the amount produced (Figure 1). After menstruation, there are days when most women notice a sensation of dryness at the vaginal orifice. As estrogen levels rise, the cervical mucus increases in quantity and elasticity and becomes clear, resembling raw egg white.[69–71] The peak symptom, the last day of the clear, stretchy, estrogenic mucus, has been shown to be within a day of ovulation for most women. With the postovulatory rise in progesterone, the mucus becomes thick and sticky or is absent. The woman is considered fertile from the first day after menstruation on which mucus is detected until 72 hours after the appearance of the peak symptom (Table 8). With experience, a woman learns to differentiate other vaginal secretions, such as an infectious discharge or seminal fluid, from normal mucus. Most women can learn this method after three cycles. The average number of days of abstinence required per cycle is 17.[69] This method of natural family planning is preferred over the BBT method for postpartum lactating women and those nearing menopause. Women who use this method are also apt to detect abnormalities in their normal mucus patterns that may be due to infections and thus are able to seek early treatment.

Symptothermal Method The symptothermal method combines BBT charting with notations of other cyclical signs of ovulation (Figure 1). These signs might include breast tenderness, intermenstrual pain (mittelschmerz), labial edema, peak symptom cervical mucus, and changes in the character and position of the cervix. Most studies on the effectiveness of this method use the thermal shift (the temperature rise after the nadir) of the BBT method to determine the postovulatory safe period, and use the cervical mucus or calendar method to determine the end of the preovulatory or postmenstrual infertile period.[71] Combinations of these methods have good predicted effectiveness; with perfect use, the annual failure rate is 2% (Table 3).

Adjunctive Contraceptive Methods

Lactational Infertility In many developing countries, breastfeeding is used as a contraceptive method for spacing the birth of children. When the infant receives only breast milk and the mother has not menstruated, protection against conception may persist for up to 6 months.[72] However, if breast feedings are supplemented with bottle feedings, lactational amenorrhea may not be a reliable form of contraception. Although menstrual periods in lactating women may be anovulatory, ovulation may also occur before the return of menses. In general, if a breastfeeding woman is sexually active, other contraceptive measures should be used no later than 5 weeks postpartum.[70]

In-Home Ovulation Prediction Tests Ovulation prediction test kits, which are designed to aid couples in conceiving, detect the surge in LH that occurs shortly before ovulation. (See Chapter 3, "In-Home Testing and Monitoring Products.") These kits detect an increase in urinary excretion of LH, which usually occurs 8–40 hours before actual ovulation. Because the life expectancy of sperm may be longer than 72 hours, these ovulation predictors do not give warning of impending ovulation with enough accuracy to be effective contraceptive agents when used alone.

Home urine assays for estrogen and pregnanediol have been developed to detect the beginning and end, respectively, of the fertile phase.[69,73] These tests can warn of impending ovulation at least 3 days before its occurrence and can also detect the rise in progesterone that signals the end of the fertile period. In one group of women using these assays, there were only four unplanned pregnancies over 55 woman-years. (This figure can be extrapolated to 7.3 pregnancies per 100 woman-years.[73]) These urine assays, when commercially available, may be used as a nonprescription method of fertility prediction for contraceptive purposes.

Advantages/Risks of Natural Family Planning

Advantages Natural family planning methods have the positive effect of encouraging communication within a relationship and may be the only truly shared contraceptive method. The cost of monitoring symptoms is minimal. Many couples like the fact that no chemicals are used in preventing conception, producing no chemical risk to the fertility or health of the couple (or to the fetus, should pregnancy occur).

Risks The risks of natural family planning methods fall into three areas. First is the risk of pregnancy: these techniques have higher pregnancy rates than most other contraceptive methods. Second is the risk of STDs because, unlike condoms or spermicides, these methods involve no barriers to such infections. However, the risk for STDs may be relatively low overall because these methods are most often practiced by couples in stable, long-term, monogamous relationships. The third and most controversial risk is that of abnormal pregnancy outcomes, such as birth defects or fetal wastage, should a couple conceive unintentionally. This risk is related to the possible association of such a conception with aged gametes (either sperm or ovum). Comparative studies have found a relative risk of 1.0–5.2 for birth defects or spontaneous abortion among those practicing natural family planning at the time of conception. At present, however, the evidence for an increased risk of abnormal pregnancy outcomes is not conclusive. This controversial issue may become clearer as surveillance continues.[74]

Ineffective/Unrecommended Methods of Contraception

Withdrawal

Coitus interruptus (withdrawal), although used intentionally by only a small percentage of couples in the United States, is more commonly practiced in some European countries[36] and in undeveloped countries around the world. The practice involves coital activity until ejaculation is imminent, followed by withdrawal of the stimulated penis and ejaculation away from the vagina or vulva. Accidental pregnancy rates with this method are in the range of 19 pregnancies per 100 couples in the first year of use.[36] Method failures (pregnancy even when the method is used correctly and consistently) are due in part to the fact that involuntary preejaculation secretions may contain millions of sperm. Disadvantages of this method include a higher pregnancy rate, a lack of protection against STDs, the requirement of considerable self-control by the man, and the potential for diminished pleasure for the couple due to interrupted lovemaking. Although this method should not be recommended, it is better than no contraceptive method.

Douching

Vaginal douches should *never* be considered a method of contraception. Under favorable conditions in the female reproductive tract, active sperm have been found in the cervical crypts and oviducts within 5 minutes after ejaculation.[70] Postcoital douching has no effect in removing sperm from the upper reproductive tract and could, in fact, force or propel sperm higher up in the tract. Because consistent users of douches have a higher incidence of pelvic infections and ectopic pregnancies,[36] it is questionable whether the practice of douching, even for personal hygiene, is of any benefit to a woman's vaginal health. (See Chapter 6, "Vaginal and Menstrual Products.")

Pharmacoeconomics of Contraceptive Products

The application of the concepts of pharmacoeconomics to contraception can be different from that seen with other drug products. The costs of the different contraceptive methods vary. If one assumes 100 acts of intercourse annually, product costs can range from $50 for the male condom to $85 for spermicides to $250 for the female condom.[75] Use of more than one method is often recommended to increase the potential for preventing unwanted pregnancies and STDs. A summary of the costs of various contraceptive products is found in Table 4.

A study comparing the costs of various contraception methods was recently conducted by Trussell et al,[76] who note that all forms of contraception are cost-effective when viewed against the costs of an undesired pregnancy. Their model, which evaluated 1- and 5-year costs for 15 contraceptive methods, included the costs of acquisition and the incidence and costs of both common side effects and pregnancy outcomes associated with each product. Pregnancy outcome costs included ectopic pregnancy; induced and spontaneous abortion; and maternity care, delivery, and newborn hospitalization for a term pregnancy.

For each method studied, the authors showed that the use of contraception was less costly than the resolution of an undesired pregnancy. As a result, part of the pharmacist's job is to educate third-party payers and patients that the up-front acquisition costs of contraceptive products can be misleading as a predictor of the economic value of a contraceptive method. Indeed, investment in a contraceptive product must be examined from the standpoint of the ability of that product to provide economic savings and societal benefits. As shown in the study by Trussell et al, each of the contraceptive products available provides the potential for economic benefit when compared with no use at all.

Differences between methods depend on the willingness of both members of a couple to use a product properly. Significant cost savings for barrier methods can be achieved by minimizing imperfect use. The pharmacist is often the health care provider who the contraceptive user contacts most frequently for the purchase of barrier contraceptives. The pharmacist's role in patient counseling can thus be enhanced by ensuring that users (and their partners) fully understand the proper use of the product.

The Pharmacist's Role in Contraceptive Selection

Reproductive health and contraceptive information may well be one of the most challenging areas of a pharmacist's practice, and one that has a profound impact on the public health and individual well-being of those being served. Thus, as the most accessible health care professionals, pharmacists can be invaluable in contributing to the reproductive health and knowledge of people in their communities.

Pharmacists should thoroughly familiarize themselves with the proper use of currently available nonprescription contraceptive products and should provide opportunities for consultation with patients by removing barriers that may prevent dialogue. Contraceptive products and information should be available in an area where the patient can browse and where the pharmacist can easily interact with the patient, such as next to or directly in front of the prescription counter. A private area for education and counseling is important if adequate discussion is to take place.

Special efforts should be made to offer contraceptive information and services to adolescents. This population group is especially likely to be uninformed or misinformed about reproductive matters. Those pharmacists who are uncomfortable discussing reproductive health with young people should refer adolescents to a clinic that specializes in services to young people, if one is available. Adolescents need clear, accurate information on all aspects of reproductive health. The pharmacist should keep in mind that printed instructions are often written above the reading level of most adolescents (as well as of many adults); therefore, verbal instructions are very important. Nonprescription methods that are particularly useful for the impulsive adolescent might include condoms and contraceptive foam in prefilled applicators.

The diaphragm, cervical cap, or natural family planning methods may be an acceptable approach to contraception for a couple in a stable relationship. The first two methods require special fitting. Natural family planning methods, especially the BBT and cervical mucus methods, require extensive training and support from those who have experience and training with these methods. The pharmacist should be supportive and available to answer questions regarding these techniques. Couples should be reminded of medications that may interfere with physical signs and symptoms. For instance, phenothiazines, aspirin, and other medications may alter body temperature,[77] and vaginal foams, gels, creams, and douches will interfere with cervical mucus. In addition to stocking spermicidal products, BBT thermometers, and monitoring charts, the pharmacist may also serve as a referral center for those desiring to use these methods of family planning. A pharmacist with the proper training might consider counseling in natural family planning as a unique practice possibility.

Condom use should be stressed as a method of disease prevention for all, including those who currently use prescription methods of birth control (eg, oral contraceptives or the IUD). Reservoir-tip and spermicidally lubricated latex condoms add additional protection against STDs and the risk of condom rupture.

Further information on reproductive health and AIDS may be found by contacting the organizations listed in Appendixes 1 and 2.

Case Studies

Case 7–1

Patient Complaint/History

SO, a 22-year-old female, comes to the pharmacy counter holding a tube of Monistat 7 vaginal cream and a box of spermicide-treated latex condoms. In the last few months, the patient has purchased the vaginal cream on several occasions. A quick review of her pharmacy profile shows that the following prescription was filled the previous week: Acyclovir 200 mg one capsule 5 times daily for 5 days.

In response to questions about her symptoms, SO describes intense vaginal itching but denies any vaginal discharge. She says that the itching, which has occurred numerous times, usually occurs after intercourse but not after every act of intercourse. Her sexual partner has no symptoms. SO also says that the itching, which she usually treats with the Monistat 7 vaginal cream, resolves in a day or so. Once when she was unable to obtain the product, the itching resolved within 2 days without treatment.

The patient and her partner use either latex condoms or vaginal spermicides for contraception; however, when she has an outbreak of genital herpes, they always use latex condoms.

Clinical Considerations/Strategies

The following considerations/strategies are provided to aid the reader in (1) determining whether treatment of the patient's condition with nonprescription medications is warranted, (2) selecting the appropriate nonprescription medication, and (3) developing a patient counseling strategy to ensure optimal therapeutic outcomes:

- Assess the appropriateness of Monistat 7 vaginal cream for treatment of the vaginal itching.
- Assess alternative causes, other than candidal vaginitis, of the vaginal itching.
- Assess the contraceptive needs of this patient and her partner.
- Suggest an alternative contraceptive product that will meet their needs for prevention of pregnancy and STDs.
- Develop a patient education/counseling strategy that will optimize proper and consistent use of the recommended contraceptive product.

Case 7–2

Patient Complaint/History

EA, a 25-year-old female who has been walking around the pharmacy casually looking at various products, seems to always stop in front of the display of contraceptive products. When approached by the pharmacist, she admits that she is looking for a product to use during sexual intercourse. During further conversation, she reveals that she and her boyfriend have a monogamous relationship. Her boyfriend, however, refuses to use a male condom; he insists that it "takes the feeling out of lovemaking."

The patient's profile shows that she has a history of hypertension, which has been treated for the past 3 years with nifedipine sustained-release tablets 90 mg once daily.

Clinical Considerations/Strategies

The following considerations/strategies are provided to aid the reader in (1) determining whether treatment of the patient's condition with nonprescription medications is warranted, (2) selecting the appropriate nonprescription medication, and (3) developing a patient counseling strategy to ensure optimal therapeutic outcomes:

- Assess the patient's desires and priorities for prevention of pregnancy versus protection from STDs.
- Assess the patient's experience with various contraceptive methods.
- Elicit the patient's opinion of which contraceptive methods are acceptable to her and her partner.
- Suggest contraceptive methods other than condoms for this patient's needs. Consider any disease-related contraindications and potential acceptance by the patient and her sexual partner.
- Develop a patient education/counseling strategy that will optimize successful use of the recommended contraceptive product(s).

Summary

Not many decisions in life are more personal or more important than the choice of a contraceptive method. Optimally, the decision should be made by both sexual partners. Because no single method is likely to be suitable throughout a person's reproductive life, it is important for all options to be presented in a clear and nonjudgmental manner. All sexually active individuals who are not in a mutually monogamous relationship should be aware that they must protect themselves and their partners from AIDS and other STDs and should choose a contraceptive method accordingly.

References

1. Eichhorst BC. Contraception. *Prim Care.* 1988 Sep; 15: 437–9.
2. Forrest JD, Fordyce RR. Women's contraceptive attitudes and use in 1992. *Fam Plann Perspect.* 1993 Jul/Aug; 25: 175–9.
3. Sophocles AM Jr, Brozovich EM. Birth control failure among patients with unwanted pregnancies: 1982–1984. *J Fam Pract.* 1986 Jan; 22: 45–8.
4. Forrest JD, Singh S. The sexual and reproductive behavior of American women, 1982–1988. *Fam Plann Perspect.* 1990 Sep/Oct; 22: 206–14.
5. Kost K, Forrest JD. Intention status of US births in 1988: differences by mothers' socioeconomic and demographic characteristics. *Fam Plann Perspect.* 1995 Jan/Feb; 27: 11–7.
6. Henshaw SK. Teenage abortion, birth and pregnancy statistics by state, 1988. *Fam Plann Perspect.* 1993 May/Jun; 25: 122–6.
7. Zabin LS, Stark HA, Emerson MR. Reasons for delay in contraceptive clinic utilization: adolescent clinic and nonclinic populations compared. *J Adolesc Health.* 1991; 12: 225.
8. Zabin LS, Kantner JF, Zelnik M. The risk of adolescent pregnancy in the first months of intercourse. *Fam Plann Perspect.* 1979 Jul/Aug; 11: 215–22.
9. Adolescent sexual behavior, pregnancy, and childbearing. In: Hatcher RA et al. *Contraceptive Technology.* 16th rev ed. New York: Irvington Publishers; 1994: 571–600.
10. Centers for Disease Control and Prevention. HIV/AIDS surveillance report 1993; 5(1):1–10.
11. Pleck JH, Sonenstein FL, Ku L. Changes in adolescent males' use of and attitudes toward condoms, 1988–1991. *Fam Plann Perspect.* 1993 May/Jun; 25: 106–9, 117.
12. Wasserheit JN. Epidemiological synergy: interrelationships between human immunodeficiency virus infection and other sexually transmitted diseases. *Sex Transm Dis.* 1992 Mar–Apr; 19: 61–77.
13. Centers for Disease Control. The second 100,000 cases of acquired immunodeficiency syndrome—United States, June 1981–December 1991. *MMWR.* 1992 Jan; 41: 28–9.
14. Ellerbrock TV et al. Epidemiology of women with AIDS in the United States, 1981 through 1990. *JAMA.* 1991; 265: 2971–5.
15. Centers for Disease Control. Update: acquired immunodeficiency syndrome—United States, 1991. *MMWR.* 1992 Jul; 41: 463–8.
16. Cates W Jr, Stone KM. Family planning, sexually transmitted diseases, and contraceptive choices: a literature update—part I. *Fam Plann Perspect.* 1992; 24: 75–84.
17. Food and Drug Administration. Counseling patients about the prevention of AIDS. *N Y State J Med.* 1988 May; 88: 264–5.
18. HIV and AIDS. In: Hatcher RA et al. *Contraceptive Technology.* 16th rev ed. New York: Irvington Publishers: 1994: 51–75.
19. Ngugi EN et al. Prevention of transmission of human immunodeficiency virus in Africa: effectiveness of condom promotion and health education among prostitutes. *Lancet.* 1988 Oct; 2: 887–90.
20. Feldblum PJ, Fortney JA. Condoms, spermicides, and the transmission of human immunodeficiency virus: a review of the literature. *Am J Public Health.* 1988 Jan; 78: 52–4.
21. Darrow WW. Condom use and use-effectiveness in high-risk populations. *Sex Transm Dis.* 1989 Jul–Sep; 16: 157–9.
22. Gotzsche PC, Hording M. Condoms to prevent HIV transmission do not imply truly safe sex. *Scand J Infect Dis.* 1988; 20: 233–4.
23. Van Griensven GJP et al. Failure rate of condoms during anogenital intercourse in homosexual men. *Genitourin Med.* 1988 Oct; 64: 344–6.
24. Centers for Disease Control. Condoms for prevention of sexually transmitted diseases. *MMWR.* 1988 Mar; 37: 133–7.
25. Rietmeijer CAM et al. Condoms as physical and chemical barriers against human immunodeficiency virus. *JAMA.* 1988 Mar; 259: 1851–3.
26. Kreiss J et al. Efficacy of nonoxynol-9 contraceptive sponge use in preventing heterosexual acquisition of HIV in Nairobi prostitutes. *JAMA.* 1992; 268: 477–82.
27. Rekart ML et al. *Nonoxynol-9: Its Adverse Effects.* Abstract #SC36. Paper presented at San Francisco: Sixth International Conference on AIDS; June 23, 1990.
28. Ilaria G et al. Detection of HIV-1 DNA sequences in pre-ejaculatory fluid. *Lancet.* 1992; 340: 1469.
29. Pudney J et al. Pre-ejaculatory fluid as potential vector for sexual transmission of HIV-1. *Lancet.* 1992; 340: 1470.
30. Deneberg R. Female sex hormones and HIV. *AIDS Clin Care.* 1993; 5: 69–71, 76.
31. Clemetson DBA et al. Detection of HIV DNA in cervical and vaginal secretions: prevalence and correlates among women in Nairobi, Kenya. *JAMA.* 1993; 269: 2860–4.

32. Sexually transmitted diseases. In: Hatcher RA et al. *Contraceptive Technology*. 16th rev ed. New York: Irvington Publishers; 1994: 77–106.
33. Henry K, Osterholm MT. Reduction of HIV transmission by use of condoms. *Am J Public Health*. 1988 Sep; 78: 1244.
34. Schirm AL et al. Contraceptive failure in the United States: the impact of social, economic and demographic factors. *Fam Plann Perspect*. 1982 Mar/Apr; 14: 68–94.
35. Moran JS et al. Increase in condom sales following AIDS education and publicity, United States. *Am J Public Health*. 1990 May; 80: 607–8.
36. Hatcher RA et al. *Contraceptive Technology*. 16th rev ed. New York: Irvington Publishers; 1994: 146–53, 179–89, 192–4, 213–8, 327–45.
37. Marc Wasserman. Personal communication on polyurethane condom. New York: Edelman Public Relations Worldwide (for Avanti); January 11, 1996.
38. Minuk GY, Bohme CE, Bowen TJ. Condoms and hepatitis B virus infection. *Ann Intern Med*. 1986 Apr; 104: 584.
39. Fisher AA. Condom dermatitis in either partner. *Cutis*. 1987 Apr; 39: 281, 284–5.
40. Provencher GC, Miller PJ. Who's responsible for condom quality? *Am J Nurs*. 1988 May; 88: 640, 643.
41. FDA develops latex condom permeability test method. *The Gray Sheet*. 1990 Dec 24; 16(52): 22.
42. How reliable are condoms? *Consumer Rep*. 1995 May; 320–5.
43. Richters J et al. Low condom breakage rate in commercial sex. *Lancet*. 1988 Dec; 2: 1487–8.
44. Russel-Brown P et al. Comparison of condom breakage during human use with performance in laboratory testing. *Contraception*. 1992 May; 45: 429–37.
45. Steiner M et al. Can condom users likely to experience condom failure be identified? *Fam Plann Perspect*. 1993 Sep/Oct; 25: 220–3, 226.
46. Trussell J, Warner DL, Hatcher RA. Condom slippage and breakage rates. *Fam Plann Perspect*. 1992 Jan/Feb; 24: 20–3.
47. Richwald GA et al. Are condom instructions readable? Results of a readability study. *Public Health Rep*. 1988 Jul–Aug; 103: 355–9.
48. Gebhart F. Pharmacists fail condom quiz, other AIDS prevention questions. *Drug Topics*. 1992 Mar; 136: 14–5.
49. Voeller B et al. Mineral oil lubricants cause rapid deterioration of latex condoms. *Contraception*. 1989 Jan; 39: 95–102.
50. White N et al. Dangers of lubricants used with condoms. *Nature*. 1988 Sep; 335: 19.
51. Clark LJ, Sherwin RP, Baker RF. Latex condom deterioration accelerated by environmental factors: I. ozone. *Contraception*. 1989 Mar; 39: 245–51.
52. Fisher AA. Condom conundrums: part 1. *Cutis*. 1991 Nov; 48: 359–60.
53. Fisher AA. Allergic contact reactions in health personnel. *Allerg Clin Immunol*. 1992 Nov; 90: 729–38.
54. Turjanmaa K, Reunala T. Condoms as a source of latex allergen and cause of contact urticaria. *Contact Dermatitis*. 1989 May; 20: 360–4.
55. Trussell J et al. Comparative contraceptive efficacy of the female condom and other barrier methods. *Fam Plann Perspect*. 1994 Mar/Apr; 26: 66–72.
56. Drew WL et al. Evaluation of the virus permeability of a new condom for women. *Sex Transm Dis*. 1990 Apr/Jun; 17: 110–2.
57. Soper DE et al. Prevention of vaginal trichomoniasis by compliant use of the female condom. *Sex Transm Dis*. 1993 May/Jun; 20: 137–9.
58. Leitch WS. Longevity of Ortho Creme and Gynol II in the contraceptive diaphragm. *Contraception*. 1986 Oct; 34: 381–93.
59. Stone KM, Grimes DA, Mageder LS. Personal protection against sexually transmitted diseases. *Am J Obstet Gynecol*. 1986 Jul; 155: 180–8.
60. Louv WC et al. A clinical trial of nonoxynol-9 for preventing gonococcal and chlamydial infections. *J Infect Dis*. 1988 Sep; 158: 518–23.
61. Niruthisard S, Roddy RE, Chutivongse S. Use of nonoxynol-9 and reduction in rate of gonococcal and chlamydial cervical infections. *Lancet*. 1992 Jun; 3: 1371–5.
62. Miller CJ et al. The effect of contraceptives containing nonoxynol-9 on the genital transmission of simian immunodeficiency virus in rhesus macaques. *Fertil Steril*. 1992 May; 57: 1126–8.
63. Voeller B. Nonoxynol-9 and HTLV-III. *Lancet*. 1986 May; 1: 1153.
64. Kestelman P, Trussell J. Efficacy of the simultaneous use of condoms and spermicides. *Fam Plann Perspect*. 1991 Sep/Oct; 23: 226–7, 232.
65. Niruthisard S, Roddy RE, Chutivongse S. The effects of frequent nonoxynol-9 use on the vaginal and cervical mucosa. *Sex Transm Dis*. 1991 Jul/Sep; 18: 176–9.
66. Mills JL et al. Are there adverse effects of periconceptional spermicide use? *Fertil Steril*. 1985 Mar; 43: 442–6.
67. Harlap S et al. Chromosomal abnormalities in the Kaiser-Permanente Birth Defects Study, with special reference to contraceptive use around the time of conception. *Teratology*. 1985 Jun; 31: 381–7.
68. Data do not support association between spermicides, birth defects. *FDA Drug Bull*. 1986; 16: 21.
69. Brown JB et al. Natural family planning. *Am J Obstet Gynecol*. 1987 Oct; 157(pt 2): 1082–9.
70. Klaus H. Natural family planning: a review. *Obstet Gynecol Survey*. 1982 Feb; 37: 128–50.
71. Gross BA. Natural family planning indicators of ovulation. *Clin Reprod Fertil*. 1987; 5: 91. Invited review.
72. Kennedy KI, Rivers R, McNeilly AS. Consensus statement on the use of breastfeeding as a family planning method. *Contraception*. 1989 May; 39: 477–91.
73. Brown JB, Holmes J, Barker G. Use of the home ovarian monitor in pregnancy avoidance. *Am J Obstet Gynecol*. 1991 Dec; 165(pt 2): 2008–11.
74. Gray RH, Kambic RT. Epidemiological studies of natural family planning. *Hum Reprod*. 1988; 3: 693.
75. The essentials of contraception: effectiveness, safety, and personal considerations. In: Hatcher RA et al. *Contraceptive Technology*. 16th rev ed. New York: Irvington Publishers; 1994: 107–38.
76. Trussell J et al. The economic value of contraception: a comparison of 15 methods. *Am J Public Health*. 1995; 85: 494–503.
77. Frazier JL, Schumock GT. Drug-induced alterations in body temperature. *P&T*. 1991 Mar; 16: 164, 271–5.

Appendix 1: Family Planning Information

In addition to the resources listed below, many states and counties have their own chapters of family planning organizations such as Planned Parenthood. Check with your local board of health or look in your local telephone directory.

- The Alan Guttmacher Institute
  120 Wall Street, 21st floor
  New York, NY 10005
  212–248–1111
  800–765–7514
- Planned Parenthood Federation of America, Inc
  810 Seventh Avenue
  New York, NY 10019
  212–541–7800
  800–829–7732 (New York only)
  800–230–7526
- The Population Council
  Office of Communications
  1 Dag Hammarskjold Plaza
  New York, NY 10017
  212–339–0500
- Population Information Program
  The Johns Hopkins University
  111 Market Place, Suite 310
  Baltimore, MD 21202
  410–659–6300
- Special Programme of Research, Development and Research Training in Human Reproduction
  World Health Organization
  Avenue Appia
  CH 1211, Geneva 27
  Switzerland

Appendix 2: AIDS Information Resources

The 15 AIDS education and training centers are listed alphabetically by state. Each center serves a geographic area and provides information and ongoing education for health care providers.

Serving Arizona, California, Hawaii, Nevada

- Pacific AIDS Education and Training Center
  University of California at San Francisco
  5110 East Clinton Way, Suite 115
  Fresno, CA 93727–2098
  Western Division: 209–252–2851
  Southern Division: 213–342–1846

Serving Colorado, Kansas, Nebraska, North Dakota, South Dakota, Utah, Wyoming

- Mountain Plains Regional AIDS Education and Training Center
  University of Colorado Health Sciences Center
  4200 East Ninth Avenue, Box A–096
  Denver, CO 80262
  303–270–5885

Serving Florida

- Florida AIDS Education and Training Center
  University of Miami
  Department of Family Medicine
  South Shore Hospital
  600 Alton Road, Suite 502
  Miami Beach, FL 33139
  305–672–2100, extension 3549

Serving Georgia

- Southeast AIDS Training and Education Center
  Emory University
  735 Gatewood Road, NE
  Atlanta, GA 30322–4950
  404–727–2929

Serving Illinois, Indiana, Iowa, Minnesota, Missouri, Wisconsin

- Midwest AIDS Training and Education Center
  University of Illinois at Chicago
  808 South Wood Street (M/C 779)
  Chicago, IL 60612–7303
  312–996–1373 or 312–996–1426

Serving Arkansas, Louisiana, Mississippi

- Delta Region AIDS Education and Training Center
  LSU Medical Center
  136 South Roman Street, 3rd floor
  New Orleans, LA 70112
  504–568–3855

Serving Connecticut, Maine, Massachusetts, New Hampshire, Rhode Island, Vermont

- New England AIDS Education and Training Center
University of Massachusetts
55 Lake Avenue North
Worcester, MA 01655
508–856–3255

Serving Kentucky, Michigan, Ohio, Tennessee

- Great Lakes to Tennessee
Valley AIDS Education and Training Center
Wayne State University
2727 Second Avenue, Room 142
Detroit, MI 48201
313–962–2000

Serving New Jersey

- New Jersey AIDS Education and Training Center
University of Medicine and Dentistry of New Jersey
Center for Continuing Education
30 Bergen Street, ADMC #710
Newark, NJ 07107–3000
201–982–3690

Serving New York and the Virgin Islands

- New York/Virgin Islands AIDS Education
and Training Center
Columbia University School of Public Health
600 West 168th Street, 7th floor
New York, NY 10032
212–305–3616

Serving Pennsylvania

- Pennsylvania AIDS Education and Training Center
University of Pittsburgh
Graduate School of Public Health
130 DeSoto Street, Room A427
Pittsburgh, PA 15261
412–624–1895

Serving Puerto Rico

- Puerto Rico AIDS Education and Training Center
University of Puerto Rico
Medical Sciences Campus
GPO 36–5067, Room A–956
San Juan, PR 00936–6067
809–756–7931

Serving Texas and Oklahoma

- AIDS Education and Training Center
for Texas and Oklahoma
The University of Texas
1200 Herman Pressler Street
PO Box 20186
Houston, TX 77225
713–794–4075

Serving Delaware, Maryland, Virginia, West Virginia, Washington DC

- Mid-Atlantic AIDS Education and Training Center
Virginia Commonwealth University
PO Box 980159
Richmond, VA 23298–0159
804–828–2447

Serving Alaska, Idaho, Montana, Oregon, Washington

- Northwest AIDS Education and Training Center
University of Washington
1001 Broadway, Suite 217
Seattle, WA 98122–4304
206–720–4250

CHAPTER 8

Cold, Cough, and Allergy Products

Karen J. Tietze

Questions to ask in patient assessment and counseling

Allergic Rhinitis

- *What symptoms do you have?*
- *Are the symptoms present year-round or during selected times of the year?*
- *What factors aggravate the symptoms?*
- *Are the symptoms better or worse at home or at work (or at school)?*
- *Does anyone in your family have a history of allergies?*
- *Do you have a fever, sore throat, cough, vomiting, or diarrhea?*
- *What prescription and nonprescription medications are you currently taking?*
- *What prescription and nonprescription medications have you taken in the past to treat your symptoms? Did any of these medications relieve your symptoms?*
- *Are you allergic to any medications?*
- *Do you have any dietary restrictions?*

Congestion

- *What are your symptoms?*
- *Is your nasal discharge thickened or discolored?*
- *What medications have you used to treat your symptoms?*
- *What other medications are you taking?*
- *Are you allergic to any medication?*
- *Have you ever experienced an adverse reaction to any medication?*
- *Have you ever experienced rebound congestion from a topical decongestant?*
- *Do you have hypertension or other cardiovascular diseases? Angle-closure or open-angle glaucoma? Diabetes? Thyroid disease? Benign prostatic hypertrophy? A seizure disorder?*
- *Are you being treated for depression? If so, are you taking isocarboxazid (Marplan), phenelzine (Nardil), or tranylcypromine (Parnate)?*
- *Are you pregnant or breast-feeding?*
- *If the medication is for a child, how old is the child?*
- *Do you participate in official sporting events?*

Allergic rhinitis is the most common atopic disease in the United States.[1,2] The common cold is the second most frequent cause of respiratory tract infection, which is the most common type of infectious disease in the United States.[3] Unfortunately, there are no cures for either allergic rhinitis or the common cold.

Although similar types of drugs are used to treat the symptoms of allergic rhinitis and the common cold, each condition is caused by distinctly different mechanisms. Therefore, different therapeutic approaches are required. This chapter provides the pharmacist with the information necessary to identify and distinguish between the common cold and allergic rhinitis as well as other disorders that may mimic them, to advise the patient on the appropriate selection and use of products, and to monitor patient response.

Anatomy and Physiology

Anatomy

The nose and the mouth are the entry points into the respiratory system. The upper respiratory system, which includes the nose, pharynx, and larynx, filters, warms, and humidifies inspired air. The lower respiratory system, which includes the trachea, bronchi, bronchioles, and alveolar sacs, directs the flow of inspired and expired air and participates in gas exchange (Figures 1 and 2). The nose contains the olfactory apparatus and has an important role in speech.

The external nose is the visible portion of the nose. The internal nose, which is not visible, is located between the cranium and the hard palate in the roof of the mouth. The nostrils (nares), separated by the nasal septum, are lined with coarse hairs (vibrissae) that filter inspired air. Each nostril ends in a cavity that is divided horizontally into the superior, middle, and inferior turbinates. These chambers increase the surface area of the nasal cavities, enhancing the ability of the nose to filter, warm, and humidify inspired air.

Four pairs of sinus cavities (frontal, maxillary, ethmoidal, and sphenoidal) are located around the nose. These cavities, which are named for the bones in which each is found, drain posteriorly into the pharynx, lighten the cranium, and serve as resonating chambers for speech.

Editor's Note: This chapter is based, in part, on a chapter with the same title that appeared in the 10th edition but was written by Bobby G. Bryant and Thomas P. Lombardi.

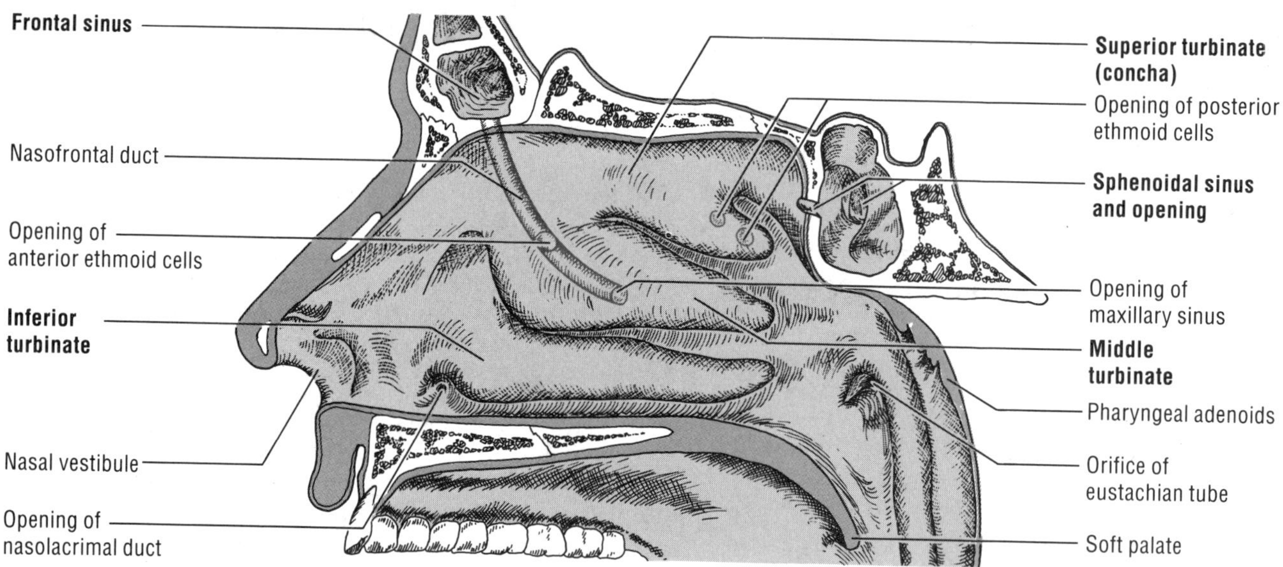

FIGURE 1 The nose and paranasal sinus. Reprinted with permission from *Medical Notes on the Common Cold.* Pub No P199–2. Research Triangle Park. NC: Burroughs Wellcome Co; 1972.

The pharynx connects the nasal cavities to the larynx and esophagus. The pharynx is divided into three areas: the nasopharynx, the oropharynx, and the hypopharynx. Each area is named for the closest anatomic structure. The nasopharynx, the area from the posterior nares to the soft palate, contains the pharyngeal tonsils (adenoids); the eustachian tubes connect the nasopharynx to the middle ears. The middle ears are closed compartments that communicate with the respiratory system via the eustachian tubes. The eustachian tubes are closed 99% of the time but open during swallowing to equilibrate atmospheric and middle ear pressures. The oropharynx, the area behind the rear opening of the mouth down to the hyoid bone, contains the palatine tonsils. The hypopharynx is the area from the hyoid bone to the esophagus and larynx. The larynx is the area below the tongue to the trachea and includes the vocal cords and the epiglottis. The epiglottis closes over the larynx during swallowing, preventing material from being aspirated into the lower respiratory tract system.

The nasal mucosa is lined with a complex, specialized membrane called the respiratory mucosa. The respiratory mucosa contains ciliated epithelial cells, nonciliated columnar epithelial cells, goblet cells, and basal cells. A basement membrane separates the respiratory mucosa from the submucosa, which contains mucous, seromucous, and serous glands. These glands secrete a variety of substances (eg, lysozyme, lactoferrin, neutral endopeptidase, secretory leukoprotease inhibitor, and secretory IgA) that provide important defenses against some inflammatory mediators, bacteria, and viruses.

The respiratory mucosa is covered by a double layer of fluid. Outermost is a thick, sticky layer that traps dust, bacteria, viruses, and other foreign materials; innermost is a thinner, more aqueous layer that contains most of the immunologic mediators. The columnar epithelial cells contain microvilli, nonmobile projections that increase cell surface area and facilitate hydration of inspired air. Cilia from ciliated epithelial cells beat in a synchronized, wavelike pattern in the aqueous mucus layer, sweeping the thicker outer layer toward the larynx, where the mucus is swallowed.

The interstitium contains lymphocytes, fibroblasts, and mast cells. The mast cells are located close to nerves and blood vessels and are clustered in the epithelium just beneath the basement membrane.

The nose is a highly vascular organ, with a greater total blood flow per cubic centimeter of tissue than the brain, liver, or muscle. The large blood flow presumably increases the efficiency of the nose in warming and conditioning inspired air. The nasal mucosa contains the usual arterial and venous circulations, many arteriovenous anastomoses, and specialized blood vessels called the cavernous sinusoids.

Physiology

Neurotransmitters

The nose is innervated by sensory, cholinergic, and sympathetic nerves. The sensory fibers respond to mechanical injury, thermal injury, temperature changes, and a variety of mediators such as histamine and bradykinin. The sympathetic nerves innervate veins and venules. The glands and the arteries that supply the glands are innervated by both sympathetic and cholinergic nerves. Sympathetic stimulation causes vasoconstriction; cholinergic

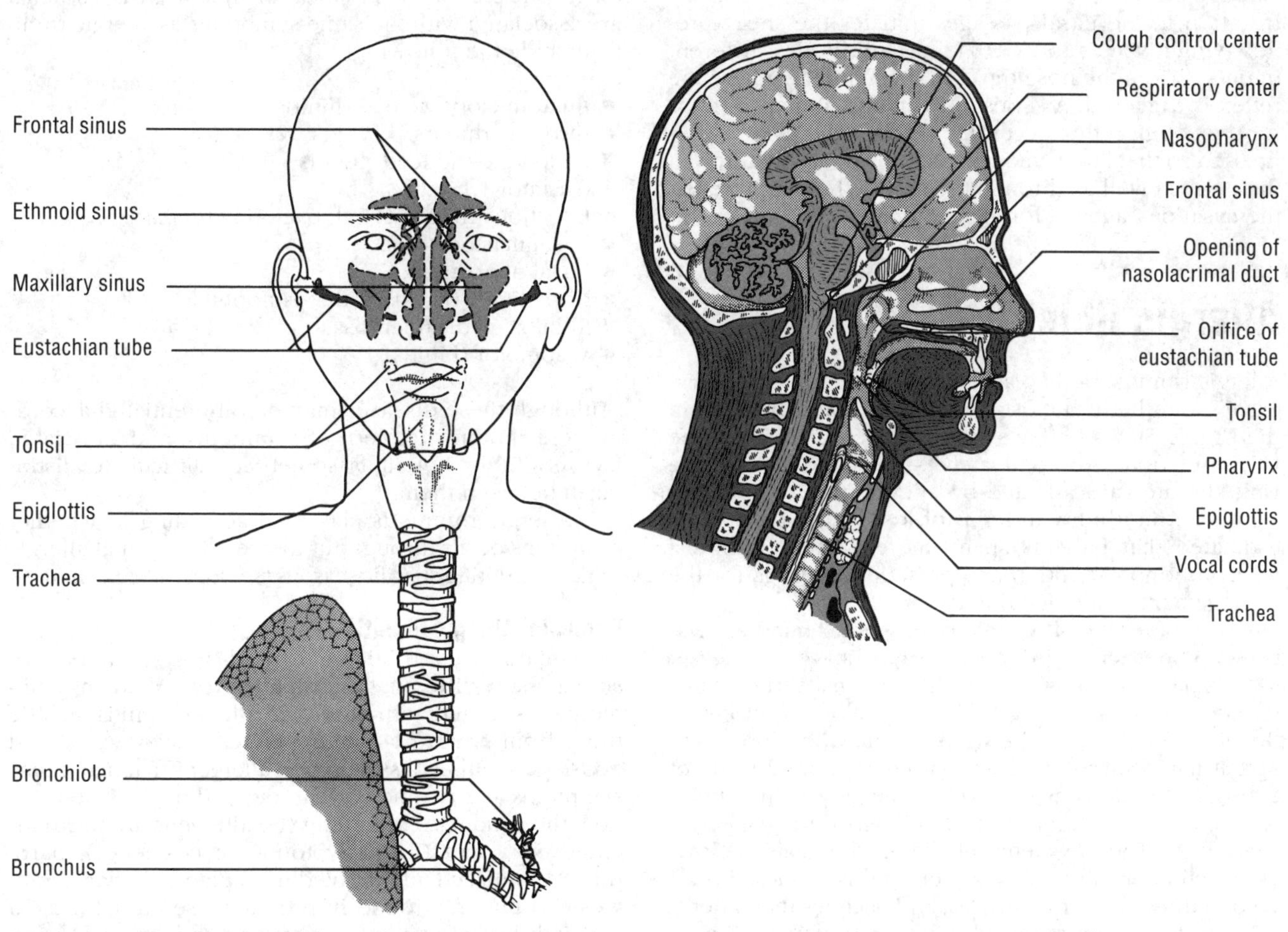

FIGURE 2 Anatomy of the respiratory passages.

stimulation causes vasodilatation. The cavernous sinusoids contain erectile tissue that becomes engorged when the sympathetic tone is reduced or when the cholinergic system is stimulated.

The sensory, cholinergic, and sympathetic nerves also respond to a variety of neuropeptide neurotransmitters, including calcitonin gene-related peptide (CGRP), substance P (SP), neurokinin A (NKA), gastrin-releasing peptide (GRP), vasoactive intestinal peptide (VIP), peptide histidine methione, and neuropeptide Y. Although the exact function of most of these neurotransmitters is not known, some functions have been identified. For example, CGRP induces vasodilatation; neuropeptide Y induces vasoconstriction; and GRP, VIP, SP, and NKA induce mucous cell and/or serous cell secretion. Future drug therapy may be targeted at these neuropeptides.

Cough Reflex

The cough reflex is an important respiratory tract defense mechanism. Coughing, which may be voluntary or secondary to the stimulation of mechanical or chemical irritant receptors located throughout the larynx and lower respiratory tract, expels mucus, cellular debris, and foreign material from the bronchi, trachea, and larynx. Stimulation of mechanical or chemical irritant receptors by foreign material, irritant gases, inflammation, and extremes of temperature initiates afferent impulses along nerve pathways to the central cough center in the medulla. The central cough center coordinates the complex cough response, which consists of a deep inspiration followed by closure of the glottis and forceful contraction of the chest wall, abdominal wall, and diaphragmatic muscles against the closed glottis. When the glottis reopens, the airways are cleared by the very high expiratory flow rates generated by the differences between intra-airway and atmospheric pressures.

Cough may be a symptom of a wide variety of unrelated diseases, including allergic rhinitis, the common cold, asthma, bronchitis, chronic obstructive pulmonary disease, pneumonia, carcinoma, and congestive heart failure. A cough may be classified as either productive or nonproductive. A productive cough is associated with the expectoration of secretions from the lower respiratory tract; a nonproductive cough is a dry cough. Coughing may be self-perpetuating in that excessive coughing further irritates tracheal and pharyngeal mucosa.

Sneeze Reflex

Irritation in the nasal passages initiates the sneeze reflex, which serves to clear the nasal passages. Afferent impulses from the nose travel to the medulla, where the reflex is triggered. A series of reactions similar to those for the cough reflex occur. In addition, the uvula is depressed so that large amounts of air pass rapidly through the nose as well as through the mouth, helping to clear the nasal passages of foreign material.

Allergic Rhinitis

Allergic rhinitis, ranked as the most common atopic disease[1,2] and the fifth most common chronic condition in the United States,[1] affects approximately 10–15% of the US population.[4] Approximately 8–10% of children in the United States are affected by allergic rhinitis, causing significant morbidity in terms of lost school days.[5] It is estimated that patients spend more than $1 billion a year on nonprescription and prescription drugs for the management of allergic rhinitis.[6]

The hallmark of allergic rhinitis is a temporal relationship between exposure to allergens and the development of nasal symptoms. Although approximately two thirds of individuals with allergic rhinitis develop symptoms of the disease before age 30, symptoms may develop at any age. It has been estimated that it takes about 2 years of exposure to allergens to develop allergic rhinitis; therefore, the disease rarely affects children during the first year of life. The prevalence of allergic rhinitis is the lowest in children under 5 years of age, is highest in the second through fourth decades, and declines thereafter.[7]

There is a genetic predisposition to developing allergic rhinitis; 60% of patients with the disease have a family history of atopy.[8] The risk of developing allergic rhinitis is 30% if one parent has a history of atopic diseases; the risk rises to 50% if both parents have atopic disease.[9] There is no association between the development of allergic rhinitis and the patient's birth month, birth order, or birth weight; the maternal age at conception; or breast-feeding.[10] Although there is no gender predilection for allergic rhinitis when all age groups are considered, boys up to age 10 are twice as likely as girls to have allergic rhinitis.[2]

Data regarding remission rates are limited. The remission rate in the only community-based study to report remission rates was 5–10% in the 4 years following diagnosis.[7] The rates were higher in males, older patients, those with recent onset of disease, and those with seasonal symptoms. In another study, approximately 10% of children were symptom free 10 years after the initial diagnosis, and about half the children were managed without medications.[11] Asthma develops in about 19% of children with allergic rhinitis and is more likely in those children presenting with perennial allergic rhinitis.[11]

Etiology

The term *rhinitis* means "inflammation of the nose." Rhinitis is considered allergic when a causative allergen can be identified. However, there are no universally accepted diagnostic criteria or classification systems. Diseases that are associated with the same symptoms as allergic rhinitis include the following:

- Anatomic obstructive rhinitis;
- Atrophic rhinitis;
- Endocrine-induced rhinitis;
- Gustatory rhinitis;
- Infectious rhinitis (viral, bacterial, fungal);
- Nasal mastocytosis;
- Nasal neoplasms;
- Nonallergic rhinitis with eosinophilia;
- Rhinitis medicamentosa;
- Vasomotor rhinitis.

Although these diseases may be differentiated according to symptoms, pattern of symptoms, and associated factors (Table 1),[12] it is sometimes difficult to distinguish between them.

Allergic rhinitis is classified according to whether symptoms occur throughout the year (perennial allergic rhinitis) or during specific seasons (seasonal allergic rhinitis).

Perennial Allergic Rhinitis

Perennial allergic rhinitis is caused by continual exposure to many different types of allergens. Allergens commonly associated with perennial allergic rhinitis include those from house dust mites, molds, cockroaches, and house pets. Other, less common allergens that may cause symptoms at any time of year, depending on when and how the products containing the allergens are used, include orris root (formerly found in cosmetics), pyrethrum (an insecticide derived from plants similar to ragweed, commonly found in products used to treat head and body lice infestations), cottonseed and flaxseed (found in animal feeds, fertilizers, hair-setting preparations, and some foods), and some vegetable gums (found in some denture adhesive powders, tooth powders, hair-setting preparations, and foods).

House dust, a mixture of lint, mites, mite feces, fibers, and insect parts, is a well-known cause of allergies. The house dust mite, a large constituent of house dust, is among the most common causes of perennial rhinitis. Patients who can associate bouts of repeated sneezing first thing in the morning with making the bed or cleaning the house are most likely allergic to the house dust mite.

Two species of house dust mites, *Dermatophagoides farinae* and *Dermatophagoides pteronyssinus*, have been identified. These organisms, found in all but the driest desert regions of the United States, thrive in carpets, bedding, and upholstery and reproduce best in the warm (65–70°F [18.3–21.1°C]), humid (>50%) environments found in most homes. The mites feed on human skin scales, an abundant food source. The mite itself is not the allergen; the main allergen is a glycoprotein found in mite feces.[13] These feces remain airborne for about 30 minutes after being disturbed. House dust mites ingest their own feces, which are coated with a glycoprotein that aids in the digestion of the fecal material. Other mite proteins and proteases are also allergenic.

Indoor and outdoor molds are another common cause of perennial allergic rhinitis. Molds grow best in warm, moist environments and are found year-round in basements and other moist indoor areas. In contrast to pollen allergens, which are removed from the air by rain, molds remain in clouds and mist. *Alternaria* and *Cladosporium* are the most common outdoor molds; *Penicillium* and *Aspergillus* are the most common indoor molds. Other molds associated with perennial allergic rhinitis include grain-associated smut and rust fungi, *Rhizopus nigricans* (black bread mold), *Saccharomyces cerevisiae* (baker's yeast), *Chaetomium*, *Curvularia*, *Helminthosporium*, *Spondylocladium*, *Stemphylium rhodotorula*, and the slime molds *Fusarium*, *Phoma*, *Pullumlaria*, and *Trichoderma*.

Allergens associated with house pets and insects are common causes of perennial allergic rhinitis. The cockroach is a major allergen in urban environments. Cat-derived allergens—proteins secreted through sebaceous glands in the skin—are small, light proteins that can stay airborne for up to 6 hours. Cat allergens can be identified in house dust for several months after the cat has been removed from the environment.

Seasonal Allergic Rhinitis

Seasonal allergic rhinitis is caused by windborne plant (eg, tree, grass, and ragweed) pollens. Plants that depend on insect pollination, such as goldenrod and dandelions, do not usually cause allergic rhinitis. The terms *hay fever* and *rose fever* relate to the seasons associated with grass and ragweed pollinosis and are not associated with fever.

Although the duration of the pollinating season varies geographically, the onset is about the same in all regions. Ragweed is the worst offender, affecting about 75% of patients with allergic rhinitis in the eastern and midwestern United States. Ragweed begins to pollinate in mid-August and persists until the first frost. Other weed pollens appear in late summer and early fall and also last until the first frost. Other common pollens include tree pollens, which appear in late March and last through May, and grass pollens, which appear in May and last through June or early July.

TABLE 1 Features of common rhinitis syndromes

	Allergic rhinitis	Infectious rhinitis	Vasomotor rhinitis	Rhinitis medicamentosa
Etiology	Allergens	Viral or bacterial	Unknown	Tachyphylaxis to topical decongestants
Symptoms	Rhinorrhea, congestion, sneezing, pruritus (nose or roof of mouth), allergic shiners, allergic salute, cough with postnasal drip, ocular itching and lacrimation	Fever[a], constitutional symptoms, mucopurulent rhinorrhea, scratchy throat, congestion, cough	Rhinorrhea, congestion	Congestion
Pattern	Perennial or seasonal	Any time	Any time	Temporal relationship with use of topical decongestants
Associated factors	Concurrent atopic disease, family history	None	Affects primarily women; precipitated by strong odors, alcohol, stress, and changes in temperature, humidity, and barometric pressure	Overuse of topical decongestants, concurrent antihypertensive therapy

[a]Rare; more common in children.

Adapted from Fireman P. Pathophysiology and pharmacotherapy of common upper respiratory diseases. *Pharmacotherapy*. 1993 Nov-Dec; 13 (16 pt 2): 101S–9S.

Pathophysiology

Immunologic Response

Patients do not experience symptoms when first exposed to an allergen. Rather, a complex series of immunologic events occurs, resulting in the creation of sensitized mast cells and mediator generation following reexposure to the allergen.[5,14,15]

Initially, the allergen is engulfed by antigen-presenting cells (macrophages, dendritic cells, and Langerhans' cells), which partially degrade the allergen and then incorporate fragments of it onto their cell surfaces. The antigen-presenting cells secrete interleukin-1 (IL-1), a growth factor that activates T lymphocytes. The activated T lymphocytes recognize the altered antigen-presenting cells and secrete a variety of mediators, including interleukin-4 (IL-4), interleukin-5 (IL-5), and histamine-releasing factor. IL-4 promotes the production of antigen-specific immunoglobulin E (IgE); IL-5 promotes B cell differentiation and induces differentiation of eosinophils; and histamine-releasing factor promotes the release of preformed mast cell mediators. The antigen-specific IgE binds to high-affinity receptors on mast cells and basophils and to low-affinity receptors on monocytes, eosinophils, and platelets. Subsequent exposure to the antigen results in mast cell degranulation and the release and synthesis of a cascade of inflammatory and irritant mediators.[5,15]

Mast cells release a variety of preformed (histamine, heparin, chondroitin sulfate, tryptase, chymotrypase, and carboxypeptidase) and newly synthesized lipid (LTB_4, LTC_4, PGD_2, platelet-activating factor) and cytokine (IL-4, IL-5, IL-6, tumor necrosis factor-alpha) mediators. Histamine, a potent vasodilator, induces mucus hypersecretion and irritates local nerves, resulting in immediate congestion, rhinorrhea, sneezing, and pruritus. These responses are amplified by leukotrienes, prostaglandins, and cytokines. The chemotactic mediators, including platelet-activating factor and LTB_4, attract neutrophils and eosinophils to the area. Eosinophils release a variety of mediators that contribute to the tissue inflammation and edema and increase the nasal reactivity.[5]

The early or immediate response to an allergen occurs within minutes following reexposure to it. Symptoms include rhinorrhea, mucus secretion, pruritus, flushing, hypotension, and smooth muscle contraction. These initial symptoms are of short duration (minutes), and corticosteroids have little or no effect on them. About half the patients with allergic rhinitis also experience a recurrence of symptoms without any additional allergen exposure.[16] This late-phase reaction, which occurs within hours of the initial symptoms, lasts hours to days and can be treated with corticosteroids. The late-phase reaction is secondary to the infiltration of the nasal mucosa with eosinophils, neutrophils, macrophages, and fibroblasts. Repeated allergen exposure results in increased sensitivity and an almost continuous mediator release.

Complications

Chronic obstruction around the sinus ostia and eustachian tubes increases the risk of sinusitis, recurrent otitis media, and eustachian tube dysfunction. Poor tympanic membrane compliance and significant hearing loss may result from fluid collections in the middle ears. Patients who develop fever, purulent nasal discharge, frequent headaches, or earache should be referred to their physicians for evaluation and treatment.

Patient Assessment

Patient assessment consists of detailed patient interviews and close observation of the patient for the presence of physical findings associated with allergic rhinitis. The pharmacist should ask the patient the questions listed at the beginning of the chapter to determine the specific symptoms experienced; the severity and pattern, if any, of those symptoms; predisposing factors; and current and past treatment regimens.

Symptoms

The major ocular symptoms include itching, lacrimation, mild soreness, puffiness, chemosis, and conjunctival hyperemia. The major nasal symptoms include nasal congestion, watery rhinorrhea, itching, sneezing paroxysms, and postnasal drip. Nasal pruritus may result if the nose is repeatedly rubbed or picked. The characteristic gesture of rubbing the tip of the nose upward with the palm of the hand is known as the "allergic salute." The major head and neck symptoms include loss of taste and smell, mild sore throat secondary to postnasal drip, earache, sinus headache, itching of the palate and throat, and repeated clearing of the throat. The major systemic symptoms include malaise and fatigue. It is important to note that uncomplicated allergic rhinitis does not cause fever, significant sore throat, vomiting, or diarrhea. The presence of these symptoms instead suggests a viral or bacterial infection; patients with these symptoms should be referred to their physicians for evaluation and treatment.

Symptom Patterns

The symptoms associated with perennial allergic rhinitis are similar but less severe than those associated with seasonal allergic rhinitis. Symptoms may be clearly associated with specific activities such as mowing the lawn, raking leaves, or vacuuming the carpet, or they may be exacerbated by nonspecific irritants such as cigarette smoke. Patients may be symptom free at work or school but extremely symptomatic in other environments. Patients should be questioned as to what factors they associate with their symptoms and what patterns their symptoms seem to show. Aggravating factors such as cigarette smoke, strong odors, and air pollution should be identified.

Physical Assessment

Patients may have "allergic shiners," which are dark circles beneath the eyes secondary to venous and lymphatic congestion. A horizontal crease across the lower third of the nose may be visible in patients who repeatedly rub their noses upward. Severe nasal obstruction may result in chronic mouth breathing, which in turn may cause changes such as a highly arched palate, an overbite, or dental malocclusion. The nasal mucosa appear pale and swollen; the nasal secretions are clear and watery. The eyes may be watery with scleral and conjunctival hyperemia, and there may be periorbital edema.[5]

TABLE 2 Symptomatic nonprescription drug treatment of allergic rhinitis

Symptoms	Treatment
Ocular itching, lacrimation, puffiness	Ophthalmic antihistamines, systemic antihistamines
Chemosis, conjunctival redness	Ophthalmic decongestants
Rhinorrhea, nasal itching, postnasal drip	Systemic antihistamines
Nasal congestion	Systemic decongestants (topical is an option but overuse potential is high)
Headache, earache, sinus pain	Systemic analgesics (decongestants may relieve sinus pain due to sinus congestion)

Diagnostic Testing

Skin tests can differentiate allergic from nonallergic reactions. Although negative results on skin tests indicate a nonallergic etiology, positive results cannot be positively associated with a specific allergen unless a relationship can be established between exposure to the allergen and the characteristic symptoms. Therefore, intensive patient histories must be obtained. Patients as young as 1–4 months can be tested; however, it takes 2–4 years of exposure to aeroallergens to develop a sensitivity to these types of allergens. Food allergies are much more common in children less than 1 year of age.

There are several different types of skin tests.[17] Scratch tests, the original skin tests, are performed by placing a drop of concentrated antigen on abraded skin; the classic wheal and flare responses indicate a positive reaction. However, scratch testing cannot quantify the reaction and is not always reproducible. Therefore, scratch testing is no longer recommended by the Allergy Panel of the American Medical Association Council of Scientific Affairs.

Other types of skin tests include the skin prick test, the intradermal skin test, and the skin endpoint titration (SET) test. The skin prick test is commonly used as the initial test for house dust mite, animal dander, mold, and pollen allergies. It involves placing a drop of antigen on the skin and puncturing the skin superficially with a needle; the localized reaction is evaluated subjectively. The intradermal skin test involves injecting a small amount of allergen intradermally; the wheal and flare responses are rated subjectively on a scale of 0–4. The SET test, which is the only quantitative skin test, involves making a series of injections with increasingly more concentrated allergen and then evaluating the reaction.

Two serologic tests are available. These tests correlate total IgE levels with severity of disease; however, there is considerable overlap between normal and abnormal serum IgE levels. The serum IgE radioallergosorbent test is recommended for patients with severe eczema or dermatographism (physical hives) in whom interpretation of skin tests would be difficult, or for patients taking long-acting antihistamines in whom the response to standard skin tests would be diminished. The paper disk radioimmunosorbent test also measures total serum IgE levels.

Other diagnostic tests may be used to diagnose allergic rhinitis and identify complications of it. Nasal cytology, as determined by microscopic evaluation of nasal secretions, helps differentiate between allergic rhinitis (elevated eosinophils) and infectious rhinitis (elevated neutrophils). Plain radiographic images are useful for imaging the maxillary sinuses; computed tomography (CT) or magnetic resonance imaging (MRI) scans are needed to image the other sinuses. Chest radiographs and pulmonary function tests may be used to rule out asthma. Flexible and rigid nasal endoscopy may be used to identify anatomical abnormalities. Audiometry and tympanometry may be used to test the hearing.

Disease Management

The first step in managing allergic rhinitis is avoidance of the offending allergens. Pharmacotherapy is used if avoidance measures are not feasible or do not adequately relieve the symptoms. Treatment is symptomatic and should be targeted at patient-specific symptoms (Table 2).

Classes of drugs used to treat allergic rhinitis include antihistamines, decongestants, anticholinergics, mast cell stabilizers, mucolytics, and corticosteroids. Immunotherapy is indicated for patients whose symptoms cannot be adequately controlled with medications or whose symptoms occur most days of the year.

Preventive Measures

Patients allergic to outdoor allergens can avoid many allergens by following pollen count reports, keeping house and car windows closed, and using air conditioners. Pollen counts—the number of pollen grains per cubic meter per 24 hours—may help patients plan outdoor activities. Low pollen counts (0–10 grains/m^3 per 24 hours) are generally associated with symptoms only in patients who are very sensitive to outdoor allergens; most patients will be symptomatic when the pollen counts are very high (>500 grains/m^3 per 24 hours).

Patients with grass allergies should not work or play in grassy areas, especially during early summer or when the grass is being mowed or raked. Patients with outdoor mold allergies should avoid mowing the lawn and raking leaves and should not disturb leaf or compost piles. Indoor mold exposure can be reduced by venting moist bathrooms and kitchens, using dehumidification, and eliminating chronically moldy areas of the indoor environment (eg, wet basements).

House dust mite exposure can be minimized by carefully controlling the indoor environment. Indoor humidity should be reduced to less than 50%. Pillows, mattresses, and box springs should be encased in plastic airtight covers that are cleaned weekly with a damp cloth. Items that collect dust, such as rugs, stuffed furniture, stuffed toys, and open bookshelves and television or stereo cabinets, should be removed from sleeping areas. All bedding, including mattress pads, should be cleaned weekly in hot water. Vacuum cleaners should be equipped with high-efficiency particulate air cleaner (HEPA) filters to avoid aerosolizing the house dust mite feces when vacuuming. Acaricides such as tannic acid and benzyl benzoate can be used to treat furniture and carpeting, but treatment needs to be repeated frequently.

Animal allergen exposures can be limited by removing pets from the household or at least by totally excluding the pet from the patient's bedroom. Weekly washing of cats will decrease the amount of cat allergen in the environment.

Air filtration devices, of which HEPA filtration devices are the most effective, can be used to remove pollen, mold spores, and cat allergens from the air; house dust mite particles are heavier and settle to the floor too quickly to be effectively reduced by air filtration. HEPA filters can be installed in the central ductwork of homes with forced air heat or can be freestanding units. Because they are expensive, however, patients should be encouraged to rent HEPA filters before investing in permanently installed devices.

TABLE 3 Structural antihistamine classification

Ethanolamines	Piperazines
Carbinoxamine maleate	Cyclizine hydrochloride
Clemastine fumarate	Cyclizine lactate
Dimenhydrinate	Hydroxyzine hydrochloride
Diphenhydramine hydrochloride	Hydroxyzine pamoate
Doxylamine	Meclizine hydrochloride
Phenyltolaxime	
Ethylenediamines	**Phenothiazines**
Pyrilamine maleate	Methdilazine
Tripelennamine citrate	Promethazine hydrochloride
Tripelennamine hydrochloride	Trimeprazine
Alkylamines	**Piperidines**
Brompheniramine maleate	Astemizole
Chlorpheniramine maleate	Azatadine maleate
Dexchlorpheniramine	Cyproheptadine
Pheniramine	Diphenylpyraline
Triprolidine hydrochloride	Phenindamine tartrate
	Terfenadine

Antihistamines

Antihistamines are first-line agents for the prophylaxis and treatment of allergic rhinitis. However, antihistamines can reduce symptoms by only about 40–60%.[18] Their usefulness is limited because they compete with just one of the mediators (histamine) produced during the allergic reaction. In addition, antihistamines directly compete with histamine for the histamine receptor; their success depends on the timing and the amount of drug available for the competition.

Histamine is the primary mediator for sneezing and pruritus; it contributes to but is not the sole mediator for mucus production, vascular permeability, and smooth muscle contraction. Therefore, antihistamines are very effective for reducing the symptoms of sneezing and itching and somewhat effective for reducing rhinorrhea, but they have no effect on nasal congestion.

Mechanism of Action Three histamine receptors have been identified.[19] Stimulation of histamine-1 receptors produces sneezing, pruritis, increased mucus production, increased vascular permeability, and smooth muscle contraction. Stimulation of histamine-2 receptors results in stomach acid secretion and is associated with vascular dilation and cutaneous reactions. Histamine-3 receptors, located in the brain, control the synthesis and release of histamine. Antihistamines used to control the symptoms of allergic rhinitis compete with histamine for binding to histamine-1 receptors. Histamine-2 blockers have been investigated but found to be ineffective and potentially harmful in that they decrease the threshold dose of histamine.[20]

Some antihistamines have additional antiallergic and anti-inflammatory properties, which appear to be agent specific. For example, azatadine, terfenadine, and ketotifen inhibit the release of some mediators[21]; cetirizine inhibits tissue eosinophil influx[22]; and terfenadine, astemizole, and cetirizine may have mild bronchodilatory properties.[23] The clinical significance of these actions is not known. The older, traditional antihistamines have varying degrees of anticholinergic, antiemetic, sedative, and local anesthetic activity.

Classification Antihistamines may be classified by chemical structure (Table 3), relative sedative properties, or generation. The second-generation, nonsedating antihistamines (astemizole [Hismanal], cetirizine, loratadine [Claritin)], and terfenadine [Seldane]) differ from the first-generation antihistamines in that they are highly specific for histamine-1 receptors and do not have any anticholinergic, antiemetic, or local anesthetic activity.[19]

Side Effects The side effects profile of antihistamines depends on the receptor activity, chemical structure, and lipophilicity of the drug. First-generation antihistamines block muscarinic cholinergic receptors. Side effects associated with cholinergic blockage include dryness of the eyes, mouth, and nose; blurred vision; urinary retention; and tachycardia. High doses of drugs that block cholinergic receptors may induce central cholinergic blockage manifested as irritability.[2] First-generation antihistamines are highly lipophilic; they cross the blood-brain barrier and are associated with significant sedation and impaired mental performance. Second-generation antihistamines are not lipophilic; they do not cross the blood-brain barrier and are less sedating than traditional first-generation antihistamines.

TABLE 4 Recommended dosage guidelines for nonprescription antihistamines

Drug	Dosage (maximum/24 h) Adults (>12 y)	Children[a]
Brompheniramine maleate	4 mg every 4–6 h (24 mg)	6–<12 y: 2 mg every 4–6 h (12 mg) 2–<6 y: 1 mg every 4–6 h (6 mg)
Chlorcyclizine hydrochloride	25 mg every 6–8 h (75 mg)	6–<12 y: 12.5 mg every 6–8 h (37.5 mg) 2–<6 y: 6.25 mg every 6–8 h (18.75 mg)
Chlorpheniramine maleate	4 mg every 4–6 h (24 mg)	6–<12 y: 2 mg every 4–6 h (12 mg) 2–<6 y: 1 mg every 4–6 h (6 mg)
Dexbrompheniramine maleate	2 mg every 4–6 h (12 mg)	6–<12 y: 1 mg every 4–6 h (6 mg) 2–<6 y: 0.5 mg every 4–6 h (3 mg)
Dexchlorpheniramine maleate	2 mg every 4–6 h (12 mg)	6–<12 y: 1 mg every 4–6 h (6 mg) 2–<6 y: 0.5 mg every 4–6 h (3 mg)
Diphenhydramine citrate	38–76 mg every 4–6 h (456 mg)	6–<12 y: 19–38 mg every 4–6 h (228 mg) 2–<6 y: 9.5 mg every 4–6 h (57 mg)
Diphenhydramine hydrochloride	25–50 mg every 6–8 h (300 mg)	6–<12 y: 12.5–25 mg every 4–6 h (150 mg) 2–<6 y: 6.25 mg every 4–6 h (37.5 mg)
Doxylamine succinate	7.5–12.5 mg every 4–6 h (75 mg)	6–<12 y: 3.75–6.25 mg every 4–6 h (37.5 mg) 2–<6 y: 1.9–3.125 mg every 4–6 h (18.75 mg)
Phenindamine tartrate	25 mg every 4–6 h (150 mg)	6–<12 y: 12.5 mg every 4–6 h (75 mg) 2–<6 y: 6.25 mg every 4–6 h (37.5 mg)
Pheniramine maleate	12.5–25 mg every 4–6 h (150 mg)	6–<12 y: 6.25–12.5 mg every 4–6 h (75 mg) 2–<6 y: 3.125–6.25 mg every 4–6 h (37.5 mg)
Pyrilamine maleate	25–50 mg every 6–8 h (200 mg)	6–<12 y: 12.5–25 mg every 6–8 h (100 mg) 2–<6 y: 6.25–12.5 mg every 6–8 h (50 mg)
Thonzylamine hydrochloride	50–100 mg every 4–6 h (600 mg)	6–<12 y: 25–50 mg every 4–6 h (300 mg) 2–<6: 12.5–25 mg every 4–6 h (150 mg)
Triprolidine hydrochloride	2.5 mg every 4–6 h (10 mg)	6–<12 y: 1.25 mg every 4–6 h (5 mg) 4–<6 y: 0.93 mg every 4–6 h (3.744 mg) 2–<4 y: 0.625 mg every 4–6 h (2.5 mg) Infants 4 mo–<2 y: 0.313 mg every 4–6 h (1.252 mg)

[a]With the exception of triprolidine hydrochloride, these products are not recommended for children under 2 years of age except under the advice and supervision of a physician.

Reprinted from Cold, cough, allergic bronchodilator, and antiasthmatic drug products for over-the-counter human use; final monograph for OTC antihistamines; final rule. *Federal Register.* 1992 Dec; 57: 58356–76.

Antihistamines have a quinidine-like effect on cardiac muscle. This can lead to prolongation of the Q-T interval. Torsade de pointes, a potentially fatal dysarrhythmia, has been reported with terfenadine and astemizole; some first-generation antihistamines may also cause this rare arrhythmia.[24] The ethylenediamines appear to be associated with more pronounced gastrointestinal side effects than other antihistamines. Astemizole and cyproheptadine (Periactin) appear to be associated with greater increases in appetite and weight gain.

Product Selection Guidelines Dosage guidelines for nonprescription antihistamines are listed in Table 4.[25] Product selection depends on the side effects profile of the drug and the patient's response to the drug. Second-generation antihistamines are currently available only by prescription and are more costly than first-generation antihistamines. Of the first-generation antihistamines, the alkylamines (chlorpheniramine, brompheniramine, and pheniramine) are the least sedating and the ethanolamines (diphenhydramine, doxylamine, and phenyltoloxamine) are the most sedating.

TABLE 5 Decongestants

Topical intranasal decongestants

Short acting (4- to 6-h duration)
Ephedrine
Epinephrine
Naphazoline
Phenylephrine
Tetrahydrozoline

Intermediate acting (8- to 10-h duration)
Xylometazoline

Long acting
Oxymetazoline

Ophthalmic decongestants
Epinephrine

Ophthalmic decongestants *(continued)*
Naphazoline
Oxymetazoline
Phenylephrine
Tetrahydrozoline

Systemic decongestants
Ephedrine
Phenylephrine
Phenylpropanolamine
Pseudoephedrine

Inhalers
Desoxyephedrine
Propylhexedrine

Tolerance, the reduced response to a drug after prolonged use, is most likely an overstated issue. Antihistamines do induce their own metabolism, but the clinical significance of this action is unknown. The loss of response that some patients report is most likely due to noncompliance, increasing antigen exposure, worsening disease, the limited effectiveness of antihistamines in severe disease, or the development of similar symptoms from unrelated diseases.[26] Despite these issues, some clinicians still recommend trying different structural classes of drugs when patients report a lack of response (see product table "Cold, Cough, and Allergy Products").

Decongestants

Decongestants are vasoconstrictive drugs that reduce nasal congestion. However, decongestants have no effect on histamine or any other mediator involved in the allergic reaction. Therefore, decongestants are commonly administered in combination with antihistamines.

The decongestants that are available for oral (systemic) and topical (intranasal and ophthalmic) administration are listed in Table 5; the advantages and disadvantages of the various topical dosage forms are listed in Table 6. Common dosages for selected systemic and topical decongestants are listed in Tables 7 and 8.[27]

Mechanism of Action Decongestants are alpha-adrenergic agonists (sympathomimetics). Stimulation of alpha-adrenergic receptors constricts blood vessels throughout the body, reduces the supply of blood to the nose, decreases the amount of blood in the sinusoid vessels, and decreases mucosal edema.[28]

Side Effects Topical decongestants are minimally absorbed; systemic side effects tend to be infrequent and minimal when they do occur. Topical decongestants may cause local irritation secondary to irritation from the propellant or vehicle or from trauma from the tip of the bottle during drug administration.

Rebound congestion (rhinitis medicamentosa), or rebound nasal mucosal edema, is a common problem when decongestants are administered topically for more than 3–5 days; it is more common with the short-acting agents than with the long-acting ones. Patients complain of a stuffy nose despite frequent doses of topical decongestants. Although the precise mechanism of this reaction has not been identified, prolonged vasoconstriction is thought to cause a secondary vasodilatation and a decreased response to vasoconstricting agents. Treatment of rebound congestion consists of slow withdrawal of the topical decongestant (one nostril at a time); replacement of the decongestant with topical normal saline, which is believed to soothe and moisten the nasal mucosa; and, if needed, topical corticosteroids and systemic decongestants.[29] The mucous membrane returns to normal in 1–2 weeks following discontinuation of the topical decongestant.

Systemic decongestants constrict all vascular beds and stimulate the central nervous system. Side effects associated with central nervous system stimulation include nervousness, irritability, restlessness, and insomnia. Potential side effects from systemic vasoconstriction include increased blood pressure, increased heart rate, irregular heart rate, and palpitations. Diseases potentially aggravated by sympathomimetics include high blood pressure, heart disease, diabetes mellitus, and hyperthyroidism. Monoamine oxidase inhibition intensifies sympathomimetic activity; oral sympathomimetics are contraindicated in patients who are taking monoamine oxidase inhibitors for the treatment of depression, other psychiatric or emotional conditions, or Parkinson's disease except under the advice and supervision of a physician.

Stimulation of alpha-adrenergic receptors with systemic decongestants may induce urinary sphincter constriction, which may interfere with urinary flow in males. Stimulation of alpha-adrenergic receptors in the eye may produce slight pupillary dilation and elevation of intraocular pressure by narrowing the anterior chamber angle, but the adverse effects on angle-closure glau-

TABLE 6 Advantages and disadvantages of topical decongestant dosage forms

Dosage form	Advantages	Disadvantages
Sprays[a]	Simple to use; fast onset of action; relatively inexpensive; large surface-area coverage	Imprecise dosage; high risk of aspiration of nasal mucus into bottle; tendency for tip of bottle to become clogged
Drops	Preferred for small children	Awkward to use; high risk of contamination of the medication from dropper; limited coverage of the nasal mucosa; easy passage into the larynx
Inhaler	Small and unobtrusive; easy to handle and carry	Unobstructed airway and sufficient airflow needed to distribute drug to nasal mucosa; limited durability of only 2–3 months even when tightly capped

[a]Metered pump sprays deliver a more precise dose.

coma are minimal; no adverse effects on open-angle glaucoma have been reported.[30]

Headache has been reported with systemic decongestants. The side effects may be more pronounced if the patient is taking other sympathomimetic medications such as systemic or inhaled beta-adrenergic agonists (albuterol, terbutaline, metaproterenol, epinephrine).

Product Selection Guidelines Product selection depends on the expected duration of treatment and the presence of concomitant disease. Patients with seasonal or allergic rhinitis generally require decongestants throughout the entire period of exposure to allergens.

Topical dosage forms include sprays, drops, and inhalers (see product table "Topical Decongestant Products"). Nasal sprays are the simplest drug delivery method and are the preferred dosage form for older children and adults. Topical decongestants are effective; however, the risk of rebound congestion greatly limits their usefulness in the management of allergic rhinitis. Topical drug administration may be used, however, to control acute symptoms on a short-term (3–5 day) basis. Nasal obstruction that is secondary to the presence of nasal polyps or enlarged inferior or middle turbinates also greatly reduces the effectiveness of topical agents. Physical abnormalities such as severe septal deviation may interfere with drug administration by blocking access to the nares.

The systemic decongestants are relatively safe to use over the long term (see product table "Cold, Cough, and Allergy Products"). Although some clinicians have raised the issue of tachyphylaxis (down regulation of the receptors), the clinical relevance is not known. It is important to note that pseudoephedrine (Sudafed) and phenylpropanolamine (various) are old drugs and are therefore exempt from Food and Drug Administration (FDA) regulations. No assumptions should be made regarding the equivalency of generic and brand-name products.

The systemic decongestants are short acting; most patients prefer sustained-action products for long-term administration. Efidac/24 (pseudoephedrine hydrochloride 240 mg) is the first of a new type of dosage form.[31] The decongestant is delivered with OROS controlled release system. The outer coating of the tablet releases an immediate dose; the remainder of the drug is contained in the inner core of the tablet and is slowly dissolved by fluid drawn into the core of the tablet osmotically from the gastrointestinal tract. Dissolved drug is slowly released through small holes in the tablet shell.

Pharmacists should question patients about the presence of concomitant diseases and the use of other medications. For example, patients with hypertension and other cardiovascular diseases, diabetes mellitus, benign prostatic hypertrophy, or hyperthyroidism should use oral sympathomimetics only under the supervision of a physician. Although the effect of the sympathomimetics on blood pressure, while in dispute, is probably minimal, patients with labile or difficult-to-control hypertension may be at a higher risk. Pseudoephedrine appears to have less effect on blood pressure than does phenylpropanolamine.[5] Short-acting products may be safer for patients with cardiovascular disease in that the duration of an adverse cardiovascular event would be relatively short.

Some of the side effects associated with the sympathomimetics (nervousness, tremor, anxiety, and dizziness) are the same symptoms associated with hyperglycemia and hypoglycemia (eg, an increase in blood glucose). This may confuse diabetic patients, who inappropriately seek treatment when the symptoms are drug related or delay seeking treatment when the symptoms are related to glycemic dysregulation.

Decongestants are considered stimulants; patients who participate in official athletic events should avoid phenylephrine (Neo-Synephrine), ephedrine (various), pseudoephedrine, and propylhexedrine (Benzedrex). Physical performance may be impaired by first-generation antihistamines (owing to their sedating and anti-

TABLE 7 Recommended dosage guidelines for nonprescription oral nasal decongestants

	Dosage (maximum/24 h)		
Drug	**Adults >12 y**	**Children 6–<12 y**	**Children 2–<6 y[a]**
Phenylephrine	10 mg every 4 h (60 mg)	5 mg every 4 h (30 mg)	2.5 mg every 4 h (15 mg)
Phenylpropanolamine	25 mg every 4 h, or 50 mg every 8 h (150 mg)	12.5 mg every 4 h, or 25 mg every 8 h (75 mg)	6.25 mg every 4 h, or 12.5 mg every 8 h (37.5 mg)
Pseudoephedrine	60 mg every 4 h (360 mg)	30 mg every 4 h (180 mg)	15 mg every 4 h (90 mg)

[a]There is no recommended dosage for children under 2 years of age except under the advice and supervision of a physician.

Reprinted from Establishment of a monograph for OTC cold, cough, allergy, bronchodilator, and antiasthmatic products. *Federal Register.* 1976 Sep; 41: 38312–424.

cholinergic effects) and by immunotherapy (owing to discomfort at site of injection).

Decongestants should be used during pregnancy only if the potential benefit justifies the potential risk to the fetus. Ephedrine, oxymetazoline (Afrin), phenylephrine, phenylpropanolamine, and pseudoephedrine are all Category C agents (ie, either studies in animals have revealed adverse effects on the fetus and there are no controlled studies in women, or studies in women and animals are not available).[32] It is not known how much decongestant is excreted into breast milk following topical or systemic administration; women who breast-feed should use the decongestants with caution.[33]

The combination ophthalmic decongestant/antihistamine of pheniramine/naphazoline (Opcon A) was recently approved for over-the-counter (OTC) sale. It is indicated for temporary relief of eye redness and itching due to airborne irritants and allergens.

Topical Anti-Inflammatory Drugs

Corticosteroids are the most potent and effective drugs available for the management of allergic rhinitis. Corticosteroids inhibit the release of preformed mediators from mast cells and basophils, suppress the synthesis of inflammatory mediators, reduce edema and inflammation, and decrease the migration of neutrophils and eosinophils into the nasal mucosa. Corticosteroids are therefore effective against all stages of the allergic response. Intranasal corticosteroid administration minimizes the risk of systemic side effects and is the route of choice most of the time. Short courses of systemic corticosteroids may be required for severe symptoms; however, systemic side effects may develop with high doses. Adverse effects associated with intranasal corticosteroids include local irritation and epistaxis.

Cromolyn sodium (Nasalcrom) inhibits the release of mediators from mast cells. It is administered intranasally and is not associated with systemic side effects, but it has to be dosed four to six times daily. Cromolyn sodium is not as effective as corticosteroids for patients with more severe symptoms and is considered an adjunctive treatment.

Expectorants and Mucolytics

Mucolytics thin mucus, making it easier to expel secretions. Mucus consists of mucin, epithelial cells, leukocytes, and various inorganic salts suspended in water. Water cannot be incorporated into mucus after the mucus has been formed, but hydration will aid in the formation of a less viscid, more liquid mucus. Hydration can be accomplished by maintaining an adequate fluid intake; steam inhalation may soothe irritated membranes. The expectorant guaifenesin (various) allegedly facilitates mucociliary transport, but its efficacy in allergic rhinitis has not been proved (see product table "Cold, Cough, and Allergy Products").

Future Drugs

Drug development is being targeted at drugs that inhibit or block the IgE-mediated reaction. Potential targets include circulating IgE, mast cell degranulation, and the target cells affected by the mediators. New antihistamines with additional properties, such as prostaglandin and leukotriene inhibition and neuropeptide activity, will continue to be developed. Topical anticholinergics are being developed to treat hypersecretory rhinitis.

Immunotherapy

Immunotherapy, previously called "desensitization" or "hyposensitization," is indicated for patients whose symptoms are not controlled by drugs, who have severe conditions or perennial symptoms, or who are allergic to allergens that are difficult to avoid. Although immunotherapy is most effective for pollen-related allergy, patients with house dust mite, animal dander, or mold allergy may obtain significant relief.

Although the exact mode of action of immunotherapy is not known, immunotherapy is thought to work by decreasing the production of IgE antibodies and stimulating the production of IgG-blocking antibodies.[4] Other proposed mechanisms include generating antigen-spe-

TABLE 8 Recommended dosage guidelines for topical nasal decongestants

Drug	Concentration (%)	Dosage (drops or sprays) Adults >12 y	Children 6–<12 y	Children[a] 2–<6 y
Ephedrine	0.5	2–3 drops/sprays not more often than every 4 h	1–2 drops/sprays not more often than every 4 h	—[b]
Naphazoline	0.05	1–2 drops/sprays not more often than every 6 h	—[c]	—[c]
	0.025	1–2 drops/sprays not more often than every 6 h	1–2 drops/sprays not more often than every 6 h	—[d]
Oxymetazoline	0.05	2–3 drops/sprays twice daily in AM and PM	2–3 drops/sprays twice daily in AM and PM	—[e]
	0.025	2–3 drop/sprays twice daily in AM and PM	2–3 drops/sprays twice daily in AM and PM	2–3 drops twice daily in AM and PM
Phenylephrine	0.5	2–3 drops/sprays not more often than every 4 h	—[f]	—[f]
	0.25	2–3 drops/sprays not more often than every 4 h	2–3 drops/sprays not more often than every 4 h	—[g]
	0.125	2–3 drops/sprays not more often than every 4 h	2–3 drops/sprays not more often than every 4 h	2–3 drops not more often than every 4 h
Propylhexedrine		2 inhalations not more often than every 2 h	2 inhalations not more often than every 2 h	—[h]
Tetrahydrozoline	0.1	2–4 drops not more often than every 3 h	2–4 drops not more often than every 3 h	—[i]
	0.05	2–4 drops not more often than every 3 h	2–4 drops not more often than every 3 h	2–3 drops not more often than every 3 h
Xylometazoline	0.1	2–3 drops/sprays every 8–10 h	—[j]	—[j]
	0.05	2–3 drops/sprays every 8–10 h	2–3 drops/sprays every 8–10 h	2–3 drops every 8–10 h

[a]There is no recommended dosage for children under 2 years of age except under the advice and supervision of a physician.

Except under the advice and supervision of a physician, the following drugs or drug concentrations are not recommended for children of the specified ages:

- [b]Ephedrine: <6 years;
- [c]Naphazoline 0.05%: <12 years;
- [d]Naphazoline 0.025%: <6 years;
- [e]Oxymetazoline 0.05%: <6 years;
- [f]Phenylephrine 0.5%: <12 years;
- [g]Phenylephrine 0.25%: <6 years;
- [h]Propylhexedrine: <6 years;
- [i]Tetrahydrozoline 0.1%: <6 years;
- [j]Xylometazoline 0.1%: <12 years;

Reprinted from Establishment of a monograph for OTC cold, cough, allergy, bronchodilator, and antiasthmatic products. *Federal Register*. 1976, Sep; 41: 38312–424.

cific suppressor T lymphocytes, and decreasing lymphokine production and mononuclear cell-derived histamine-releasing factor.[34]

Immunotherapy consists of a series of injections with extracts of the allergens identified as the cause of the symptoms. Treatment is initiated with very dilute solutions. Injections are then repeated weekly using gradually increasing concentrations of the allergen. The top "maintenance" dose is generally reached within 4–8 months; injections of this dose are repeated every 3–4 weeks for 3–5 years. Patients may improve as early as 3 months after initiation of immunotherapy. About 80% of patients have significant relief while receiving immunotherapy; approximately 60% will remain symptom free after the immunotherapy is discontinued.

Patient Counseling

Patients with allergic rhinitis generally prefer to use sustained-release products. Saline sprays may provide some relief from drying and crusting (see product table "Miscellaneous Nasal Products"). All products should be kept out of the reach of children.

Use of Antihistamines

Patients taking antihistamines need to be counseled regarding what to expect from the medication and how to use it safely. The pharmacist should emphasize the following points:

- Antihistamines provide symptomatic relief only and will not cure or prevent the disease.
- Antihistamines have no effect on the production or release of histamine. Therefore, patients with seasonal allergic rhinitis should be advised to start taking antihistamines before their specific allergy season begins, whereas patients with perennial allergic rhinitis may need to take antihistamines year-round. Compliance with long-term therapy needs to be emphasized.
- Histamine release is a nearly continuous process. Therefore, patients should be advised to take antihistamines on a schedule rather than as needed.
- Sedation associated with some agents can be minimized by (1) administering a full dose at bedtime and using minimally recommended doses combined with a decongestant during the day (some clinicians recommend using long-acting first-generation antihistamines at night only); or (2) starting with low doses and gradually increasing the dose as tolerated over a several-day period.
- Patients taking first-generation antihistamines should be advised against driving, performing tasks that require alertness, and consuming alcohol or other sedative drugs. Although less likely, sedation and/or decreased mental alertness may also occur with the second-generation antihistamines; thus, patients should be similarly advised against driving, performing tasks that require alertness, and consuming alcohol or other sedative drugs until their response to these drugs is known.
- The very young and the elderly may be more sensitive to antihistamines. First-generation antihistamines may cause paradoxical reactions such as nervousness, irritability, and restlessness in these patients.
- Antihistamines should be used during pregnancy only if the potential benefit outweighs the possible risks.
- Very little data are available regarding the appearance of antihistamines in breast milk and/or the effect of antihistamines on the infant.[33] In general, antihistamine use by breast-feeding patients is not recommended. Specifically, clemastine (Tavist) has been reported to have significant adverse effects on nursing infants.
- Antihistamines with anticholinergic properties may cause excessive drying or crusting of secretions, making it more difficult for patients with chronic bronchitis or emphysema to clear secretions.
- First-generation antihistamines may exacerbate symptoms of benign prostatic hypertrophy.
- Antihistamines may alter the results of skin and serologic testing. Therefore, patients should inform their physicians that they are taking antihistamines before scheduling any of these diagnostic tests.

Use of Decongestants

Patients using topical decongestants should be advised to limit use to no more than 3–5 days. If patients experience rebound congestion, they need to be counseled on how to withdraw from the medication. Patients who have problems sleeping can be advised to limit the use of decongestants to the daytime hours and to take an antihistamine alone before bedtime. Further, women who are pregnant or breast-feeding should not take these medications without the supervision of a physician.

Patients should also be given general guidelines on administering topical decongestants, as well as specific instructions for administering the dosage form chosen.[35]

General Administration Guidelines

- Always check the expiration date before using the product.
- Discard the product if it is discolored or if deterioration is suspected.
- Limit product use to a maximum of 3–5 days.
- Do not share the product with another person.
- Blow the nose before using the product.
- Wait at least a few minutes after administering a dose before blowing the nose.

Administration of Sprays

- Do not shake the bottle.
- Remove the cap before using the spray.
- Gently insert the tip of the bottle into one nostril.
- Keep the head upright.
- Sniff deeply while squeezing the bottle.
- Repeat with the other nostril if necessary.
- Rinse the bottle tip with hot water but do not let water enter the bottle; replace the cap.

Administration of Metered Dose Pumps

- Do not shake the bottle.
- Remove the cap, then prime the pump (depress it several times with the nozzle pointed away from the face) before using it for the first time.
- Hold the bottle with the nozzle between the first two fingers and the thumb on the bottom of the bottle.
- Gently insert the tip of the pump into the nose.
- Keep the head upright.
- Sniff deeply while depressing the pump once.
- Repeat with the other nostril if necessary.
- Rinse the spray tip with hot water but do not let water enter the bottle.
- Replace the cap.

Administration of Drops

- Squeeze the rubber bulb on the dropper to withdraw medication from the bottle.
- Tilt head back while standing or sitting, or lie on the bed with the head tilted back over the side.
- Place the drops into each nostril.
- Gently tilt the head from side to side.
- Rinse the dropper with hot water and let it air dry.

Administration of Inhalers

- Warm the inhaler in the hand.
- Remove the cap before using the inhaler.
- Inhale the vapor up one nostril at a time while occluding the other nostril.
- Sniff deeply while inhaling.
- Wipe the inhaler clean after each use.
- Replace the cap.
- Discard the inhaler after 2–3 months even if the medication can still be smelled.

Use of Corticosteroids

Topical corticosteroids should be used regularly and not on an as-needed basis. Patients should be advised that the maximal benefit may not occur until after 2–6 weeks of regular treatment.

Pediatric Considerations

Very little definitive data are available regarding specific dosing recommendations in children. In general, the FDA recommends that children age 6 to under 12 years receive one half the adult dose, children age 2 to under 6 years receive one fourth the adult dose, and children under 2 years be dosed under the supervision of a physician.[27] Because the potential consequences of airway obstruction are so severe in young children, all children under the age of 2 should be referred to a physician. These dosage recommendations, although easily understood by consumers, do not take the weight of the child into consideration. Doses may need to be modified for children who are much smaller or bigger than their usual age group.

The efficacy and side effects profile of systemic antihistamines and decongestants have not been systematically evaluated in children. Topical and systemic decongestants should not be used in young children without the advice of a physician; topical decongestants should be used for no longer than 3 days. Isotonic saline drops and the gentle aspiration of secretions with a nasal syringe can temporarily relieve nasal obstruction in infants and young children; nasal drainage may be enhanced by letting infants and young children sleep upright in car seats.

The Common Cold

Viral upper respiratory infections, generally referred to as the common cold but also known as acute infectious rhinitis, coryza, or catarrh, cause more time away from work and school than any other illness.[3] Children under 5 years of age experience four to nine episodes of upper respiratory infections per year, with the peak incidence among the 1- to 2-year-olds.[36–38] Children aged 5–9 have an annual frequency of four to six episodes, and young adults experience three to five episodes per year.[36,39] The number of episodes is higher in crowded conditions and among adults in close contact with young children.[37,39] Children in day care with seven or more children average six to seven respiratory infections per year.[38,40,41]

Etiology

The five viruses that commonly infect the upper respiratory tract include the rhinovirus types 2, 9, and 14; the coronavirus type 229E; and the respiratory syncytial virus.[42] The rhinovirus group consists of more than 100 different antigenic serotypes and accounts for 15–40% of upper respiratory infections.[42] Other, less common viruses include the influenza virus types A, B, and C; the parainfluenza virus; the adenovirus; the coxsackie virus; and the echovirus.[42]

The etiology of upper respiratory infections in children varies with age.[38] The three most common viruses in children 0–4 years of age are rhinoviruses (39%), respiratory syncytial viruses (19%), and parainfluenza (18%); the three most common viruses in children 5–18 years of age are influenza A (32%), rhinoviruses (22%), and influenza B (18%).[38] The rhinoviruses and coronaviruses, fastidious organisms that are hard to isolate, are most likely underrepresented in reports of the etiology of the common cold.

There is no single mode of transmission. Modes implicated include inhalation of the virus in sneezed aerosols or droplets, ingestion of saliva spread directly or indirectly by eating or drinking implements, and hand-to-hand contact with an infected person followed by rubbing the nose and eyes. However, it appears to be very hard to become infected by contact with infected hands or by kissing.[43,44]

Factors associated with an increased susceptibility to viral upper respiratory infections include smoking[45] and psychologic stress, as judged by the number of major stressful life events.[46] In one study, moderate alcohol consumption lowered the risk for nonsmokers but did not change the risk for smokers.[45] Cold environments and sudden chilling are not associated with an increased susceptibility to viral upper respiratory infections.[47,48]

Pathophysiology

Immunologic and Biochemical Response

Viral infection initiates a series of biochemical and immunologic events resulting in the release of numerous inflammatory mediators.[12] The inflammatory mediators induce a variety of local reactions, including increased vascular permeability, increased glandular secretion, inflammatory cell infiltration, and stimulation of neural pathways.[12] Nasal secretions contain large numbers of ciliated epithelial cells and polymorphonuclear cells; proteins, including plasma proteins (albumin and immunoglobulin G) and glandular proteins (lactoferrin, lysozyme, and secretory IgA)[49]; and kinins (bradykinin and lysyl-bradykinin).[50]

Although the local immunopathology and the exact pathogenesis of symptoms are not completely understood, the response to viral infections does not appear to involve mast cell mediators. Rather, the mediators involved in the viral response appear to be generated in the nasal mucosa. Kinins generated in the nasal mucosa may cause nasal obstruction, nasal burning, and rhinorrhea. However, other inflammatory mediators such as IL-1 are found in nasal secretions of symptomatic subjects and may be responsible for enhanced vascular permeability, the recruitment of other inflammatory cells, and the release of other proinflammatory mediators.

Complications

Virus-induced inflammatory changes in the nose may spread to contiguous structures, including the sinuses and eustachian tubes. Complications may include sinusitis, eustachian tube obstruction, middle ear effusions, and secondary bacterial infections. Complications in the lower respiratory tract may include bronchitis, bacterial pneumonia, and exacerbations of asthma and chronic obstructive pulmonary disease.

Patient Assessment

The first symptom of a cold to appear is sore throat, followed by nasal symptoms (stuffiness, rhinorrhea, postnasal drip), watering eyes, sneezing, and then cough.[42] The sequence of symptoms is the same regardless of the infecting virus; however, the timing, frequency, and severity vary with the infecting virus.[42] For example, rhinovirus infections are associated with rapidly developing symptoms that peak 2–3 days after infection; respiratory syncytial virus infections are associated with symptoms that develop very slowly over 5 or more days. The majority of patients will experience nasal symptoms regardless of the infecting virus. Fewer patients will develop headache, pyrexia, sinus pain, and myalgia, and less than 20% of patients will experience cough.[42] The exception is with respiratory syncytial viral infections, in which more than 60% of patients will experience cough.[42] Patients will be symptomatic for approximately 1–2 weeks.

It is sometimes difficult to differentiate between the symptoms of the common cold and other infections such as bacterial sore throat and influenza. Sore throats secondary to a bacterial infection differ from those associated with viral infections in terms of onset, severity of pain, and concomitant symptoms (Table 9).[51]

Influenza is generally associated with more prominent systemic symptoms (temperature above 102°F [38.8°C]; fatigue, weakness, and exhaustion) but fewer nasal symptoms (rhinorrhea, congestion, and sneezing) than the common cold (Table 10).[52,53]

Disease Management

Cold symptoms are usually self-limiting and resolve in 1–2 weeks whether treated or not. General therapeutic measures such as rest and maintaining an adequate fluid intake remain the mainstays of therapy. Treatment remains symptomatic and should be symptom specific (Table 11).

TABLE 9 Bacterial versus viral sore throats

Characteristic	Bacterial sore throat	Viral sore throat
Onset	Rapid	Slower
Soreness	Marked	Usually less severe
Constitutional symptoms	Marked	Mild
Upper and lower respiratory symptoms	Not always present	Usually present
Lymph nodes	Large, tender	Slight enlargement, not tender

Adapted from Bulteau V. Sore throat. *Med J Aust.* 1966 Nov; 2: 1053–5.

TABLE 10 Comparative symptoms of the common cold and influenza

Symptom	Common Cold	Influenza
Fever	Rare	Sudden onset; temperature >102–104°F (38.8–40°C)
Headache	Mild or absent	Prominent
Myalgia or arthralgia	Mild or absent	Prominent
Fatigue, weakness, and exhaustion	Mild or absent	Extreme
Rhinorrhea	Common	Less common
Nasal congestion	Common	Less common
Sneezing	Common	Less common
Sore throat	Common	Common
Cough	Less common; usually nonproductive	Common; persistent nonproductive
Ocular	Watery eyes	Pain on motion of eyes; photophobia; burning
Duration	5–10 days	1 wk
Complications	Sinus congestion; earache	Bronchitis; pneumonia

Reprinted from Dolan R. In: Isselbacher KJ et al, eds. *Harrison's Principles of Internal Medicine.* 13th ed. New York: McGraw-Hill, Inc; 1994: 803–7, 814–9.

Preventive Measures

There is no effective means of prevention. Numerous compounds have been investigated, but nothing has been proven safe and effective. Intranasal interferon alfa-2b appears to prevent viral shedding and diminish nasal stuffiness; however, this agent is associated with an unacceptably high risk of nasal bleeding and superficial nasal mucosa erosions.[54]

Decongestants

Decongestants, which are vasoconstrictive drugs that reduce nasal congestion, are the mainstay of treatment of the common cold. For information about the mechanism and side effects of these agents, as well as for product selection guidelines, see the discussion of decongestants in the section Allergic Rhinitis.

Analgesics and Antipyretics

Patients may complain of feeling feverish, but the common cold is rarely associated with a temperature greater than 100°F (37.8°C). Simple analgesics/antipyretics such as aspirin and acetaminophen are effective treatments. However, children and teenagers should avoid aspirin and aspirin-containing products.

TABLE 11 Symptomatic nonprescription drug treatment of the common cold

Symptom	Treatment
Nasal congestion and discharge	Decongestants
Cough	Hydration, demulcents, antitussives, expectorants, cool mist/steam vapors
Sore throat	Demulcents, saline gargles, local anesthetics, systemic analgesics
Laryngitis	Cool mist/steam vapors
Feverishness and headache	Systemic analgesics

Expectorants and Mucolytics

Expectorants are oral agents that aid in the removal of respiratory tract secretions by either increasing bronchial secretions or facilitating their expulsion. However, there are few objective data to support these claims. Increasing fluid intake to six to eight glasses (8 oz per glass) in patients who do not have fluid restrictions and maintaining adequate humidification of inspired air are important for the production and expectoration of respiratory secretions.

The FDA advisory panel has classified guaifenesin as the only monograph expectorant. All other expectorants (eg, terpin hydrate, ammonium chloride, iodides, etc) are classified as nonmonograph agents. Guaifenesin is thought to act as an expectorant by reflex gastric stimulation; however, it does not appear to thin sputum or increase the volume of secretions even at high doses.[55] Commonly cited gastrointestinal side effects are rarely associated with recommended doses.

Recommended nonprescription dosage guidelines for guaifenesin are as follows[56]:

- 200–400 mg every 4 hours (to a maximum of 2,400 mg in 24 hours) for adults;
- 100–200 mg every 4 hours (to a maximum of 1,200 mg in 24 hours) for children aged 6 to under 12 years;
- 50–100 mg every 4 hours (to a maximum of 600 mg in 24 hours) for children aged 2 to under 6 years;
- Not recommended for children under 2 years of age except under the advice and supervision of a physician.

Other ingredients of unproven effectiveness that may be added to cold products for claimed but unproven expectorant properties include beechwood creosote/potassium guaiacolsulfonate, benzoin preparations, camphor, eucalyptus oil, menthol, peppermint oil, pine tar, sodium citrate, tolu balsam, and turpentine oil.

The FDA issued a warning in 1992 regarding the use of nonprescription expectorants in children under age 12. This warning states that, unless directed by a physician, expectorants should not be given if there is a persistent or chronic cough such as occurs with asthma or if the cough is accompanied by excessive mucus.

Antitussives

Antitussives (cough suppressants) inhibit or suppress the act of coughing and are indicated for the suppression of dry, hacking, nonproductive coughs.[57,58] Tables 12 and 13 list the usual doses, dosage ranges, and administration techniques for the commonly used antitussives.

TABLE 12 Recommended dosage guidelines for nonprescription oral antitussives

	Dosage (maximum/24 h)		
Drug	**Adults >12 y**	**Children 6–<12 y**	**Children 2–<6 y**
Codeine[a,b]	10–20 mg every 4–6 h (120 mg)	5–10 mg every 4–6 h (60 mg)	1 mg/kg/day in 4 equal doses, or by ABW[c]
Dextromethorphan	10–20 mg every 4–8 h or 30 mg every 8 h (120 mg)	5–10 mg every 4 h or 15 mg every 6–8 h (60 mg)	2.5 mg every 4 h or 7.5 mg every 8 h (30 mg)
Diphenhydramine	25 mg every 4–6 h (100 mg)	12.5 mg every 6 h (50 mg)	6.25 mg every 6 h (25 mg)

[a]Codeine is not recommended for use in children under 2 years of age, who may be more susceptible to the respiratory depressant effects of codeine, including respiratory arrest, coma, and death.

[b]The FDA recommends that the labels on nonprescription agents containing codeine not give dosage information for children under 6 years of age.

[c]Codeine may be dosed by average body weight (ABW): 2 years of age (ABW of 12 kg) = 3 mg every 4–6 hours (max 12 mg); 3 years of age (ABW of 14 kg) = 3.5 mg every 4–6 hours (max 14 mg); 4 years of age (ABW of 16 kg) = 4 mg every 4–6 hours (max 16 mg); 5 years of age (ABW of 18 kg) = 4.5 mg every 4–6 hours (max 18 mg). A dispensing device such as a dropper calibrated for age or weight should be dispensed along with the product when it is intended for use in children aged 2 to under 6 years to prevent possible overdose due to improper measuring.

Source:

Cold, cough, allergy, bronchodilator, and antiasthmatic drug products for over-the-counter human use; final monograph for OTC antitussive drug products; final rule. *Federal Register.* 1987 Aug; 52: 30049–57.

Cold, cough, allergy, bronchodilator, and antiasthmatic drug products for over-the-counter human use; amendment of final monograph for OTC antitussive drug products. *Federal Register.* 1993 Oct; 58: 54232–6.

Table 13 Recommended administration guidelines for nonprescription topical antitussives for adults and children aged 2 to under 12 years[a]

Medication	Administration
Camphor ointment, 4.7–5.3%	Rub on the throat and chest as a thick layer. Applications may be repeated up to three times daily or as directed by a physician.
Menthol ointment, 2.6–2.8%	Rub on the throat and chest as a thick layer. Applications may be repeated up to three times daily or as directed by a physician.
Menthol lozenges or compressed tablets, 5–10 mg	Allow lozenge or tablet to dissolve slowly in the mouth. Repeat every hour as needed or as directed by a physician.
Camphor for steam inhalation, 6.2%	Add 1 tbsp of solution per quart of water directly to the water in a hot steam vaporizer, bowl, or washbasin; or add 1.5 tsp of solution per pint of water to an open container of boiling water. Breathe in the medicated vapors. Repeat up to three times daily or as directed by a physician.
Menthol for steam inhalation, 3.2%	Add 1 tbsp of solution per quart of water directly to the water in a hot steam vaporizer, bowl, or washbasin; or add 1.5 tsp of solution per pint of water to an open container of boiling water. Breathe in the medicated vapors. Repeat up to three times daily or as directed by a physician.

[a]For children of 2 years of age or younger, consult a physician.

Adapted from:

Cold, cough, allergy, bronchodilator, and antiasthmatic drug products for over-the-counter human use; final monograph for OTC antitussive drug products; final rule. *Federal Register.* 1987 Aug; 52: 30049–57.

Cold, cough, allergy, bronchodilator, and antiasthmatic drug products for over-the-counter human use; amendment of final monograph for OTC antitussive drug products. *Federal Register.* 1993 Oct; 58: 54232–6.

Direct-acting antitussives (codeine, dextromethorphan, diphenhydramine) depress the medullary centers of the brain, decrease the sensitivity of respiratory system cough receptors, or interrupt the transmission of cough impulses. Antitussives are sometimes used to suppress productive coughs if the cough prevents sleep or is especially bothersome. However, antitussives may be counterproductive when used to treat a productive cough because cough suppression may impair the expectoration of secretions. Thus, combination products containing cough suppressants and expectorants are irrational.

Codeine Codeine is the standard antitussive against which all other antitussives are compared. The dose required for cough suppression (10–20 mg) is less than the analgesic dose; higher doses may be used for more cough suppression.[59] Codeine, under usual conditions of use as a cough suppressant, has low-dependency potential; however, dependence may develop after prolonged use. Although codeine-containing cough products are available without prescription in some states, stringent controls are placed on their nonprescription distribution.

The most common side effects from codeine include nausea, drowsiness, lightheadedness, and constipation. Allergic reactions and pruritus may occur but are less common. Codeine's central nervous system effects are additive to those of other central nervous system depressants. Codeine has a slight drying effect on the respiratory mucosa, which may lead to the production of more viscid secretions. Codeine is contraindicated in patients in whom mucosal drying or respiratory depression may be harmful (eg, patients with chronic obstructive pulmonary disease) and in patients with known codeine allergies.

Dextromethorphan Dextromethorphan is the dextrorotatory isomer of the morphinan molecule. Dextromethorphan has no significant analgesic properties and does not depress respiration; the addiction potential is low. Some investigators believe that dextromethorphan and codeine are equipotent, others give a slight edge to codeine, and still others support dextromethorphan as the superior antitussive. Increasing the dose to 30 mg may prolong the duration of action by a few hours without changing the antitussive effects.

Dextromethorphan is generally well tolerated; drowsiness and gastrointestinal upset are the most common complaints. Larger doses in the abuse range have produced intoxication with bizarre behavior. Dextromethorphan is associated with a substance-dependence syndrome, which is probably related to high-affinity binding sites in the central nervous system. Patients taking monoamine oxidase inhibitors should not use products containing dextromethorphan without the supervision of a physician.

Diphenhydramine Diphenhydramine hydrochloride is an antitussive and an antihistamine. The antitussive effect is due to a central mechanism involving the medullary cough center. A peripheral action may contribute to the drug's effectiveness, but further studies are needed to confirm this.

The most common side effects include sedation and anticholinergic effects. Diphenhydramine hydrochloride should not be taken by individuals in whom the use of anticholinergics are contraindicated (eg, those with narrow-angle glaucoma or benign prostatic hypertrophy) or in situations in which mental alertness or physical coordination and dexterity are required (eg, driving a car or operating motor equipment). The side effects will be additive if taken with other drugs that cause sedation or reduced mental alertness (eg, antianxiety agents, sedatives, hypnotics, antidepressants, narcotics, and alcohol).

Topical Antitussives Camphor and menthol are the only two monograph topical antitussives. The antitussive action of these products is believed to occur from a local anesthetic action of the aromatic vapor. Ointments containing camphor (4.7–5.3%) or menthol (2.6–2.8%) are rubbed on the throat and chest as a thick layer; the area may be covered with a warm, dry cloth or left uncovered. Camphor and menthol are also approved for steam inhalation, and menthol is also approved in a lozenge or compressed tablet formulation (Table 14). Care should be taken to avoid the accidental ingestion of menthol- or camphor-containing ointments or solutions. Seizures may occur if camphor-containing products are ingested.

Effectiveness of Expectorants, Mucolytics, and Antitussives

The cough reflex may be blocked by agents that depress the cough center in the medulla (opiate and nonopiate depressants), by agents that inhibit efferent motor nerve impulses to the medullary center (local anesthetics), and by agents that act on the sensory nerves (demulcents/expectorants, local anesthetics). Expectorants may aid in the removal of scant secretions. Mucolytics may aid in the removal of thick, viscous secretions.

There are very few data available regarding the effectiveness of expectorants, mucolytics, and antitussives in the treatment of the common cold. Codeine and dextromethorphan are standard antitussives, but the data from limited studies specifically in patients with the common cold suggest that neither is more effective than placebo in controlling cough associated with the common cold.[60,61] Dry or annoying coughs may be treated with demulcents such as hard candy or cough drops. Cough suppressants may be tried for dry coughs that interfere with sleeping but may be ineffective. Patients should maintain an adequate fluid intake.

Anesthetics and Antiseptics

Lozenges, gargles, and sprays containing antiseptics and topical anesthetics (benzocaine and dyclonine hydrochloride) are heavily promoted for the treatment of sore throats; antiseptics are ineffective, however, against viral infections. Products containing local anesthetics may be used every 3 or 4 hours for temporary symptomatic relief. Alternatives include hard candy, which stimulates salivary flow and acts as a soothing demulcent, warm saline gargles (1–3 tsp of salt per 8–12 oz of warm water), and fruit juices.

Future Medications

The antigenic diversity of cold viruses will probably prevent the development of a cold vaccine in the foreseeable future. Biologic agents, agents that prevent viral attachment, and agents that inhibit viral replication have been investigated but do not appear to be useful.

Humidifiers

Inhalation of heated or unheated humidified air may soothe irritated airways and improve airway hydration. However, nasal hyperthermia (application of hot humidified air directly to the nasal passages) is of no benefit. Nasal hyperthermia was thought to inhibit viral replication by raising the temperature of the nasal passages, and results from initial unblinded trials were very positive. However, later controlled trials found no effect as measured by symptom scores, viral shedding, or antibody response.

Treatment Controversies

Treatment of the common cold is confusing and somewhat controversial. The confusion arises from the continued marketing of new products; the cross-marketing of products for colds, allergies, and sinus problems; and the use of numerous undefined terms (eg, fast acting, slow release, pediatric, nighttime, etc) for these products. One advertising agency found that consumers ranked the cold and allergy market as the fifth most confusing market out of 32 categories; the only markets rated more confusing were the insurance, automobile, home computer, and vacation markets.[62]

Role of Antihistamines One of the biggest controversies has to do with the use of antihistamines in treating the common cold. The common cold is caused by a viral infection that produces symptoms similar to those associated with allergies. However, histamine is not a mediator of nasal congestion or of any other cold symptom; thus, there is no pharmacologic basis for using antihistamines to treat common cold symptoms.[50,63] The anticholinergic side effects associated with first-generation antihistamines may have contributed to the perception that antihistamines reduce common cold symptoms. However, the nonsedating antihistamines have no anticholinergic effect, so their use is even more dubious.

There are few well-designed controlled studies on the use of antihistamines to treat common cold symptoms. One problem lies in defining a clinically significant response. Another is in the use of self-reported subjective evaluative parameters. Although a few investigators have concluded that antihistamines are effective in reducing common cold symptoms, all the studies contained one or more design or analysis flaws.[64–66] The 1976 report of the FDA's Advisory Review Panel on Over-the-Counter Cold, Cough, Allergy, Bronchodilator, and Antiasthmatic Products concluded that there were insufficient data to establish the effectiveness of antihistamines in the common cold.[27] One pivotal multicenter study on which subsequent FDA approval was based was a placebo-controlled study of chlorpheniramine versus placebo.[64] Although the authors concluded that chlorpheniramine was statistically better than placebo (using a P value of .1), the symptom score curves for chlorpheniramine and placebo were nearly superimposable. In contrast, antihistamines were found to be of no benefit in several other studies.[67–71] An expert panel concluded in 1987 that antihistamines do not have a place in the management of upper respiratory infections,[72] and the final monograph on nonprescription antihistamines does not include them for the common cold.[25]

Combination versus Single-Drug Therapy One of the initial decisions to be made regarding the treatment of the common cold is whether to recommend products that contain a combination of active ingredients. Recent data suggest that the majority of patients experience most of the characteristic cold symptoms during the course of a cold.[42] However, most patients do not experience all the symptoms at the same time. The advantage of individualized single-drug therapy is that effective doses of appropriate drugs can be used to treat patient-specific symptoms without exposing the patient to risks from unnecessary drugs. The disadvantage is that patients may be less compliant than they are with combination-drug therapy. The initial cost of purchasing several single-entity products is greater than the cost of purchasing one combination product; however, the patient has more dosage units available for future use. Combination-drug products may improve patient compliance, but this must be weighed against the risk of side effects from unnecessary drugs.

Role of Vitamin C The use of vitamin C to prevent or treat the common cold has been a topic of long-standing controversy since the 1940s. It has been proposed that vitamin C, an antioxidant, neutralizes the large amounts of oxidizing compounds released by neutrophils. Numerous studies have attempted to verify Linus Pauling's conclusions in the early 1970s that vitamin C reduces the incidence and severity of the common cold.[73] Knipschild, in an extensive review of 61 trials published between 1940 and 1991, concluded that vitamin C, even in gram doses per day, cannot prevent a cold.[74] However, Knipschild and other investigators have suggested that megadoses (1–4 g per day) may decrease the duration and severity of symptoms by as little as 10% or as much as 29%.[74,75]

Role of Zinc Zinc has been proposed to act as an antiviral agent. Although the data are sparse, some research suggests that the frequent administration of adequate doses of zinc in the form of lozenges may reduce the severity of symptoms if therapy is started within hours of the onset of symptoms.[76,77]

Role of Milk and Milk Products Many people believe that milk or milk products stimulate the production of mucus, but milk does not have this property.[78]

Patient Counseling

Topical and systemic nasal decongestants relieve nasal congestion and discharge; topical decongestants are very effective for short-term relief. Patients using topical decongestants should be counseled on the appropriate administration technique and advised to limit their use of these products to 3–5 days. (For more detailed information, see the patient counseling discussion in the section Allergic Rhinitis.) Patients should be referred to a physician if they have symptoms indicative of a more serious problem. These symptoms include sore throat that persists for longer than 1 week, high fever, rash, or persistent headache.

The first step in controlling cough associated with the common cold is to maintain an adequate fluid intake. The tickling sensation in the pharynx that may cause a cough may be controlled with a demulcent such as hard candy or cough drops. A cough suppressant may be indicated if the cough is dry and nonproductive, and if it interferes with work or sleep. Sore throats may be treated with demulcents, saline gargles, or local anesthetic lozenges or solutions (see product table "Sore Throat Products").

Vague complaints of headache and fever may be treated with usual doses of aspirin, acetaminophen, ibuprofen, or naproxen. (See Chapter 4, "Internal Analgesic and Antipyretic Products.") Patients should be referred to their physicians if the fever persists for more than 24 hours or if the cold symptoms do not improve in about a week.

Patients with complicating diseases and women who are pregnant or breast-feeing should not take these medications without the supervision of a physician.

Pediatric Considerations

Children with colds are often medicated with nonprescription drugs. A 1994 survey of US preschoolers found that 53.7% of 3-year-olds had been given some type of nonprescription medication in the past 30 days; 66.7% of these children had received cough or cold medications.[79] Common parental misperceptions regarding the use of these medications in children include the belief that acetaminophen or other cough and cold medications cure common colds, that cough and cold medications allow children to sleep by relieving the symptoms of the common cold, and that all fevers must be treated. The most frequent symptoms prompting the use of cough and cold medications in children are difficulty in sleeping and cough.

Despite the widespread belief that medications are effective in treating cough and cold symptoms in children, very few studies have specifically evaluated the safety and effectiveness of these medications specifically in children. Current data do not support the use of cough suppressants, expectorants, or antihistamines[60]; short-term use of decongestants may improve nasal congestion, but their use is limited by the risk of side effects.[61]

The risk of toxicity from cough and cold medications is higher in infants and young children than in adults.[80,81] The clearance and metabolism of these medications appear to vary with age and hepatic function. Children may develop mild symptoms such as irritability and drowsiness, but may also occasionally develop serious and/or paradoxical side effects such as hallucinations and psychosis.[82,83]

Acetaminophen is the analgesic and antipyretic of choice for children. Children with a history of febrile seizures should be given an antipyretic. Children and teenagers less than 15 years of age should not be given aspirin. Aspirin use during viral illnesses is associated with Reye's syndrome, a serious illness characterized by vomiting, liver damage, hypoglycemia, and progressive central nervous system damage.[84] Reye's syndrome is associated with an approximately 50% rate of mortality; some survivors are left with permanent brain damage. Acetaminophen may be dosed by age (less than 1 year, 60 mg; 1–3 years, 60–120 mg; 3–6 years, 120 mg; 6–12 years, 150–300 mg; older than 12 years, 325–650 mg)[85] or by weight (10–15 mg/kg). The dose can be repeated every 4 hours as needed.

The American Academy of Pediatrics Committee on Drugs has advised against the use of combination cough and cold medications.[86] It has also recommended that single-ingredient medications targeted at the leading symptom be selected if medications have to be used.[86] Simple, soothing, inexpensive, and safe remedies such as tea with lemon and honey, chicken soup, and hot broths should be used until definitive data are available on the efficacy and safety of cough and cold medicines in young children.[87] Supportive measures for infants include clearing the nose with a bulb syringe, positioning the infant so that the secretions drain from the nose, maintaining adequate fluid intake, increasing the humidity of inspired air, and using saline nose drops.

Case Studies

Case 8–1

Patient Complaint/History

YN, a 56-year-old female, presents to the pharmacist with symptoms of a severe viral infection of the upper respiratory tract. Her symptoms include profound nasal congestion, watery eyes, headache, malaise, and a dry, nonproductive cough. The patient reports that she feels warm; however, her oral temperature taken at 5:30 PM (about 30 minutes before her arrival) was 98.9°F (37.5°C).

YN also reveals that she has several chronic diseases, including hypertension, non–insulin-dependent diabetes, hyperlipidemia, and coronary artery disease. The patient says that her blood pressure has been in the range of 130–140 mm Hg/80–85 mm Hg for the last 6 months. Current prescription medications include hydrochlorothiazide 25 mg one tablet daily QAM for 6 years; Vasotec 10 mg one tablet daily QAM for 5 years; Micronase 10 mg one tablet daily with breakfast for 3 years; Zocor 20 mg one tablet daily QPM for last 8 months; and Nitrostat 0.4 mg one tablet (sublingual) prn for 1 month. YN selected the following nonprescription medications for the symptoms of her respiratory infection: Contac Maximum Strength 12-hour caplets; Tylenol Cold Medication; and Robitussin CF cough syrup. The patient has no known drug allergies.

Clinical Considerations/Strategies

The following considerations/strategies are provided to aid the reader in (1) determining whether treatment of the patient's condition with nonprescription medications is warranted, (2) selecting the appropriate nonprescription medication, and (3) developing a patient counseling strategy to ensure optimal therapeutic outcomes:

- Assess the appropriateness of the decongestant.
- Assess the value of the cough syrup.
- Assess the usefulness of an antihistamine in treating a viral infection of the upper respiratory tract (ie, versus an allergy-mediated clinical situation).
- Assess the ability of each patient-selected product to complicate the management of hypertension, diabetes, and coronary artery disease.
- Determine which ingredients will have little positive impact on the patient's symptoms.
- Propose a nonprescription medication regimen that is more targeted and focused to the symptoms associated with the respiratory infection.
- Develop a patient education/counseling strategy that will:
  - Support/justify changes in the patient-selected nonprescription medication regimen;
  - Optimize proper use of the alternative nonprescription medication regimen recommended by the pharmacist.

Case 8–2

Patient Complaint/History

MT, a 34-year-old male, presents to the pharmacist with symptoms of allergic rhinitis, which include moderate nasal congestion with watery rhinorrhea; sneezing paroxysms; itchy nose; and itchy, puffy, red eyes. During conversation with the patient, the pharmacist learns that these symptoms occur year-round but are worse when the patient gets up in the morning and in the spring and autumn. The patient also reveals that he is scheduled to see an allergist the following month for skin testing.

MT has mild hypertension, currently controlled by diet and exercise, and a history of repeated sinus infections for which he usually takes Bactrim DS. He selected the following nonprescription medications for his allergic rhinitis symptoms: Dristan AF tablets; Neo-Synephrine 1% ophthalmic solution; Neo-Synephrine 0.5% nasal spray; and Advil 200-mg tablets. The patient has no known drug allergies.

Clinical Considerations/Strategies

The following considerations/strategies are provided to aid the reader in (1) determining whether treatment of the patient's condition with nonprescription medications is warranted, (2) selecting the appropriate nonprescription medication, and (3) developing a patient counseling strategy to ensure optimal therapeutic outcomes:

- Assess the appropriateness of the antihistamine.
- Assess the appropriateness of the ophthalmic solution.
- Assess the appropriateness of the nasal spray.
- Assess the appropriateness of the analgesic.
- Assess the ability of each patient-selected product to complicate the management of his hypertension.
- Determine which ingredients will have little positive impact on the patient's symptoms.
- Propose a nonprescription medication regimen that is more targeted to the allergic rhinitis symptoms.

- Develop a patient education/counseling strategy that will:
  - Support/justify changes in the patient-selected nonprescription medication regimen;
  - Optimize proper use of the nonprescription medication regimen recommended by the pharmacist;
  - Optimize the patient's adherence to the antibiotic treatment regimens;
  - Minimize the patient's exposure to offending allergens;
  - Maximize the outcome of the skin testing.

References

1. Collins JG. Prevalence of selected chronic conditions: United States, 1986–1988. *Vital and Health Statistics [10]*. 1993; 182: 1–87.
2. Naclerio RM. Allergic rhinitis. *N Engl J Med*. 1991 Sep; 325: 860–9.
3. Garibaldi RA. Epidemiology of community-acquired respiratory tract infections in adults. *Am J Med*. 1985 Jun; 78(6B): 32–7.
4. Badhwar AK, Druce HM. Allergic rhinitis. *Med Clin North Am*. 1992 Jul; 76: 789–803.
5. Virant FS. Allergic rhinitis. *Pediatr Rev*. 1992 Sep; 13: 323–8.
6. Kaliner M, Lemanske R. Rhinitis and asthma. *JAMA*. 1992 Nov; 268: 2807–29.
7. Broder I et al. Epidemiology of asthma and allergic rhinitis in a total community, Tecumseh, Michigan: III. second survey of the community. *J Allergy Clin Immunol*. 1974 Mar; 53: 127–38.
8. Van Arsdel PP Jr, Motulsky AG. Frequency and hereditability of asthma and allergic rhinitis in college students. *Acta Genet*. 1959 Feb; 9: 101–14.
9. Marsh DG, Meyers DA, Bias WB. The epidemiology and genetics of atopic allergy. *N Engl J Med*. 1981 Dec; 305: 1551–9.
10. Taylor B et al. Breast feeding, eczema, asthma, and hayfever. *J Epidemiol Community Health*. 1983 Jun; 37: 95–9.
11. Linna O, Kokkonen J, Lukin M. A 10-year prognosis for childhood allergic rhinitis. *Acta Paediatr*. 1992 Feb; 81: 100–2.
12. Fireman P. Pathophysiology and pharmacotherapy of common upper respiratory diseases. *Pharmacotherapy*. 1993 Nov–Dec; 13(6pt2): 101S–9S.
13. Sporik R, Platts-Mills TAE. Epidemiology of dust-mite-related disease. *Exp Appl Acarol*. 1992 Nov; 16: 141–51.
14. Baroody FM, Naclerio RM. An overview of immunology. *Otolaryngol Clin North Am*. 1993 Aug; 26: 571–91.
15. Metcalfe DD. Mediators relevant in asthma and allergic diseases. In: Goldstein RA, moderator. Asthma. *Ann Intern Med*. 1994 Nov; 121: 701–7.
16. Naclerio RM et al. Inflammatory mediators in late antigen-induced rhinitis. *N Engl J Med*. 1985 Jul; 313: 65–70.
17. Trevino RJ, Gordon BR. Allergic rhinosinusitis: the total rhinologic disease. *Ear Nose Throat J*. 1993 Feb; 72: 116, 121–9.
18. Sutherland DC. Drug treatment for allergic rhinitis: a clinical immunologist's view. *Rhinology*. 1992; 14(suppl): 72–6.
19. Garrison JC. Histamine, bradykinin, 5-hydroxytryptamine, and their antagonists. In: Gilman AG et al, eds. *Goodman and Gilman's the Pharmacological Basis of Therapeutics*. 8th ed. New York: Pergamon Press; 1990; 575–99.
20. Heyneman CA. Histamine$_2$-antagonists in allergic disorders. *Ann Pharmacother*. 1994 Jun; 28: 742–3.
21. Togias AG et al. Demonstration of inhibition of mediator release from human mast cells by azatadine base. *JAMA*. 1986 Jan; 255: 225–9.
22. Massey WA, Lichtenstein LM. The effects of antihistamines beyond H$_1$ antagonism in allergic inflammation. *J Allergy Clin Immunol*. 1990 Dec; 86: 1019–24.
23. Gong H Jr et al. Effects of oral cetirizine, a selective H$_1$ antagonist, on allergen- and exercise-induced bronchoconstriction in subjects with asthma. *J Allergy Clin Immunol*. 1990 Mar; 85: 632–41.
24. Smith SJ. Cardiovascular toxicity of antihistamines. *Otolaryngol Head Neck Surg*. 1994 Sep; 113: 348–54.
25. Cold, cough, allergy, bronchodilator, and antiasthmatic drug products for over-the-counter human use; final monograph for OTC antihistamines; final rule. *Federal Register*. 1992 Dec; 57: 58356–76.
26. Kemp JP. Tolerance to antihistamines: is it a problem? *Ann Allergy*. 1989 Dec; 63: 621–3.
27. Establishment of a monograph for OTC cold, cough, allergy, bronchodilator, and antiasthmatic products. *Federal Register*. 1976 Sep; 41: 38312–424.
28. Leftowitz RJ, Hoffman BB, Taylor P. Neurohumoral transmission: the autonomic and somatic motor nervous systems. In: Gilman AG et al, eds. *Goodman and Gilman's the Pharmacological Basis of Therapeutics*. 8th ed. New York: Pergamon Press; 1990: 84–121.
29. Black MJ, Remsen KA. Rhinitis medicamentosa. *Can Med Assoc J*. 1980 Apr; 122: 881–4.
30. Gourley DR, McKenzie CA. Glaucoma. In: Herfindal ET, Gourley DR, Hart LL, eds. *Clinical Pharmacy and Therapeutics*. 5th ed. Baltimore: Williams & Wilkins; 1992: 813.
31. Newton GD, Pray WS, Popovich NG. New OTCs: a selected review. *Am Pharm*. 1994 Feb; NS34(2): 31–8.
32. Briggs GG, Freeman RK, Yaffe SJ, eds. *Drugs in Pregnancy and Lactation: A Reference Guide to Fetal and Neonatal Risk*. 4th ed. Baltimore: Williams & Wilkins; 1994.
33. American Academy of Pediatrics, Committee on Drugs. The transfer of drugs and other chemicals into human milk. *Pediatrics*. 1994 Jan; 93: 137–50.
34. Creticos PS, Norman PS. Immunotherapy with allergens. *JAMA*. 1987 Nov; 258: 2874–80.
35. Engle JP. Topical nasal decongestants. *Am Pharm*. 1992 May; NS32: 33–7.
36. Dingle JH, Badger GF, Jordan WS Jr. Common respiratory diseases. In: *Illness in the Home: A Study of 25,000 Illnesses in a Group of Cleveland Families*. Cleveland, Ohio: Press of Western Reserve University; 1964: 33–9.
37. Denny FW, Collier AM, Henderson FW. Acute respiratory infections in day care. *Rev Infect Dis*. 1986 Jul–Aug; 8: 527–32.
38. Monto AS, Sullivan KM. Acute respiratory illness in the community. Frequency of illness and the agents involved. *Epidemiol Infect*. 1993 Feb; 110: 145–60.
39. Monto AS, Ullman BM. Acute respiratory illness in an American community. *JAMA*. 1974 Jan; 227: 164–9.
40. Wald ER et al. Frequency and severity of infections in day care. *J Pediatr*. 1988 Apr; 112: 540–6.
41. Wald ER, Guerra N, Byers C. Upper respiratory tract infections in young children: duration of and frequency of complications. *Pediatrics*. 1991 Feb; 87: 129–33.
42. Tyrrell DAJ, Cohen S, Schlarb JE. Signs and symptoms in common colds. *Epidemiol Infect*. 1993 Aug; 111: 143–56.
43. Jennings LC et al. Near disappearance of rhinovirus along a fomite transmission chain. *J Infect Dis*. 1988 Oct; 158: 888–92.
44. D'Alessio DJ et al. Short-duration exposure and the transmission of rhinoviral colds. *J Infect Dis*. 1984 Aug; 150: 189–94.
45. Cohen S et al. Smoking, alcohol consumption, and susceptibility to the common cold. *Am J Public Health*. 1993 Sep; 83: 1277–83.
46. Cohen S, Tyrrell DAJ, Smith AP. Psychological stress and susceptibility to the common cold. *N Engl J Med*. 1991 Aug; 325: 606–12.
47. Paul JH, Freese HL. An epidemiological and bacteriological

study of the "common cold" in an isolated arctic community (Spitsbergen). *Am J Hyg.* 1933 May; 17: 517–35.

48. Douglas RG, Lindgren KM, Couch RB. Exposure to cold environment and rhinovirus common cold. *N Engl J Med.* 1968 Oct; 279; 742–7.
49. Igarashi Y et al. Analysis of nasal secretions during experimental rhinovirus upper respiratory infections. *J Allergy Clin Immunol.* 1993 Nov; 92: 722–31.
50. Proud D et al. Kinins are generated in nasal secretions during natural rhinovirus colds. *J Infect Dis.* 1990 Jan; 161: 120–3.
51. Bulteau V. Sore throat. *Med J Aust.* 1966 Nov; 2: 1053–5.
52. Dolan R. Influenza. In: Isselbacher KJ et al, eds. *Harrison's Principles of Internal Medicine.* 13th ed. New York: McGraw-Hill; 1994: 814–9.
53. Dolan R. Common viral respiratory infections. In: Isselbacher KJ et al, eds. *Harrison's Principles of Internal Medicine.* 13th ed. New York: McGraw-Hill; 1994: 803–7.
54. Monto AS et al. Intranasal interferon for seasonal prophylaxis of respiratory infection. *J Infect Dis.* 1986 Jul; 154: 128–33.
55. Kuhn JJ et al. Antitussive effect of guaifenesin in young adults with natural colds. *Chest.* 1982 Dec; 82: 713–8.
56. Cold, cough, allergy, bronchodilator, and antiasthmatic drug products for over-the-counter human use; expectorant drug products for over-the-counter human use; final monograph; final rule. *Federal Register.* 1989 Feb; 54: 8495–509.
57. Cold, cough, allergy, bronchodilator, and antiasthmatic drug products for over-the-counter human use; final monograph for OTC antitussive drug products; final rule. *Federal Register.* 1987 Aug; 52: 30049–57.
58. Cold, cough, allergy, bronchodilator, and antiasthmatic drug products for over-the-counter human use; amendment of final monograph for OTC antitussive drug products. *Federal Register.* 1993 Oct; 58: 54232–6.
59. Jaffe JH, Martin WR. Opioid analgesics and antagonists. In: Gilman AG et al, eds. *Goodman and Gilman's the Pharmacological Basis of Therapeutics.* 8th ed. New York: Pergamon Press; 1990: 503–4.
60. Eccles R, Morris S, Jawad M. Lack of effect of codeine in the treatment of cough associated with acute upper respiratory infection. *J Clin Pharm Ther.* 1992 Jun; 17: 175–80.
61. Smith MBH, Feldman W. Over-the-counter cold medications. *JAMA.* 1993 May; 269: 2258–63.
62. Meade V. Patients need advice as array of cold products grows. *Am Pharm.* 1991 Dec; NS31(12): 24–5.
63. Hendeles L. Efficacy and safety of antihistamines and expectorants in nonprescription cough and cold preparations. *Pharmacotherapy.* 1993 Feb; 13: 154–8.
64. Howard JC Jr et al. Effectiveness of antihistamines in the symptomatic management of the common cold. *JAMA.* 1979 Nov; 242: 2414–7.
65. Doyle WJ et al. A double-blind, placebo-controlled clinical trial of the effect of chlorpheniramine on the response of the nasal airway, middle ear and eustachian tube to provocation rhinovirus challenge. *Pediatr Infect Dis J.* 1988 Mar; 7: 229–38.
66. Crutcher JE, Kantner TR. The effectiveness of antihistamines in the common cold. *J Clin Pharmacol.* 1981 Jan; 21: 9–15.
67. West S et al. A review of antihistamines and the common cold. *Pediatrics.* 1975 Jul; 56: 100–7.
68. Gaffey MJ et al. Intranasally and orally administered antihistamine treatment of experimental rhinovirus colds. *Am Rev Respir Dis.* 1987 Sep; 136: 556–60.
69. Bye CE et al. Effects of pseudoephedrine and triprolidine, alone and in combination, on symptoms of the common cold. *Br Med J.* 1980 Jul; 281: 189–90.
70. Berkowitz RB, Tinkelman DG. Evaluation of oral terfenadine for treatment of the common cold. *Ann Allergy.* 1991 Dec; 67: 593–7.
71. Gaffey MJ, Kaiser DL, Hayden FG. Ineffectiveness of oral terfenadine in natural colds: evidence against histamine as a mediator of common cold symptoms. *Pediatr Infect Dis J.* 1988 Mar; 7: 223–8.
72. Bluestone CD et al. Symposium in efficacy and safety of antihistamines in the treatment of upper respiratory infection—consensus statement. *Pediatr Infect Dis J.* 1988 Mar; 7: 241–2.
73. Pauling L. The significance of the evidence about ascorbic acid and the common cold. *Proc Natl Acad Sci USA.* 1971 Nov; 68: 2678–81.
74. Knipschild P. Systemic reviews. Some examples. *Br Med J.* 1994 Sep; 309: 719–21.
75. Hemila H. Does vitamin C alleviate the symptoms of the common cold? A review of the current evidence. *Scand J Infect Dis.* 1994 Jan; 26: 1–6.
76. Eby GA, Davis DR, Halcomb WW. Reduction in duration of common colds by zinc gluconate lozenges in a double-blind study. *Antimicrob Agents Chemother.* 1984 Jan; 25: 20–4.
77. Godfrey JC et al. Zinc gluconate and the common cold: a controlled clinical study. *J Int Med Res.* 1992; 20: 234–46.
78. Pinnock CB et al. Relationship between milk intake and mucus production in adult volunteers challenged with rhinovirus-2. *Am Rev Respir Dis.* 1990 Feb; 141: 352–6.
79. Kovar MG. Use of medications and vitamin-mineral supplements by children and youths. *Public Health Rep.* 1985 Sep–Oct; 100: 470–3.
80. Gadomski A, Horton L. The need for rational therapeutics in the use of cough and cold medicine in infants. *Pediatrics.* 1992 Apr; 89: 774–6.
81. Chaplin S. Adverse reactions to sympathomimetics in cold remedies. *Adverse Drug React Bull.* 1984 Aug; 107: 396–9.
82. Sills JA, Nunn AJ, Sankey RJ. Visual hallucinations in children receiving decongestants. *Br Med J.* 1984 Jun; 288: 1912–3.
83. Kane FJ, Green BQ. Psychotic episodes with the use of common proprietary decongestants. *Am J Psychol.* 1966 Oct; 123: 484–7.
84. Hurwitz ES et al. Public health service study on Reye's syndrome and medications. *N Engl J Med.* 1985 Oct; 313: 849–57.
85. Cherry JD. The common cold. In: Feigin RD, Cherry JD, eds. *Textbook of Pediatric Infectious Diseases.* 3rd ed. Philadelphia: WB Saunders; 1992: 137–42.
86. American Academy of Pediatrics, Committee on Drugs. Use of codeine and dextromethorphan-containing cough syrups in pediatrics. *Pediatrics.* 1978 Jul; 62: 118–22.
87. Gadomski A. Rational use of over-the-counter medications in young children. *JAMA.* 1994 Oct; 272: 1063–4.

CHAPTER 9

Asthma Products

Dennis M. Williams and Timothy H. Self

Questions to ask in patient assessment and counseling

- *Has a physician diagnosed your condition as asthma? (If patient answers "no," proceed with questions for undiagnosed asthma. If "yes," proceed with questions for diagnosed asthma.)*

Undiagnosed Asthma

- *Have you had an attack or recurrent attacks of wheezing?*
- *Do you have a troublesome cough at night?*
- *Do you have a cough or wheeze after exercise?*
- *Do you have a cough, wheeze, or chest tightness after exposure to airborne allergens or pollutants?*
- *Do your colds "go to the chest" or take more than 10 days to clear up?*

Diagnosed Asthma

- *Are you under the care of a physician?*
- *Do you have a written asthma care plan?*
- *Do you have other medical problems, such as heart disease, seizures, high blood pressure, hyperthyroidism, or diabetes?*
- *What prescription or nonprescription medications are you currently taking?*
- *During the past year, how many days have you missed from school or work because of asthma?*
- *How many nights per week do you awake with asthma?*
- *In the last year, have you been to the emergency room or hospital because of asthma?*
- *Does asthma affect your ability to exercise (even brisk walking)?*
- *Have you used any asthma products in the past? If so, which ones? Were they effective? Did they cause any problems (side effects)? If so, what were they?*
- *How often during each day and each week do you use a bronchodilator inhaler for symptoms of asthma? Would you demonstrate how you use your inhaler? How do you clean it?*
- *Do you use a spacer device? If so, would you demonstrate how you use it?*
- *Do you have a peak flow meter? If so, is it a manual or electronic meter? How do you use it?*

An estimated 10 million persons in the United States, including 3 million children, have asthma. From 1982 to 1992, the reported prevalence rate increased 42% to 49.4 per 1,000 population.[1] The estimated cost of treating asthma in the United States in 1990 was approximately $6.2 billion.[2] The largest single direct medical expenditure was inpatient hospital services (emergency care), reaching almost $1.5 billion. Loss of school days was the largest single indirect cost, approaching $1 billion. In total, approximately 43% of the economic impact of asthma was potentially avoidable because it was associated with emergency room use, hospitalization, and death.

The annual age-adjusted death rate from asthma increased 40% during the period 1982–1991. In 1991, 5,106 deaths were attributed to asthma.[1] An increase in morbidity and mortality from asthma in the United States and worldwide has been a major concern and was the impetus for the National Heart, Lung, and Blood Institute (NHLBI) to establish the National Asthma Education Program, now known as the National Asthma Education and Prevention Program (NAEPP). An expert panel from the NAEPP has developed national guidelines for the diagnosis and management of asthma.[3] Subsequently, the NHLBI also sponsored the development of international guidelines and a document examining global issues in asthma management.[4,5]

Editor's Note: This chapter is based, in part, on the chapter with the same title that appeared in the 10th edition but was written by H. William Kelly and Mary Beth O'Connell.

Anatomy of the Respiratory Tract

The respiratory system, which comprises the upper and lower respiratory tracts, consists of a series of airways, starting with the nose and mouth and leading ultimately to the terminal air sacs or alveoli. The mouth and nasal passages lead to the pharynx, which branches out into the esophagus and the trachea. The trachea divides into

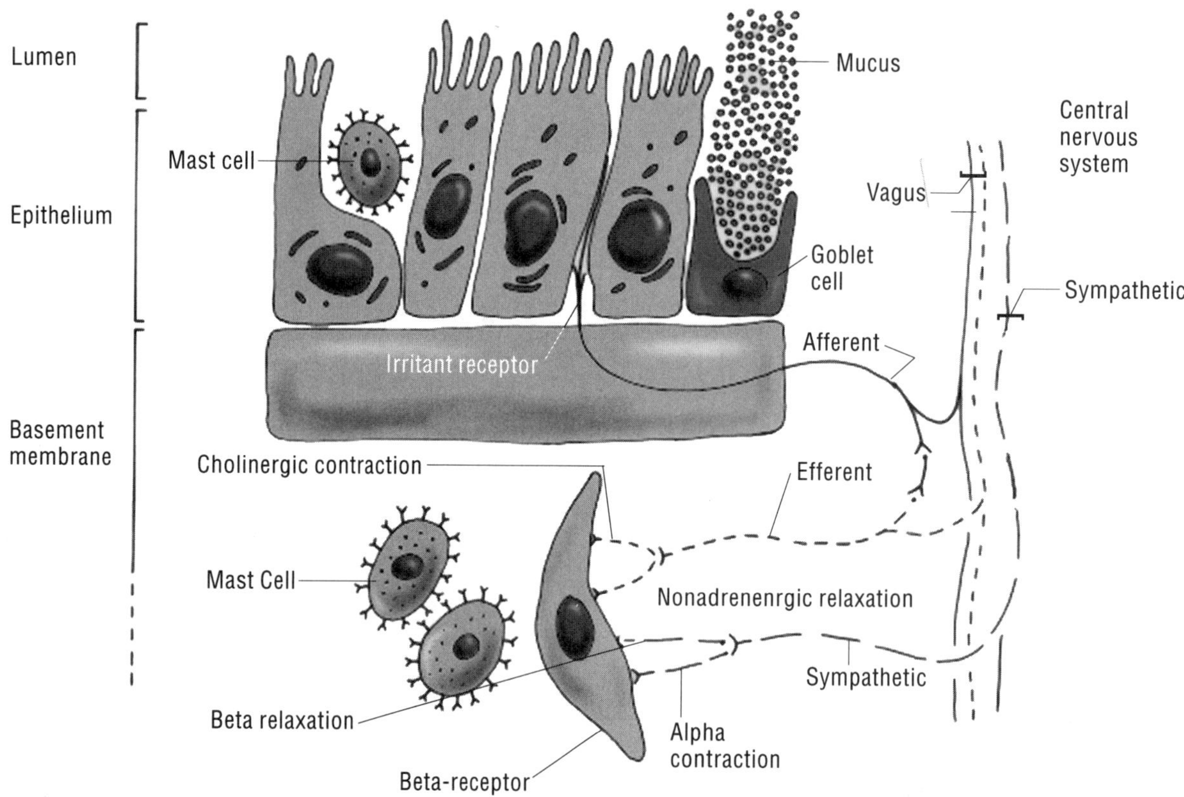

FIGURE 1 Innervation of the airways by the sympathetic, cholinergic, and nonadrenergic inhibitory systems. Mast cell concentration increases from the epithelial lumen to the submucosa. Adapted with permission from *Pharmacotherapy: A Pathophysiologic Approach*. 2nd ed. Dipiro J et al, eds. New York: Elsevier Science Publishing; 1992: 410.

the two large mainstem bronchi that supply air to the lungs. Each bronchus progressively divides into smaller airways (bronchioles), leading through the alveolar ducts to the alveoli.[6] Layers of smooth muscle are wrapped around the airways; the number of muscle layers decreases as the airways progress toward the alveoli. As an airway branches, the walls become progressively thinner. At the level of the alveoli, only a thin layer of cells surrounded by pulmonary capillaries remains.

Respiration is an exchange of gases between the alveoli and capillary blood. Inspired oxygen passes across the alveolar walls into the capillaries, whereas carbon dioxide diffuses in the opposite direction and is expired. Oxygenated blood returns through the pulmonary vein to the left side of the heart where it is pumped through the aorta to other organs.

The lungs are essentially elastic air sacs suspended in the airtight thoracic cavity. The movable walls of this cavity are formed by the sternum (breastbone), ribs, and diaphragm. The ribs are attached to the spinal vertebrae and join together at the sternum. As the thoracic cavity expands, the pressure within it becomes less than the atmospheric pressure, air enters, and the lungs expand. This process is accomplished by means of two simultaneous mechanisms. The diaphragm, a dome-shaped muscle (when relaxed) that extends upward into the thoracic cavity, contracts. As it contracts, the diaphragm becomes flattened and moves downward into the abdomen, increasing the longitudinal size of the thoracic cavity. Simultaneous contraction of the external intercostal muscles raises the ribs, causing an elevation and forward movement of the sternum and an increase in the diameter of the chest cavity. During inspiration, the diaphragm and ribs move simultaneously, expanding the thoracic cavity and thus allowing the lungs to fill with air. Expiration results from relaxation of the ventilatory muscles and the elastic recoil force of the alveoli and airways.

The nasal cavities are lined with highly vascular mucous membranes and ciliated epithelial cells interspersed with mucus-producing goblet cells. During normal inspiration, as air passes over these areas enroute to the alveoli, it is warmed, humidified, and filtered. Dust particles, bacteria, and other foreign matter are trapped in the mucus and propelled toward the pharynx by the wavelike movement of the nasal cilia; they are then deposited in the oral cavity, where they are either expelled or swallowed. The humidification and filtration processes continue as air passes through the trachea, bronchi, and bronchioles.

Bronchial smooth muscle tone and mucus secretion are under neural and humoral control (Figure 1).[7] Afferent nerves leading from irritant receptors in the

Step 4: Severe persistent asthma

Clinical features before treatment[a]	Daily medication(s) required to maintain control
Continuous symptoms Frequent exacerbations Frequent nocturnal asthma symptoms Physical activities limited by asthma symptoms PEF or FEV_1: ≤60% predicted; variability >30%	Multiple daily controller medications: high doses of inhaled corticosteroid, long-acting bronchodilator, and long-term use of oral corticosteroid

Step 3: Moderate persistent asthma

Clinical features before treatment[a]	Daily medication(s) required to maintain control
Daily symptoms Exacerbations affect activity and sleep Nocturnal asthma symptoms occur >1 time a week Daily use of inhaled short-acting $beta_2$-agonists PEF or FEV_1: >60–<80% predicted; variability >30%	Daily controller medications: inhaled corticosteroid and long-acting bronchodilator (especially for nocturnal symptoms)

Step 2: Mild persistent asthma

Clinical features before treatment[a]	Daily medication(s) required to maintain control
Symptoms occur ≥1 time a week but <1 time a day Exacerbations may affect activity and sleep Nocturnal symptoms occur >2 times a month PEF or FEV_1: ≥80% predicted; variability 20–30%	One daily controller medication; a long-acting bronchodilator could be added to anti-inflammatory medication (especially for nocturnal symptoms)

Step 1: Intermittent asthma

Clinical features before treatment[a]	Daily medication(s) required to maintain control
Intermittent symptoms occur <1 time a week Brief exacerbations lasting from a few hours to a few days Nocturnal symptoms occur <2 times a month Lung function between exacerbations is asymptomatic and normal PEF or FEV_1: ≥80% predicted; variability <20%	Intermittent reliever medication taken only as needed: inhaled short-acting $beta_2$-agonists Intensity of treatment depends on severity of exacerbation; oral corticosteroids may be required

[a]The presence of one of the clinical features of a category is sufficent to place a patient in that category.

FIGURE 2 Classification of asthma severity. Reprinted from National Heart, Lung, and Blood Institute. *Global Initiative for Asthma*. Pub No 95–3659. Bethesda, Md: US Department of Health and Human Services; 1995.

mucosal epithelium produce reflex bronchoconstriction, increased mucus production, and cough through cholinergic innervation of bronchial smooth muscle and goblet cells from the vagus nerve. Smooth muscle of the airway is only sparsely innervated by the adrenergic system; however, smooth muscle throughout the entire airway contains beta-adrenergic receptors. Alpha-adrenergic stimulation produces smooth muscle contraction that is primarily vascular, and $beta_2$-adrenergic stimulation produces smooth muscle relaxation. The nonadrenergic, noncholinergic (NANC) nervous system is the principal inhibitory system of the airways, counteracting the cholinergic excitatory system.[7] Stimulation of the NANC system through the vagus nerve primarily produces bronchodilation but can also produce bronchoconstriction. Neurotransmission through the NANC system is mediated by neuropeptides, which have not been conclusively identified. It appears that a vasoactive intestinal peptide acts as an inhibitory transmitter (resulting in smooth muscle relaxation) and that substance P acts as an excitatory transmitter.[7] Under normal circumstances, these systems assist in maintaining normal bronchomotor tone.

Epidemiology and Etiology of Asthma

The NAEPP expert panel report defines asthma as a lung disease with the following characteristics:

- Airway obstruction that is reversible (but not completely so in some patients) either spontaneously or with treatment;
- Airways inflammation;
- Increased airway responsiveness to a variety of stimuli.[3]

More than 5,000 asthma deaths were reported in 1991. The cause of the increase in mortality is multifactorial, but the increase has been greater in elderly and urban populations. Among persons aged 15–44 years, African-Americans have a death rate five times that of Caucasians. Excessive use of sympathomimetic metered-dose inhalers (MDIs) is a sign of poorly controlled asthma and has been implicated as a risk factor for asthma mortality.[8] In addition, retrospective studies of asthma deaths both outside and inside the hospital indicate that failure to appreciate the severity of illness by both patients and the medical profession has led to inadequate therapy and is a major contributing factor in most asthma-related deaths.[3] Because most asthma deaths occur outside the hospital, impaired access to medical care has also been proposed as a contributing factor.

Symptomatic asthma is more common in children, with the age of onset being under 10 years of age for 50% of all subjects.[9] The prevalence rate is slightly higher in males until puberty, at which time the gender ratio is approximately equal. Often, symptoms significantly decrease in severity as patients age, so the overall prognosis for children who develop asthma is good. Longitudinal studies indicate that 50–70% of children with asthma have a permanent or temporary symptom-free remission by adulthood.[5] However, 30% of children with asthma continue to have chronic symptoms into adulthood. Asthma is present in 3.8% of men and 7.1% of women over age 65.[10] Evidence increasingly suggests that chronic asthma may result in irreversible chronic obstruction.[9]

The precise etiology of asthma is not known; however, epidemiologic studies in families and twins suggest a genetic component.[9] Atopy is the strongest identified predisposing factor in the development of asthma. An estimated 30–50% of the population is atopic although the prevalence of asthma is much lower. Atopy in parents and children predicts an increased risk of developing asthma but is not essential; further, not all allergic patients develop asthma.[5,9]

Several causal factors that sensitize the airways and lead to the onset of asthma have been identified. The most frequent and important ones are indoor allergens, including house dust mites, furred animals, and fungi. These allergens sensitize the individual, resulting in the production of immunoglobulin E (IgE) antibodies. Outdoor allergens, including dust, pollens, and fungi, are also sensitizers. Other important sensitizers are occupational agents and drug or food additives.

Although underlying lung pathology is common to all patients with asthma, patients often differ in what incites their asthma. Once patients have been sensitized, they are susceptible to asthma triggers. Asthma is generally exacerbated by respiratory tract infections (primarily viral); inhaled allergens; inhaled air pollutants; smoking (active and passive); exercise; or occupational and industrial irritants, sulfites, or drugs. An identifiable allergen is the major precipitating factor in 35–55% of the population with asthma, and respiratory infections are a major factor in about 40%.[3,5] About 2–10% of patients with asthma develop acute asthma following ingestion of aspirin or other nonsteroidal anti-inflammatory drugs (NSAIDs).[7]

Previously, asthma patients were classified according to their predominant trigger. Regardless of whether they are classified as extrinsic (allergic) or intrinsic patients with asthma, most patients with asthma have elevated serum levels of IgE. Currently, asthma is more commonly categorized based on its severity. This classification system is described in Figure 2.

Pathophysiology of Asthma

Asthma is a chronic inflammatory disease that involves the airways and is further characterized by recurrent exacerbations. Although the cellular defect in asthma is still unknown, it is now recognized that unchecked inflammation of the airways is the principal cause of their excessive reactivity to various triggering events.[3,7,11] This bronchial hyperreactivity (BHR) is characterized by (1) smooth muscle contraction (bronchoconstriction), (2) mucus hypersecretion, (3) mucosal edema, and (4) epithelial desquamation (Figure 3). The inflammatory process in asthma is characterized by submucosal infiltration of eosinophils and lymphocytes, with epithelial shedding and hyperplasia of the basement membrane.[11] In addition, tissue mast cells increase in number and often appear to be activated.[7] Mast cell degranulation,

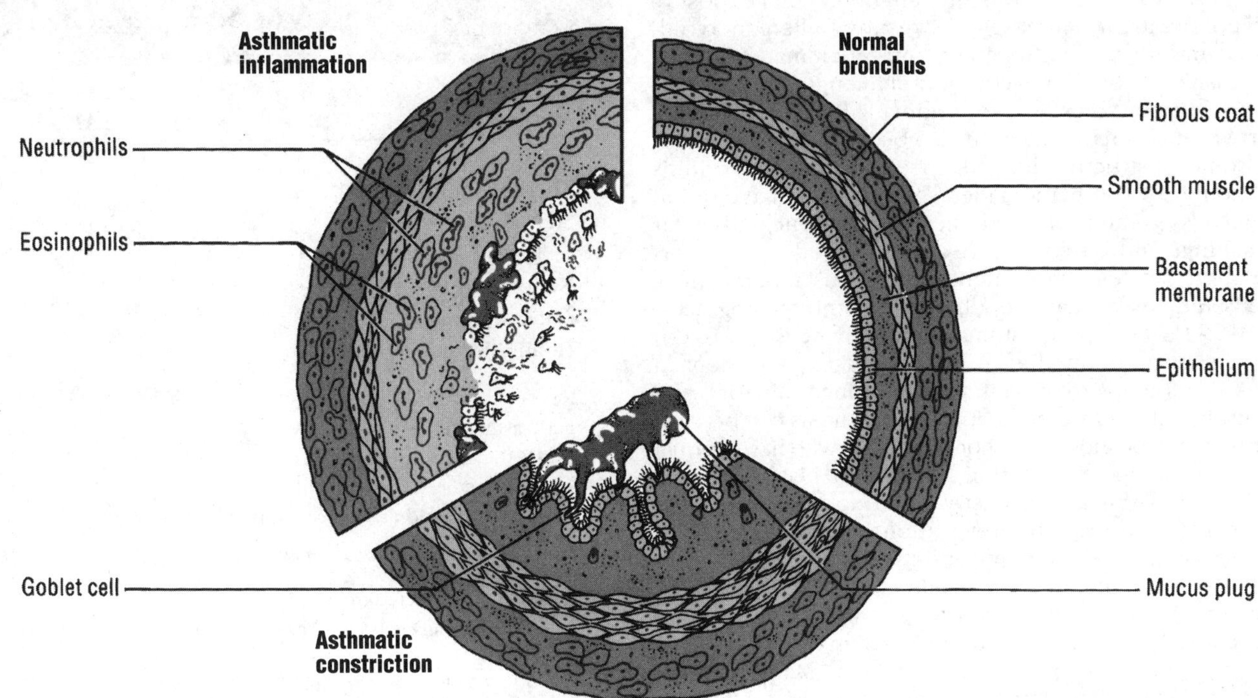

FIGURE 3 Representative illustration of the pathology found in the asthmatic bronchus compared with a normal bronchus (upper right section). Each section demonstrates how the lumen is narrowed. Edema of the basement membrane, mucus plugging, smooth muscle hypertropy, and construction contribute (lower section). Inflammatory cells producing epithelial desquamation fill the airway lumen with cellular debris and expose the airway smooth muscles to other mediators (upper left section). Adapted with permission from *Pharmacotherapy: A Pathophysiologic Approach*. 2nd ed. Dipiro J et al, eds. New York: Elsevier Science Publishing; 1992: 409.

which is produced by exercise, exposure to allergen, hyperosmolar conditions from hyperventilation, or occupational or environmental irritants, may release preformed mediators such as histamine; eosinophil chemotactic factor; platelet-activating factor; prostaglandins; and leukotrienes C-4, D-4, and E-4. The release of these mediators is known as the early asthmatic response (EAR). Although the relative importance of each mediator in the pathogenesis of asthma is still unknown, each is capable of producing bronchoconstriction; stimulating mucus secretion; increasing vascular permeability; and attracting and activating eosinophils, neutrophils, and lymphocytes.[7] The activated eosinophils are then capable of releasing toxins such as major basic protein, which can desquamate epithelium. The lymphocytes release cytokines capable of retaining and priming eosinophils in the airways as well as amplifying the effects of other mediators.[12]

The bronchial smooth muscle hypertrophy, goblet cell hypertrophy, and excessive mucus production are secondary to the ongoing inflammatory process. Although imbalances in neural control of the airways have been postulated as a primary cause of BHR, it now appears that, if such imbalances exist, they are more likely to play a role in amplifying the inflammation and bronchoconstriction.[4] When bronchial smooth muscle from patients with asthma is taken out of the inflammatory milieu of the airways, it does not react any differently to contracting or relaxing substances than does bronchial smooth muscle from patients without asthma.

The characteristic feature of the asthma patient is excessive BHR to various stimuli. The clinical severity and need for therapy correlate with the degree of BHR; acute exacerbations are associated with an increase in BHR.[13] The degree of BHR can be measured with a number of pharmacologic (histamine, methacholine), physical (cold air or hypertonic saline), or physiologic (exercise or eucapnic hyperventilation of dry air) stimuli. The standard approach is bronchoprovocation with inhaled histamine or methacholine, which are defined as "nonspecific" bronchoprovocation stimuli to differentiate them from "specific" allergen bronchoprovocation stimuli. Patients inhale increasing concentrations in doubling increments of either histamine or methacholine, and spirometric measurements are made after each increment. The provocative dose or concentration that produces a 20% drop in forced expiratory volume exhaled in 1 second (FEV_1) is calculated, and that value is used as a measure of airway reactivity.[13] A lower provocative concentration indicates greater BHR.

BHR increases following allergen exposure, viral respiratory tract infections, and environmental exposure to pollutants. It decreases as a result of allergen avoidance and therapy with certain anti-inflammatory drugs. A positive bronchoprovocation challenge is consistent with, but not diagnostic of, asthma.[13] Positive bronchoprovocation challenges can also occur in cystic fibrosis, chronic obstructive lung disease, and allergic rhinitis although symptomatic patients with asthma have quantitatively greater BHR. Studies using bronchoalveolar washings and biopsies have demonstrated a good correlation between the number of various inflammatory cells and desquamated epithelial cells and the degree of BHR.[12,13] In the past, asthma could only be diagnosed if reversibility (defined as at least a 15% improvement in FEV_1 following treatment with a bronchodilator) was present with spirometry. Now the diagnosis can be confirmed by bronchoprovocation in patients who have normal spirometry on examination but have a history consistent with asthma. Spirometry often does not correlate with BHR, so bronchoprovocation is a more sensitive indicator of airway inflammation.

Within 5 minutes of inhaling a specific allergen, patients with asthma demonstrate a drop in pulmonary function that reaches a nadir in 10–20 minutes and then spontaneously improves within 1 hour. Many patients with asthma will undergo a second response 4–12 hours later, which may persist for 2–4 hours. This response, known as the late asthmatic response (LAR), is one key factor involved in increasing BHR and maintaining that increase. The LAR occurs after inflammatory cells infiltrate the airways and is associated with an increase in BHR that does not occur with an EAR alone. Drugs that effectively block the LAR prevent the increase in BHR and, with chronic use, can lower BHR (Table 1). Because the LAR is associated with an influx of inflammatory mediators, agents that only influence EAR (eg, beta-agonists) have no significant effect on BHR or the LAR. Specific allergen avoidance can not only prevent the usual seasonal increases in BHR in patients with asthma but also lower their BHR over time.

TABLE 1 Phase activity of asthma medications

Medication	EAR	LAR
$Beta_2$-agonist	+	-[a]
Theophylline	+	-
Steroids	-	+
Cromolyn	+	+
Nedocromil	+	+
Anticholinergics	+	-
H_1-antihistamines	-	-

Key:
Early asthmatic response (EAR).
Late asthmatic response (LAR).
+ means medication inhibits this response.
- means medication does not inhibit this response.

[a]Long-acting $beta_2$-agonists may inhibit the LAR.

Information extracted from:
Lipworth BJ, McDevitt DG. *Br J Clin Pharmacol.* 1992; 33: 129–38.
Twentyman OP et al. *Lancet.* 1990 Dec 1; 336: 1338–42.

Symptoms of Asthma

By definition, asthma is episodic in nature. Periods of airway obstruction may last from a few minutes to several days. The severity of obstruction is highly variable, producing mild symptoms or rapidly progressing to respiratory failure. Patients with more severe disease may have continuous symptoms that require chronic medication for control; others may have normal pulmonary function between episodes and require only periodic medication.

Common symptoms of asthma are cough, wheezing, dyspnea (difficulty in breathing), and chest tightness. These may be present in various combinations in individual asthma patients. The classic symptom of asthma is wheezing (a fine whistling sound) on expiration; in more severe obstruction, wheezing may occur on inspiration as well. Coughing caused by stimulation of the irritant receptors is common. Chronic cough may be the only presenting symptom in some patients with asthma. Patients may have normal spirometric pulmonary function tests between episodes, but many patients with asthma have an increased bronchomotor tone, which is readily reversed with a bronchodilator drug. During attacks, patients with asthma demonstrate a marked decrease in all measures of expiratory flow rate and often complain of a tightness in their chest and of dyspnea. Because outflow of air is obstructed to a greater degree than is inflow of air, the lungs actually become overinflated and the patient has to breathe at higher lung volumes, which makes breathing more difficult. Patients then become “air hungry” and apprehensive. About 30–50% of patients with asthma complain of excessive sputum production. The sputum is usually yellowish and, upon microscopic examination, full of eosinophils. Although the airflow limitation caused by asthma has traditionally been considered completely reversible, it is now apparent that some patients develop irreversible airflow limitation over a period of several years. This is most likely related to airway wall remodeling and associated with an accumulation of inflammatory cells, edema, fibrosis, and changes in elastic properties.

Patient Assessment

As with other diseases, medical diagnosis of asthma is essential to rule out other causes of pulmonary symptoms such as physical obstruction from a tumor, congestive heart failure, and chronic bronchitis. For example, if a patient with new pulmonary symptoms describes a history of hypertension or heart disease, physician referral is critical. A patient who awakens in the middle of the night with dyspnea and cough resulting from pulmonary edema ("cardiac asthma") may have congestive heart failure. As another example, shortness of breath and chest pain in women taking oral contraceptives may be signs of pulmonary emboli rather than asthma; such patients should also be referred to a physician immediately. Patients with chronic bronchitis and emphysema experience some symptoms similar to those associated with asthma. However, these symptoms are usually continuous, not episodic, and should not be treated with nonprescription drugs except under a physician's direction. The first set of questions presented at the beginning of this chapter should be helpful in differentiating asthma from other pulmonary conditions.

Asthma is frequently unrecognized, especially in children, and therefore untreated. Pharmacists can play a major role in identifying potential patients with asthma and referring them for appropriate care. Symptoms such as recurrent wheezing, periods of dyspnea, coughing, chest tightness, and repeated respiratory tract infections warrant additional assessments to determine whether asthma is present. In some cases, however, the patients themselves make the diagnosis of asthma after several episodes of intermittent shortness of breath and wheezing.[14] Many patients have mild asthma that does not progress; in others, the condition may worsen and be accompanied by dyspnea and wheezing, cough, tachycardia, retraction of the sternocleidomastoid muscle, apprehension, chest distention, tenacious sputum, and flaring nostrils. Sinus tachycardia with a pulse rate up to 120 beats per minute is a very common finding, as is sternocleidomastoid muscle retraction in patients with severe airway obstruction.[14]

If a diagnosis of asthma has been previously established, it is important to determine the frequency and severity of symptoms and which self-treatment approaches have already been attempted. Patients need immediate medical intervention if shortness of breath makes them unable to complete a full sentence without stopping, if discomfort persists while they are at rest after using a bronchodilator, or if the bronchodilator does not completely relieve their symptoms. If a bronchodilator is being used but the dyspnea becomes worse, a severe attack may be imminent or already in progress, and the patient should see a physician immediately. Patients with progressive dyspnea and wheezing who are dependent on nonprescription products may be in danger of severe pulmonary obstruction, which may require treatment in a hospital.

Treatment

The use of nonprescription medications for the management of asthma symptoms is controversial.[15] The pulmonary-allergy advisory committee to the FDA has stated that "although the bronchodilators are generally safe for OTC use at recommended dosage and are effective in relieving the shortness of breath caused by bronchospasm, . . . it is emphasized that these preparations should not be used unless a diagnosis of asthma has been made by a physician and a dosage schedule of the OTC medication has been established by a physician. Patients with asthma may also require prescription drugs which may have serious dangers and side effects and there is, then, an added need for continued medical supervision."[16]

If indicated, nonprescription medications are clearly reserved for patients with mild, intermittent symptoms. Even in this situation, many clinicians prefer to recommend a prescription, short-acting, inhaled, selective $beta_2$-agonist (eg, albuterol) based on its greater potency, longer duration of effect, and fewer adverse effects. Clearly, potent medications, available only by prescription, are required for the treatment of moderate and severe asthma. Continued use of nonprescription products should be monitored by the pharmacist. If frequent or regular doses are required, the patient should be referred to a physician for appropriate care. Prescription therapy with an as-needed selective $beta_2$-agonist inhaler or chronic use of one of the anti-inflammatory medications (eg, inhaled corticosteroids or cromolyn) should be instituted if nonprescription drug therapy does not provide adequate symptomatic relief.[10]

The Pharmacist's Role in Managing Asthma

Opportunities for pharmacists in improving asthma care have recently been highlighted. The NHLBI published a report in the fall of 1995 titled *The Role of the Pharmacist in Improving Asthma Care*.[17,18] This document describes numerous areas of involvement for the pharmacist, including:

- Educating patients about asthma medications;
- Instructing patients in proper inhalation techniques;
- Monitoring medication use and refill intervals to identify patients with poorly controlled asthma;
- Referring patients for appropriate care;
- Assisting patients in using peak flow meters properly;
- Assisting patients in incorporating the meters in a self-management plan designed by a physician;
- Helping patients discharged from hospitals to understand their asthma management plan;
- Serving as a resource for physicians by sharing current expert guidelines about asthma management.

These areas represent an action plan for pharmacists and should be the primary focus of pharmaceutical care for the asthma patient.

To assist with the appropriate treatment plan for a specific asthma patient, the pharmacist must consider the goals of treatment, the severity of the disease, specific patient characteristics, past medical history, and the benefits and risks of the various drug classes for asthma treatment. The clinical goals of asthma treatment are to:

- Maintain normal activity levels (including exercise);
- Maintain normal or near normal pulmonary function rates;
- Prevent chronic and troublesome symptoms;
- Prevent recurrent exacerbations of asthma;
- Avoid adverse effects from asthma medications.[3]

The pharmacist should be actively involved in the patient's decision process to use nonprescription medications. It is extremely important for the pharmacist to determine the pattern of use for patients using nonprescription bronchodilator inhalers. If the underlying disease is asthma, self-treatment may delay the patient's seeking necessary medical care and result in resistant acute severe asthma attacks. Patients with symptoms that occur more often than one to two times weekly, or with nocturnal asthma, should be *strongly encouraged* to seek medical advice and to consider using a home peak flow meter (see the section Use of Peak Flow Meters in Asthma Management) for a more objective physical assessment. If the symptoms are new and the patient has not been diagnosed by a physician as having asthma, medical referral for evaluation is essential.

Stepped-Care Treatment

A stepped-care approach to asthma treatment, as outlined by the NAEPP expert panel report, may be instituted.[3] Guidelines are also available from NHBLI's *International Consensus Report on Diagnosis and Treatment of Asthma* and its *Global Initiative for Asthma*.[4,5] The latter two publications are more recent and are used by many clinicians because they include information about the role of newer therapies.

The steps in this therapeutic approach include prevention of inflammation, as-needed drug usage, chronic regular drug usage, rescue, and step-down in therapy when the condition is controlled. Integral components of this approach are patient education and evaluation of patient compliance and response.

Prevention of Inflammatory Response

The primary focus and first step of asthma therapy is prevention of the inflammatory response. Patients should be instructed on the home use of a peak flow meter so that therapy can be initiated as soon as significant obstruction is measured. If as-needed or chronic medications do not abate the asthma attack, the patient should be instructed to seek medical attention early. Caregivers and significant others of patients with asthma should also be educated on how to assess the severity of and treat asthma attacks as well as on how and when to seek medical assistance. Patients should learn what triggers their asthma attacks so that they can either avoid these triggers or premedicate appropriately prior to exposure. Patients with asthma should receive annual immunizations against influenza virus, preferably each fall, unless they have a history of adverse reactions to the vaccine.[19,20]

As-Needed Drug Therapy

The NAEPP expert panel's plan for as-needed drug therapy is as follows: mild asthma can be treated using a short-acting beta$_2$-agonist inhaler when needed.[3] The patient can use the inhaler either to prevent attacks when exposure to known triggers associated with difficulty in breathing are anticipated or to abate dyspnea. The patient should maintain a record of inhaler usage and peak flow measurements so that the need for chronic therapy can be evaluated.

Chronic Drug Therapy

For the patient with moderate asthma who has at least two episodes of asthma symptoms a week, chronic therapy with an anti-inflammatory should be initiated. The anti-inflammatory should be combined with an as-needed or a regularly scheduled inhaled bronchodilator. One issue that remains as a subject of debate is whether scheduled, chronic use of inhaled, short-acting bronchodilators leads to worsening pulmonary functions and asthma control.[8,21] Regardless of whether this is the case, short-acting, inhaled beta$_2$-agonists may be used most appropriately as needed for symptoms because the frequency of use is a good marker of adequacy of anti-inflammatory therapy.

Inhaled corticosteroids are the most potent anti-inflammatories, but issues such as long-term sequelae and use in children need to be resolved before inhaled steroids are used as first-line treatment agents in all patients. Symptoms of asthma occur more frequently at night in many patients. Strategies of management in this instance are to increase the anti-inflammatory therapy or add a longer acting bronchodilator (eg, salmeterol, sustained-release theophylline, or a sustained-release oral beta$_2$-agonist.) In young children and in adults with predominantly allergen-induced or seasonal asthma, cromolyn or nedocromil may be considered as first-line therapy. Anticholinergics have a minor role in the initial treatment of asthma and generally should be reserved for resistant patients. For moderate to severe asthma, combinations of drugs that work on the different phases of asthma (ie, inflammation and bronchoconstriction) are essential. These patients require a fast-acting agent for relief of acute symptoms (short-acting, inhaled beta$_2$-agonist) for as-needed use and an inhaled anti-inflammatory agent as a controller.

For patients with severe asthma, chronic multiple drug use is required. Chronic use of both a long-acting, inhaled beta-agonist and a high-dose inhaled corticosteroid, supplemented as needed with an additional inhaled short-acting beta$_2$-agonist, is often required. Theophylline, salmeterol, an oral beta$_2$-agonist, and oral steroids may also be needed.[3–5]

Rescue Therapy

Rescue therapy refers to the management of asthma exacerbations characterized by progressively worsening shortness of breath, cough, wheezing, or chest tightness. Exacerbations are also characterized objectively by decreases in measurable expiratory airflow (FEV$_1$ or PEFR). The primary aims of treatment are to relieve airflow limitation as quickly as possible, relieve hypoxemia, restore lung function to normal, and formulate a plan to avoid future relapses. For rescue therapy, reliever medications are required; the most commonly used agents are short-acting inhaled beta$_2$-agonists and systemic corticosteroids (eg, prednisone). Once the exacerbation is relieved, shifting attention to the chronic maintenance regimen is appropriate.

Step-Down Therapy

Asthma is a variable disorder and may improve spontaneously or as a result of therapy. Specifically, chronic treatment with anti-inflammatory therapy may reduce the severity of asthma. When asthma control is achieved and maintained for at least 3 months, it is reasonable to attempt to identify the minimum therapy required to maintain control by gradually reducing doses or discontinuing medication. Step-down therapy must be done in a stepwise fashion and symptoms and lung function must be closely monitored during the process. This approach should help reduce the occurrence of side effects and enhance patient compliance.

Use of Peak Flow Meters in Asthma Management

It is extremely important to recognize that delay in seeking medical care is a major contributing factor to asthma mortality.[3] Subjective symptoms of wheezing and dyspnea are notoriously poor measures of lung function and contribute to such delay. Certain patients have an altered perception of asthma symptoms that can result in a delay in seeking treatment when symptoms are the sole monitoring parameter. Thus, the NAEPP expert panel has recommended home monitoring of peak expiratory flow rate (PEFR) with portable peak flow meters in all patients with chronic, moderate to severe asthma.[3]

Various brands of peak flow meters are available (see product table "Asthma Auxiliary Devices"), but they all work similarly to achieve the same objective: to determine the PEFR, or the maximum rate of air flow following forced expiration. The PEFR correlates well with a patient's FEV_1 and provides an objective at-home measurement of airway obstruction. These devices are to asthma patients what home blood pressure monitors are to hypertensive patients and what blood glucose meters are to diabetic patients. Thus, proper use of these devices is important and pharmacists should ensure proper technique (Table 2). Recent evidence suggests that the performance accuracy and durability of devices vary; therefore, the pharmacist should evaluate individual products before recommending their use.[22]

The NAEPP's expert panel recommends that the patient and the physician determine the patient's best peak flow value. Once this value has been adequately determined, the "three-zone" system may be used to relate peak flow readings to asthma management (Table 3). However, this color-coded scheme, which uses a traffic light analogy, should serve as a guideline only: the patient and his or her physician should individualize the system by defining the peak flow values for each zone that will provide optimal therapy for the patient. A key point in peak flow monitoring is the establishment of the patient's baseline because this represents a more practical parameter than a population value. Until the patient's best peak flow value is determined (eg, typically after a few weeks of optimal therapy), the use of population averages (based on age, height, and gender) is helpful.[7]

TABLE 2 Correct use of peak flow meters

1. Set the meter indicator on the bottom of the scale before each forced expiration.
2. (If possible) Take all measurements while standing.
3. Make sure that the hole in the back of the meter is not covered.
4. Take a deep breath.
5. Seal the lips tightly around the mouthpiece (do not let any air leak out).
6. Rest the mouthpiece on the tongue but do not obstruct the opening of the mouthpiece with the tongue.
7. Expire hard and fast (forcefully).
8. Record the best of three efforts as the peak flow value.

Pharmacologic Agents

General Pharmacology

Asthma medications can be categorized by their ability to inhibit the EAR and/or the LAR. Medications that prevent the EAR are bronchodilators or inhibitors of mast cell mediator release.[7,11] Medications that modify the

TABLE 3 Three-zone system of asthma management

Zone	Peak flow values	Patient guideline
Green	≥80–100% of the patient's personal best, or the predicted flow value indicated by a standard chart	*Go!* Continue regular activity and regular asthma maintenance therapy
Yellow	50–80% of the patient's personal best, or the predicted flow value indicated by a standard chart	*Caution!* Patient may require additional medication or increase in regular maintenance therapy
Red	<50% of the patient's personal best, or the predicted flow value indicated by a standard chart	*Stop!* Seek medical advice or medication immediately

TABLE 4 Selected characteristics of bronchodilator drugs

Drug	Route of administration	Availability	Pharmacologic activity				Duration of action (h)
			Sympathomimetic			Anticholinergic	
			Alpha	*Beta$_1$*	*Beta$_2$*		
Albuterol[a]	Inhalation	Rx		+	+++		3–6
	Oral: tablets	Rx		+	+++		5–8
Atropine	Inhalation	Rx	—	—	—	+++	4
Bitolterol[a]	Inhalation	Rx		+	+++		4–6
Epinephrine[a]	Inhalation	OTC	+++	+++	+++		1–3
	Subcutaneous	Rx	+++	+++	+++		1–4
Ephedrine	Oral: syrup, capsules, tablets	OTC	+++	++	++		3–5
	Intramuscular, subcutaneous	Rx	+++	++	++		<1
Ipratropium	Inhalation	Rx	—	—	—	+++	4–6
Isoproterenol[a]	Inhalation	Rx		+++	+++		0.5–2
	Sublingual	Rx		+++	+++		1–2
Isoetharine[a]	Inhalation	Rx		++	+++		1–3
Metaproterenol[a]	Inhalation	Rx		+++	+++		2–4
	Oral: tablets, syrup	Rx		+++	+++		4
Pirbuterol[a]	Inhalation	Rx		+	+++		4–6
Salmeterol	Inhalation	Rx		+	+++	—	12
Terbutaline[a]	Inhalation	Rx		+	+++		3–6
	Oral: tablet	Rx		+	+++		4–8
	Subcutaneous	Rx		+	+++		1.5–4
Theophylline[b] (various salts) (sustained release)	Oral: liquid, tablets	Rx	+	++	++		8–24

+ indicates relative intensity of effect.

[a]Inhalation confers more bronchial activity than systemic administration.

[b]Although theophylline is not a sympathomimetic drug, it causes the release of endogenous catecholamines.

LAR inhibit the inflammatory response that is characteristic of asthma.[7,11] Table 1 lists the various prescription and nonprescription asthma medications according to which phase they prevent or reverse. Only those drugs that inhibit the LAR can reduce BHR. A comparison of the dosage forms, receptor activity, and duration of action of the nonprescription versus prescription bronchodilators is presented in Table 4.

Beta$_2$-agonists relieve spasms of bronchial smooth muscle caused by the EAR. When beta$_2$-receptors are stimulated by sympathomimetic amines, the enzyme adenylate cyclase is stimulated in turn and produces an increased intracellular concentration of cyclic adenosine monophosphate. In the airways, this results in smooth muscle relaxation, prejunctional inhibition of cholinergic neurotransmission, increased mucociliary clearance, reduced mucosal edema, and inhibition of mast cell mediator release.[7] The currently available short-acting beta$_2$-agonists have no significant anti-inflammatory effect and therefore have no significant effect on the LAR.

Beta-receptors found in other tissues explain the other effects seen with beta-agonist medications. Because 30–50% of cardiac beta-receptors are beta$_2$-receptors, beta$_2$-agonists can produce tachycardia by directly stimulating these receptors. Other effects of beta$_2$-receptor stimulation include peripheral vasodilation; skeletal muscle tremor; hypokalemia; uterine relaxation; increased release of glucose, lactate, pyruvate, insulin, and high-density lipoproteins from the liver and pancreas; and increased urinary excretion of magnesium, calcium, and phosphate.[23] Peripheral vasodilation from systemic beta$_2$-adrenergic stimulation decreases blood pressure and produces a compensatory increase in the heart rate to maintain cardiac output.

The nonprescription, and some prescription, beta-agonists also influence other adrenergic receptors (Table 4). The alpha-adrenergic stimulation produces bronchoconstriction, vasoconstriction, urinary retention, and mydriasis, which are not beneficial in asthma. Stimulating beta$_1$-receptors results in increased cardiovascular inotropic and chronotropic activity.

Long-term use of beta$_2$-agonists may produce minor degrees of tolerance or tachyphylaxis. Down regulation (decreased number) and a decreased affinity at the beta$_2$-receptor may develop.[24] A plateau response is reached within 2–8 weeks with no further deterioration; the duration of action is affected more than the intensity of effect.[24] However, the clinical consequence of beta$_2$-agonist tolerance appears minor in that beta$_2$-receptors in the airways are not as susceptible to tolerance as are other beta$_2$-receptors.[25] Moreover, corticosteroid therapy can prevent and reverse the tolerance.[24]

Asthma medications classified as mast cell stabilizers, anti-inflammatories, and bronchodilators other than epinephrine and ephedrine are available only by prescription. A brief review of their pharmacology follows. In-depth discussions of these medications are available in pharmacology and therapeutics textbooks. The pharmacology and role of antihistamines in asthma treatment are discussed in the section Ingredients in Nonprescription Products.

Cromolyn, a mast cell stabilizer, inhibits both the EAR and LAR.[11] This agent can be used to treat intermittent, seasonal, and chronic asthma or allergen-, sulfite-, aspirin-, and exercise-induced asthma. Further, its use may permit a reduction in the systemic steroid dose. Nedocromil, which is pharmacologically similar to cromolyn, is effective for chronic stable asthma and exercise-induced asthma; its use allows for a reduction in theophylline and beta$_2$-agonist doses.[11]

Theophylline, a methylxanthine, attenuates the bronchospasm component of the LAR but does not prevent the increase in BHR; therefore, it has no significant anti-inflammatory activity.[7,11] The FDA recently ruled that all nonprescription products containing theophylline be withdrawn (see the section Ingredients in Nonprescription Products). Anticholinergics such as atropine, glycopyrrolate, and ipratropium are also bronchodilators that have no anti-inflammatory properties. Although they are not used as primary therapy for asthma, anticholinergics may be useful in selected patients, including the elderly and patients with psychogenic asthma (eg, emotional stress can be an asthma trigger in some patients).[26]

Because asthma is predominantly an inflammatory disease, inhaled corticosteroids have become the mainstay of chronic asthma therapy.[3,4,5] These agents prevent the LAR but not the EAR. However, they have not been universally adopted as a first-line drug of choice in the pediatric patient because the long-term sequelae of corticosteroid use in children are unknown.

Ingredients in Nonprescription Products

Recent actions by the FDA and other recommendations under consideration will significantly affect the composition of nonprescription asthma products.[27] Based on lack of data concerning the efficacy of theophylline at doses available in nonprescription products, the agency has ruled that all nonprescription products containing theophylline be withdrawn. Because this agent exhibits significant intrapatient and interpatient variability in metabolism, individual dosage titration and monitoring of serum theophylline concentrations are essential. It is inconceivable how these precautionary measures could be accomplished in a patient using a nonprescription product. Theophylline has also been the subject of numerous legal challenges in personal injury cases.

With theophylline no longer available without a prescription, remaining nonprescription oral products will contain only ephedrine. However, there are increasing reports that ephedrine is being diverted to clandestine operations for use in the production of methamphetamine (see the section Ephedrine). Thus, increased record keeping is now required.[28] Finally, the worldwide phase out of chloroflurocarbon (CFC) use will affect current epinephrine-containing MDIs. Although MDIs have been granted a medical exemption allowing CFC use until the end of 1996, it is unclear whether the manufacturers of epinephrine-containing products will pursue approval of a product with an alternate propellant or an alternate delivery system. Therefore, all current nonprescription products for asthma could be unavailable within 2 years.

A hearing was held by an FDA advisory committee in November 1994 to determine if currently available prescription products might be appropriate for reclassification to nonprescription status. Cromolyn sodium and albuterol (in a dry powder formulation) were discussed.[29] Most of the testimony was not supportive of reclassifying these products. A definite possibility exists that no nonprescription products for asthma will be available in the future.

Because current asthma management emphasizes using anti-inflammatory medications as first-line therapy for moderate and severe chronic asthma and, perhaps, in mild asthma as well, the utility of currently available nonprescription therapies has been appropriately questioned. The only apparent clinically relevant effect of nonprescription asthma agents (epinephrine and ephedrine) is bronchodilation. Nonprescription bronchodilator therapy is essentially symptomatic treatment for asthma.

Epinephrine

The FDA has classified the following agents as Category I: epinephrine, epinephrine bitartrate, and epinephrine hydrochloride (racemic) in pressurized, metered-dose aerosol dosage forms and aqueous solutions equivalent to 1% epinephrine for use with hand-held rubber-bulb nebulizers (see product table "Asthma Inhalant Products").

Mechanism of Action Epinephrine has equipotent alpha, beta$_1$-, and beta$_2$-agonist effects, all of which are dose dependent. These effects are terminated as the drug is taken up by sympathetic nerve endings and surrounding tissues. Epinephrine is metabolized in the nerve endings by monoamine oxidase and in the tissues by catechol-*O*-methyltransferase (COMT). Epinephrine is ineffective when taken by mouth because nearly complete metabolism by COMT and sulfatase occurs in the gastrointestinal tract and the liver. The peak effect of epinephrine aerosol for inhalation occurs within 5–10 minutes after use; the duration of action is less than 30 minutes.

Indications For many years, subcutaneous epinephrine was the gold standard of treatment for acute bronchospasm. Its use has declined greatly because use of selective inhaled beta$_2$-agonists increased during the 1980s. Epinephrine can be used to treat periodic and acute severe bronchospasm. For periodic asthma, epinephrine is available as a nonprescription product administered by inhalation. Although the various epinephrine-containing products differ slightly in the dose delivered, no significant difference exists between prescription and nonprescription epinephrine inhalation products. Acute, severe asthma attacks can be treated by subcutaneous injection or by inhalation. However, inhalation of beta$_2$-agonists is currently considered the therapy of first choice for both indications.[3]

Contraindications Epinephrine products should not be used unless a physician has made a diagnosis of asthma, the patient has never been hospitalized for asthma, and no other medications are being taken for asthma unless directed by a physician.[30] Patients with preexisting disease or conditions such as heart disease (eg, coronary artery disease, heart failure, or cardiac rhythm disturbance), high blood pressure, thyroid disease, diabetes, or difficulty in urinating due to enlargement of the prostate should avoid self-treatment with these products except under the advice and supervision of a physician.[30] In addition, patients taking a prescription antihypertensive or antidepressant drug should consult their physician or pharmacist before using the epinephrine products.[30]

Dosage A single inhalation from epinephrine-containing inhalers contains the equivalent of 0.16–0.25 mg of epinephrine base.[30] For adults and children 4 years of age and older, the dosage recommendation adopted for metered-dose delivery systems is one inhalation followed by a second inhalation if symptoms have not been relieved after at least 1 minute;[30] usage should not then be repeated for at least 3 hours. When an aqueous solution at a concentration equivalent to 1% epinephrine base is used with a hand-held rubber-bulb nebulizer, the inhalation dosage for adults and children 4 years of age or older is one to three inhalations no more often than every 3 hours. For children under 4 years of age, no dosage recommendations exist and the physician should be consulted. The solution should not be used if it is brown or cloudy. An adult should supervise the use of these products by children to avoid underuse or overuse.

Adverse Effects Adverse effects related to epinephrine (eg, tachycardia, cardiac arrhythmia, hypertension, tremor, and anxiety) are almost always associated with the parenteral route of administration. These effects would not generally be expected by the inhalation route except in an overdose situation. Some patients may tend to overuse these products, particularly when relief of symptoms does not occur.

Precautions Epinephrine products require statements that warn against exceeding the recommended dosages unless directed by a physician. The following warnings must appear in boldface type on the package labeling:

> Do not continue to use this product, but seek medical assistance immediately if symptoms are not relieved within 20 minutes or become worse. Patients should be warned that excessive use of epinephrine-containing products may cause nervousness, rapid heart beat, and possibly adverse effects on the heart. Epinephrine may increase certain symptoms of Parkinson's disease such as tremor and rigidity.[31]

Many clinicians consider the nonselective adrenergic properties and short duration of action of epinephrine to be adequate reasons not to recommend these products. The short duration of action may increase the potential for abuse of epinephrine-containing products. Recent attention about nonprescription asthma inhalers has occurred as a result of a celebrity model's death.[32] The death was actually related to inadequate asthma therapy, highlighting the fact that nonprescription asthma products are not appropriate in most cases. These issues severely limit the utility of inhaled epinephrine products in asthma management.

Ephedrine

The status of ephedrine as a nonprescription asthma therapy has recently changed. In November of 1994, all sales of single-entity ephedrine products became subject to the record-keeping and reporting requirements of the 1988 Chemical Diversion and Trafficking Act. Purchase of an ephedrine product requires the buyer's signature and two forms of identification. Sales records should be kept for 4 years and are subject to inspection by the Drug Enforcement Administration (DEA). Ephedrine, which is available as a base, hydrochloride and sulfate salts, and racemic ephedrine hydrochloride (see product table "Asthma Oral Products"), has been used as a precursor compound in the production of methamphetamine and methcathinone (CAT). Like amphetamines, ephedrine produces the release of catecholamines in the CNS. Ephedrine, caffeine, and phenylpropanolamine are common ingredients in drugs manufactured to physically resemble amphetamine-containing dosage forms. The FDA is reviewing whether nonprescription ephedrine products should remain on the market.

Mechanism of Action Ephedrine has equivalent alpha-, beta$_1$-, and beta$_2$- activity. These effects are primarily produced indirectly through the release of norepinephrine from sympathetic nerve endings. The peak bronchodilation effect from orally administered ephedrine occurs in 1 hour and lasts about 5 hours. Tachyphylaxis or tolerance may develop with long-term use. Ephedrine is predominantly eliminated unchanged in urine. Although the average elimination half-life is 6 hours, the half-life is decreased by urinary acidification and increased by urinary alkalinization.

Indications Ephedrine is useful for treating only mild forms of seasonal or chronic asthma. Ephedrine is also FDA approved for enuresis, hypotension, nasal congestion, penile erection, rhinorrhea, and sinusitis. Ephedrine sulfate is available on a nonprescription basis for use as a single entity in a 25-mg capsule and a syrup.

Contraindications The FDA considers nonprescription ephedrine to be a safe and effective bronchodilator; however, the drug is not to be used unless a physician has made a diagnosis of asthma, the patient has never been hospitalized for asthma, and no other medications are being taken for asthma unless directed by a physician. Patients with heart disease, high blood pressure, thyroid disease, diabetes, or difficulty in urinating due to enlargement of the prostate should avoid self-treatment with these products except under the advice and supervision of a physician. In addition, patients taking a prescription antihypertensive or antidepressant drug should consult their physician or pharmacist before using the products.

Dosage The dosage recommendation for ephedrine in adults and children over 12 years of age is 12.5–25 mg every 4 hours, not to exceed 150 mg in 24 hours.[30] For children 6–12 years of age, the recommended dosage is one-half to one tablet every 3–5 hours, depending on the specific combination product; the American Medical Association suggests 3 mg/kg per day divided into four to six doses. The manufacturers suggest that a physician be consulted for use of ephedrine in children under 6 years of age. The maximum daily dosage recommended for adults is 150 mg per day.

Adverse Effects The principal adverse effects of ephedrine are CNS stimulation, sleeplessness, nausea, loss of appetite, tremors, tachycardia, and urinary retention. To prevent insomnia, ephedrine should be taken a few hours before bedtime. Reports indicate that chronic ephedrine overdosage may result in either severe cardiac toxicity or psychosis.[33,34]

Severe hypertension could develop in a patient who has been receiving ephedrine while taking a monoamine oxidase inhibitor (MAOI). The MAOI decreases the degradation and increases the storage of norepinephrine. Blood pressure may also be increased if ephedrine is taken with clonidine, procarbazine, furazolidine, and selegiline. Further, ephedrine may increase the effect of ergotamine on the heart and blood vessels[31] and decrease the blood pressure–lowering ability of guanethidine.

The effects of ephedrine may be minimized if it is taken with methyldopa or reserpine. In addition, tricyclic antidepressants may partially block the action of ephedrine.[31] Because of alkalinization of the urine, the concentrations of ephedrine may be increased with concomitant administration of acetazolamide, dichlorphenamide, or a large dose of sodium bicarbonate. The risk-benefit profile of ephedrine is poor and limits the clinical utility of ephedrine-containing products.

Precautions Labeling requirements for ephedrine-containing products include a warning statement against exceeding the recommended dosage unless directed by a physician. If symptoms are not relieved within 1 hour or become worse, the product should be discontinued and a physician consulted immediately.[30]

Antihistamines

The classic antihistamines competitively inhibit histamine at type I receptors (H_1) in vascular smooth muscle. However, most of the first-generation antihistamines also influence other receptors such as cholinergic, serotonin, and alpha-adrenergic receptors, producing adverse effects. The second-generation H_1-antagonist antihistamines (eg, terfenadine, astemizole, cetirizine, ketotifen, loratidine, and azelastine) partially prevent the EAR by blocking histamine release from the mast cell.[35] As a result, vascular permeability and prostaglandin generation are decreased, smooth muscle is relaxed, and activation of airway vagal afferent nerves is inhibited.[7]

The role of antihistamines in asthma management has also changed substantially in recent years. Historically, these agents were felt to be contraindicated in asthma patients because of the potential for excessive drying of mucous secretions secondary to anticholinergic side effects. With the introduction of less sedating antihistamines (terfenadine, astemizole, and loratidine), which may possess some mild direct antiasthma activity, this issue was revisited. The current prevailing opinion is that antihistamines are not contraindicated and may offer modest benefit for the patient with asthma and associated allergies (eg, allergic rhinitis). Although the labeling of most prescription and nonprescription antihistamine products still contain warnings about their use in patients with asthma, these products are generally considered safe. On the other hand, one report suggests that many pharmacists still advise asthma patients to avoid antihistamines.[36] In this survey, only 17% of pharmacists felt that antihistamines pose no problems for asthma patients.

Because histamine produces bronchospasm, inflammation, and edema, antihistamines have an adjunctive role in the treatment of asthma.[35] Perhaps the most important point is that good control of concurrent allergic rhinitis helps control asthma, whereas poorly controlled allergic rhinitis may worsen asthma. Some of the second-generation antihistamines, such as ketotifen, cetirizine, and azelastine, also have anti-inflammatory activity unrelated to their antihistamine activity.[35] These newer agents are lipophobic, do not cross the blood brain barrier, act more peripherally, and therefore produce less sedation than the first-generation antihistamines. Further information on available nonprescription antihistamines can be found in Chapter 8, "Cold, Cough, and Allergy Products."

Expectorants

Many asthma products contain expectorants, especially guaifenesin and potassium iodide. Guaifenesin, at proper doses, is considered to be a safe and effective expectorant. Other nonprescription expectorants, however, are probably no more effective than is adequate hydration of the patient and are therefore of questionable clinical value. A change in mucus production may be a sign of worsening asthma or infection and requires medical evaluation rather than self-assessment and self-treatment. Because of the concern for iodide toxicity, an FDA advisory panel has recommended that iodide-containing products (expectorants) be restricted to prescription status. The FDA also states that, unless ordered by a physician, guaifenesin should not be taken for a persistent or chronic cough that occurs with asthma or is accompanied by excessive sputum.[30] Further information on expectorants can be found in Chapter 8, "Cold, Cough, and Allergy Products."

Antitussives

Coughing is the major physiologic host defense mechanism for removing bronchial secretions and mucus plugs. Antitussives should generally not be used for asthma because a productive cough has a highly useful effect. The reflex cough induced by bronchospasm is often relieved by bronchodilators, not antitussives. However, nonprescription antitussives, such as codeine and dextromethorphan, are occasionally used in asthma products.

According to the FDA, codeine should not be taken by patients with a chronic pulmonary disease or shortness of breath unless directed by a physician.[30] Similarly, dextromethorphan should not be used without a physician's prescription if cough persists for longer than 1 week; tends to recur; or is accompanied by fever, rash, or persistent headache.[30] Further information on antitussives can be found in Chapter 8, "Cold, Cough, and Allergy Products."

TABLE 5 Correct inhaler technique

1. Remove dust cap.
2. Shake canister.
3. Position inhaler with mouthpiece at the bottom.
4. Tilt head back slightly.
5. Breathe out slowly.
6. Close lips on inhaler or hold inhaler 1 to 2 inches from open mouth.
7. Actuate while inhaling slowly and deeply.
8. Hold breath as long as possible, up to 10 seconds.
9. Breathe out slowly.
10. Wait 30 seconds to 1 minute before administering second inhalation.
11. If steroid inhaler is being used, rinse mouth after use.

Delivery Systems

Traditional Inhalers

As delivery systems for asthma medications, MDIs deliver approximately 10–15% of the dose to the lower airway. Thus, it is essential that proper technique be used. In a classic study, correct inhaler technique deposited only about 8.8% of medication into the lungs.[37] Incorrect inhaler technique, which can reduce drug delivery and efficacy, can result from incorrect or conflicting instruction, lack of instruction, and patient confusion and forgetfulness. Several reports suggest that knowledge about correct MDI technique among health professionals is lacking.[37–40] Education of patients and health care practitioners, as well as evaluation programs on proper inhaler technique and use of spacers, can improve therapeutic response.

Up to 89% of patients using inhalers do not perform all the drug administration steps correctly.[41] Results from two evaluations revealed that 50–79% of nonpulmonary physicians, 35–53% of medical residents, 71% of pharmacists, 43% of nurses, and 8% of respiratory technicians did not perform or identify at least four of the steps required for correct inhaler usage.[42,43] The number and nature of specific steps taught by various health care practitioners may also differ. Currently, both the closed- and open-mouth techniques are taught; however, manufacturers' package instructions are for the closed-mouth technique. Many health practitioners instruct patients on only the basic steps; others include specific complete instructions on every aspect of inhaler use. As a result of this inconsistency in education, patients may be confused on how to use inhalers.

Investigators have found that patients perform inhaler technique better when they receive written and verbal education.[44] Yet 87% of patients visiting a community pharmacy did not receive any verbal education on inhaler use.[42] In addition, a patient's inhaler technique may actually worsen over time. Therefore, repeated patient education and assessment of inhaler technique are strongly encouraged.

The steps for correct inhaler use with the open- and closed-mouth technique for MDIs are listed in Table 5. Shaking the canister distributes the drug particles evenly throughout the suspension. The open-mouth technique is advocated to decrease the amount of drug making contact with and adhering to the back of the throat; the risk with this technique, however, is that patients may miss their mouth when they spray. The slower the breath, the greater is the likelihood that the drug will reach the smaller airways. Holding the breath longer and exhaling slowly increases the amount of drug that is retained in the airways. Waiting between inhalations allows the bronchodilator to work and may increase delivery of the drug to the airways with subsequent inhalations. Because most beta$_2$-agonists begin to work within minutes after inhalation, reaching their peak effect within 5–15 minutes, beta$_2$-agonist inhalers may be used first (if as-needed use is advocated) to open the airways for other inhaled medications. When using multiple inhalers, a practical general rule is to use the fastest acting bronchodilator first, followed by the second bronchodilator (if applicable), followed by the nonbronchodilator medications.

The number of sprays remaining in the canister can roughly be determined by submerging the canister in water. When the canister is full, it will sink to the bottom of the water. When the canister is completely empty, it will float on its side on the water line. More recently, the practice of floating inhalers has been discouraged because the effect of water at the valve stem may be detrimental for some products (eg, cromolyn and nedocromil). An alternate means of determining the need for a refill is to calculate the number of days that the medication should last (when used on a regular schedule) or estimate the number of as-needed doses that an inhaler usually contains.

Nontraditional Inhalers, Spacers, and Other Devices

Because of the prevalence of suboptimal MDI technique by patients, the use of assist devices or alternative delivery systems may be considered. The most commonly used add-on spacer devices—Aerochamber, InspirEase, and Inhal-Aid—are available only by prescription. Breath-activated dry powder inhalers are being developed to decrease the usage of CFC propellants. The FDA pulmonary-allergy advisory committee heard testimony about switching Ventolin and Rotahaler to nonprescription status, but that appears unlikely to occur.

Spacers or extender devices used with MDIs can improve delivery of the drug to the airways.[45] The distance between the inhaler mouthpiece and the mouth allows the CFC to evaporate, resulting in smaller droplet sizes and greater lung deposition.[45] Use of a spacer lessens impaction of the drug on the oropharynx and thereby decreases the incidence of oral candidiasis that can occur with regular use of steroid.[41]

The Aerochamber and InspirEase spacers provide the patient with feedback on the appropriate rate of inhalation. If a whistle is heard on inhalation, it indicates that the patient inhaled too quickly. These devices also have inhalation valves to minimize drug loss from the device until the patient is ready to inhale, obviating the need for good hand-lung coordination. For best results, patients should be instructed to actuate the MDI once and inhale the drug immediately after actuating the aerosol into the device.

The inhalation technique for dry powder inhalers such as Rotahaler is significantly different from that for MDIs. After inserting the device in the mouth the patient should breathe in deeply and rapidly.

Specific Patient or Disease Considerations

Geriatric Patients

Elderly patients may have altered pharmacodynamic and pharmacokinetic responses to asthma medications. Some investigators have reported decreased beta-agonist activity in elderly patients as a result of decreased receptor number, decreased receptor affinity, or altered biochemical pathways.[46-48] Because most of the receptor studies have been in vitro or in vivo on cardiovascular and endocrine receptors, the effect of aging on beta-receptors in the lungs is largely unknown. For a given serum concentration, theophylline was found to provide a lesser degree of bronchodilation in elderly patients with asthma than in younger patients with asthma.[49] This was caused by differences in asthma severity or duration, concomitant bronchitis and emphysema, or aging. Many investigators have reported decreased theophylline elimination in elderly patients.[50] Because of the potential for lower clearances in such patients, lower doses of theophylline should be initiated and the therapy should be monitored by determining serum theophylline concentrations. Increased age is a risk factor for the development of life-threatening events (eg, seizures or cardiac arrhythmias) with theophylline overdosage. Because other prescription and nonprescription medications are used frequently, an elderly patient's medication profile should be closely scrutinized for potential drug interactions with theophylline.[51]

The percentage of elderly patients who are unable to perform correctly most of the steps required for proper inhaler use is greater than that of younger adult patients. Reasons for the elderly patients' inappropriate inhaler technique include arthritis, decreased muscle strength, dementia, inability to read or comprehend the instructions, and/or inadequate prior patient education on inhaler technique. One third of elderly patients may not have sufficient hand strength to actuate the inhaler.[52] Specialized inhaler instruction should be repeatedly given to the elderly patient. Spacers or nebulizers should be used with elderly patients who are unable to use inhalers correctly.

Pediatric Patients

Many children under the age of 5 years will not be able to use an MDI correctly; they may need nebulizers to administer their medication. Some studies suggest that children as young as 2 and 3 years of age can learn to use a spacer device.[53,54] An MDI attached to a spacer device is more convenient than a nebulizer and can be mastered by some preschool age asthma patients. Children over 8 years of age can generally use an inhaler without a spacer. The child's technique should be assessed often and the need for a spacer ascertained. Thirty percent of children who previously showed good administration technique were found to develop an incorrect technique over time.[55] Spacer devices with whistles may help a child learn the appropriate rate for breathing during an inhalation.

Concerns exist about the impact of theophylline on learning, attention, behavioral, and cognitive functions. Negative behavioral effects have not been found in all studies of theophylline's impact on these functions; in fact, improvement has been reported in some studies or in some children. Patients who appear to demonstrate a higher incidence of compromised cognitive function with theophylline may have had prior attention and achievement problems. The FDA has reviewed this issue and concluded that the evidence of theophylline-induced cognitive impairment is inconclusive.[56]

Pregnant/Lactating Patients

The use of asthma medications in a pregnant or lactating patient with asthma is based on the balance between adverse drug reactions and the sequelae of an

TABLE 6 Classification of fetal risk from asthma medications by FDA pregnancy categories[a]

Medication	Category	Medication	Category
Anti-Inflammatories		**Bronchodilators**	
Beclomethasone dipropionate	C	Albuterol	C
Cromolyn sodium	B	Atropine	C
Flunisolide	C	Bitolterol	C
Prednisone	B	Ephedrine	C
Triamcinolone	D	Epinephrine	C
		Glycopyrrolate	B
Antihistamines		Ipratropium	B
Astemizole	C	Isoproterenol	C
Brompheniramine	C	Metaproterenol	C
Chlorpheniramine	B	Nedocromil	B
Diphenhydramine	C	Pirbuterol	C
Hydroxyzine	C	Salmeterol	C
Pyrilamine maleate	C	Terbutaline	B
Terfenadine	C	Theophylline	C
Tripelennamine	B	**Decongestants**	
Triprolidine	C	Phenylephrine	C
		Phenylpropanolamine	C
		Pseudoephedrine	C
		Miscellaneous	
		Guaifenesin	C
		Iodinated glycerol	X
		Phenobarbital	D

Key to pregnancy categories:

A: Adequate studies in pregnant women have not demonstrated a risk to the fetus in the first trimester of pregnancy, and there is no evidence of risk in later trimesters.

B: Animal studies have not demonstrated a risk to the fetus, but there are no adequate studies in pregnant women. . . or. . .Animal studies have shown an adverse effect, but adequate studies in pregnant women have not demonstrated a risk to the fetus during the first trimester of pregnancy, and there is no evidence of risk in later trimesters.

C: Animal studies have shown an adverse effect on the fetus, but there are no adequate studies in humans; the benefits from the use of the drug in pregnant women may be acceptable despite its potential risks. . .or. . .There are no animal reproduction studies and no adequate studies in humans.

D: There is evidence of human fetal risk, but the potential benefits from the use of the drug in pregnant women may be acceptable despite its potential risks.

X: Studies in animals or humans demonstrate fetal abnormalities, or adverse reaction reports indicate evidence of fetal risk. The risk of use in a pregnant woman clearly outweighs any possible benefit.

[a]Regardless of the designated pregnancy category or presumed safety, no drug should be administered during pregnancy unless it is clearly needed and potential benefits outweigh potential risks.

asthma attack on the developing fetus or nursing infant. Theophylline can cause tachycardia, jitteriness, irritability, gagging, vomiting, and breathing disorders in newborns.

Information on drug safety during pregnancy has been compiled by the Collaborative Perinatal Project Study, case reports, and manufacturers' information. Information for newer medications has been obtained from the package insert. The classification of fetal risk from asthma medications can be found in Table 6.

Certain asthma medications can be delivered to a nursing infant via mother's milk. The American Academy of Pediatrics Committee on Drugs lists the following medications as potentially problematic: atropine, dexbrompheniramine maleate with *d*-isoephedrine, iodinated glycerol, pseudoephedrine, prednisone, prednisolone, terbutaline, theophylline, and triprolidine.[57] Examples of drug-related toxicities experienced by breast-fed infants include insomnia (theophylline); altered thyroid function (iodinated glycerol); and irritability, crying, and poor sleep patterns (dexbrompheniramine with isoephedrine).[57]

Exercise-Induced Asthma

Exercise-induced asthma may be treated by modifying the exercise regimen or using inhaled beta$_2$-agonists or cromolyn sodium.[58] Patients with exercise-induced asthma may minimize the adverse impact of exercise by choosing exercises that are conducted in warm, humid areas (eg, swimming); extending their warm-up period; increasing their fitness level; refraining from food ingestion 2 hours before exercise; or wearing a face mask.[58] Theophylline's efficacy in preventing exercise-induced asthma depends on its concentration; however, its efficacy is significantly less than that of inhaled beta$_2$-agonists.[3,7,12] Short-acting beta$_2$-agonist therapy should generally be administered approximately 15 minutes before the onset of exercise. Ephedrine, epinephrine, barbiturates, isoetharine, isoproterenol, metaproterenol, oral albuterol, oral terbutaline, prednisone, theophylline-ephedrine-phenobarbital combination, and ephedrine-phenobarbital combination are banned by the US Olympic Committee. The committee allows inhalation therapy with albuterol, bitoterol, pirbuterol, procaterol, terbutaline, cromolyn, ipratropium, and corticosteroids; it also allows oral therapy with theophylline, guaifenesin, and pyrilamine maleate.[31] Even though a drug is prescribed by a physician, it may not be approved by the US Olympic Committee. The patient or health care providers may consult with the committee to determine the current status of accepted drug use in amateur competitive athletic competition (800–233–0393). The rules of the National Collegiate Association of America (NCAA) and other national and international sports rules are generally consistent with guidelines established by the US Olympic Committee.

Nocturnal Asthma

In some patients, additional pharmacologic therapy may be required to provide treatment throughout the sleeping period. Long-acting inhaled beta-agonists (eg, salmeterol), sustained-release beta-agonists and sustained-release theophylline can be used to provide full coverage during the sleeping period.[12] Nocturnal symptoms of asthma may be a manifestation of airway inflammation. Because increased eosinophils and histamine levels have been measured during nocturnal asthma, most patients' nocturnal asthma will improve by increasing their daytime anti-inflammatory therapy with cromolyn or inhaled steroids.[12]

Product Selection Guidelines

Asthma represents an excellent opportunity for the pharmacist to provide pharmaceutical care for the asthma patient. The value of pharmacists' involvement in providing such service has been documented.[59,60] Identifying undiagnosed asthma, making appropriate referrals, and monitoring medication use are important components of managing the asthma patient.

Once the assessment of asthma has been confirmed, the pharmacist should ask the patient a series of questions to gather the necessary information for product choice and to determine whether the patient needs medical attention. The pharmacist may consider using a nonprescription asthma drug if the patient has never been to an emergency room or been hospitalized for asthma treatment, is not currently receiving prescription asthma medications, and does not have any of the following conditions:

- Hypertension;
- Diabetes;
- Uncontrolled thyroid disease;
- Heart disease;
- Difficulty in urinating due to an enlarged prostate.

This consideration would only be appropriate if the patient has symptoms no more than once a week and very infrequent nocturnal symptoms. The patient's pharmacy profile and use of other nonprescription medications must then be reviewed for (1) drugs that interact with any of the products available in the nonprescription drugs and (2) any allergies or hypersensitivities to the nonprescription products, including aspirin or other NSAIDs. Specific patient factors such as age, pregnancy, lactation, and finances also need to be considered. The patient's compliance with other medications may also be determined from the pharmacy profile.

Using nonprescription drugs to treat bronchospasm from asthma presents a dilemma because nonprescription bronchodilators are usually effective in only mild disease; however, mild disease can progress to more moderate to severe disease if it is not appropriately treated with anti-inflammatories. In addition, nonprescription bronchodilators may potentially mask a worsening of asthma by treating only overt symptoms. To tread this fine line can be dangerous, and the patient and the patient's family should know when to abandon self-treatment and immediately seek medical care. In most cases of death from asthma, the severity of the obstruction had been underestimated by the physician or patient. Thus, patients should be encouraged to rely more heavily on peak flow measurements in making treatment decisions.

Epinephrine and ephedrine are nonselective with short durations of activity. Ephedrine is less potent and potentially more toxic, particularly in hypertensive patients, than the newer, orally active, selective beta$_2$-agonists. The combination products prevent individualization of drug therapy; their ingredients may also produce additive adverse effects. In some patients with bronchospasm and rhinorrhea, decongestant effects may be desirable; however, these patients may be treated more effectively with an alpha-adrenergic nasal spray for the short term and with intranasal cromolyn or corticosteroids for chronic allergic rhinitis.

Patient Counseling

When counseling asthma patients, the pharmacist should provide general information about the use and storage of medications, instructions on the use and care of inhalers (if appropriate), and pertinent pharmacologic information about a patient's particular medication.

Patients should be told the following about the use and storage of medications:[31]

- Because asthma medication can produce significant toxicity with an overdose, do not exceed dosages stated on the labeling.
- Store asthma medications away from a child's access; do not store medications in damp or hot places or in direct sunlight.
- Discard outdated medications away from a child's access.
- Contact a health care practitioner if you experience decreased responsiveness to a drug; this may indicate a worsening of the asthma.

To educate patients adequately on inhaler use, pharmacists should provide demonstrations of correct technique along with both written and verbal instructions.[44] Patients should then demonstrate their inhaler technique to the pharmacist. Resources such as videotaped demonstrations are available from several pharmaceutical manufacturers.

If a patient's technique is not adequate after repeated inhaler instruction, the pharmacist should suggest the use of a spacer. If epinephrine aerosols are being used, the patient should be advised to wait at least 1 minute between inhalations. Patients should also be told that rinsing the mouth after using an inhaler (with or without a spacer) may prevent dryness of the mouth and throat as well as oral candidal infections.

Care and disposal of the canister are also important. Because of several reports of patients aspirating small objects, including coins, lodged in the mouthpiece,[61] the dust cap should be kept over the mouth piece of the inhaler. The following tips should also be discussed with the patient:

- Wash the inhaler mouthpiece daily with warm water to prevent clogging; keep the mouthpiece free of particles.
- Routinely clean and air dry inhaler devices.
- Do not puncture the unit; the contents are under pressure.
- Do not store the canister near heat (≥120°F [≥48.9°C]) or open flames.
- Do not discard canisters into fires or incinerators.
- Be aware that canisters left in freezing temperatures will release large aerosol particles after actuation. Allow the canister to come to room temperature (59–86°F [15–30°C]) before use.

An important element in educating patients about their asthma therapy is telling them which precautions to take with their medications, what side effects might occur, and what foods, beverages, and medications might contain sulfites. For example, precaution should be taken with the use of antihistamines, which may be associated with increased CNS side effects if taken with other CNS medications (eg, phenobarbital, pain medications, and alcohol).[31]

From 4–28% of patients with asthma will have bronchospasm induced by aspirin.[62] A cross-sensitivity may exist with other NSAIDs (eg, ibuprofen, ketoprofen, and naproxen). Patients should be cautioned that some nonprescription allergy, cough/cold, and analgesic preparations contain aspirin. Aspirin-sensitive patients can usually take acetaminophen as an analgesic.[62] Some patients may be aspirin sensitive and not aware of the problem because of infrequent aspirin use.

Asthma patients also need to be educated about the potential of sulfites and sulfur dioxide to elicit bronchospasm. Sulfites are used as preservatives in the pharmaceutical, food, and fermentation industries. Foods and beverages that may contain these preservatives include dried and packaged fruits and beverages; beer, wines, and other fermented beverages; salads and salad bar ingredients; guacamole and other dips; potatoes (chips or fries); cider and wine vinegars; pickled vegetables; shrimp and other seafood; and processed, preserved, and "ready to eat" foods and beverages.[63] Certain medications also contain sulfites; however, by FDA regulations, such medications must list sulfites as an ingredient in the package insert.

Finally, patients should be advised to seek immediate medical intervention if they experience any of the following:

- Inability to complete a full sentence without stopping;
- Persistent discomfort after using a bronchodilator even while at rest;
- Incomplete relief of symptoms after using a bronchodilator;
- Worsening of dyspnea after using a bronchodilator.

Various pharmaceutical companies, agencies, and foundations offer patient education materials and services. A complete list of educational material can be obtained from the National Asthma Education and Prevention Program.

Case Studies

Case 9-1

Patient Complaint/History

The mother of a 7-year-old boy named JM purchases Pedia Care Cough-Cold Formula in a liquid dosage form and then asks to speak to a pharmacist. She explains her concerns about JM's frequent "summer colds," which are characterized by wheezing, chest congestion, and a dry cough. She notes that her son often has to stop to "catch his breath" during physical activities, especially during soccer practice.

During further discussion, the pharmacist determines that JM is in good general health and that his current medications include only a children's chewable vitamin taken once daily. Further, the mother has seasonal allergies and the father is a heavy cigarette smoker.

Clinical Considerations/Strategies

The following considerations/strategies are provided to aid the reader in (1) determining whether treatment of the patient's condition with nonprescription medications is warranted, (2) selecting the appropriate nonprescription medication, and (3) developing a patient counseling strategy to ensure optimal therapeutic outcomes:

- Further assess the nature of the summer colds and any correlation between the symptoms and potential causal factors.
- Determine whether the patient has any allergies to drugs, foods, or other substances.
- Determine whether the patient's difficulty in breathing follows any predictable pattern or frequency of occurrence.
- Determine whether the difficulty in breathing has ever required a visit to a physician or hospital emergency room.
- Identify which nonprescription medication, if any, might be appropriate for providing some symptomatic relief.
- Suggest a response to the mother's choice of nonprescription medication, taking into consideration the indications for the decongestant, antihistamine, and antitussive contained in the selected medication.
- Identify any warnings, precautions, or adverse effects associated with the use of the selected medication.
- Consider the appropriateness of a medical referral.
- Develop a patient education/counseling strategy that will:
  - Ensure that the mother knows when to contact a physician about the symptoms;
  - Address the issue of the father's cigarette smoking as a confounding factor;
  - Determine the proper role of adjunctive nonprescription drug therapy;
  - Explain the proper selection and use of nonprescription drug therapy.

Case 9-2

Patient Complaint/History

PR, a 35-year-old male who has asthma, selects two Primatene Mist inhalers from the shelf and proceeds to the checkout counter. While checking out, he casually mentions to the pharmacist that his current asthma medication "doesn't work very well" and that using the Primatene Mist along with his prescription asthma medication provides the greatest relief.

PR, who was diagnosed with asthma at 10 years of age, has no other significant medical history. His patient profile lists the following current medications: Proventil (albuterol) inhaler one to two puffs q6h prn and Azmacort (triamcinolone) inhaler two puffs qid. The profile also shows that the patient has been using at least two Proventil inhalers per month for the last 5 months and that he has not had the prescription for Azmacort filled in the last 3 months. When asked to check his PEFR, the patient reports that it is 65% of his baseline value.

Clinical Considerations/Strategies

The following considerations/strategies are provided to aid the reader in (1) determining whether treatment of the patient's condition with nonprescription medications is warranted, (2) selecting the appropriate nonprescription medication, and (3) developing a patient counseling strategy to ensure optimal therapeutic outcomes:

- Assess the patient's symptoms and the status of his asthma control.
- Assess the patient's compliance with the regimen of prescribed asthma medications.
- Consider referring the patient to his local primary care physician.
- Advise the patient whether it is appropriate to use a nonprescription inhaler under the current circumstances.
- Develop a patient education/counseling strategy that will:
  - Counsel the patient on how to identify factors that precipitate asthma attacks;
  - Reinforce the proper technique in administering inhalers;
  - Ensure that the patient understands his disease and what constitutes appropriate therapy;
  - Explain the importance of strict compliance with the prescribed regimen;
  - Explain the limitations of nonprescription inhalers in treating asthma;
  - Determine the proper role, if any, of adjunctive therapy with nonprescription asthma medications;
  - Ensure that the patient knows when to contact a physician about his asthma management program.

Summary

Asthma is a chronic inflammatory disease that requires continuous care. Hyperactivity of the airways to various physical, chemical, or pharmacologic stimuli is the hallmark of asthma. Therapy is directed at preventing severe attacks and normalizing an asthma patient's lifestyle. Treatment involves drug and nondrug measures. Pharmaceutical care for asthma patients involves a multifaceted approach of education, counseling, instruction, monitoring, and encouragement. Nonprescription medications currently available for managing asthma are only suited for managing mild, infrequent symptoms. Patients whose asthma is not responding to nonprescription products should consult their physician. It may be prudent to encourage all patients with asthma to have a thorough evaluation of their condition before attempting self management with nonprescription products.

References

1. Asthma—United States, 1982-1992. *MMWR.* 1995; 43(51,52): 952–955.
2. Weiss KB, Gergen PJ, Hodgson TA. An economic evaluation of asthma in the United States. *N Engl J Med.* 1992 Mar 26; 326: 862–66.
3. National Heart, Lung, and Blood Institute, National Asthma Education Program, Expert Panel Report. *Guidelines for the Diagnosis and Management of Asthma.* Pub No 91–3042. Bethesda, Md: US Department of Health and Human Services; 1991.
4. National Heart, Lung, and Blood Institute. *International Consensus Report on Diagnosis and Treatment of Asthma.* Pub No 92–3091. Bethesda, Md: US Department of Health and Human Services; 1992.
5. National Heart, Lung, and Blood Institute. *Global Initiative for Asthma.* Pub No 95–3659. Bethesda, Md: US Department of Health and Human Services; 1995.

6. West JB. *Respiratory Physiology—the Essentials*. 3rd ed. Baltimore: Williams & Wilkins; 1985.
7. Kaliner MA, Barnes PJ, Persson CGA. *Asthma: Its Pathology and Treatment*. New York: Marcel Dekker; 1991.
8. Sears MR et al. Regular inhaled beta-agonist treatment in bronchial asthma. *Lancet*. 1990 Dec 8; 336: 1391–6.
9. Coultas DB, Samet JM. Epidemiology and natural history of childhood asthma. In: Tinkelman DG, Falliers CJ, Naspitz CK, eds. *Childhood Asthma: Pathophysiology and Treatment*. New York: Marcel Dekker; 1987: 131–57.
10. Burrows B et al. Characteristics of asthma among elderly adults in a sample of the general population. *Chest*. 1991; 100: 935–42.
11. Barnes PJ. A new approach to the treatment of asthma. *N Engl J Med*. 1989 Nov 30; 321: 1517–27.
12. Djukanovic R et al. Mucosal inflammation in asthma. *Am Rev Respir Dis*. 1990; 142: 434–57.
13. Hargreave FE, Gibson PG, Ramsdale EH. Airway hyperresponsiveness, airway inflammation, and asthma. *Immunol Allergy Clin North Am*. 1990 Aug; 10: 439–48.
14. Kelly HW, Hill MR. Asthma. In: DiPiro JT et al, eds. *Pharmacotherapy: A Pathophysiological Approach*. 2nd ed. New York: Elsevier; 1992: 408–49.
15. Gibson P et al. Association between availability of non-prescription ß^2 agonist inhalers and undertreatment of asthma. *BMJ*. 1993; 306: 1514–18.
16. Report of the FDA advisory review panel on OTC cold, cough, allergy, bronchodilator, and antiasthma drug products. *Federal Register*. 1976; 41: 38312.
17. National Heart, Lung, and Blood Institute, National Asthma Education and Prevention Program.National Heart, Lung, and Blood Institute, National Asthma Education and Prevention Program. *The Role of the Pharmacist in Improving Asthma Care*. NIH Pub No 95–3280. Bethesda, Md: US Department of Health and Human Services; 1995.
18. National Heart, Lung, and Blood Institute, National Asthma Education and Prevention Program. The role of the pharmacist in improving asthma care. *Am J Health-Sys Pharm*. 1995; 52: 1411–16.
19. Immunization Practices Advisory Committee. Update on adult immunizations. *MMWR*. 1991; 40(RR-12): 42–4.
20. Immunization Practices Advisory Committee. Prevention and control of influenza recommendations. *MMWR*. 1991; 40(RR-6): 1–14.
21. Van Schayck CP et al. Bronchodilator treatment in moderate asthma or chronic bronchitis: continuous or on demand? A randomized controlled trial. *Br Med J*. 1991 Dec 7; 303: 1426–7.
22. Jackson AC. Accuracy, reproducibility, and variability of portable peak flowmeters. *Chest*. 1995; 107:648–51.
23. Lipworth BJ. Risks versus benefits of inhaled ß^2-agonists in the management of asthma. *Drug Safety*. 1992; 7: 54-70.
24. Kelly HW. New ß^2-adrenergic agonist aerosols. *Clin Pharm*. 1985; 4: 393–403.
25. Lipworth BJ, Struthers AD, McDevitt DG. Tachyphylaxis to systemic but not to airway response during prolonged therapy with high dose inhaled salbutamol in patients with asthma. *Am Rev Respir Dis*. 1989; 140: 586–92.
26. Neild LE, Cameron IR. Bronchoconstriction in response to suggestion: its prevention by inhaled anticholinergic agent. *Br Med J*. 1985; 290: 674.
27. Cold, cough, allergy, bronchodilator, and antiasthmatic drug products for over-the-counter human use; combination bronchodilator drug products containing theophylline; final rule. *Federal Register*. 1995 Jul; 60(144): 38636–42.
28. New reporting requirements for ephedrine take effect. *Am J Health-Syst Pharm*. 1995; 52: 10.
29. *FDC Reports*. 1994; 2(28): 3–4.
30. Cold, cough, allergy, bronchodilator, and antiasthma drug products for over-the-counter human use. *Federal Register*. 1991 Apr 1; 190-7.
31. *USP DI 1995 Advice for the Patient. Vol II*. Rockville, Md: US Pharmacopeial Convention; 1995.
32. Gorman C. Asthma! the hidden killer. *Time*. 1995; 146(6): 56.
33. Van Mieghem W, Stevens E, Cosemans J. Ephedrine-induced cardiopathy. *Br Med J*. 1978; 1: 816.
34. Roxanas MG, Spalding J. Ephedrine abuse psychosis. *Med J Aust*. 1977; 2: 639–40.
35. Holgate ST, Finnerty JP. Antihistamines in asthma. *J Allergy Clin Immunol*. 1989; 83: 537–47.
36. Lantner R, Tobin MC. Pharmacist advice to asthmatics regarding antihistamine use. *Ann Aller*. 1991;66: 411.13.
37. Newman SP et al. Deposition of pressurized aerosols in the human respiratory tract. *Thorax*. 1981; 36: 52–5.
38. Kelly HW. Correct aerosol medication use and the health professions: Who will teach the teachers? *Chest*. 1993; 104(6): 1648–9.
39. Kesten S, Zive K, Chapman KR. Pharmacist knowledge and ability to use inhaled medication delivery systems. *Chest*. 1993; 104: 1737–42.
40. Interiano B, Guntupalli KK. Metered dose inhalers: Do health providers know what to teach? *Arch Intern Med*. 1993; 153: 81–5.
41. Toogood JH et al. Use of spacers to facilitate inhaled corticosteroid treatment of asthma. *Am Rev Respir Dis*. 1984; 129: 723–9.
42. Mickle TR et al. Evaluation of pharmacists' practice in patient education when dispensing a metered-dose inhaler. *DICP Ann Pharmacother*. 1990; 24: 927–30.
43. Guidry GG, Brown WD, Stogner SW, et al. Incorrect use of metered-dose inhalers by medical personnel. *Chest*. 1992; 101: 31–3.
44. Self TH et al. The value of demonstration and role of the pharmacist in teaching the correct use of pressurized bronchodilators. *Can Med Assoc J*. 1983; 128: 129–31.
45. Konig P. Spacer devices used with metered-dose inhalers: breakthrough or gimmick? *Chest*. 1985; 88: 276–84.
46. Schocken DD, Roth GS. Reduced beta-adrenergic receptor concentrations in aging man. *Nature*. 1977; 267: 856–8.
47. Stressman J et al. Deterioration of beta-receptor-denylate cyclase function in elderly, hospitalized patients. *J Gerontol*. 1984; 39: 667–72.
48. Vestal RE, Wood AJJ, Shand DG. Reduced ß-adrenoceptor sensitivity in the elderly. *Clin Pharmacol Ther*. 1979; 26: 181–6.
49. Chandler MHH, Clifton GD, Burki NK, et al. Pulmonary function in the elderly: response to theophylline bronchodilation. *J Clin Pharmacol*. 1990; 30: 330–5.
50. Edwards DJ, Zarowitz BJ, Slaughter RL. Theophylline. In: Evans WE, Schentag JJ, Jusko WJ, eds. *Applied Pharmacokinetics*. 3rd ed. Vancouver, Wash: Applied Therapeutics. 1992; 13–1 to 13-38.
51. Sims JA, doPico GA, Reed CE. Bronchodilating effect of oral theophylline-ephedrine combination. *J Allergy Clin Immunol*. 1978; 62: 15–21.
52. Armitage JM, Williams SJ. Inhaler technique in the elderly. *Age Ageing*. 1988; 17: 275-8.
53. Croft RD. 2 year old asthmatics can learn to operate a tube spacer by copying their mothers. *Arch Dis Childhood*. 1989; 64: 742.
54. Sly RM et al. Delivery of albuterol aerosol by aerochamber to young children. *Ann Allergy*. 1988; 60(5): 403.
55. Lee H, Evans HE. Evaluation of inhalation aids of metered-dose inhalers in asthmatic children. *Chest*. 1987; 91: 366–9.
56. Nicklas RA. Theophylline, school performance, and Food and Drug Administration [letter]. *Pediatrics*. 1989; 83: 146–7.

57. American Academy of Pediatrics Committee on Drugs. Transfer of drugs and other chemicals into human milk. *Pediatrics.* 1989; 84: 924–36.

58. Pierson WE. Exercise-induced bronchospasm in children and adolescents. *Pediatr Clin North Am.* 1988; 25: 1031–40.

59. Im J. Evaluation of the effectiveness of an asthma clinic managed by an ambulatory care pharmacist. *Calif J Hosp Pharm.* 1993; 5: 5–6.

60. Pauley TR. Magee MJ, Gury JD. Pharmacist-managed, physician directed, asthma management program reduces emergency department visits. *Ann Pharmacother.* 1995; 29: 5–9.

61. Hannan SE et al. Foreign body aspiration associated with the use of an aerosol inhaler. *Am Rev Respir Dis.* 1984; 129: 1025–27.

62. Slepian IK, Mathews KP, McLean JA. Aspirin-sensitive asthma. *Chest.* 1985; 87: 386–91.

63. Mathison DA, Stevenson DD, Simon RA. Precipitating factors in asthma: aspirin, sulfites, and other drugs and chemicals. *Chest.* 1985; 87: 50S–4S.

CHAPTER 10

Sleep Aid and Stimulant Products

M. Lynn Crismon and Donna M. Jermain

Questions to ask in patient assessment and counseling

Sleep Aid Products

- *How long have you had trouble sleeping?*
- *How severe is your sleep disturbance?*
- *Do you generally have trouble falling asleep? Do you wake up frequently or too early?*
- *Do you feel rested when you awake in the morning?*
- *Do you have trouble functioning or staying alert during the day?*
- *How often do you take naps?*
- *What do you think is causing your sleep problem?*
- *Has there been increased stress in your life lately?*
- *Do you have any health problems or physical complaints?*
- *What prescription and nonprescription medications do you take?*
- *How often and at what times during the day do you drink coffee or other caffeinated beverages? Alcoholic beverages?*
- *Do you smoke?*
- *Have you ever been treated for psychiatric problems?*
- *Would you describe yourself as a nervous or anxious person?*
- *Have you felt depressed or disinterested in your usual activities?*
- *Have you ever been told you snore loudly or are a restless sleeper?*
- *What methods or medications have you used to treat insomnia thus far? How long did you use them? Were they effective?*

Stimulant Products

- *Why do you want to use this product?*
- *How long do you intend to use this product?*
- *Have you ever used a stimulant product before? Did you experience any adverse effects?*
- *Do you regularly consume coffee, tea, cola, or other caffeinated beverages? Have you experienced adverse effects from drinking them?*
- *What other medications, prescription and nonprescription, do you take?*
- *Are you under a physician's care? What types of medical problems do you have?*
- *Do you have anxiety, irritability, or any other nervous condition?*
- *Do you have problems sleeping? (If patient has problems sleeping, see sleep aid questions.)*
- *Are you pregnant or breast-feeding?*
- *Do you smoke cigarettes or chew tobacco?*
- *Do you drink alcohol? If so, how much and how often?*

Sleep Aids

Insomnia is one of the most common patient complaints, ranking third behind headache and the common cold. Annually, approximately one third of all Americans report at least occasional difficulty sleeping, and about 10–20% of the US population experiences insomnia to an extent that can be classified as "always or severe." More than 2.5% of adult Americans use a prescription sleep aid medication, and more than 3% buy a nonprescription sleep product.[1–3] The prevalence of sleep complaints is increased among the elderly, and it is estimated that approximately 35% of all sleep aid prescriptions are written for older people.[1] Despite these figures, it is estimated that only a small percentage of patients with a sleep disorder actually verbalize their complaints to a physician.[4] This, combined with frequent misuse of sleep aids and the availability of nonprescription agents, makes insomnia a disorder of significant concern for the pharmacist.

Insomnia is not a disease. It is a symptom or patient complaint for which there are no precise criteria or definitions. Patients may complain of difficulty falling asleep (sleep latency insomnia), frequent nocturnal awakening, early morning awakening, or poor quality of sleep. There is no ideal duration of sleep, and patients complaining of a sleep disturbance may actually sleep for the same length of time as other individuals who feel they sleep well. However, these patients usually report that it takes them more than 30 minutes to fall asleep, and their sleep duration is less than 6–7 hours nightly.[1] Moreover, their perceived sleep pattern and quality of daytime functioning may be more important than their duration of sleep. Thus, patients with insomnia are those who feel they sleep poorly at night and function poorly during the day.

Sleep Physiology

Physiologically, sleep can be categorized into different stages by using the sleeping electroencephalogram (EEG) in conjunction with electro-oculography and electromyography. Stage 1 sleep is a transitional stage, which occurs as the patient falls asleep; the EEG resembles the waking state more than sleep. Stage 2 sleep, in which approximately 50% of sleep time is spent, is light sleep. Stages 3 and 4, collectively known as deep sleep or delta sleep, are characterized by the patterns of delta (slow frequency) waves on the EEG. Rapid eye movement (REM) sleep is neither light nor deep. It is characterized by the body being more physiologically active than during other sleep stages while skeletal muscles are actively inhibited. The EEG shows an increase in high frequency waves; the eyes move rapidly from side to side; and the blood pressure, heart rate, temperature, respirations, and metabolism are increased.[2,5]

Upon falling asleep, one progresses through the four stages of sleep and reaches the first REM period in about 70–90 minutes. This time, from falling asleep to the first REM period, is referred to as the REM latency. The first REM period is of short duration, usually 5–7 minutes. The sleep cycle then repeats about every 90 minutes, with each progressive REM period becoming longer and the time in deep sleep becoming shorter.[2,5] Although the effects of medication on the sleep stages are thought to be important, their relative importance on the different stages of sleep is unclear. However, prolonged suppression of REM sleep may result in psychologic and behavioral changes.

Sleep physiology changes with increasing age. Among elderly persons, less time is spent in stage 4 and REM sleep, the total duration of sleep becomes shorter, sleep becomes more shallow and disrupted, the number of nocturnal awakenings increases, and sleep latency usually remains normal.

Sleep Disorders

Although insomnia is the most common cause of difficulty in sleeping, patients with other sleep disorders may also seek a nonprescription sleep aid from the pharmacist. Among these disorders are sleep apnea, narcolepsy, nocturnal myoclonus, and restless legs syndrome.

Insomnia

Based on the duration of the sleep disturbance, insomnia can be classified as transient, short term, or chronic.[2,6] It is extremely important that the pharmacist ask the patient questions to determine the etiology and duration of the insomnia. Although nonprescription sleep products have not been extensively evaluated, it is assumed they work best in transient and short-term insomnia.

Transient insomnia is usually situational and is commonly caused by environmental changes or life stresses

TABLE 1 Drugs that may exacerbate insomnia

Drugs that may cause insomnia	Drugs that may produce withdrawal insomnia
Alcohol	**Alcohol**
Antidepressants Buproprion Monoamine oxidase Serotonin-specific reuptake inhibitors Tricyclic antidepressants Venlafaxine	**Antihistamines**
Antihypertensives Beta blockers (especially propanolol) Clonidine Diuretics (at bedtime) Methyldopa Reserpine	**Barbiturates**
Hypnotic use (chronic)	**Benzodiazepines**
Nicotine	**Hypnotics (miscellaneous)** Bromides Chloral hydrate Ethchlorvynol Glutethimide
Sympathomimetic amines Amphetamines Appetite suppressants Beta-adrenergic agonists Caffeine Decongestants (eg, phenylpropanolamine, phenylephrine)	**Monoamine oxidase inhibitors**
Miscellaneous Anabolic steroids Antineoplastics Corticosteroids Histamine$_2$-receptor antagonists Levodopa Methysergide Oral contraceptives Phenytoin Quinidine Theophylline Thyroid preparations	**Tricyclic antidepressants**
	Miscellaneous Amphetamines Cocaine Marijuana Opiates Phencyclidine

TABLE 2 Etiology of chronic (long-term) insomnia

Medical problems	Psychiatric problems (30–70% of cases)
Pain	Anxiety disorder
Angina pectoris	Bipolar disorder
Arthritis	Dementia
Cancer	Depression
Chronic pain syndromes	Posttraumatic stress disorder
Cluster headaches	Schizophrenia
Migraine	Substance abuse
Peptic ulcer/gastro-intestinal reflux	**Sleep disorders**
Postoperative pain	Sleep apnea
Respiratory difficulty	Nocturnal myoclonus
Asthma	Delayed sleep phase syndrome (night-shift workers)
Bronchitis	Drug-related insomnia
Chronic obstructive pulmonary disease	Psychophysiologic insomnia (idiopathic insomnia)
Congestive heart failure	Restless legs syndrome
Other medical problems	
Constipation	
Epilepsy	
Hyperthyroidism	
Nocturia	
Parkinson's disease	
Peptic ulcer disease	
Renal insufficiency	
Tachyarrhythmias	

such as travel, hospitalization, or anticipation of an important or stressful event. Transient insomnia is often self-limiting, lasting less than 1 week. However, if more severe stresses are present (eg, divorce, the death of a loved one, or the loss of a job), transient insomnia may become short-term insomnia, usually lasting 1–3 weeks.[2,7] Unless it is managed appropriately, short-term insomnia may progress to chronic insomnia.

Chronic or long-term insomnia lasts from more than 3 weeks to years and is often the result of medical problems, psychologic dysfunction, or substance abuse.[4,6] An estimated 60% of cases of chronic insomnia are secondary to psychiatric disorders, with depression being the most common.[3] Individuals with psychophysiologic insomnia have a type of chronic insomnia that is thought to result from faulty sleep habits present during transient or short-term insomnia that have progressed to chronic insomnia. For example, the elderly often take daytime naps, which may contribute to nocturnal sleep disturbance. Thus, it is critical to identify the problem that is responsible for long-term insomnia if the sleep disturbance is to be appropriately managed.[3,7]

Sleep Apnea

Sleep apnea is characterized by patient and family complaints of poor sleep quality, gasping, snoring, and daytime fatigue and sedation. This disorder, which occurs more often among the elderly,[2] appears to be more common in men; the stereotype is the middle-aged, overweight, hypertensive male. Although it is usually caused by some form of airway obstruction, sleep apnea may be produced through central nervous system (CNS) mechanisms. Significant morbidity is associated with obstructive sleep apnea, and the disorder is cited as being linked with 38,000 cardiovascular deaths annually.[2]

Narcolepsy, Nocturnal Myoclonus, and Restless Legs Syndrome

Narcolepsy is characterized by daytime sleep attacks, cataplexy (sudden loss of muscle tone), hypnagogic hallucinations, and sleep paralysis. The patient with nocturnal myoclonus experiences jerky leg movements throughout the night. This patient may only perceive poor-quality sleep and daytime fatigue; however, the bed partner can confirm the presence of muscle jerks. Restless legs syndrome is manifested by an uncomfortable feeling in the calves and thighs and irresistible leg movements in the evening hours. Patients may not be able to fall asleep until 2 or 3 am. Nocturnal myoclonus and restless legs syndrome may occur concomitantly, and like sleep apnea, they also occur more often among the elderly.[2] Patients who complain of any of these types of symptoms should be referred to a physician, preferably a sleep specialist, for a thorough evaluation. Formal assessment by a sleep laboratory, including sleep studies, can be extremely useful in evaluating patients with chronic sleep dysfunction.[1,2]

TABLE 3 Principles of good sleep hygiene

1. Follow a regular sleep pattern: go to bed and arise at about the same time daily.
2. Make the bedroom comfortable for sleeping. Avoid temperature extremes, noise, and lights.
3. Make sure the bed is comfortable.
4. Engage in relaxing activities prior to bedtime.
5. Exercise regularly but not late in the evening.
6. Use the bedroom only for sleep and sexual activities, and not as an office, game room, etc.
7. If tense, practice relaxation exercises.
8. If hungry, eat a light snack, but avoid eating meals or large snacks immediately prior to bedtime.
9. Eliminate daytime naps.
10. Avoid caffeine use after noon.
11. Avoid alcohol or nicotine use later in the evening.
12. If unable to fall asleep, do not become anxious; leave the bedroom and participate in relaxing activities until tired.

Patient Assessment

Regardless of the etiology of the disorder, sleep-deprived individuals are highly symptomatic and their quality of life is negatively affected. In a telephone survey of 691 untreated insomniacs, 83% reported being "easily upset, irritated, or annoyed"; 80% reported feeling "blue, down in the dumps, or depressed"; 78% said they were "too tired to do things"; and 59% admitted having "more general trouble remembering things," among other complaints.[8]

The pharmacist should evaluate the patient carefully before deciding whether to recommend a nonprescription product. Questions such as those at the beginning of this chapter should be asked regarding sleep habits, medical disorders, psychiatric disorders, medications (Table 1), psychologic or situational stresses, or other problems that may be responsible for the sleep disturbance. Medical and psychiatric problems (Table 2) are often associated with long-term insomnia, and the underlying problem needs to be addressed. This issue is particularly relevant for the elderly. Numerous medications and recreational drugs may induce sleep disturbance, and the pharmacist should perform a careful history on the patient to rule out the possibility of drug-induced sleep dysfunction. If, during questioning of a patient, the pharmacist discovers a medical, psychiatric, or drug-induced reason for the insomnia, or if the patient has long-term insomnia, the pharmacist should not recommend a nonprescription sleep aid but should instead encourage the patient to see a physician for a complete evaluation. Whether a sleep product is recommended or not, however, the pharmacist should counsel the patient regarding measures to improve sleep hygiene (Table 3).

Sleep Aid Products

The primary indication for nonprescription sleep aids is the symptomatic management of transient and short-term insomnia. Antihistamines are the most common nonprescription treatment for insomnia; however, a phytomedicinal product valerian and the hormone melatonin are also marketed as sleep aids (see product tables "Sleep Aid Products" and "Herbal and Phytomedicinal Products").

Antihistamines

When the Food and Drug Administration (FDA) issued its final monograph on over-the-counter (OTC) sleep aids in 1989, the antihistamine diphenhydramine (hydrochloride or citrate) was the only agent on the list deemed safe and effective for nonprescription use.[9,10] Although the safety of another antihistamine, doxylamine, has not been fully established and no published studies supporting the efficacy of doxylamine as a sleep aid are currently available, the FDA has allowed it to remain on the market.[10] However, products containing pyrilamine maleate, potassium or sodium bromide, and scopolamine hydrobromide have been removed from the market.[7] Under an agreement between the Nonprescription Drug Manufacturers Association and the FDA, clinical trials are currently under way to assess the efficacy and safety of acetaminophen-diphenhydramine products. The FDA is requiring that the study population be composed of patients who require both an analgesic and a sleep aid.[11]

TABLE 4 Selected pharmacokinetic and clinical properties of nonprescription hypnotics

	Diphen-hydramine	Doxy-lamine
Time to maximum plasma concentration	1–4 h	2–3 h
Maximum sedation	1–3 h	N/A
Protein binding	80–85%	N/A
Elimination half-life	2.4–9.3 h	10 h
Duration of sedation	3–6 h	N/A
Bioavailability	26–61%	N/A

Key: N/A means not available.

Source:
AHFS Drug Information. 92: 2–5, 17–20.
Clin Pharmacol Ther. 1980; 28: 229–34.
Clin Pharmacol Ther. 1989; 45: 15–21.
Clin Pharmacol Ther. 1978; 23: 375–82.

Both diphenhydramine and doxylamine are members of the ethanolamine group of antihistamines. Although the exact mechanism by which the ethanolamines affect sleep is unclear, it is probably related to their affinity for histamine$_1$ and muscarinic receptors.[10]

Pharmacokinetics Selected clinical and pharmacokinetic properties of diphenhydramine and doxylamine are summarized in Table 4. Both drugs are well absorbed from the gastrointestinal (GI) tract and have short to intermediate half-lives. Diphenhydramine is metabolized in the liver through two successive *N*-demethylations, and its apparent half-life may be prolonged by a factor of approximately 1.5 in patients with chronic liver disease.[12,13] A positive relationship exists between diphenhydramine plasma concentrations and drowsiness and cognitive impairment. Significant drowsiness has been shown to last from 3 to 6 hours after a single 50-mg dose of diphenhydramine whereas impairment in performance on psychomotor tests lasts from 2 to 4 hours.[14,15] How this may be extrapolated to nightly dosing of diphenhydramine is unclear; however, it may indicate that patients can be assured that their ability to perform tasks requiring mental alertness and cognitive ability will not be impaired for any longer than they feel drowsy.

Patient ethnicity may account for differences in drug effect. One study indicates that Asians have lower diphenhydramine peak plasma concentrations, more rapid clearance, and less subjective sedation than Caucasians.[12] Thus, Asians may require as much as 1.7 times more diphenhydramine than Caucasians to experience the same level of sedation. Asian patients who do not respond to 25- and 50-mg doses of diphenhydramine may be advised to try a 75-mg nightly dose.

Efficacy Of the published clinical trials with diphenhydramine, most but not all indicate efficacy, particularly in decreasing sleep latency.[1] In one study, diphenhydramine 50 mg and triazolam 0.25 mg, when administered in the morning after a good night of sleep, had similar effects on decreasing sleep latency.[16] Fifty milligrams of diphenhydramine appears to be the optimal adult dose, and with the possible exception of Asian patients, doses greater than 50 mg are not more efficacious as a sleep aid but do increase the potential for adverse effects. Patients who have never been treated with sleep aids tend to respond better to diphenhydramine than previously treated individuals.[17] In a study of elderly nursing home patients, subjects rated both diphenhydramine 50 mg and temazepam 15 mg as more effective than placebo in inducing sleep.[18] Although these patients reportedly tolerated diphenhydramine well, the possibility of anticholinergic side effects should not be overlooked. However, because no published efficacy and safety studies are available documenting the value of doxylamine as a sleep aid, only diphenhydramine should be recommended to patients for such use at the present time.

Interestingly, the results of a telephone survey of insomniac patients in four major US cities question the usefulness of nonprescription sleep aids. Sleep aid users who responded to newspaper advertisements announcing a survey of consumer opinions concerning sleep products were questioned about multiple aspects of hypnotic effects. These consumers reported nonprescription sleep aids to be less effective in improving nighttime or daytime symptoms of insomnia than three marketed benzodiazepine sleep aids.[8] Although the results of clinical trials have suggested that nonprescription products are effective in treating sleep latency insomnia, the authors of this study concluded that "OTC sleep aids provide some relief from insomnia, but from a benefit-risk perspective, their net benefits are meager."[8] Of nocturnal symptoms, "frequent awakenings" is the symptom reported to respond best, but even then this was so for only 26% of 310 respondents. In addition, 11% of nonprescription sleep aid users reported experiencing more morning grogginess while taking the nonprescription product than before taking it. However, when asked the following question—"Taking into account both the positive effects on your sleep and daytime functioning and any negative effects you may have experienced, would you take this medication again for the same purpose?"—61% of nonprescription sleep aid users answered affirmatively. The results of telephone surveys need to be considered differently than those of clinical trials, but they do lend some useful consumer information. That is, although consumers report some satisfaction regarding nonprescription sleep aid use, it is not as high as that reported by users of prescription sleep aids.

Although poorly studied, tolerance to the hypnotic effects of diphenhydramine appears to result with repeated use. With the exception of Asians, adult patients should be advised not to exceed 50 mg nightly, and all patients should limit their use of diphenhydramine to no more than 7–10 consecutive nights. For patients with transient or short-term insomnia—assuming there are no underlying problems—reestablishing the normal sleep cycle with sleep aids should assist in normalizing sleep patterns. Patients complaining of continuing insomnia after 10 days of nonprescription sleep aid use and good sleep hygiene measures should be referred to a physician for a more thorough evaluation.

Adverse Effects/Toxicity In addition to sedation, the intended effect when these drugs are used as sleep aids, the primary side effects of diphenhydramine and doxylamine are anticholinergic in nature.[10] Commonly occurring adverse effects include dry mouth and throat, constipation, blurred vision, and tinnitus. Older male patients should be asked about prostatic hypertrophy and difficulty urinating. Narrow- (closed-) angle glaucoma is also a contraindication. Patients with cardiovascular disease (eg, angina or rhythm disturbance) may be particularly susceptible to the anticholinergic adverse effects of ethanolamine sleep aids. If these problems exist, diphenhydramine should not be recommended. In addition, a patient's concomitant medication regimen should be reviewed before a pharmacist recommends diphenhydramine. A patient who is taking other anticholinergics should be alerted to the potential for additive side effects.

Patients should be cautioned not to drive an automobile or operate machinery until their response to the drug is known. They should also be warned of the additive CNS depressant effects of alcohol and encouraged not to drink alcoholic beverages while taking these drugs. Some patients may develop excitation from diphenhydramine and other highly anticholinergic antihistamines. Symptoms include nervousness, restlessness, agitation, tremors, insomnia, delirium, and, in rare cases, seizures. This occurs more often in children, elderly patients, and patients with organic mental disorders. Elderly patients older than 80 years of age and with acute physical disorders or dementia seem particularly susceptible to developing delirium from even modest doses of diphenhydramine.[19]

Antihistamine dosage excess can result in anticholinergic toxicity.[20] This may occur as a result of drug interactions, the purposeful ingestion of a large amount, or individual sensitivity. Anticholinergic toxicity is particularly common in children, in whom the symptoms are usually more severe. CNS anticholinergic toxicity is one of the primary presenting features of antihistamine excess. Patients may be anxious, excited, delirious, hallucinating, or stuporous; in more severe cases, coma or seizures may occur. Other physical signs may include dilated pupils, flushed skin, hot and dry mucous membranes, and elevated body temperature. Tachycardia is common, and in severe cases, rhabdomyolysis, dysrhythmias, cardiovascular collapse, and death may occur.

The primary treatment of anticholinergic toxicity includes emesis with syrup of ipecac to decrease drug absorption if ingestion is acute. If the patient is stuporous or comatose, gastric lavage and activated charcoal may be used; activated charcoal should be followed by 240 mL of a magnesium sulfate solution to hasten GI elimination. Patients should receive general supportive care such as hydration, antipyretics, a cooling blanket if needed, and maintenance of vital signs, including ventilatory support.[21] Seizures should be treated with standard anticonvulsants such as diazepam. Despite the potential pharmacologic rationale, physostigmine is not recommended as first-line therapy in anticholinergic toxicity because of its narrow therapeutic index and short duration of action.

Use during Pregnancy/Lactation The safety of antihistamines during pregnancy has not been clearly established.[10] Therefore, the benefit-to-risk ratio of using these drugs during pregnancy should be carefully evaluated. Doxylamine was formerly marketed as a prescription combination product for the treatment of morning sickness during pregnancy. However, the manufacturer voluntarily removed this combination from the market in 1976 following allegations of teratogenicity. Although it is not possible to prove conclusively that doxylamine is not teratogenic, epidemiologic studies indicate that the possibility of such a relationship is remote.[10] Nevertheless, rather than recommending a nonprescription product, pharmacists should advise pregnant women to consult their physician regarding any sleep disturbance.

There appears to be an increased risk of CNS side effects from antihistamine use in neonates. For this reason, and because such drugs may inhibit lactation, pharmacists should recommend that nursing mothers not use antihistamines for sleep.

Miscellaneous Products

L-Tryptophan The efficacy of L-tryptophan in treating insomnia has not been clearly established. Some studies have demonstrated hypnotic efficacy; others have not.[1,22]

Although often touted by health food stores in 1- to 3-g doses as being a safe and natural way to induce sleep, L-tryptophan is not an innocuous product. More than 1,500 cases of eosinophilia-myalgia syndrome (EMS), including at least 27 deaths, were reported in patients taking contaminated L-tryptophan before the FDA, in 1990, recalled all products containing L-tryptophan except protein supplements, infant formulas, and parenteral and enteral nutritional products.[1,18] EMS was thought to be caused by contamination with 1-1′-ethylidene-bis[tryptophan] (EBT) in the manufacturing process. However, animal studies have suggested that large doses of noncontaminated tryptophan may also cause EMS on unusual occasions owing to abnormalities in metabolism.[1,23]

The symptoms of EMS develop over several weeks. Primary symptoms are myalgia, which may be severe and incapacitating, and fatigue. Other symptoms may include shortness of breath, cough, skin rash, arthralgia, muscle weakness, and peripheral edema. In a few severe cases, congestive heart failure, dysrhythmias, pneumonia, vasculitis, ascending polyneuropathy (similar to Guillain-Barré syndrome), and scleroderma-like skin changes have been reported. Clinical symptoms are accompanied by eosinophilia, often with more than 1,000 cells per cubic millimeter. The natural course of EMS is unpredictable. Although some patients' symptoms will remit when L-tryptophan is discontinued, others will develop into some of the more severe symptoms described above.[1]

In addition to EMS, L-tryptophan has been associated with causing "serotonin storm" when used in combination with serotonin reuptake or monoamine oxidase inhibitors. Symptoms of this drug interaction include agitation, restlessness, aggressiveness, tremor, hyperthermia, diarrhea, and cramping.[1] L-tryptophan should not be initiated in combination with one of these agents in outpatients. Given its questionable efficacy and known adverse effects, pharmacists should be reluctant to recommend L-tryptophan as a sleep aid.

Valerian Valerian is an herbal remedy, most commonly coming from the plant *Valeriana officinalis* L. It has been used for some time in several European countries as a sleep aid, and there is increasing interest in the United States as well. Germany has adopted a monograph for valerian as a sleep aid, and in the United Kingdom it has approval as a "traditional herbal remedy" for use in poor sleep.[24,25] (See Chapter 35, "Herbs and Phytomedicinal Products.")

Pharmacodynamically, synaptosome studies indicate that valerian increases the release of gamma-aminobutyric acid (GABA), a mechanism that suggests potential use as an anxiolytic or sedative.[26] However, in spite of manufacturer claims of efficacy and safety, there are few published and well-controlled clinical studies upon which to base an evaluation of valerian. One study of 14 elderly individuals complaining of poor sleep showed that valerian 405 mg taken orally three times daily increased the amount of time in slow wave or delta sleep but had no effect on time to fall asleep, total sleep time, or patient's perception of sleep quality.[27]

Valerian is not included in the 1989 FDA-approved monograph on nonprescription sleep aids; however, the European-American Phytomedicines Coalition is recommending approval of a monograph for valerian based upon the European approvals.[24,25] At the present time, there is inadequate available information for a pharmacist to make rational decisions regarding the clinical use of valerian. Pharmacists should not recommend the use of valerian to their patients as a sleep aid or sedative until there is more information available regarding its dosage, efficacy, safety, interaction potential, and instructions for appropriate use.

Melatonin Melatonin, an endogenous hormone produced by the pineal gland, has multiple functions in the body, many of which are poorly understood. Although it is primarily secreted at night, melatonin's physiologic effects on sleep are largely unknown.[28] Its secretion, however, appears to be related to the neuroendocrine-gonadal axis.[29] Melatonin shifts circadian rhythm by a mechanism that is nearly opposite to that of light exposure.[30] When administered in the morning, melatonin delays the circadian rhythm; conversely, administration of this agent in the evening advances the circadian rhythm. Melatonin also decreases body temperature and mental alertness. These findings have aroused interest in examining the effects of this hormone in sleep disorders, especially sleep phase shifts, jet lag, and mood disorders.

The hypnotic/sedative effects of physiologic doses of melatonin have been examined in normal male volunteers.[28] In this study, doses of either 0.3 mg or 1 mg decreased both sleep latency and REM latency as compared with placebo. The effects on time to fall asleep were most pronounced in those individuals who had longer sleep latencies (ie, >20 min); further, no residual effects on alertness were noted the next morning. These findings support a hypothesis that physiologic doses of melatonin are associated with sleep induction.

This hormonal sleep aid has also been used at supraphysiologic or pharmacologic doses. Although these doses are not well studied, some, but not all, reports showed at least partial improvement in sleep parameters.[28,31,32] Some of the patients had severe sleep disorders, including delayed sleep phase insomnia. In the latter disorder, melatonin's effects appear to be reversible after drug discontinuation. The reports also indicate that time of administration may influence melatonin's effects.

The hormone has also been purported to be effective in treating symptoms of jet lag. In a double-blind, placebo-controlled trial in international flight attendants, melatonin 5 mg taken daily for 5 days, beginning on the day of departure, was shown by retrospective self-report to decrease jet lag and sleep disturbance.[33] In contrast, subjects who started taking the sleep aid 3 days before the flight actually did worse than the placebo group.

Some experts recommend caution with the use of melatonin because its optimal dose and time of administration have not been determined.[34] Further, potential drug interactions, side effects, and toxicity, particularly with long-term use, are not known. If recommending melatonin for use in a patient with insomnia, the pharmacist should stipulate that only physiologic doses of 0.1–1 mg should be taken 1–2 hours before the desired bedtime. Patients should also be cautioned not to drive or operate machinery after taking the sleep aid. Pharmacists should be aware that these recommendations are made without benefit of the FDA's review of data to determine if the agent is efficacious and safe in treating insomnia. The previous experience with L-tryptophan is an example of the potential adverse outcomes of unbridled enthusiasm for the medicinal use of unapproved agents.

Alcohol Ethanol is a CNS depressant that has been used for centuries for both its sedative and disinhibiting properties. However, alcohol does not have the positive effects on sleep that many people believe it to have. After occasional evening consumption of one or two drinks, alcohol is effective in decreasing sleep latency. However, with heavy or continuous consumption, alcohol disrupts the sleep cycle. Although sleep latency decreases, the patient usually begins to experience restless sleep and often awakens within 2–4 hours. The total duration of sleep also decreases. Moreover, after alcohol is discontinued, rebound insomnia is likely to occur.[35] Chronic alcoholics usually have marked disorganization of their sleep cycle, with shortened REM periods and delta sleep.

Alcohol is present in some nonprescription combination cold products, such as NyQuil, which contains 25% alcohol by volume. Products of this type are marketed and sometimes recommended by physicians and pharmacists to induce sleep. Data are limited, however, regarding their efficacy and safety as sleep aids. They

TABLE 5 Approximate caffeine content of selected beverages and foods

Beverage or food	Caffeine content (mg)
Coffee (5 oz)	
Brewed, automatic drip	60–180
Brewed, percolator	40–170
Instant	30–120
Decaffeinated, instant	1–5
Decaffeinated, brewed	2–5
Tea (5 oz)	
Brewed, imported brands	25–110
Brewed, US brands	20–90
Instant	25–50
Iced (12 oz)	67–76
Soft drinks (12 oz)	
Mountain Dew	54
Coca-Cola	45.6
Diet Coke	45.6
Dr Pepper	39.6
Sugar-Free Dr Pepper	39.6
Big Red	38.4
Sugar-Free Big Red	38.4
Pepsi-Cola	38.4
Diet Pepsi	36
7-Up	0
Sunkist Orange	0
Ginger ale	0
Chocolate cake (1/16 of 9-in. cake)	13.8
Chocolate ice cream (2/3 c)	4.5
Chocolate pudding, instant (1/2 c)	5.5
Chocolate milk beverage (8 oz)	2–7
Chocolate-flavored syrup (1 oz)	4
Milk chocolate (1 oz)	1–15
Dark chocolate, semisweet (1 oz)	5–35
Baker's chocolate (1 oz)	26
Cocoa beverage (5 oz)	2–20

Source:
JAMA. 1984 Aug; 252: 803–6.
FDA Consumer. 1984 Mar; 18: 14–6.
Hosp Pharm. 1984 Apr; 19: 257–67.

contain multiple ingredients, which increases the risk of side effects and interactions with other drugs. At least four cases of liver injury, possibly due to the alcohol-acetaminophen combination, have been reported with Nyquil.[36]

Alcohol has negative effects on patients with sleep apnea. As little as 3 oz (two shots) of 80-proof ethanol may increase the frequency and severity of apneic episodes, even in patients with mild apnea.[37] Furthermore, alcohol has even been reported to cause apnea in normal individuals.[38]

Approximately 10–15% of chronic insomniacs have problems with substance abuse, especially alcohol abuse.[4] Patients who abuse alcohol are also frequent abusers of other CNS depressants, including benzodiazepines. The pharmacist must acquire the patient's medication history to evaluate the possibilities both of additive CNS depression between alcohol and other medications and of substance abuse. Patients should be questioned regarding their alcohol use before a nonprescription sleep aid is recommended; those who drink regularly should instead be referred to a physician. Patients who inquire about using alcohol as a sleep aid should be advised to limit such use to one or two drinks on an occasional basis. Most clinicians advise that alcohol never be used as a sleep aid or an adjunct to a sleep aid program.

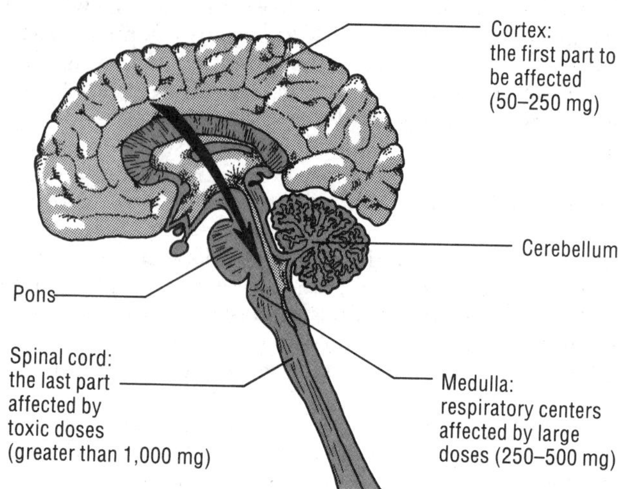

FIGURE 1 Sites of action of caffeine in the central nervous system. (The arrow indicates the progression of the effect.)

Stimulant Products (Caffeine)

Caffeine is the only FDA-approved stimulant for nonprescription use (see product table "Stimulant Products"). Nearly 80% of the US adult population consumes caffeine daily, thus making it one of the most popular drugs.[39] Many children also consume caffeine. For example, mean caffeine intake in children 6–11 months old is 4.2 mg per day; in children 6–17 years old, it increases to 43 mg per day.[40] In adults, mean caffeine intake is 186 mg per day (approximately two cups of coffee daily or the equivalent). Daily caffeine intake correlates with age.

Caffeine is a common ingredient in coffee, tea, soft drinks, and chocolate products[39] (Table 5). It is also present in many prescription and nonprescription drugs, including headache and cold remedies, menstrual pain relief products, diet aids, and stimulant preparations. Caffeine concentrations vary among the products; generally, stimulants contain the highest concentrations, averaging 100–200 mg per tablet.

Physiologic Effects

Central Nervous System Effects

Caffeine is the most potent methylxanthine in terms of CNS stimulation, even at low plasma concentrations. As caffeine plasma concentrations increase, the cortex, then the medulla, and lastly the spinal cord are stimulated (Figure 1). Caffeine doses of 50–200 mg can increase alertness and decrease fatigue and drowsiness. At higher doses (200–500 mg), caffeine may produce tremulousness, nervousness, headache, and irritability. High plasma concentrations may also cause excitement, tinnitus, insomnia, and restlessness.

Caffeine's effect on sleep may be dose dependent, but it varies greatly among individuals. Caffeine appears to increase stage 2 sleep and decrease delta sleep. Thus, it may increase awakenings and arousability although tolerance may develop to these effects.

Caffeine also has varying effects on mood. Aggressive behavior has been reported to decrease with caffeine reduction. Caffeine may exacerbate anxiety, thus potentially worsening symptoms in patients with anxiety or panic disorder.[41] Depression has been reported in persons consuming large amounts of caffeine (five cups of coffee a day or more).[41] However, it is difficult to know whether depressed patients self-medicate with caffeine or whether caffeine produces depression. Increased caffeine intake has been linked to a worsening in the behavioral symptoms of moderate to severe premenstrual syndrome.[42]

Cardiovascular Effects

Pharmacologic effects of caffeine on the cardiovascular system have long been debated. Caffeine stimulates heart muscle; however, this action is often opposed by simultaneous medullary vagal stimulation. The resultant heart rate changes are variable. As the caffeine dose is increased, the myocardium stimulation overcomes the vagal effect and increased cardiac activity is noted.

Blood Pressure Caffeine causes systemic release of norepinephrine, epinephrine, and renin, causing alterations in blood pressure.[39] However, recent studies suggest that caffeine does not produce persistent increases in blood pressure because tolerance develops quickly.[43] Even in individuals who do not regularly consume caffeine, the increased blood pressure resulting from caffeine ingestion rapidly returns to normal. Thus, hypertensive patients can continue to consume moderate amounts of caffeine.

Coronary Heart Disease Several reports have suggested that heavy caffeine consumption is associated with coronary heart disease.[39,44] One prospective study involving 1,130 male medical students followed for 19–35 years noted a positive dose-response relationship between caffeine consumption and coronary heart disease.[44] However, another prospective study over 2 years and involving 45,589 men with no history of cardiovascular disease found no association between coffee consumption and the risk of coronary heart disease or stroke.[45]

Cardiac Rate/Rhythm The effect of caffeine on cardiac rate and rhythm, and the possible development of arrhythmias have been studied. In 34 normal adults, high caffeine doses were not associated with any significant change in cardiac rate or rhythm.[46] Moderate caffeine intake, 300–450 mg per day, did not increase the severity or frequency of arrhythmias in normal individuals, in ischemic heart disease patients, or in patients with preexisting serious ventricular ectopy.[47] In contrast, an increased incidence of spontaneous ventricular ectopic beats was noted in persons with preexisting ventricular ectopic beats who received 1 mg of caffeine per kilogram of body weight.[48] Thus, in both healthy individuals and in heart disease patients, the role of moderate amounts of caffeine in cardiac arrhythmias is unclear. In very high concentrations, however, caffeine may cause sinus tachycardia, paroxysmal supraventricular tachycardia, ventricular arrhythmias, or hypotension.[39,49]

Cholesterol Concentration Caffeine may also contribute to adverse changes in lipid metabolism.[39] Some epidemiologic studies suggest a link between coffee consumption and increased total and low-density lipoprotein cholesterol concentrations.

Miscellaneous Effects

Caffeine affects the respiratory, endocrine, GI, and renal systems. Caffeine is a bronchodilator, but it is only about 40% as potent as theophylline,[39] and it may increase the respiratory rate. Endocrine effects include increases in renin, cortisol, free fatty acids, blood glucose concentrations, and the metabolic rate. Effects on the GI system include increases in gastric acid and pepsin secretion. Caffeine may either decrease or have no effect upon lower esophageal sphincter pressure, and it relaxes smooth muscle in the biliary and GI tract. It also reduces mesenteric and liver blood flow, the latter by up to 19%. Finally, caffeine has a mild diuretic effect by increasing the glomerular filtration rate and inhibiting sodium tubular reabsorption.

Caffeine has been linked to decreased fertility. One study of 104 women attempting pregnancy noted that women were half as likely to become pregnant if more caffeine than the equivalent of one cup of coffee per day was consumed compared with intake of less than this amount.[50] Another study found similar results in 6,303 women.[51]

Pharmacokinetics

Caffeine is rapidly and completely absorbed from the GI tract, and peak plasma concentrations occur 30–60 minutes after ingestion. Caffeine crosses the blood brain barrier rapidly and has a volume of distribution of 0.5–0.8 L/kg of body weight. It is extensively metabolized in the liver by the microsomal cytochrome P-450 system, primarily through oxidative demethylation and hydroxylation. Furthermore, no significant first-pass effect exists. Paraxanthine, theobromine, and theophylline are active metabolites of caffeine. In adults, the average half-life of caffeine is 4–6 hours. In smokers, the half-life is shorter; in patients with chronic liver disease and in pregnant women, the half-life is extended. In neonates, the half-life may be as long as 100 hours because neonates primarily eliminate caffeine unchanged by the kidneys until they are 3 months old. The half-life of caffeine in elderly patients is not significantly different from that in younger adults.

Indications

Caffeine is commercially available as the sole ingredient in most CNS stimulant products as well as one of the ingredients in many combination products such as headache remedies. Used as a CNS stimulant, caffeine is marketed as a product to help fatigued patients stay awake and to restore mental alertness. Oral doses of 100–200 mg are needed to achieve mild CNS stimulation in adults. If a timed-release caffeine preparation is used, the dose should not be taken less than 6 hours before bedtime. The recommended adult dose of timed-release products is 200–250 mg. Before recommending caffeine as a CNS stimulant, however, the pharmacist should ask the patient a number of questions (outlined at the beginning of this chapter) that address the etiology of the patient's fatigue and the patient's medical or psychiatric problems, current medications, dietary caffeine consumption, and intended use of the product. Based on the paucity of data supporting the efficacy of caffeine and the well-known effects of caffeine excess, pharmacists should carefully consider whether caffeine products should be recommended to improve daytime alertness.

Adverse Effects

The primary adverse events associated with caffeine are CNS stimulant effects and GI irritation. Adverse CNS effects include insomnia, nervousness, restlessness, excitement, tinnitus, muscular tremor, headache, lightheadedness, and mild delirium. These effects are more pronounced in children. Adverse GI effects include nausea, vomiting, diarrhea, and stomach pain. Other adverse effects include diuresis, extrasystoles, palpitations, and tachycardia. Further, prolonged consumption of caffeine can result in dependence whereas excessive consumption can result in toxicity.

Dependence/Withdrawal

Physical dependence may result from prolonged caffeine consumption; withdrawal symptoms can occur following abrupt cessation.[39] The most common withdrawal symptoms are fatigue and headache. Anxiety, nausea, vomiting, impaired psychomotor function, irritability, restlessness, lethargy, and, less commonly, yawning and rhinorrhea are also noted. Withdrawal symptoms generally occur 12–24 hours after cessation of caffeine ingestion, peak in 20–48 hours, and may persist for a week. A throbbing headache, the typical symptom, results from the rebound vasodilatation that occurs following abrupt withdrawal. Some suggest that there is a distinct clinical withdrawal syndrome consisting of headache, lethargy, and depression.[52]

Caffeine withdrawal is included as a research proposal in the appendix of the *Diagnostic and Statistical Manual of Mental Disorders* 4th edition (*DSM-IV*). Investigators, however, have suggested that caffeine meets criteria for drug dependence. Caffeine is a reinforcer: it produces withdrawal symptoms, tolerance, and intoxication. Further research will determine whether caffeine is added to the list of agents producing drug dependence.

Toxicity

Serious symptomatology can occur after caffeine overdose. Caffeinism, the ingestion of high caffeine doses (>250 mg), can produce symptoms mimicking anxiety. The diagnostic criteria for caffeinism include recent caffeine consumption of more than 250 mg and at least five of the following symptoms: nervousness, restlessness, insomnia, excitement, diuresis, facial flushing, muscle twitching, GI disturbance, tachycardia or cardiac arrhythmia, "rambling" flow of thought and speech, psychomotor agitation, or periods of inexhaustibility.[53] Five caffeine overdose deaths have been reported in patients who ingested caffeine-containing nonprescription products.[54] Four of the five cases were successful suicide attempts, and the fifth was an accidental death secondary to drug abuse. The lethal dose in adults is 150–200 mg/kg of body weight.[55]

The primary management of caffeine toxicity includes general supportive care. For an acute ingestion, emesis should be initiated with ipecac unless the patient is obtunded, comatose, or convulsing. A cathartic such as magnesium sulfate, magnesium citrate, sodium sulfate, or sorbitol should be given with or without charcoal. If the patient is stuporous or comatose, gastric lavage and activated charcoal should be used. Patients should receive general supportive care such as hydration, antipyretics, and maintenance of vital signs, including ventilatory support and electrocardiogram monitoring. Antacids such as aluminum hydroxide gel can be used for GI irritation. Seizures should be treated with intravenous diazepam and, if they recur, with phenytoin or phenobarbital. For extremely high caffeine serum concentrations, exchange transfusion or hemoperfusion may be considered.

Drug Interactions/ Laboratory Test Interferences

Drug interactions between caffeine and other agents may be clinically significant. Patients should be informed that caffeine's metabolism is inhibited by disulfiram, mexiletine, cimetidine, norfloxacin, enoxacin, ciprofloxacin, and oral contraceptives containing estrogen; and that alcohol acutely inhibits the metabolism of caffeine.[39,56–58] In addition, caffeine may decrease iron absorption, although the clinical significance of this interaction is unclear; patients should be instructed to take iron 1 hour before or 2 hours after caffeine consumption.

GI distress is increased when nonsteroidal anti-inflammatory drugs, aspirin, corticosteroids, or alcohol is administered along with caffeine. Blood pressure may be increased when caffeine and phenylpropanolamine are coadministered. Monoamine oxidase inhibitors in combination with caffeine are of particular concern because patients may develop potentially life-threatening cardiac complications. Caffeine does not typically affect the efficacy of medications used to treat hypertension but may interfere with the therapeutic benefit of antiarrhythmic agents. Furthermore, caffeine and diazepam coadministered have antagonizing effects, depending on the dose of the two agents and the specific task behavioral tests used.[59,60] For example, caffeine antagonizes diazepam-induced impairment of psychomotor performance and sedation but does not antagonize diazepam-induced impairment of delayed recognition memory performance or immediate recall.[59] Alternatively, diazepam antagonizes caffeine-induced restlessness, alertness, arousal, and tension.

Caffeine may cause false-positive diagnostic tests for both pheochromocytoma and neuroblastoma because it causes elevations in urine concentrations of vanillylmandelic acid, catecholamines, and 5-hydroxyindoleacetic acid. Also, serum uric acid concentrations may be falsely elevated.

Therapeutic Concerns

Pediatric Considerations

Although there appear to be no behavioral problems reported in normal children consuming caffeine, there is no indication that children have been intentionally given caffeine as a stimulant.

Geriatric Considerations

In the elderly, caffeine consumption may be a factor in subjective insomnia. Caffeine has been studied for prevention of postprandial hypotension; however, in the best-designed study, caffeine was not found to be efficacious. Caffeine has also been studied as a potential risk factor for developing osteoporosis. The studies suggest that if calcium intake/balance is maintained, caffeine does not pose a risk for osteoporosis.

Use during Pregnancy/Lactation

Teratogenic Effects The safety of caffeine during pregnancy is a significant issue because caffeine is often consumed by pregnant women and freely crosses the placenta. Based on the teratogenic effects of caffeine in rodents, the FDA issued a warning in 1980 advising pregnant women to limit or avoid caffeine consumption.[61] However, no consistent teratogenic effects have been reported in animal studies that used massive caffeine doses.[62]

Possible teratogenic mechanisms are uncertain, but three hypotheses are proposed. Caffeine may interfere with fetal cell growth by increasing cyclic adenosine monophosphate (cAMP).[63] Because it structurally resembles adenine and guanine, caffeine may directly alter nucleic acids, resulting in chromosome abnormalities. Or caffeine may restrict uteroplacental circulation through vasoconstriction, resulting in fetal hypoxia.

Data on caffeine's teratogenic effect in humans are limited to a few studies, most of which rely on questionnaires or interviews.[64] Based on these limited data, caffeine's teratogenic potential appears to be dose related.[62] One study found an increased risk for late first- and second-trimester spontaneous abortions in women consuming at least 151 mg of caffeine daily.[63] However, the study noted that larger amounts of caffeine were consumed by mothers who were also relatively heavy alcohol users and smokers, both of which practices are known to increase the risk for spontaneous abortion.[65,66]

Caffeine intake of more than 300 mg per day is associated with intrauterine growth retardation and infants of low birth weight.[64,67] These findings are not surprising because caffeine at doses of 200 mg significantly decreases placental blood flow through vasoconstriction within the placental villi,[67] and any decrease in uteroplacental circulation is significantly correlated with decreased fetal growth. Increased fetal breathing activity was noted in mothers consuming two cups of regular or decaffeinated coffee[68]; similar results were found in mothers consuming more than 500 mg of caffeine per day.[69] Consumption of six or more cups of coffee daily during pregnancy has been associated with spontaneous abortion, stillbirth, low birth weight, breech presentation, and decreased activity and muscle tone of neonates.[62] Cleft palate, electrodactyly, and interventricular septal defect have been noted in infants of mothers consuming eight or more cups of coffee per day.[62,70] Furthermore, three cases of arrhythmias have occurred in infants whose mothers ingested large amounts of caffeine.[71]

Although anecdotal case reports suggest adverse fetal effects in mothers ingesting caffeine, case-control studies involving infants with congenital malformations suggest no relationship.[72–74] In a prospective study of 286 mothers, caffeine intake was not associated with an increased incidence of breech birth, miscarriage, premature birth, or caesarian section deliveries.[75] Nor was a relationship noted between caffeine intake and low birth weight in several large prospective and retrospective studies.[76,77] Overall, information is incomplete and the data are conflicting, but no direct correlations can be made between caffeine consumption and birth defects.[64] However, it is prudent to recommend limiting caffeine intake to 300 mg per day or less because decreases in birth weight are reported to occur when intake exceeds this amount.[64,67]

Concentration in Breast Milk Caffeine passes into breast milk; however, the caffeine concentration in breast milk is only 1% of the mother's plasma concentration.[64] Peak caffeine concentrations in breast milk occur within 1 hour of consumption, but infant caffeine plasma concentrations are not correlated with the levels in breast milk. No adverse effects have been reported in infants of nursing mothers consuming 200–336 mg per day of caffeine, although wakefulness and irritability have been noted in infants of nursing mothers consuming 600 mg per day. Caffeine, whether from medicinal or food sources, should be ingested immediately after nursing to avoid high maternal plasma and milk concentrations. To avoid the potential for caffeine accumulation in the infant, consumption should be moderate, especially when mothers are nursing infants younger than 4 months of age.

Usage Considerations in Neonates

Liver metabolic pathways, including the cytochrome P-450 system, are immature in the neonate. Thus, newborns metabolize caffeine very slowly and may accumulate toxic caffeine plasma concentrations. The rate of caffeine elimination increases as liver metabolic function matures. Caffeine clearance and half-life are correlated directly with gestational age.[78] If caffeine is used therapeutically in neonates, dosing intervals should be 24 hours in infants under 1 month old, 12 hours in infants 1–2 months old, 8 hours in infants 2–4 months old, and 6 hours for infants over 4 months old.[78]

Malignancy

Clinical studies proposing an association between caffeine intake and increased risk of breast cancer provide conflicting and nonconclusive results.[79–81] The causal relationship between caffeine ingestion and bladder and pancreatic cancers has been evaluated. A case-control study of 75 patients with bladder cancer and 142 control patients found no association between caffeine intake and the risk of bladder cancer.[82] Earlier studies suggest that the relative risk of developing pancreatic cancer is 2.7 (95% confidence intervals = 1.6, 4.7) in persons consuming three or more cups of coffee per day[83]; however, later studies do not support this conclusion.[84–86] Thus, no conclusive data exist to suggest that caffeine ingestion is associated with any malignancy.

Benign Breast Disease

As results from various studies have been inconsistent, the possibility of a relationship between benign breast disease and caffeine is controversial.[80] Case-control studies suggest no such association.[87,88] Fibrocystic breast disease, however, may be associated with caffeine consumption.[87] Some investigators have noted the complete resolution of benign breast nodules, tenderness, pain, and nipple discharge once women with fibrocystic disease eliminated caffeine from their diet.[89]

Guidelines for Patient Education and Counseling

Pharmacists should be aware of the various prescription and nonprescription products containing caffeine. Dietary caffeine consumption may be substantial; thus, patients should be advised of the additive effects of dietary and medicinal caffeine. This is particularly important for elderly patients, who may be more sensitive to the stimulant effects of caffeine and may present with nervousness, anxiety, insomnia, and irritability. Elderly patients who are receiving other CNS stimulants should ingest caffeine with caution. Agents such as theophylline, decongestants, amantadine, tricyclic antidepressants, and appetite suppressants added to caffeine may result in disorientation, delirium, and a host of other adverse effects.

Patients need to be advised of the possible drug

interactions, as outlined above, that may occur with caffeine. The combination of caffeine and alcohol ingestion needs to be addressed. Caffeine does not antagonize the effect of alcohol, improve a person's driving ability, or lessen any of the detrimental effects of alcohol. Contrary to folklore, caffeine will not "sober up" a person intoxicated on alcohol.

Caffeine is contraindicated in patients with known hypersensitivity to the drug. It should be used cautiously in patients who have or have had peptic ulcer disease, and in patients with symptomatic cardiac arrhythmias and palpitations. Also, high-dose caffeine intake may result in a hyperglycemic event as it may increase blood glucose concentrations. Lower doses should be used in patients with renal dysfunction. Caffeine has been shown to worsen mental status in some patients with psychiatric disorders, and it should be used cautiously in this population.

Again, pharmacists should ask themselves whether there is any reason to recommend caffeine-containing products. Although caffeine is commonly used, its use should not be encouraged by health professionals, and it should never be recommended as a substitute for adequate sleep and rest.

Case Studies

Case 10–1

Patient Complaint/History

JC, a 28-year-old accountant, presents to the pharmacist with a complaint of difficulty in sleeping for the past two nights. The patient, who is averaging only 5 hours of sleep instead of his usual 8, relates that once he falls asleep, he does not awake until the alarm goes off. He requests something to help him fall asleep.

During further conversation, the patient reveals that he is giving a very important business presentation in 4 days; he seems to be "stressed out" about the presentation. He goes on to say that over the past week he has increased his caffeine consumption from the usual one cup of coffee with breakfast and lunch to two cups of coffee with each meal. JC has no known drug allergies and occasionally takes ibuprofen for muscle aches; he does not smoke and most weekends drinks only a few beers.

Clinical Considerations/Strategies

The following considerations/strategies are provided to aid the reader in (1) determining whether treatment of the patient's condition with nonprescription medications is warranted, (2) selecting the appropriate nonprescription medication, and (3) developing a patient counseling strategy to ensure optimal therapeutic outcomes:

- Identify factors that may be causing the sleep problems.
- Identify principles of good sleep hygiene that may resolve the sleep problems.
- Determine whether the patient has previously used any nonprescription sleep aid products.
- Assess the value of therapy with a nonprescription sleep aid product; list the advantages and disadvantages of such therapy.
- Identify key points about the nonprescription products (eg, adverse effects, onset of action, duration of use) to discuss with the patient.
- Identify symptoms whose occurrence would warrant the patient contacting a pharmacist or physician.
- Develop a patient education/counseling strategy that will:
  - Explain the importance of good sleep hygiene;
  - Explain the advantages and disadvantages of any nonprescription medications used to treat the sleep problem.

Case 10–2

Patient Complaint/History

DK, a 25-year-old college student, presents to the pharmacist with a complaint of not being able to stay awake at night. Indicating the box of NoDoz in her hand, she asks if the medication will help her stay up at night. During further discussion, she reveals that she has several finals to take during the next week.

DK also reveals that she was diagnosed as mildly hypertensive last year and has been taking Dyazide daily for the past year; she has a history of mitral valve prolapse. In addition to ibuprofen for occasional headaches, she takes the oral contraceptive Tri-Levlen 21 one tablet daily for 21 days, 7 days off. The patient, who is allergic to penicillin, reports that she does not smoke and drinks alcohol in moderation during social events.

When asked about her diet and caffeine consumption, DK admits to drinking on average two cups of coffee with breakfast, two diet colas during the afternoon, and one glass of tea with dinner. She also eats a chocolate candy bar every afternoon.

Clinical Considerations/Strategies

The following considerations/strategies are provided to aid the reader in (1) determining whether treatment of the patient's condition with nonprescription medications is warranted, (2) selecting the appropriate nonprescription medication, and (3) developing a patient counseling strategy to ensure optimal therapeutic outcomes:

- Assess the appropriateness of the patient using NoDoz to help stay awake.
- Assess the potential for drug-drug, drug-disease, and drug-dietary interactions if the patient were to take the NoDoz.
- Determine whether the patient has used nonprescription stimulant products before.
- Propose a response to the patient's original question: Will NoDoz help her stay awake at night?
- Develop a patient education/counseling strategy that will:
  - Ensure that the patient understands the importance of the drug-drug, drug-disease, and drug-dietary interactions that might occur if NoDoz is taken;
  - Ensure that the patient understands what symptoms she may experience if she ingests too much caffeine and what she should do about them.

Summary

Sedating antihistamines such as diphenhydramine are effective in treating occasional transient or short-term insomnia, particularly if the sleep disturbance is primarily related to difficulty falling asleep. Because little information is available regarding the hypnotic effects of doxylamine, the herbal remedy valerian, or the hormone melatonin, only diphenhydramine should be recommended as a sleep aid at the present time. Before recommending a nonprescription agent, the pharmacist should question the patient carefully regarding the characteristics and possible etiologies of the sleep disturbance. A patient who appears to have long-term insomnia or sleep disturbance caused by an underlying disorder should be referred to a physician for further evaluation. The patient should also be questioned regarding medical disorders or concomitant medications that may interact with diphenhydramine, and should be counseled regarding diphenhydramine's side effects and particularly the additive effects of alcohol. The patient should be advised that nonprescription sleep aids are intended for short-term use and that a physician should be consulted if sleep problems persist beyond 7–10 nights. Regardless of whether a nonprescription product is recommended, the pharmacist should emphasize the importance of maintaining healthy sleep habits to ensure a good night's sleep.

Caffeine is present in many foods, beverages, and drug products. Moderate use is generally considered safe, and no conclusive data exist linking regular caffeine use with various cardiovascular diseases, teratogenic effects, or cancer. However, pregnant or nursing patients and patients with cardiac dysfunction should consume caffeine with moderation, if at all.

Patients should be advised of several issues related to the use of nonprescription stimulants containing caffeine. First, caffeine toxicity may occur if higher than recommended doses are ingested. Second, stimulant products will not reverse alcohol impairment. Third, stimulant use should be discontinued if rapid pulse, dizziness, or heart palpitations occur. Finally, stimulant products are not intended as a substitute for normal sleep. If fatigue persists or recurs, the patient should consult a physician.

References

1. Eggert AE, Crismon ML. Dealing with insomnia, the evaluation and treatment of sleep disorders. *Am Druggist.* 1992; 205(5): 83–96.
2. Farney RJ, Walker JM. Office management of common sleep-wake disorders. *Med Clin North Am.* 1995; 79: 391–414.
3. Pagel JF. Treatment of insomnia. *Am Fam Physician.* 1994; 49: 1417–21.
4. Lechky O. Questions about sleep should be routine part of patient visits, physician says. *Can Med Assoc J.* 1993; 149: 1296–8.
5. Bixler EO, Vela-Bueno A. Normal sleep: patterns and mechanisms. *Semin Neurol.* 1987; 7: 227.
6. Gillin JC, Byerly WF. The diagnosis and management of insomnia. *N Engl J Med.* 1990; 322: 239.
7. Becker PM, Jamieson AO, Bown WD. Insomnia, use of a "decision tree" to assess and treat. *Postgrad Med.* 1993; 93: 66–85.
8. Balter MB, Uhlenhuth EH. The beneficial and adverse effects of hypnotics. *J Clin Psychiatry.* 1991; 52(7, suppl): 16–23.
9. FDA announces standards for nonprescription sleep-aid products and expectorants. *Clin Pharm.* 1989 Jun; 8: 388.
10. Antihistamine drugs. In: McEvoy GK, ed. *AHFS Drug Information 95.* Bethesda, Md: American Society of Hospital Pharmacists; 1995: 2–5, 17–20.
11. NDMA task force to sponsor acetaminophen/diphenhydramine clinicals. *F-D-C Rep.* 1992 Jan 27; T&G–12.
12. Spector R et al. Diphenhydramine in Orientals and Caucasians. *Clin Pharmacol Ther.* 1980; 28: 229–34.
13. Meridith CG et al. Diphenhydramine disposition in chronic liver disease. *Clin Pharmacol Ther.* 1984; 35: 474–9.
14. Gengo F, Gabos C, Miller JK. The pharmacodynamics of diphenhydramine-induced drowsiness and changes in metal performance. *Clin Pharmacol Ther.* 1989; 45: 15–21.
15. Carruthers SG et al. Correlation between plasma diphenhydramine level and sedative and antihistamine effects. *Clin Pharmacol Ther.* 1978; 23: 375–82.
16. Roehrs T, Zwyghuizen-Doorenbos A, Roth T. Sedative effects and plasma concentrations following single doses of triazolam, diphenhydramine, ethanol and placebo. *Sleep.* 1993; 16: 301–5.
17. Kudo Y, Kurihara M. Clinical evaluation of diphenhydramine hydrochloride for the treatment of insomnia in psychiatric patients: a double-blind study. *J Clin Pharmacol.* 1990; 30: 1041–8.
18. Meuleman JR et al. Evaluation of temazepam and diphenhydramine as hypnotics in a nursing-home population. *Drug Intell Clin Pharm.* 1987; 21: 716.
19. Tejera CA et al. Diphenhydramine-induced delirium in elderly hospitalized patients with mild dementia. *Psychosomatics.* 1994; 35: 399–402.
20. Koppel C, Ibe K, Tenczer J. Clinical symptomatology of diphenhydramine overdose: an evaluation of 136 cases in 1982 to 1985. *Clin Toxicol.* 1987; 25: 53–70.
21. Nash W. Treating diphenhydramine overdose. *Nursing.* 1994; 24: 33.
22. Schneider-Helmert D, Spinweber CL. Evaluation of L-tryptophan for treatment of insomnia: a review. *Psychopharmacology.* 1986; 89: 1–7.
23. Kamb ML et al. Eosinophilia-myalgia syndrome in L-tryptophan exposed patients. *JAMA.* 1992; 267: 77–82.
24. American Vitamin Products petitions for valerian OTC monograph status. *F-D-C Rep.* 1994 Aug 22; 12–3.
25. Valerian monograph status as OTC nighttime sleep aid sought. *F-D-C Rep.* 1994 Jun 27; 15–6.
26. Santos MS et al. Synaptosomal GABA release as influenced by valerian root. *Arch Int Pharmacodyn Ther.* 1994; 327: 220–31.
27. Schulz H, Stolz C, Muller J. The effect of valerian extract on sleep polygraphy in poor sleepers: a pilot study. *Pharmacopsychiatry.* 1994; 27: 147–51.
28. Zhdanova IV et al. Sleep-inducing effects of low doses of melatonin ingested in the evening. *Clin Pharmacol Ther.* 1995; 57: 552–8.
29. Webb SM, Puig-Domingo M. Role of melatonin in health and disease. *Clin Endocrinol.* 1995; 42: 221–34.
30. Lewy AJ et al. Melatonin shifts human circadian rhythms according to a phase-response curve. *Chronobiol International.* 1992; 9: 380–2.
31. Alvarez B et al. The delayed sleep phase syndrome: clinical and investigative findings in 14 subjects. *J Neurol Neurosurg Psychiatr.* 1992; 55: 665–70.
32. Dawson D, Encel N. Melatonin and sleep in humans. *J Pineal Research.* 1993; 15: 1–12.
33. Petrie K et al. A double-blind trial of melatonin as a treatment for jet lag in international cabin crew. *Biol Psychiatr.* 1993; 33: 526–30.

34. Butler RN. A wake-up call for caution. If insomnia is the patient's problem, is over-the-counter melatonin the cure? *Geriatrics*. 1996; 51: 14–5.
35. Roth R et al. Pharmacological effects of sedative-hypnotics, narcotic analgesics, and alcohol during sleep. *Med Clin North Am*. 1985; 69: 1281.
36. Foust RT et al. Nyquil-associated liver injury. *Am J Gastroenterol*. 1989; 84: 422–5.
37. Scrima L et al. Increased severity of obstructive sleep apnea after bedtime alcohol ingestion: diagnostic potential and proposed mechanism of action. *Sleep*. 1982; 5: 318.
38. Tasan VC et al. Alcohol increases sleep apnea and oxygen desaturation in asymptomatic men. *Am J Med*. 1981; 71: 240.
39. Benowitz NL. Clinical pharmacology of caffeine. *Annu Rev Med*. 1990; 41: 277–88.
40. Graham DM. Caffeine—its identity, dietary sources, intake and biological effects. *Nutr Rev*. 1978 Apr; 36: 97–102.
41. Clementz GL, Dailey JW. Psychotropic effects of caffeine. *Am Fam Physician*. 1988 May; 37: 167–72.
42. Rossignol AM, Bonnlander H. Caffeine-containing beverages, total fluid consumption, and premenstrual syndrome. *Am J Public Health*. 1990 Sep; 80: 1106–10.
43. Myers MG. Effects of caffeine on blood pressure. *Arch Intern Med*. 1988 May; 148: 1189–93.
44. LaCroix AZ et al. Coffee consumption and the incidence of coronary heart disease. *N Engl J Med*. 1986 Oct; 315: 977–82.
45. Grobbee DE et al. Coffee, caffeine, and cardiovascular disease in men. *N Engl J Med*. 1990 Oct; 323: 1026–32.
46. Newcombe PF et al. High-dose caffeine and cardiac rate and rhythm in normal subjects. *Chest*. 1988 Jul; 94: 90–4.
47. Myers MG. Caffeine and cardiac arrhythmias. *Ann Intern Med*. 1991 Jan; 114: 147–50.
48. Sutherland DJ et al. The effect of caffeine on cardiac rate, rhythm, and ventricular repolarization. *Chest*. 1985 Mar; 87: 319–24.
49. Pentel P. Toxicity of over-the-counter stimulants. *JAMA*. 1984 Oct; 252: 1898–1903.
50. Christianson RE, Oechsli FW, van den Berg BJ. Caffeinated beverages and decreased fertility. *Lancet*. 1989 Feb; 1: 378.
51. Wilcox A, Weinberg C, Baird D. Caffeinated beverages and decreased fertility. *Lancet*. 1988 Dec; 2: 1453–6.
52. Strain EC et al. Caffeine dependence syndrome. *JAMA*. 1994 Oct; 272: 1043–8.
53. Organic mental syndromes and disorders. In: Spitzer RL, ed. *Diagnostic and Statistical Manual of Mental Disorders*. 3rd ed, rev. Washington, DC: American Psychiatric Association; 1987: 138–9.
54. Garriott JC et al. Five cases of fatal overdose from caffeine-containing "look-alike" drugs. *J Anal Toxicol*. 1985 May/Jun; 9: 141–3.
55. *Poisindex*. Vol 72. Englewood, Colo: Micromedex; 1992.
56. Fazio A. Caffeine, oral contraceptives, and over-the-counter drugs. *Arch Intern Med*. 1989 May; 149: 1217–8.
57. Healy DP et al. Interaction between oral ciprofloxacin and caffeine in normal volunteers. *Antimicrob Agents Chemother*. 1989 Apr; 33: 474–8.
58. Harder S, Fuhr U, Staib AH. Ciprofloxacin-caffeine: a drug interaction established using in vivo and in vitro investigations. *Am J Med*. 1989 Nov; 87(5A): 89S–91S.
59. Roache JD, Griffiths RR. Interactions of diazepam and caffeine: behavioral and subjective dose effects in humans. *Pharmacol Biochem Behav*. 1987 Apr; 26: 801–12.
60. Ghoneim MM et al. Pharmacokinetic and pharmacodynamic interactions between caffeine and diazepam. *J Clin Psychopharmacol*. 1986 Apr; 6: 75–80.
61. Caffeine and pregnancy. *FDA Drug Bull*. 1980 Nov; 10: 19–20.
62. Al-Hachim GM. Teratogenicity of caffeine; a review. *Eur J Obstet Gynecol Reprod Biol*. 1989; 31(3): 237–47.
63. Srisuphan W, Bracken MB. Caffeine consumption during pregnancy and association with late spontaneous abortion. *Am J Obstet Gynecol*. 1986 Jan; 154: 14–20.
64. Berger A. Effects of caffeine consumption on pregnancy outcome—a review. *J Reprod Med*. 1988 Dec; 33: 945–56.
65. Harlap S, Shiono PH. Alcohol, smoking, and incidence of spontaneous abortions in the first and second trimester. *Lancet*. 1980 Jul; 2: 173–6.
66. Kline J et al. Drinking during pregnancy and spontaneous abortion. *Lancet*. 1980 Jul; 2: 176–80.
67. Fenster L et al. Caffeine consumption during pregnancy and fetal growth. *Am J Public Health*. 1991 Apr; 81: 458–61.
68. Salvador HS, Koos BJ. Effects of regular and decaffeinated coffee on fetal breathing and heart rate. *Am J Obstet Gynecol*. 1989 May; 160(pt 1): 1043–7.
69. McGowan J et al. The effects of long- and short-term maternal caffeine ingestion on human fetal breathing and body movements in term gestations. *Am J Obstet Gynecol*. 1987 Sep; 157: 726–9.
70. Jacobson MF, Goldman AS, Syme RH. Coffee and birth defects. *Lancet*. 1981 Jun; 1: 1415–6.
71. Oei SG, Vosters RPL, van der Hagen NLJ. Fetal arrhythmia caused by excessive intake of caffeine by pregnant women. *Br Med J*. 1989 Mar; 298: 568.
72. Kurppa K et al. Coffee consumption during pregnancy. *N Engl J Med*. 1982 Jun; 306: 1548.
73. Rosenberg L et al. Selected birth defects in relation to caffeine-containing beverages. *JAMA*. 1982 Mar; 247: 1429–32.
74. Kurppa K et al. Coffee consumption during pregnancy and selected congenital malformations: a nationwide case-control study. *Am J Public Health*. 1983 Dec; 73: 1397–9.
75. Watkinson B, Fried PA. Maternal caffeine use before, during, and after pregnancy and effects upon offspring. *Neurobehav Toxicol Teratol*. 1985; 7: 9–17.
76. Brooke OG et al. Effects on birth weight of smoking, alcohol, caffeine, socioeconomic factors, and psychosocial stress. *Br Med J*. 1989 Mar; 298: 795–801.
77. Linn S et al. No association between coffee consumption and adverse outcomes of pregnancy. *N Engl J Med*. 1982 Jan; 306: 141–5.
78. Pons G et al. Developmental changes of caffeine elimination in infancy. *Dev Pharmacol Ther*. 1988; 11(5): 258–64.
79. Wolfrom D, Welsch CW. Caffeine and the development of normal, benign and carcinomatous human breast tissues: a relationship? *J Med*. 1990; 21(5): 225–50.
80. Lubin F, Ron E. Consumption of methylxanthine-containing beverages and the risk of breast cancer. *Cancer Lett*. 1990 Sep; 53: 81–90.
81. Lubin F et al. Coffee and methylxanthines and breast cancer: a case-control study. *J Natl Cancer Inst*. 1984 Mar; 74: 569–73.
82. Najem GR et al. Life time occupation, smoking, caffeine, saccharine, hair dyes and bladder carcinogenesis. *Int J Epidemiol*. 1982; 11(3): 212–7.
83. MacMahon B et al. Coffee and cancer of the pancreas. *N Engl J Med*. 1981 Mar; 304: 630–3.
84. Hsieh CC, MacMahon B, Yen S. More on coffee and pancreatic cancer. *N Engl J Med*. 1987 Feb; 316: 484.
85. Hsieh CC et al. Coffee and pancreatic cancer. *N Engl J Med*. 1986 Aug 28; 315: 587–8.
86. Hiatt RA, Klatsky AL, Armstrong MA. Pancreatic cancer, blood glucose and beverage consumption. *Int J Cancer*. 1988; 41(6): 794–7.
87. Boyle CA et al. Caffeine consumption and fibrocystic breast disease: a case-control epidemiologic study. *J Natl Cancer Inst*. 1984 May; 72: 1015–9.
88. Lubin F et al. A case-control study of caffeine and methylxanthines in benign breast disease. *JAMA*. 1985 Apr; 253: 2388–92.
89. Minton JP et al. Response of fibrocystic disease to caffeine withdrawal and correlation of cyclic nucleotides with breast disease. *Am J Obstet Gynecol*. 1979 Sep; 135: 157–8.

CHAPTER 11

Acid-Peptic Products

Julianne B. Pinson and C. Wayne Weart

Questions to ask in patient assessment and counseling

- *Can you describe the pain? How severe is it?*
- *Are there any other signs and symptoms that accompany this pain?*
- *How long have you had this pain?*
- *Is the pain constant or does it come and go?*
- *Where and when does the pain occur? Do you experience it immediately after meals or several hours later? Does the pain wake you up at night?*
- *Is the pain worse when you lie down? When you bend over?*
- *Is the pain relieved by food? Do certain foods, coffee, or carbonated beverages make it worse?*
- *Do you drink alcohol? How much? Is the pain worse after drinking alcohol?*
- *Have you lost any weight?*
- *Have you vomited blood or black material that looks like coffee grounds?*
- *Have you noticed red blood in the stool, or have the stools been black or tarry?*
- *Have you had any difficulty or pain when swallowing?*
- *Have you seen a health care provider about these symptoms? If so, what did your health care provider tell you to do?*
- *Have you previously used an antacid or histamine$_2$-receptor antagonist to treat this pain? Which one? How were you taking the product? Did it relieve the pain?*
- *What prescription and nonprescription drugs do you regularly take? Have you recently taken aspirin, naproxen sodium, or ibuprofen-containing products?*
- *Do you smoke? How much?*
- *Have you or has anyone in your family ever had an ulcer?*
- *Do you have any medical problems such as diabetes or kidney or heart disease? Are you currently under a health care provider's care for any medical conditions?*
- *Are you on any special diets such as a low-salt diet?*

Twenty-five percent of adults in the United States report having at least one episode of dyspepsia in an average 2-week period.[1] Self-care is an important part of the management of upper abdominal pain and discomfort, as reflected in annual sales of antacids exceeding $1 billion.[2] Considering the frequency of gastrointestinal (GI) complaints, the popularity of antacids, antireflux agents, and antiflatulents is not surprising. Antacids are useful for the short-term relief of indigestion, heartburn, and excessive eating and drinking, as well as for the relief of symptoms associated with gastroesophageal reflux disease (GERD) and peptic ulcer disease (PUD). The recent shift of the histamine$_2$-receptor antagonists (H_2RAs) to nonprescription status is expected to have a substantial impact on the self-care of GI complaints; it is estimated that these agents will be taken much as antacids are currently taken. The pharmacist should first be able to distinguish between those patients who are appropriate for self-treatment and those who need medical attention, and then be able to select appropriate antacids, H_2RAs, and/or antiflatulent products for patients with mild GI complaints.

Physiology of the Upper Gastrointestinal Tract

A basic understanding of the physiology of the esophagus, stomach, and duodenum (Figure 1) is essential to understanding the pathophysiology of GI disorders and the drugs used to treat them.

The esophagus is a hollow tube, approximately 18–25 cm long, which serves as a conduit between the pharynx and the stomach.[3] The esophagus is closed at both ends by the upper esophageal sphincter and the lower esophageal sphincter (LES). The LES is an area of specialized smooth muscle located at the lower end of the esophagus, about 2–5 cm above the junction where the stomach meets the esophagus. When at rest, the LES is contracted, creating a high-pressure zone that prevents the passage of stomach contents into the esophagus.[3] When swallowing occurs, the LES relaxes and allows food to pass freely into the stomach from the esophagus.

The stomach is divided into four anatomic regions: the cardia, fundus, body, and antrum. Little is known about the function of the cardia, the smallest region of the stomach. The body and fundus, which comprise the largest part of the stomach, contain the cells responsible for acid and pepsin secretion: parietal cells and chief cells. Parietal cells secrete hydrochloric acid and intrinsic factor (required for vitamin B_{12} absorption), whereas chief cells secrete pepsinogen, a precursor of pepsin.

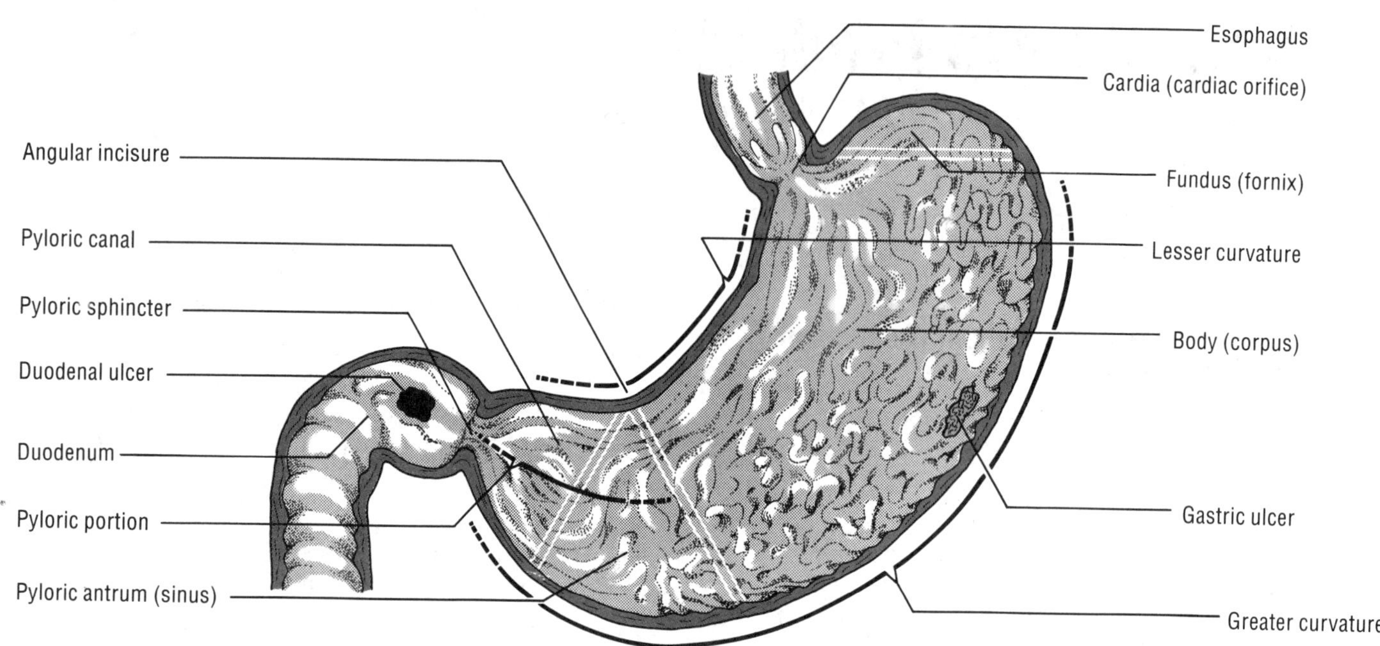

FIGURE 1 Sites of duodenal and gastric ulcers. Adapted from Netter FH. *The Ciba Collection of Medical Illustrations*. Vol 3, part II. New York: Ciba Pharmaceutical Company; 1962: 49, 52.

The antrum contains gastrin cells, which secrete the hormone gastrin into the circulation.

Gastric Acid Secretion

Gastric acid serves several important functions. Acid and pepsin are powerful proteolytic substances that hydrolyze protein and other foods so they can be absorbed by the intestine; thus, gastric acid aids in the digestion and absorption of food. In addition, gastric acid kills most bacteria in the stomach and helps to maintain a stable stomach environment.

The outer membrane of the parietal cell has receptors for (1) histamine released from mast cells in the stomach, (2) acetylcholine released from nerve endings in the stomach, and (3) gastrin, which reaches the parietal cell through the circulation. When any of these substances comes into contact with its receptors on the parietal cell, calcium and cyclic adenosine monophosphate (cAMP) concentrations within the cell increase.[4] The increased levels of calcium and cAMP activate the hydrogen/potassium (H^+/K^+) adenosine triphosphatase enzyme, which is located on the parietal cell and is referred to as the proton pump. When stimulated, the proton pump secretes hydrogen ions in the stomach lumen in exchange for potassium. The proton pump can respond directly to calcium and cAMP as well as indirectly to histamine, acetylcholine, and gastrin. Thus, the proton pump is the final common pathway for acid secretion from any stimuli.

The parietal cell serves as the target for pharmacologic inhibition of acid secretion. Anticholinergic agents inhibit acid secretion by occupying the acetylcholine receptor. H_2RAs reduce acid secretion by blocking the histamine receptor. Because the proton pump is the final step in acid secretion, proton pump inhibitors abolish acid secretion regardless of the stimulus.

Pepsinogen is released by the chief cells of the body and fundus in response to much the same stimuli as acid from the parietal cell—that is, vagal stimulation, histamine, and acetylcholine. In the presence of acid, pepsinogen is hydrolyzed to the active proteolytic enzyme pepsin. Pepsin is active when pH ranges from 1.8 to 3.5 and is inactivated when pH exceeds 5.[5]

The rate and amount of acid that the parietal cell secretes depend on whether the stomach has been stimulated or is in the basal state. Both basal and stimulated acid outputs vary considerably among individuals and are generally higher in men than in women. Basal acid secretion follows a circadian rhythm, with peak secretion occurring in the evening and lowest secretion in the morning.[5]

Gastric Mucosal Barrier

The gastric mucosa is equipped to withstand the acidic environment of the stomach through a combination of defense and repair mechanisms that are collectively called the gastric mucosal barrier. A major component of this barrier is the epithelial cells that line the entire surface of the stomach as well as the duodenum. These cells secrete both mucus and bicarbonate to form a protective mucus gel layer between the gastric lumen and the mucosa.[4] The high-viscosity mucus limits the penetration of hydrogen ions across the mucosa, while the bicarbonate allows a pH gradient to develop between the acidic stomach lumen and the more alkaline surface of the mucosa. The mucus-bicarbonate layer thus acts as a physical and chemical barrier to prevent diffusion of hydrogen ions across the mucosa. When this mucosal barrier is disrupted, rapid mucosal blood flow removes any hydrogen ion that has diffused across the barrier. When damage does occur, the epithelial cells have a unique ability to repair themselves quickly through rapid cell turnover. This process, known as restitution or reconstitution, is aided by the delivery of oxygen and other nutrients to the cells by the mucosal blood supply.[4]

Prostaglandins are also a vital component of the gastric mucosal barrier. Prostaglandin E_2 is synthesized by the gastric mucosa and works to enhance its protective mechanisms.[4] Prostaglandins inhibit gastric acid secretion from the parietal cells as well as increase mucus and bicarbonate secretion from the epithelial cells. Prostaglandins also help maintain mucosal blood flow and thus help remove back-diffused hydrogen ions.

Acid-Peptic Disorders

The maintenance of normal, healthy gastroduodenal mucosa is often described as a balance between the aggressive forces of acid and pepsin and the defensive forces of the gastric mucosal barrier.[4,5] As long as the gastric mucosal barrier is healthy and intact, the stomach is protected from acid and pepsin. When this barrier is disrupted, however, acid and pepsin predominate and mucosal injury or ulceration occurs. Although acid and pepsin play a critical role in the pathogenesis of acid-peptic diseases, a breakdown in mucosal defense is equally important in determining whether disease will occur. Virtually all factors implicated in the etiology of these diseases affect this critical balance by increasing aggressive factors, impairing mucosal defenses, or altering both sides of the balance.

Peptic Ulcer Disease

PUD is a group of chronic disorders characterized by ulcerating mucosal lesions in the upper GI tract. The most common sites of PUD are the duodenum and the stomach. Duodenal ulcers (DUs) characteristically occur in the first portion of the duodenum, or the duodenal bulb, and are usually from 1 mm to 1 cm in diameter. Most gastric ulcers (GUs) occur in the antrum of the stomach and are surrounded by a widespread area of chronic gastritis.[4,6] DUs typically affect persons 25–55 years of age while the peak incidence of GUs occurs around 55–65 years of age.[5]

Pathogenesis

Current understanding of the pathogenesis of PUD has undergone a revolution over the past several decades. Acid was previously thought to be the most important factor in the development of peptic ulcers, giving rise to the common phrase "No acid, no ulcer." However, only about 30–50% of patients with DUs secrete excess acid, whereas GU patients secrete normal or less than normal amounts.[4] Today, it is recognized that although acid must be present for ulcers to develop, it does not usually cause ulcers in the absence of factors that disrupt the gastric mucosal barrier. The two most important factors that disturb this barrier and thus promote ulcer development are *Helicobacter pylori* and nonsteroidal anti-inflammatory drugs (NSAIDs).

Helicobacter pylori *H pylori* is a gram-negative aerobic bacillus that colonizes the epithelial cells lining the surface of the stomach, where it causes inflammation and potential ulceration. The organism may also adhere to islands of gastric epithelium, or gastric metaplasia, in the duodenum or other areas of the GI tract.[4,7,8] *H pylori* has a unique ability to survive in the normal gastric mucosa by burrowing under the mucus-bicarbonate layer, where it is protected from acid. The bacterium produces large amounts of urease, an enzyme that generates bicarbonate and ammonium from urea, thus neutralizing the lethal effects of gastric acid.[4,7,8] It is thought that *H pylori* produces an enzyme that degrades gastric mucus, thus exposing the gastric epithelium and making it an easy target for back-diffused hydrogen ions. However, numerous mechanisms of damage have been proposed, and further studies are needed to clarify their contribution to the pathogenesis of PUD.[7]

Since 1982, when *H pylori* was first isolated from patients with gastritis, overwhelming epidemiologic and clinical evidence has been published that implicates the organism in the etiology of PUD. Virtually all patients (95–100%) with DUs and more than 95% of patients with GUs that are not caused by NSAIDs harbor the organism.[4,6] Recently, a National Institutes of Health (NIH) Consensus Development Panel declared that infection with *H pylori* is a prerequisite for the development of ulcers in the absence of other precipitating factors (eg, NSAIDs, hypersecretory conditions).[7]

PUD has historically been viewed as a chronic disease characterized by numerous recurrences. The dictum "Once an ulcer, always an ulcer" was derived from observations that up to 80% of ulcer patients relapsed within 1 year of initial healing with conventional therapy (eg, H_2RAs or sucralfate).[4] However, mounting evidence demonstrates dramatic reductions in recurrence rates in patients in whom *H pylori* has been eradicated.[3–8] Indeed, unless reinfection occurs, it is rare for an ulcer to recur once the organism has been cleared. The fact that *H pylori* eradication can alter the natural course of PUD is perhaps the strongest evidence for a causative role of the organism in this disorder.

NSAIDs NSAIDs are the most common cause of ulcers in patients who are not infected with *H pylori*. It is estimated that 14 million Americans use NSAIDs chronically and that 25% of these chronic users will develop an ulcer.[4,9] Most NSAID-induced ulcers occur in the stomach; GUs are at least four times more likely than DUs.[4] NSAIDs produce a dual insult to the gastric mucosa by (1) causing direct, topical damage and (2) inhibiting prostaglandin synthesis. The risk of developing NSAID-induced ulcers and/or complications increases with advancing age, previous history of peptic ulcer or GI bleeding, higher doses of NSAIDs, concomitant cardiovascular disease, and concomitant use of corticosteroids.[4,9] Patients taking other ulcerogenic medications (eg, methotrexate, cyclophosphamide, azathioprine) or medications that predispose them to bleeding (eg, warfarin) with an NSAID may also be more likely to develop an ulcer. Some studies have found that smoking and heavy intake of alcohol also increase the risk for NSAID-induced ulceration.[4]

Other Factors Several other factors have been implicated in the development of peptic ulcers. Smoking doubles the incidence of PUD, increases ulcer recurrence, and reduces ulcer healing with H_2RAs.[4] A genetic influence is supported by the fact that first-degree relatives of patients with PUD have a two- to threefold risk of developing the disease.[4] However, this observation may stem from the clustering of *H pylori* within families rather than from genetic factors. Alcohol is not a proven risk factor for PUD except in patients with cirrhosis.[4] Although stress and psychologic factors are widely believed to contribute to PUD, there is no clearly established ulcer-type personality, and this relationship remains controversial.[4,5]

Signs and Symptoms

The most frequent symptom of PUD is epigastric pain (in the upper abdomen). This pain is often described as burning, annoying, or gnawing, or as a dull ache resembling hunger pain.[4] The pain is usually relieved within 5–10 minutes of eating or taking antacids. About 50–80% of ulcer patients report being awakened with pain at night, usually between midnight and 3:00 AM, when gastric acid secretion is maximal and food that could buffer the acid is absent.[3] The pain is usually not present in the morning on awakening. Nausea and vomiting, diarrhea, a sense of fullness, and abdominal distention are fairly common with GUs but less so with DUs. For these reasons, weight loss is common in patients with GUs (benign and malignant) and may be profound (up to 30–50 lb). However, because symptoms overlap, DUs and GUs often cannot be distinguished without diagnostic testing.

Although most patients with PUD have symptoms, there is very poor correlation between these symptoms and ulceration. This is especially true of patients with NSAID-associated ulcers, more than half of whom are asymptomatic. In fact, 60–80% of such patients have a major hemorrhage or perforation as the first clinical sign that an ulcer is present.[10,11] Asymptomatic disease is particularly likely in elderly patients.

The most common complication of PUD is bleeding, which occurs in about 20% of all patients.[4] Bleeding may occur at all ages but is more common in patients over age 60. Other major complications include perforation, penetration, and gastric outlet obstruction. Complications from GUs are associated with higher morbidity and mortality rates than those from DUs, probably because GUs tend to occur in older persons.[4,5]

Treatment

Patients who describe a history and symptoms consistent with PUD or NSAID-induced gastropathy should be referred to a health care provider rather than self-medicate with antacids or H_2RAs. This is especially important for elderly patients and/or those with symptoms suggestive of ulcer complications such as severe, intractable pain; blood in stools; nausea; or vomiting coffee grounds–like material. Patients who have experienced significant weight loss should also be advised to consult a health care provider since this may be a sign of complicated PUD and/or gastric malignancy.

Use of Prescription Drugs Traditionally, the goals of therapy for PUD have been to promote ulcer healing, relieve pain, prevent complications, and prevent recurrences. Since the introduction of cimetidine in 1977, H_2RAs have been the preferred agents to achieve these goals because of their efficacy, patient acceptance, and favorable side effects profile. At equipotent doses administered twice daily or once at bedtime, H_2RAs can be expected to heal about 85–90% of DUs in 8 weeks and about 80–90% of GUs after 8–12 weeks of therapy.[4] When used as maintenance therapy, these agents are effective at reducing recurrence rates of ulcers. Sucralfate is as effective as the H_2RAs in healing and reducing recurrence rates of DUs but is not approved for healing or maintenance of GUs. Ulcer healing may also be accomplished with proton pump inhibitors, which tend to achieve faster symptomatic relief and healing rates than H_2RAs.

Eradication of Helicobacter pylori Increasingly, the goals for PUD are being met by eradication of *H pylori*, which is now viewed by many as a cure for PUD. The recent NIH Consensus Panel recommended that ulcer patients with *H pylori* infection be treated with antibiotics in addition to antisecretory agents, regardless of whether the patients are suffering from the initial presentation of the disease or from a recurrence.[7] Triple drug therapy with tetracycline, bismuth subsalicylate (BSS), and metronidazole produces eradication rates of nearly 90%.[7] Other regimens currently being used for *H pylori* eradication include combinations of antisecretory agents such as H_2RA or proton pump inhibitors with antibiotics such as amoxicillin, clarithromycin, metronidazole, or tetracycline.[4,7,8] Successful eradication of *H pylori* modestly reduces time to ulcer healing, enhances healing of refractory ulcers, and substantially reduces the rate of ulcer recurrence (to <10% per year).[7]

Use of Antacids Although antacids are no longer used routinely to heal ulcers, they were the mainstay of therapy for PUD until the late 1970s, when H_2RAs became available. It was not until 1977, however, that antacids were actually proven effective in healing ulcers.[12] High doses of a liquid aluminum-magnesium antacid given seven times a day (1 and 3 hours after each meal and at bedtime) were shown to heal 78% of DUs in 4 weeks. The rationale for this intensive dosing regimen was the assumption that it was necessary to keep the gastric pH continuously elevated throughout the day. Several studies have found such high-dose antacid regimens (560–1,008 mEq acid-neutralizing capacity [ANC] per day) to be comparable to standard doses of H_2RAs in healing both DUs and GUs.[13,14] Antacids also heal most small NSAID-induced ulcers within 12 weeks, whether or not NSAIDs are continued.[13] Additionally, at least two studies have found that antacids given two to four times daily effectively reduce the rate of DU relapse.[13]

Recent interest in the mucosal protective effects of antacids has prompted studies to examine the potential of lower doses of antacids in healing ulcers. Several studies have found that doses as low as 120–200 mEq per day of buffering capacity produce DU healing rates equivalent to those found in studies using the higher traditional doses.[13,14] The buffering capacity of such doses is modest at best. Other studies have demonstrated medium (414 mEq ANC per day) or lower doses of antacids to be comparable to standard doses of H_2RAs[15,16]; however, frequency of dosing in these studies has been six to seven times a day—an inconvenient schedule for patients. Several studies have shown that neither this frequency of administration nor high doses of antacid are necessary to promote healing.[13,17] In most of these studies, antacid tablets (120 mEq per day) given four times daily (1 hour after meals and at bedtime) healed DUs more effectively than placebo and as effectively as cimetidine. Similar doses of antacids have healed GUs better than placebo.[18] To date, only full doses of antacids have been shown to heal NSAID-induced ulcers effectively.

Despite an equal ability to heal ulcers, antacids are not favored as first-line therapy over prescription agents for PUD. Standard high-dose regimens for healing ulcers are 80–160 mEq ANC taken 1 and 3 hours after meals and at bedtime. Antacids should be given 1 hour after meals because food buffers gastric acid for about an hour. When given 1 and 3 hours after meals, antacids will neutralize acid for approximately 2 hours. In this way, the gastric pH is continuously elevated throughout the day. However, achieving this goal requires taking 1–2 tbsp seven times a day of a liquid that is often unpalatable. These high doses often cause changes in bowel habits (eg, diarrhea) and are inconvenient and expensive. If additional studies substantiate the effectiveness of low-dose antacids, those regimens may prove more acceptable to patients. Low-dose antacids would also offer a cost-effective alternative for healing ulcers and might be considered a practical therapeutic option for PUD.

Currently, the primary role of antacids in PUD is to provide additional pain relief for patients already taking prescription agents for healing, maintenance, or eradication of *H pylori*. However, whether antacids relieve ulcer pain better than placebo has been difficult to determine from clinical trials. A significant problem in interpreting results of these trials is the large placebo response (up to 50%) observed in patients.[4] Accordingly, some ulcer patients report significant pain relief from antacids while others do not.

When antacids are recommended for supplemental pain relief, patients should be advised to take doses providing 40–80 mEq neutralizing capacity. These doses may be taken on an as-needed basis and may be titrated upward if needed. Because antacids can reduce the bioavailability of H_2RAs, doses should be separated by 1–2 hours.[19,20] Most patients will need supplemental antacids for pain relief only for the first 7–14 days of treatment. However, healing cannot be expected before 4–6 weeks for DUs and often takes longer for GUs.[4] Pharmacists should educate patients regarding the poor correlation between pain relief and ulcer healing. Patients should also be made aware that the potential for undertreatment exists if they do not continue their antiulcer regimens for the full treatment duration even when their symptoms have resolved. Conversely, the lack of pain relief with an agent does not mean that an ulcer is not healing properly. Patients who are taking antacids or other medications and whose pain has not yet resolved should contact their health care providers, but should not discontinue their medication even though they feel their ulcer is not healing.

Use of Nonprescription H_2-Receptor Antagonists Currently, nonprescription H_2RAs are not approved for the healing or maintenance of PUD, nor are they indicated for symptomatic relief of pain associated with ulcers. Patients wishing to self-medicate with these agents should be questioned about their symptoms, history of GI disorders, and use of prescription medications. Some patients may not understand that nonprescription H_2RAs are simply lower doses of the prescription agents they are already taking. If patients are already receiving antisecretory agents (ie, prescription H_2RAs, proton pump inhibitors) for ulcer healing or maintenance, it is unlikely that the addition of nonprescription doses of H_2RAs will provide any significant additive benefit.

It is possible that patients may take more than the recommended doses of the nonprescription H_2RAs in an attempt to treat ulcers with prescription doses they have previously used. This type of manipulation should be actively discouraged because medical supervision is necessary to confirm the diagnosis, rule out other serious disorders and complications, and monitor the success of therapy. An additional risk in increasing doses is the increased potential for drug interactions with cimetidine, given that cimetidine inhibits drug metabolism in a dose-dependent fashion.

Although antacids may alleviate dyspeptic symptoms associated with NSAID use, they have not been found to prevent the development of NSAID ulcers.[9,21] Since prescription doses of H_2RAs do not appear to prevent NSAID-induced GUs, nonprescription H_2RAs cannot be expected to prevent them, either. It is possible, however, that H_2RAs would relieve dyspeptic symptoms associated with NSAID use. Considering the poor correlation between symptoms and NSAID damage, it is unclear whether suppressing these symptoms with antacids will benefit patients or mask signs of serious mucosal injury. It is not possible to predict with a high degree of accuracy who will develop an NSAID-induced ulcer.[4] However, it is prudent for the pharmacist to refer patients with NSAID-associated dyspeptic symptoms for medical evaluation if they are at high risk for, or would not tolerate, complications of an NSAID-induced ulcer. Such patients include the elderly, smokers, those using corticosteroids concomitantly, those with a history of PUD or GI bleeding, those using high doses of NSAIDS, and those with concomitant cardiovascular disease.[4,9] Otherwise, antacids or H_2RAs taken as needed may provide adequate symptomatic relief and allow for continued NSAID therapy.

Nondrug Measures Since the 1940s, special diets have been recommended for the management of PUD. These diets have typically consisted of bland foods given in multiple small feedings throughout the day. However, there appears to be no benefit with such diets.[4] Although food relieves ulcer pain and buffers gastric acid for approximately 30–60 minutes, each meal results in an increased acid load for several hours. Therefore, patients should be encouraged to eat three meals a day of their own choosing and should avoid eating snacks at night, which will increase nocturnal acid secretion. The restriction of spicy foods does not speed ulcer healing, but patients should avoid foods that cause dyspeptic symptoms. Because they increase acid secretion significantly, coffee (both caffeinated and decaffeinated), caffeine-containing beverages, and alcohol are the only items that ulcer patients should eliminate from their diets.[4] Additionally, ulcer patients should be encouraged to stop smoking.

The frequent ingestion of milk has traditionally been recommended to buffer acid in patients with PUD. However, milk is a very poor buffering agent, and the calcium and protein in milk actually stimulate acid secretion.[4] Despite its historical popularity, the use of milk for ulcer disease is without scientific basis and should not be encouraged.

Gastroesophageal Reflux Disease

The reflux of gastric contents into the esophagus, or gastroesophageal reflux, is generally a benign physiologic process that occurs in normal individuals. In fact, virtually everyone experiences multiple episodes of gastroesophageal reflux throughout the day, particularly after meals. Most of these episodes are unnoticed and do not cause symptoms or mucosal damage to the esophagus. However, gastroesophageal reflux does produce symptoms in some individuals and may cause tissue damage to the esophagus, oropharynx, larynx, and respiratory system.[22] Patients who suffer symptoms or tissue damage as a result of gastroesophageal reflux are said to suffer from GERD. What distinguishes patients with GERD from those with normal physiologic reflux is the frequency and duration of reflux episodes, resulting in related signs and symptoms and/or esophageal tissue damage.

The most common form of GERD is reflux esophagitis, which develops when there is prolonged contact of the acidic contents of the stomach with esophageal tissue. This contact may produce a broad range of damage, such as inflammation, hyperplasia, esophageal erosions, or ulcerations.[22] The typical complaint of patients with reflux esophagitis is heartburn, which is probably one of the most common symptoms a pharmacist is asked to treat. The incidence of heartburn is high in the American population: 7% of adult Americans experience it daily and 45% experience it at least once a month.[23] Most individuals with GERD have only mild and sporadic symptoms. Accordingly, most patients do not seek medical attention from a physician but rather seek symptomatic relief from antacid products. Pregnant women experience GERD frequently, with about 25% complaining of heartburn daily. However, patients with heartburn do not necessarily have reflux esophagitis, given that 60–70% of patients complaining of heartburn do not have mucosal injury to the esophagus.[23]

Pathogenesis

Like that of PUD, the pathogenesis of GERD can be described as an imbalance between aggressive and protective factors. The aggressive side of this balance is determined by the noxious quality of the gastric contents that reflux into the esophagus. Most patients with GERD secrete normal or greater than normal amounts of gastric acid and thus have acidic refluxates. The factors that normally protect the esophagus from this acid refluxate include (1) antireflux barriers that limit the rate of reflux, (2) clearance mechanisms that limit the duration of contact of refluxate with the epithelium, and (3) esophageal mucosal resistance that minimizes epithelial damage from noxious gastric contents.[22]

The major barrier that prevents the passage of stomach contents into the esophagus is the LES. Normal individuals experience transient relaxations of the LES multiple times throughout the day. Patients with GERD, however, tend to have more transient relaxations of the LES and thus reflux more often than healthy individuals. Many patients with GERD also have a weak, or hypotonic, LES.[22,24] In such patients, the high pressure in the stomach creates enough force to overcome the weak squeeze of the LES and allows reflux to occur. Many factors may promote reflux by reducing LES tone, delaying gastric emptying, increasing acid secretion, or impairing the gastroesophageal pressure gradient (Table 1).

After reflux occurs, the symptoms and degree of damage depend on the duration of contact between the gastric contents and the esophageal mucosa.[24] The esophagus normally clears the refluxate by one to two peristaltic contractions induced by swallowing. Gravity speeds up this process when the patient is upright, but it does not operate when the patient is lying down.[22] The residual acid refluxate in the esophagus is then neutralized by bicarbonate-rich saliva that has been swallowed. A defect in one or both of these processes may lead to increased contact time with refluxed material and the development of esophagitis. These mechanisms are impaired during sleep, when there is neither swallowing nor salivation and when clearance by gravity is not operative. Thus, prolonged acid exposure may occur during sleep and predispose patients to esophagitis.[22,24]

Although the esophagus does not have a well-defined mucosal barrier like the stomach and duodenum have, its cells are structurally designed to limit penetration of hydrogen ions into the epithelium.[22] However, the contribution of cellular defense mechanisms to GERD is currently uncertain.

Signs and Symptoms

The classic symptom of GERD is heartburn, or pyrosis, occurring in more than half of patients with this disorder.[25] Heartburn is usually described by the patient as a burning sensation or pain located in the lower chest (substernal area). The pain may radiate up into the chest, to the back, and, less often, into the throat.[25] Most patients complain of heartburn soon after meals and upon lying down at bedtime, and they may be awakened from sleep because of the pain. Heartburn may also occur when the patient bends or stoops over and after some forms of exercise. Some patients have brief episodes of heartburn that are readily relieved by antacids or simple dietary measures; others have persistent and severe symptoms that disrupt their daily lives. The severity of the symptoms of GERD does not correlate well with the severity of esophageal mucosal damage.

TABLE 1 Factors that promote gastroesophageal reflux disease

Reduced lower esophageal sphincter tone

Smoking

Beverages and foods
- Alcohol
- Caffeine
- Chocolates
- Fatty, greasy foods
- Spearmint
- Peppermint

Medications
- Anticholinergic agents
- $Beta_2$-agonists
- Calcium channel antagonists
- Diazepam
- Dopamine
- Estrogen
- Meperidine
- Morphine
- Nitrates
- Progesterone
- Prostaglandins
- Tricyclic antidepressants

Delayed gastric emptying

Anticholinergic medications
Overeating
Motility disorder

Increased acid secretion

Smoking

Beverages and foods
- Alcohol
- Citrus fruits
- Coffee
- Garlic
- Milk
- Onions
- Soda
- Spicy foods
- Tomatoes, tomato-based foods

Hypersecretory conditions
- Duodenal ulcers
- Endocrine adenomas
- Zollinger-Ellison syndrome

Impaired gastroesophageal pressure gradient

Supine body position
Obesity
Tight-fitting clothing

Adapted from *Pepcid AC New Product Bulletin*. Washington, DC: American Pharmaceutical Association; August 1995.

Some patients with GERD may complain of chest pain that is not typical of heartburn. Atypical chest pain due to reflux is difficult to distinguish from anginal chest pain due to ischemic heart disease.[22] Like anginal pain, this atypical chest pain may be sharp or dull and may radiate widely, extending into the neck or arms.

Other symptoms of reflux disease may occur with or without heartburn. Regurgitation is an extension of the reflux process, with gastric contents entering the mouth. Patients complain of an acid, burning, or bitter taste and may refer to this problem as "sour stomach."[25] Patients with delayed gastric emptying often complain of bloating, early satiety, belching, and nausea. Dysphagia, which is a sensation of slow or blocked passage of food from the mouth to the esophagus, may indicate an esophageal stricture (narrowing of the esophageal lumen), cancer, or motility disorder. Odynophagia, or pain on swallowing, may occur and usually suggests severe mucosal damage in the esophagus.[25]

Complications of GERD include acute and chronic bleeding from esophageal ulcers, esophageal strictures, and pulmonary complications (eg, cough, bronchitis, pneumonia) resulting from the aspiration of refluxed material into the upper airways and lungs. Approximately 10–15% of patients with erosive esophagitis develop Barrett's esophagus.[22] Barrett's esophagus is associated with midesophageal strictures, esophageal ulcers, and histologic changes in the lower esophageal mucosa that may become cancerous in 5–10% of patients.[24]

Treatment

The pharmacist will often be the first health care professional encountered by patients with GERD. Thus, the pharmacist has a unique opportunity and responsibility to ensure that patients' symptoms are appropriate for self-medication. Any patient who describes difficulty or pain when swallowing may have developed complications from GERD and should be referred to a health care provider for evaluation. Gastric cancer might be suspected in patients who report significant, unintentional weight loss or in patients older than 45 years who report a new onset of symptoms. Patients whose symptoms are suggestive of anginal pain, such as crushing chest pain that worsens with physical activity, also warrant referral. The reader is directed to the Patient Assessment section for more information regarding the clinical differences between ischemic and reflux-type pain.

The management of GERD may be viewed as a stepped-care approach, with antacids, nonprescription H_2RAs, and nondrug measures forming the basis for the first step (Figure 2). These measures may help to alleviate symptoms in patients with mild to moderate GERD but cannot be expected to heal damaged esophageal mucosa or prevent complications.[24]

Use of Antacids Antacids have long been the mainstay for patients needing symptomatic relief for mild to moderate GERD. They reduce the aggressive factors in GERD by neutralizing gastric acid and increasing the pH of refluxed gastric contents. As a result, the refluxed contents are not as damaging to the esophageal mucosa. Antacids also strengthen defensive forces because gastric alkalinization increases LES pressure.

Antireflux surgery	**Phase 3:** Refractory disease
Lansoprazole 30 mg/day Omeprazole 20–40 mg/day *or* Cimetidine 800 mg bid or 400 mg qid Ranitidine 150 mg qid Famotidine 40 mg bid Nizatidine 150 mg bid *and/or* Cisapride 10–20 mg ac & hs *or* Metoclopramide 10–20 mg ac & hs	**Phase 2B:** Severe mucosal damage
Cimetidine 400 mg bid or 300 mg qid Ranitidine 150 mg qid Famotidine 20 mg bid Nizatidine 150 mg bid *and/or* Metoclopramide 10–20 mg ac & hs *or* Cisapride 10–20 mg ac & hs	**Phase 2A:** Persistent symptoms Mucosal damage
Diet modification Weight loss Elevate head of bed Avoid drugs that decrease LES tone Restrict smoking and alcohol Avoid lying down after eating Avoid tight-fitting clothes *and* Antacids ± alginic acid 40–80 mEq ANC pc & hs *or* Cimetidine 200 mg bid Famotidine 10 mg bid Ranitidine 75 mg bid Nizatidine 75 mg bid	**Phase 1:** Mild/occasional symptoms Do not seek medical help

Lower esophageal sphincter (LES); acid neutralizing capacity (ANC).
Before meals (ac); after meals (pc); bedtime (hs); twice daily (bid); four times daily (qid).

FIGURE 2 Stepped-care approach to managing gastroesophageal reflux disease.

It is thought that the primary reason people take antacids is for heartburn and acid indigestion. Yet studies examining the benefit of antacids in treating GERD have reached conflicting results. At least three controlled studies found antacids superior to placebo for symptomatic relief, but two studies failed to find a significant benefit of antacids over placebo.[13,24] In those patients whose symptoms are relieved by antacids, relief usually occurs rapidly, within 5–15 minutes after administration, and can be expected to last from 1 to 3 hours, depending on the gastric emptying rate. Because of this short duration, patients taking antacids for GERD may need to take four to five doses throughout the day for adequate symptomatic relief. Similarly, antacids cannot be expected to neutralize acid adequately throughout the night. Nor have antacids been found to heal eroded esophageal mucosa adequately, as healing rates as low as 13–41% have been reported.[13]

Patients seeking relief from GERD with antacid therapy have used numerous dosage regimens. Treatment ranging from high doses of liquid aluminum-magnesium antacids (80–160 mEq ANC given seven times daily) to low doses of antacid tablets (14–30 mEq ANC/tablet) taken as needed have been reported to provide symptomatic relief.[13,26] Given this variability, it is reasonable to advise patients to begin with 40–80 mEq as needed for symptoms. If necessary, these doses may be titrated to a scheduled regimen, such as 40–80 mEq after meals and at bedtime.

Some antacid products also contain alginic acid. Alginic acid works by reacting with sodium bicarbonate and saliva to form a viscous solution of sodium alginate, which floats on the surface of gastric contents. When reflux occurs, sodium alginate rather than acid is refluxed and irritation is minimized. Products containing alginic acid are not as effective when patients are supine; therefore, patients receiving such products should be instructed not to lie down immediately after taking them. Similarly, it follows that products containing alginic acid are best suited for use throughout the day, whereas antacids may be taken throughout the day and/or at bedtime.

Use of Nonprescription H_2-Receptor Antagonists Like antacids, the nonprescription H_2RAs ranitidine, cimetidine, and famotidine are approved for the relief of heartburn, acid indigestion, and sour stomach. Famotidine and cimetidine, however, are also approved for *prevention* of these symptoms associated with food and beverages. The nonprescription form of nizatidine is approved *only for the prevention* of these symptoms. By decreasing gastric acid secretion, H_2RAs reduce the damaging potential of the refluxed gastric contents. While H_2RAs do not strengthen LES tone or reduce the frequency of reflux episodes, the refluxate is less damaging because it is less acidic.

To date, data supporting the use of famotidine 10 mg in the management of heartburn are limited. In a large controlled trial, patients were randomized to self-medicate with famotidine (5 mg, 10 mg, or 20 mg), aluminum-magnesium hydroxide antacid (11 mEq/tablet), or placebo for the relief of spontaneous, individual heartburn episodes.[27] Overall, after 4 weeks of treatment, heartburn episodes were relieved by all three doses of famotidine and by antacids, but not by placebo. None of the regimens, however, healed esophageal erosions.

An unexpected finding from this trial was that the onset of symptomatic relief with famotidine and antacids was similar, approximately 1½ hours for both. However, patients were instructed to report relief only when symptoms were completely, not partially, resolved. Based on kinetic parameters and clinical experience with these agents, some symptomatic relief should be expected within 15 minutes of antacid administration, whereas H_2RAs may not offer relief for 1–2 hours after administration.

The ability of famotidine 10 mg to prevent heartburn was studied in patients who could identify specific foods or beverages that provoked their symptoms.[28] In this study, patients were randomized to take famotidine (5 mg, 10 mg, or 20 mg) or placebo 1 hour before a test meal consisting of chili and red wine. In the first hour after the meal, heartburn severity was similar among the patients receiving placebo and famotidine. For the remainder of the time, however, heartburn was significantly milder in the patients receiving all three doses of famotidine than in those receiving placebo. Although other trials support the use of famotidine 10 mg and cimetidine 200 mg for the management of heartburn, the results are currently on file with the manufacturer and have not been published.[29,30]

Medical Referral When patients have pain that does not respond to conservative treatment with lifestyle modifications, antacids, and/or nonprescription H_2RAs, they should be referred for medical evaluation. Antacids and nonprescription doses of H_2RAs are unlikely to provide sufficient relief for patients with moderate to severe GERD, and certainly will not provide it for patients with complications. For such patients, successful healing and/or maintenance of GERD depends on achieving complete acid suppression for as long as possible.[31,32] This is not possible with antacids or nonprescription doses of H_2RAs. In contrast to PUD, moderate to severe GERD requires very high doses of prescription H_2RAs or proton pump inhibitors because damaged mucosa in the esophagus is more difficult to heal than that in the duodenum. Some patients may benefit from the addition of a prokinetic agent that stimulates esophageal motility, such as cisapride, metoclopramide, or bethanechol. Patients with recurring disease require maintenance therapy with full doses of H_2RAs, proton pump inhibitors, or antireflux surgery to restore competence of the LES.

Nondrug Measures Whereas dietary and lifestyle modifications have little proven benefit in treating PUD, conservative nondrug measures are considered a cornerstone of therapy for GERD. Before directing the patient to an acid-peptic product, the pharmacist should educate the patient regarding these lifestyle changes. Some patients with mild GERD can be managed with such measures alone and without pharmacologic intervention. Those who respond to antacids or nonprescription H_2RAs should still be educated about lifestyle modifications since these changes may significantly reduce or eliminate symptoms.

Nonpharmacologic interventions for patients with GERD attempt to reduce or eliminate factors that promote reflux. Because esophageal defenses are impaired during sleep, special effort should be made to improve esophageal clearance and to reduce the duration of nocturnal reflux.[22,24] Patients should be instructed to elevate the head of the bed 6 in. either with blocks or by placing a foam wedge under the patient's head. Patients should not try to raise the head of the bed by sleeping on pillows because this will cause them to bend at the waist and will actually increase intragastric pressure. Eating the evening meal at least 3 hours before going to bed to allow adequate time for gastric emptying also reduces reflux during sleep. Dietary suggestions for GERD are to (1) avoid foods that reduce LES tone (eg, chocolate, mints, and fats), (2) avoid foods that are direct irritants (eg, citrus juice, tomato products, and coffee), (3) reduce the size of meals, and (4) avoid lying down after meals (Table 1). Patients with GERD should be encouraged to stop smoking and limit their alcohol intake. Obese patients with GERD may have symptomatic improvement if they lose weight and avoid wearing tight-fitting clothing. It may be helpful to advise patients to avoid aerophagic habits, such as chewing gum, sucking on hard candy, or drinking carbonated beverages. Finally, patients with GERD should be questioned about the use of drugs that decrease LES pressure. When a drug is implicated in causing reflux, switching to a drug with similar therapeutic benefit but without an effect on the LES should be considered.

Gastritis

The term *gastritis* is often used too loosely to describe virtually any condition in the stomach. Of the various conditions usually described as gastritis, the one common feature is inflammation of the gastric mucosa. Gastritis may be classified as either acute erosive gastritis or chronic nonerosive gastritis.[4,33] Acute erosive gastritis is a short-lived inflammatory process characterized by superficial erosions or ulcerations of the stomach. Chronic nonerosive gastritis refers to the presence of gastric mucosal inflammation over an extended period without associated mucosal erosion or ulceration. Chronic nonerosive gastritis is classified into two types based on the anatomical location in the stomach. Type A gastritis is an autoimmune disease characterized by chronic inflammation of the acid-secreting mucosa of the fundus and body of the stomach.[33] Type B gastritis, which is more common, affects the mucus-secreting epithelial cells that line the antrum of the stomach.

Pathogenesis

The agents most often responsible for causing acute gastritis erosions are alcohol, aspirin, and other NSAIDs. Because pure ethanol is lipid soluble, it penetrates the gastric mucosal barrier and may cause acute mucosal erosions and hemorrhages.[4] The extent of damage appears to correlate with the ethanol concentration consumed. Acute mucosal injury does not appear to occur at ethanol concentrations of less than 10% (20 proof) but does occur when concentrations exceed 20% (40 proof).[4]

Type B gastritis is generally believed to be caused by *H pylori*.[7,33] Type B gastritis is more important because of the company it keeps (ie, DUs and GUs) rather than because of the symptoms it produces. GUs that are not associated with NSAIDs almost always occur within an area of chronic gastritis rather than in normal mucosa. *H pylori*–associated gastritis is also present in more than 99% of patients with DUs.[4,6,7]

Signs and Symptoms

Most patients with acute erosive gastritis are asymptomatic. A few patients complain of epigastric pain or discomfort, typically of a burning nature. Patients may also experience anorexia, nausea, and vomiting. The most common complication of acute erosive gastritis is upper GI bleeding. Most patients who bleed will have signs and symptoms of acute blood loss (hematemesis, melena, hypotension, or tachycardia). Less commonly, patients may have chronic bleeding, which may be detected by more subtle signs (black tarry stools, guaiac-positive stools, and symptoms of iron deficiency anemia).

Most patients with Type B gastritis do not have symptoms, but some patients may experience chronic dyspeptic symptoms. When symptoms do occur, they are likely to be epigastric pain, heartburn, anorexia, and vomiting.[34] Gastritis is slow in progression, may last for years or decades, and rarely heals spontaneously.

Treatment

Acute erosive gastritis usually heals spontaneously within a few days when the offending agent or condition is removed. Removing the cause of the condition, therefore, is the most important step in managing acute erosive gastritis; pharmacologic agents are rarely needed. Controlled studies supporting the benefit of antacids or H_2RAs in relieving symptoms are not generally available, but these agents are often offered to patients to provide symptomatic relief. Patients subjectively appear to obtain relief from antacids after a bout of heavy alcohol drinking or other conditions in which acute erosive gastritis is suspected. Thus, provided there is no evidence of bleeding, it is reasonable to recommend an antacid for such patients. In the absence of controlled trial data, it is logical to recommend standard doses (ie, 40–80 mEq ANC 1 and 3 hours after meals and at bedtime). The use of nonprescription H_2RAs for symptoms related to gastritis has not been evaluated.

Nonulcer Dyspepsia

Dyspepsia is a vague, misunderstood term that literally means "bad digestion." Clinicians and patients use this term to describe any abdominal discomfort, including epigastric pain, heartburn, nausea, bloating, belching, and indigestion. Patients are said to have nonulcer dyspepsia when they present with symptoms that prompt a clinician to believe an ulcer is present but no ulcer is found on evaluation.

Pathogenesis of Nonulcer Dyspepsia

The role of acid in the development of nonulcer dyspepsia is uncertain since most studies indicate that acid secretion is normal in these patients.[35] Studies have not found a clear relationship between nonulcer dyspepsia and *H pylori*, stress, emotions, personality, food, environmental factors (eg, smoking, alcohol, caffeine), genetic factors, or other diseases.[35,36] Until any of these factors is proven to be a pathogenetic feature, nonulcer dyspepsia remains a disease in search of a cause.

Signs and Symptoms of Nonulcer Dyspepsia

The typical patient with nonulcer dyspepsia presents with a chronic history (>3 months) of widespread abdominal symptoms, usually in relation to meals.[36] These symptoms are most often epigastric pain and nausea without vomiting, but they may include belching, indigestion, heartburn, bloating, and abdominal distention. Patients do not typically lose weight, and they may look surprisingly healthy given the magnitude and duration of symptoms they describe.[36] Nonulcer dyspepsia is a chronic condition that may persist over many years and become very troublesome for patients. However, it is generally a benign disease that is not associated with complications. There is no evidence that it leads to PUD or any other disorder.

Treatment of Nonulcer Dyspepsia

Antacids have been used to treat dyspepsia since the first century AD, when crushed coral (calcium carbonate) was given to patients complaining of such symptoms. Despite the widespread use of antacids for dyspeptic symptoms, however, there is little objective proof of their benefit. Neither high doses of liquid aluminum-magnesium antacid (400 mEq ANC per day, given 1 and 3 hours after meals and at bedtime) or low doses of aluminum-magnesium tablets (120 mEq ANC per day, given 1 hour after meals and at bedtime) have proven superior to placebo in controlled trials.[13,35] Controlled trials with prescription H_2RAs have yielded inconsistent results, and there are no published trials with nonprescription H_2RAs.

Intestinal Gas

A common patient complaint heard by pharmacists is that of intestinal gas, which may present as excessive belching, abdominal discomfort, bloating, and/or flatulence. Despite the frequency of such symptoms, their pathogenesis is poorly understood and treatment is far from satisfactory (see the section Antiflatulents).

Patient Assessment

The most valuable service the pharmacist can provide to patients with GI complaints is to determine whether their symptoms are amenable to self-treatment or need medical attention. Patients presenting with dyspeptic symptoms should be carefully questioned to rule out pain related to ischemic heart disease, complications of GERD or PUD, or other serious conditions that warrant medical attention. Important clues in determining the nature of the problem include:

- The type, severity, and location of the pain;
- Whether the pain radiates;
- The presence of other symptoms, such as nausea, vomiting, bloody stools, weight loss, or pain or difficulty on swallowing;
- Whether symptoms are exacerbated by certain foods, lying down, or exercise;
- Whether the symptoms are relieved by food, antacids, or H_2RAs;
- Medication history;
- Personal and family history of acid-peptic disorders.

Distinguishing between anginal pain and pain due to GERD may be difficult, if not impossible, when judgment is based solely on a patient's clinical presentation. However, the pharmacist should ask specific questions to determine whether the classic features of ischemic pain are present. Although both types of pain may radiate into the jaw and arm, severe, crushing chest pain, especially if accompanied by sweating, strongly suggests ischemic pain and possibly myocardial infarction. Pain that is exacerbated by physical activity or exercise but that subsides with rest or nitroglycerin is consistent with anginal pain rather than with GERD. When a patient's medication profile includes calcium channel antagonists, nitrates, and/or beta-blockers, the pharmacist should certainly suspect ischemic disease. However, the ability of calcium channel antagonists and nitrates to lower LES tone may also worsen GERD and confuse the clinical picture. Ischemic pain should also be suspected when a patient describes pain that has not responded to antacids or H_2RAs within a reasonable amount of time. After questioning the patient, if ischemic pain is clearly evident or if the type of pain cannot be determined and there are reasonable grounds to suspect angina, the pharmacist should refer the patient for immediate medical evaluation. Even then, numerous diagnostic tests may be necessary to determine the cause of the pain.

Patients who describe pain or difficulty in swallowing may have developed complicated GERD (eg, esophageal stricture, Barrett's esophagus) and will require medical evaluation. Those who describe severe, incapacitating pain may be suffering from complicated PUD, acute pancreatitis, gallbladder disease, or a number of other serious disorders that warrant referral. Significant, unintentional weight loss should always be taken seriously as it often accompanies malignancies. Finally, vomiting blood or material that looks like coffee grounds (hematemesis) or producing black tarry stools with a distinctive foul odor (melena) are serious signs, both of which signal acute blood loss and indicate that bleeding is occurring or has recently occurred. By the time melena develops, the patient has already lost at least 200 mL of blood.[37] Thus, it is essential that pharmacists give prompt attention to such complaints. Complaints and/or symptoms for which patients should be referred to a physician are summarized as follows[30]:

- Known allergy to H_2RAs;
- Possibility of being pregnant;
- Severe abdominal or back pain;
- Unexplained weight loss;
- Abdominal pain or heartburn that is unresponsive to antacid or nonprescription H_2RAs within 2 weeks or that recurs soon after stopping;
- Chest pain that is indistinguishable from heartburn;
- Difficulty or pain on swallowing;
- Presence or history of vomiting blood;
- Black, tarry bowel movements (if not taking iron or bismuth subsalicylate);
- Fever (temperature >100°F, [37.8°C]);
- Blood in urine;
- Elderly patients taking NSAIDs with the following risk factors for NSAID-induced ulceration and complications: concomitant use of corticosteroids, history of PUD, history of GI bleeding, concomitant cardiovascular disease, high doses of NSAIDs, smoking;
- Children younger than 12 years of age.

It is always important to question the patient about the use of both prescription and nonprescription drugs, paying special attention to the pattern of NSAID use. If the patient is taking a nonprescription drug, the brand name should be specified because patients may not be aware that certain combination products contain aspirin or ibuprofen. Because of the frequent asymptomatic nature of NSAID-induced ulcers, especially in elderly patients, it is not possible for the pharmacist to determine whether such an ulcer has developed. However, studies clearly indicate that risk factors for NSAID ulceration are (1) advanced age, (2) duration of NSAID use, (3) concomitant use of corticosteroids, (4) concomitant cardiovascular disease, and (5) history and/or complications of PUD. Based on these factors, if the pharmacist deems the patient at high risk for an NSAID-induced ulcer, it is prudent to refer the patient for medical evaluation.

Based on a patient's signs and symptoms, it may not be possible for the pharmacist to distinguish pain related to PUD from reflux-type pain. However, any patient describing classic symptoms of PUD (burning epigastric pain that is relieved by food) should be directed to a health care provider to confirm the diagnosis and initiate treatment with prescription agents.

Once serious disorders and complications have been ruled out, the pharmacist should assess whether the patient's symptoms are related to minor acid-peptic disorders such as heartburn or acid indigestion. The patient should be questioned about the relationship of the pain to eating because pain related to GERD usually occurs immediately after meals and can often be linked to specific foods, overeating, or overconsumption of alcohol. The pain is typically described as an uncomfortable, burning sensation in the upper chest area, and it is likely to have been relieved by antacids in the past. The pain may also be worsened by lying down or bending over, and it may waken patients at night. Patients who describe this type of pain are appropriate candidates for self-treatment with nonprescription acid-peptic products. In this regard, pharmacists will play a vital role in ensuring the safe transition of the H_2RAs to nonprescription status.

If antacids or H_2RAs are recommended in any of these situations and the patient does not experience prompt relief, the pharmacist should refer the patient to a physician for further evaluation. Similarly, symptoms that are relieved by these products but return often probably warrant medical attention.

Pharmacologic Agents

Healing and/or maintenance of peptic ulcers, NSAID-induced ulcers, severe GERD, and/or acute erosive esophagitis is accomplished with prescription doses of H_2RAs, sucralfate, or proton pump inhibitors, or by eradication of *H pylori* with antibiotic agents in combination with antisecretory medications. The primary aim of nonprescription medications in the treatment of acid-peptic disorders is to provide symptomatic relief, either alone or in conjunction with prescription medications (see product tables "Antacid and Antireflux Products" and "Histamine II Receptor Antagonists").

Antacids

Antacids neutralize gastric acid secreted by the parietal cells. Antacids only neutralize existing acid; they do not affect the amount or rate of gastric acid secreted. Antacids increase pH in both the stomach and the duodenal bulb, with a greater effect on duodenal pH than on gastric pH. Antacids do not neutralize all stomach acid; with usual therapeutic doses, they do not raise and cannot maintain gastric pH over 4–5.[26] However, when the pH is increased from 1.3 to 2.3, 90% of acid is neutralized, and at a pH of 3.3, 99% is neutralized.[26]

Antacids also inhibit the conversion of pepsinogen to pepsin, which depends on the degree of acid neutralization. Pepsin is most active at a pH of 1.8–3, and progressive inhibition occurs as gastric pH increases.[5,26] At a pH of 4 or greater, pepsin activity is completely inhibited. Additionally, aluminum-containing antacids have been reported to bind pepsin.[26]

Various other pharmacologic actions of antacids have been reported. Antacids that contain aluminum hydroxide have a strong binding capacity for bile salts with an affinity comparable to that of cholestyramine.[38] Magnesium hydroxide and aluminum phosphate antacids also appear to bind bile salts but not as strongly as aluminum. Aluminum antacids appear to delay gastric emptying, presumably because the aluminum ion relaxes the smooth muscle of the stomach. Alkalinization of gastric contents by antacids generally increases LES tone, which may partially account for its benefit in GERD. Additionally, antacids have been shown in one study to suppress *H pylori* infection, but this finding has not been reproduced in other trials.[39]

Antacids may have healing and protective actions beyond and independent of their neutralizing capacities. Animal studies have found antacids to stimulate several components of the gastric mucosal barrier, including bicarbonate and mucus secretion, mucosal cell regeneration, and mucosal blood flow.[13] Because antacids act locally and do not penetrate the mucosa, they may enhance these mechanisms by increasing the release of prostaglandins. One of the few studies in human gastric mucosa demonstrated an increase in mucosal prostaglandins after low-dose antacid therapy.[40]

Potency

The potency of antacids should be expressed in terms of mEq of ANC—that is, the amount of acid buffered per dose over a specified period. The Food and Drug Administration (FDA) requires that an antacid product neutralize at least 5 mEq per dose and must maintain the pH over 3.5 for 10 minutes in an in vitro test.[2] Any ingredient in a product must contribute at least 25% of the total ANC of the product to be called an antacid.

The neutralizing capacities of antacid products vary considerably, depending on the product's ingredient(s), formulation, and manufacturer (Table 2). Because the neutralizing capacity of 15 mL of liquid antacid may vary from 6 mEq in a low-potency formulation to 60 mEq in a concentrated or high-potency formulation, equal volumes of antacids are not equipotent. Consequently, antacids should be dosed according to the mEq ANC rather than by the volume or number of tablets. Aluminum-magnesium combination products offer adequate neutralizing capacity with the least potential for side effects.

Onset and Duration of Action

An antacid's onset of neutralizing action depends on how fast the product dissolves in gastric acid. Sodium bicarbonate and magnesium hydroxide dissolve quickly at gastric pH and provide a rapid buffering effect. Aluminum hydroxide and calcium carbonate dissolve slowly in stomach acid, and it may take 10–30 minutes for any significant neutralization to take place. Antacid suspensions generally dissolve more easily in gastric acid than do tablets or powders.

An antacid's duration of action depends on how long the product remains in the stomach, which is determined by gastric emptying time. If taken on an empty stomach, antacids are rapidly emptied from the stomach and have a duration of action of only 20–40 minutes.[41] However, gastric emptying is greatly slowed by the presence of food; thus, antacids taken after meals leave the stomach more slowly. When taken 1 hour after meals, antacids may neutralize acid for up to 3 hours. Sodium bicarbonate and magnesium hydroxide have the shortest duration of neutralizing action, while aluminum hydroxide and calcium carbonate have the longest. Combination aluminum-magnesium antacids have an intermediate duration of neutralizing action.

Formulation

The formulation of an antacid is important for neutralizing capacity as well as for patient acceptance and compliance. The most popular antacid formulations, liquids (suspensions) and tablets, differ significantly with regard to neutralizing capacity and patient acceptance.

TABLE 2 Potency of antacid products

Antacid suspensions	mEq ANC per mL[a]	Equivalent volume[b]
Riopan Extra Strength	6	13.3
Extra Strength Maalox Plus	5.8	13.8
Maalox-TC	5.44	14.7
Mylanta II	5.08	15.7
Gelusil-II	4.8	16.7
Camalox	3.7	21.6
AlternaGEL	3.2	25
Riopan Plus	3	26.7
Milk of Magnesia	2.8	28.6
Maalox	2.66	30
Mylanta	2.54	31.5
Di-Gel	2.45	32.7
Gelusil	2.4	33.3
Basaljel	2.4	33.3
Titralac Plus	2.2	36.4
Kolantyl Gel	2.1	38.1
Amphojel	2	40
Gaviscon	0.8	100

Antacid tablets	mEq ANC per tablet[a]	Equivalent number of tablets[b]
Maalox TC	28	3
Riopan Plus 2	30	3
Extra Strength Maalox	23.4	4
Mylanta II	23	4
Gelusil-II	21	4
Camalox	18	5
Amphojel (600 mg)	16	5
Riopan Plus	13.5	6
Temp	14.4	6
Tums E-X	15	6
Basaljel	13	7
Mylanta	11.5	7
Maalox Plus	11.4	7
Tums	10	8
Gelusil	11	8
Maalox	9.7	9
Rolaids Sodium-Free	8.5	10
Titralac	7.5	11
Gaviscon	0.5	160

[a]Acid-neutralizing capacity (ANC), as stated by the product's manufacturer.
[b]Equivalent volumes (mL) or number of tablets calculated to provide 80 mEq ANC.

Because only dissolved antacid can react with hydrogen ions, the dissolution rate or ease of solubility is an important determinant of ultimate neutralizing capacity. Antacid suspensions are formulated with smaller particles than tablets; therefore, they provide a larger surface area and are more rapidly and effectively dissolved in gastric acid. Moreover, antacid suspensions are already in a form to dissolve and react with acid, whereas tablets must be chewed so they will disintegrate and dissolve in stomach fluids. Because of these differences, suspensions are more potent than tablets of the same antacid on a milligram-for-milligram basis.

Despite the higher potency, many patients find liquid antacids unpalatable or cumbersome and prefer to take tablets. Some patients may prefer to alternate tablets during the day at work with liquids at night at home. Patients should be instructed to chew antacid tablets thoroughly and follow with a full glass of water to ensure maximum therapeutic benefit.

Other formulations of antacids include lozenges, chewing gums with antacid coating, and effervescent tablets and powders to be dissolved in water. These formulations do not offer any advantages over liquids and tablets in either neutralizing capacity or patient acceptance.

Palatability

Because antacids often must be taken frequently and in large amounts, their taste, or palatability, is a critical factor in determining patient compliance. A taste test performed with 19 liquid antacids failed to find any overwhelming favorites.[42] Mylanta II has been well accepted in several taste tests, but there is much individual variation. More recently, 14 aluminum-magnesium antacid suspensions were evaluated for smell, taste, texture, and aftertaste.[43] In this comparison, overall palatability was highest for Mylanta Cherry Creme and Mylanta Double Strength Cool Mint Creme, while Riopan Plus 2 and Di-Gel Lemon Orange were ranked lowest. Unfortunately, it is unlikely that any scientific study can resolve the issue of taste for all patients because taste preference is an individual matter.

General recommendations for improving taste tolerability of antacids include refrigerating the product and using high-potency liquid antacids, which can be taken in smaller quantities. However, patients should be advised not to freeze antacid suspensions because this may result in coarse particles that are less reactive to acid. Some patients may prefer flavored tablets if an equivalent neutralizing capacity can be provided with a reasonable number of tablets.

Primary Ingredients

All antacids are basic compounds that react with gastric acid to form a salt and water. Four primary neutralizing compounds are found in antacid products: sodium bicarbonate, calcium carbonate, aluminum salts (hydroxide, phosphate), and magnesium salts (hydroxide, chloride). All antacid products contain at least one of these ingredients, which differ significantly in potency, GI side effects, systemic complications, and drug interactions. Most of these properties are determined by the metal cation of the antacid and the degree of its systemic absorption.

Sodium Bicarbonate Sodium bicarbonate is a potent, highly soluble compound that reacts almost instantaneously with acid in the stomach to produce sodium chloride, carbon dioxide, and water. The chemical reaction is $NaHCO_3 + HCl \rightarrow NaCl + H_2O + CO_2$. The loss of carbon dioxide as a gas makes the reaction irreversible. Sodium bicarbonate differs from other antacids in that it is a systemic antacid, meaning that it is completely absorbed into the systemic circulation and can alter systemic pH. When sodium bicarbonate is taken orally, gastric acid is neutralized by exogenous antacid instead of by endogenous bicarbonate in the intestinal lumen. Because sodium chloride does not react with bicarbonate in the small intestine, this endogenous bicarbonate is "left over" in the small intestine, where it is absorbed into the systemic circulation. Thus, the amount of sodium bicarbonate taken orally equals the amount that is absorbed into the blood. In patients with normal renal function, this excess bicarbonate is rapidly excreted by the kidneys. However, in patients with poor renal function, sodium bicarbonate can accumulate and cause a clinically significant metabolic alkalosis, or it can offset the metabolic acidosis of renal failure.

A particular form of the systemic alkalosis caused by high doses of sodium bicarbonate is the milk-alkali syndrome. This syndrome can occur whenever there is high intake of calcium combined with any factor producing alkalosis. Many reports involve calcium carbonate as the sole source of both calcium and alkali. Sodium bicarbonate can cause alkalosis (and the milk-alkali syndrome) when ingested with calcium but not when ingested alone.

The risk of milk-alkali syndrome was greater in the past, when antacid regimens were routinely prescribed with hourly administration of milk for patients with peptic ulcers. Although such regimens are considered antiquated and are no longer recommended, the milk-alkali syndrome may be important in pregnant women, for whom milk or calcium intake is emphasized, as well as in postmenopausal women taking large doses of supplemental calcium salts. Other risk factors for the development of the syndrome include factors that may worsen or prolong alkalosis, such as vomiting, gastric aspiration, hypokalemia, and dehydration. Because thiazide diuretics inhibit calcium excretion and increase calcium absorption, they may be involved in the production of hypercalcemia in the milk-alkali syndrome.

Presenting symptoms of the milk-alkali syndrome include hypercalcemia, alkalosis, irritability, headache, vertigo, nausea, vomiting, weakness, and myalgia. If calcium and alkali ingestion continues, neurologic symptoms (eg, memory loss, personality changes, lethargy, stupor, coma) may develop.[26] Renal dysfunction occurs early in the course of the disorder and is present in all stages of the syndrome. Most of the symptoms and biochemical abnormalities are reversed rapidly after calcium and alkali ingestion is discontinued; however, renal damage may be irreversible.

Another problem occurring as a result of systemic absorption of sodium bicarbonate is sodium overload. Because each gram of sodium bicarbonate contains 12 mEq of sodium, normal doses deliver large quantities of sodium into the systemic circulation. Accordingly, sodium bicarbonate is contraindicated in patients with edema, congestive heart failure, renal failure, and cirrhosis and in those on low-salt diets. Hypertensive patients should also avoid the therapeutic use of sodium bicarbonate, even on a short-term basis. For other patients, the sodium load may cause the less dangerous yet troublesome side effects of fluid retention and weight gain.

Baking soda consists of 100% sodium bicarbonate, and baking powder contains sodium bicarbonate as the active ingredient. Some commercial combination products contain effervescent sodium bicarbonate and aspirin. These effervescent preparations may cause gastric distention and flatulence as a result of carbon dioxide being lost during the chemical reaction of sodium bicarbonate and gastric acid. Ingestion of large doses of combination sodium bicarbonate-aspirin products after heavy alcohol ingestion may lead to hematemesis and melena in some patients.

Because of the risks of systemic alkalosis and sodium overload, sodium bicarbonate should be used only for short-term relief of symptoms of overeating or indigestion. It is not recommended for the treatment of PUD, and it is contraindicated for chronic therapy.

Calcium Carbonate Calcium carbonate dissolves more slowly in the stomach than sodium bicarbonate does, but it produces a potent and more prolonged neutralization of gastric acid. It reacts with gastric acid to produce calcium chloride, carbon dioxide, and water. The reaction is $CaCO_2 + 2HCl \rightarrow CaCl_2 + H_2O + CO_2$. Unlike sodium chloride, which is formed from the reaction of sodium bicarbonate and gastric acid, about 90% of calcium chloride reacts with bicarbonate in the small intestine to form insoluble calcium salts. Because these calcium salts are excreted in the feces and not absorbed, calcium carbonate is considered a nonsystemic antacid. However, about 10% of the calcium chloride does not react with intestinal bicarbonate; this small percentage of leftover endogenous bicarbonate is reabsorbed into the systemic circulation.

Clinically significant alkalosis from calcium carbonate ingestion does not usually develop. However, as previously discussed, calcium carbonate may cause or contribute to the development of the milk-alkali syndrome.

When calcium carbonate serves as the source of both calcium and alkali, the risk of the syndrome is increased by prolonged administration of calcium carbonate, the concomitant ingestion of milk fortified with vitamin D (which increases the intestinal absorption of calcium), renal impairment, and dehydration with electrolyte imbalance.

Although the amount of calcium that does not react with intestinal bicarbonate and is absorbed systemically is minimal (10%), enough may be absorbed after several days of high-dose antacid ingestion to cause hypercalcemia. Hypercalcemia is characterized by neurologic symptoms, renal calculi, and reduced renal function. These side effects are rare in healthy patients, and they do not appear to occur in patients with normal renal function if daily consumption of calcium carbonate is less than 20 g. However, patients with impaired renal function may develop hypercalcemia from as little as 4 g per day. This adverse effect becomes a concern when calcium carbonate is used to bind phosphate in patients with renal failure.

Calcium carbonate has been noted to cause acid rebound, which is a sustained hypersecretion of gastric acid after antacid has been emptied from the stomach. Increased gastric acid secretion begins within 2 hours after administration of calcium carbonate and may last for 3–5 hours. This effect has been reported after large doses (4–8 g) as well as after single small doses (500 mg). Acid rebound caused by calcium carbonate is particularly pronounced after meals.[26] The mechanism for this effect is not well defined but may be related to a local effect of calcium ions on gastric mucosa in addition to hypergastrinemia.[44] Despite evidence that acid rebound occurs, there is no evidence that it is clinically significant. Acid rebound has not been shown to delay ulcer healing, and no studies suggest that calcium carbonate is inferior to other antacids in the treatment of acid-peptic disorders.

It is widely believed that calcium carbonate causes constipation. However, published reports of patients with PUD indicate that calcium carbonate may act as a laxative, increasing fecal bulk in some patients and causing diarrhea in others.[45] Because PUD itself may be constipating, it may be that the constipation noted in patients taking calcium carbonate for PUD may be a consequence of the ulcer rather than of the calcium.

Aluminum Aluminum hydroxide is slowly dissolved in the stomach, where it reacts with gastric acid to form aluminum chloride and water. The reaction is $Al(OH)_3 + 3HCl \rightarrow AlCl_3 + 3H_2O$. In the small intestine, aluminum chloride reacts with bicarbonate to form a series of poorly absorbed basic aluminum salts. Because most of the aluminum chloride reacts with intestinal bicarbonate, very little endogenous bicarbonate is left over, and systemic alkalosis is a minimal risk.

Although the formation of insoluble salts limits aluminum absorption, about 17–30% of the aluminum chloride formed is absorbed.[41] In patients with normal renal function, this aluminum chloride is rapidly excreted by the kidneys. However, patients with impaired renal function who take aluminum antacids chronically may fail to clear the aluminum, resulting in hyperaluminemia and accumulation of aluminum in other tissues.

Aluminum-containing antacids, except for aluminum phosphate, bind phosphate in the gut, forming insoluble phosphate salts that are excreted in the feces. The result is reduced intestinal phosphate absorption. This effect is beneficial in patients with chronic renal failure who have increased serum levels of phosphorous. However, use of aluminum-containing antacids as phosphate binders in renal failure patients is associated with serious risks. Elevated aluminum concentrations have been reported in the bone, muscle, and brain tissue of such patients.[46] Aluminum is neurotoxic and has been associated with the development of encephalopathy in uremic patients on hemodialysis who are taking aluminum antacids.[26,46] However, the relationship between aluminum and this "dialysis dementia" is not well supported. The primary concern with use of aluminum antacids in patients with renal failure is that too much phosphate will be bound by the antacid. The resulting phosphorous depletion can cause calcium to be resorbed from bone, leading to osteomalacia.

In patients with normal renal function, the reduction in phosphate absorption caused by aluminum antacids may lead to clinically significant phosphate depletion. Phosphorous depletion is characterized by anorexia, malaise, and muscle weakness. If severe and prolonged, it may lead to osteomalacia, osteoporosis, and fractures. Although uncommon, phosphorous depletion may occur as early as the second week of therapy and has been reported with dosages of aluminum hydroxide as low as 30 mL three times daily.[47] Although hypophosphatemia is not a concern with most patients taking antacids, it is more likely to occur in those taking large doses of aluminum hydroxide for prolonged periods and in those with inadequate dietary intake of phosphorous.[41] Other patients at risk for hypophosphatemia include elderly persons, alcoholics, and those with diarrhea or malabsorption syndromes. Hypophosphatemia can be reversed by administering phosphate supplements or increasing phosphate in the diet.

The most frequent side effect of aluminum-containing antacids is constipation. Antacids containing aluminum hydroxide have been reported to cause intestinal obstruction, hemorrhoids, fissures, and fecal impaction.[41] Patients predisposed to obstruction include those with reduced bowel motility, dehydration, and fluid restriction. Constipation from aluminum is dose related but can be managed with stool softeners or laxatives, or with combination aluminum-magnesium antacids.

Although aluminum may be administered in several different salt forms (hydroxide, carbonate, phosphate, or aminoacetate), the hydroxide salt is the most potent buffer and is used most often. In comparison with magnesium hydroxide, calcium carbonate, and sodium bicarbonate, however, aluminum hydroxide has a relatively low ANC.

Magnesium Like sodium bicarbonate, magnesium hydroxide reacts with gastric acid to produce a potent, short-acting neutralizing action. The reaction is $Mg(OH)_2 + 2HCl \rightarrow MgCl_2 + 2H_2O$. Most of the magnesium chloride formed reacts with bicarbonate in the small intestine, thus minimizing the risk of systemic alkalosis. However, about 5–10% of the magnesium chloride is absorbed and rapidly excreted by the kidneys in patients with

Mg = diarrhea
Al^{+3} = constipation

normal renal function. As with other antacids, the risk of cation absorption and toxicity is significant only in patients with impaired renal function.

Although magnesium toxicity from antacids is rare and occurs primarily in patients with significant renal failure, it can produce life-threatening complications. Magnesium is a strong central nervous system (CNS) depressant and may cause depressed reflexes, muscle paralysis, nausea, vomiting, hypotension, respiratory depression, coma, and death. Magnesium toxicity can also cause severe cardiac depression, seen clinically as hypotension and bradyarrhythmias. Cardiotoxicity does not usually occur until there is severe hypermagnesemia (10–15 mEq/L; normal is 1.8–2.4 mEq/L) in patients with renal dysfunction.[48] Considering these risks, magnesium antacids should not be used in patients with marked renal failure (ie, those with creatinine clearance <30 mL/min). If they are, doses of magnesium exceeding 50 mEq per day should be used cautiously and only under the supervision of a health care provider, who should monitor electrolytes regularly.[41]

The most frequent and limiting side effect of magnesium-containing antacids is diarrhea, which may be severe enough to cause fluid and electrolyte imbalances. Any magnesium hydroxide that does not react with gastric acid is converted in the small intestine to soluble but poorly absorbed magnesium salts. These nonabsorbable salts cause an osmotic gradient that is at least partially responsible for the diarrhea associated with magnesium. One study suggests that the laxative effect of magnesium hydroxide is associated with increased output of prostaglandin E_2 in the stool.[49] However, whether these prostaglandins actually cause the diarrhea associated with magnesium therapy requires further study.

Diarrhea associated with magnesium-containing antacids is dose related. The incidence of diarrhea from magnesium ranges from 4% in patients taking low-dose antacids (144 mEq per day) to 76% in patients taking higher doses (1,064 mEq per day). Diarrhea caused by magnesium may differ from diarrhea from other causes in that it does not bring on abdominal cramps or nocturnal bowel movements.[49] Efforts to minimize this diarrhea include using combination aluminum-magnesium antacid products or alternating aluminum-magnesium therapy with an aluminum-only antacid.

Although the hydroxide salt is used most often, other magnesium salts with antacid properties are the oxide (which is converted to hydroxide in water), carbonate, and trisilicate. The ANC of magnesium salts is greater than that of aluminum hydroxide but less than that of sodium bicarbonate and calcium carbonate.

Aluminum-Magnesium Combinations Many commercially available antacid products contain a mixture of aluminum and magnesium. Because constipation from aluminum and diarrhea from magnesium are dose related, combining these two agents allows for potent ANC with lower doses of each agent. In theory, the constipating effect of aluminum should balance the diarrheal effect of magnesium, and vice versa. However, the optimal ratio between magnesium and aluminum to achieve this balance has not been found in any commercially available product. Diarrhea appears to be the predominant effect, regardless of the ratio, if doses of magnesium hydroxide exceed 8.5 g per day. Indeed, up to three fourths of patients taking these combination products experience diarrhea; constipation is rarely reported.

The risk of side effects other than those affecting the GI system are not reduced with combination products. To the contrary, the presence of both salts introduces the possibility of side effects from absorption of two cations. Thus, patients taking combination products may experience hypermagnesemia, hyperaluminumemia and toxicity, hypophosphatemia, or metabolic alkalosis. As with either agent alone, these risks appear to be of concern primarily in patients with reduced renal function.

Magaldrate is a chemical mixture of aluminum and magnesium hydroxides that is converted to aluminum and magnesium ions in hydrochloric acid. Magaldrate has a lower ANC than a physical mixture of aluminum and magnesium hydroxides. Because the presence of aluminum is not readily recognized from the term *magaldrate,* the pharmacist should take care not to recommend magaldrate as a non–aluminum-containing product.

Additional Ingredients

Most antacid products contain excipient ingredients that may be clinically important in certain patients. In addition, many products contain ingredients that do not have antacid properties but are used by manufacturers to meet unique advertising claims.

Sugars Some antacids contain considerable amounts of sugars or saccharin. When taken occasionally or in small doses, the sugar content is not great enough to cause clinical problems. However, when taken in large amounts over long periods, enough sugar is ingested to alter glucose control in patients with labile diabetes. When recommending an antacid for diabetic patients, the pharmacist should consider the sugar content. Unfortunately, this information is not required to be listed on the product labeling. An additional concern with the sugar content of antacids is the possibility of tooth decay with extended use.

Sodium Most antacids contain sodium as an impurity, but the amount differs considerably among products. Because of the risks of sodium to certain patients, the sodium content in antacids has been reduced significantly over the past several years. Many antacid products have been developed that contain less than 0.04 mEq (1 mg) sodium per 5 mL, or no sodium at all. These products should be used in patients with hypertension, congestive heart failure, renal failure, edema, or cirrhosis, and in those on salt-restricted diets. The usual amount of sodium allowed in sodium-restricted diets is 2–4 g per day. Antacids containing more than 5 mEq (115 mg) sodium in the total daily dose should not be recommended without first consulting with the patient's health care provider. Obviously, antacids containing sodium bicarbonate have the largest quantities of sodium and should not be used in these patients.

Simethicone See the discussion of simethicone in the section Antiflatulents.

Alginic Acid Alginic acid is combined with sodium bicarbonate and other antacids in several commercial products. The addition of alginic acid to antacids appears to be effective in relieving symptoms of GERD. Some studies suggest that this combination is superior to antacids alone.[13,22,24] As discussed previously, alginic acid works by reacting with sodium bicarbonate and saliva to form a viscous solution of sodium alginate. This viscous solution floats on the surface of gastric contents so that, when reflux occurs, sodium alginate rather than acid is refluxed and irritation is minimized. When using antacid-alginic acid combination tablets, patients should understand that the tablets must be chewed to be effective and should be followed by a glass of water so that the viscous foam (sodium alginate) can float on water in the stomach. In addition, patients should be aware that the formulation only works when they are in the upright position and therefore must not be taken at bedtime or just before they lie down.[50]

The use of alginic acid-containing products is not indicated for acid-peptic diseases other than GERD because the amount of antacid ingredients included does not provide sufficient ANC to be useful. The FDA considers alginic acid to be of questionable value.

Antacid-Drug Interactions

Antacid-drug interactions have been reported with more than 30 classes of drugs. Although most of these interactions are not clinically important, some may be significant enough to result in clinical treatment failures with one or both drugs (Table 3).

Antacids interact with drugs by a variety of mechanisms. Intraluminal interactions occur when an antacid chelates another drug or adsorbs another drug onto its surface.[51] Antacids can also interfere with the absorption and elimination of drugs by increasing gastric pH and urine pH, respectively. Although all antacids may interact in these ways, some are more likely to cause these changes than others. Factors that influence whether an antacid interacts with another drug include the valence of the cation in the antacid, the dose used, the chronicity of dosing, and, most important, the timing of the administration or consumption of the antacid in relation to the other drug.

Intraluminal Interactions The most significant drug interactions with antacids are those in which antacids containing divalent (Ca^{2+}, Mg^{2+}) or trivalent (Al^{3+}) cations chelate or bind certain other drugs and reduce their absorption. Antacids containing magnesium hydroxide or magnesium trisilicate appear to have the greatest potential for drug binding, whereas those containing aluminum hydroxide and calcium carbonate have an intermediate ability.[41]

Probably the most well known drug interaction with antacids is that of tetracycline. Polyvalent metallic cations have a strong affinity for tetracycline, resulting in the formation of a chelate. This insoluble compound cannot penetrate the intestinal mucosa for absorption. When antacids are coadministered with tetracycline, response to the antibiotic may vary depending on the extent of chelation. Antacids containing aluminum, magnesium, or calcium are strong inhibitors of tetracycline absorption and have been reported to reduce bioavailability by 50% to more than 90%.[19] Chelation with antacids has also been reported with other tetracyclines, including doxycycline, demeclocycline, and oxytetracycline.[19] Although not reported, this interaction is likely to occur with minocycline as well. Patients taking any form of tetracycline who need an antacid should be advised not to take antacids until at least 2 hours after tetracycline administration.

The metal cations of antacids also have a strong ability to chelate quinolone antibiotics, which may result in impaired GI absorption. Significant reductions (up to 90%) in bioavailability and peak plasma concentrations of ciprofloxacin have been reported with magnesium- and aluminum-containing antacids, as well as with calcium carbonate.[19,20,51] Significant reductions in peak serum concentrations have also occurred with ofloxacin, norfloxacin, temafloxin, lomefloxacin, and enoxacin.[19] The magnitude of this interaction is influenced by the length of time separating the antacid and the quinolone, as well as by the order of drug administration.[51] Although definite guidelines do not exist, available data suggest that if antacids are to be used with quinolones, they should be separated by at least 2 hours, and preferably by 4–6 hours. If doses can only be separated by 2 hours, giving the quinolone before the antacid may minimize the potential for serious interaction.[20,51]

Modest reductions in the absorption of H_2RAs have been documented with concurrent administration of antacids, but conflicting results exist. Although the antacid is suspected of binding the H_2RAs, the precise mechanism is unknown. Single doses of magnesium-aluminum combination antacids have decreased the absorption of cimetidine, ranitidine, famotidine, and nizatidine.[19] However, several studies have failed to find this interaction. Although the clinical significance of this interaction is probably minimal, it is prudent to administer the H_2RA 1–2 hours before the antacid.[19,20]

Drugs Affected by Increased Gastric pH Because antacids increase gastric pH, they can interfere with the absorption of drugs requiring an acidic environment for dissolution or absorption. Significant reductions in ketoconazole have been reported with the concomitant administration of antacids.[51] If concomitant administration of these agents cannot be avoided, they should be separated by at least 2 hours. Theoretically, antacids could interfere with the action of sucralfate, which is thought to need an acidic environment to dissociate and form the viscous gel that binds to gastric and duodenal mucosa. Although antacids have diminished the binding of sucralfate to GUs in animals, it is not known whether they interfere significantly with the binding of sucralfate in humans.[26] Until more is known about this interaction, it is wise to give antacids at least 30 minutes apart from sucralfate.

Drugs Affected by Increased Urine pH By increasing the urine pH, antacids may affect the elimination of certain acidic or basic drugs whose renal clearance depends on the urine pH. This interaction is particularly pronounced with sodium bicarbonate, the strongest urinary alkalinizer of all antacids. Other antacids have also been shown to increase urinary pH significantly in the following order: aluminum-magnesium combination > magnesium hydroxide > calcium carbonate.[29] Antacids that contain

TABLE 3 Antacid–drug interactions

Drug	Antacids: Al	Mg	Al–Mg	$CaCO_3$	$NaHCO_3$	Effect	Mechanism	Clinical implication
Allopurinol	✓					↓ absorption in 3 patients on chronic hemodialysis with failure to reduce uric acid	Unknown	Monitor patient for ↓ allopurinol response. Separate doses by ≥2 h
Amphetamine					✓	↓ urinary excretion, allowing potential for retention & intoxication	↓ renal clearance due to ↑ urine pH	Avoid concurrent use
Antibiotics								
Nitrofurantoin	✓					↓ rate & extent of absorption		Separate doses by ≥2 h
Tetracycline and quinolones	✓	✓	✓	✓		↓ absorption (up to 90%), resulting in ↓ serum and urine concentrations	Chelation	May result in treatment failures. Separate doses by ≥2 h, preferably 4–6 h
Anticoagulants		✓				↑ absorption of dicumarol by 50%; no effect on warfarin absorption	Chelation	Patients needing antacids & anticoagulants should receive warfarin
Anticonvulsants								
Phenytoin		✓	✓			↓ rate & extent of absorption with large doses of antacid; no effect with small doses	Unknown	Monitor phenytoin effects/levels
Valproic acid	✓	✓	✓			↑ absorption by 12%	Unknown	Potential for valproic acid toxicity
Beta-blockers								
Propranolol	✓					↓ bioavailability by 50% in 4 of 5 subjects; no effect in another study	Delay in gastric emptying	Clinical significance of long-term therapy not assessed
Metoprolol			✓			↑ bioavailability by 25% after single dose in 6 healthy volunteers	Interference with first-pass metabolism	Probably not significant
Atenolol	✓		✓	✓		↓ bioavailability from 37–51%		May be clinically significant; separate doses by at least 1 h
Benzodiazepines							Unknown	May result in delay in sedative effect. Important only in acute anxiety with single doses, not in chronic dosing
Diazepam	✓		✓			↑ absorption & ↑ sedative effects; ↓ rate, but not extent, of absorption		
Chlordiazepoxide			✓			↓ rate, but not extent, of absorption		
Clorazepate			✓			↓ rate & extent of absorption		
Captopril			✓			↓ absorption by 42% in 10 healthy volunteers	Unknown	No evidence of compromised efficacy
Chlorpromazine			✓			↓ absorption & serum concentration; ↓ therapeutic response reported	Adsorption	Monitor for ↓ therapeutic response. Separate doses by ≥2 h
Corticosteroids							Adsorption	Evidence conflicting & clinical significance questionable
Dexamethasone		✓				↓ absorption		
Prednisone	✓		✓			↓ absorption in one study, but not confirmed		

Drug	Antacids: Al	Mg	Al–Mg	$CaCO_3$	$NaHCO_3$	Effect	Mechanism	Clinical implication
Digoxin	✓	✓	✓			↓ absorption of digoxin up to 30% in some reports, but no effect in others. May be more likely to occur with tablets than capsules	Adsorption	Clinical significance uncertain. Monitor patients for ↓ digoxin effect when antacids are given concurrently. Space doses to avoid possible interaction
H_2RAs						↓ absorption & peak concentration by 10–40%; clinical failures not reported	Adsorption	Separate doses by at least 1–2 h
Cimetidine	✓							
Ranitidine	✓		✓					
Famotidine			✓					
Nizatidine			✓					
Iron	✓	✓		✓	✓	↓ absorption by 50–60%	↓ iron solubility due to chelation or ↑ gastric pH	May interfere with patient's response to iron replacement therapy. Separate doses by ≥2 h
Isoniazid	✓	✓				↓ absorption, particularly with aluminum antacids	Delayed gastric emptying due to aluminum	Separate doses by ≥1 h
Ketoconazole	✓		✓		✓	↓ ketoconazole absorption	↑ gastric pH	Separate doses by ≥2 h
Levodopa			✓			↑ absorption in some patients, but effect is variable	↑ gastric emptying due to antacids, thus more levodopa delivered to small intestine for absorption	May be clinically useful in certain patients with delayed gastric emptying. Monitor patient response when adding or stopping antacid
NSAIDs								
Aspirin			✓	✓		↓ serum concentrations by 30–70%	↑ renal clearance due to ↑ urine pH	Monitor serum salicylate levels & observe symptoms when sustained levels are important (eg, rheumatoid arthritis, systemic lupus erythematosus)
Enteric-coated aspirin						Premature rupture of enteric coating & dissolution in the stomach	↑ gastric ph	Separate doses in patients at risk for NSAID gastropathy
Indomethacin	✓	✓				Delayed absorption & possible ↓ peak concentrations	Adsorption	Not clinically important
Naproxen			✓					
Diflunisal	✓		✓					
Pseudoephedrine						↑ rate, but not extent, of absorption in 6 healthy volunteers		Clinical significance unknown
Quinidine		✓	✓	✓		↑ serum concentrations; toxicity has been reported	↓ renal clearance due to ↑ urine pH	Use with caution. Monitor levels & patient response
Sodium polystyrene sulfonate		✓	✓	✓		Metabolic alkalosis	Antacid binds resin instead of intestinal HCO_3, resulting in ↑ reabsorption of HCO_3	Concurrent use may be dangerous. Separate doses by ≥2 h
Sucralfate						↓ dissolution & possible loss of efficacy	↑ gastric pH	Separate doses by ≥30 min
Theophylline						↑ & ↓ in rate, but not extent, of absorption observed, depending on the theophylline preparation	Unknown	Not important in chronic dosing

Key:
✓ indicates interactions reported in humans. However, interactions may be likely with other antacids in which interactions are not yet reported.

↑ = increased; ↓ = decreased.

Information extracted from:

Gugler R, Allgayer H. *Clin Pharmacokin*. 1990; 18 (3): 210–9.
Gibaldi M et al. *Clin Pharmacol Ther*. 1974; 16: 520–5.
Tatro DS, ed, *Drug Interaction Facts*. St Louis: Facts and Comparisons Division, J B Lippincott; 1990.
Hansten PD, Horn JR. *Drug Interactions*. 6th ed. Philadelphia: Lea & Febiger; 1989.

only aluminum hydroxide do not appear to increase urine pH.

Aspirin and salicylates are weakly acidic drugs that become ionized in alkaline urine, thus accelerating their renal clearance. Antacid-induced urine pH changes can decrease steady-state plasma salicylate levels by almost one half.[20] In contrast, the renal excretion of basic drugs such as quinidine and amphetamines may be significantly reduced by antacids.[19] Increased drug concentrations and effects may result from such interactions. In fact, quinidine toxicity has been documented to occur as a result of an increase in urine pH.[20] Concurrent use of these drugs with antacids should be avoided or closely monitored.

Miscellaneous Uses of Antacids

Overindulgence/Hangover The FDA has long recognized antacids as being safe and effective for the symptomatic relief of heartburn, sour stomach, or acid indigestion. However, patients often take antacids for a wide variety of GI complaints, many of which do not fit these indications. One of the most common reasons people take antacids is for relief of symptoms associated with overeating or excessive indulgence in alcohol. A previous review by the FDA concluded that antacids are safe for the relief of immediate postprandial upper abdominal discomfort, but no data supported their efficacy for this indication. More recently, the FDA has reviewed nonprescription oral products for the relief of symptoms associated with overindulgence in food and drink and has endorsed the use of antacids for such purposes.[52] Thus, along with indications for heartburn, sour stomach, and acid indigestion, antacid product labeling may include the statement "and upset stomach associated with these symptoms" or "associated with overindulgence in food and drink." The FDA has also approved antacid-acetaminophen combination products for the relief of symptoms associated with hangover or overindulgence in food and drink. Finally, it has reversed a previous recommendation and placed in Category II (not generally recognized as safe and effective) all combination products for hangover that contain both an antacid and caffeine.[52]

Phosphate-Binding Effects The phosphate-binding effects of antacids are often used clinically to lower serum phosphate in patients with chronic renal failure. Aluminum hydroxide has been the standard phosphate binder for many years. When added to dietary phosphate restriction, aluminum hydroxide in dosages of 1.9–4.8 g given three to four times daily significantly reduces serum phosphate concentrations in these patients. However, patients with chronic renal failure may absorb significant amounts of aluminum, resulting in osteomalacia. Recognition of the risks of aluminum accumulation has prompted the use of other antacids, particularly calcium salts, for this indication. Many studies have shown calcium carbonate in doses of 8–12 g per day to be a safe and effective phosphate binder in 70–80% of patients receiving chronic dialysis.[53] However, long-term use of calcium carbonate in this setting is limited by the development of hypercalcemia and GI intolerance (diarrhea and constipation). Calcium citrate has been used successfully on a short-term basis as a phosphate binder,[54] but its long-term safety and efficacy for this indication have not been established.

Cholesterol-Lowering Effects Recognition of the bile salt–binding properties of aluminum antacids has prompted investigation into the potential lipid-lowering potential of antacids.[55] Because aluminum antacids bind bile acids as strongly as cholestyramine, it is possible that aluminum hydroxide acts like cholestyramine to lower cholesterol. Because bile salts are bound and enterohepatic circulation is interrupted, more cholesterol is converted in the liver to bile acid, and hepatic cholesterol is depleted. This prompts the liver to make more low-density lipoprotein cholesterol receptors, thus clearing cholesterol faster and reducing serum cholesterol. A recent study showed that 4 months of treatment with an aluminum-magnesium antacid significantly reduced serum low-density lipoprotein cholesterol and, to a lesser extent, high-density lipoprotein cholesterol in hypercholesterolemic patients. However, far more data are needed to establish antacids as a therapeutic modality in treating hyperlipidemia.[55]

Reconstitution of Didanosine Didanosine (Videx), which is indicated for the treatment of adult and pediatric human immunodeficiency virus infection, is rapidly degraded at acidic pH. Therefore, all oral forms of the drug contain antacid to increase gastric pH and allow for maximal absorption.[41] The pediatric powder for oral solutions does not contain an antacid and must be reconstituted by the pharmacist with a high-potency liquid antacid. The product labeling specifies that either Mylanta Double Strength Liquid or Maalox TC Suspension be mixed with the didanosine powder to reach the final dispensing concentration.[41]

H_2-Receptor Antagonists

The introduction of the first H_2RA, cimetidine, in 1977 revolutionized the treatment of acid-peptic disorders. Since that time, new and more potent H_2RAs have been developed, and four H_2RAs are currently available for prescription use in the United States: cimetidine, ranitidine, famotidine, and nizatidine. In 1995, famotidine, cimetidine, and ranitidine were reclassified from prescription-only to nonprescription status in the United States. A nonprescription form of nizatidine was subsequently approved in May 1996. The oral doses approved for nonprescription use—famotidine 10 mg (up to 20 mg per day), cimetidine 200 mg (up to 400 mg per day), ranitidine 75 mg (up to 150 mg per day), and nizatidine 75 mg (up to 150 mg per day)—are substantially lower than those indicated in the management of PUD and GERD (see product table "Histamine II Receptor Antagonists").

H_2RAs work in acid-peptic diseases by reducing aggressive forces rather than by enhancing mucosal defenses. H_2RAs inhibit gastric acid secretion by competitively blocking H_2-receptors on the parietal cell. While all phases of acid secretion are suppressed, H_2RAs generally inhibit basal and nocturnal acid secretion to a greater extent than they do meal-stimulated acid secretion. Antisecretory activity usually begins within 1 hour

TABLE 4 Comparison of nonprescription H_2-receptor antagonists

	Cimetidine (Tagamet-HB)	Ranitidine (Zantac-75)	Nizatidine (Axid AR)	Famotidine (Pepcid-AC)
Nonprescription dosage form	100 mg tablet	75 mg tablet	75 mg tablet	10 mg tablet
Relative potency	1	4–8	4–8	20–50
Oral bioavailability	60–80%	50–60%	90–100%	40–50%
Elimination half-life	1.5–2.5 h	2–3 h	1–2 h	2.5–4 h
Urinary excretion of oral dose	50%	30%	>90%	30%
Dosages for treatment of heartburn, sour stomach, acid indigestion	200 mg bid prn, up to twice daily; also approved for prevention of these conditions	75 mg bid prn, up to twice daily	75 mg bid prn, up to twice daily; approved only for prevention of these conditions	10 mg bid prn, up to twice daily; also approved for prevention of these conditions
Mechanisms/potential for drug interactions				
Inhibit cP450 enzymes[a]	+++	+	—	—
Increase gastric pH[b]	+	+	+	+
Change renal elimination[c]	+++	++	—	—
Inhibit gastric alcohol dehydrogenase[d]	+	+	+	—

Key:

\+ indicates degree of potential for drug interactions.

— indicates no potential for drug interactions.

[a]Monitor serum levels and adverse effects if cimetidine is given with theophylline, phenytoin, or warfarin. Use caution if cimetidine is administered with tricyclic antidepressants, lidocaine, quinidine, benzodiazepines, or tacrine.

[b]H_2RAs may significantly decrease bioavailability of itraconazole, ketoconazole, enoxacin, and cefpodoxime proxetil. Avoid concomitant administration or administer antibiotic when antisecretory effect of H_2RA is lowest.

[c]Avoid concomitant administration of cimetidine and ranitidine with procainamide, or monitor levels of procainamide and *N*-acetylprocainamide.

[d]H_2RAs may increase alcohol concentrations slightly, but clinical significance appears to be minimal.

of administration and persists for 6–12 hours.[30] The duration of antisecretory effect reported for oral nonprescription doses of cimetidine (200 mg) and famotidine (10 mg) is 6 hours and 8–10 hours, respectively.[31,56] The duration of this effect for oral nonprescription doses of ranitidine (75 mg) and nizatidine (75 mg) is approximately 6–8 hours. Both the degree and the duration of acid suppression achieved with H_2RAs depend upon the dose.[57] Therefore, both the reduction in acid output and the duration of effect are significantly lower with nonprescription doses of H_2RAs, than with prescription doses of these agents.

The H_2RAs are not equipotent on a milligram-for-milligram basis. Famotidine is at least 20–50 times more potent than cimetidine on a molar basis. Ranitidine and nizatidine, which are approximately equipotent, are 4–10 times more potent than cimetidine.[4] Although nonprescription doses have not been directly compared, cimetidine 300 mg appears to inhibit gastric acid secretion to the same degree as famotidine 5 mg and nizatidine 75 mg.[26] Extension of this observation suggests that famotidine 10 mg, nizatidine 75 mg, and ranitidine 75 mg are more potent than cimetidine 200 mg. Whether the lower potency of the nonprescription dose of cimetidine will confer a clinical disadvantage for patients with mild GERD is unknown.

The pharmacokinetic profiles of the H_2RAs are all very similar in healthy, normal volunteers (Table 4). These drugs are all rapidly absorbed from the small intestine, with peak concentrations occurring from 1 to 3 hours after oral administration.[4] Their bioavailability is not affected by food but, as previously discussed, may be reduced modestly by antacids.[19,20] For all H_2RAs, elimination occurs by a combination of renal and hepatic metabolism, with renal elimination being the most important for nizatidine. Although prescription doses of H_2RAs must be reduced in patients with renal impairment and/or elderly patients, this is not the case for approved nonprescription doses. Dosage adjustment is not necessary in patients with liver disease who have normal renal function.

Adverse Effects

As a class, the H_2RAs are among the most studied and hence the safest agents ever marketed. They have been administered to nearly 30 million people and have rarely caused serious side effects; their overall incidence of side effects is less than 3%.[4] The most common adverse effects reported with standard doses of H_2RAs are headache, drowsiness, constipation, diarrhea, nausea, vomiting, and abdominal pain/discomfort.[4,5,46] Despite a clinical impression that CNS reactions occur more often with cimetidine, there is no evidence that such effects are more common with one H_2RA than with another[30]; serious CNS reactions, including confusion, dizziness, agitation, and hallucinations, have occurred with all the H_2RAs but are extremely rare in ambulatory patients. Hematologic effects (thrombocytopenia, leukopenia, neutropenia, anemia) and mild, reversible elevations in hepatic aminotransferase enzymes have also been reported with all the H_2RAs; however, the incidence of these reactions is very low.[4,5] Small reductions in blood pressure and heart rate have been reported with oral H_2RAs, but clinically important hypotension and bradycardia are generally associated with rapid intravenous infusions of these drugs.[30]

Cimetidine is unique among the H_2RAs in its ability to cause impotence and gynecomastia. These antiandrogenic effects result from the ability of cimetidine to displace dihydrotestosterone from androgen binding sites and to inhibit the cytochrome P-450 metabolism of estradiol.[4,5] However, this effect occurs primarily in men receiving large doses (>3 g per day) for hypersecretory conditions, and it is reversible upon discontinuation or changing to another H_2RA. These reactions would be highly unlikely at cimetidine doses approved for nonprescription use.

The extensive safety profile of prescription doses of H_2RAs suggests that the lower nonprescription doses will be well-tolerated and safe. To date, the most frequent adverse effects reported by patients receiving famotidine 10 mg include headache, dizziness, nausea, and diarrhea.[31] Similarly, patients receiving cimetidine 200 mg complained most often of headache, diarrhea, and nausea.[56] The incidence of these reactions was less than 10% and usually not different from that with placebo.[31,56]

The toxic:therapeutic dose ratio for all four H_2RAs appears to be very high.[30] Ingestion of up to 10–20 g of cimetidine has caused only minimal and transient adverse effects. However, serious CNS effects have been reported after acute ingestion of 20–40 g cimetidine, and two deaths have been reported in adults who ingested more than 40 g.[26] There is limited experience with ranitidine overdose, but acute ingestion of up to 18 g has not caused serious toxicity. Famotidine overdose has not been documented, and there is no evidence of serious toxicity in patients receiving more than 800 mg famotidine daily for hypersecretory conditions.[26] To date, there is very little information on nizatidine overdose in humans.

Drug Interactions

Of the H_2RAs, cimetidine has the greatest potential to interact with other drugs. Because cimetidine binds to several isoenzymes of the cytochrome P-450 enzyme system, it impairs the hepatic metabolism of drugs that are normally cleared by this system. The magnitude of inhibition depends on numerous factors, including the cimetidine dose, the age of the patient, and the patient's hepatic enzyme status.[51] In adults with normal renal function, cimetidine doses lower than 400 mg per day do not generally cause clinically important increases in serum concentrations of other drugs.[20] However, even small increases in concentrations of drugs that are eliminated by nonlinear kinetics and/or have a narrow therapeutic range may be important. In this regard, concomitant administration of cimetidine is of particular concern with theophylline, phenytoin, and warfarin.

In one study, low-dose cimetidine (300 mg at bedtime) inhibited theophylline clearance by 12%, while another trial demonstrated cimetidine 400 mg per day to reduce theophylline clearance by 14%.[51,56] By comparison, larger doses of cimetidine (1,200–1,600 mg per day) may reduce theophylline clearance by as much as 35%.[51] The effects of low-dose cimetidine on phenytoin metabolism have not been examined specifically. However, an earlier study found cimetidine 400 mg per day to inhibit phenytoin clearance by 10.2% as compared with 21.2% with cimetidine 1,200 mg per day.[56] In 15 patients receiving maintenance warfarin therapy, cimetidine doses of 100 mg or 200 mg twice daily increased the prothrombin ratio by 1% and 9%, respectively.[56] These changes were considered small and clinically insignificant.

Considering these data, the magnitude of changes occurring in drug metabolism with nonprescription doses of cimetidine is likely to be small. However, the potential for adverse clinical consequences exists, particularly in elderly patients whose renal function may be declining and who are likely to be taking multiple medications. The potential for drug interactions will also be magnified if patients exceed the recommended dosage. Accordingly, the product label for nonprescription cimetidine includes a warning for patients who take theophylline, phenytoin, or warfarin to consult a physician before taking the product. When cimetidine is added or stopped in a patient receiving one of these drugs, theophylline or phenytoin levels and international normalized ratios should be monitored and doses adjusted accordingly. Although inhibition of drug metabolism may begin within 24 hours of initiating cimetidine therapy, the maximum increase in object drug concentration will not occur until the new steady state is reached.[51] Other drugs whose metabolism may be inhibited by cimetidine include the tricyclic antidepressants, benzodiazepines, beta-blockers, calcium channel blockers, lidocaine, and quinidine.[19,20,51]

When patients who are taking theophylline, cimetidine, or warfarin wish to self-medicate with an H_2RA, it may be simpler and more cost-effective to recommend one other than cimetidine. While ranitidine also binds to cytochrome P-450 enzymes, it does so with much less affinity than cimetidine and the potential for drug interactions is much lower. Famotidine and nizatidine do not bind appreciably to the system and therefore do not inhibit the metabolism of other drugs.

Like antacids, all the H_2RAs can affect the bioavailability of certain drugs by raising gastric pH. Standard doses of cimetidine and ranitidine have been noted to increase the absorption of nifedipine, resulting in enhanced antihypertensive effect.[51] Cimetidine reduces GI inactivation of pancreatic enzymes, causing reductions of steatorrhea in patients receiving both agents. Conversely, concomitant administration of H_2RAs has been reported to reduce the bioavailability of enoxacin, cefpodoxime proxetil, itraconazole, and ketoconazole by 26%, 40%, 51%, and 95%, respectively.[51] It is important to note, however, that these studies involved prescription doses of H_2RAs. Currently, there are no data to determine whether these interactions occur with nonprescription H_2RAs, or to what extent. In the absence of such data, it is wise to avoid concomitant administration of H_2RAs with these agents. If this is not possible, the antibiotic should be administered when the antisecretory effect of the H_2RA is at a minimum (ie, 6–10 hours after a dose).[51]

Standard doses of cimetidine and ranitidine may compete for renal tubular secretion and thus impair the renal elimination of basic compounds such as procainamide and its metabolite, *N*-acetylprocainamide (NAPA).[19,51] The magnitude of this interaction appears to be greater with cimetidine than with ranitidine and, in both cases, depends upon the dose of the H_2RA. The potential for nonprescription cimetidine and ranitidine to interact with procainamide has not been assessed. Famotidine does not alter the serum concentration of procainamide or NAPA, and studies with nizatidine are not available.[51] Thus, patients receiving procainamide and wishing to self-medicate with H_2RAs may best be treated with famotidine.

Cimetidine, ranitidine, and nizatidine have been shown to inhibit gastric alcohol dehydrogenase, the enzyme responsible for the first-pass metabolism of alcohol.[19] Famotidine does not inhibit this enzyme. In small numbers of patients under specific experimental conditions, standard doses of cimetidine, ranitidine, and nizatidine have increased blood alcohol concentrations, resulting in higher levels of intoxication than those achieved with alcohol alone.[19,51] The magnitude of this interaction is very small and appears to be related to the H_2RA dose as well as to the amount and timing of the alcohol.[51] Other studies dispute these results, finding no interaction between H_2RAs and alcohol at all. Accordingly, the FDA Advisory Committee on Gastrointestinal Drugs recently concluded that a labeling change for the H_2RAs was not necessary at this time because the elevations in blood alcohol concentrations have yet to be proven to be clinically significant.[58] Given the uncertainty of this reaction with prescription doses of H_2RAs, it is unlikely that nonprescription doses will interact significantly with alcohol.

The approval of nonprescription H_2RAs follows many years of controversy regarding the safety of such a switch. A major concern has been that patients with dyspeptic symptoms due to gastric cancer, angina, or complicated acid-peptic disorders may self-medicate with H_2RAs, thus delaying diagnosis and appropriate medical care.[1,30] The potential for undertreatment of PUD or esophagitis exists as well, as the H_2RAs may provide pain relief without actually healing the ulcer.[1] However, these concerns are neither new nor unique to H_2RAs as patients with dyspeptic symptoms have had the option to self-medicate with antacids for years.[30,56] The product labeling for H_2RAs, like that for antacids, recommends that they not be taken for longer than 2 weeks without consulting a physician. If these recommendations are followed, a 2-week delay in diagnosis is not likely to affect the prognosis of gastric cancer or other acid-peptic disorders. Other critics believe the nonprescription doses of H_2RAs are much too low to be useful for patients with significant symptoms and suggest that these agents will serve only as expensive antacids.[59]

Another concern regarding the switch to nonprescription status is the potential for rare but serious adverse reactions, which occur at a frequency of 1 in 100,000 cases with H_2RAs.[30] Given this frequency, it is estimated that if 50 million people switched from antacids to nonprescription H_2RAs, approximately 500 serious reactions would occur in 1 year.[30] The other major safety concern is the potential for drug interactions with cimetidine. As discussed, the magnitude of such interactions is likely to be small, but it may be important for some patients and should not be overlooked.

Despite these arguments, the availability of nonprescription H_2RAs offers the convenient option of self-care for patients with dyspeptic symptoms, and may especially benefit patients in underserved areas where there is a shortage of health care providers.[30] There may be significant cost savings as well in the form of reduced physician visits and avoidance of prescription dispensing fees. Overall, the extensive safety record of the H_2RAs supports the shift to nonprescription status. In Denmark, where cimetidine and ranitidine have been available without a prescription for nearly 5 years, the incidence of adverse effects reported with these agents has been extremely low (six significant adverse effects in 2 years).[60] However, this incidence may be underestimated as it was derived from voluntary reporting.

Clearly, the consequences of the shift of H_2RAs to nonprescription status in the United States are uncertain, and there is some risk involved. Pharmacists can minimize this risk by recognizing and triaging patients who are at risk for serious GI disease, by guiding patients at risk for cimetidine-drug interactions to other agents, and by counseling and educating patients about the appropriate use of these agents.

Bismuth

Bismuth compounds have been used to treat various GI disorders for more than 200 years. These compounds have recently attracted attention because of their ability to suppress *H pylori* infection and their potential for cytoprotection. Bismuth subsalicylate (BSS) (Pepto Bismol) is the only nonprescription bismuth compound available in the United States. BSS was once called an antacid but has no measurable ANC. Currently, it is indicated only for common diarrhea, traveler's diarrhea, and occasional relief of upset stomach or upper GI symptoms. Although BSS has been shown to coat the mucosal lining in animals, it does not appear to form a protective coating in human mucosa and is not recognized as a gastric mucosal protectant. It is generally believed that the benefit of BSS in treating peptic ulcers is derived almost entirely from its ability to suppress *H pylori*.

The major concern with the use of the bismuth salts is the potential for systemic bismuth absorption and toxicity, the primary manifestation of which is neurotoxicity. Most reports of bismuth neurotoxicity have been related to other bismuth salts, such as the subnitrate and the subgallate. In the many years in which BSS has been used as an occasional nonprescription medication, only a few cases of neurotoxicity have been reported.[4] Bismuth compounds react with hydrogen sulfide to produce bismuth sulfide, a highly insoluble black salt responsible for the darkening of the tongue or grayish black stools.[4] This side effect should not be confused with melena, in which the stools become black and tarry because of GI blood loss.

Antiflatulents

Although several antiflatulent products are available for nonprescription use, their use is largely empiric and evidence supporting their benefit is limited (see product table "Antiflatulent Products").

Simethicone

Simethicone, a mixture of inert silicon polymers, is used as a defoaming agent to relieve gas. Simethicone acts in the stomach and intestine to reduce the surface tension of gas bubbles embedded in mucus in the GI tract. As surface tension changes, the gas bubbles are broken or coalesced so that they can be eliminated more easily by belching or passing flatus.[41] The FDA considers simethicone safe and effective as an antiflatulent agent, but simethicone has no activity as an antacid.

The ability of simethicone to reduce intestinal gas is equivocal. While several controlled trials have found it to relieve gas, others have failed to show its efficacy.[61,62] Nonetheless, the use of simethicone may be encouraged on a trial basis as some patients subjectively report benefit from it. Moreover, since it is not absorbed from the GI tract, simethicone has no known systemic side effects and its safety has been well documented.[61]

Many antacid products contain a combination of simethicone and antacids, but use of both agents is often unnecessary and the efficacy of such combination products has not been well studied. The use of a combination product may be rational for patients with acid-peptic disorders who have symptoms related to gas (eg, upper GI bloating, pressure, fullness, flatulence). However, one study reported that the addition of simethicone to an aluminum-containing antacid adsorbed the antacid, thereby reducing the bioavailability of both agents.[63]

alpha-Galactosidase

Another product more recently approved for use as an antiflatulent is Beano, a solution of the enzyme alpha-galactosidase. This enzyme, which is derived from the *Aspergillus niger* mold and classified as a food, is said to break down oligosaccharides before they can be metabolized by colonic bacteria.[64] Since high-fiber foods contain large amounts of oligosaccharides, Beano is recommended as a prophylactic treatment of intestinal gas symptoms produced by high-fiber diets (eg, whole grains, lentils, broccoli, peas, cabbage).[65] The recommended dose is three to eight drops added to the first bite of the offending food. A five-drop dose contains greater than 175 units of galactose.[42] The solution should be added after the food has cooled because food temperatures higher than 130°F may inactivate the enzyme.[65]

To date, at least three controlled trials have found alpha-galactosidase to significantly reduce flatulence in patients fed oligosaccharide-containing foods.[64,65] However, patient numbers were small, and evidence for this product's efficacy is far from conclusive.

The safety of alpha-galactosidase also remains to be determined. Although this enzyme has been used in food processing for years and is regarded as safe by the FDA, the amount contained in Beano is probably much greater than that in processed foods.[65] One patient developed an intestinal perforation after taking Beano for several weeks, but a causal relationship was not established and there have been no similar reports.[65] Because the enzyme produces galactose, patients with galactosemia should not use this product. Similarly, diabetic patients should be cautioned about the use of the enzyme, which may produce 2–6 g of carbohydrates per 100 g of food. Allergic symptoms are also possible in patients allergic to molds.[65]

Other Drugs

Sucralfate is the only agent approved for the treatment of PUD that does not reduce or neutralize gastric acid. Although it is currently available only by prescription, sucralfate may be approved for nonprescription use in the future. Sucralfate is a complex salt of sucrose sulfate and aluminum hydroxide that dissolves in stomach acid, releases aluminum, and forms a viscous gel. This viscous substance has a strong negative charge and binds electrostatically to any positively charged chemical groups, such as proteins at the base of an ulcer. In its active form, sucralfate binds to defective mucosa and forms a barrier that protects the ulcer from the destructive forces of acid and pepsin. Numerous other cytoprotective mechanisms have been demonstrated in vitro, but whether these effects occur in human GI mucosa and are clinically significant is not known.[4]

Compliance with sucralfate is rarely compromised because of side effects; however, the large tablet size and multidose regimen may be inconvenient for some patients. Patients who find the large tablets difficult to swallow may find it easier to suspend the tablets in a glass of water or use the suspension form. Patients should be advised to take sucralfate on an empty stomach, about 30 minutes before meals. This is when the stomach is most acidic and the potential for sucralfate dissolution is greatest.[26]

Numerous other agents that are useful for the management of acid-peptic disorders are available only by prescription. These agents include prescription-dose H_2RAs, proton pump inhibitors (omeprazole, lansoprazole), misoprostol, cisapride, and various antibiotics in combination with antisecretory drugs. Although anticholinergic agents reduce acid secretion, the high incidence of side effects associated with these drugs precludes their usefulness for acid-peptic disorders. A detailed discussion of these agents is beyond the scope of this chapter.

Product Selection Guidelines

With the approval of nonprescription H_2RAs, the pharmacist will often be asked to choose between these agents and antacids, both of which are indicated for the relief of acid indigestion, sour stomach, and heartburn. Since there is no evidence that either type of product is more effective than the other for such indications, the choice should be based on patient factors and individual preferences. Thus, the patient should be questioned about the relative importance of the onset and duration of symptomatic relief, preference for product formulation, use of prescription medications, and history of response with antacids. Antacids are preferred for patients seeking rapid symptomatic relief because they provide immediate relief whereas H_2RAs provide relief within 1–2 hours. On the other hand, a longer duration of relief may be more important to patients who find taking multiple doses of antacids throughout the day inconvenient or undesirable. H_2RAs, which provide relief for 6–10 hours, depending on the agent, will be preferred for such patients. Patients who find antacids unpalatable may prefer H_2RAs, whereas patients who have difficulty swallowing tablets may be better treated with antacid suspensions or chewable antacid tablets.

The patient's medication history is important in selecting an acid-peptic product. Clearly, antacids and cimetidine have the greatest potential to cause drug interactions, and patients taking numerous medications may best be treated with one of the other H_2RAs. Lastly, financial restraints may dictate the choice of agents as antacids are substantially less expensive; if used at the recommended doses for 2 weeks, the cost of H_2RAs is approximately four times that of antacids.

Currently, only antacids are indicated for supplemental pain relief in patients taking prescription agents for healing or maintenance of PUD. Because most patients with PUD will already be taking antisecretory agents, the addition of nonprescription H_2RAs is unlikely to provide a significant benefit. In patients with severe GERD and/or reflux esophagitis, neither antacids nor nonprescription doses of H_2RAs are likely to provide additional benefit to prescription antisecretory medications.

Selection of Antacids

When an antacid is to be used, selection of a particular product should be guided by consideration of the chemical properties of the ingredients, the GI and systemic side effects of the ingredients, potency, formulation, taste, drug interactions, and cost. High-potency antacids are generally preferred since smaller amounts can neutralize large amounts of gastric acid, thereby reducing the amount of medication the patient must take. Care should be taken to select a formulation that is palatable to the patient because a product that tastes good is almost a prerequisite to successful antacid therapy. Unfortunately, clear guidelines for palatability do not exist, and the patient's personal history of antacid use may be the best indicator of what he or she considers acceptable.

Contents to consider before selecting an antacid for a patient include sodium, lactose, potassium, magnesium, and sugar. In general, all antacids pose a risk of systemic side effects or electrolyte imbalances in patients with chronic renal failure. Specifically, products containing large amounts of sodium (ie, sodium bicarbonate) or more than 50 mEq per day of magnesium are to be avoided in such patients. Similarly, sodium bicarbonate antacids should be avoided in patients with congestive heart failure, hypertension, or edema, or in patients on low-salt diets. Lactose content should be evaluated when choosing an antacid for patients with lactose intolerance, whereas sugar content is important to evaluate for diabetic patients.

Patients complaining of constipation, which is common in elderly patients, or hemorrhoids should be given antacids containing magnesium or magnesium-aluminum combinations. Conversely, patients with a history of diarrhea (eg, Crohn's disease, irritable bowel syndrome) should avoid magnesium-containing antacids and may best be treated with aluminum-only antacids.

The patient's medication history should be reviewed carefully when selecting an antacid product. However, the most significant drug interactions (ie, with tetracycline, quinolones) have been reported with aluminum-magnesium combinations as well as with calcium-containing antacids.

Apart from listing amounts of certain excipient ingredients, the antacid product labeling contains little information that is helpful to the pharmacist in choosing an antacid for a patient. A listing of the quantity of active ingredients is voluntary, and the milliequivalent ANC provided per dose is not specified.

A final consideration in antacid product selection is cost. Although most antacids are relatively inexpensive, the cost may vary considerably when the ANC of each is compared. As with all antacid ingredients, the cost should be calculated for equipotent, not equivolume quantities.

Selection of H_2-Receptor Antagonists

Currently, there are no data to support either superior efficacy or the side effects profile of one H_2RA over another when used for heartburn, acid indigestion, and sour stomach. The duration of acid suppression reported for cimetidine 200 mg (6 hours) may be shorter than that of the other nonprescription H_2RAs. Whether this difference is clinically important is not yet known.

Although significant drug-drug interactions at low doses of cimetidine are unlikely, patients receiving medications that have known interactions with cimetidine may be better managed with famotidine, ranitidine, or nizatidine.

The nonprescription H_2RAs are substantially less expensive than the prescription H_2RAs, but some patients may still prefer the prescription ones as many managed care reimbursement schemes will not cover the cost of nonprescription medications. There is no significant cost difference among the nonprescription H_2RAs.

Although a specific H_2RA may be labeled for treatment only, prevention only, or treatment and prevention of heartburn, sour stomach, or indigestion, it is likely that all the nonprescription H_2RAs are effective in both preventing and treating these conditions.

Selection of Antiflatulents

The selection of an antiflatulent product should be guided by the pattern of symptoms, cost, and concurrent disease states. Since alpha-galactosidase is intended for use as a preventive measure, patients experiencing symptoms of gas who need immediate relief or patients who cannot associate their symptoms with certain foods will be better managed with simethicone. Patients who anticipate gas from certain foods may add alpha-galactosidase to their food for prophylaxis, and/or they may prefer to have simethicone on hand to take as needed. If used on a regular basis, alpha-galactosidase is more cost-effective than simethicone. Finally, because alpha-galactosidase produces carbohydrates, patients with galactosemia or diabetes should avoid this product and use simethicone instead.

Therapeutic Considerations in Special Populations

Geriatric Patients

An appreciation for the special concerns of elderly patients with GI complaints is essential to the pharmacist for several reasons. First, antacid use is heaviest in this age group. The frequent purchase of antacids appears to begin around age 45 and increases with age so that 20–25% of people older than 65 years take antacids.[66,67] Frequent use of acid-peptic products by elderly patients is to be expected because many GI disorders occur more often in this age group. The elderly have an increased incidence of GUs, NSAID-induced ulcers, and Type B (*H pylori*) gastritis. Although their incidence of GERD is not greater, elderly patients often take drugs that re-[illegible]e LES tone and predispose them to this disorder. In addition, constipation is an extremely common complaint in the elderly, who often use magnesium-containing antacids as a laxative rather than as therapy for acid-peptic disorders.

Not only are acid-peptic disorders more common in the elderly, but so too are complications such as perforations and bleeding from peptic ulcers. Furthermore, mortality rates are high in this population when complications occur: more than one third of elderly patients with peptic ulcer complications die.[68] Mortality rates increase with multiple medical illnesses, delay in diagnosis and treatment, and use of NSAIDs. In fact, elderly NSAID users are four times more likely to die from peptic ulcers or GI bleeding than are nonusers.[69]

Because of these risks, the pharmacist's ability to assess the need for medical intervention in an elderly patient with GI complaints is very important. However, this task can be difficult because symptoms of PUD in elderly patients are very different from those seen in younger patients and can even be quite misleading. Many elderly patients with ulcers, and most patients with NSAID-induced ulcers, have no symptoms at all. The pharmacist should not expect the elderly patient with an ulcer to complain of classic burning epigastric pain; if symptoms are present, they are more likely to be vague abdominal discomfort, weakness, dizziness, anorexia, and severe weight loss.[69] It is very common for a perforation or bleeding to be the first sign that an ulcer is present, especially in those taking NSAIDs.[10,11] Therefore, regardless of whether pain or other symptoms are present, the elderly patient should be questioned about signs or symptoms of these complications. An adequate drug history, especially with regard to NSAID use, should be obtained as well. Because delayed diagnosis and treatment may result in significant morbidity or even mortality in elderly patients, the pharmacist should have an increased awareness of the risk factors for GI diseases in this population and should evaluate even vague or minor complaints. If the pharmacist cannot determine that the symptoms are related to overeating, eating spicy foods, or occasional reflux, it is wise to refer the elderly patient to a physician for further evaluation.

Selection of an antacid product for an elderly patient should be guided by the same principles used in choosing antacids for any patient population. However, the pharmacist should realize that elderly patients are less likely to tolerate a large sodium load, more likely to experience side effects from antacids, and more likely to be taking a drug that can interact with antacids. Because constipation is a troublesome and frequent occurrence in elderly patients, magnesium-containing antacids should be recommended provided the patient does not have severe renal impairment. Antacids containing only aluminum hydroxide are not good choices for elderly patients with constipation and have been reported to cause hypophosphatemia and resultant bone changes in this population.[68] On the other hand, these patients may be more likely to have diarrhea from magnesium or calcium carbonate antacids, and fluid-electrolyte disturbances are more dangerous in elderly patients than in younger persons. Patients should be aware that diarrhea and constipation are possibilities from antacid use and should be encouraged to switch antacids if these side effects occur. Because many elderly patients are on low-salt diets owing to hypertension or congestive heart failure, they should avoid sodium bicarbonate, even for short-term use. Doses of antacids do not need to be altered in elderly patients because of age-related changes in drug elimination, but may need to be reduced because of side effects.

Elderly patients with acid-peptic complaints may be safely treated with nonprescription H_2RAs. Despite clinical impressions that adverse CNS effects occur more often in this population, there is no evidence to support this idea in ambulatory patients.[68] The nonprescription doses of H_2RAs are low enough that dosage reductions are not necessary to compensate for age-related reductions in elimination and metabolism. The most important concern is that elderly patients are more likely to be taking medications that interact with cimetidine and possibly ranitidine.

Pregnant/Lactating Patients

Because 30–50% of pregnant women have symptomatic gastroesophageal reflux, they often seek advice from the pharmacist about the safe use of antacids.[70] Heartburn in pregnancy occurs most commonly in the third trimester and is a recurrent problem for more than 75% of women who experienced reflux symptoms in preceding pregnancies.[70] Antacids have not produced teratogenic effects and are generally considered safe in pregnancy as long as chronic high doses are avoided. There have been reports of magnesium-, calcium-, or aluminum-containing antacids causing hypermagnesemia, hypomagnesemia, hypercalcemia, and increased tendon reflexes in fetuses and neonates whose mothers were using these antacids chronically in high doses.[70,71] In addition, it is best not to recommend sodium bicarbonate to pregnant women because of the risks of systemic alkalosis and the sodium load leading to edema and weight gain.

Controlled data regarding the safety of H_2RA use in pregnancy are limited. Cimetidine readily crosses the placenta, and in one study produced antiandrogenic effects and feminization of male rat pups who were exposed in utero.[70–72] However, data collected by the manufacturer in 50 pregnant women receiving prescription doses of cimetidine failed to reveal any teratogenic effects.[70] To date, no teratogenic effects of ranitidine or famotidine have been reported in humans, either.[72] Clinical experience with nizatidine is too limited to draw any conclusions, but data in animals do not suggest any adverse effects. Cimetidine, ranitidine, and famotidine have received FDA pregnancy risk category B ratings while nizatidine has a pregnancy risk category of C. Despite their apparent safety, there is more clinical experience with the use of antacids in pregnancy than there is with H_2RAs. For this reason, pregnant women seeking a nonprescription product for an acid-peptic disorder should be directed to use antacids rather than H_2RAs unless a health care provider has instructed her otherwise.

To date, there are no reports linking simethicone to congenital defects.[72] Simethicone has been assigned a pregnancy risk category of C. Data regarding the safety of alginic acid or alpha-galactosidase in pregnancy are not available.

Neither aluminum nor magnesium hydroxide enters breast milk significantly, and no problems have been reported in lactating women.[71] Although cimetidine is concentrated in breast milk, adverse effects on breast-feeding newborns have not been observed, and the American Academy of Pediatrics considers cimetidine compatible with breast-feeding.[73] Famotidine, ranitidine, and nizatidine have also been demonstrated in human breast milk. Data regarding the use of alginic acid, simethicone, or alpha-galactosidase in breast-feeding women are not available.[72]

Pediatric Patients

Gastroesophageal reflux occurs commonly in infants and children. Signs and symptoms in such patients include vomiting, chest pain, irritability, feeding refusal, belching, hoarseness, hiccups, and apnea.[74] Antacids, with or without alginic acid, have been widely used in pediatric patients for this disorder as well as for esophagitis and PUD.[74] Despite the widespread use of antacids, however, their safety in pediatric patients has not been clearly established. Data from one study suggest that infants with normal renal function may experience an elevation of plasma aluminum levels while receiving doses of aluminum-containing antacids that are assumed to be safe.[75] Indeed, two recent cases of rickets in infants were attributed to phosphate depletion resulting from the prolonged use of aluminum-containing antacids.[76]

Although many cases of reflux in infants are benign, important complications can occur, including failure to thrive, esophageal strictures, Barrett's esophagus, intraesophageal polyps, and associated pulmonary diseases. Considering the serious nature of these complications and the inability of pharmacists to assess such problems, as well as the potential for harmful effects, any parents or caregivers who are seeking to use antacids for infants or children should be referred to their physicians or pediatricians for further evaluation.

Ranitidine, cimetidine, and famotidine have all been shown to be effective and have been used in the treatment of acid-peptic disorders in infants and children.[77] However, because the nonprescription H_2RAs are not available in liquid formulations, they are not useful for pediatric patients. These products are not to be used in children younger than 12 years unless directed by a physician.

Several pediatric formulations of simethicone are indicated for the relief of intestinal gas. These products, which contain 40 mg simethicone per 0.6 mL suspension, are often promoted and used to relieve gas associated with colic. Earlier studies found simethicone to be beneficial in infantile colic, but deficiencies in the study designs limit the validity of their conclusions. More recent, carefully controlled trials have not found simethicone superior to placebo for intestinal gas and/or infantile colic.[78] Although its efficacy is questionable, simethicone is not absorbed from the GI tract and is considered safe for use in infants and children.[26,41]

The safety and efficacy of alpha-galactosidase have not been evaluated in infants and children. Therefore, this product should not be used in pediatric patients until data are available to support such use.

Patient Counseling

Antacid/Antacid-Alginic Acid Combinations

The patient who purchases an antacid product should be given the following specific advice:

- Patients using antacids for relief of indigestion, upset stomach, or heartburn should take 40–80 mEq as needed. Some patients may experience relief from a scheduled dose, such as 40–80 mEq immediately after meals and at bedtime.
- Patients should not eat within 3 hours of going to bed; further, they should elevate the head of the bed 6–8 in. with blocks.
- Patients should not lie down for approximately 3 hours after eating.
- Patients should avoid smoking, caffeine, alcohol, fatty foods, tomato-based foods, chocolate, and peppermint/spearmint.
- Patients should avoid wearing tight-fitting clothing.
- If obese, patients should lose weight.
- Patients with PUD who are using antacids for supplemental ulcer pain relief should take 40–80 mEq ANC as needed for symptoms. If an H_2RA is being taken concomitantly, it should be given 1–2 hours before the antacid to avoid a possible reduction in H_2RA bioavailability.
- In general, patients should be advised not to take more than 500–600 mEq ANC of antacid per day.
- Antacids should not be taken for longer than 2 weeks. If they do not relieve symptoms promptly or if symptoms return often, a health care provider should be contacted.
- If a product with alginic acid is recommended, the patient should drink a glass of water after taking it and wait 1–2 hours before lying down or going to bed. Patients should understand that alginic acid products are best suited for daytime use.
- Because antacids may cause constipation or diarrhea, the patient should seek advice on switching antacids if one of these side effects develops.
- Patients on low-salt diets should know the amount of sodium in an antacid product and take only those products with a low sodium content. Patients with renal or cardiac disease should also be wary of potassium and magnesium content.
- Antacid tablets are not as potent as liquids. Patients who find liquids bulky and difficult to carry may take antacid tablets during the day at work and more potent liquids at night.
- Chewable antacid or antacid-alginic acid tablets should be chewed thoroughly and followed with a full glass of water. Effervescent tablets should be dissolved completely in water and the bubbles should subside before the patient drinks the liquid.
- Patients should space doses of antacids at least 2 hours apart from interacting drugs, such as tetracyclines, iron, and digoxin. When possible, antacids should be spaced at least 4–6 hours apart from quinolone antibiotics; if spaced only 2 hours apart, the quinolone should be given first.

H_2-Receptor Antagonists

The patient who purchases an H_2RA should be given the following specific advice:

- H_2RAs are not antacids, and they work differently to relieve acid-related symptoms. Moreover, nonprescription H_2RAs are the same medications as prescription H_2RAs but are simply lower doses.
- Patients using famotidine for relief of heartburn should take one tablet as soon as symptoms occur. If relief is not experienced within 1 hour, another tablet may be taken (up to a maximum of two tablets within a 24-hour period). However, patients using cimetidine to relieve heartburn should take two tablets when symptoms occur; this dose may be repeated up to a maximum of four tablets (400 mg) per day. Patients using ranitidine or nizatidine should take one tablet when symptoms occur; if necessary, this dose may be repeated up to a maximum of two tablets within a 24-hour period. Patients should also be educated about lifestyle modifications that may alleviate GERD (see previous section Antacids).
- In patients who anticipate heartburn or indigestion, one dose of any of the H_2RAs can be taken 1 hour before eating.
- H_2RAs should not be taken for more than 2 weeks continuously except under the advice and supervision of a health care provider. Patients whose symptoms do not resolve with H_2RAs or who experience difficulty swallowing or persistent abdominal pain should consult a health care provider.
- H_2RAs should not be given to children younger than 12 years of age, pregnant women, or lactating women without the advice of a health care provider.
- The most common side effects reported with nonprescription doses of H_2RAs are headache, dizziness, nausea, and diarrhea.
- Patients who are taking phenytoin, theophylline, or warfarin and who wish to take cimetidine 200 mg should consult their health care providers before taking the product. Alternatively, patients should be advised to take famotidine, ranitidine, or nizatidine.

Antiflatulents

The patient who purchases an antiflatulent product should be given the following specific advice:

- Patients using simethicone should take one tablet after meals and at bedtime. Patients should not take more than 500 mg simethicone per 24 hours.
- Dosage recommendations for simethicone drops for infants younger than 2 years of age are 0.3 mL four times daily after meals and at bedtime. To facilitate administration, the suspension may be mixed with 1 oz of cool water, infant formula, or other liquid. Children older than 2 years of age should be given 0.6 mL four times daily after meals and at bedtime.

- Patients using alpha-galactosidase solution should add three to eight drops to the first bite of the offending food. Because high temperatures (>130°F) may inactivate the enzyme, the solution should be added after the food has cooled, and patients should be advised not to cook with the product.
- Patients using alpha-galactosidase tablets may be instructed to swallow, chew, or crumble two to three tablets with the first bite of problem foods. One tablet is equivalent to five drops of alpha-galactosidase solution (175 units galactose). For larger meals, more tablets may be used.

Case Studies

Case 11–1

Patient Complaint/History

MM, a 20-year-old overweight female, presents to the pharmacist with a complaint of substernal pain that has been present for the past 2 weeks. During questioning about the pain, the pharmacist learns that it occurs after meals and when the patient lies down. The patient reports that she takes two Tums tablets at each episode of pain.

In response to questions about her diet, the patient reveals that she often eats fast-foods, usually eats a Milkyway candy bar after dinner, and drinks one cup of coffee in the morning as well as several glasses of fruit juice during the day. Further, she is often so tired after work that she goes to sleep 30 minutes after dinner.

The patient's other current medications include Centrum one tablet daily QAM and Monostat 7 one applicatorful hs for 7 days (she is currently on day 3 of therapy). MM, who is allergic to penicillin, smokes one pack of cigarettes a day and occasionally drinks beer.

Clinical Considerations/Strategies

The following considerations/strategies are provided to aid the reader in (1) determining whether treatment of the patient's condition with nonprescription medications is warranted, (2) selecting the appropriate nonprescription medication, and (3) developing a patient counseling strategy to ensure optimal therapeutic outcomes:

- Assess the possible causes of the substernal pain.
- Recommend dietary and lifestyle changes to decrease the pain.
- Assess the appropriateness of self-medication with a nonprescription H_2-receptor antagonist.
- Determine the appropriate response to the patient's clinical situation.
- Develop a patient education/counseling strategy that will:
  - Ensure that the patient understands the importance of the dietary and lifestyle modifications;
  - Ensure that the patient understands the proper use of the recommended nonprescription medications;
  - Ensure that the patient knows when to contact a health care provider.

Case 11–2

Patient Complaint/History

RJ, a 46-year-old female, presents to the pharmacist with a complaint of fatigue. She goes on to explain that for the past week she has been unable to perform her usual daily half-mile swim. Two weeks ago, she noticed a dull ache in her upper abdomen that was more pronounced at night and when she was hungry. The pain caused her to eat more often, increasing her weight by 4 lb. RJ's sister, who has a duodenal ulcer, recommended ALternaGEL for the stomach pain. Since taking the ALternaGEL, the patient has felt the stomach pain only at night.

Questions about the patient's lifestyle and dietary habits reveal that RJ smokes a pack of cigarettes a day, drinks a glass of wine with dinner every night, and drinks four cups of coffee during the day. When asked about the presence of other medical conditions, the patient explains that she was diagnosed with osteoarthritis of the right knee 5 years ago and that she has had occasional constipation for the past week. Her current medications include Motrin 400 mg q6h prn for pain; Fer-In-Sol 60 mg one capsule daily QAM; Centrum once daily QAM; Aristospan 10 mg intraarticular once a month; Ex-Lax 90 mg one tablet prn for constipation; and ALternaGEL 30 mL qid prn for pain.

Clinical Considerations/Strategies

The following considerations/strategies are provided to aid the reader in (1) determining whether treatment of the patient's condition with nonprescription medications is warranted, (2) selecting the appropriate nonprescription medication, and (3) developing a patient counseling strategy to ensure optimal therapeutic outcomes:

- Assess the possible causes of the fatigue and abdominal pain.
- Determine the appropriateness of treating the abdominal pain with ALternaGEL.
- Assess the effect of cigarette smoking, ethanol, and caffeine on this patient's condition.
- Determine an appropriate response to the clinical situation.
- Develop a patient education/counseling strategy that will:
  - Ensure that the patient understands the importance of discontinuing cigarette smoking and modifying her diet;
  - Ensure that the patient knows when to contact a health care provider.

Summary

The safe and effective use of acid-peptic products starts with the pharmacist's ability to distinguish between patients who are appropriate for self-treatment and those who need to be referred to a health care provider. The pharmacist should take care in selecting a safe acid-peptic product for a particular patient by evaluating a patient's symptoms, age, history, concomitant disease states, and concomitant medications.

To date, there is no evidence to support the superior efficacy of antacids or nonprescription H_2RAs for heartburn, sour stomach, or indigestion. Until such data are available, the choice of agents for such indications may best be dictated by practical issues, such as ease of use, frequency of administration, duration of effect, potential for adverse effects, and cost. Many patients will prefer H_2RAs because they are easier to use, more palatable, and less likely to cause troublesome GI side effects than antacids. However, antacids provide faster symptomatic relief and are substantially less expensive than H_2RAs. Patients who may be taking a medication that has the potential to interact with cimetidine should instead take famotidine, ranitidine, or nizatidine. The pharmacist should instruct the patient not to take the product for more than 2 weeks, at which time the patient should be referred to a health care provider if symptoms persist.

Although there is little objective evidence of antacid effectiveness for many acid-peptic disorders, their widespread and long-term use by patients can be viewed as a statement of their efficacy. Patients with symptoms of mild heartburn, indigestion, or sour stomach may be relieved by any antacid. Therapy can be initiated with 40–80 mEq ANC of a liquid antacid or with 2–4 g of sodium bicarbonate or calcium carbonate. Patients with heartburn may benefit from a product containing alginic acid but should be educated as to the proper use of the product.

The transfer of H_2RAs to nonprescription status continues to spark controversy and uncertainty. Critics maintain that nonprescription availability of these agents will mask acid-peptic symptoms, possibly delaying diagnosis of serious GI disorders. However, this possibility currently exists with antacids, which have been used for decades on an as-needed basis for similar indications. Another major concern is the potential for drug interactions with cimetidine, although the magnitude of such interactions is likely to be small given the low dose of cimetidine approved for nonprescription use. These risks can be minimized by pharmacists, who have a unique opportunity to identify and refer patients who should not take H_2RAs and to educate patients about the appropriate use of these agents. With proper triage and education of patients, the nonprescription H_2RAs can reduce health care costs and should provide a welcome alternative to antacids for patients with heartburn and minor GI complaints.

Knowledge of GI diseases is advancing rapidly, and changing with it is the role of antacids and antisecretory agents (ie, H_2RAs). As the association of *H pylori* with acid-peptic disorders grows stronger, the roles of acid neutralization and suppression become secondary to eradication of *H pylori* with antibiotics. Antacids continue to be used widely for short-term relief of mild GI complaints; however, the nonprescription availability of H_2RAs will undoubtedly affect the popularity of antacids for such indications. The impact of the nonprescription H_2RAs on this market may not be fully realized for many years. To continue the safe and effective use of acid-peptic products, pharmacists should understand the value of these agents in relation to other therapies for acid-peptic disorders and be informed of advances that affect the use of these products.

References

1. Gonzalez ER, Grillo JA. Over-the-counter histamine$_2$-blocker therapy. *Ann Pharmacother.* 1994 Mar; 28: 392–5.
2. Cramer T. When do you need an antacid? *FDC Consumer.* 1992 Jan-Feb; 19–22.
3. Biancani P, Behar J. Esophageal motor function. In: Yamada T, Alpers DH, Owyang C, eds. *Textbook of Gastroenterology.* 2nd ed. Philadelphia: JB Lippincott; 1995: 158–80.
4. Isenberg JI et al. Acid-peptic disorders. In: Yamada T, Alpers DH, Owyang C, eds. *Textbook of Gastroenterology.* 2nd ed. Philadelphia: JB Lippincott; 1995: 1347–429.
5. Berardi RR. Peptic ulcer disease and Zollinger-Ellison syndrome. In: DePiro JT et al, eds. *Pharmacotherapy: A Pathophysiologic Approach.* New York: Elsevier Science Publishing Co; 1992: 511–32.
6. Sung JJY et al. Antibacterial treatment of gastric ulcers associated with *Helicobacter pylori. N Eng J Med.* 1995 Jan; 332: 139–42.
7. NIH Consensus Development Panel on *Helicobacter pylori* in Peptic Ulcer Disease. *Helicobacter pylori* in peptic ulcer disease. *JAMA.* 1994 Jul; 272: 65–9.
8. Partipilo ML, Woster PS. The role of *Helicobacter pylori* in peptic ulcer disease. *Pharmacotherapy.* 1993; 13: 330–9.
9. Silverstein FE et al. Misoprostol reduces serious gastrointestinal complications in patients with rheumatoid arthritis receiving nonsteroidal anti-inflammatory drugs. *Ann Intern Med.* 1995 Aug; 123: 241–9.
10. Larkai EN et al. Gastroduodenal mucosa and dyspeptic symptoms in arthritic patients during chronic nonsteroidal anti-inflammatory drug use. *Am J Gastroenterol.* 1987; 82: 1153–8.
11. Armstrong CP, Blower AL. Non-steroidal anti-inflammatory drugs and life-threatening complications of peptic ulceration. *Gut.* 1987; 28: 527–37.
12. Peterson WL et al. Healing of duodenal ulcer with an antacid regimen. *N Engl J Med.* 1977; 297: 341–5.
13. Ching CK, Lam SK. Antacids. Indications and limitations. *Drugs.* 1994; 47: 305–17.
14. Sewing K. Efficacy of low-dose antacids in the treatment of peptic ulcers: pharmacological explanation. *J Clin Gastroenterol.* 1991; 13(suppl 1): S134–S138.
15. Weberg R et al. Low-dose antacids or cimetidine for duodenal ulcer? *Gastroenterology.* 1988 Jun; 95: 1465–9.
16. Weberg R et al. Duodenal ulcer healing with four antacid tablets daily. *Scand J Gastroenterol.* 1985; 20: 1041–5.
17. Nauert C, Caspary WF. Duodenal ulcer therapy with low-dose antacids: a multicenter trial. *J Clin Gastroenterol.* 1991: 13(suppl 1): S149–S154.
18. Berstad A, Weberg R. Antacids for peptic ulcer: do we have anything better? *Scand J Gastroenterol.* 1986; 21(suppl 125): 32–6.
19. Tatro DS, ed. *Drug Interaction Facts.* St Louis: JB Lippincott, Facts and Comparisons Division; 1995.
20. Hansten PD, Horn JR, eds. *Drug Interactions & Updates Quarterly 13.* Vancouver, Wash: Applied Therapeutics. 1993.
21. Sievert W et al. Low-dose antacids and nonsteroidal anti-inflammatory drug-induced gastropathy in humans. *J Clin Gastroenterol.* 1991; 13(suppl 1): S145–S148.
22. Orlando RC. Reflux esophagitis. In: Yamada T, Alpers DH, Owyang C, eds. *Textbook of Gastroenterology.* 2nd ed. Philadelphia: JB Lippincott; 1995: 1214–42.
23. Richter JE. Gastroesophageal reflux: diagnosis and management. *Hosp Pract.* 1992 Jan; 59–66.

24. Welage LS. Gastroesophageal reflux. In: DePiro JT et al, eds. *Pharmacotherapy: A Pathophysiologic Approach*. New York: Elsevier Science Publishing Co; 1993: 495–510.

25. Traube M. The spectrum of the symptoms and presentations of gastroesophageal reflux disease. *Gastroenterol Clin North Am*. 1990 Sep; 19: 609–17.

26. McEvoy GI, Litvak K, Welsh OH, eds. *AHFS Drug Information*. Bethesda, Md: American Society of Health-System Pharmacists; 1995.

27. Simon TJ et al. Self-directed treatment of intermittent heartburn: a randomized, multicenter, double-blind, placebo-controlled evaluation of antacid and low doses of an H_2-receptor antagonist (famotidine). *Am J Ther*. 1995; 2: 304–13.

28. Gottlieb S et al. Efficacy and tolerability of famotidine in preventing heartburn and related symptoms of upper gastrointestinal discomfort. *Am J Ther*. 1995; 2: 314–9.

29. Gibaldi M, Grundhofer B, Levy G. Effect of antacids on pH of urine. *Clin Pharmacol Ther*. 1974; 16: 520–5.

30. Feldman M. Pros and cons of over-the-counter availability of histamine$_2$-receptor antagonists. *Arch Intern Med*. 1993 Nov; 153: 2415–24.

31. *Pepcid AC Product Monograph*. Fort Washington, Pa: Johnson & Johnson Merck Consumer Pharmaceuticals; 1995.

32. Howden CW et al. The rationale for continuous maintenance treatment of reflux esophagitis. *Arch Intern Med*. 1995 Jul; 155: 1465–71.

33. Weinstein WM. Gastritis. In: Sleisinger J, Fordtan JS, eds. *Gastrointestinal Disease*. 5th ed. Philadelphia: WB Saunders; 1993: 545–71.

34. Veldhuyzen van Zanten SJO et al. Can gastritis symptoms be evaluated in clinical trials? An overview of treatment of gastritis, nonulcer dyspepsia and campylobacter-associated gastritis. *J Clin Gastroenterol*. 1989 May; 11: 496–501.

35. Talley NJ. Nonulcer dyspepsia. In: Yamada T, Alpers DH, Owyang C, eds. *Textbook of Gastroenterology*. 2nd ed. Philadelphia: JB Lippincott; 1995: 1446–55.

36. Shaffer EA. Nonulcer dyspepsia. A complex spectrum of disorders. *Can Fam Physician*. 1992 Mar; 38: 466, 470–1.

37. Liebeman DA, Melnyk CS. Gastrointestinal hemorrhage. In: Gitnick G, ed. *Principles and Practice of Gastroenterology and Hepatology*. New York: Elsevier Science Publishing Co; 1988: 1542–63.

38. Kivilaakso E. Antacids and bile salts. *Scand J Gastroenterol*. 1982; 17(suppl 75): 16–9.

39. Berstad A et al. Antacids reduce *Campylobacter pylori* colonization without healing the gastritis in patients with nonulcer dyspepsia and erosive prepyloric changes. *Gastroenterology*. 1988 Sep; 95: 619–24.

40. Preclik G et al. Stimulation of mucosal prostaglandin synthesis in human stomach and duodenum by antacid treatment. *Gut*. 1989; 30(2): 148–51.

41. Olin B, ed. *Drug Facts & Comparisons*. St Louis: JB Lippincott; 1995.

42. Schneider RP, Roach AC. An antacid testing: the relative palatability of 19 liquid antacids. *South Med J*. 1976 Oct; 69: 1312–3.

43. Bahal-O'Mara N, Force RW, Nahata MC. Palatability of 14 over-the-counter antacids. *Am Pharm*. 1994 Jan; NS34: 31–5.

44. Hade JE, Spiro HM. Calcium and acid rebound: a reappraisal. *J Clin Gastroenterol*. 1992; 15(1): 37–44.

45. Clemens JD, Feinstein AR. Calcium carbonate and constipation: a historical review of medical mythopoeia. *Gastroenterology*. 1977 May; 72: 957–61.

46. Piper DW. A comparative overview of the adverse effects of antiulcer drugs. *Drug Safety*. 1995; 12: 120–38.

47. National Institutes of Health. Over-the-counter antacid preparations can have adverse effects on bone. *JAMA*. 1977; 238: 1018.

48. Herzog P, Holtermuller KH. Antacid therapy—changes in mineral metabolism. *Scand J Gastroenterol*. 1982; 17(suppl 75): 56–62.

49. Donowitz M, Rood RP. Magnesium hydroxide: new insights into the mechanism of its laxative effect and the potential involvement of prostaglandin E_2. *J Clin Gastroenterol*. 1992 Jan; 14: 20–6.

50. Castell DO, Dalton CB, Becker D. Alginic acid decreases postprandial upright gastroesophageal reflux. Comparison with equal-strength antacid. *Dig Dis Sci*. 1992 Apr; 37: 589–93.

51. Welage LS, Berardi RR. Drug interactions with antiulcer agents: considerations in the treatment of acid-peptic disease. *J Pharm Pract*. 1994 Aug; 7: 177–95.

52. FDA changes approach to hangovers. *NDMA Executive Newsletter*. 1992 Jan; 1–92: 1–2.

53. Mayo M, Middleton RK. Calcium carbonate in hyperphosphatemia. *DICP, Ann Pharmacother*. 1991 Sep; 25: 945–7.

54. Wasan SM. Phosphate binders in hyperphosphatemia of chronic renal failure. *DICP, Ann Pharmacother*. 1991 Sep; 25: 942–5.

55. Sperber AD et al. The effect of an antacid containing aluminum hydroxide on plasma cholesterol and lipoproteins. *Curr Ther Res*. 1988; 77: 986–90.

56. *SmithKline Beecham Consumer Healthcare Tagamet HB Product Monograph*. June 1995.

57. Schentag JJ, Goss TF. Pharmacokinetics and pharmacodynamics of acid-suppressive agents in patients with gastroesophageal reflux disease. *Am J Hosp Pharm*. 1993 Apr; 50(suppl 1): S7–10.

58. H_2 blocker interaction with alcohol is not clinically significant. *FDC Rep Pink Sheet*. 1993 Mar 22; 55: 10–1.

59. Douds AC. Over the counter H_2 receptor antagonists. *Br Med J*. 1994 Oct; 309: 1156.

60. Andersen M, Schou JS. Safety implications of the over-the-counter availability of H_2-antagonists. *Drug Safety*. 1993; 8: 179–85.

61. Van Ness MM, Cattau EL. Flatulence: pathophysiology and treatment. *Am Fam Physician*. 1995 Apr; 31: 198–208.

62. Friis H, Bode S, Gudmand-Hoyer E. Effect of simethicone on laculose-induced H_2 production and gastrointestinal symptoms. *Digestion*. 1991; 49: 227–30.

63. Stead JA, Wilkins RA, Ashford JJ. In vitro and in vivo defoaming action of three antacid preparations. *J Pharm Pharmacol*. 1978; 30: 350–2.

64. Ganiats TG et al. Does Beano prevent gas? A double-blind crossover study of oral alpha-galactosidase to treat dietary oligosaccharide intolerance. *J Fam Pract*. 1994 Nov; 39: 441–5.

65. Abramowica M, ed. alpha-galactosidase to prevent gas. *Med Lett Drugs Ther*. 1993; 35: 30.

66. DP Hamacher & Associates. Antacids and antidiarrheals. *NARD J*. 1989 Nov; 111: 145–6.

67. Stewart RB, Hale WE, Marks RG. Antacid use in an ambulatory elderly population. *Dig Dis Sci*. 1983 Dec; 28: 1062–9.

68. Holt PR. Approach to gastrointestinal problems in the elderly. In: Yamada T, Alpers DH, Owyang C, eds. *Textbook of Gastroenterology*. Philadelphia: JB Lippincott; 1995; 1: 968–87.

69. Griffin MR, Ray WA, Schaffner W. Nonsteroidal anti-inflammatory drug use and death from peptic ulcer in elderly persons. *Ann Intern Med*. 1988 Sep; 109: 359–63.

70. Baron TH, Ramirez B, Richter JE. Gastrointestinal disorders during pregnancy. *Ann Intern Med.* 1993 Mar; 118: 366–75.

71. Smallwood RA et al. Safety of acid-suppressing drugs. *Dig Dis Sci.* 1995 Feb; 40(suppl): 63S–80S.

72. Briggs GG, Freeman RK, Yaffe SJ. *Drugs in Pregnancy and Lactation.* 4th ed. Baltimore, Md: Williams & Wilkins; 1994.

73. American Academy of Pediatrics, Committee on Drugs. The transfer of drugs and other chemicals into human milk. *Pediatrics.* 1994; 93: 137–50.

74. Glassman M, George E, Grill B. Gastroesophageal reflux in children. Clinical manifestations, diagnosis, and therapy. *Gastroenterol Clin North Am.* 1995 Mar; 24: 71–98.

75. Tsou VM et al. Elevated plasma aluminum levels in normal infants receiving antacids containing aluminum. *Pediatrics.* 1991 Feb; 87: 148–51.

76. Pivnick EK et al. Rickets secondary to phosphate depletion. A sequela of antacid use in infancy. *Clin Pediatr.* 1995 Feb; 34: 73–8.

77. Kelly DA. Do H_2 receptor antagonists have a therapeutic role in childhood? *J Pediatr Gastroenterol.* 1994; 19: 270–6.

78. Metcalf TJ et al. Simethicone in the treatment of infant colic: a randomized, placebo-controlled, multicenter trial. *Pediatrics.* 1994 Jul; 94: 29–34.

CHAPTER 12

Laxative Products

Clarence E. Curry, Jr, and Demetris Tatum-Butler

Questions to ask in patient assessment and counseling

- *Why do you feel you need a laxative?*
- *Are you experiencing or have you experienced abdominal discomfort or pain, bloating, weight loss, nausea, or vomiting?*
- *What other symptoms do you have?*
- *Are you currently being treated by a health care provider for any illness?*
- *Have you recently had abdominal surgery?*
- *Are you pregnant?*
- *How often do you normally have a bowel movement? Have you noticed a change in frequency?*
- *How would you describe your bowel movements? Has the nature of your bowel movements recently changed in any way?*
- *Has the appearance of your stools changed? In what way?*
- *How long has constipation been a problem?*
- *Have you attempted to relieve the constipation by eating more cereals, bread with a high fiber content, fruits, or vegetables?*
- *How much physical exercise do you get?*
- *How many glasses of water or other fluids do you drink each day?*
- *Have you previously used laxatives to relieve constipation?*
- *Are you using a laxative now? How often and how long have you used a laxative?*
- *Have you had any unwanted effects from laxatives, such as diarrhea or stomach pain?*
- *Are you currently taking any medication other than laxatives? If so, what prescription and nonprescription medications are you currently taking?*
- *Are you allergic to any medication?*

Extensive media advertising suggests that having clockwork-like bowel movements somehow enhances physical well-being and social acceptability. Laxative products are purchased in a variety of places and their use is common. Overall laxative sales in the United States during 1994 amounted to more than $725 million.[1]

By definition, a laxative facilitates the passage and elimination of feces from the colon and rectum. Despite numerous recognized indications for the use of laxatives, however, many people use them inappropriately to alleviate what they consider to be constipation.

Physiology of the Gastrointestinal Tract

The digestive and absorptive functions of the gastrointestinal (GI) system involve the intestinal smooth muscle, visceral reflexes, and GI hormones (Figure 1). Nearly all absorption of solids (>94%) occurs in the small intestine; relatively little occurs in the stomach.

The function of the colon is to allow for the orderly elimination from the body of nonabsorbed food products, desquamated cells from the gut lumen, and detoxified and metabolic end products. The colon functions to conserve fluid and electrolytes so that the quantity that is eliminated represents about 10% of what was presented to it in a 24-hour period. In addition, the colon has the capacity (as does the kidney) to absorb certain electrolytes because of differences in osmotic pressure.[2] If approximately 6 L of fluid per day are ingested and supplied by secretions of the GI tract, about 1.5%, or 90 mL, will be excreted with the feces.

Tonic contractions of the stomach churn and knead food, and large peristaltic waves start at the fundus and move food toward the duodenum. The time it takes the stomach contents to empty into the duodenum is regulated by autonomic reflexes or a hormonal link between the duodenum and the stomach. Carbohydrates are emptied from the stomach most rapidly, proteins more slowly, and fats are emptied the slowest. Vagotomy and fear tend to lengthen gastric emptying time; excitement generally shortens it. Most factors that increase gastric emptying time also inhibit the secretion of hydrochloric acid and pepsin. When the osmotic pressure of the stomach contents is higher or lower than that of the plasma, gastric emptying time is increased until isotonicity is achieved.

The mixture and passage of the contents of the small and large intestines are the result of four muscular movements: pendular, segmental, peristaltic, and vermiform. Pendular movements result from contractions of the longitudinal muscles of the intestine, which pass up and down small segments of the gut at the rate of about 10 contractions per minute. Pendular movements mix rather than propel the contents. Segmental movements result from contractions of the circular muscles and occur at about the same rate as pendular movements. Their primary function is also mixing. Pendular and segmental movements are caused by the intrinsic contractility of

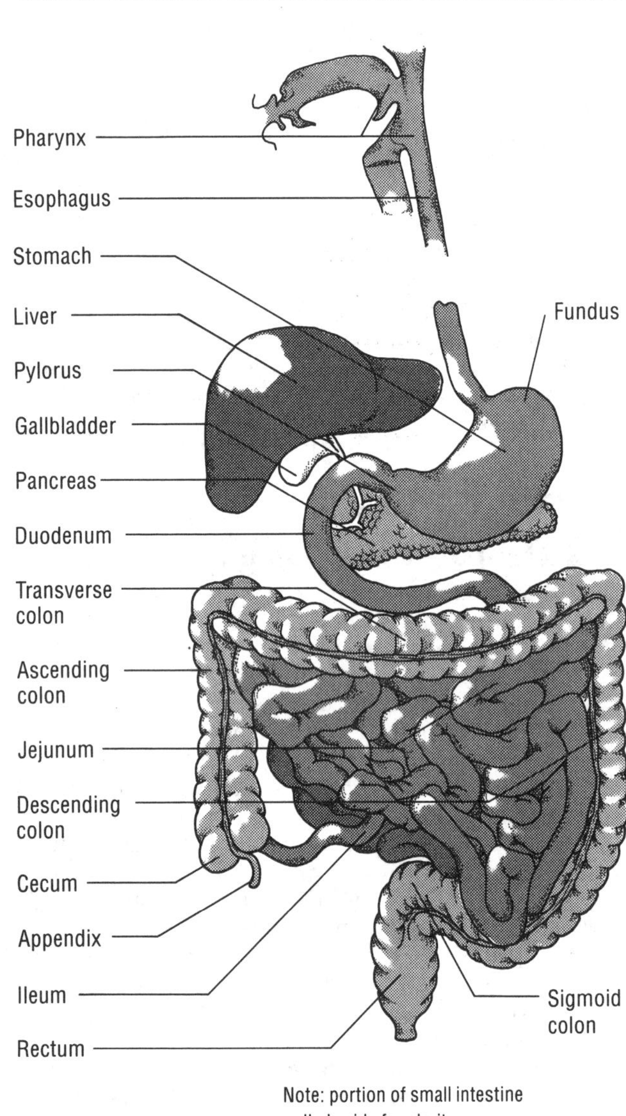

Note: portion of small intestine pulled aside for clarity.

smooth muscle and occur in the absence of innervation of intestinal tissue.

Peristaltic movements propel intestinal contents by circular contractions that form behind a point of stimulation and pass along the GI tract toward the rectum. The contraction rate ranges from 2 to 20 cm per second. These contractions require an intact myenteric (Auerbach's) nerve plexus, which apparently is located in the intestinal mucosa. Peristaltic waves move the intestinal contents through the small intestine in about 3.5 hours. Vermiform (wormlike) movements occur mainly in the large intestine (colon) and are caused by the contraction of several centimeters of the colonic smooth muscle at one time. In the cecum and ascending colon, the contents retain a fluid consistency, and peristaltic and antiperistaltic waves occur frequently. However, the activity of the transverse, descending, and sigmoid segments of the colon is very irregular, and here, through further water absorption, the contents become semisolid.

Three or four times a day, a strong peristaltic wave (mass movement) propels the contents about one third (38 cm) the length of the colon. When initiated by a meal, the mass movement is referred to as the gastrocolic reflex. This normal reflex seems to be associated with the entrance of food into the stomach and the subsequent distention of the stomach, and it is very strong in infants. The sigmoid colon serves as a storage place for fecal matter until defecation. The GI tract normally functions involuntarily in a coordinated manner.

The act of defecation involves multiple physiologic processes, but it is basically the rectal passage of accumulated fecal material. The fecal material from the sigmoid colon is propelled into the rectum by a mass peristaltic movement, which often occurs at breakfast time in persons with normal eating habits. This movement results in a desire to defecate because somatic impulses are sent to the defecation center in the sacral spinal cord. The defecation center then sends impulses to the internal anal sphincter, causing it to relax; this causes intra-abdominal pressure to increase as the muscles of the abdominal wall tighten, and a Valsalva maneuver forces the stool down. Voluntary relaxation of the exter-

TABLE 1 Drugs that may induce constipation

Analgesics (including NSAIDs)
Anesthetics
Antacids (calcium and aluminum compounds)
Anticholinergics (including felbamate and gabapentin)
Anticonvulsants
Antidepressants
Barium sulfate
Benzodiazepines (especially alprazolam and estazolam)
Bismuth
Diuretics
Ganglionic blockers
Hematinics (especially iron)
Hyperlidemia agents (eg, cholestyramine, pravastatin, and simvastatin)
Hypotensives (eg, agiotensin-converting enzyme inhibitors, beta-blockers, and calcium channel blockers)
Laxative excess
Monoamine oxidase inhibitors
Metallic intoxication (arsenic, lead, mercury, phosphorus)
Muscle paralyzers
Opiates
Parasympatholytics
Parkinsonism agents (eg, bromocriptine and selegiline)
Psychotherapeutic drugs (eg, phenothiazines, butyrophenones)

Adapted with permission from Fordtran JS, Sleisenger M, eds. *Gastrointestinal Disease*. Philadelphia: WB Saunders; 1993: 844.

TABLE 2 Metabolic and endocrine disorders associated with constipation

Metabolic disorders
Diabetic ketoacidosis
Diabetic neuropathy
Hypokalemia
Porphyria
Type I (Portuguese) and II (Indiana) amyloid neuropathy; sporadic primary amyloidosis
Uremia

Endocrine disorders
Enteric glucagon excess
Hypercalcemia: pseudohypoparathyroidism, hyperparathyroidism, milk–alkali syndrome, carcinomatosis
Hypothyroidism
Panhypopituitarism
Pheochromocytoma

Adapted with permission from Fordtran JS, Sleisenger M, eds. *Gastrointestinal Disease*. Philadelphia: WB Saunders; 1993: 844.

nal anal sphincter occurs, followed by elevation of the pelvic diaphragm, which lifts the anal sphincter over the fecal mass, allowing the mass to be expelled. Defecation, a spinal reflex, either is voluntarily inhibited by keeping the external sphincter contracted or is facilitated by relaxing the sphincter and contracting the abdominal muscles. Children usually defecate after meals; in adults, however, habits and cultural factors may determine the "proper" time for defecation.

Pathophysiology of the Lower Gastrointestinal Tract

Alteration in motor activities is responsible for various disorders in the small intestine. Distention or irritation of the small intestine can cause nausea and vomiting; the duodenum is most sensitive to irritation. Motility in the small intestine is intensified when the mucosa is irritated by bacterial toxins, chemical or physical irritants, and mechanical obstruction.

Pain from various causes, including gallbladder disease, appendicitis, and regional ileitis, may inhibit GI reflexes. As a result, functional obstruction may occur in the small intestine and with it, symptoms of acute intestinal blockage.

Large masses of fecal material tend to accumulate in a greatly dilated rectum. This is especially true in older individuals. The loss of tonicity in the rectal musculature may be caused by ignoring or suppressing the urge to defecate. It also may be caused by degeneration of nerve pathways concerned with defecation reflexes.

Painful lesions of the anal canal, such as ulcers, fissures, and thrombosed hemorrhoidal veins, impede defecation by causing a spasm of the sphincter and promoting voluntary suppression of defecation to avoid pain. The normal rectal mucosa is relatively insensitive to cutting or burning. However, when it is inflamed, it becomes highly sensitive to all stimuli, including those acting on the receptors mediating the stretch reflex. A constant urge to defecate in the absence of appreciable material in the rectum may occur with an inflamed rectal mucosa.[3]

Constipation

Constipation is generally defined as a decrease in the frequency of fecal elimination and is characterized by the difficult passage of hard, dry stools. It usually results from the abnormally slow movement of feces through the colon with a resultant accumulation in the descending colon.

Etiology

Causes of constipation are numerous (Tables 1–4). Idiopathic constipation often begins in childhood or adolescence. Elderly persons often suffer constipation owing to inappropriate diet, lack of exercise, or lack of muscle tone in the colon. Dietary issues related to the development of constipation include insufficient fluid intake, low-fiber content of the diet, and excessive ingestion of foods (eg, processed cheese) that harden stools.

TABLE 3 Conditions associated with neurogenic constipation

Peripheral
Aganglionosis (Hirschsprung's disease)
Autonomic neuropathy: paraneoplastic, pseudo-obstruction
Chagas' disease
Ganglioneuromatosis:
- Multiple endocrine neoplasia, type 2B
- Primary
- von Recklinghausen's disease

Hyperganglionosis
Hypoganglionosis

Central medulla
Cauda equina tumor
Meningocele (anterior or posterior)
Multiple sclerosis
Shy–Drager syndrome
Tabes dorsalis
Trauma to the medulla
Trauma to nervi erigentes

Brain
Cerebrovascular accidents
Parkinson's disease
Tumors

Reprinted with permission from Fordtran JS, Sleisenger M, eds. *Gastrointestinal Disease*. Philadelphia: WB Saunders; 1993: 845.

TABLE 4 Diseases of the large intestine associated with constipation

Lesions of the colon

Stenotic obstruction
Extraluminal
- Chronic volvulus
- Hernias
- Tumors

Luminal
- Chronic amebiasis
- Corrosive enemas
- Diverticulitis
- Endometriosis
- Ischemic colitis
- Lymphogranuloma venereum
- Strictures
- Surgery
- Syphilis
- Tuberculosis
- Tumors

Muscular abnormalities
Dermatomyositis
Diverticular disease
Myotonic dystrophy
Segmental dilatation of the colon
Systemic sclerosis

Lesions of the rectum
Internal rectal prolapse
Rectocele
Surgical stricture (EEA anastomosis)
Tumors
Ulcerative proctitis

Lesions of the pelvic floor
Descending perineum syndrome

Lesions of the anal canal
Anal fissure
Anterior ectopic anus
Mucosal prolapse
Stenosis

Reprinted with permission from Fordtran JA, Sleisenger M, eds. *Gastrointestinal Disease*. Philadelphia: W B Saunders; 1993: 847.

Constipation of recent onset suggests a possible organic or drug-induced cause. Constipation is often a problem in patients with ulcerative colitis that is limited to the rectum: when such patients experience diarrhea, the use of antidiarrheal agents can result in colonic dilation and the accumulation of hard stool in an area of bowel not affected by disease.[4,5] Constipation of organic origin may be caused by numerous pathologic conditions, including hypothyroidism, megacolon, stricture, or lesions (benign or malignant). Laxatives are contraindicated in such cases; instead, proper diagnosis and medical treatment should be obtained.

Symptoms

If constipation does occur, symptoms of varying degrees of severity may develop. Typical symptoms include anorexia, dull headache, lassitude, low back pain, abdominal distention, and lower abdominal distress. Abdominal discomfort and an inadequate response to an increasing variety and dosages of laxatives are common complaints. The frequency of bowel movements in humans generally ranges from three times a day to three times a week.[6] Individuals in the latter category are usually symptom free and do not have any specific abnormality related to their individual pattern of defecation. Therefore, constipation cannot be defined solely in terms of the number of bowel movements in any given period. Regularity is what is "regular" or typical for the individual who experiences none of the classic symptoms of constipation.

Patient Assessment

The pharmacist should obtain as much lifestyle and medical information as possible before making any recommendations for preventing or treating constipation. Appropriate information allows the pharmacist to make rational recommendations based on knowledge of the patient, the problem, and the product, as well as on the pharmacist's own judgment and experience. Because laxative products are both widely used and abused, the pharmacist can also provide a valuable service by educating patients about the appropriate use of laxatives.

A fundamental question is for what purpose the patient intends to use a laxative product. Not all people purchasing a laxative are constipated. A laxative might be needed to evacuate the bowel prior to an upcoming radiologic or endoscopic examination of the colon, or it may be purchased for a friend or a relative. It is important to know why the patient believes a laxative is necessary.

If symptoms have persisted for more than 2 weeks or have recurred after previous dietary or lifestyle changes or laxative use, the patient should be referred to a physician. Patients who admit to blood in the stool should be referred to a physician to rule out colon cancer or other significant disease. Any patient who has an established disease or surgery affecting the GI tract presents a particular concern because laxative products very possibly may affect their condition adversely. The pharmacist should obtain accurate information regarding all comorbidity and should refer the patient to a physician when insufficient information or any doubt exists regarding the patient's disease status.

As previously noted, the "healthy" population experiences from three bowel movements a day to three bowel movements a week, and individuals who fall outside this range might be classed as unusual but not always abnormal. Thus, the frequency of bowel movements may not be the most relevant concern; consistency of the stool, difficulty in elimination, and accompanying symptoms are also important characteristics of constipation.

The pharmacist should always inquire about the patient's current and past use of laxative products. The patient may be using one or more such products already, and improper use may be either preventing the desired effect or producing laxative dependency. The possibility of laxative abuse should also be considered. An in-depth knowledge of the patient's history of laxative use provides the pharmacist with information about the frequency and severity of constipation, prior patterns of medication use, effective or ineffective products, and the use of home remedies. Depending on the pharmacist's findings, referral to a physician may be necessary.

The pharmacist should exercise caution when recommending laxatives for patients who are receiving prescription drug products. Laxative preparations may interact adversely with other drugs that pass through the GI tract; the resulting effect could be decreased absorption of those other drugs. Drugs with constipating side effects (eg, calcium- or aluminum-containing antacids, narcotic analgesics, and drugs with anticholinergic activity) may counteract the therapeutic effects of laxatives or require their use. Tricyclic antidepressants and certain calcium channel blockers are two frequently used groups of prescription drugs that have persistently caused constipation in many patients. A clinical condition known as the narcotic bowel syndrome is characterized by chronic abdominal pain, nausea and vomiting, abdominal distention, constipation, and at least one occurrence of intestinal pseudo-obstruction.[7] When narcotics are discontinued and narcotic bowel syndrome does not abate, patients may require continuous subcutaneous infusions of metoclopramide.[8] Such a condition might occur in a cancer patient or in other patients who require chronic administration of large doses of narcotics. Some drugs, such as magnesium-containing antacids, prostaglandins (eg, misoprostol), and antiadrenergic drugs, may produce laxative side effects (eg, diarrhea). Pharmacists must assess all drug use and foster the rational selection of appropriate laxatives.

In some cases, treatment for another medical condition may relieve symptoms of constipation. In perianal disease, for example, constipation is usually the result of the patient's unwillingness to defecate because of the pain encountered. In such a case, medical or surgical treatment removes the barrier to normal defecation. Similarly, conditions such as hypothyroidism or depression may be responsible for constipation, which can be eliminated if these underlying medical conditions are treated successfully. Patients who have gastric esophageal reflux disease and constipation and who are receiving cisapride may have their constipation eliminated and are likely to experience diarrhea.

Treatment

Nondrug Measures

Constipation that does not have an organic etiology can often be alleviated with lifestyle modifications such as increased fiber in the diet, adequate fluid intake, and exercise. It is commonly thought that increasing dietary fiber enhances regularity; fiber improves bowel function by adding bulk and softening the stool. Both insoluble fiber (such as whole grain breads, prunes, raisins, and corn) and soluble fiber (such as beans, oat bran, barley, peas, carrots, citrus fruits, and apples) have been thought to be instrumental in this regard. But while this approach is useful for many people, it is not a panacea for all cases of constipation. Some people simply do not respond to the addition of fiber, the initial use of which may also lead to an increase in flatulence.

In conjunction with fiber, an increase in the intake of fluids, especially water, helps alleviate constipation. Recommendations for daily fluid consumption vary widely and range from 32 to 128 oz. Although most see additional fluid as expanding and softening the fiber, thereby leading to improved stool evacuation, microbial action on the fiber may account for the effect.[9]

Because constipation often afflicts sedentary persons, the importance of exercise to the body cannot be discounted. While any concentrated regular exercise is good, aerobic exercise is best. Regular walking, running, or swimming, among other forms of exercise, may help to alleviate constipation.

Finally, for those persons who achieve a beneficial effect from one of these measures, heeding the urge to pass the stool is paramount or the ultimate result will be the same as before. When these measures prove ineffective, however, a laxative may be indicated.

Pharmacologic Agents

The ideal laxative would (1) be nonirritating and nontoxic; (2) act only on the descending and sigmoid colon; and (3) produce a normally formed stool within a few hours, after which its action would cease and normal bowel activity would resume. Because a laxative that precisely meets these criteria is not currently available, proper selection of a laxative depends on the etiology of the constipation.

Laxative drugs have been classified according to their chemical structure, site of action, intensity of action, or mechanism of action. The most meaningful classification is the mechanism of action, whereby laxatives are classified as bulk forming, emollient, lubricant, saline, hyperosmotic, and stimulant (Table 5)(see product table "Laxative Products").

Bulk-Forming Laxatives

Because they most closely approximate the physiologic mechanism in promoting evacuation, bulk-forming products are the recommended choice as initial therapy for most forms of constipation. These laxatives are natural and semisynthetic hydrophilic polysaccharides and cellulose derivatives that dissolve or swell in the intestinal fluid, forming emollient gels that facilitate passage of the intestinal contents and stimulate peristalsis. They are usually effective in 12–24 hours but may require as long as 3 days in some individuals.

Polysaccharides and Cellulose Derivatives Bulk-forming laxatives are derived from agar, plantago (psyllium) seed, kelp (alginates), and plant gums including tragacanth, chondrus, and karaya (*Sterculia*). The synthetic cellulose derivatives—methylcellulose and carboxymethyl cellulose sodium—are being used more often, and many

TABLE 5 Classification and properties of laxatives

Agent	Dosage form	Daily dosage range: Adult	Daily dosage range: Pediatric (age, y)	Site of action	Approximate time required for action	Systemic absorption
Bulk-forming						
Methylcellulose	Solid	4–6 g	1–1.5 g (>6)	Small and large intestines	12–72 h	No
Carboxymethyl cellulose sodium	Solid	4–6 g	1–1.5 g (>6)	Small and large intestines	12–72 h	No (laxative) Yes (sodium)
Malt soup extract	Solid, liquid, powder	12–64 g	6–32 mL (1 mo–2 y)	Small and large intestines	12–72 h	—
Polycarbophil	Solid	1–6 g	0.5–1.0 g (<2) 1–1.5 g (2–5) 1.5–3.0 g (6–12)	Small and large intestines	12–72 h	No
Plantago seeds	Solid	2.5–30 g	1.25–15 g (>6)	Small and large intestines	12–72 h	No
Emollient						
Docusate calcium	Solid	0.05–0.36 g	0.025 g (<2) 0.05–0.150 g (≥2)	Small and large intestines	12–72 h	Yes
Docusate sodium	Solid	0.05–0.36 g	0.02–0.05 g (<2) 0.05–0.15 g (≥2)	Small and large intestines	12–72 h	Yes
	Liquid	50–240 mg	10–40 mg (<3) 20–60 mg (3–6) 40–120 mg (6–12)	—	—	—
Docusate potassium	Solid	100–300 mg	100 mg (≥6) at bedtime	Colon	2–15 min	—
Lubricant						
Mineral oil	Liquid (oral)	14–45 mL	10–15 mL (>6)	Colon	6–8 h	Yes, a minimal amount
Saline						
Magnesium citrate	Liquid	240 mL	0.5 mL/kg	Small and large intestines	0.5–3 h	Yes
Magnesium hydroxidc	Liquid	15–40 mL	0.5 mL/kg	Small and large intestines	0.5–3 h	
Magnesium sulfate	Solid	10–30 g	2.5–5.0 g (2–5) 5.0–10.0 g (≥6)	Small and large intestines	0.5–3 h	Yes
Dibasic sodium phosphate	Solid (oral) Solid (rectal)	1.9–3.8 g 3.8 g	1/4 adult dose (5–10) 1/2 adult dose (≥10) 1/2 adult dose (>2)	Small and large intestines Colon (rectal)	0.5–3h 2–15 min	Yes
Monobasic sodium phosphate	Solid (oral)	8.3–16.6 g	1/4 adult dose (5–10) 1/2 adult dose (≥10)	Small and large intestines	0.5–3 h	Yes
	Solid (rectal)	16.6 g	1/2 adult dose (>2)	Colon	2–15 min	
Sodium biphosphate	Solid (oral)	9.6–19.2 g	1/4 adult dose (5–10) 1/2 adult dose (≥10)	Small and large intestines	0.5–3 h	Yes
	Solid (rectal)	19.2 g	1/2 adult dose (>2)	Small and large intestines	2–15 min	—
Hyperosmotic						
Glycerin	Solid (rectal)	3 g	1–1.5 g (<6)	Colon	0.25–1 h	—
	Liquid (rectal)	Not recommended	1–1.5 g/kg or 40 g/m^2	—	—	—

TABLE 5 *continued*

Agent	Dosage form	Daily dosage range: Adult	Daily dosage range: Pediatric (age, y)	Site of action	Approximate time required for action	Systemic absorption
Stimulant						
Anthraquinones	Solid	0.12–0.25 g	Not recommended (<6)	Colon	8–12 h	Yes
Aloe		120–200 mg (≥15)	80–120 mg (8–14)			
Cascara sagrada	Fluidextract (aromatic)	2–6 mL	1/2 adult dose (2–11)	Colon	6–8 h	Yes
	Solid	0.3–1.0 g (daily)	Consult physician (<2)			
Senna	Solid	0.5–2.0 g	1/8 adult dose (>2)	Colon	6–10 h	Yes
	Fluidextract	2.0 mL				
	Syrup	8.0 mL	1/4 adult dose (1–6)			
	Fruitextract	3.4–4.0 mL	1/2 adult dose			
	Suppository	1 at bedtime	1/2 adult dose (children >60 lb)			
Calcium salt of sennosides A and B	Solid	12–24 mg	20 mg (≥6) at bedtime	Colon	6–10 h	Yes
Diphenylmethane stimulants						
Bisacodyl	Solid (oral)	10–30 mg	5–10 mg (>6)	Colon	6–10 h	Yes
	Solid (rectal)	10 mg	5 mg (<2) 10 mg (≥2)	Colon	15–60 min	Yes
Phenolphthalein	Solid	0.03–0.27 g	Not recommended (<2) 0.015–0.020 g (2–6) 0.03–0.06 g (>6)	Colon	6–8 h	Yes
	Liquid	60–194 mg at bedtime	1 mg/kg or 30 mg/m^2	—	—	—
Miscellaneous						
Castor oil	Liquid	15–60 mL	1–5 mL (<2) 5–15 mL (2–12)	Small intestines	2–6 h	Yes

preparations that contain these drugs also contain stimulant and/or fecal-softening laxative drugs (eg, docusate). These synthetic colloidal materials have a high degree of uniformity and can be readily compressed into tablets.

Calcium Polycarbophil Calcium polycarbophil, the calcium salt of a synthetic polyacrylic resin, has a marked capacity for binding water. It is often used to treat constipation associated with irritable bowel syndrome and diverticular disease. The maximum calcium content of this agent is approximately 150 mg (7.6 mEq) per tablet. Ingestion of the recommended therapeutic doses may increase the risk of hypercalcemia in susceptible patients, so caution should be used in such patients. The US recommended daily allowance of calcium is 1,000–1,300 mg for adults. (See Chapter 19, "Nutritional Products.") A recent National Institutes of Health Conference indicated that up to 2,000 mg per day of calcium, from all sources, appears safe for most individuals.[10]

Malt Soup Extract Another bulk-forming laxative, malt soup extract, is obtained from barley and contains maltose protein, potassium, and amylolytic enzymes. An interesting aspect of this agent is that it reduces fecal pH, which may contribute to its laxative activity.

Indications/Contraindications Bulk-forming laxatives may be indicated for people on low-residue diets that cannot be corrected; postpartum women; elderly patients; and patients with colostomies, irritable bowel syndrome, or diverticular disease.

Failure to consume sufficient fluid with a bulk laxative decreases drug efficacy and may result in intestinal or esophageal obstruction. Therefore, bulk-forming laxatives may be inappropriate for persons who must severely restrict their fluid intake, such as those with significant renal dysfunction.

Adverse Effects Esophageal obstruction has occurred in elderly persons, in patients who have difficulty swallowing, and in patients with strictures of the esophagus after they ingested a bulk laxative that had been chewed or taken in dry form. Symptoms of esophageal obstruction include chest pain, vomiting, excessive salivation, and an inhibited swallowing reflex that may precipitate choking. In addition, there have been reports of acute bronchospasm associated with the inhalation of dry hydrophilic mucilloid,[11] as well as of hypersensitivity reactions including swollen, watery eyes and skin rash. Because of the danger of fecal impaction or intestinal obstruction, the bulk-forming laxatives should not be taken by individuals with intestinal ulcerations, stenosis, or disabling adhesions. Diarrhea, abdominal discomfort, flatulence, and excessive loss of fluid can also occur. However, when taken properly, these agents have few systemic side effects because they are not absorbed.

Usage Considerations Choosing among the different bulk products is a matter of personal preference. It is more important that each dose be taken with a full glass of fluid (at least 240 mL, or 8 oz). The dose should be adjusted as directed until the required effect has been obtained. In addition to being relatively safe, bulk-forming laxatives are appropriate for long-term therapy. The dextrose content of some of the commercial products should be evaluated for usage by diabetic patients and other patients on carbohydrate-restricted diets. Likewise, sugar-free bulk-forming agents containing aspartame should be avoided by patients suffering from phenylketonuria.

The hydrophilic colloid bulk laxatives are not absorbed systemically and do not seem to interfere with the absorption of nutrients. When given as a powder or as granules, bulk laxatives should be mixed with pleasant-tasting fluids and administered with a full (8-oz) glass of fluid. Most people prefer juices, sugar-free fruit drinks, or soft drinks to water because such fluids help mask the gritty tastelessness of some bulk-forming laxatives; however, some newer formulations have been introduced that claim to have no gritty taste.

Emollient Laxatives

Docusate sodium, formerly known as dioctyl sodium sulfosuccinate, is an anionic surfactant that, when administered orally, increases the wetting efficiency of intestinal fluid and facilitates admixture of aqueous and fatty substances to soften the fecal mass. It is commonly known as a stool softener. Other fecal-softening laxatives are docusate calcium and docusate potassium (both anionic surfactants). In many cases of fecal impaction, a solution of docusate is added to the enema fluid. Docusate does not retard absorption of nutrients from the intestinal tract.

Indications Orally administered emollient laxatives are best suited to prevent the development of constipation and are of little or no value in treating long-standing constipation, especially in elderly and debilitated patients. Thus, their value when used in proper doses is more prophylactic than therapeutic. Emollient laxatives may be used for up to 1 week without physician consultation. Emollient laxatives are indicated in cases of acute perianal disease to soften and inhibit painful elimination of stool or when avoidance of straining at the stool is desirable (eg, after rectal or abdominal surgery, labor and delivery, or myocardial infarct). Emollient laxatives do not stimulate bowel movements when used alone but do achieve this purpose when combined with stimulant laxatives. Fecal-softening emollient laxatives are usually effective in 1–2 days but may take as long as 3–5 days in some individuals. Liquid formulations may be more palatable if mixed with juices or milk. Fluid intake should be increased to facilitate softening of stools.

Patients with abdominal hernia, severe hypertension, or cardiovascular disease should not strain to defecate; neither should patients who are immediately postpartum, or who have undergone or are about to undergo surgery for hemorrhoids or other anorectal disorders. An emollient or fecal-softening laxative is indicated in such cases, but its use should be avoided if nausea and vomiting, symptoms of appendicitis, or undetermined abdominal pain exist.

Adverse Effects By facilitating the absorption of other poorly absorbed substances such as mineral oil, emollient laxatives, when administered concomitantly, may increase the toxicity of those substances.[12] Docusate and its congeners are claimed to be nonabsorbable, nontoxic, and pharmacologically inert. However, it has been postulated that the detergent (surfactant) properties of docusate facilitate transport of other substances across cell membranes. Consequently, a Food and Drug Administration (FDA) advisory panel recommended that these laxatives carry the following warning statement: "Do not take this product if you are presently taking a prescription drug or mineral oil."[13]

Lubricant Laxatives

Liquid petrolatum (mineral oil) and certain digestible plant oils such as olive oil soften fecal contents by coating them, thus preventing colonic absorption of fecal water. Emulsified products are used to increase palatability. There is little difference in their cathartic efficacy although emulsions of mineral oil penetrate and soften fecal matter more effectively than nonemulsified preparations.

Indications Liquid petrolatum is beneficial when used judiciously in cases requiring the maintenance of a soft stool to avoid straining (eg, when there has been hernia, aneurysm, hypertension, myocardial infarct, or cerebrovascular accident, or after a hemorrhoidectomy or abdominal surgery). However, routine use of liquid laxatives in these cases is probably not indicated; instead, stool softeners such as docusate sodium are probably better agents for preventing constipation.

Adverse Effects The adverse effects and toxicity of mineral oil are associated with repeated and prolonged use. Significant absorption of mineral oil may occur, especially if emulsified products are used. The oil droplets may reach the mesenteric lymph nodes and may also be present in the intestinal mucosa, liver, and spleen, where they elicit a typical foreign-body reaction.

Lipid pneumonia may result from the oral ingestion and subsequent aspiration of mineral oil, especially when the patient reclines. The pharynx may become coated with the oil, and droplets may reach the trachea and the posterior part of the lower lobes of the lungs. Because aspiration into the lungs is possible, mineral oil should not be administered at bedtime or to very young, elderly, or debilitated patients.

The role of mineral oil in impairing the absorption of fat-soluble nutrients is uncertain. Mineral oil may impair the absorption of vitamins A, D, E, and K; impaired vitamin D absorption may affect the absorption of calcium and phosphates. Mineral oil should not be taken with meals because it may delay gastric emptying. Additionally, it should not be given to pregnant patients because it can decrease the availability of vitamin K to the fetus. Patients taking oral anticoagulants should use mineral oil with caution because the potentially decreased absorption of vitamin K may increase the blood-thinning property of the anticoagulant.

When large doses of mineral oil are taken, the oil may leak through the anal sphincter and produce anal pruritus (pruritus ani), cryptitis, and other perianal conditions. This leakage can be avoided by reducing or dividing the dose, or by using a stable emulsion of mineral oil. Prolonged use should be avoided. Because surfactants tend to increase the absorption of otherwise "nonabsorbable" drugs, mineral oil should not be taken with emollient fecal softeners.[14]

Saline Laxatives

The active constituents of saline laxatives are relatively nonabsorbable cations and anions such as magnesium and sulfate ions. Sulfate salts are considered to be the most potent of this category of laxatives. The wall of the small intestine, acting as a semipermeable membrane to the magnesium, sulfate, tartrate, phosphate, and citrate ions, retains the highly osmotic ions in the intestine. The presence of these ions draws water into the intestine, causing an increase in intraluminal pressure. This increased pressure exerts a mechanical stimulus that increases intestinal motility.

However, different mechanisms independent of the osmotic effect may be partially responsible for the laxative properties of the salts. Saline laxatives produce a complex series of reactions, both secretory and motor, on the GI tract. For example, the action of magnesium sulfate on the GI tract is similar to that of cholecystokinin-pancreozymin. There is evidence that this hormone is released from the intestinal mucosa when saline laxatives are administered.[14] This release in turn favors accumulation of fluid and electrolytes within the intestinal lumen.

Indications Saline laxatives are indicated for use only when acute evacuation of the bowel is required, as when preparing for endoscopic examination or eliminating drugs in suspected poisonings. Saline laxatives have no place in the long-term management of constipation.

In some cases of food or drug poisoning, saline laxatives are used in purging doses. Magnesium sulfate is recommended except in cases of depressed central nervous system activity or renal dysfunction. Liquid preparations may be more palatable if chilled prior to administration, but that is not possible in acute medical emergencies.

Adverse Effects In some cases, the choice of a saline laxative may result in serious adverse effects. As much as 20% of the administered magnesium ion may be absorbed from magnesium salts. If renal function is normal, the absorbed ion can be eliminated without consequence. However, if renal function is markedly impaired, or if the patient is a newborn or is elderly, toxic concentrations of the magnesium ion could accumulate with resulting intoxication.[15] Hypotension, muscle weakness, and electrocardiographic changes may indicate a toxic effect of magnesium. In addition, excessive serum magnesium levels exert a depressant effect on the central nervous system and neuromuscular activity. Other adverse effects include abdominal cramping, excessive diuresis, nausea, vomiting, and dehydration.

Precautions Phosphate salts are available in oral and rectal dosage forms. The typical oral dose contains 96.5 mEq of sodium and therefore should be administered with caution to patients on sodium-restricted diets. When phosphate salts are given as an enema, up to 10% or more of the sodium content may be absorbed. Rectal phosphate products are used to prepare the bowel for a barium enema and for the elimination of fecal impaction. However, cathartics containing sodium may be toxic to individuals with edema, congestive heart disease, or renal failure; phosphates will accumulate with impaired renal function and should be avoided in such patients. The use of phosphate salts in children under 2 years of age can result in hypocalcemia, tetany, hypernatremia, dehydration, and hyperphosphatemia. Because dehydration may occur with the repeated use of hypertonic solutions of saline cathartics, phosphate salts should not be used by those who cannot tolerate fluid loss. In patients who are not fluid restricted, oral phosphate salts should be followed by at least one full glass of water to prevent dehydration.

Hyperosmotic Laxatives

Glycerin has been available for many years in suppository form to be used for lower bowel evacuation. Its laxative capability is caused by the combination of glycerin's osmotic effect with the local irritant effect of sodium stearate. Rectal irritation may occur with its use.

Use of glycerin suppositories in infants and adults usually produces a bowel movement within 30 minutes.

In infants, the physical manipulation and insertion of a solid rectal mass will usually initiate the reflex to defecate. Adverse reactions and side effects from glycerin suppositories are minimal.

The customary rectal dose of glycerin considered to be safe and effective for adults and for children older than 6 years of age is 3 g as a suppository or 5–15 mL as an enema. For infants and for children under 6 years of age, the dose is 1–1.5 g as a suppository or 2–5 mL as an enema.[13]

Stimulant Laxatives

Stimulant laxatives are conveniently classified according to their chemical structure and pharmacologic activity. These laxatives are thought to increase the propulsive peristaltic activity of the intestine by local irritation of the mucosa or by a more selective action on the intramural nerve plexus of intestinal smooth muscle, thus increasing motility. It has been suggested that these laxative products stimulate secretion of water and electrolytes in either the small or large intestine or both, depending on the specific laxative.[16] Intensity of action is proportional to dosage, but individually effective doses vary. All stimulant laxatives may produce griping, colic, increased mucus secretion, and, in some people, excessive evacuation of fluid. Listed doses and dosage ranges are only guides to determining the optimal individual dose.

Anthraquinone Stimulants Anthraquinone laxatives include aloe, cascara sagrada, casanthranol, senna, aloin, danthron, rhubarb, and frangula. The drugs of choice in this group are the cascara, casanthranol, and senna compounds. Rhubarb, aloe, and aloin, which are very irritating, should not be recommended. The properties of each anthraquinone laxative vary somewhat, depending on the anthraquinone content and the speed with which the active principles are liberated. The anthraquinones are hydrolyzed by colonic bacteria into active compounds.

The precise mechanism by which peristalsis is increased is unknown. The cathartic activity of anthraquinones is limited primarily to the colon. Anthraquinones usually produce their action 8–12 hours after administration but may require up to 24 hours.

The active principles of anthraquinones are absorbed from the GI tract and subsequently appear in body secretions, including human milk. However, the practical significance of this event in nursing infants is poorly defined. After taking a senna laxative, postpartum patients have reported a brown discoloration of breast milk and subsequent catharsis by their nursing infants. A study with constipated postpartum breast-feeding women receiving a senna laxative reported that 17% of their infants experienced diarrhea.[17] Preparations of senna are more potent than those of cascara and can produce considerably more abdominal cramping.

Chrysophanic acid, a component of rhubarb and senna that is excreted in urine, colors acidic urine yellowish-brown and colors alkaline urine reddish-violet. The pharmacist should warn patients that a number of prescription and nonprescription medications and some foods produce either alkaline or acidic urine and may produce this effect.

The prolonged use of anthraquinone laxatives, especially cascara sagrada, can result in a harmless, reversible melanotic pigmentation of the colonic mucosa (melanosis coli), which is usually found on sigmoidoscopy, colonoscopy, or rectal biopsy.

The liquid preparations of cascara sagrada are more reliable than the solid forms. Aromatic cascara sagrada fluidextract is less active and less bitter than cascara sagrada fluidextract. Magnesium oxide, used in the preparation of aromatic cascara fluidextract, removes some of the bitter and irritating principles from the crude drug.

In 1987, the FDA announced the total recall of a formerly popular stimulant laxative known as danthron. Danthron, a breakdown product of the glycosides of senna, is an anthraquinone with actions similar to those of the natural anthraquinones. It was withdrawn from the market because of reports of its tendency to produce liver tumors in rats.[18]

Diphenylmethane Stimulants The most commonly used diphenylmethane laxatives are bisacodyl and phenolphthalein.

Bisacodyl, administered in a combination of either tablets and suppositories or tablets and enemas, has been recommended for cleaning the colon before GI surgery, endoscopy, or radiography. Bisacodyl is effective in patients with colostomies, and it may reduce or eliminate the need for irrigations.

Bisacodyl acts in the colon on contact with the mucosal nerve plexus. Stimulation is segmented and axonal, producing contractions of the entire colon. Bisacodyl's action is independent of intestinal tone, and the drug is minimally absorbed systemically (approximately 5%).[19] Action on the small intestine is negligible. A soft, formed stool is usually produced 6–10 hours after oral administration and 15–60 minutes after rectal administration.

Adverse effects, which come with chronic, regular use (abuse), include metabolic acidosis or alkalosis, hypocalcemia, tetany, loss of enteric protein, and malabsorption. The suppository form may produce a burning sensation in the rectum. No systemic or adverse effects on the liver, kidney, or hematopoietic system have been observed following administration.

Enteric-coated bisacodyl tablets prevent irritation of the gastric mucosa and therefore should not be broken, crushed, chewed, or administered with agents that increase gastric pH such as antacids, histamine$_2$-receptor antagonists, or proton pump inhibitors.

Phenolphthalein is effective in small doses and is tasteless, making it desirable for use in candy, wafer, and chewing gum dosage forms. When ingested, it passes through the stomach unchanged and is dissolved in the intestine by bile salts and the alkaline intestinal secretions. As much as 15% of the dose is absorbed; the rest is excreted unchanged in the feces.

This drug exerts its stimulating effect primarily on the colon. Although the exact mechanism of action is not known, phenolphthalein appears to alter multiple steps of the absorptive process. It is usually active 6–8 hours after administration.

Part of the absorbed phenolphthalein is secreted into the intestinal tract along with bile. The resulting enterohepatic cycle may prolong the action of phenolphthalein for 3 or 4 days. Because bile must be present for phenolphthalein to be effective, the drug does not relieve constipation in patients who have obstructive jaundice.

Phenolphthalein is usually nontoxic. However, at least two types of allergic reactions may follow its use. In susceptible individuals, a large dose may cause diarrhea, colic, cardiac and respiratory distress, or circulatory collapse. The other reaction is a polychromatic rash that ranges from pink to deep purple. The eruptions may be as small as a pinhead or as large as the palm of the hand. Itching and burning may be moderate or severe. If the rash is severe, it may lead to vesication and erosion, especially around the mouth and genital areas. Patients should be advised to report any rash to the physician or the pharmacist. Other skin reactions, including toxic epidermal necrosis and bullous eruptions, may occur and appear to be related to sunlight exposure.[20]

Osteomalacia caused by impaired absorption of vitamin D and calcium is one untoward effect that has been attributed to excessive phenolphthalein ingestion.[14] Phenolphthalein abuse can mimic Bartter's syndrome by inducing juxtaglomerular cell hyperplasia with secondary hyperaldosteronism. This is characterized by hypokalemic alkalosis and marked renin increase in the absence of hypertension.[21]

Some of the absorbed drug appears in the urine, which is colored pink to red if it is sufficiently alkaline. Similarly, the drug excreted in the feces causes a red coloration if the feces are sufficiently alkaline. This effect may be alarming, so the patient should be forewarned.

Castor Oil Castor oil is used in situations requiring a thorough evacuation of the GI tract; it is seldom used routinely for constipation. Castor oil's laxative action is produced by ricinoleic acid, which is produced when castor oil is hydrolyzed in the small intestine by pancreatic lipase. Its exact mechanism of action is unknown. However, its laxative effect appears to depend primarily on cyclic adenosine monophosphate–mediated fluid secretion and not on an increased peristalsis caused by the irritant effect of ricinoleic acid.[22]

Castor oil, a glyceride, may be absorbed from the GI tract and is probably metabolized like other fatty acids. Because the main site of action is the small intestine, its prolonged use may result in excessive loss of fluid, electrolytes, and nutrients.

Castor oil is most effective when administered on an empty stomach, and it produces an evacuation within 2–6 hours after ingestion. Because a laxative effect occurs quickly, the drug should not be given at bedtime. The most commonly used products containing castor oil are the more palatable emulsions. When plain castor oil is used, it may be administered with fruit juice or a carbonated beverage to mask its unpleasant taste.

Indications Stimulant laxatives, such as castor oil and bisacodyl, are often used before radiologic or endoscopic examination of the GI tract and before GI surgery, when thorough evaluation of the bowel is crucial. Bisacodyl may be administered orally or rectally and used instead of an enema for emptying the colon and rectum before proctologic or colonic examination.

In general, stimulant laxatives may be used as initial drug therapy in patients with simple constipation, but they should not be used for more than 1 week. The dose should be within the recommended dosage range (Table 5).

Adverse Effects Major hazards of stimulant laxative use are severe cramping, electrolyte and fluid deficiencies, enteric loss of protein, malabsorption resulting from excessive hypermotility and catharsis, and hypokalemia. Stimulant laxatives are effective but should be recommended cautiously; because the intensity of their activity is proportional to the dose used, a large enough dose of any stimulant laxative can produce unwanted and sometimes dangerous adverse effects. Nevertheless, these laxatives are frequently used by those who self-medicate for constipation. Stimulant laxatives are abused and such abuse can lead to "cathartic colon," a poorly functioning colon.[20] Patients should be advised that the dose may need to be individualized to obtain the appropriate effect.

Precautions Stimulant laxatives should be used with caution when symptoms of appendicitis (abdominal pain, nausea, and vomiting) are present, and they should not be used at all when the diagnosis of appendicitis is made.

Dosage Forms

Laxative products are available in a wide array of dosage forms, most of them for oral use. This variety probably yields the most benefits for pediatric and geriatric patients. Many of the dosage forms enhance patient acceptability and perhaps make laxative use more pleasant. However, laxatives available as chewing gum, wafers, effervescent granules, and chocolate tablets may not be thought of as drug products and thus are more likely to be misused and abused. Enemas and suppositories are dosage forms often used for laxative administration.

Enemas Enemas are used routinely to prepare patients for surgery, child delivery, and GI radiologic or endoscopic examination and to treat certain cases of constipation. The enema fluid determines the mechanism by which evacuation is produced. Tap water and normal saline create bulk by an osmotic volume effect; vegetable oils lubricate, soften, and facilitate the passage of hardened fecal matter; soapsuds produce defecation by their irritant action. However, prolonged rectal irritation may occur after soap enemas, which have also led to reports of anaphylaxis, rectal gangrene, and serious fluid loss secondary to acute colitis.[23] Therefore, soap enemas are not recommended for use.

The popular sodium phosphate-sodium biphosphate enemas (eg, Fleet) fall into the category of saline laxatives. They are usually effective evacuants in preparing patients for surgical, diagnostic, or other procedures involving the bowel. These agents are more efficient and effective than tap water, soapsuds, or saline enemas. Because they can alter fluid and electrolyte balance significantly if used on a prolonged basis, chronic use of these products is not warranted in the control of constipation.

A properly administered enema cleans only the distal colon, most nearly approximating a normal bowel movement. Proper administration requires that the diagnosis, the enema fluid, and the technique of administration be correct. Improperly administered, an enema can produce fluid and electrolyte imbalances. Enema fluids have caused mucosal changes or spasm of the intestinal wall. Water intoxication has resulted from the use of tap water or soapsud enemas in the presence of megacolon. A misdirected or inadequately lubricated nozzle may cause abrasion of the anal canal and rectal wall or colonic perforation.

Patients should be advised to follow all directions carefully when using these products. The patient should lie or be placed on the left side with knees bent or in the knee-to-chest position. If the patient is in a sitting position, use of an enema clears only the rectum of fecal material. The solution should be allowed to flow into the rectum slowly; if the patient is uncomfortable, the flow is probably too fast. One pint (500 mL) or less of properly introduced fluid usually produces adequate evacuation if it is retained until definite lower abdominal cramping is felt. As long as 1 hour may be needed for the entire procedure.

Suppositories Bisacodyl suppositories are promoted as replacements for enemas when the distal colon requires cleaning. Suppositories that contain bisacodyl are promoted for postoperative, antepartum, and postpartum care and are adequate in the preparation for proctosigmoidoscopy. Although bisacodyl suppositories are prescribed and used more often than other suppositories, some clinicians still prefer enemas as agents for cleaning the lower bowel.

Therapeutic Considerations in Special Populations

Pediatric Laxative Use

Laxatives are often given to children according to what the parents believe should be normal bowel habits. As a result, indiscriminate use of laxatives may occur. Bowel movement patterns vary widely in children, and constipation can be a complex problem that is often difficult to detect and manage. Parents should observe their child for frequency of bowel movements, difficulty in passing stools, pain during bowel movements, and the child's withholding of stools. Any deviation from the child's usual pattern should be noted. Infants and children appear to show a decreasing frequency of bowel movements with increasing age. Normally, neonates may pass more than four bowel movements a day during the first week of life. This declines to approximately one to two bowel movements a day by 4 years of age. Constipation can occur in infants who have one to two daily bowel movements and is often unrecognized as such. Infants whose frequency of bowel movements is less than average in the first weeks of life may be prone to develop chronic constipation in later years.[24–26]

A number of factors can alter a child's bowel habits, including emotional distress, febrile illness, family conflict, dietary changes (eg, human to cow milk), or environmental changes, such as a move or recent travel. The pharmacist must consider such factors when determining whether constipation exists.[27]

TABLE 6 Suggested pediatric dosages of commonly used nonprescription laxatives

Agent	Patient's age	Dosage
Malt soup extract (Maltsupex)	Breast-fed infant	5–10 mL in 2–4 oz of water or fruit juice twice daily
	Bottle-fed infant	7.5–30 mL in day's total formula, or 5–10 mL in every second feeding
Corn syrup (Karo Syrup)	Infant	Same as that of malt soup extract
Milk of magnesia	>6 mo	1–3 mL/kg of body weight per day, in one to two doses
Mineral oil	>6 y	10–15 mL at bedtime
Senna syrup (Senokot)	1–5y	5 mL at bedtime; maximum 5 mL twice daily
	5–13 y	10 mL at bedtime; maximum 10 mL three times daily

Adapted with permission from Loening-Baucke V. Elimination disorders. In: Greydanus DE, Walraich ML, eds. *Behavioral Pediatrics.* New York: Springer-Verlag; 1992: 280–97.

As with adults, increasing both fluids and the bulk content of the child's diet may improve bowel habits and decrease frequency of constipation. Simply increasing the amount of fluid or sugar in the formula may be corrective in the first few months of life. After this age, better results are obtained by adding or increasing the amounts of high-fiber cereal, vegetables, and fruits. Sugar-water solutions (fruit juice or soda) often diminish the child's appetite for solid foods and should be administered in moderation. The child should be encouraged to drink water, and excessive milk intake should not be considered a substitute. Unbuttered popcorn is a good bulk-containing snack for children.

If medications are indicated in children under 5 years of age, glycerin suppositories may initiate the defecation reflex with an onset usually within 15–60 minutes. Malt soup extract is relatively safe for infants under 2 months of age. Dark corn syrup (1–2 tsp per feeding) or milk of magnesia (beginning with ½ tsp) may be useful for fecal impaction. Bisacodyl may be used for moderate to severe constipation. In general, stimulants should probably be avoided, as should excessive use of enemas. Enemas are not usually recommended for children under 2 years of age. Senna and mineral oil should be administered only on the advice of a physician. When successful bowel evacuation cannot be achieved with oral supplementation or enemas, pediatricians may prescribe a balanced polyethylene glycol-electrolyte solution (eg, Golytely or Colyte) to be administered orally. Children may find such a solution more palatable if it is chilled.[28]

The pharmacist should always consider a child's age when recommending laxative products (Table 6). The route of administration and the taste of oral products may be especially significant in children. The use of laxatives may be avoided in older children if they are encouraged to establish a regular pattern of bowel movements and adhere to suggested dietary guidelines.

Geriatric Laxative Use

Constipation is a common complaint of many elderly persons. It may progress with age, and prolonged and excessive laxative use is not uncommon in this population. Many elderly persons have been laxative dependent for many years. However, because of the physiologic effects of chronic laxative use on the intestine, laxative dependency is often difficult to manage. Thus, proper education about laxative products and advice on product selection and use are particularly crucial for the elderly patient.

Constipation in elderly persons can result from a number of factors, including failure to establish a time habit; insufficient fluid and/or bulk intake; abuse of stimulant laxatives, which can result from an attempt to regulate bowel activity; and immobility. Constipation in this population is often associated with a prolonged transit time through the colon and a decreased perception of the need to defecate, which is often precipitated by conditions such as neuromuscular disorders, confusion, and depression.[29–31] Elderly patients often strain to pass hard stools, which may predispose them to serious complications, including cardiovascular problems and hemorrhoids. In addition, geriatric patients tend to have multiple diseases and take multiple medications, some of which may contribute to the development of constipation and, in some cases, chronic constipation. Such agents include sedatives; hypnotics; antispasmodics; antidepressants; antipsychotics; calcium-, aluminum-, and iron-containing products; and calcium channel blockers.[30] Laxative preparations can increase the rate at which other drugs pass through the GI tract by increasing GI motility, which then decreases absorption and the effectiveness of concurrently administered medications.

Elderly patients are particularly sensitive to shifts in fluid and electrolytes. Use of any laxative that alters the fluid and electrolyte balance, particularly saline-type laxatives, may be inappropriate in certain elderly patients. Such laxatives can place patients, particularly those who are on diuretics or have decreased fluid intake, at risk for adverse effects.

For geriatric patients without a history of constipation, a thorough investigation should be conducted to determine whether acute cases of constipation have resulted from new or old diseases or from the use of medications. The colon in the elderly can lack normal tone, resulting in an overreliance on oral laxatives or rectal enemas.

A low-residue diet, a diet consisting mainly of soft foods, or the poor chewing of food may be associated with the development of constipation in this age group. If any of these factors exist, the pharmacist should consider corrective action in the patient's lifestyle or current drug therapy before recommending a laxative.

It has been suggested that an acute episode of constipation be treated with plain water or saline enemas.[29,31,32] Soapsud enemas should be avoided because they can be irritating and can cause serious complications.[31,33] Sodium phosphate and biphosphate enemas are effective. Polyethylene glycol-electrolyte solutions, commonly used as bowel preparations for GI procedures, have been safely used for acute management of constipation in elderly patients suffering from cardiac or renal disease.[29,31] Dietary fiber should be increased by including bran, fruits, and vegetables in the diet (Table 7). However, the pharmacist should advise patients that increasing bran in the diet may lead to erratic bowel habits, flatulence, and abdominal discomfort during the first few weeks. It is suggested that excess bran be avoided in patients with hypocalcemia or low serum iron as well as in patients confined to bed.[29,31,32]

For elderly patients requiring laxatives, bulk-forming agents are generally preferred; onset is usually in 2–3 days. Sugar-free products (eg, Konsyl, Serutan, and various Metamucil products) are recommended for diabetic patients.[31] Glycerin suppositories and orally administered lactulose are safe and have been used successfully in elderly patients[31]; lactulose may be of particular benefit to those who are bedridden.[31] Some health care providers may recommend chronic stimulant laxatives in certain situations, but these products should not be generally recommended in all elderly patients. The pharmacist should exercise caution when recommending magnesium-containing products to patients with renal failure because of the risk of hypermagnesemia. The pharmacist should be similarly cautious when recommending sodium-containing products to patients with cardiovascular disease because of the potential for sodium overload. Mineral oil can cause malabsorption of fat-soluble vitamins or lipid pneumonia if it is aspirated, so its use should be avoided.

Recommendations of laxative use in this population should be patient specific because the elderly have complicating pathology and multiple disease states and are often vulnerable to medications. Even though bulk-forming agents are often successfully used in this population, a complete and thorough history should aid in the selection of the most appropriate product.

Laxative Use in Pregnancy

Constipation is common in pregnancy, often because the increasing size of the uterus causes compression of the colon. However, the primary reason is probably a reduction in intestinal muscle tone, which contributes to a decrease in peristalsis.[34] In addition, prenatal vitamin and mineral supplements that contain iron and calcium tend to be constipating.

One study showed a 31% incidence of constipation in pregnancy, with 65% of these women self-treating with either diet or laxatives and without professional advice.[17] Most types of laxatives appear to be effective in pregnancy. However, because of such adverse ef-

TABLE 7 **Provisional dietary fiber table**

Food	Analytical method[a]	Fiber (g) per 100 g	Calories per 100 g	Serving size	Fiber (g) per serving	Calories per serving
Breakfast cereals						
All-Bran	1	29.9	249	1/3 c (1 oz)	8.5	71
Bran Buds	1	27.7	258	1/3 c (1 oz)	7.9	73
Bran Chex	1	16.2	319	2/3 c (1 oz)	4.6	91
Cheerios-type	1	3.8	391	1 1/4 c (1 oz)	1.1	111
Corn Bran	1	19.0	346	2/3 c (1 oz)	5.4	98
Cornflakes	1	1.1	389	1 1/4 c (1 oz)	0.3	110
Cracklin' Bran	1	15.1	382	1/3 c (1 oz)	4.3	108
Crispy Wheats n' Raisins	1	4.6	349	3/4 c (1 oz)	1.3	99
40% Bran-type	1	13.4	325	3/4 c (1 oz)	4.0	93
Frosted-Mini Wheats	1	7.6	359	4 biscuits (1 oz)	2.1	102
Graham Crackos	1	6.1	361	3/4 c (1 oz)	1.7	102
Grape-Nuts	1	4.8	357	1/4 c (1 oz)	1.4	101
Heartland Natural Grain, plain	1	4.7	434	1/4 c (1 oz)	1.3	123
HoneyBran	1	11.1	341	7/8 c (1 oz)	3.1	97
Most	1	12.4	337	2/3 c (1 oz)	3.5	95
Nutri-Grain, barley	1	5.8	372	3/4 c (1 oz)	1.7	106
Nutri-Grain, corn	1	6.2	381	3/4 c (1 oz)	1.8	108
Nutri-Grain, rye	1	6.4	359	3/4 c (1 oz)	1.8	102
Nutri-Grain, wheat	1	6.3	360	3/4 c (1 oz)	1.8	102
Oatmeal, regular, quick, and instant, cooked	4,5	0.9	62	3/4 c (1 oz)	1.6	108
100% Bran	1	29.6	269	1/2 c (1 oz)	8.4	76
100% Natural Cereal, plain	1	3.7	470	1/4 c (1 oz)	1.0	133
Raisin Bran-type	1	11.3	312	3/4 c (1 oz)	4.0	115
Rice Krispies	1	0.2	395	1 c (1 oz)	0.1	112
Shredded Wheat	1	9.3	359	2/3 c (1 oz)	2.6	102
Special K	1	0.8	390	1 1/3 c (1 oz)	0.2	111
Sugar Smacks	1	0.9	373	3/4 c (1 oz)	0.4	106
Tasteeos	1	3.5	393	1 1/4 c (1 oz)	1.0	111
Total	1	7.2	352	1 c (1 oz)	2.0	100
Wheat Chex	1	7.4	367	2/3 c (1 1/3 oz)	2.1	104
Wheat germ	1	14.3	386	1/4 c (2 oz)	3.4	108
Wheaties	1	7.0	349	1 c (1 oz)	2.0	99
Wheat 'n' Raisin Chex	1	6.6	343	3/4 c (1 1/3 oz)	2.5	130
Fruits						
Apple (w/o skin)	2,3,4	2.1	57	1 med	2.7	72
Apple (w/skin)	2	2.5	59	1 med	3.5	81
Apricot (dried)	6	8.1	238	5 halves	1.4	42
Apricot (fresh)	2,3	1.7	48	3 med	1.8	51
Banana	2,4	2.1	92	1 med	2.4	105
Blueberries	2	2.7	51	1/2 c	2.0	39
Cantaloupe	3	1.0	24	1/4 melon	1.0	30
Cherries, sweet	2,3	1.2	72	10	1.2	49
Dates	3,4	7.6	275	3	1.9	68
Grapefruit	2,3,4	1.3	32	1/2	1.6	38
Grapes	3,4	1.3	63	20	0.6	30
Orange	2,4	2.0	47	1	2.6	62
Peach (w/skin)	4	2.1	43	1	1.9	37
Peach (w/o skin)	2,3	1.4	43	1	1.2	37
Pear (w/skin)	4	2.8	59	1/2 large	3.1	61

TABLE 7 *continued*

Food	Analytical method[a]	Fiber (g) per 100 g	Calories per 100 g	Serving size	Fiber (g) per serving	Calories per serving
Pear (w/o skin)	2,3,4	2.3	59	1/2 large	2.5	61
Pineapple	2,3	1.4	49	1/2 c	1.1	39
Plums, Damsons	2,4	1.7	60	5	0.9	33
Prunes	3,4	11.9	239	3	3.0	60
Raisins	3,4	8.7	300	1/4 c	3.1	108
Raspberries	3,4	5.1	57	1/2 c	3.1	35
Strawberries	2,3	2.0	30	1 c	3.0	45
Watermelon	2	0.3	26	1 c	0.4	42
Juices						
Apple	2	0.3	47	1/2 c (4 oz)	0.4	56
Grape	2	0.5	51	1/2 c (4 oz)	0.6	64
Grapefruit	2	0.4	41	1/2 c (4 oz)	0.5	51
Orange	2	0.4	45	1/2 c (4 oz)	0.5	56
Papaya	2	0.6	57	1/2 c (4 oz)	0.8	71
Vegetables						
Cooked						
Asparagus, cut	2,3	1.5	20	1/2 c	1.0	15
Beans, string, green	2,3,4	2.6	25	1/2 c	1.6	16
Broccoli	2,4	2.8	26	1.2 c	2.2	20
Brussel sprouts	2,3	3.0	36	1/2 c	2.3	28
Cabbage, red	4	2.0	20	1/2 c	1.4	15
Cabbage, white	4	2.0	20	1/2 c	1.4	15
Carrots	2,3,4	3.0	31	1.2 c	2.3	24
Cauliflower	3,4	1.7	22	1/2 c	1.1	14
Corn, canned	2,3	2.8	83	1/2 c	2.9	87
Kale, leaves	3	2.6	34	1/2 c	1.4	22
Parsnip	3,4	3.5	66	1/2 c	2.7	51
Peas	2,3,4	4.5	71	1/2 c	3.6	57
Potato (w/skin)	4	1.7	93	1 med	2.5	106
Potato (w/o skin)	3,4	1.0	93	1 med	1.4	97
Spinach	2,4	2.3	23	1/2 c	2.1	21
Squash, summer	2,4	1.6	14	1/2 c	1.4	13
Sweet potatoes	2,3	2.4	141	1/2 med	1.7	80
Turnip	3,4	2.2	23	1/2 c	1.6	17
Zucchini	4	2.0	12	1/2 c	1.8	11
Raw						
Bean sprout, soy		2.6	46	1/2 c	1.5	13
Celery, diced	3,4	1.5	8	1/2 c	1.1	10
Cucumber	3,4	0.8	15	1/2 c	0.4	8
Lettuce, sliced	3,4	1.5	12	1 c	0.9	7
Mushrooms, sliced	3	2.5	28	1/2 c	0.9	10
Onions, sliced	3,4	1.3	23	1/2 c	0.8	33
Pepper, green, sliced	3,4	1.3	23	1/2 c	0.5	9
Tomato	3,4	1.5	22	1 med	1.5	20
Spinach	2	4.0	26	1 c	1.2	8
Legumes						
Baked beans, tomato sauce	3	7.3	121	1/2 c	8.8	155
Dried peas, cooked	3,4	4.7	115	1/2 c	4.7	115
Kidney beans, cooked	3	7.9	118	1/2 c	7.3	110
Lentils, cooked	3	3.7	97	1/2 c	3.7	97
Lima beans, cooked/canned	2	5.4	75	1/2 c	4.5	64
Navy beans, cooked	6,3	6.3	118	1/2 c	6.0	112

continued

TABLE 7 *continued*

Food	Analytical method[a]	Fiber (g) per 100 g	Calories per 100 g	Serving size	Fiber (g) per serving	Calories per serving
Breads, pastas, and flours						
Bagels	1	1.1	264	1 bagel	0.6	145
Bran muffins	1	6.3	263	1 muffin	2.5	104
Cracked wheat	1	4.1	246	1 slice	1.0	62
Crisp bread, rye	1	14.9	376	2 crackers	2.0	50
Crisp bread, wheat	1	12.9	376	2 crackers	1.8	50
French bread	1	2.0	291	1 slice	0.7	102
Italian bread	1	1.0	278	1 slice	0.3	83
Mixed grain	1	3.7	235	1 slice	0.9	59
Oatmeal	1	2.2	253	1 slice	0.5	63
Pita bread (5")	1	0.9	273	1 piece	0.4	123
Pumpernickel bread	1	3.2	207	1 slice	1.0	66
Raisin bread	1	2.2	267	1 slice	0.6	67
White bread	1,4	1.6	279	1 slice	0.4	78
Whole wheat bread	1,4	5.7	243	1 slice	1.4	61
Pasta and rice (cooked)						
Macaroni	1,5	0.8	111	1 c	1.0	144
Rice, brown	3,5	1.2	119	1/2 c	1.0	97
Rice, polished	1,4,5	0.3	109	1/2 c	0.2	82
Spaghetti (regular)	1,5	0.8	111	1 c	1.1	155
Spaghetti (whole wheat)	1,5	2.8	111	1 c	3.9	155
Flours and grains						
Bran, corn	4	62.2				
Bran, oat	3	27.8				
Bran, wheat	1,3,4,5	41.2				
Rolled oats	4,5	5.7				
Rye flour (72%)[b]	4	4.5	350			
Rye flour (100%)[b]	4	12.8	335			
Wheat flour:						
Brown (85%)[b]	3,4	7.3	327			
White (72%)[b]	3,4	2.9	333			
Wholemeal (100%)[b]	3,4	8.9	318			
Nuts						
Almonds	4	7.2	627	10 nuts	1.1	79
Filberts	3	6.0	634	10 nuts	0.8	90
Peanuts	3	8.1	568	10 nuts	1.4	105

Dietary fiber values are averages compiled from literature sources. Users of the table are advised to read the accompanying manuscript to understand fully the derivation and meaning of the values.

[a]The numbers in this column refer to the analytical method used to obtain the mean dietary fiber value, as follows:

1. Neutral detergent fiber
2. Neutral detergent fiber plus water-soluble fraction
3. Southgate procedure
4. Total dietary fiber procedure
5. Englyst, nonstarch polysaccharide (NSP)

[b]The number in parentheses refers to the extraction rate of the flour. White-type breads and household flour are made with 72% flour; 85% extraction flour was consumed in the United States before World War II.

Reprinted from Lanza E, Butrum RR. *J Am Diet Assoc*. 1986; 86: 732.

fects as possible loss of vitamin absorption caused by mineral oil, premature labor brought on by the irritant effects of castor oil, or possible dangerous electrolyte imbalances with osmotic agents, pregnant women should probably use only bulk-forming or emollient laxatives.[35] Although stimulant laxatives should generally be avoided during pregnancy, at least one report indicates that some stimulants may be acceptable for use during the lactation period if precautions are taken.[36] Senna and related anthraquinones have been used during breast-feeding despite a lack of information regarding their concentration in breast milk. Bisacodyl appears in breast milk in trace amounts but may not pose problems for the infant.[36] If these products are used, the infant should be carefully observed for diarrhea. Saline cathartics should probably be avoided during pregnancy and lactation because appreciable GI absorption can occur in the mother. Toxicity occurring from excessive use of a saline cathartic such as magnesium sulfate could be significant, considering that such toxicity could result in diarrhea, drowsiness, hypotonia, and respiratory difficulty.

Pregnant women should be counseled on proper diet, adequate fluid intake, and reasonable exercise.[34] If these measures do not alleviate or prevent the development of constipation, a laxative preparation may be appropriate. In some instances, the pharmacist should consult with the woman's health care provider, especially if any doubt exists regarding the provider's desire for the patient to have a laxative. Laxatives may also have to be administered postpartum to reestablish normal bowel function that may have been lost because of perineal pain. Other indications include ileus secondary to colonic dilatation in a decompressed abdomen, laxness of the anal sphincter and abdominal musculature, low fluid intake, and administration of enemas during labor. In addition, hemorrhoids in the period after delivery may be aggravated, if not caused, by constipation.

Laxative Abuse

Routine, chronic use of most laxative preparations is considered laxative abuse and should be avoided if at all possible. Although we often have a stereotypic view of the laxative abuser, that person is not always elderly. For example, some adolescents, college students, and young adults (especially women) use laxatives for weight control.[37,38] Such abuse is often part of a pattern of "purging behavior," which also may include self-induced vomiting. These persons may suffer from bulimia nervosa or anorexia nervosa.

Excessive use of laxatives can cause diarrhea and vomiting, leading to fluid and electrolyte losses, especially hypokalemia, which may result in a general loss of tone of smooth and striated muscle. Clinical features of laxative abuse include:

- Factitious diarrhea;
- Electrolyte imbalance (eg, hypokalemia, hypocalcemia, and hypermagnesemia);
- Osteomalacia;
- Protein-losing enteropathy;
- Steatorrhea;
- Cathartic colon;
- Liver disease.

Cathartic colon, which develops after years of laxative abuse, is difficult to diagnose. In a study of seven hospitalized female patients, 26–65 years of age, the chief admitting complaints were abdominal pain and diarrhea, the number of hospital admissions ranged from 2 to 11, and the total number of days spent in the hospital ranged from 58 to 202.[39] The diagnosis of laxative abuse was difficult because the patients invariably denied taking laxatives, and none of the colonic tissue characteristics usually associated with excessive laxative use was observed on sigmoidoscopy or radiologic examination. With such patients, psychiatric intervention provided the only viable means to establish patient actions.

Diarrhea can be a serious consequence of the overuse of laxative products, especially irritant laxatives. The prolonged misuse of laxatives can produce morbid anatomic changes in the colon. In a study of 12 chronic stimulant laxative users, the primary anatomic changes were mucosal inflammation, loss of intrinsic innervation, atrophy of smooth muscle coats, and pigmentation of the colon.[40] Most users had been taking laxatives regularly for 30–40 years. In such cases, the transverse colon is often pendulous, the sigmoid section is highly dilated, and the muscle layers are thin and contain excess adipose tissue, indicating some tissue atrophy.

Laxative abuse can usually be classified as either habitual or surreptitious. The habitual abuser often believes that a daily bowel movement is a necessity and uses a laxative to accomplish this end. Such patients may freely admit to this practice because they believe regular laxative use to be entirely correct and natural. On the other hand, surreptitious abuse is similar to other illnesses. Surreptitious abusers tend to manifest various psychiatric disturbances. Confronting this type of abuser does not usually help resolve the problem, and psychiatric intervention should be encouraged. To assess the abuser, the diagnostic process must include effective detection methods. This may include a *potassium hydroxide* test of the stool to detect phenolphthalein, or a stool osmolarity test to detect salines and colonoscopy to detect melanosis coli. Although not always practical, urine samples may be analyzed for the presence of the most commonly used laxatives.[41]

Once the abuse has been adequately substantiated, it may be possible to wean the patient off the laxative before permanent bowel damage occurs and to regularize the patient's bowel habits with a high-fiber diet supplemented by bulk-forming laxatives as needed. After an abuser is withdrawn from one or more laxatives, several months may be required to retrain the bowel to work in regular, unaided function. Affected patients should be educated about laxative abuse. The information provided should describe types of laxatives and their harmful effects. Patients should be advised that constipation, weight gain, bloating, or abdominal distention may occur following the end of laxative abuse. These persons should be encouraged to exercise, increase dietary fiber, and maintain adequate fluid intake. The pharmacist should also encourage them to discuss their attitudes about laxative abuse and should be prepared to answer any questions that arise in such discussions.

Product Selection Guidelines

When considering the use of any laxative to treat constipation, the pharmacist should remember that normal defecation empties only the rectum and the descending and sigmoid branches of the colon. The preparation chosen should duplicate the normal physiologic process as nearly as possible. Most stimulant products have the potential to promote catharsis—that is, a complete emptying of the entire colon. However, the laxative user who is unaware of this effect may take another laxative dose on the first or second postlaxative day, thereby maintaining a completely empty colon. Thus, when it is necessary to use a laxative to treat constipation, the recommended initial choice is most often a bulk-forming product.

Acute constipation is the primary indication for self-treatment with a nonprescription laxative. However, nonprescription laxative products are also prescribed or indicated for patients preparing for diagnostic GI procedures and radiography. A physician should supervise the use of laxatives during treatment for perianal disease (pre- or postoperatively), during conditions in which straining is undesirable (eg, postoperative or postmyocardial infarct), or for chronic constipation. Because defecation has been found to alter hemodynamics, straining to defecate may result in blood pressure surges or cardiac rhythm disturbances. In patients who had previously experienced a myocardial infarct, straining to defecate has resulted in death from emboli, ventricular rupture, and cardiogenic shock.

The pharmacist should also recognize the situations in which laxative use is inappropriate. For example, laxatives are not recommended to treat constipation associated with intestinal pathology or secondary to laxative abuse unless bowel retraining has been successful. Laxatives also are not a cure for functional constipation and therefore are of only secondary importance in treating this condition. Attention should be directed first to questions relating to diet, fluid intake, physical activity, and any underlying pathology that may be producing constipation as a symptom.

Laxative products whose maximum daily dose contains more than 15 mEq (345 mg) of sodium, 25 mEq (975 mg) of potassium, 50 mEq (600 mg) of magnesium, or 90 mEq (1800mg) of calcium should not be used in kidney or liver disease, heart failure, hypertension, or other conditions requiring sodium, potassium, magnesium, or calcium restriction. Any product containing dextrose should be used with caution in labile diabetic patients because glycemic control may be lost, and products containing aspartame should be avoided in patients with phenylketonuria.

Patient Counseling

The most useful approach in counseling the person who requests a laxative product for self-treatment should first include a discussion of dietary habits (adequate fiber and fluids), physical exercise, the ability to respond to the urge to defecate, and general emotional well-being. Although it is well recognized that these factors may be largely responsible for problems associated with constipation, people may not understand how these factors may affect the development of constipation and how they can return a person to a relatively normal state of bowel function without laxative intervention.

A diet consisting of plenty of fluids (four to six 8-oz glasses a day) and high-fiber foods will help prevent chronic constipation. Caution regarding fluid intake must be used with patients on fluid restriction. Dietary fiber is that part of whole grain, vegetables, fruits, and nuts that resists digestion in the GI tract (Table 7). Food fiber content, which is expressed in terms of crude fiber residue after treatment with dilute acid and alkali, has a significant effect on bowel habits. Because fiber holds water, stools tend to be softer, bulkier, and heavier in persons with a higher fiber intake, and they probably pass through the colon more rapidly.

Along with a high-fiber diet, the pharmacist may encourage regular, mild exercise such as walking, provided the patient's cardiovascular system is healthy and mild exercising presents no apparent health risk owing to other pathology. Exercise in any form improves muscle tone, but exercise using the abdominal muscles is the most beneficial in maintaining or improving intestinal muscle tone.

The patient should be advised not to ignore the urge to defecate and should allow adequate time for elimination. A relaxed, unhurried atmosphere can be very important in aiding elimination. The patient should be encouraged to set a regular pattern for bathroom visits. Having a specific time set aside for elimination may help the body adjust itself to producing a regular stool.

When counseling the patient on rational laxative use, the pharmacist should stress the following points:

- Laxative agents should not be used regularly; more natural methods such as diet, exercise, and fluid intake should be used to foster regular bowel movements.
- The use of a laxative to treat constipation should be only a temporary measure; once regularity has returned, laxative use should be discontinued.
- Laxatives are not designed for long-term use; if they are not effective after 1 week, a physician should be consulted.
- If a skin rash appears after the patient has taken a laxative containing phenolphthalein, the product should be discontinued and a physician should be contacted.
- Saline laxatives should not be used daily, nor should they be administered orally to children under 6 years of age or rectally to infants under 2 years of age.
- The dose of a stimulant product should be individualized for appropriate effect.
- Mineral oil should be avoided in children under 6 years of age, and it should not be used in conjunction with emollient laxatives, during pregnancy, in elderly patients, and in patients taking anticoagulants.
- Castor oil should not be used to treat constipation.
- Enemas and suppositories must be administered properly to be effective.

- Laxatives should not be used in the presence of abdominal pain, perianal lesions, nausea, vomiting, bloating, or cramping without consulting a physician.
- Laxatives containing phenolphthalein or senna may discolor urine; laxatives containing phenolphthalein may discolor feces and urine pink to red, depending on the alkalinity.

Case Studies

Case 12–1

Patient Complaint/History

QA, a 66-year-old recently retired landscaper, walks up to the pharmacy counter with two products in hand: Fleet Mineral Oil Enema and Kondremul. He explains that he is having a difficult time deciding between the two products. He also notes that he cannot remember being constipated since he became an adult. For occasional constipation during adolescence, his mother always gave him mineral oil. "It always seemed to work," he says.

During questioning about his symptoms, the patient remarks that he should have come to the pharmacy 4 days ago; however, thinking that a good night's sleep would solve the problem, he picked up Benadryl capsules at a convenience store and has taken them for 3 nights. The patient reports that he is sleeping well but has had only one small bowel movement in 9 days.

After hearing the patient's description of his symptoms and attempted self-treatment, the pharmacist pulls up the patient's profile. The profile lists gouty arthritis, hypertension, and hyperlipidemia as chronic medical conditions for which the patient takes Capoten 25 mg bid; colchicine 0.6 mg bid; and Pravachol 10 mg bid, which was begun 3 weeks earlier. The patient has no known allergies.

Clinical Considerations/Strategies

The following considerations/strategies are provided to aid the reader in (1) determining whether treatment of the patient's condition with nonprescription medications is warranted, (2) selecting the appropriate nonprescription medication, and (3) developing a patient counseling strategy to ensure optimal therapeutic outcomes:

- Determine whether this patient has constipation.
- Assess the appropriateness of the active ingredient (mineral oil) in the patient-selected nonprescription products.
- Assess the appropriateness of the dosage forms selected by the patient.
- Assess the usefulness of dietary and lifestyle changes.
- Consider the patient's age as a factor in recommending a nonprescription product.
- Assess whether the patient's current drug therapy could play a role in the development of constipation.
- Develop a patient education/counseling strategy that will:
  - □ Ensure that the patient understands the importance of the dietary and lifestyle modifications;
  - □ Ensure that the patient understands the proper use of the recommended nonprescription medications;
  - □ Ensure that the patient knows when to contact a health care provider.

Case 12–2

Patient Complaint/History

SD, a 34-year-old mother of two small children (ages 2 and 5 years), is 7 months pregnant. Her managed care plan requires that she obtain any chronic or long-term medication (more than a month's supply) from a mail-order program. Because the patient obtains her prenatal vitamins by mail order, she calls the hotline counseling number for advice about her constipation. She asks, "What nonprescription product should I take to relieve my constipation? I've been having a bowel movement about every 4 or 5 days, and it's difficult to pass. I have some milk of magnesia and this product that contains something called cascara. Is it all right to use them?"

The patient's profile lists iron deficiency anemia and irritable bowel syndrome as current medical conditions. Current medications include Natalins one tablet daily and Vitron-C one tablet bid with meals. The patient has no known allergies.

Clinical Considerations/Strategies

The following considerations/strategies are provided to aid the reader in (1) determining whether treatment of the patient's condition with nonprescription medications is warranted, (2) selecting the appropriate nonprescription medication, and (3) developing a patient counseling strategy to ensure optimal therapeutic outcomes:

- Determine whether this patient has simple constipation.
- Assess whether the patient's current drug therapy could play a role in the development of constipation.
- Assess the usefulness of dietary and lifestyle changes.
- Assess the appropriateness of the laxative products that the patient has at home.
- Recommend appropriate nonprescription medications to manage this patient's constipation.
- Develop a patient education/counseling strategy that will:
  - □ Ensure that the patient understands the importance of the dietary and lifestyle modifications;
  - □ Ensure that the patient understands the proper use of the recommended nonprescription medications;
  - □ Ensure that the patient knows when to contact a health care provider.

Summary

The widespread misuse and abuse of nonprescription laxatives is evidence of the need for professional consultation and patient education. Successful treatment of constipation depends on careful identification of the cause. To determine whether self-treatment or medical referral is indicated, the pharmacist needs to know the case history and current symptoms. If the case history discloses a sudden change in bowel habits that has persisted for 2 weeks, the pharmacist should refer the patient to a physician immediately. However, if the constipation can be treated without physician intervention, knowledge of the many available products is essential.

For most cases of simple constipation, proper diet, exercise, and adequate fluid intake will be helpful. Therapy with any laxative product should be limited in most cases to short-term use (1 week). If no relief has been achieved after 1 week of proper laxative therapy, use of the product should be discontinued and a physician consulted.

References

1. *Drug Topics*. 1995; 139(9): 55.
2. Carey WD. Colon physiology: a review. *Cleve Clin J Med*. 1977; 44: 73.
3. Netter FH. *The Ciba Collection of Medical Illustrations*. Vol 3, part 2. Summit, NJ: Ciba Pharmaceuticals; 1962: 98.
4. Jacknowitz AI. Ulcerative colitis and its treatment. *Am J Hosp Pharm*. 1980; 37: 1635.
5. Gattuso JM, Kamm MA. Review article: the management of constipation in adults. *Aliment Pharmacol Ther*. 1993; 7: 487–500.
6. Connell AM et al. Variation of bowel habit in 2 population samples. *Br Med J*. 1965; 2: 1095.
7. Sandgren JE, McPhee MS, Greenberger NJ. Narcotic bowel syndrome treated with clonidine. *Ann Intern Med*. 1984; 101: 331–4.
8. Bruera E et al. Continuous sc infusion of metoclopramide for the treatment of narcotic bowel syndrome. *Cancer Treatment Rep*. 1987; 71: 1121–2.
9. Cummings JH. Fermentation in the human large intestine: evidence and implications for health. *Lancet*. 1983; 1: 1206.
10. Optimal calcium intake. National Institutes of Health Consensus Development Conference Statement. National Institutes of Health; September 1994. Abstract.
11. Gross R. Acute bronchospasm associated with inhalation of psyllium hydrophilic mucilloid. *JAMA*. 1979; 241: 1573.
12. Wald A. Constipation in elderly patients: pathogenesis and management. *Drugs and Aging*. 1993; (3): 220–31.
13. Proposed monograph of the panel on the safety and efficacy of laxatives, antidiarrheals, antiemetics and emetics, part II. *Federal Register*. 1975; 40(56): 12907, 12911–2.
14. Gattuso JM, Kamm MA. Adverse effects of drugs used in the management of constipation and diarrhea. *Drug Safety*. 1994; 10(1): 47–65.
15. Mofenson HC, Caraccio TR. Magnesium intoxication in a neonate from oral magnesium hydroxide laxatives. *J Toxicol Clin Toxicol*. 1991; 29(2): 215–22.
16. Muller-Lissner SA. Adverse effects of laxatives: fact and fiction. Pharmacology. 1993; 47(suppl 1): 138–45.
17. Greenhalf JO, Leonard HS. Laxatives in the treatment of constipation of pregnant and breast feeding infants. *Practitioner*. 1973; 210: 259.
18. Gilbertson WE, Lessing M. Danthron alarm, FDA response: crucial OTC drug control. *Milit Med*. 1988; 153: 487–8.
19. Brunton LL. Agents affecting gastrointestinal water flux and motility, digestants and bile acids. In: Gilman AG et al., eds. *The Pharmacological Basis of Therapeutics*. 8th ed. New York: Pergamon Press; 1990: 921.
20. Pietrusko RG. Use and abuse of laxatives. *Am J Hosp Pharm*. 1977; 34: 291.
21. Fleisher N et al. Chronic laxative-induced hyperaldosteronism and hypokalemia stimulating Bartter's syndrome. *Ann Intern Med*. 1969; 70: 791.
22. Binder HJ, Dobbins JW, Whiting DS. Evidence against importance of altered mucosal permeability in ricinoleic acid induced fluid secretion. *Gastroenterology*. 1977: 72: 1029.
23. Pike BF et al. Soap colitis. *N Engl J Med*. 1971; 285: 217.
24. Pettei MJ. Chronic constipation. *Pediatr Ann*. 1987; 16(10): 796–800, 804–6, 811–3.
25. Lemoh JN. Frequency and weight of normal stools in infancy. *Arch Dis Child*. 1979; 54: 719.
26. Weaver LT. The bowel habits of young children. *Arch Dis Child*. 1984; 59: 649.
27. Loening-Baucke V. Constipation in children. *Curr Opinion Pediatr*. 1994; 6: 556–61.
28. Loening-Baucke V. Management of chronic constipation in infants and toddlers. *Am Fam Physician*. 1994; 49: 2397–406.
29. Brandt LJ. Constipation in the elderly. *Pract Gastroenterol*. 1987 Mar/Apr; 11(2): 31–6.
30. Wald AW. Constipation and fecal incontinence in the elderly. *Semin Gastr Dis*. 1994; 5(4): 179–88.
31. Rosseau P. Treatment of constipation in the elderly. *Postgrad Med*. 1988; 83(4): 339–40, 343–5, 349.
32. Brandt LJ. *Gastrointestinal Disorders of the Elderly*. New York: Raven Press; 1984: 261–367.
33. Rosseau P. No soapsuds enemas. *Postgrad Med*. 1988; 83(4): 352–3.
34. Biggs JSG, Vesey EJ. Treatment of gastrointestinal disorders of pregnancy. *Drugs*. 1980; 19: 70.
35. Hart LH. Constipation and diarrhea. In: Young LY, Koda-Kimble MA, eds. *Applied Therapeutics: The Clinical Use of Drugs*. 4th ed. Vancouver, Wash: Applied Therapeutics; 1989: 112.
36. Chaplin S et al. Drug excretion in human breast milk. *Adv Drug React*. 1982; 1: 255.
37. Vanin JR, Saylor KE. Laxative abuse: a hazardous habit for weight control. *J Am Coll Health*. 1989 Mar; 37(5): 227–30.
38. Halmi KA, Falk JR, Schwartz E. Binge-eating and vomiting: a survey of a college population. *Psychol Med*. 1981; 11(4): 697–706.
39. Babb RR. Constipation and laxative abuse. *West J Med*. 1975; 122: 93.
40. Smith B. Pathologic changes in the colon produced by anthraquinone purgatives. *Dis Colon Rectum*. 1973; 16: 455.
41. deWolff FA. A screening method for establishing laxative abuse. *Clin Chem*. 1981; 27: 914.

CHAPTER 13

Antidiarrheal Products

R. Leon Longe

Questions to ask in patient assessment and counseling

- *How long have you had diarrhea (≥2 days)?*
- *Was the onset of diarrhea sudden?*
- *How often do the episodes of diarrhea occur?*
- *What is the character of the stool (ie, its consistency, odor, and color)?*
- *Do your stools contain blood or mucus?*
- *Is the diarrhea associated with other symptoms such as fever, weakness, loss of appetite, vomiting, dizziness, rapid heart rate, gas, or abdominal pain?*
- *Have you tried any antidiarrheal treatments or products? Which ones? How effective were they?*
- *How old are you?*
- *How often do you normally have a bowel movement?*
- *Have other family members experienced similar symptoms?*
- *Have you changed your diet recently?*
- *Can you relate the onset of diarrhea to a specific cause such as a particular meal or food (eg, milk product) or drug?*
- *Have you recently traveled to a foreign country or a border area of the United States?*
- *Have you recently consumed nonchlorinated water such as that from a river, pond, or lake?*
- *Are you currently taking or have you recently taken any prescription or nonprescription medications? Which ones?*
- *Do you have diabetes, heart or blood vessel disease, or any other chronic medical condition?*

The frequency of normal bowel movements varies with the individual. Some healthy adults may have as many as three well-formed stools a day; others may defecate once every 2 or more days.[1] Except for vegetarians, who consume a fiber-rich diet and thus may produce daily stools of more than 300 g, the mean daily fecal weight loss is 100–150 g. An increase to 200–300 g may be interpreted as diarrhea.

Diarrhea is a symptom that is characterized by abnormal frequency or consistency of stools. It may be acute or chronic in nature. Its presence may signal either a gastrointestinal (GI) or non-GI disease. Most often diarrhea is due to an enteritis or colitis of noninfectious or infectious etiology. A major feature of diarrhea is the excretion of a relatively large volume of water normally reabsorbed from the gut. Disruption of intestinal water absorption of even a few hundred milliliters may bring on diarrhea. The approach to treatment depends on recognizing the cause of diarrhea.

Physiology of the Intestines

The small and large intestines consist of a long, hollow tube surrounded by layers of smooth muscle. These include a thick, circular layer on the mucosal side of the intestine; a thinner, longitudinal layer on the serosal side; and a third layer of both circular and longitudinal muscle fibers. Active contractions of the various muscles control intestinal tone. As a rule, this tone is maintained with little energy, so the intestinal musculature stays relatively free from fatigue and remains capable of performing normally.

Small Intestine

The small intestine, a convoluted tube about 6.4 m long, has three sections: the duodenum, jejunum, and ileum. It begins at the pylorus of the stomach and ends at the cecum. Although the digestive process begins in the mouth, the small intestine is the primary site of digestion, absorption of nutrients, and retention of waste material. These activities depend on normal musculature, neurologic innervation, muscular tone, and digestive enzymes.

A mucous layer protects and lubricates the walls of the intestines. Mucus is released from goblet cells interspersed among the columnar epithelial cells (enterocytes) in the intestines. This secretion is increased by local irritation from foods or stimulant cathartics or stress. The mucus is more viscous in the upper portion of the small intestine than it is in the colon, and it forms a protective physical barrier to the intestinal lining, thus reducing contact with irritating substances, bacteria, and viruses. The alkalinity of the mucus contributes further to protection of the intestinal lining as it neutralizes acidic dietary and bacterial products.

Normal intestinal motility and peristalsis are maintained by smooth muscles and intrinsic nerves. The vagus and parasympathetic pelvic nerves stimulate intestinal motility and secretion, whereas sympathetic innervation inhibits these activities. Extrinsic autonomic innervation influences the strength and frequency of intestinal move-

TABLE 1 Electrolyte and water content of normal and diarrheal feces

Components	Normal	Diarrheal
Bicarbonate[a]	30	30–45
Chloride[a]	15	20–40
Potassium[a]	90	35–60
Sodium[a]	40	25–50
Water[b]	0.1–0.2	3–10

[a]mEq/L.
[b]L/24 h.

Adapted from Longe RL, DiPiro JT. In: *Pharmacotherapy: A Pathophysiologic Approach*. New York: Elsevier Science Publishing; 1989.

ments and mediates reflexes by which activity in one part of the intestine influences another.

Eating causes the lumen of the small and large intestines to distend and the smooth muscle layers to contract. Normally, segmental contractions of the circular muscles are accompanied by a decrease in the propulsive activity of the gut. This process mixes and retains food in the lumen and increases its duration of exposure to digestive elements, thus enhancing digestion and absorption.

Normally, about 9 L of digestive fluid enter the GI tract daily. Of these, approximately 8 L are reabsorbed in the small intestine. The large intestine reabsorbs about 850 mL of the remaining liter, leaving about 150 mL to be excreted in the stool each day.

Approximately 3–5 L of stomach fluid containing electrolytes and nutrients enter the small intestine every 24 hours. Reabsorption reduces the quantity that reaches the large intestine to an isotonic semiliquid substance, chyme, which consists primarily of unabsorbed, undigested food residue; nutrients; electrolytes; water; and bacteria. Ileal chyme has an average electrolyte content of 140 mEq/L sodium, 70 mEq/L bicarbonate, 8 mEq/L potassium, and 60 mEq/L chloride. Stool electrolyte content is 30 mEq/L bicarbonate, 15 mEq/L chloride, 90 mEq/L potassium, and 40 mEq/L sodium.[2] Stool is generally stored in the sigmoid colon until defecation.

Colon

The colon, which is about 1.5 m long, is composed of the cecum, ascending colon, transverse colon, descending colon, and sigmoid colon. It has two primary functions: absorption and storage. The first two thirds of the colon facilitates absorption, and the remaining third functions as a storage area. The proximal half (ascending and transverse parts) of the colon reduces chyme to a semisolid substance called feces, or stool. Stool is a 75% water and 25% solid material containing unabsorbed food residue and minerals, bacteria, desquamated epithelial cells, and a small quantity of electrolytes (Table 1).

The colon is structured like the small intestine, with both circular and longitudinal muscles. The longitudinal muscles are shorter than the underlying colonic tissue and tend to draw the colon into sacs. The segments of the circular musculature further divide the colon into sausagelike units known as haustra. Through segmented contractions, the haustra help churn colonic contents and assist in the absorption of water. Should the frequency or intensity of these segmental contractions decrease, the predominance of propulsive forces of the longitudinal musculature may lead to diarrhea. Without circular muscle contractions, abnormal mass colonic movements may occur in which the colon contracts to half its normal length and resembles a smooth, hollow tube without segmented units. As noted above, colonic motor activity is increased by parasympathetic stimulation and inhibited by sympathetic stimulation.

Peristaltic waves propel feces to the rectum. Normal bowel movements begin with the stimulation of stretch receptors in the rectum by feces. The external anal sphincter controls voluntary defecation.

In the colon, bacteria produce enzymes necessary for the degradation of waste products, synthesize certain vitamins, and generate ammonia. *Bacteroides* species and anaerobic *Lactobacillus* species comprise much of the colonic bacterial flora. Organisms such as Enterobacteriaceae species (eg, *Escherichia coli*), hemolytic *Streptococcus*, *Clostridium* species, and yeasts may also be present in the colon but represent only a small portion of the normal flora. Many factors such as diet, intestinal pH, coexisting disease, and drugs may influence the relative proportion of these organisms. If these potential pathogens are allowed to overgrow or if their normal balance is disrupted, they may cause serious symptoms and complications.

Diarrhea

Variability in the causes of diarrhea makes identification of the pathophysiologic mechanisms difficult. A complete medical assessment, including clinical laboratory evaluation, may be required to identify the cause. The etiology may be psychogenic, neurogenic, surgical, endocrine, irritative, osmotic, dietary, allergenic, malabsorptive, infectious, or inflammatory (Figure 1).

Mechanisms of Diarrhea

The development of diarrhea may involve four general pathophysiologic mechanisms: decreased absorption, increased secretion, excessive exudation, and motility alterations (Tables 2 and 3). These mechanisms classify diarrhea into four clinical groups: osmotic, secretory, exudative, and motility disorder. The most common clinical types of diarrhea are osmotic and secretory.

During normal functioning of the intestines, a balance between absorption and secretion is maintained. Water absorption in the intestines is passive and depends on the electrolytes and selected solutes (ie, sodium chloride, glucose, small peptides, and amino acids). As these substances are absorbed, water accompanies

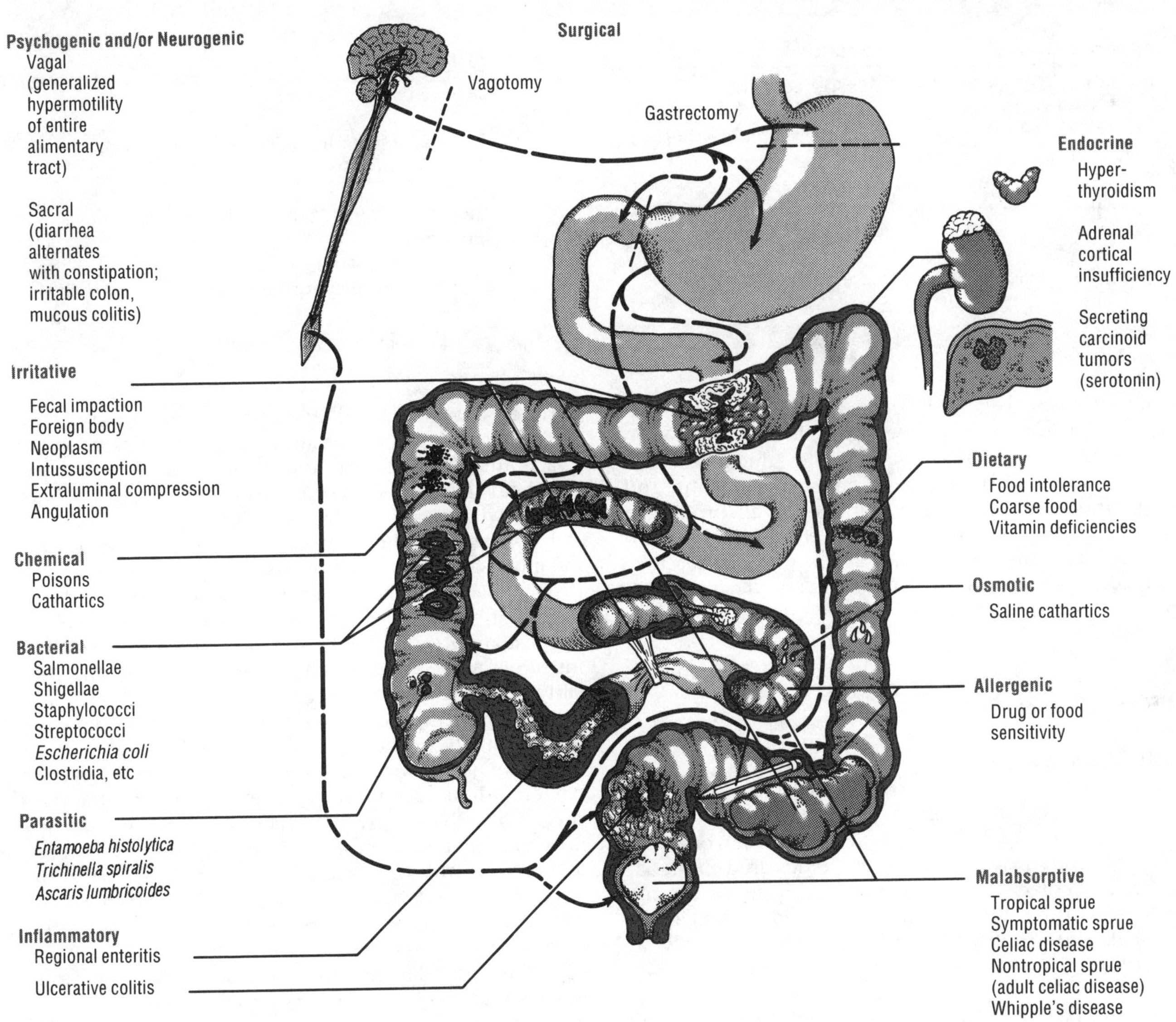

FIGURE 1 Etiology of diarrhea. Adapted from Netter FN. *The Ciba Collection of Medical Illustrations* Vol 1. New York: Ciba Pharmaceutical Co; 1962: 99.

their movement to maintain an isotonic state. Generally, 1 L of water is absorbed with about 150 mEq of sodium chloride.[3] There are also secretory mechanisms at work balancing iso-osmotic pressure.

Several intestinal ion-transport mechanisms regulate the normal transfer of electrolytes and other solutes[4]; these mechanisms play a primary role in maintaining the balance between absorption and secretion. Sodium transport is the primary ion-transport mechanism that controls water movement. Intracellular sodium movement across the brush border occurs by electrogenic and neutral mechanisms. Enterocytes have an active sodium-potassium adenosine triphosphatase pump throughout the intestines.[4] This pump moves sodium into the enterocyte and potassium out of it. Another transport mechanism occurs with the cotransport of sodium-glucose and sodium-amino acids into the enterocyte. Another identified transport mechanism is linking of sodium with the luminal exchange of hydrogen.

Chloride movement maintains electrical neutrality. Chloride is transferred from the interstitial space into the enterocyte and is secreted through the brush border into the intestinal lumen. Chloride secretion is increased by intracellular release of cAMP, cyclic guanosine monophosphate, and calcium. Chloride also moves from the intestinal lumen in exchange for bicarbonate.

Various intracellular and extracellular regulators (eg, cyclic adenosine monophosphate [cAMP], calmodulin, hormones, and neurotransmitters) can modify the normal functioning of intestinal ion transport.[4] Hormones

TABLE 2 Clinical classification of diarrhea

Type	Mechanism	Typical causes
Osmotic	Unabsorbed solute	Lactase deficit, magnesium antacid excess
Secretory	Increased secretion of electrolytes	*Escherichia coli* infection, ileal resection, thyroid cancer
Exudative	Defective colonic absorption, outpouring of mucus and/or blood	Ulcerative colitis, Crohn's disease, shigellosis, leukemia
Motility disorder	Decreased contact time	Irritable bowel syndrome, diabetic neuropathy

such as vasopressin, atrial natriuretic factor, aldosterone, and glucocorticoids have variable effects on various intestinal segments. For example, glucocorticoids enhance sodium absorption in the small intestine and colon, and aldosterone enhances sodium absorption in the colon. Neurotransmitters (eg, acetylcholine, serotonin, somatostatin) have either absorptive or secretory effects. Acetylcholine has primarily secretory effects whereas somatostatin has absorptive effects.

Types of Diarrhea

Acute Diarrhea

Acute diarrhea is characterized by a sudden onset of abnormally frequent, watery stools accompanied by weakness, flatulence, pain, and possibly fever or vomiting. Acute diarrhea may be infectious, toxic, drug induced, or dietary in origin. It may occur as the result of various acute or chronic illnesses. In the United States, infectious diarrhea is usually viral in origin, especially in children.

Food-Borne Diarrhea Although the causative agent is often not readily identifiable, pathogens most commonly responsible for producing diarrhea in the United States are *Shigella* sp, *Salmonella* sp, *Campylobacter* sp, *Staphylococcus* sp, *Bacillus cereus,* and Norwalk viruses.[5] Some organisms cause diarrhea through an enterotoxin (toxigenic *E coli* and *Staphylococcus aureus*). Others (*Shigella, Salmonella, Yersinia, Campylobacter jejuni,* and invasive *E coli*) directly invade the mucosal epithelial cells. Patients with diarrhea caused by toxin-producing agents usually present clinically with a watery diarrhea, which primarily involves the small intestine. Such patients experience an abrupt onset of large-volume watery stools, variable nausea, vomiting, cramps, and possibly a low-grade fever. If the large intestine is the site of attack, invasive organisms produce a dysentery-like syndrome. This syndrome is characterized by fever, abdominal cramps, tenesmus (straining), and the frequent passage of small-volume stools that may contain blood and pus.

An attentive and thorough history regarding food intake during the week prior to the onset of diarrhea is essential in identifying a probable cause. For example, staphylococci grow rapidly in food (especially salads, custard, sausage, ham, dairy products, and poultry), producing a toxin. Upon ingestion, the toxin quickly (within 1–2 hours) provokes an attack of vomiting with some diarrhea. In contrast, the incubation period for salmonellae, which are harbored on raw foods and particularly on eggs, is 12–24 hours. These microbes invade the mucosal layer to disrupt absorptive-secretory mechanisms. Fever, malaise, muscle aches, and profound epigastric or periumbilical discomfort with severe anorexia suggest an infectious, inflammatory disease of the large intestine. Severe periumbilical pain, vomiting, and possibly diarrhea may be experienced with viral gastroenteritis, and symptoms usually persist for 2–3 days before gradually subsiding.

Campylobacter species are another cause of acute bacterial diarrhea.[6] With an onset of 2–4 days, the diarrhea is usually limited to 1 week. If supportive therapy fails to manage symptoms, erythromycin may be used to eradicate the organism. *Yersinia enterocolitica* and *Yersinia pseudotuberculosis* are isolates of bacterial diarrhea, and symptoms of this self-limiting infectious process may persist for 1–3 weeks.

The acute diarrhea that may develop among tourists visiting foreign countries or US border areas with warm climates and poor sanitation is usually caused by bacterial enteropathogens. Enterotoxigenic *E coli* is the most common infecting organism in traveler's diarrhea, a secretory diarrhea acquired, for the most part, via contaminated food or water. After ingestion of the causative organism, which is found usually in foods such as fruits, vegetables, raw meat, and seafood and less commonly in the local water (and ice cubes), the bacteria produces two plasmid-mediated enterotoxins, known as heat-labile toxin and heat-stable toxin. These toxins cause a diarrheal disorder characterized by a sudden onset of loose stools (usually within 3–7 days of arrival), nausea, occasional vomiting, abdominal cramping, bloating, malaise, and possibly a low-grade fever. Traveler's diarrhea is also a self-limiting illness[7,8]; patients may experience between three and eight (or more) watery stools per day, and symptoms usually subside over 3–5 days.

Infectious diarrhea may be treated with fluid and electrolytes. Often the illness is self-limiting, and normal function of the alimentary tract is restored with or without treatment in 24–72 hours. If the patient has a persistent case of infectious diarrhea, a specific

TABLE 3 Pathophysiologic classification of chronic diarrhea

Decreased absorption

Small intestine
Generalized malabsorption
- Mucosal damage (celiac disease)
- Impaired intraluminal digestion (pancreatic insufficiency)
- Bacterial overgrowth (bile salt deconjugation and mucosal injury—scleroderma)

Specific malabsorption
- Enzyme deficiency (disaccharidases)
- Transport defect (chloridorrhea glucose–galactose malabsorption)
- Unabsorbed solute (magnesium, lactulose)

Colon
Idiopathic inflammatory bowel disease
- Ulcerative colitis
- Crohn's disease

Specific inflammatory bowel disease
- Amebiasis
- Ischemic colitis
- Radiation colitis

Increased secretion

Small intestine
Dumping syndrome
Gastric hypersecretion (Zollinger–Ellison syndrome)
Endogenous secretagogues (vasoactive intestinal peptide, prostaglandins, serotonin)

Colon
Unabsorbed fatty acids
Bile acids (failure of ileal reabsorption)
Unabsorbed carbohydrates (lactase deficiency)

Motility disturbances (decreased mixing activity)

Small intestine and colon
Carcinoid syndrome
Postvagotomy diarrhea
Hyperthyroidism
Diabetic visceral neuropathy
Scleroderma

Colon
Irritable bowel syndrome

Malabsorption syndromes

Failure of digestion
Decreased pancreatic enzymes
Impairment of bile acid micelle formation
Bacterial overgrowth
Inadequate mixing of food, bile, and pancreatic enzymes
Gastrojejunostomy

Failure of absorption
Inadequate absorptive surface
- Intestinal bypass surgery

Damaged absorbing surface
Celiac disease

Biochemical defect without anatomic alteration
Lactase deficiency

Infiltration of intestinal wall
Crohn's disease

Impaired lymph and blood flow
Developmental abnormality
Lymphatic obstruction
Tuberculosis
Mesenteric vascular insufficiency
Fluid-secreting tumor (large villose adenoma)

Adapted from Harvey et al. *The Principles and Practice of Medicine*. 22nd ed. San Mateo, Calif, and Norwalk, Conn: Appleton and Lange; 1988; 814, 823.

anti-infective such as doxycycline, trimethoprim-sulfamethoxazole, or one of the fluoroquinolones may be indicated (Table 4).

Food-Induced Diarrhea Food intolerance can also provoke diarrhea. Such intolerance may be the result of a food allergy or of ingestion of foods that are excessively fatty or spicy or that contain a high amount of roughage or many seeds.

Carbohydrates in the diet commonly include the disaccharides, lactose and sucrose, which are normally hydrolyzed to monosaccharides by the enzyme lactase. When disaccharides such as sucrose and lactose are not hydrolyzed, they pool in the lumen of the intestine, where they not only ferment but also produce an osmotic imbalance and pH change. The resulting hyperosmolarity draws fluid into the intestinal lumen, resulting in diarrhea. Enzymatic activity of lactase may be reduced in intestinal disorders such as infectious diarrhea and GI allergy. Acute viral diarrhea may cause a temporary milk intolerance at all ages. Infants born with a lactase deficiency and adults who develop one are intolerant of whole milk and milk-based products (eg, ice cream). Milk and ice cream may be particularly problematic because of the lactose content.

Viral Gastroenteritis Diarrhea and vomiting are common clinical problems in infants and young children. Although

TABLE 4 Infectious diarrheas and their treatment

Type	History	Symptoms	Treatment	Prognosis
Bacterial				
Salmonella sp	Ingestion of improperly cooked or refrigerated poultry and dairy products, immunocompromised host	Onset of 24–48 hours, diarrhea, fever, and chills	Fluid and electrolytes; no antibiotics	Self-limiting
Shigella sp	Ingestion of contaminated vegetables or water, immunocompromised host	Onset of 24–48 hours, nausea, vomiting, diarrhea	Fluid and electrolytes; antibiotics (cotrimoxazole, ampicillin, ciprofloxacin/norfloxacin)	Self-limiting
Enterotoxigenic *Escherichia coli* (traveler's diarrhea)	Ingestion of contaminated food or water, recent travel outside the United States or to a US border area	Onset of 8–72 hours, watery diarrhea, fever, abdominal cramps	Fluid and electrolytes; in moderate or severe cases, antibiotics (cotrimoxazole, fluoroquinolones)	Self-limiting
Campylobacter jejuni	Ingestion of contaminated water, fecal–oral route, immunocompromised host	Nausea, vomiting, headache, malaise, fever, watery diarrhea	Fluid and electrolytes; in severe or persistent diarrhea, antibiotics (erythromycin, fluoroquinolones)	Self-limiting
Clostridium difficile	Antibiotic-associated diarrhea	Watery or mucoid diarrhea, high fever, cramping	Water and electrolytes; discontinuation of offending agent; oral metronidazole, oral vancomycin, bacitracin, cholestyramine	Good, if treated

the etiology may be difficult to determine, the illness is often caused by a viral infection of the intestinal tract.

Rotaviruses have been implicated as the cause of approximately 50% of all infantile gastroenteritis.[9] Children aged 6–24 months are most susceptible to this viral infection. Respiratory illnesses such as otitis media or tonsillitis may occur concurrently. The peak infectious period is during the winter months. Spread is by the fecal-oral route. Clinical features include a 12- to 48-hour incubation period, vomiting, watery diarrhea, and a low-grade fever. The illness tends to be self-limiting, lasting 5–8 days, and treatment is usually restricted to symptomatic therapy.

Norwalk viruses have also been implicated in children and adults, with signs and symptoms resembling those of rotaviruses. The diarrhea is sudden and is often accompanied by a low-grade fever, malaise, mild nausea, and abdominal cramps. The diarrhea usually lasts 2–3 days. Like rotavirus infections, most outbreaks occur in the winter months. The virus is usually transmitted by contaminated water or food. Community-wide outbreaks may result when municipal water supplies become contaminated.

In children, particularly infants, acute diarrhea may cause severe and possibly dangerous dehydration and electrolyte imbalance; children under 2 years of age are most likely to suffer complications requiring hospitalization. In newborns, water may make up 75% of total body weight; water loss in severe diarrhea may be 10% or more of body weight. After 8–10 bowel movements within a 24-hour period, a 2-month-old infant could lose enough fluid to cause circulatory collapse and renal failure. Moderate to severe diarrhea in infants requires evaluation by a health care provider.[10]

Protozoal Diarrhea *Giardia lamblia* and *Entamoeba histolytica* are protozoa associated with acute diarrhea. Giardiasis is an infection of the small intestine most commonly involving children, travelers, institutionalized patients, and hikers who drink from streams or ponds. Symptoms may be absent or mild. Following a 1- to 3-day incubation, symptoms may include sudden onset of watery

TABLE 4 *continued*

Type	History	Symptoms	Treatment	Prognosis
Staphylococcus aureus	Ingestion of improperly cooked or stored food	Nausea, vomiting, watery diarrhea	Fluid and electrolytes; no antibiotics	Self-limiting
Protozoal				
Giardia lamblia	Ingestion of water contaminated with human or animal feces, travel outside the United States, immunocompromised host	Chronic watery diarrhea	Metronidazole, quinacrine, furazolidone	Good, if treated
Cryptosporidia	Travel outside the United States, AIDS, immunocompromised host	Chronic watery diarrhea	Fluid and electrolytes	Self-limiting, except in AIDS or other immunocompromised patients
Entamoeba histolytica	Travel outside the United States, fecal-soiled food or water, immunocompromised host	Chronic watery diarrhea	Fluid and electrolytes; metronidazole; iodoquinol	Good, except for immunocompromised patients
Viruses				
Rotaviruses	Infects infants, fecal–oral spread	Vomiting, fever, nausea, acute watery diarrhea	Vigorous fluid and electrolyte replacement; no antibiotics	Self-limiting
Norwalk	Infects all ages	"24-hour flu," vomiting, nausea, headache, myalgia, fever, watery diarrhea	Fluid and electrolytes; no antibiotics; bismuth subsalicylate; loperamide	Self-limiting

stool, abdominal cramps, flatulence, and epigastric pain. Although quinacrine, 100 mg taken orally three times a day for 5–7 days, is effective therapy in most adults,[11] metronidazole (Flagyl), 250 mg taken orally three times a day for 5–7 days, is equally effective and is better tolerated.

E histolytica causes amebiasis in areas with poor sanitation and among institutionalized patients, travelers, and migrant workers. The illness is characterized by severe crampy pain, tenesmus, and dysentery within 3–10 days. Metronidazole, 750 mg taken orally three times a day for 10 days, is generally effective against this protozoan.

Drug-Induced Diarrhea All antibiotics can produce adverse GI symptoms, but severity depends largely on the specific antibiotic, its spectrum, and the dose and duration of therapy. Commonly prescribed antibiotics that have a broad spectrum of activity against aerobic and anaerobic organisms (eg, ampicillin and numerous other penicillins, clindamycin, erythromycin, azithromycin, clarithromycin, trimethoprim-sulfamethoxazole, the tetracyclines, the fluoroquinolones, and the cephalosporins) can produce diarrhea as a side effect.[12]

Antibiotic-associated diarrhea (AAD) may be caused by an overgrowth of an antibiotic-resistant bacterial or fungal strain or of toxin-producing *Clostridium difficile*. Intestinal microorganisms other than *C difficile* that tend to proliferate during antibiotic therapy include *S aureus*, *Pseudomonas aeruginosa*, *Streptococcus faecalis*, *Candida albicans*, and selected species of *Salmonella* and *Proteus*. Any antibiotic can cause AAD, and the disease can begin during or several weeks after treatment. AAD may be self-limiting with antibiotic discontinuation.

C difficile may also cause antibiotic-associated pseudomembranous colitis.[13] Although *C difficile* produces at least two identified toxins, A and B, only A has been shown to cause diarrhea. These bacteria can be spread to other persons, so enteric isolation precautions are recommended. The diagnosis is suggested by a test for the toxins in the stool, although the toxins have been found in patients without AAD. The watery or greenish-mucoid diarrhea usually starts during antibiotic treatment, but it can begin up to 4 weeks after the antibiotic has been discontinued. The offending antibiotic must be discontinued and *C difficile* eradicated. Relapses are common and can be treated with the same antibiotic if the microorganisms have been shown to be susceptible. Oral vancomycin (125 mg four times daily for 7–10 days) or oral metronidazole (250 mg three times a day for 7–10 days) is usually prescribed for adults.[14,15] Metronidazole is often the preferred initial antibiotic because it is less expensive than vancomycin and patients do not develop vancomycin-resistant *Enterococcus*. Treatment in children is less well defined. Bacitracin or rifampin may be used in treatment failure. Exchange resins, such as cholestyramine, bind the toxins but do not eradicate *C difficile* and so are used to treat only mild cases.

Medications such as laxatives, misoprostol, olsalazine, anticancer agents, quinidine, and colchicine may cause diarrhea. Drugs that cause the retention of electrolytes and water in the intestinal lumen (eg, mannitol, sorbitol, and lactulose) may produce a hyperosmolar, osmotic diarrhea. Certain antacid laxative preparations contain magnesium; depending on the dose taken and the individual's susceptibility, magnesium-containing preparations may induce diarrhea. Drugs that affect the autonomic control of normal intestinal motility, such as certain antihypertensive agents with sympatholytic activity (eg, guanethidine, methyldopa, and reserpine), may also cause diarrhea. Generalized cramping and diarrhea may follow the use of a prokinetic drug such as bethanecol, metoclopramide, or cisapride.

AIDS-Associated Diarrhea Patients with acquired immunodeficiency syndrome (AIDS) and individuals infected with human immunodeficiency virus (HIV) are known to be susceptible to many intestinal infections that produce diarrhea as one of their manifestations. An estimated 80% of AIDS patients will experience a diarrheal infection at some time in their illness.[16] These immunocompromised patients may be infected with bacteria, fungi, parasites, viruses, and protozoal organisms. Common stool isolates are *Cryptosporidium*, *C difficile*, *Isospora belli*, *G lamblia*, and *E histolytica*.[17]

Following a 1- to 3-day incubation, fever and a sudden onset of explosive watery stool begin. Abdominal cramps also occur frequently. No currently available antimicrobial has been shown to be effective in diarrhea caused by *Cryptosporidium*. *Isospora* infections are managed with trimethoprim-sulfamethoxazole. Quinacrine and metronidazole are the treatments of choice for proven *G lamblia* diarrhea in adults and older children.[16] For empiric therapy of suspected giardiasis, metronidazole may offer advantages relative to its tolerability, side effect profile, and effects on other causes of persistent diarrhea. For managing giardiasis in small children, a pediatric liquid formulation of furazolidone is available.

E histolytica infection, which produces acute amebic dysentery, is characterized by severe crampy pain, tenesmus, and dysentery within 3–10 days of infection. Metronidazole, 750 mg taken orally three times a day for 10 days, combined with iodoquinol, 650 mg taken orally three times a day for 20 days, is recommended therapy and is generally effective.[18]

Chronic Diarrhea

Chronic diarrhea is the long-term (lasting more than 4 weeks), abnormally frequent passage of poorly formed or watery stools. Its etiology is often multifactorial and therefore may be difficult to diagnose (Table 3). Chronic diarrhea may be caused by a disease of the small or large intestine or the stomach, or it may be a secondary manifestation of a systemic disease. The pharmacist should refer patients with persistent or recurrent diarrhea for medical care; a definitive diagnosis can generally be made only after a health care provider carefully evaluates the patient's history, performs a physical examination, and orders and receives proper laboratory reports.

Clinicians differentiate chronic diarrhea into organic or functional causes. Organic causes originate within the intestines while functional causes originate outside the intestines but disrupt intestinal functions. According to Donowitz et al,[19] criteria pointing to an organic cause of diarrhea are:

- Less than 3 months' duration;
- Weight loss of more than 5 kg;
- High erythrocyte sedimentation rate;
- Low hemoglobin concentration;
- Low serum albumin;
- Predominately nocturnal diarrhea;
- Continual rather than intermittent diarrhea;
- Average daily stool weight of greater than 400 g.

A common cause of chronic diarrhea of unknown origin is laxative abuse. Many people believe that a daily bowel movement is essential for good health. This belief is seriously flawed and may lead to the abuse of laxatives (particularly irritant/stimulant laxatives), which itself may create a serious health problem from iatrogenic chronic diarrhea. Chronic laxative use may result in serious fluid and electrolyte loss, protein wasting (hypoalbuminemia), and melanosis coli. (See Chapter 12, "Laxative Products.") Recovery requires laxative withdrawal, bowel training, psychologic counseling, and, on rare occasions, hospitalization.

Patients who abuse laxatives fall into five types: hysterical patients, patients with Munchausen syndrome, patients with eating disorders (ie, bulimia, anorexia nervosa), patients with psychogenic disorders, and victims of child abuse with laxatives.[19] These patients, and, in the case of the last group, those inflicting the abuse, are extremely deceptive and hide their abusive behavior.

In recent years, chronic abuse of laxatives in weight control programs has become a problem. The laxative abuser usually complains of weight loss and diarrhea. Upon questioning, however, the patient may deny laxative abuse. Thus, the inappropriate use of laxatives may not be discovered until other potential causes of the chronic diarrhea are ruled out. A hospitalized patient's diarrhea may stop only to recur at home. To identify the laxative abuser, the practitioner must take a thorough drug history and should monitor for frequent laxative purchases. Sometimes, screening tests for laxatives may be the only way to detect laxative abuse. (See Chapter 12, "Laxative Products.")

Psychogenic factors are associated with chronic diarrhea. For example, stress-related diarrhea, which may increase the flow of parasympathetic impulses to the GI tract, is usually characterized by small, frequent stools and abdominal pain. The stools may be watery and may follow a normal bowel movement or appear shortly after eating. The diarrhea may alternate with constipation. Patients complaining of chronic diarrhea that appears to be psychogenic in origin should be referred to medical care.

Some patients who suffer from persistent diarrhea are aware of the cause and can manage the condition symptomatically. For example, many persons with diabetes who have evident neuropathy experience chronic diarrhea. (See Chapter 18, "Diabetes Care Products and Monitoring Devices.") However, individuals who experience persistent or recurrent diarrhea and are unaware of its cause should seek prompt medical attention. Conditions such as cancer of the stomach or colon or an endocrine tumor may be the source of the diarrhea.[20] One of the seven danger signals of cancer is a change in bowel habits. In both sexes, cancer of the colon and rectum is frequently reported. The American Cancer Society estimates that three of every four patients with cancer of the GI tract could be saved by early diagnosis and proper treatment.

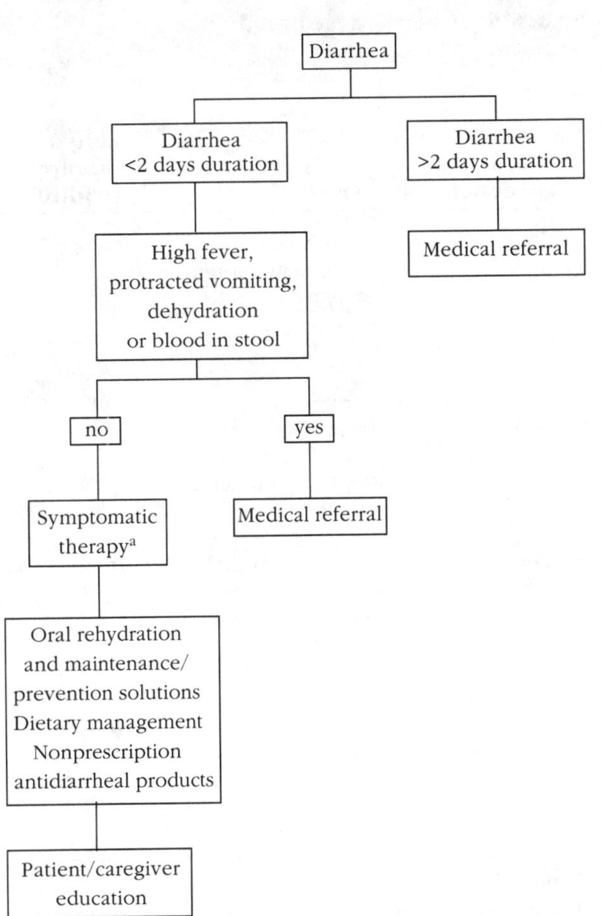

[a]If diarrhea is not resolved in 2 days of therapy or if condition worsens, patient should seek medical care.

FIGURE 2 Diarrhea evaluation and decision making.

Patient Assessment

Evaluation of the patient's responses to the questions presented at the beginning of this chapter should enable the pharmacist to assess the patient's condition and recommend a proper course of action, which may include self-treatment or referral to a health care provider. This triage function requires the pharmacist to differentiate symptoms and make clinical judgments. Figure 2 is a decision tree for managing diarrhea.

The pharmacist should acquire a history of the patient's present illness before recommending self-treatment. The following four groups of patients with either acute or chronic diarrhea should be referred to a health care provider for a complete diagnostic evaluation:

- Children under 3 years of age;
- Persons who have multiple medical conditions;
- Persons with a medical history of chronic illness such as AIDS, diabetes mellitus, or heart disease;
- Pregnant women.

Other medical conditions that generally suggest the need for health care provider referral include:

- The presence of bloody or mucoid stools;
- Moderate to severe abdominal tenderness or cramping;
- High fever (≥101°F or 38°C);
- Evidence of moderate or severe dehydration (Table 5);
- Loss of greater than 5% of total body weight;
- Diarrhea that has lasted 2 or more days.

Clinical judgment must be used in evaluating these patients. For example, access to medical treatment may not be readily available, and temporary self-treatment may be needed until a medical appointment can be arranged.

A properly conducted medication history may help detect drug-induced diarrhea. The pharmacist should determine the self-treatments that have been tried, the patient's age, the symptoms, the date of onset, and the characteristics of stools (number, consistency, odor, and appearance). When a drug is implicated as a cause of diarrhea, the pharmacist should refer the patient to a health care provider because the patient may need to continue taking the drug even though it is causing problems.

Alcohol abuse, diverticulitis, emotional problems, gastritis, irritable bowel syndrome, peptic ulcer disease, and ulcerative colitis or regional enteritis are some frequently reported past medical problems. Patients with a history of chronic GI disease should also be referred to a health care provider for care.

The patient needs to be monitored for signs of volume depletion. The most accurate assessment of fluid balance is body weight; however, the premorbid weight is seldom known for comparison. As detailed in Table 5, the signs and symptoms of mild dehydration (≤5% weight loss) are increased thirst and slightly dry mouth (especially under the tongue). Moderate (6–9% weight loss)

TABLE 5 Diarrhea treatment chart

Degree of dehydration (fluid deficit)	Signs[a]	Rehydration therapy (within 4 h)	Replacement of stool fluid losses	Dietary therapy[b]
Mild (3–5%)	Slightly dry buccal mucous membranes; increased thirst	ORS[c] 50 mL/kg	10 mL/kg or 1/2–1 cup of ORS for each diarrheal stool	Human milk feeding, half- or full-strength lactose-containing milk, or undiluted lactose-free formula
Moderate (6–9%)	Sunken eyes; sunken fontanelle; loss of skin turgor; dry buccal mucous membranes	ORS 100 mL/kg	Same as above	Same as above
Severe (≥10%)	Signs of moderate dehydration with one of the following: rapid thready pulse, cyanosis, cold extremities, rapid breathing, lethargy, coma	Intravenous fluids (lactated Ringer's solution); 20 mL/kg per hour until pulse, perfusion, and mental status return to normal; then 50–100 mL/kg of ORS	Same as above	Same as above

[a]If no signs of dehydration are present, rehydration therapy is not required. Maintenance therapy and replacement of stool losses should be undertaken.

[b]Infants and children who receive solid food can continue their usual diet, but foods high in simple sugars and fats should be avoided.

[c]Oral rehydration solution (ORS).

Reprinted from Centers for Disease Control and Prevention. The management of acute diarrhea in children: oral rehydration, maintenance, and nutritional therapy. *MMWR.* 1992; 41(RR-16): 14.

dehydration findings are skin tenting with poor turgor and dry buccal mucous membranes. With severe dehydration (≥10% weight loss), the patient shows signs of hypoperfusion (ie, hypovolemic shock): lethargy; altered mental state (eg, confusion); extremely poor skin turgor and prolonged tenting; orthostatic hypotension with tachycardia; oliguria; rapid, deep breathing (ie, metabolic acidosis); slow capillary refill in the fingernail bed and cool, clammy skin.[21] Additionally, the patient should be asked about vomiting, high and/or prolonged fever, and the nature and amount of fluid intake, which may further contribute to the volume depletion.

Findings of moderate to severe volume depletion include complaints of dizziness, fainting, or near fainting; they may also include postural (orthostatic) hypotension, defined as a drop in the systolic and/or diastolic pressure by greater than 15–20 mm Hg upon moving from a lying to an upright position. Normally, the diastolic pressure remains the same or slightly increases and the systolic pressure drops slightly upon arising. If the blood pressure drops, the pulse should be checked simultaneously; the pulse rate should increase as the blood pressure drops. Failure of the pulse to rise could suggest that the problem is neurogenic (eg, diabetic patients with peripheral neuropathy) or that the patient is taking a beta-blocker. The presence of orthostatic hypotension indicates that the patient has lost 1 or more liters of vascular volume and should be referred for medical care.

Stool character gives valuable information about diarrhea. For example, undigested food particles in the stool suggest small bowel irritation; black, tarry stools may indicate upper GI bleeding; and red stools suggest possible lower bowel or hemorrhoidal bleeding or perhaps simply the recent ingestion of red food such as beets or of drug products such as rifampin. Diarrhea originating from the small intestine is probably characterized by a marked outpouring of fluid high in potassium and bicarbonate. A pasty or semisolid loose stool suggests diarrhea associated with a colon disorder. Yellowish stool may indicate the presence of bilirubin and a potentially serious pathology of the liver.

TABLE 6 Comparison of electrolyte-glucose concentrations of solutions commonly administered at home

Clear liquids	Sodium (mEq/L)	Potassium (mEq/L)	Bicarbonate (mEq/L)	Glucose (g/L)	Osmolarity (mM/L)
Cola	2	0.1	13	50–150 glucose and fructose	550
Ginger ale	3	1	4	50–150 glucose and fructose	540
Apple juice	3	20	0	100–150 glucose and fructose	700
Chicken broth	250	5	0	0	450
Tea	0	0	0	0	5
Gatorade	20	3	3	45 glucose and other sugars	330

Reprinted from Centers for Disease Control and Prevention. The management of acute diarrhea in children: oral rehydration, maintenance, and nutritional therapy. *MMWR.* 1992; 41(RR-16): 6.

Treatment

Treatment goals are to (1) prevent excessive fluid and electrolyte loss and acid-base disturbance; (2) manage secondary conditions causing diarrhea; (3) provide symptomatic relief; and (4) identify and treat the cause, if possible. Symptomatic relief generally is adequate for simple functional diarrhea that is only temporary, self-limiting, and uncomplicated. Because diarrhea is a symptom, however, symptomatic relief must not be interpreted as a cure for the underlying cause.

Many nonprescription products are available to assist in managing diarrhea. The pharmacist should exercise caution in recommending their use; however, certain diarrhea-producing diseases might be serious or treated more effectively with agents specific for the underlying cause. Pregnant women and the frail elderly with diarrhea should be referred to their physician for fluid and electrolyte management. Table 4 summarizes the primary causes of diarrhea and some of the more standard approaches to treatment.

Prophylaxis and Management of Infectious (Traveler's) Diarrhea

According to a review by DuPont and Ericsson, four criteria should be considered when advising a potential traveler[22]: the importance of the trip, the person's underlying health, the person's wishes, and the person's willingness to follow dietary restrictions. Prophylaxis of traveler's (infectious) diarrhea is controversial. The 1985 National Institutes of Health Conference on Traveler's Diarrhea recognized the prophylactic value of antibiotics and bismuth subsalicylate, but it considered the emergence of microbial resistance and the risk of side effects too great to recommend prophylaxis with either product.[23] If a prophylactic drug is used, it should be started on the first day of arrival and taken continuously, including 1–2 additional days after the person's return to the United States. However, prophylaxis should not continue for more than 3 weeks, even if the person's travel is still in progress.

Many remedies have been tried to prevent traveler's diarrhea; however, antibiotics are the most effective drugs available. Travelers likely to be exposed to excessive sun should be advised to use sunscreen if they are prescribed antibiotics that may produce photosensitivity reactions (eg, sulfonamides and tetracyclines). Doxycycline (100 mg daily) has been effective in preventing traveler's diarrhea. Trimethoprim-sulfamethoxazole (160–800 mg twice daily) has also been shown to prevent this disorder or to attenuate symptoms when the offending organism is enterotoxigenic *E coli*, *Salmonella* sp, or *Shigella* sp.[24] Norfloxacin (400 mg daily), ofloxacin (300 mg daily), and ciprofloxacin (500 mg daily) are effective in preventing diarrhea although the therapy is expensive.[22,25] Generally, many infectious disease experts do not recommend drug prophylaxis but tell travelers to begin treatment when signs or symptoms first appear.[23]

Traveler's diarrhea may be managed with fluid and electrolyte replacement. Antibiotics such as trimethoprim-sulfamethoxazole, norfloxacin, ciprofloxacin, and trimethoprim have been used successfully in therapy and are more effective than placebo. Loperamide (Diar Aid, Imodium A-D) has also been shown to be an effective treatment. For symptomatic management, loperamide (a 4-mg loading dose followed by 2 mg taken orally after each loose stool, not to exceed 16 mg per day) plus a fluoroquinolone antibiotic (eg, ciprofloxacin 500 mg taken twice daily, ofloxacin 300 mg taken twice daily, or norfloxacin 400 mg taken twice daily) may be effective.[26]

Bismuth subsalicylate (Pepto-Bismol) has been shown to be effective in both preventing and treating symptoms of traveler's diarrhea.[27] Its apparent mechanism of action is to inhibit intestinal secretions. The adult prophylactic dosage is 30 mL or two tablets taken four times a day with meals and at bedtime during the first 2 weeks of travel. During bouts of acute diarrhea, the adult treatment dose is 30 mL or two tablets and should be taken every 30 minutes for five doses. No more than eight doses should be taken in any 24-hour period. Package labeling should be consulted with regard to dosing pediatric patients.

TABLE 7 Oral rehydration solutions

	WHO-ORS[a]	Pedialyte	Rehydralyte	Infalyte	Resol
Osmolarity (mOsm/L)	333	249	304	200	269
Carbohydrates (g/L)[b]	20	25	25	30[c]	20
Electrolytes (mEq/L)					
Sodium	90	45	75	50	50
Potassium	20	20	20	25	20
Chloride	80	35	65	45	50
Citrate	30	30	30	34	34
Calcium	—	—	—	—	4
Magnesium	—	—	—	—	4
Phosphate	—	—	—	—	5

[a]World Health Organization oral rehydration solution.
[b]Carbohydrate is glucose.
[c]Rice syrup solids.

Reprinted with permission from *Med Lett.* 1991 Nov; 33: 107–10.

Fluid and Electrolyte Replacement

Depending on the patient's fluid and electrolyte state, treatment may be carried out in two phases: rehydration and maintenance. Rehydration replaces lost water and electrolytes to restore the normal body composition. After rehydration therapy is completed, electrolyte solutions are given to maintain the normal body composition. If the patient is not volume depleted, only maintenance of fluid and electrolytes (ie, replacement of volume losses) is needed.

Correction of fluid loss and electrolyte imbalance is very important. The secretory and absorptive mechanisms appear to function separately; therefore, an oral sugar-electrolyte solution can be absorbed during diarrhea.[28] In mild to moderate diarrhea, oral fluids can be safely prescribed if the patient is not vomiting. Administering fluids without electrolytes—the so-called clear liquids diet—is potentially dangerous because of the risk of inducing hyponatremia or causing osmotic diarrhea. Table 6 lists common household products used in clear liquids. They either are hypertonic from excess sugar or lack electrolytes. If these products are used for rehydration or maintenance therapy, it is important to dilute them to one-half strength to avoid osmotic diarrhea.

In developing countries, the World Health Organization (WHO) recommends an oral replacement fluid that contains, per liter, glucose 20 g, sodium 90 mEq, potassium 20 mEq, citrate 30 mEq, and chloride 80 mEq.[29] The WHO oral rehydration solution (WHO-ORS) was developed to manage cholera diarrhea, which occurs rarely in the United States. In the United States, several such products are available (see product table "Oral Rehydration Solutions"), but they differ slightly from the WHO-ORS (Table 7). The American Academy of Pediatrics (AAP) recommends that oral solutions not have more than 75–90 mEq/L of sodium for rehydration and 40–60 mEq/L of sodium for maintenance.[30] To lessen the risk of carbohydrate-induced osmotic diarrhea, the ratio of carbohydrate to sodium should not exceed 2:1.

Commercial ORS products are convenient and safe because they are premixed (Table 7). These products are either for rehydration or maintenance/preventive management. They can be used for maintenance therapy if water, lactose-free infant formula, breast milk, or low-carbohydrate juice is also given to prevent hypernatremia. Rehydralyte is the only product meeting the AAP recommendation for rehydration; all others are preventive/maintenance solutions. To improve electrolyte and water absorption and reduce the risk of glucose-induced osmotic diarrhea, the duration of illness, and the volume of stools, various substrates (ie, complex carbohydrates and large proteins) have been studied.[31–35] Infalyte, a rice syrup-electrolyte solution, is the only product with a complex carbohydrate nutrient source; all others use glucose. However, when Infalyte was compared with a glucose-based ORS, duration of illness and total stool output were not different.[27]

Although oral rehydration therapy has saved millions of infants and children in developing countries, it has not been the primary therapeutic method for managing acute diarrhea in the United States. There are several reasons for this: administration is labor intensive; parents must be carefully educated to follow instructions in preparation and administration; and if the child is hospitalized, parents expect intravenous therapy. However, intravenous therapy also has risks, such as phlebitis, infection, and fluid-electrolyte imbalance, and it is more expensive. With emphasis on avoiding or reducing hospital costs, oral rehydration therapy may have an important cost-effective benefit.

Management of Diarrhea in Infants and Children

The Centers for Disease Control and Prevention (CDC) published recommendations addressing management of diarrhea in infants and children.[21] Managing acute diarrhea in these patients requires fluid-electrolyte rehydration and maintenance and nutritional therapy. Table 5 outlines the CDC-recommended dietary management of fluid and electrolytes by degree of dehydration.

During the initial pediatric patient assessment, the health care provider should determine the degree of dehydration and check for plausible diarrhea causes. The most common symptoms of acute gastroenteritis are vomiting, loose stools, and fever. However, these are nonspecific findings associated with many other childhood diseases such as acute otitis media, bacterial sepsis, meningitis, pneumonia, and urinary tract infections.

As mentioned previously, after the degree of volume depletion has been determined, management is carried out in two phases: rehydration and maintenance with nutritional support.[21] For mild dehydration, an ORS with 50–90 mEq/L of sodium is given at 50 mL/kg over a 2- to 4-hour period. For example, a 10-kg mildly dehydrated person should receive a total volume of 2,500 mL over 2–4 hours. After 2–4 hours, the hydration status should be reassessed, and if the patient remains dehydrated, rehydration should continue. For moderate dehydration, the ORS should be given as it is for mild dehydration but increased to 100 mL/kg over 2–4 hours. For severe dehydration, intravenous rehydration should be administered. Once the patient can tolerate oral therapy, the ORS can be used to replace parenteral therapy.

After the rehydration phase, fluid losses must be replaced to maintain normal balance. A maintenance ORS should have 40–60 mEq/L of sodium. A rehydration solution (50–90 mEq/L sodium) can be used if low-sodium fluids are added to avoid hypernatremia. For each diarrheal stool, 10 mL/kg of solution should be given with each diarrheal episode; if the patient is also vomiting, an additional 2 mL/kg of solution per episode is needed to replace losses.

Besides fluid and electrolyte imbalances, there can also be dietary consequences that need to be addressed in the management of acute diarrhea in this population. Once rehydration is complete, food may be reintroduced while oral solutions are given for maintenance. In older infants and children, the AAP recommends that feeding should be reintroduced within the first 24 hours of onset and should include low-carbohydrate juice, rice cereal, bananas, potatoes, and other lactose-free, complex carbohydrate–rich foods.[30] The AAP recommends gradual reintroduction of milk-based bottle feeding, but breast-feeding should resume immediately after rehydration. Foods to be avoided are fatty foods and those rich in simple sugars, which can cause osmotic diarrhea.

In infants and children, antimotility and adsorbent drugs have not been shown to alter the outcomes of acute nonspecific diarrhea. Moreover, reliance on drugs shifts the focus away from fluid-electrolyte and nutritional support and leads to potentially dangerous side effects without additional benefits. Since intestinal viruses are the leading cause of self-limiting acute gastroenteritis in children and infants, antibiotics are not routinely recommended.

Pharmacologic Agents

In the United States, most acute nonspecific diarrheal causes are self-limiting in nature. Some health care providers recommend loperamide or adsorbents in acute diarrhea. With the exception of loperamide and bismuth subsalicylate in traveler's diarrhea, however, scientific evidence is lacking to prove that pharmacologic agents reduce stool frequency or duration of disease.[36] Nevertheless, when used according to labeling, nonprescription antidiarrheals may provide relief and usually do no harm (see product table "Antidiarrheal Products"). Fluid, electrolyte, and nutritional therapies are the most important components to managing diarrhea.

Antiperistaltic Agents

Opiates and opiate-like agents exert a direct musculotropic effect on and inhibit propulsive movements in the small and large intestines. Hyperperistalsis is diminished and the passage of intestinal contents slows, allowing reabsorption of water and electrolytes. In the usual oral antidiarrheal dosages, addiction liability is low for acute diarrheal episodes because the opiate or opiate derivative is not well absorbed orally and is only used short term. The low dose given produces an effective action in the GI tract without causing analgesia or euphoria. However, acute overdose or chronic use, as in ulcerative colitis, increases the risk of physical dependency. Opiate derivatives are central nervous system (CNS) depressants, and excessive sedation may be a problem in patients taking other CNS depressants with the antidiarrheal medication. Thus, the FDA has removed opiates (eg, paregoric) and opiate derivatives from nonprescription products.

Loperamide, an effective antidiarrheal agent in traveler's diarrhea, nonspecific acute diarrhea, and chronic diarrhea associated with inflammatory bowel disease, possesses a more favorable side effect profile than opiate and opiate-like agents. It slows intestinal motility and produces a positive movement of electrolytes and water through the gut. Like other antiperistaltic drugs, it should be used for no more than 48 hours in acute diarrhea. Loperamide is supplied as 2-mg caplets or 1 mg per 5 mL liquid. The usual nonprescription adult dosage is 4 mg initially and then 2 mg after each loose bowel movement, not to exceed 8 mg per day. Package labeling should be consulted for dosage guidelines in pediatric patients. Loperamide should never be recommended for children under 2 years of age.

Antiperistaltic drugs (eg, diphenoxylate, opiate derivatives, and loperamide) are effective in relieving cramps and stool frequency. However, they may worsen the effects of invasive bacterial infection (enteroinvasive *E coli*, *Salmonella*, *Shigella*) and may cause toxic megacolon in antibiotic-induced diarrhea in pseudomembranous colitis. These drugs should be used with caution in patients presenting with fecal leukocytes, fever, or a recent history of antibiotic use, as well as in cases of diagnosed acute ulcerative colitis.

Adsorbents

The nonprescription GI adsorbents are attapulgite, kaolin, and pectin. These agents are being reviewed by the FDA's Office of OTC Drug Evaluations for possible reclassification and labeling changes. The evidence for kaolin alone is better than that for the combination of kaolin and pectin in acute nonspecific diarrhea. Although combination products containing pectin are on the market, the FDA may decide to remove pectin from adsorbent combination products. Other labeling changes under review include a drug interaction warning not to administer kaolin concurrently with other oral medications and a recommendation that kaolin not be used in children under 12 years of age. Attapulgite is also being evaluated for safety and efficacy. Pharmacists should be aware that these are proposed labeling and category classification changes and should review the final monograph when available.

Adsorbents are the nonprescription antidiarrheal preparations prescribed most often. Adsorbents are generally used to treat mild nonspecific acute diarrhea. Because large doses are generally used, most commercially available products are formulated as flavored liquid suspensions to improve palatability.

Adsorption is not selective, and when adsorbents are given orally, they may adsorb nutrients and digestive enzymes as well as toxins, bacteria, and various noxious materials in the GI tract. They may also have the undesirable effect of adsorbing drugs in the GI tract. Although the systemic absorption of an orally administered drug from the GI tract is expected to be compromised during a diarrheal episode, absorption may be further hampered by the concomitant administration of an antidiarrheal adsorbent. Thus, a clinical judgment must be made regarding when the patient will take medications other than the antidiarrheal preparations. Depending on the medication involved, the usual rate and site of absorption, and the absolute necessity of getting specific and consistent blood levels of the drug, a change in the dose or dosage interval may be required. Sometimes, it might be better to administer the drug parenterally (if available by injection) until the diarrheal episode is over and the adsorbent drugs are discontinued.

Following initial treatment, most antidiarrheal preparations containing adsorbents are taken after each loose bowel movement until the diarrhea is controlled or the maximum daily dosage is reached. The total amount of adsorbent taken may be quite large if the diarrheal episodes recur in rapid succession over several hours. Because there is negligible systemic absorption of the adsorbent drug, the most common side effects associated with adsorbents include constipation, bloating, and fullness.

Polycarbophil

Polycarbophil is a synthetic polyacrylic resin that acts as an absorbent. Because of its ability to absorb up to 60 times its original weight in water, it has been recommended in the treatment of both diarrhea and constipation. Polycarbophil is metabolically inert, and no systemic toxicity has been shown. Side effects, which are mild and infrequent, include dose-related epigastric pain and bloating. The effective adult oral antidiarrheal dose of polycarbophil is 4–6 g per day in divided doses. Adults should chew two 500-mg tablets four times a day, children 6–12 years of age should chew one 500-mg tablet three times a day, and children 3–6 years of age should chew one 500-mg tablet two times a day. Use in children under 3 years of age is not recommended without the advice of a health care provider.

Bismuth Subsalicylate

The antidiarrheal mechanisms of action of bismuth subsalicylate are reported to be "by normalizing fluid movement by an antisecretory mechanism and by binding bacterial toxins and antimicrobial activity."[37] Bismuth subsalicylate (Pepto-Bismol) is available as 262.5 mg per (original and cherry-flavored) tablet, 262.5 mg per swallowable caplet, 262.5 mg per 15 mL, or 525 mg per 15 mL (maximum strength). The usual adult dosage is 30 mL every 30–60 minutes as needed, to a maximum of eight doses in a 24-hour period. To determine pediatric dosages for children, the package directions for the appropriate age should be followed. Bismuth subsalicylate is not recommended for children under 2 years.

Bismuth subsalicylate dosage forms contain various amounts of salicylate. Methylsalicylate (oil of wintergreen) is used as a flavoring agent in the suspension dosage form and the original tablets. The suspension dosage form (262.5 mg/15 mL) contains 130 mg of salicylate whereas the original tablets (262.5 mg) contain 102 mg of salicylate. Further, the caplets (262.5 mg) and cherry-flavored tablets (262.5 mg) contain 99 mg of salicylate. The salicylate may be a problem if the patients are taking aspirin or other salicylate-containing drugs. Toxic levels of salicylate may be reached even if the patient follows dosing directions on the label for each drug. Thus, patients who are sensitive to aspirin should not use bismuth subsalicylate. Children and teenagers who have or are recovering from chicken pox or flu are at risk of aspirin-induced Reye's syndrome, a rare but serious illness.

This product may also interact adversely with oral anticoagulants, methotrexate, probenecid, and any other drug that potentially interacts with aspirin. Also, serum salicylate concentrations may exert an antiplatelet effect. Harmless black-stained stool may occur, which should not be confused with melena; harmless darkening of the tongue may occur as well. Mild tinnitus is a side effect that may be associated with moderate to severe salicylate toxicity. If diarrhea is seen with high fever or continues beyond 24 hours, the patient should seek medical care. The product is contraindicated for nursing or pregnant women without medical advice. Bismuth is radiopaque and may interfere with radiographic intestinal studies.

Digestive Enzymes

For patients with lactase enzymatic deficiency, lactase enzymes are available as SureLac, Lactaid, Dairy Ease, and Lactrase. These preparations may be added to milk products or taken with milk at mealtimes to prevent osmotic diarrhea.

Product Selection Guidelines

A complete history obtained with a review of the medication record must be assessed before a product is selected. The most important data to evaluate are the presence of high fever, the duration of illness, the presence of blood in the stool, and the fluid-electrolyte status. Figure 2 outlines an algorithm for deciding to recommend self-medication or refer for medical care.

If the patient meets the criteria for self-medication, the degree of dehydration is the next most important assessment. Oral rehydration followed by maintenance electrolyte therapy with appropriate dietary management has been described in the section Fluid and Electrolyte Replacement. The pharmacist should select either an ORS or a maintenance product. If no signs of dehydration are present, rehydration therapy is not needed; preventive therapy with a maintenance ORS may be all that is necessary to replace stool losses. Early administration of an ORS at home is vital if hospitalization is to be avoided. For infants and children, educating parents on the appropriate use of an ORS and diet is very important preventive care. For families with infants, the CDC recommends a home supply of ORS.

Nonspecific antidiarrheals have limited value and lack scientific evidence in acute diarrheal illnesses. With suspected infectious diarrhea, antibiotics may be indicated and should be managed by a health care provider.

Uncomplicated acute diarrhea usually improves within 24–48 hours. If the condition remains the same or worsens, the pharmacist should recommend that the patient seek medical care. Moderately or severely volume-depleted patients (especially infants and children) need medical care. Immediate referral to a health care provider is also required if the patient is severely dehydrated, has a high fever, has protracted vomiting, has blood in the stool, is chronically ill, or is immunocompromised.

If a nonspecific antidiarrheal is used, the pharmacist should review label contents to determine the appropriate dosage based on the patient's age, the maximum number of doses per 24 hours, auxiliary administration instructions (eg, shake the product before using), the proper method of storage, potential drug interactions, side effects, diseases for which the drug is contraindicated, and the maximum duration of treatment before seeking medical help.

Case Studies

Case 13–1

Patient Complaint/History

A mother presents to the pharmacist complaining that her 3-year-old daughter JC has diarrhea, dry mouth, stomach cramps, and nausea and has not been urinating as usual. She goes on to say that the child has had a fever of 99°F (37.2°C) for the past 12 hours but has received no medication for it. Although the mother has given JC clear liquids for the past 8 hours, the child is still complaining of dry mouth and diarrhea. The mother asks if she should use Pepto-Bismol to treat the diarrhea.

During further conversation with the mother, the pharmacist learns that JC was recently diagnosed with otitis media and the flu. The physician prescribed a 7-day course of antibiotic therapy for the otitis media but said the flu was most likely viral in origin. JC, who completed the therapy the day before, did not experience diarrhea while on the antibiotic. When asked about the diarrhea, the mother responds that it is watery and that the symptoms started suddenly about 12 hours ago. She adds that the child has not vomited.

JC weighs 38 lb and has no known drug allergies.

Clinical Considerations/Strategies

The following considerations/strategies are provided to aid the reader in (1) determining whether treatment of the patient's condition with nonprescription medications is warranted, (2) selecting the appropriate nonprescription medication, and (3) developing a patient counseling strategy to ensure optimal therapeutic outcomes:

- Assess the possible cause(s) of the patient's signs and symptoms.
- Recommend an appropriate treatment plan for the diarrhea.
- Recommend dietary measures for treatment of the diarrhea.
- Assess the appropriateness of treating the diarrhea with Pepto-Bismol.
- Develop a patient education/counseling strategy that will:
  - Ensure that the mother understands the importance of oral rehydration and dietary therapy for treatment of diarrhea in a child;
  - Ensure that the mother knows when to contact the physician about the child's diarrhea.

Case 13–2

Patient Complaint/History

KD, a 21-year-old male college student, presents to the pharmacist with complaints of watery loose stools, nausea, muscle aches, and abdominal cramps. Unable to keep down his breakfast of a bowl of cereal, he has not tried to eat anything else. He is not dizzy and does not feel faint.

Although the patient looks ill, he has a deep tan. When asked about the tan, KD responds that he just returned from Cancun 2 days ago. In response to queries about consumption of water or iced beverages, the patient admits to ordering a soda with ice at the airport in Cancun. When asked about his current medication use, he admits to taking a tablespoon of Kaopectate a couple of hours earlier and to taking an occasional ibuprofen for muscle aches related to playing volleyball.

Clinical Considerations/Strategies

The following considerations/strategies are provided to aid the reader in (1) determining whether treatment of the patient's condition with nonprescription medications is warranted, (2) selecting the appropriate nonprescription medication, and (3) developing a patient counseling strategy to ensure optimal therapeutic outcomes:

- Assess the possible cause and pathogenesis of the patient's signs and symptoms.
- Recommend appropriate treatment options for these signs and symptoms.

- Assess the appropriateness of treatment with Kaopectate and other nonprescription medications.
- Determine how long it should take to resolve the patient's condition.
- Develop a patient education/counseling strategy that will:
  - Ensure that the patient understands the importance of the recommended treatment;
  - Ensure that the patient knows when to contact a physician.

Summary

Diarrhea is often considered a trivial disorder, but it can be a symptom of a more serious underlying disease. The condition can be either acute or chronic. Acute diarrhea is characterized by a sudden onset of loose stools in a previously and otherwise healthy patient. Chronic diarrhea is characterized by persistent or recurrent episodes of loose stools accompanied by anorexia, weight loss, and weakness. Simple diarrhea can usually be treated by supportive care and/or a nonprescription drug or oral hydration product.

The debilitating effect of persistent diarrhea is due largely to loss of water through excretion resulting in an imbalance of both fluids and electrolytes. The replacement of these important substances is an integral part of diarrhea therapy, particularly in infants, children, and frail elderly persons. This replacement can be accomplished with appropriate intravenous fluids or with oral sugar-electrolyte formulations.

Patients who appear volume depleted, weak, dizzy, or hypotensive should be referred to a health care provider, as should all patients with severely acute, uncontrolled, or chronic complaints involving the GI tract. For minor acute problems such as food or drink intolerance, however, relief may be provided by a nonprescription product such as loperamide.

References

1. Connell AM, Hilton C, Irvine G. Variation of bowel habits in two population samples. *Br Med J.* 1965; 2: 1095–9.
2. Diem K, Lenthner C. *Scientific Tables.* 7th ed. Basile, Switzerland: Ciba-Geigy Ltd; 1970: 657–8.
3. Gray GM. Acute diarrhea. In: Dale DC, Federman DD, eds. *Scientific American Medicine.* New York: Scientific American; 1992: 1–16.
4. Field M, Rao MC, Chang EB. Intestinal electrolyte transport and diarrheal disease. *N Engl J Med.* 1989 Sep 21; 321(pt 1): 800–6.
5. Archer DL, Young FE. Contemporary issues: diseases with a food vector. *Clin Microbiol Rev.* 1988; 1: 377–98.
6. Cover TL, Blaser MJ. The pathobiology of campylobacter infections in humans. *Annu Rev Med.* 1989; 40: 269–85.
7. Levine MM. *Escherichia coli* that cause diarrhea: enterotoxigenic, enteropathogenic, enteroinvasive, enterohemorrhagic, and enteroadherent. *J Infect Dis.* 1987; 155: 377–89.
8. Field M, Rao MC, Chang EB. Intestinal electrolyte transport and diarrheal disease. *N Engl J Med.* 1989 Sep 28; 321(pt 2): 879–83.
9. Christensen ML. Human viral gastroenteritis. *Clin Microbiol Rev.* 1989; 2(1): 51–89.
10. Feld LG, Kaskel FJ, Schoeneman MJ. The approach to fluid and electrolyte therapy in pediatrics. *Adv Pediatr.* 1988; 35: 497–536.
11. Sanford JP. *Guide to Antimicrobial Therapy 1994.* Dallas: Antimicrobial Therapy; 1994: 76.
12. Gross MH. Management of antibiotic-associated pseudomembranous colitis. *Clin Pharm.* 1985; 5: 304–10.
13. Qualman SJ et al. *Clostridium difficile* invasion and toxin circulation in fatal pediatric pseudomembranous colitis. *Am J Clin Pathol.* 1990; 94: 410–6.
14. Fekety R et al. Treatment of antibiotic-associated *Clostridium difficile* colitis with oral vancomycin: comparison of two dosage regimens. *Am J Med.* 1989; 86: 15–9.
15. Teasley OG, Gerdine ON, Olsen MM. Prospective, randomized study of metronidazole versus vancomycin for clostridium-associated diarrhea and colitis. *Lancet.* 1983; 2: 1043–6.
16. Langhon BE et al. Prevalence of enteric pathogens in homosexual men with and without acquired immunodeficiency syndrome. *Gastroenterology.* 1988; 94: 984–93.
17. Tanowitz HB, Simon D, Wittner M. Gastrointestinal manifestations. *Med Clin North Am.* 1992; 76: 45–62.
18. Antiprotozoal drugs. In: Bennett DR, ed. *Drug Evaluations Annual 1995.* Chicago: American Medical Association; 1995: 1753.
19. Donowitz M, Kokke FT, Saidi R. Evaluation of patients with chronic diarrhea. *N Engl J Med.* 1995; 332: 725–9.
20. Fedorak RH, Field M, Chang EB. Treatment of diabetic diarrhea with clonidine. *Ann Intern Med.* 1985; 102: 197–9.
21. Centers for Disease Control and Prevention. The management of acute diarrhea in children: oral rehydration, maintenance, and nutritional therapy. *MMWR.* 1992: 41(RR-16): 1–20.
22. DuPont HL, Ericsson CD. Prevention and treatment of traveler's diarrhea. *N Engl J Med.* 1993; 328: 1821–7.
23. Traveler's diarrhea. Consensus conference. *JAMA.* 1985; 253: 2700–4.
24. Ebert SC et al. ASHP therapeutics guidelines on nonsurgical antibiotic prophylaxis. *Clin Pharm.* 1990; 9: 423–45.
25. Ericsson CD et al. Ciprofloxacin or trimethoprim-sulfamethoxazole as initial therapy for travelers' diarrhea. *Ann Intern Med.* 1987; 106: 216–20.
26. Advice for travelers. *Med Lett.* 1994 May: 41.
27. Gorbach SL. Pathophysiology of gastrointestinal infections: the role of bismuth subsalicylate. *Rev Infect Dis.* 1990; 12: 53–119.
28. Pizarro D et al. Rice-based oral electrolyte solutions for the management of infantile diarrhea. *N Engl J Med.* 1991; 324: 517–21.
29. Avery ME, Snyder JD. Oral therapy for acute diarrhea. *N Engl J Med.* 1990; 323: 891–4.
30. American Academy of Pediatrics Committee on Nutrition. Use of oral fluid therapy and post-treatment feeding following enteritis in children in a developed country. *Pediatrics.* 1985; 75: 358–61.
31. Islam A et al. Is rice-based oral rehydration therapy effective in young infants? *Arch Dis Child.* 1994; 71: 19–23.
32. Maulén-Radován I, Brown KH, Acosta MA, Fernandex-Varela H. Comparison of a rice-based, mixed diet versus a lactose-free, soy-protein isolate formula for young children with acute diarrhea. *J Pediatr.* 1994; 125(5): 699–706.
33. Fayad IM et al. Comparative efficacy of rice-based and glucose-based oral rehydration salts plus early reintroduction of food. *Lancet.* 1993; 342: 772–5.
34. Rautanen T et al. Randomized double-blind trial of hypotonic oral rehydration solutions with and without citrate. *Arch Dis Child.* 1994; 70: 44–6.
35. Thillainayagam AV et al. Evidence of a dominant role for low osmolality in the efficacy of cereal-based oral rehydration solutions: studies in a model of secretory diarrhoea. *Gut.* 1993; 34: 920–5.
36. *Federal Register.* 1990 Nov; 55: 46914–21.
37. *Physicians' Desk Reference.* 49th ed. Montvale, NJ: Medical Economics; 1995: 1912.

CHAPTER 14

Hemorrhoidal Products

Benjamin Hodes

Questions to ask in patient assessment and counseling

- *What are your symptoms?*
- *How long have your symptoms been present? Do they recur?*
- *Are your symptoms associated with straining at a bowel movement?*
- *Have you noticed any bleeding? Describe it.*
- *What improves or worsens your symptoms?*
- *Have you treated your symptoms without the use of medication? What nondrug measures have you used?*
- *Have you previously used any nonprescription or prescription drugs for these symptoms?*
- *Do you take laxatives regularly? If so, which ones and how often?*
- *What other medications do you take?*
- *Have you recently changed your diet or amount of fluid intake?*
- *Are you now or have you recently been pregnant?*
- *Do you often experience constipation or diarrhea?*
- *Do you have any other medical conditions such as heart failure, liver disease, inflammatory disease of the intestine, or varicose veins?*

Anorectal diseases, including hemorrhoids, are annoying, discomforting, and potentially serious. Several of these diseases are not amenable to self-treatment and require medical attention; however, many of their symptoms can be self-treated, as can other relatively minor anorectal disorders. The pharmacist should carefully evaluate any symptoms reported by the patient. Many nonprescription products are available for symptomatic relief of the burning, pain, itching, inflammation, irritation, swelling, and general discomfort of hemorrhoids.

Anatomy and Physiology

With respect to anorectal diseases, three parts of the body are of concern: the perianal area, the anal canal, and the lower portion of the rectum (Figure 1).

The perianal area (about 7 cm in diameter) is the portion of the skin and buttocks immediately surrounding the anus. The presence of sensory nerve endings makes this area very sensitive to pain. Perianal tissue differs from most other skin tissue in that it is constantly moist and occluded.

The anal canal (about 4 cm long) is the channel connecting the end of the gastrointestinal tract (rectum) with the outside of the body. The lower two thirds of the canal is covered by modified anal skin, which is structurally similar to the skin covering other parts of the body. The canal contains sensory nerve endings as well as pressure receptors, which allow for the perception of distention pain.

Two powerful sphincter muscles that encircle the anal canal control the passage of fecal material. The external sphincter, located at the bottom of the anal canal, is a voluntary muscle. The internal sphincter, which allows passage into the anal canal, is an involuntary muscle. Both sphincters lie under the tissues of the anal canal and extend downward. Under normal conditions, the external sphincter is closed and prevents the involuntary passage of feces or discharges.

In healthy individuals, the skin covering the anal canal serves as a barrier against absorption of substances into the body. Therefore, treatment applied to this area can be expected to manifest only local effects. If disease is present, the loss of protective oils or breaks in the surface may alter the character of the skin covering the canal, thereby diminishing the skin's protective capabilities.

The point in the mid-upper anal canal at which the skin lining changes to mucous membrane is the dentate or pectinate line, also known as the anorectal line.

The most prominent parts of the vasculature in the region above and below the anorectal line are the three hemorrhoidal arteries and the accompanying veins. Veins and arteries above the anorectal line are referred to as internal; those below, as external. In normal and healthy individuals, conglomerates of highly vascularized anchoring connective tissues, referred to as anal cushions, are found in three locations above the anorectal line: left lateral, right posterior, and right anterior.[1]

Anal crypts are normal pocketlike formations located on the internal side of the anorectal line. They face upward and, because of their position, sometimes retain small amounts of fecal material that may cause irritation. This irritation may lead to infection and foster the development of anorectal disease.

Investigators commonly distinguish between rectal mucosa and anal mucosa and consider the anorectal line to be the upper end of the anal canal. For purposes of this chapter, the appearance of the mucosal region will be considered the beginning of the rectal area.

The rectum (about 12–15 cm long) is the lower end of the gastrointestinal tract and extends from the anorectal line up to the sigmoid colon. It is lined with semi-

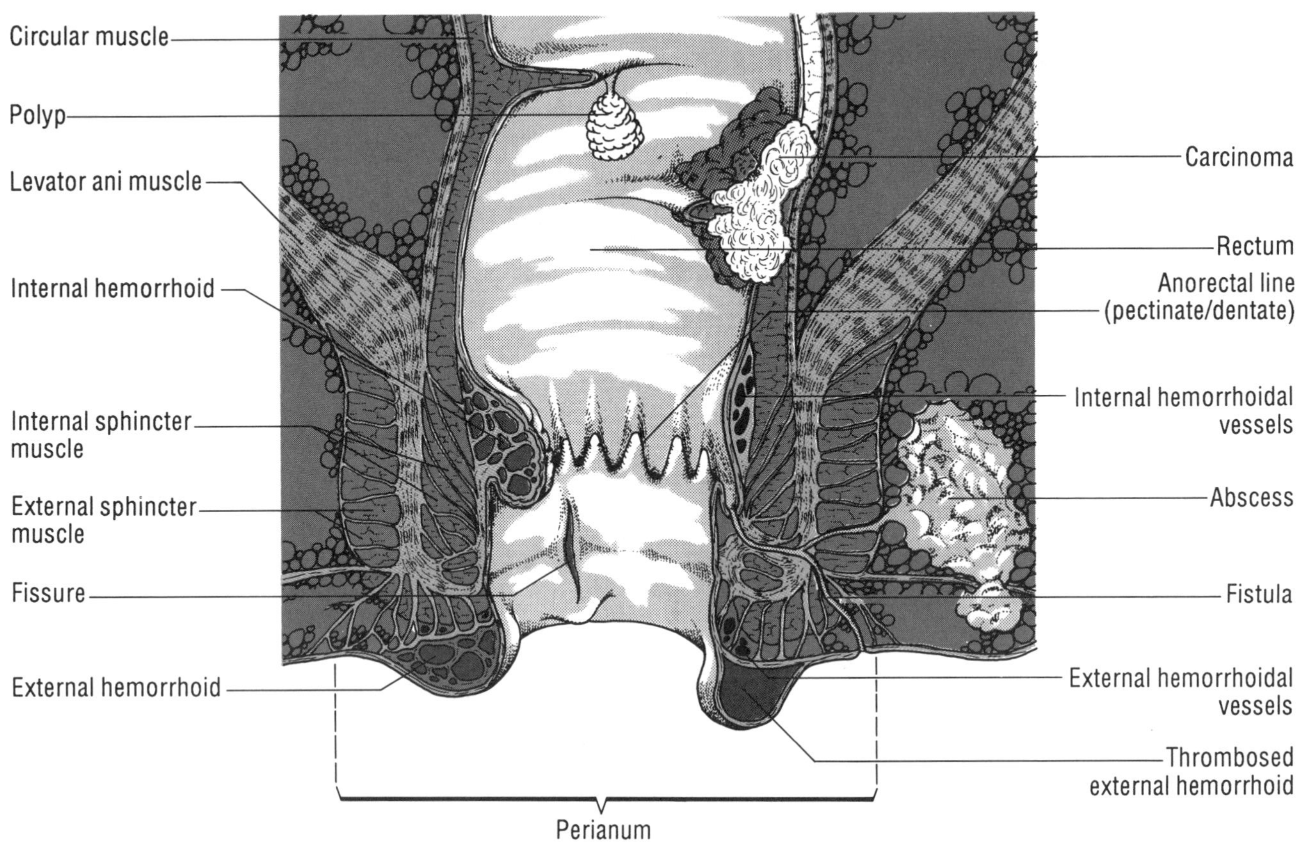

FIGURE 1 Selected disease states in anorectal region.

permeable mucous membranes, is highly vascularized, and contains no sensory pain fibers. Like the anal canal, however, it does contain pressure receptors. And like the skin of the anal canal, the mucous membranes in the rectum protect the body from invasion by the bacteria present in feces.

Because of the plexus of hemorrhoidal vessels located beneath the rectal mucosa and the paths followed by the blood returning to the heart through the hemorrhoidal veins, substances absorbed through the rectal mucous membranes may enter the systemic circulation without passing through the liver. This possibility is important in evaluating the potential systemic toxicity of locally applied drugs. The rectal pH, which ranges from neutral to basic, is important in determining the extent to which substances in the rectum are absorbed.

Anorectal Disorders

Types of Anorectal Disorders

Hemorrhoids

Hemorrhoids (also known as piles) are abnormally large, bulging, symptomatic conglomerates of hemorrhoidal vessels, supporting tissues, and overlying mucous membranes or skin of the anorectal area.

Hemorrhoidal disease appears most often in persons 20–50 years of age.[1] Responses to a national health questionnaire in 1990 showed a 4.4% prevalence of hemorrhoids in the United States.[2] Many factors have been implicated in the etiology of hemorrhoidal disease; these factors include heredity, erect posture, pregnancy, prolonged standing or sitting, lack of dietary bulk, heavy lifting with straining, constipation, and diarrhea.[2] Common denominators are physiologic vulnerability and high resting pressure on the anus.[2] Symptomatic hemorrhoids develop only in susceptible individuals; although controversial, heredity may be a factor in their formation, and socioeconomic and cultural factors (eg, diet and lifestyle) may be precipitants, but data are not consistent.[2] Evidence points to a lack of association between amount of fiber intake and prevalence of hemorrhoids.[3] Straining at defecation, which in turn leads to increased pressure within the hemorrhoidal vessels, may also precipitate the formation of hemorrhoids, as may certain bowel habits, such as prolonged sitting on the toilet during bowel movements.[2]

Pregnancy is by far the most common cause of hemorrhoids in young women. The gravid uterus produces increased pressure in the middle and interior hemorrhoidal vessels. Labor may also intensify the hemorrhoidal condition and produce intense symptoms after delivery. Pelvic tumors may give rise to hemorrhoids by a similar process.

Hemorrhoids are classified according to their location[1] (Figure 1). This classification system includes three major types of hemorrhoids: internal, external, and internal-external.

Internal Hemorrhoids Internal hemorrhoids occur above the anorectal line, where they are further classified according to location (eg, left lateral, right posterior, or right anterior). They develop when three "cushions" that are considered normal anatomic structures[4] become engorged and protrude into the anal canal. With deterioration of connective tissue caused by aging and other factors, these cushions become loosened from their submucosal anchoring, gradually become elongated, and descend toward the anus.[5] Because of this weakening, the veins also become distended. As the loose anal lining descends, the hemorrhoids and weakened cushions become increasingly exposed and susceptible to increased pressure from straining or trauma resulting from constipation. Engorgement of the blood vessels may eventually result in clot formation, swelling, erosion of the lining and vessel wall, and bleeding.[5] In support of this etiology, microscopic analysis of hemorrhoidectomy specimens has revealed fragmented supportive connective tissue.[6] After repeated episodes of straining with a relaxed sphincter, the hemorrhoids dilate and ultimately descend below the anorectal line and outside the anal sphincter. Eventually, they become permanently prolapsed and enlarged.

Internal hemorrhoids can also be classified according to a four-degree system. First-degree hemorrhoids do not move from the anal canal. Second-degree hemorrhoids can descend into the anal canal and return spontaneously. Hemorrhoids that can be returned manually into the anus are referred to as third degree. Fourth-degree hemorrhoids are prolapsed and cannot be reintroduced into the anus.

External Hemorrhoids External hemorrhoids are recognized as a swelling of the skin and associated blood vessels around the rim of the anus.[7] There are two types of external hemorrhoids, thrombosed and cutaneous, both of which occur below the anorectal line. A thrombosed hemorrhoid is a hemorrhoidal vein either in the anal canal or adjacent to the anus that contains a blood clot or thrombus. Such hemorrhoids may be quite painful. The clot may vary in size from that of a pea to that of a walnut. Cutaneous hemorrhoids, which consist of fibrous connective tissue covered by anal skin, are located outside the anal sphincter at any point on the circumference of the anus. They may result either from a previously thrombosed external hemorrhoid in which the clot has become organized and been replaced by connective tissue[5] or from uneven healing of skin following a hemorrhoidectomy. External hemorrhoids are covered by highly innervated skin, and when this skin is stretched by a thrombosis, sudden and severe pain can result.

Internal-External Hemorrhoids Internal and external hemorrhoids sometimes occur together. Also known as mixed hemorrhoids, they appear as baggy swellings. The following types occur.

- *Prolapsed.* A prolapsed hemorrhoid is characterized by pain until the prolapse is reduced; blood, which is bright red, may or may not be present.
- *Without prolapse.* A hemorrhoid without prolapse may be characterized by bleeding but not by pain.
- *Strangulated.* A strangulated hemorrhoid is one that has prolapsed to such a degree and for so long that its blood supply is occluded by the anal sphincter's constricting action; it is very painful and usually becomes thrombosed.

Other Types of Anorectal Disorders

Some potentially serious anorectal disorders, including fissures, fistulas, inflammatory bowel diseases, and tumors, may present hemorrhoidal-like symptoms and should not be self-treated. Patients should be promptly referred to a physician if any of the following conditions are suspected:

- *Abscess:* a painful swelling in the perianal or anal canal area caused by a bacterial (primarily staphylococcal) infection and resulting in the formation of a localized area of pus;
- *Anal fistula:* a channel-like lesion near the anus, associated with swelling, pain, intermittent discharge, and pruritus and usually resulting from an anorectal abscess;
- *Anal fissure:* a slitlike ulcer in the anal canal lining, which may be painful, may exist alone or in conjunction with hemorrhoids, and often causes bleeding (as evidenced by bright red blood on toilet tissue);
- *Condyloma latum:* a firm, wartlike, usually painless lesion, and one of the secondary lesions of syphilis;
- *Condyloma acuminata:* venereal warts, usually sexually transmitted, that appear as multiple, polymorphic, painless lesions in the genital or perianal region;
- *Cryptitis:* inflammation and hypertrophy of the anal crypts, a condition that probably originates in an anal gland and is primarily characterized by pain aggravated by defecation;
- *Malignant neoplasm:* a serious disease, often characterized by constipation, in which bleeding and pain may be associated with malignant anal tumors (the most common of which is squamous cell carcinoma), which are usually unnoticeable and located in the rectum;
- *Polyps:* benign or malignant rectal tumors that are characterized by bleeding and, rarely, by a mass protruding through the anus or a feeling of fullness or pressure in the rectum.

Signs and Symptoms of Anorectal Disease

Itching, burning, inflammation, pain, and swelling are usually considered signs and symptoms of minor anorectal disease. Discomfort, a vague and generalized uneasiness, may result from any or all of these symptoms. If these symptoms are caused by hemorrhoids rather than by a more serious anorectal disease, they may be relieved by self-treatment. Bleeding, seepage, protrusion, prolapse, and thrombosis should not be self-treated, both because a more serious disorder may be masked and because no appropriate nonprescription therapy is available.

Itching

Itching, or pruritus, occurs as a manifestation of mild inflammation associated with many anorectal disorders. Itching, one of the most common symptoms of anorectal disease, may be secondary to swelling, irritation caused by dietary factors, parasitic diseases (eg, pinworms), or moisture in the anal area. Pruritus ani refers to persistent itching in the anal and perianal areas that occurs even in the presence of good hygiene.

Itching is typically associated with hemorrhoidal disease when there is mucous discharge from prolapsing internal hemorrhoids. Sensitivity to fabrics; dyes and perfumes in toilet tissue; detergents; local treatment, including products used to treat hemorrhoidal symptoms; and fecal contents are common causes of itching. Fungal infections, parasites, allergies, and associated anorectal pathologic lesions may also cause itching. Oral broad-spectrum antibiotic therapy may trigger itching as a result of infection secondary to the overgrowth of nonsusceptible organisms, particularly fungi. Chronic oral intake of mineral oil can lead to pruritus ani. Itching may also be attributed to a psychologic cause on rare occasions.

Burning

Burning, a common symptom of anorectal disease, suggests a somewhat greater degree of irritation of the anorectal sensory nerves than that associated with itching. The burning sensation may range from a feeling of warmth to a feeling of intense heat and may be constant or associated with defecation.

Inflammation

Inflammation, a tissue reaction distinguished by heat, redness, pain, and swelling, is often caused by trauma, allergy, or infection. Swelling is caused by an accumulation of excess fluid associated with engorged hemorrhoids or hemorrhoidal tissue. The inflammation itself, but not the underlying cause, may be relieved by self-treatment.

Acute inflammation of the anal tissue may cause pain. Pain is experienced consistently and predictably with acute external hemorrhoids; this pain, which is steady and aching, is usually worsened by standing or defecating. Chronic external hemorrhoids, on the other hand, often exhibit no pain. Similarly, because of the absence of sensory nerve endings above the anorectal line, uncomplicated internal hemorrhoids rarely cause pain as well. However, when strangulation, thrombosis, or ulceration occurs, pain may be severe.[5] Patients with severe, persistent pain should be referred to a physician.

Bleeding

Bleeding is almost always associated with internal hemorrhoids and may occur before, during, or after defecation. Painless bleeding during defecation is the most common symptom of hemorrhoids.[1] However, bleeding may also indicate the presence of serious anorectal disease (eg, abscess, fistula, cancer, colitis, or diverticulitis), so it should not be self-treated.

The amount of bleeding experienced with hemorrhoids often varies and is not necessarily related to the amount of hemorrhoidal tissue present. When bleeding occurs from an external hemorrhoid, it is typically due to an acute thrombosis accompanied by rupture. Pain often accompanies such bleeding, although a patient may experience some relief of the pain with the onset of the bleeding. Blood from hemorrhoids is usually bright red and covers the fecal matter or toilet paper. Bleeding is stimulated by defecation but may occur as an "oozing," which will soil underclothes. The chronic blood loss associated with bleeding hemorrhoids infrequently produces severe anemia.

Seepage

Seepage, the involuntary passing of fecal material or mucus, is caused by an anal sphincter that does not close completely because of pain, swelling, or inflammation. This symptom cannot be self-treated, and the patient should be referred to a health care provider.

Protrusion

Protrusion, a frequent sign or symptom of uncomplicated internal and external hemorrhoids, is defined as the projection of hemorrhoidal or rectal tissue outside the anal canal. The rectal protrusion may vary in size and usually appears after defecation, prolonged standing, or unusual physical exertion. It is painless except when thrombosis, infection, or ulceration is present. Strangulation of a protruding hemorrhoid by the sphincter may lead to thrombosis. Additionally, when contraction of the anal sphincter interferes with blood flow from a prolapsed internal or mixed hemorrhoid, a painful lump may develop, also resulting in thrombosis. If, using digital manipulation, this prolapsed hemorrhoid is returned to an area above the anal sphincter before thrombosis occurs, the pain and lump usually disappear. However, when defecation occurs, both the pain and the lump are likely to recur. Permanently prolapsing internal hemorrhoids cause a mucoid discharge, which in turn may lead to perianal irritation, itching, pain, and swelling. Self-treatment is not appropriate and should not be encouraged.

Thrombosis

Thrombosis within a hemorrhoid is a common complication. Abrupt onset of severe, constant pain in the anal area, accompanied, for example, by a grape-sized lump, is a sign that thrombosis of a mixed or external hemorrhoid may have occurred. If untreated, the burning pain persists for about 5–7 days, diminishing in intensity after the first day. A hard, tender lump at the site of the pain typically appears; after the second day, this lump slowly dissipates and eventually leaves a skin tag.

If a thrombosed hemorrhoid persists, gangrene and ulcers may develop on its surface. This condition may lead to an oozing of blood as well as to hemorrhaging, particularly when the patient is defecating or standing. If the clot remains exposed, infection may occur and an abscess or fistula may result.

If the thrombosed hemorrhoid resides entirely above the anorectal line (a pure internal hemorrhoid), there may be minimal pain because of the lack of sensory nerve supply. Patients are likely to be unaware that such a hemorrhoid is present unless there are sudden changes in bowel habits.

Assessment

By questioning the patient, the pharmacist should be able to determine whether self-treatment of an anorectal condition is desirable and, if so, which nonprescription drug product is suitable.

The first step in the assessment process is to determine the nature of the signs and symptoms. Bleeding (bright red), pain, itching, and prolapse are most common. Abdominal symptoms, seepage, prolapse, blood in the stool, persistent or severe itching, or severe and persistent pain could indicate another potentially serious medical problem that cannot be self-treated, in which case the patient should be advised to see a health care provider promptly. If the patient has not used any medication previously, the pharmacist should determine if there are any contributing factors such as diarrhea or constipation, obesity, cardiovascular disease, hepatic disease, pregnancy, and chronic cough. The pharmacist should also determine causative or precipitating factors, such as bowel habits, physical exertion, prolonged sitting or standing at work, insufficient fiber or liquids in the diet, constipating medications, and laxative abuse. Based on information received in the assessment process, the pharmacist may either recommend an appropriate nonprescription product for the temporary relief of minor anorectal symptoms (itching, burning, pain, inflammation or swelling, or discomfort) or refer the patient to a health care provider for further medical evaluation.

Treatment

Nondrug Measures

Cleansing the anorectal area with mild, unscented soap and water regularly and after each bowel movement helps to relieve hemorrhoidal symptoms and may prevent recurrence of perianal itching. Practical means of cleansing after a bowel movement include the use of commercially available hygienic and lubricated wipes or pads. Patients should be advised to blot or pat rather than rub the irritated perianal area with these wipes. This advice also applies to the use of toilet tissue, which should be unscented, uncolored, and soft.

Sitz baths are often useful in relieving hemorrhoidal symptoms, especially after bowel movements, and in promoting good hygiene. Patients should sit in warm water (110°–115°F [43.3°–46.1°C]) two to three times a day for 15 minutes. Plastic sitz baths, which fit over the toilet rim for convenient patient use, are easily cleaned and are available at pharmacies and from medical supply vendors.

Surgical and Nonsurgical Treatments

Large and prolapsed hemorrhoids are often treated with surgery (hemorrhoidectomy). Nonsurgical treatments for hemorrhoids include injection of sclerosing agents, rubber band ligation, dilation of the anal canal and lower rectum, cryosurgery, electrocoagulation, infrared photocoagulation, and bipolar diathermy.

Pharmacologic Agents

The nonprescription pharmacologic agents recommended to relieve symptoms of anorectal disease include local anesthetics; vasoconstrictors; protectants; astringents; wound-healing agents; antiseptics; keratolytics; anticholinergics; and analgesics, anesthetics, and antipruritics (see product table "Hemorrhoidal Products"). Products containing an excessive number of agents may not be optimally effective because of potential interaction among ingredients.

Local Anesthetics

Local, topical anesthetics temporarily relieve pain, burning, itching, and discomfort by preventing the transmission of nerve impulses. Use of these products should be limited to the perianal region or the lower anal canal for two reasons. First, symptoms within the rectum generally are not relieved by topical anesthetics because of the lack of rectal sensory nerve fibers there.[8] Second, local anesthetics may be rapidly absorbed through the rectal mucosa and cause potentially toxic systemic effects, whereas absorption through the perianal skin would not be particularly rapid, even if the skin is abraded.

Local anesthetics may produce allergic reactions, both locally and systemically. Such reactions may cause burning and itching that are indistinguishable from symptoms of the anorectal disease being treated. If symptoms return after cessation of therapy, a health care provider should be contacted.

The following local anesthetics have met the Food and Drug Administration (FDA) safety and efficacy standards for use in hemorrhoidal preparations. These preparations are applied to the perianal or lower anal canal regions.

Benzocaine When used externally in the base form, benzocaine is safe and effective in concentrations of 5–20% applied up to six times a day.[9] The most common adverse reaction to topical benzocaine is sensitization.

Benzyl Alcohol When used externally, benzyl alcohol is effective in concentrations of 5–20% and may be applied up to six times a day.[9]

Dibucaine Dibucaine and dibucaine hydrochloride are considered pharmacologically equivalent for external use as local anesthetics in concentrations of 0.25–1% applied up to three or four times a day.[9]

Dyclonine Dyclonine hydrochloride is effective for external use in concentrations of 0.5–1% and may be applied up to six times a day.[9]

Lidocaine Lidocaine is effective for external use in concentrations of 2–5% and may be applied up to six times a day.[9]

Pramoxine Pramoxine hydrochloride may be used externally as a topical aerosol foam, ointment, cream, or jelly (water-miscible base). The concentration typically used as a local anesthetic is 1%.[9] Adverse effects are rare, and pramoxine hydrochloride exhibits less cross-sensitivity than do most other local anesthetics because, unlike them, it is not chemically derived from lidocaine or procaine. Pramoxine-containing anorectal products may be applied up to five times a day.

Tetracaine Tetracaine and tetracaine hydrochloride are effective when used externally in concentrations of 0.5–1% and may be applied up to six times a day.[9]

Vasoconstrictors

Vasoconstrictors are chemical agents structurally related to the naturally occurring catecholamines, epinephrine and norepinephrine. Applied locally in the anorectal area, vasoconstrictors stimulate the alpha-adrenergic receptors in the vascular beds, causing constriction of the arterioles and a modest and transient reduction of swelling. They also relieve itching, discomfort, and irritation, in part because they produce a slight anesthetic effect by an unknown mechanism. Although it has been demonstrated that locally applied vasoconstrictors promptly alter the blood supply to the mucosa, the FDA does not recognize or approve the use of these products to control minor bleeding.[10] Because rectal bleeding may be a sign of a more serious disease, a health care provider should be consulted.

The FDA has concluded that potentially serious side effects, including the elevation of blood pressure, the risk of producing cardiac arrhythmia, nervousness, tremor, sleeplessness, and aggravation of symptoms of hyperthyroidism, are less likely to occur when vasoconstrictors are used locally in recommended dosages.[10] Because of the slight possibility of systemic adverse reactions from their topical application, these products should be avoided in patients who have diabetes, hyperthyroidism, hypertension, and difficulty urinating because of an enlarged prostate, and in those patients who are taking monoamine oxidase inhibitors, tricyclic antidepressants, or a prescription drug for high blood pressure. Some topical anorectal products containing ephedrine sulphate may cause nervousness, tremor, sleeplessness, nausea, and loss of appetite.

Four vasoconstrictors are approved for external use for itching, discomfort, swelling, and irritation: ephedrine sulfate, epinephrine hydrochloride, epinephrine base, and phenylephrine hydrochloride. Ephedrine sulfate and phenylephrine hydrochloride are also recommended for internal (intrarectal) use.[9] However, data are insufficient to establish the safety and effectiveness of epinephrine base for intrarectal use. Selected facts about the use of vasoconstrictors to manage the signs and symptoms of uncomplicated hemorrhoids are discussed in the following sections.

Ephedrine Sulfate Ephedrine sulfate, which is readily absorbed through mucous membranes in the rectum, has a more prolonged effect than epinephrine and acts on both alpha- and beta-adrenergic receptors. The hypertensive effects of ephedrine are potentiated by monoamine oxidase inhibitors as well as by tricyclic antidepressants. When ephedrine is applied topically, its onset of action ranges from a few seconds to 1 minute and its duration of action is 2–3 hours. The recommended concentration, in the final dosage form, is 0.1–1.25% applied up to four times a day.[9]

Epinephrine Epinephrine hydrochloride and epinephrine base are effective only when they are used externally because epinephrine is inactivated at the pH of the rectum (which ranges from neutral to basic). Epinephrine is absorbed from the mucous membranes and acts on both alpha- and beta-adrenergic receptors. The recommended concentration, in the final dosage form, is 0.005–0.01% applied up to four times a day.[9]

Phenylephrine Phenylephrine hydrochloride is believed to relieve itching caused by histamine release and reduces congestion in the anorectal area. It acts primarily on the alpha-adrenergic receptors and produces vasoconstriction by a direct effect on receptors rather than by norepinephrine displacement. The recommended dosage, in the final dosage form, is 0.25% applied up to four times a day.[9]

Protectants

Protectants prevent irritation of the anorectal area and water loss from the stratum corneum by forming a physical barrier on the skin. Protection of the perianal area from irritants such as fecal matter leads to a reduction in irritation, itching, burning, and discomfort. Little or no absorption of protectants occurs.

Absorbents, adsorbents, demulcents, and emollients are included in the protectant classification. Many substances classified as protectants are also used as vehicles, bases, and carriers of pharmacologically active substances (eg, vasoconstrictors and local anesthetics).

The protectants recommended for use are aluminum hydroxide gel (in moist conditions only), cocoa butter, glycerin in aqueous solution, hard fat (cocoa butter substitutes, hydrogenated cocoglycerides, and hydrogenated palm kernel glycerides), kaolin, lanolin, mineral oil, white petrolatum, petrolatum, and topical starch. All these protectants are recommended for external and internal (intrarectal) use with the exception of glycerin, which is recommended for external use only. Protectants recommended only when used in combination with one, two, or three other protectants and subject to limitations are calamine, zinc oxide, cod liver oil, and shark liver oil.[9] Calamine (based on the zinc oxide content of calamine) and zinc oxide must not exceed 25% (weight to weight) per dosage unit. For either cod liver oil or shark liver oil to be considered effective as a protectant, the product must contain an amount of the oil such that a daily dose provides 10,000 USP units of vitamin A and 400 USP units of cholecalciferol.[9] Protectants may be applied up to six times a day or after each bowel movement.

If a protectant is used in a nonprescription preparation, it should make up at least 50% of the dosage unit; if two to four protectants are used, their total concentration should represent at least 50% of the whole. Adequate thickness to prevent water loss from the epidermis determines the amount of protectant required. With the exception of cod liver oil and shark liver oil, any protectant ingredient used in combination should contribute at least 12.5% by weight. Glycerin is approved in a 20–45% (weight-to-weight) aqueous solution so that the final product contains not less than 10% and not more than 45% glycerin (weight to weight). Any combination product containing glycerin must contain at least this minimum amount of glycerin.[9] Hard fat is defined according to the official *National Formulary* monograph and, according to the FDA's designation of "hard fat" in the over-the-counter anorectal drug product monograph, includes Witepsol ingredients (cocoa butter substitutes, hydrogenated cocoglycerides, and hydrogenated palm kernel glycerides).[9,11]

Adverse reactions to protectants as a class are minimal. Wool (lanolin) alcohols may cause allergies and are probably responsible for most cases of lanolin allergy.[10]

Bismuth salts are not approved as protectants.[12] Bismuth subnitrate is not considered safe because it may be absorbed, producing toxic symptoms from the bismuth ion as well as from the nitrate ion. The effectiveness of bismuth oxide, bismuth subcarbonate, wool alcohols, and bismuth subgallate as protectants in the anorectal area has not been established.

Astringents

Applied to the skin or mucous membranes for a local and limited effect, astringents coagulate the protein in skin cells, thereby protecting the underlying tissue and decreasing cell volume. When appropriately used, astringents contribute to drying by lessening mucous and other secretions. This drying effect helps relieve local anorectal irritation, discomfort, itching, and burning.

Calamine and zinc oxide in concentrations of 5–25% are recommended as astringents for both external and internal use when applied up to six times a day or after each bowel movement.[9] Zinc, a heavy metal, acts as a protein precipitant and provides an astringent effect. Witch hazel (hamamelis water) in a concentration of 10–50% is recommended as an astringent for external use in anorectal disorders; its effectiveness is owing primarily to its alcohol content (14%). The FDA concluded that witch hazel provides temporary relief of itching, discomfort, irritation, and burning,[9] and is safe and effective for external use when applied up to six times a day or after each bowel movement. Witch hazel is incorporated in several commercially available rectal pads or wipes that are advertised as being useful for hemorrhoids. Recommended products should be limited to those containing the appropriate concentration of an astringent ingredient.

Wound-Healing Agents

Several ingredients in nonprescription hemorrhoidal products are claimed to be effective in promoting wound healing or tissue repair in anorectal disease. In this regard, skin respiratory factor, a water-soluble extract of brewer's yeast, also referred to as live yeast cell derivative (LYCD), has been the subject of considerable controversy. Because products containing LYCD do not meet acceptable standards of safety and efficacy,[12] reformulation of products such as Preparation H and Wyanoids was required in September 1994. Peruvian balsam, vitamin A, and vitamin D lack demonstrated effectiveness as wound healers.[8] Cod liver oil and shark liver oil have not demonstrated any value as hemorrhoidal wound healers[12]; however, they possess conditional value as protectants in hemorrhoidal products.[8] Currently, there is no approved wound-healing agent.

Antiseptics

Antiseptics generally inhibit the growth of microorganisms. Some nonprescription anorectal products contain compounds intended for use as antiseptics. However, because of the large numbers of microorganisms in feces, it is unlikely that applying antiseptics to the anorectal area provides a degree of antisepsis greater than that achieved by washing the area with mild soap and water. There is no compelling evidence that antiseptic use prevents anorectal infection.

Compounds claimed to have antiseptic properties include boric acid, boric acid glycerite (boroglycerin), hydrastis, phenol, benzalkonium chloride, cetylpyridinium chloride, benzethonium chloride, resorcinol, and sodium salicylic acid phenolate. Serious questions remain about the safety and effectiveness of these compounds as antiseptics in products designed to relieve the symptoms of hemorrhoids; therefore, they are currently not approved for use as antiseptics in anorectal products.

Keratolytics

Keratolytics cause desquamation and debridement or sloughing of epidermal surface cells. By fostering cell turnover and loosening surface cells, keratolytics may help to expose underlying tissue to therapeutic agents. Used externally, they are somewhat useful in reducing itching and discomfort although their exact mechanism of action is not known. Because mucous membranes contain no keratin layer, the intrarectal use of keratolytics is not justified and may cause harm.

The two keratolytics recommended for external use in hemorrhoidal products are aluminum chlorhydroxy allantoinate (alcloxa) and resorcinol.[9] The dosage ranges established by the FDA are up to six 2-g applications per day of a 0.2–2% ointment for alcloxa and of a 1–3% ointment for resorcinol. Precipitated and sublimed sulfur do not meet safety or efficacy standards for either internal or external use in anorectal preparations.[8]

Anticholinergics

Anticholinergics inhibit or prevent the action of acetylcholine, the transmitter of cholinergic nerve impulses. Because anticholinergics act systemically, they are not effective in ameliorating the local symptoms of anorectal disease.

Products containing atropine and belladonna extract are not considered safe and effective for use in the anorectal area.

Analgesics, Anesthetics, and Antipruritics

To promote consistency in the rulemaking process, the FDA has redesignated as "analgesic, anesthetic, and antipruritic" several ingredients that were formerly classified as "counterirritants."[8] This nomenclature was adopted to conform with the FDA pharmacologic designations of the active ingredients despite the inherent redundancy of the terms *anesthetic* and *antipruritic* as defined in this section.

In the anorectal area, a topically applied drug that relieves pain, discomfort, and burning by depressing cutaneous sensory receptors is defined as an analgesic, anesthetic drug. Similarly, a topically applied drug that relieves itching by depressing cutaneous sensory receptors is defined as an antipruritic drug.[8]

Menthol (0.1–1%), juniper tar (1–5%), and camphor (0.1–3%) are safe and effective for external use in the anorectal area and may be applied up to six times a day.[9] Camphor (greater than 3–11%), turpentine oil (rectified) (6–50%), and menthol (1.25–16%) are not considered safe and effective for anorectal use.[8]

Corticosteroids

Topically applied corticosteroid-containing products have the potential to reduce itching and pain by producing lysosomal membrane stabilization and antimitotic activity.[13] Nonprescription topical corticosteroid-containing products are indicated for temporary relief of minor external anal itching due to minor irritation or rash.[8] Currently, however, there are no approved nonprescription combinations of a corticosteroid with another active ingredient for anorectal use.

Bulk-Forming Laxatives

Because constipation is a precipitating factor in hemorrhoidal disease, patients may be advised to consider using bulk-forming or emollient laxatives. (See Chapter 12, "Laxative Products.") Ingredients commonly found in these products include barley malt extract, methylcellulose, docusate salts, and psyllium hydrocolloid. Patients must strictly follow directions for proper use to prevent adverse effects and increase efficacy. Adequate fluid intake should also be encouraged.

Miscellaneous Pharmacologic Agents

Collinsonia (stoneroot), *Escherichia coli* vaccines, lappa (burdock), leptandra (culver's root), and mullein are ingredients that have been included in nonprescription hemorrhoidal products and do not fall within the previously discussed pharmacologic classifications. Products containing these ingredients are not considered safe and effective and will have to be reformulated.[12]

A summary of the indications for nonprescription anorectal pharmacologic agents is presented in Table 1.

Biopharmaceutical Considerations

The bioavailability of drugs from anorectal dosage forms is determined by complex interactions involving physicochemical, physiologic, manufacturing, dosage form, dosage, and application variables. Since the FDA did not require final formulation testing in situ, the precise relationship between theoretical bioavailability considerations and the therapeutic effectiveness of anorectal dosage forms remains to be established. Absorption from anorectal dosage forms involves release from the vehicle, dissolution into the surrounding medium, diffusion to a membrane, and penetration of the membrane. The rate at which a drug diffuses from its base depends on a number of factors, including the vehicle pH, the drug concentration, the dissociation constant of the drug, the presence of surfactants, and the drug's particle size. Most drugs used in hemorrhoidal products are basic amines (local anesthetics and vasoconstrictors). The un-ionized base is soluble in lipid ointment bases; the salt form is not. Salt forms from weak bases are converted to the un-ionized base at tissue pH. The un-ionized form penetrates the lipid tissue barriers such as nerve membranes.

The solubility of the drug and its partitioning in a vehicle largely determine the drug's release rate from the vehicle. If a drug has a greater affinity for the vehicle than for the surrounding medium, a relatively slow release rate is expected. Conversely, if a drug has a greater affinity for the surrounding medium than for the vehicle, a relatively rapid release rate occurs. Ephedrine sulfate dissolved in an oleaginous base such as cocoa butter is released relatively rapidly into a surrounding aqueous medium.

In the case of oleaginous bases, the rate-limiting step in absorption seems to be the release of the drug from its vehicle and the dissolution of the drug in the surrounding fluid. For a water-soluble or water-miscible base (polyethylene glycol), a water-soluble drug form is preferred to facilitate absorption, given that the absorption rate appears to be controlled, at the pH of the anorectal region, by the transfer of the drug through the mucosa.

In ointments, creams, and suppositories, additives such as viscosity-increasing agents or surfactants are of-

TABLE 1 Indications for the use of nonprescription anorectal pharmacologic agents

Signs/ Symptoms	Analgesic/ Anesthetic/ Antipruritic	Vaso-constrictor	Pro-tectant	Astringent	Local Anesthetic	Kerato-lytic	Cortico-lytic
Discomfort	yes	yes	yes	yes	yes	yes	no
Irritation	no	yes	yes	yes	no	no	no
Itching	yes	yes	yes	yes	yes	yes	yes
Pain	yes	no	no	no	yes	no	no
Swelling	no	yes	no	no	no	no	no
Burning	yes	no	yes	yes	yes	no	no

ten required to achieve a high-quality product. Surfactants may increase or decrease drug absorption and should be appropriately tested for safe and effective drug delivery.

The drug absorption rate of an anorectal product may be affected by the manufacturing process. For example, the release rates associated with cocoa butter may vary according to the temperature at which the cocoa butter is melted. This effect may be explained by the polymorphic nature of cocoa butter.

Dosage Forms

Drugs for the treatment of anorectal symptoms are available in many dosage forms. For intrarectal use, suppositories, creams, ointments, gels, and foams are available; applicators, fingers, and pile pipes are used to facilitate their application. Creams, ointments, gels, pastes, wipes, pads, liquids, and foam are used externally.

Although there are considerable pharmaceutical differences among ointments, creams, pastes, and gels, the therapeutic differences are not significant. The term *ointment* is thus used here to refer to all semisolid preparations designed for external or intrarectal use in the anorectal area. Although a suppository is defined as a solid dosage form, it differs very little from semisolids in its vehicle formulation.

The primary function of an ointment base is the safe and efficient delivery of the active ingredients. Yet ointments also possess inherent protectant and emollient properties.

When used externally, ointments should be applied as a thin covering to the perianal area and the anal canal. For intrarectal use, ointments can be inserted with pile pipes or fingers. Pile pipes have the advantage over fingers in that the drug product may be introduced into the rectal mucosa, where the potential for systemic absorption is greatest and where a finger cannot reach. For most efficient use, the pile pipe should have lateral openings, as well as a hole in the end, to allow the drug product to cover the greatest area of rectal mucosa. The pile pipe should be lubricated before insertion by spreading the ointment around the pipe tip.

The lubricating effect of a suppository may ease straining at defecation. However, because of disadvantages, suppositories are not generally recommended as a dosage form in treating anorectal disease symptoms. In prone patients, suppositories may leave the affected region and ascend into the rectum and lower colon. If the patient remains prone after inserting a suppository or an ointment, the active ingredients may not be evenly distributed over the rectal mucosa. Suppositories and ointments are relatively slow acting because they must melt to release the active ingredient.

Foam products present no proven advantage over ointments; theoretically, however, they provide more rapid release of active ingredients. Their disadvantages include the difficulty in establishing that the foam remains in the affected area and the fact that the size of the foam bubbles determines the concentration of active ingredient available.

Since the FDA did not require in situ testing of anorectal products in their final dosage form, the therapeutic differences among the various dosage forms, if any, are not known. Products containing approved ingredients in appropriate doses are probably therapeutically similar when used to treat indicated signs and symptoms. Whatever differences may exist are most likely owing to patient preference for a specific dosage form.

Product Selection Guidelines

Patient Considerations

Knowledge of a patient's present medical condition, medical history, medication profile, and socioeconomic factors is necessary to determine how an individual may respond to self-treatment. First, the pharmacist must determine whether the patient has signs and symptoms amenable to self-treatment. Then the pharmacist should decide on a suitable anorectal product, if any, taking into account what other diseases the patient may have, what medications the patient may be taking, whether the patient is able to insert the medication, and any other factors, such as diet or cost of the product, that may affect treatment.

Pregnant and nursing women should use only products recommended for external use except for the recommended protectants, which may be used internally. Children with hemorrhoids or other anorectal disease should be referred to a health care provider.

Product Considerations

Nonprescription anorectal preparations are intended to provide temporary symptomatic relief of the burning, itching, pain, swelling, irritation, and discomfort of anorectal disorders. A wider range of products is available by prescription for use in treating other anorectal diseases.

In recommending an appropriate nonprescription product, the pharmacist should consider the type and amount of ingredients and the dosage form. A product that contains recommended ingredients in an appropriate combination at safe and effective dosage levels should be offered. For intrarectal use, the only approved ingredients are vasoconstrictors, protectants, and astringents. A pile pipe of an appropriate length (5 cm [2 in.]), with a well-lubricated and flexible tip and with holes on the sides, may be used to apply an ointment-type product. Suppositories are not generally recommended for use as a dosage form for the self-treatment of hemorrhoids.

As a general rule, products containing the least number of recommended ingredients should be suggested. Those with one or a few specific ingredients are most likely to minimize undesirable interactions and maximize effectiveness. In general, scented and tinted products should be avoided. Symptoms should be managed as specifically as possible. Shotgun therapy is generally best avoided.

In evaluating nonprescription anorectal products, the pharmacist should attempt to ensure that the vehicle is appropriate for anorectal use and that the active ingredient(s) will be properly released from the formulation. The FDA has not demanded final formulation testing to assess the appropriateness of specific vehicles for anorectal preparations.

Patient Counseling

The pharmacist should emphasize the importance of good health care, sufficient fiber and liquids in the diet, and proper hygiene of the anorectal area in helping to prevent and alleviate symptoms of anorectal disease. Specific advice should include the following guidelines:

- For maximum effect, nonprescription anorectal products should be used after, rather than before, bowel movements.
- If seepage, bleeding, black tarry stools, protrusion, or severe pain occurs, a health care provider should be contacted as soon as possible.
- Products designed only for external anorectal use should not be inserted into the rectum.
- Products to be used externally in the anorectal area should be applied sparingly.
- Patients should be warned that certain people may develop allergic or hypersensitivity reactions to anorectal products that contain recommended concentrations of approved ingredients. Should redness, irritation, swelling, pain, or other signs and symptoms develop or worsen, use of the product should be discontinued and a health care provider consulted.
- Patients should be advised on how to insert a pile pipe or a suppository and how to apply a foam dosage form. If insertion of a product into the rectum causes pain, use of the product should be discontinued and a health care provider consulted promptly.
- Patients with cardiovascular disease, diabetes, hypertension, or hyperthyroidism, or patients experiencing difficulty urinating, should not generally use a topical anorectal product containing a vasoconstrictor.
- Patients taking prescription drugs to treat hypertension or depression should not use an anorectal product containing a vasoconstrictor without consulting a health care provider.
- Patients should be warned that products containing ephedrine sulfate may cause nervousness, tremor, sleeplessness, nausea, and loss of appetite.
- Patients using an anorectal product containing aluminum hydroxide gel or kaolin should be informed that, for these products to come in contact with the skin, any previously used petrolatum containing or greasy ointment should be removed.
- Patients should be advised that only products containing approved ingredients should be used.
- If possible, before any nonprescription anorectal product is applied, the anorectal area should be washed with mild soap and warm water, rinsed thoroughly, and gently dried by patting or blotting with toilet tissue or a soft cloth.
- If bleeding occurs, or if symptoms worsen or do not improve after 7 days of self-treatment, a health care provider should be consulted promptly.

Cleansing the anorectal area with moistened, unscented, and uncolored toilet tissue or a wipe after defecation is recommended. Sitz baths are an alternative nondrug approach for managing mild symptoms of uncomplicated anorectal disease. The importance of maintaining normal bowel function by eating a well-balanced diet that includes roughage, drinking adequate amounts of fluid, and avoiding excessive laxative use should be emphasized as a means of preventing anorectal disease. A diet high in fiber and fluid will promote the formation of easily passed stools, thereby preventing constipation and the accompanying straining. Patients with symptomatic hemorrhoids may experience a significant reduction in bleeding and pain within a few weeks after beginning the regular use of a bulk laxative. Stool softeners such as docusate may also be useful in preventing the straining that may lead to or aggravate hemorrhoids. (See Chapter 12, "Laxative Products.") Also, if possible, prescription and nonprescription drugs that may cause constipation should be avoided.

Case Studies

Case 14–1

Patient Complaint/History

AB, a 55-year-old male, presents to the pharmacist with complaints of irritation and itching of the rectal area. Indicating the A-Caine ointment in his hand, the patient asks if the product is "any good." When questioned about his symptoms, AB responds that he has not noticed any bleeding, swelling, or soreness of the rectal area.

The patient profile shows that AB takes Dyazide one capsule every other day for mild hypertension and Synthroid 0.2 mg once daily; his thyroid gland was removed more than 30 years ago because of cancer. Other medications include Metamucil 1 tbsp in 8 oz water bid for fiber and Dulcolax one tablet prn for constipation. AB, whose job requires that he stand most of the day and lift heavy boxes, took two Dulcolax tablets last week for constipation.

Clinical Considerations/Strategies

The following considerations/strategies are provided to aid the reader in (1) determining whether treatment of the patient's condition with nonprescription medications is warranted, (2) selecting the appropriate nonprescription medication, and (3) developing a patient counseling strategy to ensure optimal therapeutic outcomes:

- Assess the possible cause(s) of the symptoms.
- Determine the appropriateness of treatment with the A-Caine ointment.
- Recommend an appropriate nonprescription medication treatment regimen for the rectal irritation and itching.
- Develop a patient education/counseling strategy that will:
  - Ensure that the patient understands how to apply the recommended nonprescription mediation;
  - Ensure that the patient knows when to contact a health care provider.

Case 14–2

Patient Complaint/History

FD, a 23-year-old female who is 7 months pregnant, presents to the pharmacist with a complaint of rectal itching. When questioned about the presence of additional symptoms, the patient responds that she has not noticed any pain, burning, swelling, or soreness of the rectal area. She admits to occasional strain when she moves her bowels; her job as a secretary requires that she sit for long periods.

In response to queries about current medication use, FD reports that she takes Stuartnatal 1+1 one tablet daily, ferrous sulfate 325 mg one tablet daily, and docusate sodium one tablet daily.

Clinical Considerations/Strategies

The following considerations/strategies are provided to aid the reader in (1) determining whether treatment of the patient's condition with nonprescription medications is warranted, (2) selecting the appropriate nonprescription medication, and (3) developing a patient counseling strategy to ensure optimal therapeutic outcomes:

- Assess the possible cause(s) of the rectal itching.
- Recommend an appropriate nonprescription medication treatment regimen.
- Recommend an appropriate nonpharmacologic treatment plan.
- Assess the possible adverse effects associated with the recommended nonprescription treatment regimen.
- Develop a patient education/counseling strategy that will:
  - Ensure that the patient understands how to apply the recommended nonprescription medication;
  - Ensure that the patient knows when to contact a health care provider.

Summary

For external use, an ideal hemorrhoidal formulation would contain a vasoconstrictor, a local anesthetic, and one to four recommended protectants totaling at least 50% of the formulation. Another appropriate formulation might contain a vasoconstrictor; a protectant; and an analgesic, a local anesthetic, or an antipruritic. Either of these combinations should be effective in relieving the itching, irritation, burning, swelling, discomfort, and pain associated with hemorrhoids.

For internal use, a model product would contain an appropriate astringent (eg, calamine or zinc oxide), a vasoconstrictor (eg, ephedrine sulfate or phenylephrine hydrochloride), and one to four recommended protectants totaling at least 50% of the formulation. An ointment-type dosage form applied with a suitable pile pipe is recommended. This product should relieve the itching, swelling, discomfort, soreness, and irritation associated with hemorrhoids.

When used externally, products containing benzocaine (5–20%) in a polyethylene glycol base would be expected to be effective in relieving itching, burning, discomfort, soreness, and pain associated with hemorrhoids. For intrarectal use, a product consisting of 100% petrolatum is appropriate to recommend and is safe for pregnant women to use.

The pharmacist should make clear to the patient that if symptoms worsen or do not improve after 7 days of self-treatment, or if bleeding, protrusion, or seepage occurs, a physician should be consulted as soon as possible.

References

1. Cocchiara JL. *Post Grad Med.* 1991; 89 (1): 149, 150.
2. Loder PB et al. *Br J Surg.* 1994; 81: 946–954.
3. Johanson JF, Sonnenberg A. *Dis Colon Rectum.* 1991; 34: 585–591.
4. Thompson WHF. *Br J Surg.* 1975; 62: 542–52.
5. Schrock TR. In: Sleisenger R, ed. *Gastrointestinal Diseases.* Philadelphia: WB Saunders and Fortron; 1993: 1500, 1502.
6. Smith LE. *Gastroenterol Clin North Am.* 1987; 16: 83.
7. Dennison AR et al. *Surg Clin North Am.* 1988; 68(6): 1402.
8. *Federal Register.* 1988; 53: 30759, 30777, 30779, 32592.
9. *Federal Register.* 1990; 55: 31778, 31780.
10. *Federal Register.* 1980; 45: 35621, 35635.
11. *The United States Pharmacopoeia XXII and the National Formulary XVII.* Rockville, Md: United States Pharmacopeial Convention; 1989: 1931.
12. *Federal Register.* 1993; 58: 46748.
13. *AMA Drug Evaluations Annual 1995.* Chicago: American Medical Association; 1995: 1228.

CHAPTER 15

Anthelmintic Products

Kathryn K. Bucci

Questions to ask in patient assessment and counseling

- *Who is the patient? (Who is this for?)*
- *Why do you think you or your child might have worms?*
- *Have you seen any worms in stools?*
- *Describe your symptoms. Have you had any nausea, diarrhea, abdominal pain, rectal itching, or weight loss? Do you become fatigued easily?*
- *How long have the symptoms been present?*
- *Are other members of your family or close contacts also affected?*
- *Have you seen a physician for this problem?*
- *Has the problem occurred in the past? How was it treated? Did the treatment work?*
- *If the patient is not an adult, what is the age and approximate weight of the patient?*
- *If the patient is female, is she pregnant or breast-feeding?*
- *Have you traveled out of the country? If so, where and when?*

Anthelmintics are used to treat worm (helminthic) infections. The incidence of helminthic infections may exceed 90% in areas where sanitation is insufficient, water is not clean, waste disposal is inefficient, rodents and insects are poorly controlled, economic conditions are poor, or preventive medicine practices are inadequate.[1] Worm infections are primarily parasitic, and the use of immunosuppressive drugs and the spread of acquired immunodeficiency syndrome (AIDS) are resulting in infections by previously unfamiliar parasites in various settings. Additionally, increases in world travel and immigration have escalated the spread of helminthic infections. Such infections may produce serious health problems, particularly in tropical regions, as they reduce resistance to disease, impair physical development in children, decrease occupational productivity, and thus result in the general debilitation of large populations.

Helminthic infections in the United States can be serious, but their impact is not generally widespread; therefore, they do not pose a major societal threat. Endemic nematode (roundworm) infections include enterobiasis (caused by pinworms), ascariasis, anisakiasis, trichinosis, and infections caused by whipworms and hookworms. Other worms that parasitize humans are cestodes (tapeworms) and trematodes (flukes). In contrast, *Giardia intestinalis* (formerly *G lamblia*), a protozoan, represents the most important cause of parasitic diarrheas in the United States.[2] (See Chapter 13, "Antidiarrheal Products.") Table 1 lists selected human helminthic infections and agents, their sources, and their most common signs and symptoms.

Intestinal parasitic infection should always be carefully regarded; however, symptoms of such infection during pregnancy require special attention. Parasitic infections during pregnancy may (1) impair fertility, (2) injure the mother's health, (3) injure the fetus, (4) induce premature labor and/or delivery, and (5) infect the neonate. Care requires risk and benefit considerations for the mother and the fetus.

Patient Assessment

The use of nonprescription medications in the treatment of helminthic infections is limited, given that the one nonprescription anthelmintic currently on the market (pyrantel pamoate) is indicated only for pinworms. Despite this limitation, the pharmacist is often the first person called upon when a patient suspects a helminthic infection. The pharmacist should be aware of the signs, symptoms, and preferred treatment of common helminthic infections in order to counsel patients appropriately and refer them to a physician if necessary. In either case, the health care provider must be both factual and sensitive since most people find the thought of a worm infection very disturbing.

The first indication of a helminthic infection may be a worm passed with a stool; often, however, such worms are not detected. Vegetable material, mucus strands, or other artifacts may look like worms. Patients should be advised to place a suspected worm in a container with tap water and take it to a health care provider or laboratory for identification.

If children are showing any of the common signs of pinworm infection, parents should be advised to observe the skin of the child's perianal region at night for adult worms. If pinworms are observed in one child, the whole family should be treated and appropriate hygiene methods initiated.

Editor's Note: This chapter is based, in part, on the chapter with the same title that appeared in the 9th edition but was written by John M. Kinsella.

TABLE 1 Common human helminthic infections in the United States

Class/Genus and species	Common name	Source of infection	Signs and Symptoms
Nematoda			
Ancylostoma duodenale, Necator americanus	Hookworm	Contact with contaminated soil; larvae are ingested or penetrate the skin on contact	Anemia caused by blood loss (0.15 mL per worm per day); indigestion, anorexia, headache, cough, vomiting, diarrhea, weakness, urticaria at the site of entry into the skin
Ascaris lumbricoides, Ascaris suum	Roundworm	Ingestion of eggs through contact with fecally contaminated soil	Mild cases may be asymptomatic; GI discomfort, pain, diarrhea; intestinal obstruction in severe cases; occasionally, bile or pancreatic duct may be obstructed; allergic reactions
Enterobius vermicularis	Pinworm, seatworm, threadworm, oxyurid	Ingestion of eggs by fecal contamination of hands, food, clothing, and bedding; reinfection is common; the most common worm infestation in the United States, especially in schoolchildren	Indigestion; intense perianal itching, especially at night, resulting in loss of sleep, irritability and fatigue in children; scratching may cause infection
Trichuris trichiura	Whipworm	Ingestion of eggs through contact with fecally contaminated soil	Mild cases may be asymptomatic; insomnia, loss of appetite, diarrhea, anemia; in severe cases, colitis, proctitis, prolapsed rectum
Anisakis and *Pseudoterranova*	None	Eating raw or poorly cooked fish	Tingling throat, abdominal pain, fever, nausea, vomiting, diarrhea
Cestoidea			
Taenia saginata	Beef tapeworm	Eating poorly cooked infected beef	No characteristic symptoms; digestive upset, diarrhea, anemia, dizziness vary with the degree of infestation
Taenia solium	Pork tapeworm	Eating poorly cooked infected pork	Similar to beef tapeworm infestation; self-infection with eggs may lead to cysts in eye, brain, heart, other organs
Diphyllobothrium latum	Fish tapeworm	Eating raw or inadequately cooked fish	Similar to beef tapeworm infestation
Hymenolepis nana	Dwarf tapeworm	Eating food contaminated with human feces	Similar to beef tapeworm infestation

Enterobiasis

Enterobiasis, or oxyuriasis, is commonly called pinworm, seatworm, or threadworm infection. The intestinal infection in humans is caused by *Enterobius vermicularis*.

Unlike many helminthic infections, enterobiasis is not limited to rural and poverty-stricken areas but also occurs in urban communities and infects individuals from all socioeconomic strata. *E vermicularis* is most common in temperate climates but is widely distributed and is especially prevalent among schoolchildren. Pinworm infection is the most common helminthic infection in the United States.

The female adult pinworm measures 8–13 mm in length; the adult male is about 2–5 mm in length. Adult worms inhabit the first portion of the large intestine and seldom cause damage to the intestinal wall. The mature female usually stores eggs in her body until several thousand accumulate. She then migrates down the colon and out the anus, deposits 10,000 to 11,000 sticky eggs in the perianal region, and dies. Within a few hours, infective larvae develop within the eggs. If the eggs are then transferred to the mouth, most commonly on the fingers of a child who scratches the anal area, the cycle begins again. Within 15–43 days of egg ingestion, the larvae are released, they mature, and newly developed gravid females migrate to the anal area and again discharge eggs, continuing the cycle.

The most common ways of transmitting pinworm infection in children are probably direct anus-to-mouth transfer of eggs by contaminated fingers and ingestion of food that has been handled by soiled hands. Reinfection may occur readily because eggs are often found under the fingernails of infected children who have scratched the anal area. Eggs dislodged from the perianal region into the environment may survive for as long as 3 weeks, and they can be inhaled and swallowed if they become airborne. Eggs may also be spread by house dust; on the coats of family pets; or through contaminated objects such as bedding, cups, toothpaste, and doorknobs.[3]

Signs and Symptoms

Patients with minor infections of enterobiasis may be asymptomatic. The most important and most frequent symptom is usually an irritating itching in the perianal and perineal regions. This itching typically occurs at night when the gravid female deposits her eggs. Scratching to relieve the itching may lead to a secondary bacterial infection of the area. Nervousness, inability to concentrate, and lack of appetite are often observed in children infected with pinworms. Worms also occasionally enter the female genital tract and become encapsulated within the uterus or fallopian tubules, or they may migrate into the peritoneal cavity, resulting in the formation of granulomas.

The physical signs and symptoms are not the only misery-inducing effects of pinworms. Parents are often dismayed to find worms near the anus of a child, and this psychologic trauma or "pinworm neurosis" must also be considered one of the harmful effects of enterobiasis.[4] Patients need to be assured that pinworms are common and that no social stigma is attached to their occurrence.

Perianal itching is a symptom of many conditions and is often mistakenly attributed to pinworm infection.[5] Seborrheic dermatitis, atopic eczema, tinea cruris, psoriasis, lichen planus, and neurodermatitis may produce severe itching when the perianal region is involved. An allergic or contact dermatitis may result from soaps or ointments used by the patient in an attempt to alleviate the initial mild symptoms of pinworm infestation. Ointments containing local anesthetics are well-known sensitizers and should be suspected of contributing to the problem. Other parasitic infestations that induce itching, such as scabies and pediculosis pubis, may involve the perianal skin in addition to larger areas of the body. Candidiasis may be the cause of pruritus ani, especially in patients with diabetes mellitus or a suppressed immune system. Other causes of pruritus include excessive vaginal discharge and urinary incontinence in women and excessive sweating during hot weather. When mineral oil is used as a laxative, it tends to leak and produce increased moisture and perianal itching.

Treatment

Treatment of pinworm infection should begin with an accurate assessment. The presence of pinworms can be determined by either of two methods. One method is to cover the end of a cotton swab or tongue depressor with tape (sticky side out) and apply this end to the perianal area. The presence or absence of eggs is confirmed by examining the tape under the microscope. Collection of eggs can be done at home, but inspection and evaluation must be done in a laboratory or health care provider's office. Another method used frequently by parents is visual inspection of the anal area with a flashlight an hour or so after the child has gone to bed. Female pinworms can be seen emerging from the anus to deposit their eggs.

In the past, gentian violet was the only nonprescription medication available for treatment of pinworm infections. However, genetic toxicity data indicate that gentian violet interacts with DNA in cultured cells, suggesting a potential carcinogenic effect. Even though the evidence for this is not conclusive, the Food and Drug Administration (FDA) has declared gentian violet a "nonmonograph ingredient." The dye is no longer marketed as an anthelmintic and should not be used.[6]

Pyrantel pamoate (eg, Antiminth Oral Suspension) was first used in veterinary practice as a broad-spectrum drug for pinworms, roundworms, and hookworms. Because of its effectiveness and lack of toxicity, it became an important drug for treating certain helminthic infections in humans (see product table "Anthelmintic Products").[7] Pyrantel pamoate is a depolarizing neuromuscular agent that paralyzes and kills the worms.

The FDA accepted the recommendation to move pyrantel pamoate from prescription-only to nonprescription status when used for the treatment of pinworms.[8] Although this product is readily available, helminthic infections other than those caused by pinworms should be diagnosed and treated by a physician.

Guidelines for the proper use of pyrantel pamoate are as follows:

- Side effects are uncommon. If, however, a patient experiences persistent abdominal cramps, nausea, vomiting, anorexia, diarrhea, headache, drowsiness, or dizziness after taking this medication, a physician should be consulted.
- Patients who are pregnant or nursing or who have liver disease should not take this product unless directed by a physician.

- For adults and children, a single dose of 5 mg/lb or 11 mg/kg is recommended, not to exceed 1 g. A dosage schedule by weight is included with the product.
- The drug may be taken at any time of the day, with or without meals.
- When one individual in a household has pinworms, the entire household should be treated at the same time. Infants under 2 years of age or children who weigh less than 25 lb should not be treated without first consulting a physician.
- The liquid formulation, which contains 50 mg/mL, should be shaken well before the dose is measured. The measuring device provided with the package should be used.
- The recommended dosage should not be exceeded.
- A repeat course of therapy may be undertaken under the direction of a physician.
- If any worms other than pinworms are present before or after treatment, a physician should be consulted.

The following nondrug measures are recommended to prevent reinfections:

- The bed linens, bedclothes, towels, and underwear of the infected individual and the entire family should be washed. Such items should not be shaken because this can spread eggs into the air.[3] A daily morning shower is encouraged to remove eggs deposited in the perianal region during the night.
- Disinfectants should be used daily on toilet seats and bathtubs.
- The area around beds, curtains, and elsewhere in the bedroom where the concentration of eggs is likely to be the greatest should be vacuumed frequently.
- Close-fitting shorts under one-piece pajamas should be worn at night to prevent migration of worms and harm from scratching.
- After an infected child goes to the bathroom, the child's fingers should be scrubbed with soap and a brush. The child's nails should be trimmed regularly to prevent the harboring of eggs and hand-to-mouth reinfection (autoinoculation).
- Hands should be washed frequently, especially before meals and after using the toilet.

Ascariasis

Ascariasis is caused by *Ascaris lumbricoides*, also referred to as giant roundworm. This species is distributed worldwide and infects more than a billion people; however, it is most prevalent in warm, moist areas such as the tropics, Southeast Asia, Central and South America, and some parts of the southeast United States.[9] The adult ascarids are 15–35 cm long and live in the small intestine. The female eggs are passed in the feces and develop into infective larvae in the soil. Although mature larvae in the shell remain viable in the soil for many months, the eggs do not hatch until they are ingested by humans. Initial infection commonly occurs in children who play outside and ingest mature eggs in contaminated soil.[9] On ingestion, the larvae are released in the small intestine. They penetrate the intestinal wall, migrate via the bloodstream to the lungs, travel up the respiratory tree to the epiglottis where they are swallowed, and develop into adults in the small intestine. Entire households can be infected with the parasite.[9]

Although *A lumbricoides* has been primarily a problem of the southeastern United States, recent information indicates that swine ascaris, *Ascaris suum*, which usually occurs in northern states such as New Hampshire, Washington, and Montana, is also infective to humans.[10] *A suum* is more common in children and usually does not develop to the egg-laying stage. Instead, the immature worm, which is about 15 cm long, is rejected and passed out with the stool. Because of the possible presence of *A suum*, the use of pig manure in home gardens should be discouraged. Pharmacists should consider that this type of infection is present if a patient mentions that a large worm has been passed.

Signs and Symptoms

The larvae and adults of ascarids are capable of extensive migration and therefore induce diverse symptoms involving the respiratory and gastrointestinal (GI) tracts. Although many infected patients are asymptomatic, the most common symptoms caused by ascarid infections are vague abdominal discomfort and abdominal colic.[11] Occasionally nausea, vomiting, bloating, diarrhea, or weight loss is present. Children characteristically have fever and may lose weight or fail to grow. These signs and symptoms may mislead clinicians into suspecting that the patient has an abdominal tumor, peptic ulcer disease, or some other serious medical condition. Migration of the worms may cause an intestinal obstruction that may lead to intestinal perforation, suppurative cholangitis, cholecystitis, liver abscess, pancreatitis, appendicitis, or peritonitis.

Patients with minor infestations may be asymptomatic, whereas severe infestations can cause symptoms that may be mistaken for a variety of respiratory and GI diseases. Migration of the larvae through the lungs may cause a cough; in fact, the larvae may be coughed up and seen in the sputum. Fever and pulmonary infiltrate may also accompany this pulmonary syndrome.

Allergic reactions such as asthma, hay fever, urticaria, or conjunctivitis may also result from absorption of toxins from the worm.

Treatment

Nutritional supplementation is the first therapeutic step in treatment. The drug of choice for treating ascarid infections is mebendazole (100 mg taken twice a day for 3 days) or pyrantel pamoate (11 mg/kg in a single dose, not to exceed 1 g).[12] Cure rates typically exceed 99% with drugs. The treatment of swine ascariasis is unnecessary if the worm has already been passed, but the physician may prescribe a course of treatment for the patient's peace of mind in case more worms are present.

Hookworm Infection

Worldwide, 1 billion people are infected by hookworms.[13] In the United States, hookworm infection in humans is caused by *Necator americanus.* When hosts walk barefoot over contaminated soil, the infective larvae rapidly penetrate the intact skin.[14] From there the larvae enter the bloodstream and are carried to the lungs. They then enter the alveoli, ascend the trachea to the throat, are swallowed, and pass into the small intestine, where they develop into mature adults. The adult worms, which are about 10 mm long, attach themselves to the small intestine. Their eggs are excreted in the feces and then mature and hatch in warm, moist soil.

Signs and Symptoms

When the hookworm larvae penetrate exposed skin, an erythematous maculopapular rash and edema with severe itching may persist for several days. The lesions most commonly occur on the feet, particularly between the toes, and are called ground itch. Dog and cat hookworm larvae may also penetrate human skin and cause a similar condition, but they do not progress to the pulmonary or intestinal stages.

Severe infections may produce dyspnea, cough, congestive heart failure, or fever when the larvae migrate through the lungs. Mild intestinal infections may be asymptomatic; moderately severe infections may result in indigestion, dizziness, headache, anemia, weakness, fatigue, palpitations, nausea, or vomiting. In advanced cases, there is epigastric pain, abdominal tenderness, chronic fatigue, and alternating constipation and diarrhea. The epigastric pain is relieved by eating foods high in bulk or fiber.[11] These symptoms may be mistaken for those of other respiratory and GI disorders.

A major clinical manifestation of hookworm infection is iron deficiency anemia resulting from the loss of blood (as much as 0.15 mL per worm each day), which the adult worm extracts while it is attached to the intestinal mucosa.[1] Malnourished children and some menstruating women are especially prone to anemia, depending on the severity of the infection. Even people with adequate iron intake may become anemic if the hookworm infection is severe enough to cause a blood loss that cannot be compensated for by the body's normal erythropoietic mechanisms.

Treatment

The correction of hookworm-induced anemia (if present) with oral iron supplements is strongly encouraged. Mebendazole (100 mg taken twice a day for 3 days) or pyrantel pamoate (11 mg/kg, not to exceed 1 g, for 3 days) may be used to treat hookworm infections.[12]

Whipworm

Whipworms (*Trichuris trichiura*) are 30–50 mm in length. Shaped like whips, these worms have a threadlike anterior end and a thick posterior end. The anterior end is burrowed into the mucosa of the ileocecal area. Eggs excreted in the feces mature in warm, shady soil in about 21 days. When swallowed, the eggs hatch in the small intestine and the larvae enter the Lieberkühn's crypts. After molting, they reenter the lumen and migrate to the ileocecal area, maturing in about 3 months. Like roundworms, whipworms are acquired through ingestion of feces-contaminated food or water.[14]

Signs and Symptoms

Infections of fewer than 100 worms rarely cause clinical symptoms. Trauma to the intestinal epithelium and submucosa caused by these worms can, however, cause chronic blood in the stool, resulting in anemia. Secondary bacterial infection may result in colitis, proctitis, or, in extreme cases, prolapse of the rectum. Symptoms of whipworm infection include insomnia, loss of appetite, urticaria, flatulence, and prolonged diarrhea.[1]

Treatment

Mebendazole (100 mg taken twice daily for 3 days), is the preferred treatment for trichuriasis (whipworm infection) in adults and children.[12] No nonprescription drugs are available for treating this infection.

Anisakiasis

Because of the recent popularity of raw fish dishes such as sushi, previously rare anisakid infections have become a growing problem in the United States, especially on the West Coast and in Hawaii.[15] This parasite is acquired by ingesting raw, lightly salted or pickled, or inadequately cooked saltwater fish containing infected larvae.[10] Larval *Anisakis* nematodes, which are infective to marine mammals such as seals and sea lions, may cause moderate to severe intestinal problems when ingested by humans. Pacific red snapper and Pacific salmon have a particularly high prevalence of infection by these nematodes.[16]

Signs and Symptoms

Larvae of some anisakid species do not invade the intestinal mucosa but wander into the oropharynx or esophagus, causing a tingling sensation. These larvae, which are up to 3 mm long, are often coughed up within 48 hours of ingestion, causing the patient considerable anxiety and fear. Other species penetrate the wall of the stomach or intestine, resulting in symptoms that mimic diseases such as acute appendicitis, ulcer, or cancer. Because no eggs are produced, stool examination is of no use, so diagnosis of anisakiasis may depend on endoscopic examination or even laparotomy.[14]

Treatment

Anthelmintics are apparently ineffective in killing anisakid larvae. The only definitive treatment in severe cases is surgical resection of the inflamed intestine. Patients should be warned of the dangers of eating raw or poorly cooked fish, especially fish from areas where marine mammals are prevalent. Freezing fish at 1.4°F (−17°C) for 24 hours will kill any larvae present.

Cercarial Dermatitis

Cercarial dermatitis, or swimmers' itch, is caused by flukes of the genera *Trichobilharzia* and *Ornithobilharzia*, which are normally blood parasites of ducks and muskrats. Eggs of these worms, when released into water, infect various species of snails, which, in turn, release a free-swimming infective stage called a cercaria. These cercariae are capable of penetrating human skin, where they are rapidly killed by an immune reaction.

Signs and Symptoms

Inflammation resulting from the cercariae produces a local erythema, a minute macule at the site of penetration, and an intense itching. Because hundreds of cercariae may penetrate, the result is a generalized fiery rash. Cases usually occur in spring and summer in both freshwater and saltwater areas where migratory waterfowl and large snail populations are present.

Treatment

Treatment of swimmers' itch should be symptomatic because the condition generally subsides in 24–48 hours. Antihistamines and topical corticosteroids reduce the local immune response, and warm baths are helpful in combating the itching.

Public Health Recommendations

Preventive measures to minimize possible exposure to helminthic infections include (1) avoiding poorly cooked beef, pork, and fish (especially fish from areas where marine mammals are present); (2) eating sushi from a reputable establishment and avoiding sushi prepared at home; (3) avoiding walking barefoot in areas prone to hookworms; and (4) avoiding swimming in areas conducive to swimmers' itch. In this regard, pharmacists are in an ideal position to inform patients of behaviors that may increase their risk of helminthic infections.

Case Studies

Case 15–2

Patient Complaint/History

A mother presents to the pharmacist with her 5-year-old daughter CD and asks for assistance in selecting a hemorrhoid cream for the child. The mother explains that the child has intense perianal itching, especially at night. Physical observation reveals that the child has dark circles under her eyes and seems exceptionally fidgety.

Clinical Considerations/Strategies

The following considerations/strategies are provided to aid the reader in (1) determining whether treatment of the patient's condition with nonprescription medications is warranted, (2) selecting the appropriate nonprescription medication, and (3) developing a patient counseling strategy to ensure optimal therapeutic outcomes:

- Ask the mother if other family members or close personal contacts have similar symptoms.
- Ask the mother if she has seen worms in the child's stool. If not, ask her to consider visual inspection of the child's anal area after the child has gone to bed.
- Determine the child's weight.
- Suspecting pinworms as the cause of the symptoms, select an appropriate nonprescription product and its dose based on the child's weight and age.
- Counsel the mother about the proper administration and possible adverse effects of the recommended product.
- After reassuring the mother that pinworms are common, counsel her about treatment of family members and methods to prevent reinfection (eg, the child's personal hygiene, household measures).

Case 15–2

Patient Complaint/History

JS, a 30-year-old male, presents to the pharmacist and asks assistance in selecting a product for diarrhea. When questioned about his symptoms, the patient reveals that his bouts of diarrhea, which are often accompanied by nausea and abdominal pain, are fairly debilitating. He goes on to say that the diarrhea interferes with his work and his leading boy scout troops on outings.

Clinical Considerations/Strategies

The following considerations/strategies are provided to aid the reader in (1) determining whether treatment of the patient's condition with nonprescription medications is warranted, (2) selecting the appropriate nonprescription medication, and (3) developing a patient counseling strategy to ensure optimal therapeutic outcomes:

- Determine whether the patient has traveled recently and whether he drinks water from lakes or streams without taking adequate measures to decontaminate the water.
- Determine whether family members or close personal contacts have had similar symptoms.
- Determine whether the patient has lost weight or whether other symptoms are present.
- Refer this patient to a health care provider.

Summary

The pharmacist should be familiar with common helminthic infections, their symptoms, and their treatment. Enterobiasis (pinworm infection) is the only helminthic infection that should be treated with a nonprescription drug, although pyrantel pamoate is a secondary drug in treating ascariasis (roundworm infection). Self-medication should be discouraged for all helminthic infections other than enterobiasis. The clinical manifestations of these parasitic diseases may be characteristic of so many other illnesses that attempting self-diagnosis not only is difficult but may result in neglect of a more serious condition. The availability of effective, relatively safe, easy-to-take prescription drugs that can eradicate many helminthic infections should be reason enough to avoid self-medication. The pharmacist should encourage the patient to consult a physician for treatment when helminths other than pinworms are suspected.

References

1. Schmidt GD, Roberts LS. *Foundations of Parasitology*. 2nd ed. St. Louis: CV Mosby; 1981: 2, 448, 473.
2. Rosenblatt JE. Antiparasitic agents. *Mayo Clin Proc*. 1992; 67: 276–87.
3. Jones JE. Pinworms. *Am Fam Physician*. 1988; 38(3): 159–64.
4. Garcia LS, Bruckner DA. *Diagnostic Medical Parasitology*. New York: Elsevier Science Publishers; 1988: 153.
5. Schrock TL. Diseases of the anorectum. In: Sleisenger MH, Fordtran JS, eds. *Gastrointestinal Disease: Pathophysiology, Diagnosis, Management*. 5th ed. Philadelphia: WB Saunders; 1993: 1505–6.
6. *Federal Register*. 1980; 45: 59548.
7. Gilman AG et al, eds. *The Pharmacological Basis of Therapeutics*. 8th ed. New York: Pergamon Press; 1990: 969–70.
8. *Federal Register*. 1986; 51: 27756.
9. Summers L, Johnson CA. Ascariasis. *Am Fam Physician*. 1990; 42(4): 999–1002.
10. Lord WD, Bullock WL. Swine ascaris in humans. *N Engl J Med*. 1982; 306: 1113.
11. Owen RL. Parasitic diseases. In: Sleisenger MH, Fordtran JS, eds. *Gastrointestinal Diseases: Pathophysiology, Diagnosis, Management*. 5th ed. Philadelphia: WB Saunders; 1993: 1207–8.
12. Drugs for parasitic infections. *Med Lett Drugs Ther*. 1993; 35: 111–22.
13. Hoetz PJ, Pritchard DI. Hookworm infection. *Sci Am*. 1995; 68.
14. Embil JA, Embil JM. Gastrointestinal parasitic infections. *Can Fam Physician*. 1988; 34: 619–26.
15. Deardorff TL, Keyes SG, Fukumura T. Human anisakiasis transmitted by marine food products. *Hawaii Med J*. 1991; 50: 9–16.
16. McKerrow JH, Sakanari J, Deardorff TL. Anisakiasis: revenge of the sushi parasite. *N Engl J Med*. 1988; 319: 1228–9.

CHAPTER 16

Emetic and Antiemetic Products

Gary M. Oderda and Jenifer C. Jennings

Questions to ask in patient assessment and counseling

Emetics

- *Do you want the emetic for immediate or possible future emergency use?*
- *If for immediate use, have you spoken to a poison control center?*
- *For whom is the medication? How old is the patient?*
- *What substance was taken? How long ago did the ingestion occur? How much was taken?*
- *Has the patient already been given something for the ingestion?*
- *What symptoms is the patient showing? Is the patient conscious and alert?*
- *Does the patient have any chronic or acute illnesses that may affect the poisoning?*
- *Is the patient taking any nonprescription or prescription medications?*

Antiemetics

- *Do you know what caused the nausea and vomiting?*
- *For whom is the medication? How old is the patient?*
- *Is the patient pregnant?*
- *Is the patient diabetic?*
- *How long has the nausea or vomiting been present?*
- *Have you noted blood in the vomitus? Is the blood red or does it resemble coffee grounds?*
- *Have you noted other signs or symptoms such as abdominal pain, headache, or diarrhea?*
- *What medications is the patient currently taking?*
- *Is the patient receiving or has the patient recently received radiation therapy or cancer chemotherapy?*
- *Does the patient have other medical problems?*

Severe nausea and the realization that one is about to vomit are two of the more common unpleasant symptoms an individual may experience. Vomiting (emesis) can be caused by travel (ie, motion sickness) or pregnancy. However, vomiting is also an important defense mechanism by which the body attempts to rid itself of a variety of toxins and poisons.

Nonprescription emetic medications are used to induce vomiting, primarily in the treatment of a poisoning. Nonprescription antiemetics are used to prevent or control the symptoms of nausea and vomiting that are primarily due to motion sickness, pregnancy, and mild infectious diseases. Some nonprescription antiemetics are promoted for the relief of such vague symptoms as "upset stomach," indigestion, and distention associated with food overindulgence. However, their value in treating these complaints is not well documented.

Nausea and vomiting associated with radiation therapy; cancer chemotherapy; and serious metabolic, central nervous system (CNS), gastrointestinal (GI), and endocrine disorders are not covered in this chapter because they are not appropriate conditions for self-medication but instead require referral to a health care provider and appropriate management.

The Vomiting Process

Vomiting is a complex process involving both the CNS and the GI system. Nausea, an unpleasant sensation that is vaguely associated with the epigastrium and abdomen, usually precedes vomiting. Retching is a strong, involuntary effort to vomit.

The vomit reflex is mediated by a "vomiting center" located in the medulla of the brain. The vomiting center itself does not carry out the function of vomiting; rather, it coordinates the activities of other neural structures to produce a patterned response. The vomiting center receives stimuli from peripheral areas, such as the gastric mucosa, in addition to areas within the CNS itself. Stimulation of the chemoreceptor trigger zone (CTZ), which is the afferent pathway to the vomiting center, is responsible for its activation and may be involved in eliciting nausea and vomiting from a variety of causes. Centrally acting emetics (eg, codeine, morphine) work primarily by stimulating the CTZ whereas centrally active antiemetics (eg, phenothiazines) inhibit it. In addition to stimuli from the CTZ, the vomiting center also receives impulses from the GI tract and the labyrinth apparatus in the ear. Stimuli are then sent via a cranial nerve to the abdominal musculature, stomach, and esophagus to initiate vomiting.

Vomiting begins with a deep inspiration, the closing of the glottis, and the depression of the soft palate. A forceful contraction of the diaphragm and abdominal musculature occurs, producing an increase in intrathoracic and intra-abdominal pressure that compresses the stomach and raises esophageal pressure. The stomach and esophageal musculature relax, and the positive intrathoracic and intra-abdominal pressure moves stomach contents into the esophagus and mouth. Regurgitation is the casting up of stomach contents without oral expulsion. Several cycles of reflux into the esophagus occur before actual vomiting begins.[1] Vomitus is expelled from the esophagus by a combination of increased intrathoracic pressure and reverse peristaltic waves.[1] Normally, the glottis closes off the trachea and prevents the vomitus from entering the airway; however, aspiration of the vomitus can occur in patients with CNS depression or an absent or impaired gag reflex.

Overstimulation of the labyrinth (inner ear) apparatus produces the nausea and vomiting of motion sickness. The three semicircular canals in the labyrinth on each side of the head are responsible for maintaining equilibrium. Postural adjustments are made when the brain receives nervous impulses initiated by the movement of fluid in the canals. Motion sickness may be produced by unusual motion patterns in which the head is rotated on two axes simultaneously. Mechanisms other than stimulation of the semicircular canals are also important. Erroneous interpretation of visual stimuli by stationary subjects, such as occurs when one watches a film taken from a roller coaster or an airplane that is doing aerobatics or when one simply extends one's head upward while standing on a rotating platform, can produce motion sickness. Some individuals are more tolerant of the effect of a particular type of motion than are others, but no one is immune. Individuals can also vary in their susceptibility to various kinds of motions, such as flying and boat riding. But regardless of the type of stimulus-producing event, motion sickness is much easier to prevent than to treat once it has already begun.

One half of all pregnant women experience nausea, and about one third suffer from vomiting.[1] However, the mechanism of vomiting or "morning sickness" associated with pregnancy has not been established. Increased levels of chorionic gonadotropin have been implicated as a cause of morning sickness because levels of this hormone are highest during early pregnancy, when nausea and vomiting are most common.[2] Other research suggests that there is no relationship between chorionic gonadotropin levels and morning sickness.[3] Nausea and vomiting due to pregnancy are difficult symptoms to treat. In part, this is because no agent seems to be completely effective, but, more important, it is because the potential for teratogenic effects dictates that drug use during pregnancy be restricted whenever possible.[2]

Acute transient attacks of vomiting in association with diarrhea are very common. This symptom is often observed with viral gastroenteritis, a common acute infectious disease that is usually harmless and self-limiting and that may affect any age group.

Vomiting is a symptom produced not only by benign processes but also by serious illnesses. The practitioner should be aware that patients may use nonprescription antiemetics to self-treat the early stages of a serious illness. Knowledge of the patient's drug history is also important in assessing the cause of nausea and vomiting as these symptoms are common side effects of most oral medications and some parenteral and topical drugs. Nausea and vomiting may also be caused by cancer chemotherapy or may indicate such diverse disorders as those listed in Table 1. Frequent vomiting, particularly in young women, may indicate an eating disorder that may be associated with ipecac abuse and should be evaluated by a health care provider. Vomiting may produce complications that include dehydration, aspiration, malnutrition, electrolyte and acid-base abnormalities, and Mallory-Weiss syndrome tears of the esophagus resulting in blood in the vomitus.

Emetics

Emetics induce vomiting and are used to remove potentially toxic agents from the stomach. Emetics are used most commonly to treat poisoning.

Incidence of Poisoning

Unintentional poisonings occur most often in children under 5 years of age and are a leading cause of injury-related hospitalizations in preschoolers even though fatalities among preschoolers have declined significantly over the past 30 years. During 1993, 64 poison centers throughout the United States, serving a population of 181.3 million, submitted 1,751,476 cases to the American Association of Poison Control Centers' Toxic Exposure Surveillance System (TESS).[4] Fifty-six percent of these poison exposures (982,917) and 4.3% of the deaths (27/626) were in children less than 6 years of age.[4] However, mortality data alone do not adequately describe the problem because many poisonings result in significant morbidity and mortality that are not reported to poison centers.

Baseline Information for Poison Management

It is often difficult to decide whether a patient should be referred directly to an emergency treatment facility or given a nonprescription emetic and managed at home. Obtaining a reliable history, identifying the agent, and accurately assessing the patient's condition are critical steps to take in making this decision. Knowing the telephone number of the nearest poison control center is extremely important. A list of poison centers is printed in the appendix at the end of this chapter. All ingestions in which moderate to severe toxicity is possible must be referred to an emergency treatment facility. If minimal toxicity (no serious or life-threatening symptoms) is anticipated, the administration of a nonprescription emetic at home by a competent adult may be all that is necessary. Many ingestions reported to poison control centers fall into this category. For example, a child who ingests aspirin at 150–300 mg/kg of body weight can usually be treated at home by emesis induced with ipecac syrup and appropriate follow-up. If an emetic is indicated, the pharmacist should also determine whether there are any contraindications to its use and whether the emetic can be administered safely outside an emer-

TABLE 1 Primary causes of nausea and vomiting

System /Category and pathophysiology	System /Category and pathophysiology
Primary central nervous system disease	**Gastrointestinal disease**
Elevated intracranial pressure	Peptic ulcer
Neoplasm	Reflex esophagitis
Infection	Biliary tract disease
Epilepsy	Hepatic disease
Vascular diseases	Gastroenteritis
Arteriosclerosis	Appendicitis
Embolism	Functional disorders
Vasculitis	Aerophagia
Migraine	Pyloroduodenal spasm
Psychologic suggestion	Mechanical or paralytic obstruction
Metabolic and endocrine disease	**Genitourinary disease**
Diabetic ketoacidosis	Endometritis
Lactic acidosis	Parametritis
Starvation ketosis	Salpingitis
Hypothyroidism	Obstructive uropathy
Uremia	Pyelonephritis
Adrenal insufficiency	Renal calculi and stones
Chemical and drug-induced toxicity	**Labyrinthine disease**
Direct effect on chemoreceptor trigger zone	Infection
Opiates	Vascular disturbance
Digitalis glycosides	Meniere's disease
Cancer chemotherapy	Motion sickness
Radiation sickness	
Food poisoning	
Other drug toxicity or withdrawal	
Direct effect on stomach	
Drug-induced gastritis	
Irradiation enteritis	
Ethanol toxicity or withdrawal	

Adapted from Mellencamp E, Wang RIH. The patient with nausea, I: causes. *Drug Ther* (Hosp). 1977; 2: 62–9.

gency treatment facility. Thus, to assess whether a nonprescription emetic should be administered in the home or the patient should be referred to a health care facility, the pharmacist should obtain the following information.

Patient's Name and Location

If talking with the patient or caretaker by phone, the practitioner should first ask for the caregiver's and the patient's name, location, and telephone number in case the call is cut off. This also allows for follow-up by the pharmacist or poison control center staff.

Name of Product Ingested

The pharmacist can determine the identity and the amount of each ingredient from the name of the ingested product. The product label or container, if available, may list ingredients as well as the name of the manufacturer or distributor. The potential toxicity of each ingredient must be investigated.

Amount Ingested

The amount ingested is often difficult to determine. A child may be found with an empty bottle of medication, and the parent may be unable to determine how full the bottle was before ingestion. Parents often underestimate the amount consumed or provide unreliable information. For example, a parent may report that a child has taken only two digoxin tablets, basing that estimation on the fact that the child was alone for only a short period or that the tablets have an unpleasant taste.

Drugs can be both therapeutic agents and poisons, depending on the dose. Thus, a 2-year-old who takes two iron-containing multiple vitamin tablets would require no treatment; the same child who takes 15 adult ferrous sulfate tablets may be severely poisoned.

Time since Ingestion

The time since ingestion is important to know because an emetic is useful only if a substantial amount of the ingested substance remains in the stomach. Thus, an emetic is not recommended if several hours have elapsed after ingestion of quickly absorbed agents such as alcohols, yet its use may be appropriate several hours after ingestion of agents that are slow to leave the stomach, such as salicylates. Drugs that slow gastric emptying and GI motility include opiates, anticholinergics such as atropine and scopolamine, and drugs that have anticholinergic activity, such as antihistamines, antidepressants, and phenothiazines.

Signs and Symptoms

Certain signs and symptoms contraindicate the use of emetics. For example, if CNS depression, lethargy, somnolence, ataxia, hallucinations, or seizures are present, an emetic should not be used because it could have serious toxic effects such as convulsions or respiratory depression (see the section Contraindications to Emesis). Patients with these signs and symptoms must be referred to a health care provider or emergency room for immediate medical evaluation and treatment.

Other Illnesses or Medication Use

It is important to consider the impact of preexisting illnesses or therapeutic prescription or nonprescription medications on the toxicity expected or on recommendations for therapy. For example, patients with a preexisting seizure disorder, particularly if it is not well controlled, would not be good candidates for ipecac syrup use at home (see the section Contraindications to Emesis). Patients who chronically take theophylline would be at higher risk from an additional theophylline ingestion and would need to be referred to an emergency department after ingesting lower doses than would individuals who take the same single acute dose of theophylline.

Patient's Age and Weight

Information on the toxicity of an agent is generally provided on a dose-per-body weight (mg/kg) basis. Thus, knowledge of the patient's weight is often needed to determine appropriate treatment. The patient's age may also help to determine the appropriateness and dose of an emetic.

Prior Treatment

The practitioner must determine if any first aid or other procedure has been performed. Some procedures, such as the use of salt water as an emetic, may actually cause toxicity, resulting in such conditions as hypernatremia and convulsions. Sticking the finger down the patient's throat to stimulate gagging is also ineffective and potentially harmful (see the section Other Methods to Induce Emesis). Such effects would influence further treatment recommendations.

Treatment of Poisoning

Treatment of poisoning depends primarily on basic management principles, including prevention of absorption and provision of supportive care. Support of vital functions, especially respiratory and cardiovascular, is critical. Treatment of specific signs and symptoms such as seizures is also important, as are other specific actions, including emptying the stomach and administering agents such as adsorbents, cathartics, or antidotes. Stomach contents may be removed by mechanical lavage or administration of an emetic such as ipecac syrup. Both types of treatment are more effective if undertaken shortly after the ingestion of the poison. However, these treatments do not replace symptomatic and supportive care; many patients will detoxify themselves and survive with *only* such care.

Gastric Lavage

Gastric lavage is a procedure in which a tube is placed into the stomach through the mouth or nose and the esophagus. Fluid is then instilled into the tube, allowed to mix with stomach contents, and removed by suction or aspiration.

Ipecac Syrup

Of the 1,751,476 cases reported to TESS during 1993, 64,805 used ipecac syrup.[4] Ipecac syrup is the emetic of choice (see product table "Emetic Products"). It is prepared from ipecac powder, a natural product derived from the plant *Cephaelis ipecacuanha* or *C acuminata*, and contains approximately 2.1 g of powdered ipecac per 30 mL. Vomiting is probably produced by both a local irritant effect on the GI mucosa and a central medullary effect (stimulation of the CTZ). The central effect is probably caused by emetine and cephaeline, two alkaloids present in ipecac.

When a patient asks to purchase ipecac syrup, the pharmacist should determine whether it is to be used immediately to treat a poison ingestion or kept in the home as a first-aid measure. If the purchase is for immediate use, the pharmacist should determine whether that use is appropriate and whether the local poison center or other medical adviser has been contacted. If the answer is no in either case, the pharmacist should contact the poison center to alert it of the problem and receive instructions on how to manage the ingestion and instruct the purchaser.

If the ipecac is purchased for a possible future ingestion, the pharmacist should discuss poison prevention with the patient, distribute poison prevention materials, and provide the telephone number of the nearest poison control center (see Appendix, "Major Poison Control Centers"). Additionally, the purchaser should be advised that, whenever possible, ipecac syrup should not be given without first consulting a poison control center, pharmacist, or health care provider.

Dosages For children 1 year of age and older, the recommended dose of ipecac syrup is 15 mL (1 tbsp), and this dose can be repeated once if vomiting has not occurred within 20 minutes. Children from 6 months to 1 year of age may be given 5–10 mL (1–2 tsp). Although home use of ipecac in children under 1 year of age is controversial, the product has been shown to be safe and effective.[5] For adolescents and adults, the initial dose is 15–30 mL and it can be repeated once, if necessary. Ipecac syrup is virtually 100% effective at inducing vomiting when 15 mL or more is given.[6]

Fluid Administration Fluid administration is generally recommended immediately after the ipecac dose. Children should be given 4–8 oz of fluid; adults should receive 12–16 oz. One study of adult volunteers given a 15-mL ipecac dose suggests that it takes longer to induce vomiting when milk is given after the ipecac than when water is given.[7] However, two studies of overdosed children given either milk or water after ipecac showed no difference in time needed for vomiting to occur.[8,9] Thus, the use of clear fluids (eg, water, juice, or soda) is preferred because administration of milk offers no apparent advantages over that of clear fluids, and milk may obscure examination of the vomitus for evidence of tablets and capsules. Vomiting should occur within 15–20 minutes. If it does not, the initial dose of ipecac syrup should be repeated.

Whether fluids are given before or after ipecac or whether the fluids are tepid (104°F or 40°C) or cold (50°F or 10°C) does not appear to affect the time for vomiting to occur in adults.[10] Although no scientific evidence exists, patients who are ambulatory seem to vomit more quickly than those who are not; therefore, children should be encouraged to play quietly rather than recline, and adults should be encouraged to move around.

If the patient is to be brought to an emergency facility or health care provider's office for follow-up, the patient should vomit into a bucket or other container and that container should be brought to the treatment facility as well so the vomitus can be inspected for evidence of the poison. It is not necessary or advisable to wait for the patient to vomit before setting out for a health care facility; a container should be taken along in case the patient vomits en route.

Ipecac Toxicity Toxicity following ipecac syrup administration is rare. After therapeutic doses are given, diarrhea and slight CNS depression are common; mild GI upset may last for several hours following emesis. Clinical experience has shown that ingestion of 30 mL of ipecac syrup (the largest amount available without a prescription in a single unit of purchase) is safe in children over 1 year of age. The death of a 14-month-old child following the administration of less than 30 mL given for an ingestion of amaryllis leaves was not a direct result of the pharmacologic effects of ipecac but rather was due to a congenital anomaly.[11] In larger doses, ipecac is cardiotoxic and may cause hypotension, bradycardia, atrial fibrillation, ventricular fibrillation, and death.[12] A fatal intracerebral hemorrhage was reported in an 84-year-old woman given a therapeutic dose of ipecac syrup and activated charcoal following a nontoxic dose of boric acid.[13]

Several cases of chronic ipecac poisoning by proxy have been reported; in these cases, parents have repeatedly given ipecac syrup and have sought medical attention for repeated vomiting.[14] This has been described as a form of Munchausen's syndrome by proxy.[14] Most patients demonstrate recurrent GI effects, including grossly bloody stools, and other effects such as cardiomyopathy.[14]

Fluidextract of ipecac is 14 times stronger than ipecac syrup and should no longer be found in any pharmacy. Severe toxicity and death have occurred when fluidextract of ipecac was given by mistake.[15]

Pharmacists must be aware that ipecac syrup is used inappropriately by some bulimic patients to remove food from the stomach and lose weight. This practice is particularly dangerous because it brings about a drug-induced fluid and electrolyte imbalance and cardiotoxicity. However, the abuse problem does not warrant removing 1-oz (30-mL) bottles of ipecac syrup from nonprescription status.[16] Pharmacists should question any person buying ipecac syrup regularly to be certain it is being purchased for its appropriate use, and they should view with suspicion frequent purchases by the same person.

Expiration Date Using drugs beyond their stated expiration date is generally not recommended. If, however, parents have an expired container of ipecac syrup and it is the only ipecac available, should it be used? A study demonstrated no difference in the percentage of patients who vomited or in the amount of time lapsed before vomiting when ipecac was used by the expiration date as opposed to after that date.[17] The ipecac used in this study ranged from 1 month to 16 years beyond the expiration date.

Drug Interactions The only potential drug interaction with ipecac syrup involves activated charcoal. Activated charcoal is used as an adsorbent in many poisoning cases. When it is administered with ipecac, the concern has been that the ipecac may be adsorbed by the charcoal, thus delaying or preventing emesis. In addition, the adsorptive capacity of the charcoal could be reduced. However, a prospective study disproved these concerns.[18] In fact, there is no scientific evidence to support the fact that administering ipecac syrup at the same time as or after activated charcoal inhibits vomiting. This combination is not recommended, however, since patients given ipecac are very likely to vomit the activated charcoal.

Ipecac versus Gastric Lavage Several studies have compared the efficacy of ipecac treatment and gastric lavage in removing gastric contents. One study found ipecac to be superior in removing salicylates from 20 patients 12–20 months of age[19]; another found it superior in removing a toxic dose of aspirin from two adults.[20] A third study determined that ipecac was three times as effective as gastric lavage when treatment was delayed.[21] However, prospective studies using markers including thiamine, technetium Tc 99m, and cyanocobalamin in overdosed patients found that gastric lavage was superior to induced emesis.[22–24] Concerns relating to methodologic interpretation leave study results unresolved.[25] Saetta and Aminton found intragastric solids remaining in 38.5% of patients who vomited following administration of ipecac syrup and in 88.2% of patients following gastric lavage.[26] In a follow-up study, however, when Saetta et al administered barium-impregnated polyethylene pellets to poisoned patients immediately prior to gastric lavage or ipecac syrup,[27] 58.5% of the pellets were retained following ipecac syrup as compared with 51.5% following gastric lavage. Moreover, the number of pellets in the small intestine at the end of the procedure was greater in both the ipecac and gastric lavage groups than it was in an untreated control

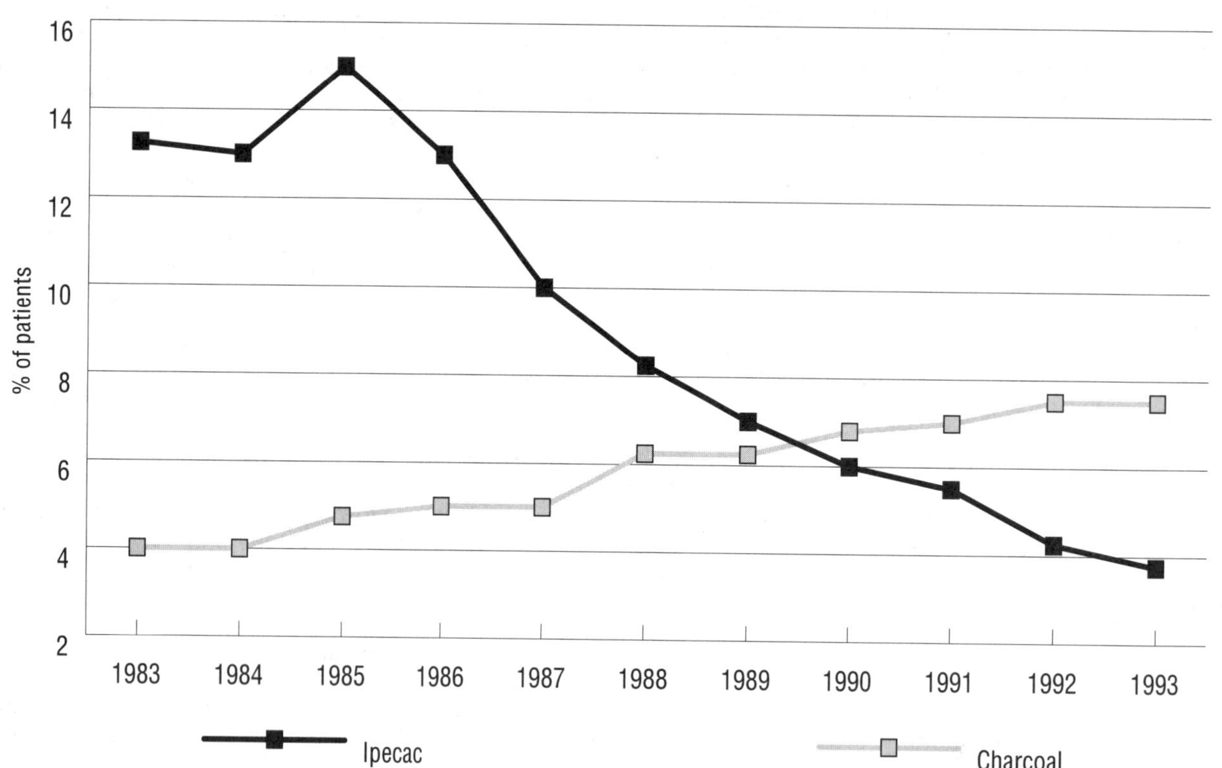

FIGURE 1 Use of ipecac and activated charcoal in poisoned patients, 1983–1993. Reprinted with permission from Litovitz TL et al. 1993 Report of the American Association of Poison Control Centers Toxic Exposure Surveillance System. *Am J Emerg Med.* 1994; 12: 546–84.

group. These studies thus suggest that neither ipecac nor gastric lavage effectively empties the stomach and that, in fact, both procedures may enhance movement of gastric contents into the small intestine. This reinforces the importance of administering activated charcoal to poisoned patients.

In general, ipecac syrup, when used with appropriate instruction and follow-up, is the only safe and effective in-home method of induced emesis. Not only can it prevent emergency room visits, but in those cases when treatment in the hospital is necessary, it also allows for earlier administration and vomiting. In the hospital setting, however, both induced emesis and gastric lavage are often used. Some hospitals prefer lavage over ipecac, particularly for adults; others have stopped using GI decontamination in favor of activated charcoal alone.

Activated Charcoal

Over the past 10 years, the use of ipecac syrup in poison management has decreased significantly while the use of activated charcoal has dramatically increased (see Figure 1).[4] Activated charcoal is an effective adsorbent for most drugs and chemicals (see product table "Gastric Decontaminant Products"). It is usually administered as a water slurry of 60–100 g of activated charcoal for adults or 15–30 g of activated charcoal for children in a minimum of 8 oz of water. (A larger dose of charcoal may require more than 8 oz of water to be the proper consistency for administration orally or by gastric tube.) The slurry can be prepared by adding water to a container with activated charcoal and shaking it. Because measuring the correct amount of charcoal is difficult, preweighed packages are available.

Activated charcoal products premixed with water, the cathartic sorbitol, or water and carboxymethylcellulose are also commercially available. When multiple doses of activated charcoal are being given, a cathartic should be given only with the first dose. Pharmacists should check premixed charcoal products to see if they contain sorbitol; if they do, other cathartics should not be given and the sorbitol-containing product should be given only initially. If the activated charcoal does not contain sorbitol, a single dose of a saline cathartic such as magnesium sulfate or magnesium citrate may be administered after charcoal administration if bowel sounds are present. This process speeds elimination of the charcoal drug complex.

Optimally, activated charcoal should be given as soon as possible after ingestion. However, it has sometimes been shown to be effective even when administration has been delayed by several hours. There is no systemic toxicity or maximum dose limit. Repeat doses of activated charcoal are recommended to interrupt enterohepatic recycling by binding agents (eg, phenobarbital or theophylline) secreted into the GI tract. Contrary to popular belief, burnt toast is not a substitute for activated charcoal and is not indicated in the treatment of poisoning.

TABLE 2 Compounds known to be effectively bound by activated charcoal in man or animals

Oral-activated charcoal inhibits absorption of the following chemicals from the gastrointestinal tract[a]

Acetaminophen	Methyl salicylate
Aconitine	Nadolol
d-Amphetamine	Nicotine
Aspirin	Nortriptyline
Atropine	Paraquat
Barbital	Pentobarbital
Benzene	Phencyclidine
Carbamazepine	Phenobarbital
Chlordane	Phenylbutazone
Chloroquine	Phenylpropanolamine
Chlorpheniramine	Phenytoin
Chlorpromazine	Propantheline
Chlorpropamide	Propoxyphene
Digoxin	Quinine
Doxepin	Salicylamide
Ethchlorvynol	Secobarbital
Ethylene glycol	Sodium salicylate
Glutethimide	Sodium valproate
Hexachlorophene	Strychnine
Kerosene	Theophylline
Malathion	Tetracycline
Mefenamic acid	Tolbutamide
Mercuric chloride	Yohimbine

Multiple oral doses of activated charcoal accelerate body clearance of the following drugs[b]

Carbamazepine	Phenobarbital
Dapsone	Phenylbutazone
Digitoxin	Theophylline
Nadolol	

[a]Based on controlled experimental investigations in man or experimental animals.

[b]Not necessarily clinically significant.

Adapted with permission from Ellenhorn M, Barceloux D, eds. *Medical Toxicology: Diagnosis and Treatment of Human Poisoning*. 1st ed. New York: Elsevier Science Publishing; 1988: 59.

Although not effective for all ingestions, activated charcoal can reduce absorption of many poisons such as analgesics (eg, salicylates, acetaminophen, or propoxyphene), sedatives, hypnotics, and tricyclic antidepressants (Table 2). In the past, a "universal antidote" mixture of activated charcoal, magnesium oxide, and tannic acid was used. However, this combination is ineffective because the adsorptive capacity of the charcoal is diminished as some of the tannic acid is adsorbed by the charcoal. The remaining tannic acid may produce significant dose-related toxicity.

The possible benefits of ipecac or gastric lavage over activated charcoal in preventing absorption from the GI tract and toxicity are unclear. Two studies in human volunteers used near-therapeutic doses of drugs or simulated drug overdoses.[28,29] Two other studies used a prospective clinic trial design to compare use of activated charcoal alone with that of activated charcoal plus either gastric lavage or ipecac in overdose patients treated in an emergency room.[30,31] In general, both pairs of studies showed no added benefit of gastric lavage or ipecac plus activated charcoal over charcoal alone in hospital-treated patients. Kulig et al did show a benefit for early gastric lavage (within 1 hour of the exposure) and activated charcoal, as compared with activated charcoal alone.[30] In the home, however, activated charcoal is not a viable substitute for ipecac syrup because it is difficult for parents to administer a therapeutic dose to children successfully. Ipecac syrup is intended primarily for patients who will be treated at home and for pediatric patients treated in a hospital setting who will not be given activated charcoal.

Other Methods to Induce Emesis

Vomiting may be induced in numerous ways. Ipecac syrup, however, is the only safe and effective emetic. Home remedies (emetics) other than ipecac produce erratic and unpredictable results, are often ineffective, and are sometimes dangerous.

Liquid dishwashing detergent, which contains anionic and nonionic surfactants, has been studied as an emetic agent.[32] Its effectiveness could not be determined because many patients refused to drink any or all of it; however, those who did drink most of the administered solution vomited. Liquid dishwashing solution should not replace ipecac syrup unless ipecac cannot be obtained quickly. The pharmacist must be aware that the ingredients in liquid dishwashing detergent are subject to frequent reformulation and that toxic ingredients may be included; therefore, the pharmacist should check with a poison control center or manufacturer before recommending a given product. Automatic dishwasher products and laundry detergents contain caustic ingredients and must never be used as emetics.

Salt water is an unpalatable, unreliable, and potentially dangerous emetic. Salt solutions may be quite toxic because of sodium absorption; severe hypernatremia may result, and the use of salt as an emetic has produced fatalities in children and adults.[33,34] It is estimated that 1 tbsp (15 mL) of salt contains about 250 mEq of sodium. If retained and absorbed, this amount could raise the serum sodium level by 25 mEq/L in a healthy 3-year-old child with an estimated total body water of 10 L. Thus, salt water should *not* be used under any circumstances.

Mustard water is an unreliable and unpalatable emetic that should not be routinely recommended.

Copper sulfate has been used as an emetic. It acts by producing direct gastric irritation that leads to reflex stimulation of the vomiting center. Based on the available data, copper sulfate is an effective emetic. However, concerns about copper absorption and its potential toxicity[35] preclude recommending this agent to induce emesis.

Apomorphine, an opiate analog, produces rapid emesis. However, it is available only by prescription and must be given parenterally. Apomorphine may produce or worsen CNS and respiratory depression. Naloxone given intravenously can usually reverse these effects. In several cases, however, significant respiratory and/or CNS depression that is unresponsive to naloxone has developed in patients given apomorphine.[36]

Finally, vomiting can be mechanically induced by giving the patient fluids and then manually stimulating the gag reflex at the back of the throat with either a blunt object or a finger. The percentage of persons who vomit following this procedure is low, however, and the mean volume of vomitus is small compared with that induced by ipecac syrup.[37] Thus, lack of efficacy and potential injury to the patient make mechanically induced vomiting a poor choice.

Contraindications to Emesis

CNS Depression or Seizures

Efforts to induce vomiting should not be attempted in patients who are lethargic or comatose because these patients are at high risk of aspirating gastric contents while vomiting. There is also a high risk of aspiration if vomiting occurs while a patient is experiencing a seizure. Similarly, emetics are generally not recommended when patients have taken agents that may produce a rapid decrease in the level of consciousness (eg, antidepressants) or may rapidly produce seizures (eg, camphor or amphetamines). The stimulation of vomiting may enhance the epileptogenic potential of the poison.

Caustic Ingestions

Patients who have ingested a caustic substance should *not* be made to vomit. Caustic agents are strong acids or bases that can severely burn the mucous membranes of the GI tract, including the mouth, esophagus, and stomach. Should vomiting occur, the esophagus and oral cavity would be reexposed to the caustic agent and more damage could occur. In addition, if the esophagus is already damaged, the force of vomiting could cause esophageal or gastric perforation.

When ingestion of a caustic agent is suspected, the patient, if conscious and able to drink, should immediately be given water or milk to dilute the agent. Attempts to neutralize the agent using an acid or base would generate heat and produce more serious injury and must therefore be avoided. Most patients who have ingested a caustic agent should be immediately referred to a medical facility.

Controversial Use of Emetics

Antiemetic Drug Ingestion

Use of emetics in cases of acute overdose of antiemetic medications is controversial. There is a theoretical concern that if an emetic is not given soon after the antiemetic has been ingested, a significant emetic failure rate may result. In practice this does not appear to be a problem.[38] If an emetic is given and vomiting does not occur, gastric lavage may be necessary to remove the ingested antiemetic substance.

Hydrocarbon Ingestion

Patients who have ingested aliphatic hydrocarbons (eg, kerosene, gasoline, or furniture polish) traditionally have not been given emetics because induced vomiting was thought to increase the likelihood of pulmonary aspiration, leading to alveolar irritation and pneumonitis. Studies have since shown that aspiration is not likely to occur when vomiting is induced; however, emptying the stomach of aliphatic hydrocarbons is generally not necessary. This is because the systemic toxicity caused by these agents does not appear to be directly related to their absorption but rather to postaspiration hypoxia. However, when a potentially dangerous chemical such as a pesticide is dissolved in a hydrocarbon base, the use of ipecac syrup is generally considered appropriate.

A retrospective study of patients who had ingested petroleum distillates revealed that a lower percentage of patients developed aspiration pneumonitis when vomiting was induced with ipecac than when gastric lavage was used or vomiting occurred spontaneously.[39] Other research has also shown that aspiration pneumonitis is less likely to occur, and is less severe when it does occur, in ipecac-treated patients than in those who receive gastric lavage.[40] Based on these findings, practitioners should use ipecac instead of gastric lavage for alert patients who have ingested a hydrocarbon and for whom gastric removal is necessary. The administration of ipecac syrup in such cases should be conducted in a hospital.

Antiemetics

Nausea and vomiting are signs and symptoms common to many minor as well as serious disorders. Most minor nausea and vomiting, such as that which occur with motion sickness or overeating, are self-limiting symptoms that require minimal therapy.

Many patients choose to self-medicate their nausea and vomiting with various nonprescription products to avoid a medical office visit. However, the pharmacist should be cautious about recommending self-medication for these symptoms and should ask appropriate questions to determine whether referral to a health care provider is indicated.

Patient Assessment

In assessing the patient's complaint, the pharmacist should determine:

- The age of the patient;
- The onset and duration of signs and symptoms;
- The nature of precipitating factors;
- A complete history of recent medication use and of food and liquid ingestion;
- Any signs and symptoms other than nausea and vomiting (eg, fever);
- Any current chronic or acute medical conditions.

Signs and symptoms or medical conditions associated with nausea and vomiting that necessitate referral to a health care provider include:

- Blood in the vomitus;
- Abdominal pain or distention;

- Prolonged nausea and vomiting (>24–48 hours), especially for children under 1 year of age, or projectile vomiting;
- Dehydration;
- Weight loss of more than 5% of body weight;
- Fever;
- Severe headache;
- Change in behavior or alertness;
- Pregnancy;
- Presence of diabetes or other medical conditions that may be affected by lack of nutritional intake or missed doses of oral medications;
- Recent trauma, particularly a significant head injury;
- Suspected poisoning.

The following are some important considerations in determining the appropriate use of an antiemetic product.

Children

Vomiting in newborns can result from a number of serious abnormalities, including obstruction of the GI tract, neurologic disorders, and neuromuscular control disorders, and it may rapidly lead to acid-base disturbances and dehydration. Dehydration and electrolyte disturbances occur more often in children and, if not appropriately managed, may result in death. Thus, referral to a health care provider is recommended for further evaluation of any vomiting in newborns.

Regurgitation or spitting up, whereby milk appears to spill gently from the mouth, is common in infants. Often the causes are simple, such as overfeeding, too rapid feeding, ineffective burping, swallowing air, and laying the infant down after feeding, as well as immaturity of the esophageal sphincters. Regurgitation generally should not cause concern and does not require medical attention.

One of the more common causes of vomiting in children is acute viral gastroenteritis. However, acute onset of vomiting in children can also be secondary to head trauma, toxic ingestion, CNS infection, and GI obstruction. Treatment of gastroenteritis is directed primarily at preventing and correcting dehydration and electrolyte disturbances. Lost fluids should generally be replaced within 24 hours. Oral rehydration solutions may be used in mild cases. If severe diarrhea or vomiting persists for more than 24–48 hours, the child should be referred to a health care provider for evaluation and for parenteral fluid and electrolyte replacement.[41]

The use of antiemetics in children is controversial, in part, because most antiemetic studies have been conducted with adult patients. Some clinicians question the wisdom and value of treating children with antiemetics in an acute, self-limiting disorder. It is suggested that vomiting in gastroenteritis is a host defense process that sheds the pathogen and should therefore not be suppressed. However, recurrent or protracted vomiting can lead to marked dehydration and electrolyte imbalance that cannot be ignored, especially in small children. The patient should be observed for signs of dehydration. These include dry oral mucous membranes, sunken eyes with or without sunken fontanel, decreased urine output (ie, no wetting for 8–12 hours or more), no tears when crying, decreased skin turgor with tenting, weight loss, and unusual listlessness, sleepiness, or tiredness. If any of these signs are present, the child should be referred to a health care provider.[42]

If a child is vomiting, the following steps can be taken to prevent dehydration:

- Stop all feeding for 1 hour.
- Start clear liquids (ie, oral rehydration solutions). After 12 hours of well-tolerated clear liquids, start half-strength formula and light solids.
- If half-strength formula or light solids are well tolerated, resume the child's regular diet.
- If the child vomits after any of these steps, start again with clear liquids.

However, the child's health care provider should be contacted if[42]:

- The child is less than 1 year of age;
- The child refuses to drink;
- The child has not urinated in the past 8–12 hours;
- The child appears lethargic or is crying;
- Weight loss or dehydration occurs;
- Vomiting occurs with each feeding;
- Vomiting is repeatedly projectile;
- Vomitus contains red, black, or green fluid;
- Vomiting is associated with diarrhea, distended abdomen, fever, or severe headache;
- Vomiting occurs following a head injury;
- Poisoning is suspected.

Pregnancy

Nausea, with or without vomiting, may be one of the earliest symptoms of pregnancy. A woman who experiences nausea and vomiting, and who has no other symptoms except a missed menstrual period and perhaps weight gain, should be referred for a pregnancy test and follow-up. Women who report nausea and vomiting during pregnancy generally suffer from these symptoms in the early part of the day—hence, the term "morning sickness." However, some pregnant women experience these symptoms in the afternoon or evening, and a small number of women experience morning sickness throughout the day.

Nausea and vomiting during the first trimester of pregnancy is often worrisome to the patient. These symptoms, which may be mild to severe, should be taken seriously and the patient reassured. However, because teratogenicity is a major consideration during pregnancy, most health care providers are reluctant to prescribe any medication for a pregnant woman unless it is absolutely necessary. Indications for nonprescription antiemetics approved by the Food and Drug Administration (FDA) do not include the treatment of nausea and vomiting associated with pregnancy. A number of nonpharmacologic approaches can be recommended instead, including eating small, frequent meals; lowering the fat content of meals; ingesting crackers before arising in the morning; lying down; and avoiding precipitating factors. If nausea and/or vomiting continue despite such measures, patients should be referred to their health care providers.[43]

Motion Sickness

Motion sickness occurs when visual and vestibular stimuli are not in accord. The symptoms consist of pallor, yawning, restlessness, nausea, and then vomiting. Although anyone can experience motion sickness, some individuals are more likely to be affected than others, and susceptibility appears to vary with age. Infants are generally least likely to experience it whereas children aged 2–12 years are more likely to do so. In young children, motion sickness associated with car travel may be minimized by placing the child in a car seat. The resulting elevation and position is sufficient to allow vision out of the front window and may prevent the disorder. Antihistamines are the primary nonprescription agents used to prevent or control motion sickness.

Overeating

For complaints of nausea associated with excessive or disagreeable food or beverage intake, avoidance or moderation of consumption may prove beneficial. Otherwise, antacids, bismuth-containing products, and H_2-antagonists are indicated for the relief of heartburn, indigestion, and upset stomach associated with dietary overindulgence. (See Chapter 11, "Acid-Peptic Products.")

Food Poisoning

Signs and symptoms associated with food poisoning usually include vomiting in addition to diarrhea, abdominal cramps, and possible fever.[41] Symptomatic treatment is often recommended. This consists of fluid and electrolyte replacement, dietary modification, and antidiarrheal products when appropriate. A diet of clear liquids and simple carbohydrates is recommended for the first 24 hours. The patient can return to a regular diet when it can be tolerated.[44] Food poisoning typically resolves within 24–36 hours. However, if symptoms continue beyond this period, referral to a health care provider for evaluation is recommended.[41] The use of nonprescription antidiarrheal agents for infectious diarrhea is not appropriate without a specific medical recommendation.[44] (See Chapter 13, "Antidiarrheal Products.")

Current Medication Use

Many medications, such as cancer chemotherapeutic agents, narcotics, antibiotics, and estrogens, are known to cause nausea and vomiting as an adverse side effect. Other medications, such as digitalis or theophylline, may produce nausea and vomiting as a sign of toxicity. In these situations, nonprescription antiemetics are not indicated. The patient should instead be referred to a health care provider.

Other Medical Problems

Bulimia (binge-purge behavior) is a psychologic disorder in which patients attempt to control their weight by repeated vomiting and the chronic use of emetics (most commonly ipecac syrup). These patients should be referred for medical and psychologic management of the underlying problems.[45] Patients with other chronic medical conditions such as diabetes, which could be affected by the lack of adequate nutritional intake or by missed doses of medication, should also be referred to their health care providers. In addition, any patient who exhibits severe nausea, vomiting, and abdominal pain or who has forceful, bloody, or protracted vomiting should receive medical attention immediately, as should adults in whom vomiting persists for more than 2 days.

Ingredients in Nonprescription Products

Antacids

Antacids neutralize gastric acidity, increasing the pH of the stomach and duodenum. Antacids are therefore indicated for the symptomatic relief of upset stomach associated with gastric acidity. This includes complaints of heartburn, dyspepsia, and acid indigestion. For relief of these symptoms, 15 mL of most antacids should be taken 30 minutes after meals and at bedtime. Because antacids may impair the absorption of many medications, patients should be counseled not to take potentially interacting oral medications within 1–2 hours of the antacid dose. The available nonprescription antacid products contain various combinations of ingredients such as magnesium hydroxide, aluminum hydroxide, calcium carbonate, and magnesium carbonate. (See Chapter 11, "Acid-Peptic Products," for a thorough review of antacid pharmacotherapy.)

H_2-Receptor Antagonists

H_2-receptor antagonists provide symptomatic relief of heartburn, dyspepsia, and indigestion by inhibiting the secretion of gastric acid. The FDA has recently approved lower nonprescription doses of these agents for these acid-peptic indications. (See Chapter 11, "Acid-Peptic Products.")

Antihistamines

Antihistamines are the primary nonprescription agents used as antiemetics (see product table "Antiemetic Products"). These agents depress labyrinth excitability and therefore are effective, to varying degrees, for the prevention and control of motion sickness. The available nonprescription antihistamine preparations that are classified as safe and effective for the prevention and treatment of nausea, vomiting, or dizziness associated with motion sickness include meclizine (Bonine), cyclizine (Marezine), dimenhydrinate (Dramamine), and diphenhydramine (Benadryl). These antihistamines should be taken at least 30–60 minutes before departure for travel and continued during travel.

Drowsiness with therapeutic doses of antihistamines can occur and is the most common side effect. Patients should be cautioned not to drive a vehicle, operate hazardous machinery, or engage in tasks requiring a high degree of mental alertness and physical dexterity while using these products. The effects are additive to those of other CNS depressants such as alcohol, tranquilizers, hypnotics, and sedatives. In large doses, these agents may also produce anticholinergic adverse effects, including blurred vision, dry mouth, and urinary retention. Antihistamines should be used with caution in patients with asthma, narrow-angle glaucoma, obstructive disease of the GI or genitourinary tracts, or benign prostatic hypertrophy. As for the nonsedating antihistamines, astemizole (Hismanal) and terfenadine (Seldane), which do not readily cross into the CNS, astemizole is considered to be ineffective in alleviating motion sickness, and there are no reports on the usefulness of terfenadine for this indication.[46]

Meclizine and Cyclizine Meclizine and cyclizine are members of the piperazine group of antihistamine compounds.

The adult dosage of meclizine is 25–50 mg once a day. The drug has a relatively long duration of action and may be administered every 24 hours. If possible, the initial dose should be taken 1 hour prior to travel. Meclizine is not recommended for children under 12 years of age.

The adult dosage of cyclizine is 50 mg every 4–6 hours, not to exceed 200 mg in 24 hours. The pediatric dosage for children 6–12 years of age is 25 mg every 6–8 hours, not to exceed 75 mg in 24 hours. Cyclizine has a shorter duration of action than meclizine and therefore requires more frequent dosing. The initial dose of cyclizine should be taken approximately 1 hour prior to travel. Cyclizine is not recommended for children under 6 years of age.

In 1965, the FDA required that products containing meclizine and cyclizine carry a warning against their use during pregnancy. This warning was based on animal studies and anecdotal case reports, which suggested that the drugs might have teratogenic potential. Subsequent epidemiologic studies of pregnant women have not shown an increase in fetal deaths or malformations with exposure to these drugs during the first trimester[47]; therefore, the warning regarding possible teratogenic effects during pregnancy is not required. However, none of these agents has an FDA-approved indication for the management of nausea and vomiting associated with pregnancy. All antihistamines appear to have a low risk of teratogenicity but should be reserved for pregnant women who have severe nausea and vomiting that are unresponsive to nonpharmacologic measures.[48] Pregnant women should always consult their health care providers before taking any medication.

Doxylamine Doxylamine, an antihistamine of the ethanolamine class, was originally in the combination product Bendectin (10 mg doxylamine and 10 mg pyridoxine [see the section Pyridoxine]). Although the FDA had approved this product for the treatment of nausea and vomiting in pregnancy. Bendectin was withdrawn from the market by its manufacturer in 1983 because of the high cost of defending against lawsuits that claimed that birth defects occurred in infants whose mothers had taken the drug. However, the ingredients, doxylamine and pyridoxine, remain available as nonprescription products, and many health care providers continue to recommend these agents for pregnant women whose nausea and vomiting do not respond to nonpharmacologic management. Doxylamine and pyridoxine are not considered to be teratogenic.

Diphenhydramine Diphenhydramine, another antihistamine of the ethanolamine class, is safe and effective for the prevention and treatment of motion sickness. The recommended dosage for adults is 25–50 mg every 4–6 hours, not to exceed 300 mg in 24 hours. The recommended dosage for children 2–6 years is 6.25 mg every 4–6 hours. For children aged 6–12 years (>20 lbs or 9.1 kg), the dosage is 12.5–25 mg every 4–6 hours, not to exceed 150 mg in 24 hours.

Dimenhydrinate Dimenhydrinate, the 8-chlorotheophyllinate salt of the antihistamine diphenhydramine, is also safe and effective for the prevention and treatment of nausea and vomiting associated with motion sickness. The usual adult dosage is 50–100 mg every 4–6 hours, not to exceed 400 mg in 24 hours. The dosage for children 2–6 years is 12.5–25 mg every 6–8 hours, not to exceed 75 mg in 24 hours. For children aged 6–12 years, the dosage is 25–50 mg every 6–8 hours, not to exceed 150 mg in 24 hours.

Pyridoxine

Pyridoxine (vitamin B_6) is a water-soluble B complex vitamin that is essential in the human diet. Uncontrolled studies in the 1940s suggested that pyridoxine might be effective in treating nausea and vomiting associated with pregnancy. Although the American Medical Association Council on Drugs stated in 1979 that there was no conclusive evidence that pyridoxine was effective for this indication, a more recent controlled study using 25 mg of pyridoxine given orally every 8 hours produced significant improvement in women who complained of severe nausea and vomiting during pregnancy.[49] However, the specific mechanism of action of pyridoxine is unknown.[49] Pyridoxine was included in the formulation of Bendectin, which was withdrawn from the market in 1983.

Phosphorated Carbohydrate Solution

Phosphorated carbohydrate solution (Emetrol, Calm-X, Nausetrol) is a mixture of levulose (fructose), dextrose (glucose), and phosphoric acid (see product table "Antiemetic Products"). Phosphoric acid is added to adjust the pH of the commercial product to between 1.5 and 1.6. This hyperosmolar carbohydrate product is indicated for nausea and vomiting associated with upset stomach caused by intestinal flu, food indiscretions, and emotional upset. Theoretically, this mixture has the potential to inhibit gastric emptying and reduce gastric tone through the high osmotic pressure exerted by the solution of simple sugars. Phosphorated carbohydrate solution has been used in attempts to alleviate the nausea and vomiting associated with pregnancy. This product however shows no advantage over other products for this problem.

The usual adult dosage of the phosphorated carbohydrate is 15–30 mL (1–2 tbsp) at 15-minute intervals until vomiting ceases. No more than five doses should be taken in 1 hour. The solution should not be diluted, and the patient should not consume other liquids for 15 minutes after taking a dose. If vomiting does not cease after five doses, a health care provider should be contacted. Large doses of fructose may cause abdominal pain and diarrhea. Thus, phosphorated carbohydrate should not be used by individuals with hereditary fructose intolerance. Practitioners should also be aware of the product's high glucose content and of associated problems in persons with diabetes.

Bismuth Salts

Bismuth salts have been used for centuries for various GI complaints such as upset stomach, indigestion, nausea, and diarrhea. Bismuth subsalicylate (Pepto-Bismol) is available as a nonprescription suspension and chewable tablet for the relief of nausea associated with dyspepsia, heartburn, and fullness (gas) caused by overindulgence in food and drink. Bismuth is proposed to act by coating the gastric mucosa. Bismuth salts are poorly absorbed from the GI tract although the amount of bismuth subsalicylate included in nonprescription preparations may lead to the absorption of some salicylate. In patients who are taking other salicylate-containing products or who have renal insufficiency, salicylate levels may be increased. Patients taking bismuth-containing products should be counseled that the mouth, tongue, and stool may temporarily appear gray-black or black. Also, patients should avoid bismuth subsalicylate if they are taking medications that may interact adversely with salicylates. Bismuth subsalicylate should *never* be recommended for children with viral influenza or chickenpox because of concern about development of Reye's syndrome. (See Chapter 11, "Acid-Peptic Products.")

Oral Rehydration Solutions

Dehydration secondary to vomiting and diarrhea is a result of a net loss of extracellular fluid that is composed of sodium, chloride, potassium, water, and bicarbonate. Signs and symptoms of dehydration include dry mouth, excessive thirst, little or no urination, dizziness, and lightheadedness. Patients should be evaluated for dehydration if they have severe vomiting or diarrhea that persists for more than 24 hours in children or 48 hours in adults.[41,42]

Replacement of fluid should mimic extracellular fluid losses. Because active glucose absorption in the small bowel promotes sodium absorption, oral rehydration therapy is based on the use of glucose to increase sodium absorption and allow for rapid replacement of extracellular fluid.[50] Oral electrolyte mixtures for rehydration include Pedialyte, Ricelyte, Infalyte, Rehydralyte, Resol, and Naturalyte (see product table "Oral Rehydration Solutions"). Although not as osmotically or chemically balanced, gelatin water, sports drinks, fruit juices, and carbonated beverages can also be administered. However, while these products are adequate energy sources, they are too low in sodium, potassium, and chloride to produce a rapid and significant therapeutic response to severe dehydration with electrolyte depletion. Use of homemade sugar-water or salt-water solutions should be discouraged.

In a child with vomiting, the fluid should be given very slowly, starting with 5–10 mL every 10 minutes. The quantity of fluid may be increased as tolerated. If vomiting and diarrhea stop after 12–24 hours of clear liquids, the child should be gradually returned to a regular diet over the next 2 or 3 days.[41] (See Chapter 13, "Antidiarrheal Products.")

Acupressure Wristbands

The use of acupressure therapy to treat nausea and vomiting is based on the ancient Chinese theory of the vital force, Chi. For centuries, the Chinese have used the Nei Kuan point, located on the inner forearm just above the wrist, to relieve the signs and symptoms of nausea and vomiting. Several studies have investigated the use of acupressure therapy in this regard.[51–53] These studies suggest a beneficial effect and have resulted in the availability of acupressure wristbands. The acupressure wristbands (SeaBands and Travel Aides) are marketed for the prevention of motion sickness. Controlled studies have also demonstrated a positive patient response in suppressing pregnancy-related nausea and vomiting.[51–53] Acupressure wristbands offer an alternative to the pharmacologic management of nausea and vomiting and should be considered by those patients who wish to avoid the adverse effects associated with antihistamines.

Case Studies

Case 16–1

Patient Complaint/History

The parent of a 2-year-old girl, TD, presents to the pharmacist with questions about managing the child's nausea and vomiting, which started the night before. During questioning of the parent about the child's symptoms, the pharmacist learns that TD refused to eat lunch and dinner on the previous day and began vomiting around bedtime. Six episodes of vomiting occurred during the period from bedtime to this morning. The child was able to drink small amounts of liquids between episodes of vomiting. The parent requests a recommendation for a nonprescription antiemetic.

During his questioning, the pharmacist also determines that the child has no medical problems and takes no chronic medications. Although the child occasionally receives acetaminophen as needed, she has not taken it in the past 24 hours because her temperature is 98.6°F (37°C).

Clinical Considerations/Strategies

The following considerations/strategies are provided to aid the reader in (1) determining whether treatment of the patient's condition with nonprescription medications is warranted, (2) selecting the appropriate nonprescription medication, and (3) developing a patient counseling strategy to ensure optimal therapeutic outcomes:

- Assess the appropriateness of giving the child an antiemetic. If appropriate, recommend a nonprescription product.
- Assess the need for medical referral.
- Recommend the appropriate steps in managing this child's nausea and vomiting.
- Develop a patient education/counseling strategy that will:
  - Optimize proper use of the recommended nonprescription antiemetic;
  - Provide advice on which signs/symptoms require medical referral.

Case 16–2

Patient Complaint/History

The parents of an 18-month-old boy, RB, call the pharmacy because they found their son with an open prescription vial of amitriptyline hydrochloride. They want to know if the child's ingestion of the medication could cause problems and what they should do. When asked about the amount of medication ingested, the parents respond that they are not sure. They report that RB seems drowsy but that it also his usual nap time.

Clinical Considerations/Strategies

The following considerations/strategies are provided to aid the reader in (1) determining whether treatment of the patient's condition with nonprescription medications is warranted, (2) selecting the appropriate nonprescription medication, and (3) developing a patient counseling strategy to ensure optimal therapeutic outcomes:

- Obtain additional history on the medication exposure, including the time of the exposure, other specific symptoms, and an estimate of the amount of medication ingested.
- Obtain information about the toxicity of amitriptyline hydrochloride, particularly as it relates to this exposure.
- Perform a preliminary assessment of the toxicity of the exposure.
- Contact the nearest poison control center to obtain a consultation.
- Assess the appropriateness of the parents observing the child at home, administering ipecac syrup, or taking the child to a health care facility. After assessing these alternatives, provide the parents with the appropriate recommendation(s).
- After resolution of the acute episode, develop an educational program that will help the parents prevent future drug or poison exposures.

Summary

Nonprescription emetic and antiemetic products are intended for use in the treatment of self-limiting conditions.

Emetics are useful in cases of poisoning; they serve to remove gastric contents and to prevent further absorption of the ingested agent. Ipecac syrup is the safest and most effective nonprescription emetic for this purpose. It should be kept in all homes with young children (a 1-oz [30-mL] bottle for each child under 5 years of age) and used with the guidance of a poison control center or health care provider if an ingestion occurs. The pharmacist should ascertain why an emetic (ipecac syrup) is being purchased and provide appropriate guidance in its use, suggesting referral if necessary.

Antiemetics are useful in limited situations but should always be used with caution because of the potential danger of masking the symptoms of more severe disease. The pharmacist should ascertain why an antiemetic is being purchased and suggest referral if necessary. Chronic unsupervised use of antiemetics, especially for an upset stomach, should be discouraged, and the patient should be encouraged to seek additional medical evaluation for continuous discomfort. Overuse or misuse of nonprescription antiemetics may result in adverse effects, toxicity, or delayed diagnosis and treatment of serious medical conditions.

References

1. Lee M, Feldman M. Nausea and vomiting. In: Sleisenger MH, Fordtran JS, eds. *Gastrointestinal Disease: Pathophysiology, Diagnosis, Management*. 5th ed. Philadelphia: WB Saunders; 1993: 509–23.
2. Cunningham FG et al, eds. *Williams Obstetrics*. 19th ed. Norwalk, Conn: Appleton and Lange; 1993: 265.
3. Soules MR et al. Nausea and vomiting of pregnancy: role of human chorionic gonadotropin and 17-hydroxyprogesterone. *Obstet Gynecol*. 1980; 55: 696–700.
4. Litovitz TL et al. 1993 Report of the American Association of Poison Control Centers Toxic Exposure Surveillance System. *Am J Emerg Med*. 1994; 12: 546–84.
5. Litovitz T et al. Safety and efficacy of ipecac administration in children younger than 1 year of age. *Pediatrics*. 1985; 76: 761.
6. Robertson WO. Syrup of ipecac—a fast or slow emetic? *Am J Dis Child*. 1972; 103: 58.
7. Varipapa RJ, Oderda GM. Effect of milk on ipecac induced emesis. *N Engl J Med*. 1977; 296: 112.
8. Grbcich PA et al. Does milk delay the onset of ipecac induced emesis? *Vet Hum Toxicol*. 1986; 28: 499.
9. Klein-Schwartz W et al. The effect of milk on ipecac-induced emesis. *J Toxicol Clin Toxicol*. 1991; 29: 505–11.
10. Spiegel RW et al. The effect of temperature of concurrently administered fluid on the onset of ipecac induced emesis. *Clin Toxicol*. 1979; 14: 281.
11. Robertson WO. *Syrup of ipecac associated fatality: a case report*. *Vet Hum Toxicol*. 1979; 21: 87.
12. McLeod J. Ipecac intoxication—use of a cardiac pacemaker in management. *N Engl J Med*. 1963; 268: 146.
13. Klein-Schwartz W et al. Ipecac use in the elderly: the unanswered question. *Ann Emerg Med*. 1984; 13: 1152.
14. Johnson JE et al. Hemorrhagic colitis and pseudomelanosis coli in ipecac ingestion by proxy. *J Pediatr Gastroenterol Nutr*. 1991; 12: 501.
15. Smith RR, Smith DM. Acute ipecac poisoning: report of a fatal case and review of the literature. *N Engl J Med*. 1964; 265: 23.
16. Litovitz T. In defense of retaining ipecac syrup as an over-the-counter drug. *Pediatrics*. 1986; 82: 514.
17. Grbcich PA et al. Expired ipecac syrup efficacy. *Pediatrics*. 1986; 78: 1085.
18. Freedman GE et al. A clinical trial using ipecac and activated charcoal concurrently. *Ann Emerg Med*. 1987; 16: 164.
19. Boxer L et al. Comparison of ipecac induced emesis with gastric lavage in the treatment of acute salicylate ingestion. *J Pediatr*. 1969; 74: 800.
20. Goldstein L. Emesis vs lavage for drug ingestion. *JAMA*. 1969; 208: 2162.
21. Arnold F Jr et al. Evaluation of the efficacy of lavage and induced emesis in treatment of salicylate poisoning. *Pediatrics*. 1959; 23: 286.
22. Auerbach PS et al. Efficacy of gastric emptying: gastric lavage vs emesis induced with ipecac. *Ann Emerg Med*. 1986; 15: 692.
23. Vasquez TE et al. Efficacy of ipecac-induced emesis for emptying gastric contents. *Clin Nucl Med*. 1988; 13: 638.
24. Tandberg D et al. Ipecac induced emesis vs gastric lavage: a controlled study in normal adults. *Am J Emerg Med*. 1986; 4: 205.
25. Litovitz T. Emesis vs lavage for poisoning victims. *Am J Emerg Med*. 1986; 4: 294.
26. Saetta JP, Aminton DN. Residual gastric content after gastric lavage and ipecacuanha-induced emesis in self-poisoned patients. *J R Soc Med*. 1991; 84: 35–8.
27. Saetta JP et al. Gastric emptying procedures in the self-poisoned patients: are we forcing gastric contents beyond the pylorus? *J R Soc Med*. 1991; 82: 274–6.

28. Curtis RA et al. Efficacy of ipecac and activated charcoal/cathartic on salicylate absorption in a simulated overdose. *Arch Intern Med.* 1984; 144: 48.
29. Neuvonen PJ et al. Comparison of activated charcoal and ipecac syrup in prevention of drug absorption. *Eur J Clin Pharmacol.* 1983; 24: 557.
30. Kulig K et al. Management of acutely poisoned patients without gastric emptying. *Ann Emerg Med.* 1985; 14: 562.
31. Merigian KS et al. Prospective evaluation of gastric emptying in the self-poisoned patient. *Am J Emerg Med.* 1990; 8: 479.
32. Geiseker DR, Troutman WG. Emergency induction of emesis using liquid detergent product: a report of 15 cases. *Clin Toxicol.* 1981; 18: 283.
33. Barer J et al. Fatal poisoning from salt used as an emetic. *Am J Dis Child.* 1973; 125: 899.
34. DeGenaro F, Nyhan W. Salt—a dangerous antidote. *J Pediatr.* 1971; 78: 1048.
35. Stein RS et al. Death after cupric sulfate. *JAMA.* 1976; 235: 801.
36. Schofferman J. A clinical comparison of ipecac and apomorphine use in adults. *J Am Coll Emerg Phys.* 1976; 5: 22.
37. Dabbous IA et al. The ineffectiveness of mechanically induced vomiting. *J Pediatr.* 1965; 66: 952.
38. Manoguerra AS, Krenzelok EP. Rapid emesis from high dose ipecac syrup in adults and children intoxicated with antiemetics and other drugs. *Am J Hosp Pharm.* 1978; 35: 1360.
39. Molinas S. A note on the use of ipecac syrup by poison control centers. Washington, DC: National Clearinghouse for Poison Control Centers, Public Health Service; 1966.
40. Ng RC et al. Emergency treatment of petroleum distillate and turpentine ingestion. *Can Med Assoc J.* 1974; 111: 537.
41. Brownlee HJ. Family practitioner's guide to patient self-treatment of acute diarrhea. *Am J Med.* 1990; 88: 27S–29S.
42. Book LS. Vomiting and diarrhea. *Pediatrics.* 1984; 74(suppl): 950–4.
43. Kousen M. Treatment of nausea and vomiting in pregnancy. *Am Fam Physician.* 1993 Nov; 48: 1279–83.
44. Johnson PC, Ericsson CD. Acute diarrhea in developed countries. *Am J Med.* 1990; 88(suppl 6A): 5S–9S.
45. Beumont PJV, George GCW, Smart DE. "Dieters" and "vomiters and purgers" in anorexia nervosa. *Psychol Med.* 1976; 6: 617–22.
46. Mitchelson F. Pharmacological agents affecting emesis. A review. *Drugs.* 1992; 43(3): 295–315.
47. Shapiro S et al. Antenatal drug exposure to doxylamine succinate and dicyclomine hydrochloride (Bendectin) in relation to congenital malformations, perinatal mortality rate, birth weight, and intelligence quotient score. *Am J Obstet Gynecol.* 1977; 128: 480–5.
48. Leathem AM. Safety and efficacy of antiemetics used to treat nausea and vomiting in pregnancy. *Clin Pharm.* 1986; 5: 660–8.
49. Sahakian V et al. Vitamin B_6 is effective therapy for nausea and vomiting of pregnancy: a randomized, double-blind placebo-controlled study. *Obstet Gynecol.* 1991; 78: 33–6.
50. Balisteri WF. Oral rehydration in acute infantile diarrhea. *Am J Med.* 1990; 88: 30S–33S.
51. Hyde E. Acupressure therapy for morning sickness. A controlled clinical trial. *J Nurse Midwifery.* 1989; 34(4): 171–8.
52. DeAloysio D, Penachioni P. Morning sickness control in early pregnancy by Neiguan point acupressure. *Obstet Gynecol.* 1992; 80: 852–4.
53. Stainton MC, Neff EJA. The efficacy of SeaBands for the control of nausea and vomiting in pregnancy. *Health Care Women Int.* 1994; 15(6): 563–75.

Appendix: Major Poison Control Centers

Alabama

- Alabama Poison Center
  408–A Paul Bryant Drive
  Tuscaloosa, AL 35401
  205–345–0600 (Administration)
  800–462–0800 (Alabama only)
- Regional Poison Control Center
  Children's Hospital of Alabama
  1600 Seventh Avenue South
  Birmingham, AL 35233
  205–939–9201
  205–933–4050
  800–292–6678 (Alabama only)

Alaska

- Anchorage Poison Control Center
  Providence Hospital Pharmacy
  PO Box 196604
  Anchorage, AK 99519–6604
  907–261–3193 (Administration)
  800–478–3193

Arizona

- Arizona Poison and Drug Information Center
  Health Sciences Center
  1501 North Campbell, Room 1156
  Tucson, AZ 85724
  602–626–6016 (Tucson)
  800–362–0101 (Arizona only)
- Samaritan Regional Poison Center
  Teleservices Department
  1441 North 12th Street
  Phoenix, AZ 85006
  602–253–3334

Arkansas

- Arkansas Poison and Drug Information Center
  College of Pharmacy-UAMS
  4301 West Markham Street, Slot 522
  Little Rock, AR 72205
  501–661–6161

California

- Central California Regional Poison Control Center
  Valley Children's Hospital
  3151 North Millbrook Avenue
  Fresno, CA 93703
  209–445–1222
  800–346–5922 (central California only)

- Los Angeles Regional Drug and Poison Information Center
  LAC/USC Medical Center, GH Room 1107 A&B
  1200 North State Street
  Los Angeles, CA 90033
  213–226–2246
- San Diego Regional Poison Center
  UCSD Medical Center
  200 West Arbor Drive
  San Diego, CA 92103–8925
  619–543–6000
  800–876–4766 (619 area code only)
- San Francisco Regional Poison Center
  San Francisco General Hospital
  1001 Potrero Avenue, Building 80, Room 230
  San Francisco, CA 94110
  415–476–6600 (Administration)
  800–523–2222
- Santa Clara Valley Medical Center
  Regional Poison Center
  750 South Bascom Avenue, Suite 310
  San Jose, CA 95128
  408–299–5112
  800–662–9886 (California only)
- UC Davis Regional Poison Control Center
  2315 Stockton Boulevard, Room 1511
  Sacramento, CA 95817
  916–734–3692
  800–342–9293 (northern California only)

Colorado

- Rocky Mountain Poison and Drug Center
  8802 East 9th Avenue
  Denver, CO 80220–6800
  303–629–1123 (Colorado only)

Connecticut

- Connecticut Poison Control Center
  University of Connecticut Health Center
  263 Farmington Avenue
  Farmington, CT 06030-5365
  800–343–2722 (Connecticut only)
  860–679–3456 (outside Connecticut)

District of Columbia

- National Capital Poison Center
  George Washington University Hospital
  3201 New Mexico Avenue, NW, Suite 310
  Washington, DC 20016
  202–625–3333
  202–362–8563 (TTY)

Florida

- Florida Poison Information Center - Jacksonville
  University of Florida Health Science Center - Jacksonville
  655 West Eighth Street
  Jacksonville, FL 32209
  904–549–4480
  800–282–3171 (Florida only)
- Florida Poison Information Center - Miami
  University of Miami, School of Medicine
  Department of Pediatrics
  PO Box 0169601 (R–131)
  Miami, FL 33101
  800–228–3171
- Florida Poison Information Center and Toxicology Resource Center
  The Tampa General Hospital
  PO Box 1289
  Tampa, FL 33601
  813–253–4444 (Tampa only)
  800–282–3171 (Florida only)

Georgia

- Georgia Poison Control Center
  80 Butler Street, SE
  PO Box 26066
  Atlanta, GA 30335–3801
  404–616–9000
  800–282–5846 (Georgia only)
  404–616–9287 (TDD)

Hawaii

- Hawaii Poison Center
  Kapiolani Women's and Children's Medical Center
  1319 Punahou Street
  Honolulu, HI 96826
  808–941–4411 (Pacific basin)

Illinois

- Chicago and Northeastern Illinois Regional Poison Control Center
  Rush-Presbyterian–St Luke's Medical Center
  1653 West Congress Parkway
  Chicago, IL 60612
  312–942–5969
  800–942–5969 (Illinois only)
- St Johns Hospital Regional Poison Control Center for Central and Southern Illinois
  800 East Carpenter
  Springfield, IL 62769
  217–753–3330
  800–543-2022 (Illinois only)

Indiana

- Indiana Poison Center
  Methodist Hospital of Indiana, Inc
  I–65 and 21st Street
  PO Box 1367
  Indianapolis, IN 46206
  317–929–2323
  317–929–2336 (TTY/TTD)
  800–382–9097 (Indiana only)

Iowa

- Mid-Iowa Poison and Drug Information Center
  Iowa Methodist Medical Center
  1200 Pleasant Street
  Des Moines, IA 50309
  515–241–6254
  800–362–2327 (outside Des Moines, Iowa only)
- St Luke's Poison Center
  St Luke's Regional Medical Center
  2720 Stone Park Boulevard
  Sioux City, IA 51104
  712–277–2222
  800–352–2222 (statewide WATS)

Kansas

- Mid–America Poison Control Center
  University of Kansas Medical Center
  Department of Pharmacy, Room B–400
  3901 Rainbow Boulevard
  Kansas City, KS 66160–7231
  913–588–6633
  800–332–6633 (Kansas only)

Kentucky

- Kentucky Regional Poison Center of Kosair Children's Hospital
  315 East Broadway
  PO Box 35070
  Louisville, KY 40232–5070
  502–629–7270
  800–722–5725 (Kentucky only)

Louisiana

- Louisiana Drug and Poison Information Center
  Northeast Louisiana University
  Sugar Hall
  Monroe, LA 71209–6430
  800–256–9822 (Louisiana only)
  318–362–5393
- Terrebone General Medical Center
  936 East Main Street
  Houma, LA 70360
  504–873–4069

Maine

- Maine Poison Control Center
  Maine Medical Center
  22 Bramhall Street
  Portland, ME 04102
  207–871–2950
  800–442–6305 (Maine only)

Maryland

- Maryland Poison Center
  20 North Pine Street
  Baltimore, MD 21201
  410–528–7701
  800–492–2414 (Maryland only)

Massachusetts

- Massachusetts Poison Control System
  300 Longwood Avenue
  Boston, MA 02115
  617–232–2120 (Boston area)
  800–682–9211 (Massachusetts only)
  617–735–6089 (TDD)

Michigan

- Bixby Medical Center Poison Center
  818 Riverside Avenue
  Adrian, MI 49221
  517–263–2412
- Blodgett Regional Poison Center
  1840 Wealthy Street, SE
  Grand Rapids, MI 49506–2968
  800–632–2727 (616 area code only)
  800–356–3232 (TTY)
- Poison Control Center
  Children's Hospital of Michigan
  3901 Beaubien Boulevard
  Detroit, MI 48201
  313–745–5711

Minnesota

- Hennepin Regional Poison Center
  Hennepin County Medical Center
  701 Park Avenue South
  Minneapolis, MN 55415
  612–347–3141
- Minnesota Regional Poison Center
  St Paul–Ramsey Medical Center
  640 Jackson Street
  St Paul, MN 55101
  612–221–2113
  800–222–1222 (Minnesota only)

Mississippi

- Forrest General Hospital
  400 South 28th Avenue
  PO Box 16389
  Hattiesburg, MS 39402
  601–288–4235
- Mississippi Regional Poison Control Center
  University of Mississippi Medical Center
  2500 North State Street
  Jackson, MS 39216
  601–354–7660

Missouri

- Cardinal Glennon Children's Hospital
  Regional Poison Center
  1465 South Grand Boulevard
  St Louis, MO 63104
  314–772–5200
  800–366–8888
- Children's Mercy Hospital
  2401 Gillham Road
  Kansas City, MO 64108
  816–234–3430

Nebraska

- The Poison Center
  8301 Dodge Street
  Omaha, NE 68114
  402–390–5555 (local)
  800–955–9119 (Nebraska and Wyoming only)

New Hampshire

- New Hampshire Poison Information Center
  1 Medical Center Drive
  Lebanon, NH 03756
  603–650–8000

New Jersey

- New Jersey Poison Information and Education System
  201 Lyons Avenue
  Newark, NJ 07112
  800–962–1253

New Mexico

- New Mexico Poison and Drug Information Center
  University of New Mexico
  Albuquerque, NM 87131–1076
  505–843–2551
  800–432–6866 (New Mexico only)

New York

- Central New York Poison Control Center
  750 East Adams Street
  Syracuse, NY 13210
  315–476–4766
- Finger Lakes Regional Poison Center
  University of Rochester Medical Center
  601 Elmwood Avenue
  Box 777
  Rochester, NY 14642
  716–275–5151
  800–333–0542
- Hudson Valley Poison Center
  Phelps Memorial Hospital Center
  701 North Broadway
  North Tarrytown, NY 10591
  914–366–3030
  800–336–6997
- Long Island Regional Poison Control Center
  Winthrop University Hospital
  259 First Street
  Mineola, NY 11501
  516–542–2323
- New York City Poison Center
  455 First Avenue, Room 123
  New York, NY 10016
  212–340–4494
  212–764–7667
  212–689–9014 (TDD)
- Western New York Regional Poison Control Center at Children's Hospital of Buffalo
  219 Bryant Street
  Buffalo, NY 14222
  716–878–7654

North Carolina

- Carolinas Poison Center
  Carolinas Medical Center
  1000 Blythe Boulevard
  PO Box 32861
  Charlotte, NC 28232–4000
  800–848–6946
- Catawba Memorial Hospital Poison Control Center
  810 Fairgrove Church Road
  Hickory, NC 28602
  704–322–6649
- Duke Regional Poison Control Center
  Duke University Medical Center
  Box 3007
  Durham, NC 27710
  7919–684–8111
  800–672–1697 (North Carolina only)
- Triad Poison Center
  1200 North Elm Street
  Greensboro, NC 27401–1020
  919–574–8105 (local)
  800–953–4001 (North Carolina only)

North Dakota

- North Dakota Poison Information Center
  720 Fourth Street North
  Fargo, ND 58122
  701–234–5575
  800–732–2200 (North Dakota only)

Ohio

- Akron Regional Poison Center
  1 Perkins Square
  Akron, OH 44308
  216–379–8562
  800–362–9922 (Ohio only)
  216–258–3066 (TTY)
- Bethesda Poison Control Center
  Bethesda Hospital
  2951 Maple Avenue
  Zanesville, OH 43701
  614–454–4221
- Central Ohio Poison Center
  700 Children's Drive
  Columbus, OH 43205
  800–762–0727 (Dayton area)
  800–682–7625 (central Ohio)
- Cincinnati Drug and Poison Information Center
  231 Bethesda Avenue, ML #144
  Cincinnati, OH 45267–0144
  513–558–5111
  800–872–5111 (Ohio and Cincinnati area)
- Greater Cleveland Poison Control Center
  2074 Abington Road
  Cleveland, OH 44106
  216–231–4455

Oklahoma

- Oklahoma Poison Control Center
  Children's Memorial Hospital
  940 Northeast 13th Street
  Oklahoma City, OK 73104
  405–271–5454

Oregon

- Oregon Poison Center
  Oregon Health Sciences University
  3181 Soutwest Sam Jackson Park Road
  Portland, OR 97201
  503–494–8968
  800–452–7165 (Oregon only)

Pennsylvania

- Central Pennsylvania Poison Center
  University Hospital
  The Milton S Hershey Medical Center
  Hershey, PA 17033
  800–521–6110
- Pittsburgh Poison Center
  One Children's Place
  3705 Fifth Avenue
  Pittsburgh, PA 15213
  412–681–6669
- The Poison Control Center Serving the Greater Philadelphia Metropolitan Area
  One Children's Center
  34th and Civic Center Boulevard
  Philadelphia, PA 19104–4303
  800–722–7112

Rhode Island

- Rhode Island Poison Center
  593 Eddy Street
  Providence, RI 02903
  401–444–5727

South Carolina

- Palmetto Poison Center
  University of South Carolina
  College of Pharmacy
  Columbia, SC 29208
  803–765–7359
  800–922–1117 (South Carolina only)

South Dakota

- McKennan Poison Center
  800 East 21st Street
  Sioux Falls, SD 57117–5045
  605–336–3894
  800–952–0123 (South Dakota only)
  800–843–0505 (Iowa, Minnesota, Nebraska, and North Dakota)

Tennessee

- Middle Tennessee Regional Poison Center
  1161 21st Avenue South
  501 Oxford House
  Nashville, TN 37232–4632
  615–322–6435
  800–288–9999
  615–322–0157 (TDD)
- Southern Poison Center, Inc
  847 Monroe Avenue, Suite 230
  Memphis, TN 38163
  901–528–6048

Texas

- Central Texas Poison Center
  2401 South 31st Street
  Temple, TX 76508
  817–774–2005
- Montgomery County Poison Control Center
  Medical Center Hospital
  504 Medical Center Boulevard
  Conroe, TX 77305
  409–788–8044
- North Texas Poison Center
  PO Box 35926
  Dallas, TX 75043
  214–590–5000
  800–441–0040 (Texas only)
- Texas State Poison Center
  University of Texas Medical Branch
  Galveston, TX 77555–1075
  409–765–1420 (Galveston)
  713–654–1701 (Houston)

Utah

- Utah Regional Poison Control Center
  410 Chipeta Way, Suite 230
  Salt Lake City, UT 84108
  801–581–2151
  800–456–7707 (Utah only)

Vermont

- Vermont Poison Center
  Fletcher Allen Healthcare
  111 Colchester Avenue
  Burlington, VT 05401
  802–658–3456

Virginia

- Blue Ridge Poison Center
  Blue Ridge Hospital
  Box 67
  Charlottesville, VA 22901
  804–924–5543
  800–451–1428 (Virginia only)
- Virginia Poison Center
  Virginia Commonwealth University
  Box 522 MCV Station
  Richmond, VA 23298–0522
  804–786–9123
  800–552–6337 (Virginia only)

Washington

- Washington Poison Center
  PO Box C5371
  Seattle, WA 98105–0371
  206–526–2121
  800–732–6985 (Washington only)

West Virginia

- West Virginia Poison Center
  3110 MacCorkle Avenue, SE
  Charleston, WV 25304
  304–348–4211 (local)
  800–642–3625 (West Virginia only)

Wisconsin

- Poison Center of Eastern Wisconsin
  Children's Hospital of Wisconsin
  PO Box 1997
  Milwaukee, WI 53201
  414–266–2222
  800–815–8855 (Wisconsin only)
- University of Wisconsin Hospital Regional Poison Center
  600 Highland Avenue, E5/238 CSC
  Madison, WI 53792
  608–262–3702

CHAPTER 17

Ostomy Care Products

Michael L. Kleinberg

Questions to ask in patient assessment and counseling

- *What type of ostomy do you have? Where is it located?*
- *How long have you had the ostomy?*
- *Why did you need an ostomy?*
- *Do you irrigate and/or use a pouch?*
- *What type of appliance are you using?*
- *What is the stoma size?*
- *Do you have problems with the skin surrounding the stoma?*
- *Have you noticed any change in the contents of your fecal discharge or urinary output?*
- *Are you experiencing any problems related to your ostomy, such as diarrhea or gas?*
- *Are you having any problems with odor or gas control?*
- *Are you taking any prescription or nonprescription medications or vitamins?*

Ostomy Care

An ostomy is the surgical formation of an opening or outlet through the abdominal wall for the purpose of eliminating waste. It is usually made by passing the colon, small intestine, or ureters through the abdominal wall. The opening of the ostomy is called the stoma. Ostomies may be permanent or temporary and are performed in individuals of all ages, from neonates to the elderly. Reasons for performing ostomies include congenital anomalies, a wide range of acquired conditions (eg, inflammatory bowel disease, cancer, radiation damage), and trauma.[1,2] Approximately 90,000 ostomies are created annually in the United States, and more than 1 million patients have established stomas.[3]

An understanding of the digestive process is important because ostomy surgery interrupts this process. The particular problems associated with each type of ostomy are directly related to the phase of digestion that is interrupted. Major functions of the digestive system include the digestion and absorption of foodstuffs and the absorption of water. Digestion begins in the mouth and continues in the stomach and small intestine; water absorption takes place in the large intestine. (The anatomy of the lower digestive tract and the urinary tract is shown in Figure 1.) (See Chapter 11, "Acid-Peptic Products," and Chapter 13, "Antidiarrheal Products.")

The idea of cutting into the abdominal cavity and creating an artificial opening is not new. This type of surgery was first suggested in 1710 by a French physician, Alexis Littre.[4] Since that time, the technique of ostomy surgery has been refined greatly. The surgical creation of a stoma is only the first step in the rehabilitation of an ostomate (a person with an ostomy). Complete recovery depends on how well ostomy patients understand and adjust to their changed medical and physical circumstances.

Ostomy surgery necessitates the use of an appliance designed to collect the waste material normally eliminated through the bowel or bladder. Because each ostomy patient is different, one patient may benefit from a particular type of appliance whereas another may develop problems with it. The ostomy patient should know how to apply and fit an appliance that affords maximum benefit. It should be recognized that appliance needs may change over time.

Pharmacy involvement in ostomy care is important. The American Pharmaceutical Association identifies ostomy care as an area in which the pharmacist plays a clinical role in direct patient care. Procurement and distribution of ostomy supplies and patient counseling are necessary services that can be provided by the pharmacist. Pharmacists who are involved in ostomy care must be familiar with the various types of ostomies and with the use and maintenance of the appliances for each type of surgery. They should also be prepared to provide patients with information on special needs related to ostomy care, such as skin care, diet, fluid intake, and drug therapy.

Types of Ostomies

Several types of ostomies are performed regularly. They include ileostomy, in which the entire colon and possibly part of the ileum are removed; colostomy (ascending, transverse, descending, and sigmoid), in which the colon is partially removed; and urostomy, or urinary diversion, in which the bladder may be removed.

The normal stoma is shiny, wet, and dark pink or red in color. The stoma does not contain nerve fibers, so it does not transmit pain or other sensations. It may bleed slightly if irritated or rubbed, such as during cleaning;

Editor's Note: This chapter is based, in part, on the chapter with a similar title that appeared in the 10th edition but was written by Michael L. Kleinberg and Moya J. Vazquez.

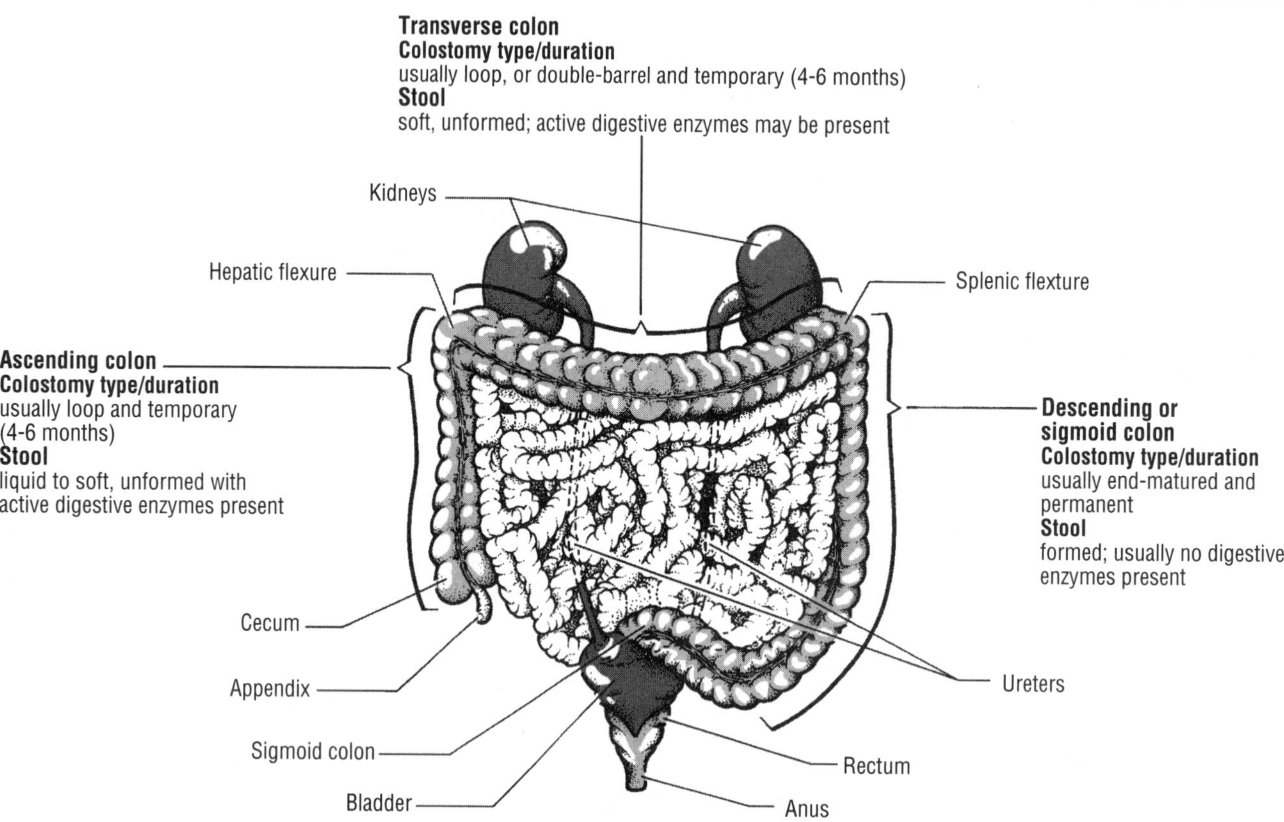

FIGURE 1 Anatomic drawing of the lower digestive and urinary tracts, which depicts the location and permanence of colostomies. Adapted with permission from *Am J Nurs.* 1977; 77(3): 443.

however, the bleeding should not be prolonged, nor should the discharge be bloody. In the adult, the stoma is usually 3/4–2 inches in size, depending on the portion of the bowel or urinary tract used. The stoma gradually shrinks after surgery and reaches its permanent size within several months.

Special problems affecting patients often depend on the location of the ostomy. Skin irritation and electrolyte and fluid imbalance cause more problems in ostomates with a fluid or semisoft stoma discharge. This is a factor for ileostomates, for ascending and transverse colostomates, and for urostomates. Urostomates and ileostomates may also experience an increased incidence of kidney and gallbladder stone formation. Constipation may be a problem in patients with descending and sigmoid colostomies. These and other complications that may occur are addressed in the following sections.

Ileostomy

An ileostomy is a surgically created opening between the ileum and the abdominal wall. Reasons to have ileostomy surgery include ulcerative colitis, Crohn's disease, trauma, familial polyposis, and necrotizing enterocolitis. The two most common disorders requiring ileostomy surgery—ulcerative colitis and Crohn's disease—are inflammatory conditions affecting the intestines. Ulcerative colitis affects the large intestine and rectum. Its clinical course is often prolonged, with the patient experiencing remissions and exacerbations. Crohn's disease may involve any part of the gastrointestinal tract. As the disease progresses, the bowel wall thickens, causing the lumen to narrow. Obstruction may result, requiring surgery. Patients with these diseases may develop debilitating extraintestinal manifestations. In an acute episode, toxic megacolon and perforation are possible. These conditions require surgery. The entire colon is surgically removed, and the ileum is brought to the surface of the abdomen (Figure 2A).

It should be mentioned that a total proctocolectomy, which results in an ileostomy, is considered a cure for the ulcerative colitis patient. Because of the possibility of recurrence, the same surgical procedure is used less often in patients with Crohn's disease. Mortality for elective surgery for ulcerative colitis is in the range of 0–2%; for emergency surgery, mortality is about 4–5%; and for toxic megacolon, it increases to 17%. A major complication of any surgical procedure is infection, either in the wound or in the intra-abdominal cavity. The most common late complication of ileostomy surgery is intestinal obstruction, which occurs in about 10% of ileostomy patients.

An ileostomy usually begins functioning within 36–72 hours after surgery.[2] An effluent may be present, but this does not necessarily indicate that peristalsis has

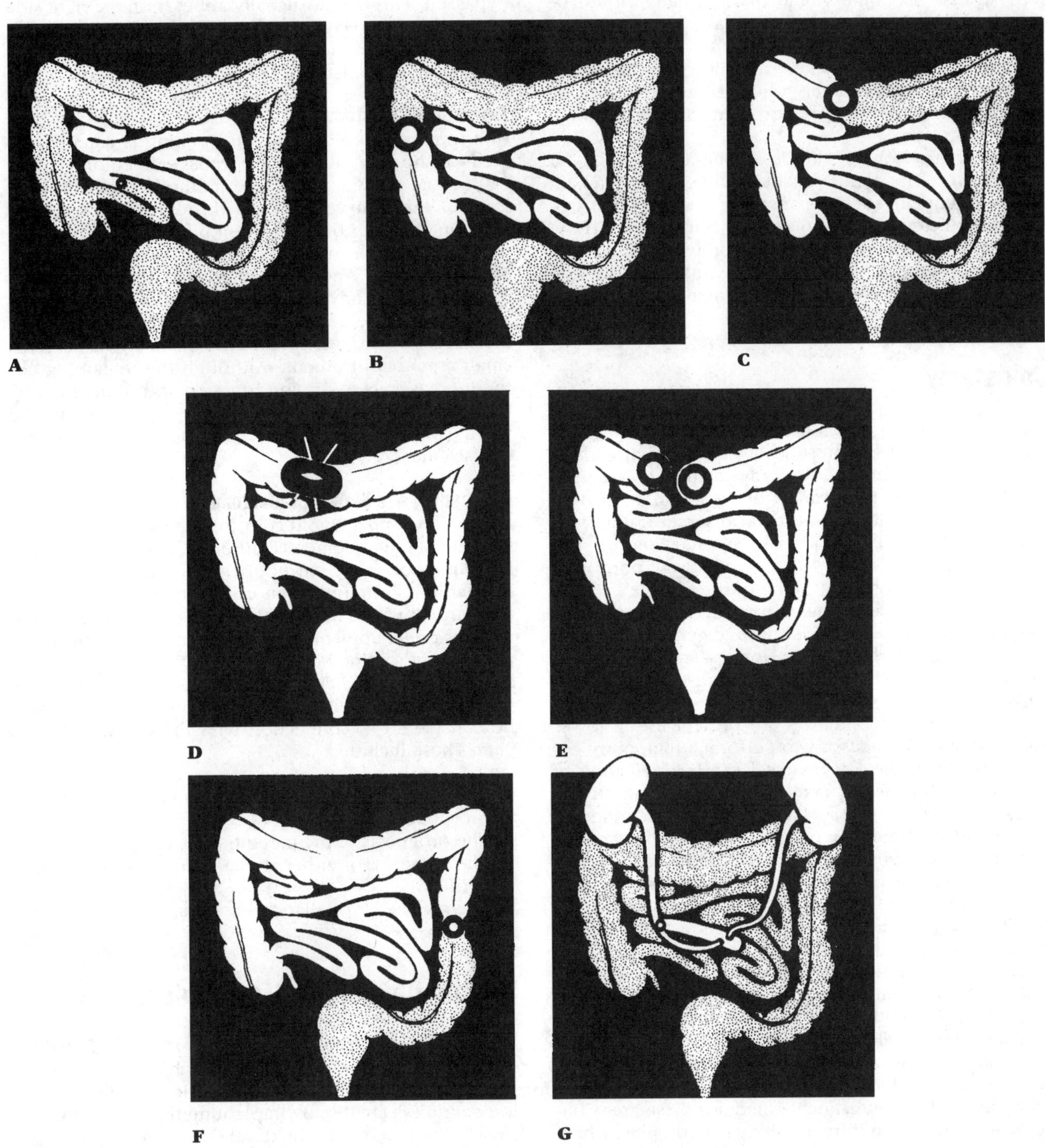

FIGURE 2A–G Types of ostomies: A, ileostomy; B, ascending colostomy; C, transverse colostomy; D, loop ostomy; E, double-barrel colostomy; F, descending or sigmoid colostomy; G, ileal conduit. Adapted from the *Hollister Ostomy Reference Chart*, ©Copyright 1978, 1979, 1980, Hollister, Inc (all rights reserved); and Wuest JR. *J Am Pharm Assoc*. 1975; NS15: 626.

returned. Initially, the discharge is liquid. As the small bowel adapts, more fluid is absorbed and the discharge may become semisoft. The discharge is liquid to semisoft because it contains fluid that normally would be absorbed from the large bowel. When the colon is removed, the body loses the capacity to reabsorb water. Therefore, ileostomates must maintain adequate fluid intake to compensate for this water loss, especially during the initial postoperative period characterized by high output.

Excoriation of the skin is a common problem for ileostomates. The continuous flow of liquid or semisoft discharge contains active pancreatic enzymes that irritate unprotected skin and digest the skin protein. However, diligent hygiene and special protective measures can help prevent these problems. Because patients with standard ileostomies are never continent, an appliance must be worn at all times.

Colostomy

A colostomy is the creation of an artificial opening using part of the large intestine or colon. Major indications for performing a colostomy include obstruction of the colon or rectum, cancer of the colon or rectum, genetic malformation, diverticular disease, trauma, radiation colitis, and loss of anal muscular control. The three types of colostomies are named for the portion of the bowel that is brought to the outside of the body to form the stoma: ascending colostomies, transverse colostomies (further subdivided into temporary loop colostomies, double-barrel colostomies, and permanent stoma colostomies), and descending or sigmoid colostomies (Figure 1).

When certain conditions are present in the lower bowel, it may be necessary to perform a temporary colostomy so that the lower bowel can heal. Healing of the diseased bowel may take several weeks, months, or years. Eventually, the colon and rectum are reconnected and bowel continuity is restored. A permanent colostomy is formed when the rectum is removed. A colostomy, permanent or temporary, may be made in any part of the colon.

The type of colostomy the surgeon will perform depends on the condition being treated. If the disease entity is cancer, the section of bowel may be resected without a colostomy. If the lesion is in the lower rectum, however, the entire rectum is removed, resulting in a permanent colostomy. The most common disease that may result in a colostomy is diverticulitis. It presents as small balloon-like areas or outpouchings in the lining of the large intestine. Sometimes these areas become irritated and rupture, resulting in peritonitis, which usually requires emergency surgery. To protect the perforated section and the suture line when this area is surgically removed, a temporary colostomy may be performed. The opening can be made at any point in the bowel above the lesion. The more proximal the colostomy, the more watery and frequent the output will be. When the disease process is resolved and the suture line is healed, a comparatively minor operation is performed to restore the continuity of the large intestine and close the colostomy.

Ascending Colostomy

In an ascending colostomy, the ascending colon is retained but the rest of the large bowel is removed or bypassed. This ostomy usually appears on the right side of the abdomen (Figure 2B). Its discharge is semiliquid because the fluid has not been reabsorbed. The patient must wear an appliance continuously.

Transverse Colostomy

In a transverse colostomy, an opening is usually created on the right side of the transverse colon (Figure 2C) in one of two ways. One method entails lifting a loop of the transverse colon through the abdominal incision. A rod or bridge is then placed under the loop to give additional support (Figure 2D) and is removed after a few days. Another method is to divide the bowel completely and have two openings (double-barrel colostomy) (Figure 2E). In this case, the proximal stoma discharges fecal material and the distal stoma secretes small amounts of mucus. Although the remaining colon increases its hydrating function with time, the discharge generally stays semisoft. An appliance must be worn continuously in patients who have transverse colostomies.

Descending and Sigmoid Colostomies

Descending and sigmoid colostomies usually are on the left side of the abdomen (Figure 2F). They can be made as double- or single-barrel openings. Because the fecal discharge is firm and often can be regulated by irrigation, an appliance may not be needed. However, many patients prefer appliances to irrigation. A long-term complication of routine bowel irrigation in some patients is a loss of bowel tonicity. When this occurs, the bowel is unable to function without irrigation. Several factors should be considered in connection with the decision to irrigate. These include:[5]

- The capability of the patient to manage the irrigation procedure;
- The prognosis of the patient;
- The presence of either stomal stenosis or peristomal hernia;
- The presence of radiation enteritis.

Urinary Diversions (Urostomies)

Urinary diversions are performed as a result of bladder loss or dysfunction usually caused by cancer, neurogenic bladder, or genetic malformation. An ileal or colon conduit is created by implanting the ureters into an isolated loop of bowel, the distal end of which is brought to the surface of the abdomen (Figure 2G). An appliance must be worn continuously. In another procedure, a ureterostomy, the ureters are detached from the bladder and brought to the outside of the abdominal wall. This procedure is performed less frequently because the ureters tend to narrow unless they have been dilated permanently by previous disease. Urinary stomas should function immediately following surgery. It should be noted that mucous shreds will be present if the bowel is used to create the diversion.[2]

Continent Diversions

The objective of a continent diversion is to construct a reservoir inside the body, usually from a section of intestinal, urinary, or gastric mucosa, to accommodate fecal or urinary discharge.[6]

Continent Ileostomy

Researchers are continually working on ways to render the ileostomate continent. One procedure, developed by Dr Nils Kock of Sweden, may be an alternative for those who meet certain criteria.[7] The surgeon creates a pouch internally, made from 35–50 cm of ileum. An intussusception of the bowel is used to create a "nipple" that renders the patient continent for stool and flatus. The distal limb of the ileum is brought to the abdomen. A flush stoma is made just above the hairline. The pouch is emptied by inserting a catheter through the nipple into the pouch. At first, the pouch holds approximately 75 mL. It stretches with use so that 6 months postoperatively it can hold 600–800 mL without discomfort or danger. At this time, the pouch needs to be drained only three or four times a day.

Restorative Proctocolectomy

Restorative proctocolectomy involves sparing the rectum of those with ulcerative colitis or familial polyposis. The mucosa is stripped from the rectum, rendering it free of disease. An internal pouch is created from the small bowel, but without a nipple valve. The distal end of the ileum is then pulled through the rectum and attached. Thus, the sphincter is preserved and no ostomy is necessary. Because of the different ways the internal pouch can be constructed, one may hear this operation described as an S or J pouch. Recipients of this procedure have more frequent bowel movements and may experience some perianal skin irritation.

Because the diseases and conditions requiring ileostomy surgery are found primarily in persons 15–25 years of age, the advantages of this operation are obvious. For those in the prime of their athletic, social, and sexual lives, the absence of an external pouch allows a speedy adjustment and rehabilitation. Not everyone is a candidate for this surgery, however. Among the factors taken into consideration are the patient's age (ideally, between 15 and 50), intelligence, motivation, other handicaps, and general health, including the absence of Crohn's disease.

Continent Urostomy

Dr Kock has developed an operation to render urinary diversion patients continent. It is very much like the continent ileostomy described above, except that the ureters are inserted into the proximal limb of the ileum leading into the isolated internal ileal pouch, and an additional nipple valve is created at the proximal opening of the pouch. This keeps the urine from refluxing into the kidneys, thus lessening the chance of infection. Other continent urinary operations, such as the Indiana pouch, have been devised, but they are all similar in that the pouch is drained by a catheter.

Appliances and Accessories

The appliance is an extremely important aspect of the ostomate's well-being. The ostomate has lost a normal body function; the appliance takes over that lost function and almost becomes a part of the body. The type of appliance depends on the type of surgery performed. Patients with regulated colostomies (those who irrigate routinely with no output from the stoma between irrigations) may wear closed-end appliances, a stoma cover or cap, or a gauze square. Those with unregulated colostomies and ileostomies usually wear open-end appliances to allow frequent emptying. Although appliances are available for infants, some ostomies in infants are managed with a diaper instead if the effluent is not caustic to the skin. Because water will not enter the stoma, it is not necessary to cover it while swimming, bathing, or showering. However, the new pouch adhesives allow the patient to keep the system in place during these activities, if desired.

The ostomy pouching system is composed of a pouch that is secured to the skin by an adhesive skin barrier. The ideal ostomy system should be leakproof, ordorprof, comfortable, easily manipulated, inconspicuous, inexpensive, and safe.[8] Unfortunately, no one appliance meets all of these criteria. (See Appendix 1 at the end of this chapter for a list of major manufacturers of ostomy products and accessories; see also the product tables "Ostomy Appliances" and "Ostomy Accessories.")

Adult and adolescent patients must be taught all the self-care skills required to maintain the stoma, including sizing the stoma, cutting a pouch or skin barrier to fit the stoma, applying paste or powder, cleaning the skin, applying the pouch, removing the pouch, and emptying the pouch. The patient must be prepared for stoma functioning at any time during the pouch changing procedure.[2,9]

For several weeks after the ostomy procedure, patients often need assistance in changing the pouch. If the stoma is poorly placed, there are complications; if the patient is debilitated, routine assistance may be required. Ostomy needs are often difficult or embarrassing for patients and their families to discuss, especially initially. Self-esteem is often damaged in patients with an ostomy; therefore, when assisting the patient with ostomy needs, the pharmacist must take special care to avoid verbal or facial expressions that might convey negative feelings regarding the procedure.

Pouching Equipment

The surgical technique used to create the stoma influences the pouching equipment required, the complexity of the pouching procedure, and the risks of stomal and peristomal complications (eg, necrosis, stenosis, hernia). In the past, most ostomy appliances were reusable. The advantages of reusable appliances are their durability, availability in numerous configurations, and relatively low cost. Their disadvantages are that they require cleaning before each use and that they are heavy, tend to retain odor, and often require a separate skin barrier. Reusable appliances may still be the best choice for some patients because of the many modalities available for treatment.

Most ostomates are now fitted with odorproof, lightweight, disposable appliances. Most of these appliances incorporate a skin barrier in each flange, eliminating the need for a separate skin barrier. The disposable equipment is available in one- and two-piece systems. The two-piece system allows the patient to center the flange easily and to change the pouch, if desired, without removing the flange from the skin. The one-piece system is very flat; it has no ring that might be noticeable through clothes. It is also easy to apply and is generally more pliable and adaptable to different abdominal contours. Reusable and disposable appliances are available in both transparent and opaque styles and in various sizes. The pouch opening may be sizable or presized. If sizable, the stoma pattern is traced onto the skin barrier wafer surface of the pouch and cut out before applying.

Newer one-piece convexity pouches are available with oval openings that fit flush with the skin, allowing the contents to flow into the pouch without leaking onto the skin. Flushable one-piece pouches also are available for use by patients with colostomies. They are not practical for patients with ileostomies or urostomies, however, because of the frequency of output.

The pouch should be emptied when it is one-third to one-half full to prevent leakage. With a two-piece system, the closed-end pouch is simply removed from the flange for easy emptying. Some patients using the two-piece system alternate the use of two pouches. The full pouch is removed, replaced by a second pouch, emptied, washed, and then reused when the second pouch is changed. One-piece closed-end systems are removed and disposed of once or twice daily, while those that are drainable can be left in place as long as they are comfortable and there is no leakage. The flange and skin barrier may be left in place for 3–7 days, depending on the condition of the skin and skin barrier. Although activities such as swimming or playing tennis may decrease the wear time of the pouch, this should not discourage participation in physical activities.

Belts

Special belts attached to various appliances give additional support. Belts are made for specific appliances and generally are not interchangeable. Not all ostomates need to wear belts. Indications for use are a deeply convex faceplate, poor wearing time, activity (especially in children), heavy perspiration, and personal preference. Belts may cause ulcers if worn too tight. To be effective, the belt must be kept even with the belt hooks. If the belt slips up around the waist, it may cause poor adherence and possibly a cut of the stoma.

Skin Barriers

Skin barriers are intended to protect the skin immediately adjacent to the stoma from the stoma discharge. They also correct imperfections in the skin surface, allowing the appliance to fit securely. Skin barriers, powders, and pastes are available for special skin problems. The powder is used on weeping skin. The paste (which is not a glue but has a pasty consistency) is used to seal around the stoma and to fill in creases in the skin. (Skin barrier paste is generally required only in patients who have problems with leakage or have uneven contours.) These products produce a flat surface for application of other skin barriers.

Solid wafer skin barriers are preattached to the pouch (one-piece system) or provided separately (two-piece system) and may be custom cut (sizable) or precut (presized). The opening in the skin barrier wafer should match the size and shape of the stoma. To apply a skin barrier, the patient should apply a bead of skin barrier paste around the stoma or directly to the edge of the skin barrier wafer, apply the skin barrier wafer to wrinkle-free skin, and then press the skin barrier around the stoma to improve adherence.

Solid wafer skin barriers may melt if exposed to high temperatures. Therefore, during the summer, especially when traveling, the solid wafer skin barrier should be put in an insulated box (ice is not required) to minimize the risk of melting.

Skin Protective Dressings

A waterproof dressing can be applied to the skin in a thin film, which might be described as a chemical bandage. After application, the product leaves a thin protective layer on the skin that aids in the removal of adhesive tape and absorbs the stress normally applied to the top layers of the skin when the ostomy appliance is removed. Although these dressings promote skin protection, they do not replace skin barriers. When the skin is reddened but unbroken, these preparations briefly protect the skin from the contact agent causing the redness. They also can help to protect the skin around a draining wound. These dressings come in varying forms: gel, bottle (with brush), spray can, roll-on, and wipe-on packets.

Transparent, semipermeable dressings come in many sizes, from one used for intravenous sites to a complete body wrap. These dressings are transparent, sterile materials that are sticky on one side; they can be used as a dressing, as a second skin to which appliances are affixed, or as a prophylactic for preventing skin irritation. They take some dexterity to apply, however, and two persons may be needed to apply larger pieces.

Cleansing and Special Skin Care Products

The stoma and surrounding skin are best cleansed with plain water. If soap is used, it should be rinsed off thoroughly and the skin dried before a new pouching system is applied. Moisturizers and lanolin-containing products should be avoided because they prevent the pouching system from adhering to the skin.

Several companies manufacture products especially for the incontinent patient or others at high risk of excoriation. The products include a gentle liquid cleaner that renders output odorless, a cream that can be rubbed into the skin and to which the appliance will adhere, and an ointment that is not water soluble and gives high-grade protection to vulnerable areas where pouching is not appropriate.

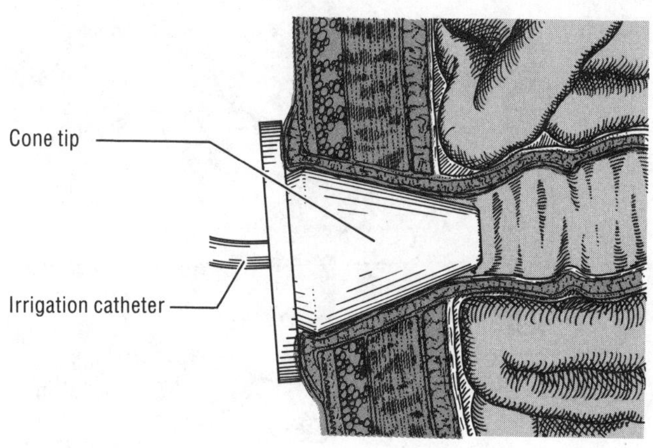

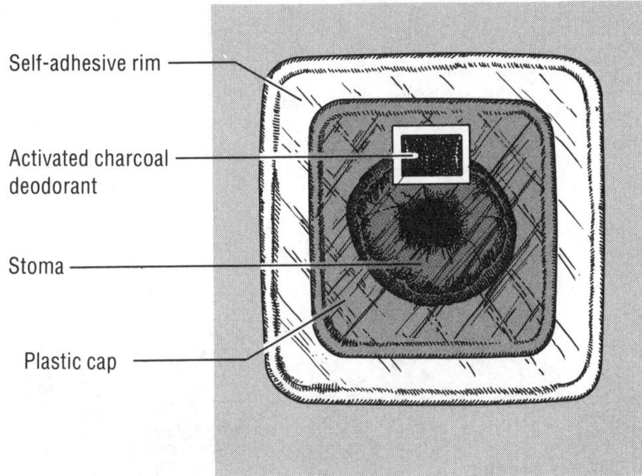

FIGURE 3 Colostomy irrigation set. A cone-tipped irrigator is preferred to a plain catheter to avoid possibility of false passage and bowel perforation. Adapted with permission from *Clinical Symposia*, illustrated by John A. Craig, MD, ©Copyright 1978 CIBA-GEIGY Corporation (all rights reserved).

Tape

Hypoallergenic tape supports appliances. A strip may be applied across the top, bottom, and sides of the faceplate, with half on the faceplate and half on the skin. Waterproof tape may be used during swimming or bathing.

Irrigating Sets

In patients who are candidates for irrigation, control can be maintained without a pouch. A good candidate for irrigation is an adult patient with a colostomy distal to the splenic flexure who does not have a history of irritable bowel or a disabling handicap. For the process to be safe and effective, a colostomy irrigation set, rather than a standard enema set, should be used. This set consists of a reservoir for the irrigating fluid, a tube, a graduated clamp, a soft catheter, and a dam or cone (Figure 3). Perforation of the bowel is a serious complication of irrigation, but it has almost been eliminated by use of a cone, which is inserted ½–1 inch into the colostomy. In patients who are not able to use a cone, the catheter should not be inserted more than 2 inches past the dam. Although introducing water into the bowel stimulates peristalsis, control (ie, at least 24 hours without any output) is rarely achieved unless the colostomate instills and holds in a prescribed amount of water. Therefore, the dam takes the place of the absent sphincter, allowing the patient to hold in the water.

Frequency of irrigation depends somewhat on the colostomate's normal bowel habits. After control is achieved, the patient may wear a security pouch or a piece of gauze, stoma cover, or cap over the stoma. Irrigation is not necessary for health; it is merely one method of management.

Deodorizers

With properly fitted, disposable, odorproof pouches, deodorizers are not required as often as they are with the reusable systems. In most cases, regular changing of the appliance is all that is needed to prevent odor. Oral deodorizers (internal or systemic) or those inserted into the pouch (external or local) can be used to reduce stool odor. Oral deodorizers, which are most often used in patients with colostomies, include bismuth subgallate and chlorophyllin copper complex. Liquid concentrates are available as companion products of most ostomy devices; they can be placed directly into the pouch to neutralize odor. A common household remedy is to add one capful of mouthwash to the pouch. Specially formulated bathroom sprays are also available. Ostomates sometimes place aspirin tablets in the pouch to control odor, but this practice should not be used because aspirin may irritate the stoma and cause ulceration.

In addition to local methods of odor control, devices are available that fit directly on the pouch to filter and control gas and odors. One such commercial device is a charcoal filter.

Fitting and Application

Measuring the stoma to determine the proper fit of an appliance is an important part of ostomy care. An appliance with an opening smaller than the stoma may cause abrasion of the stoma and poor wearing time. An appliance with an opening larger than necessary, even with a snug-fitting skin barrier, may allow skin excoriation and hyperplasia formation. Considerations in fitting the appliance include body contour, stoma location, skin creases and scars, and type of ostomy. The lack of uniformity in types of ostomies and ostomy equipment makes it difficult to give standard instructions for application. Some procedures for applying different types of appliances and their accessories (Figure 4) are discussed in greater detail

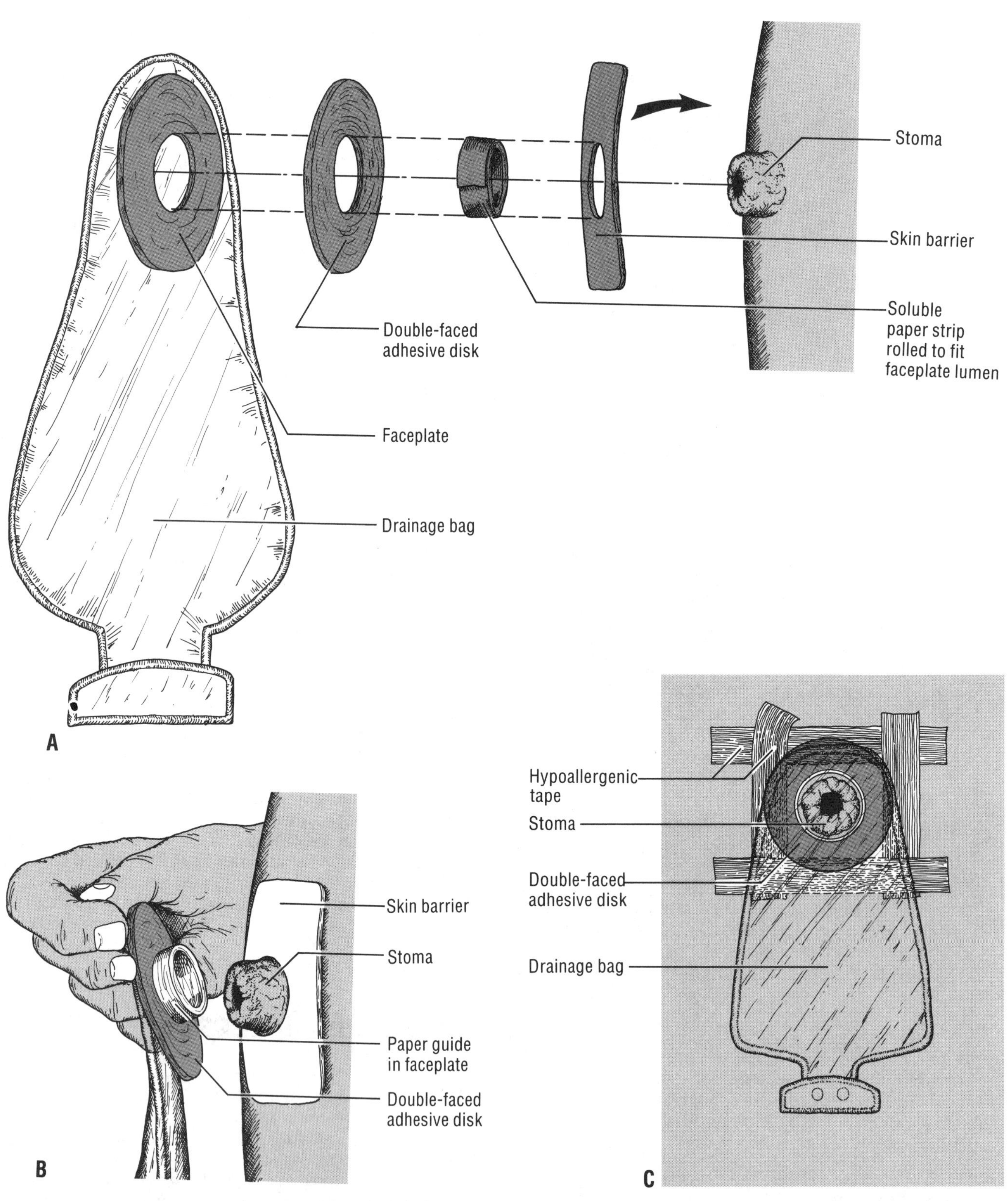

FIGURE 4A–C Components of an ileostomy appliance: A, drainable bag and skin barrier; B, after skin barrier is affixed to skin, the appliance is placed, using paper strip guide to align faceplate lumen over stoma; C, hypoallergenic tape placed around faceplate in "picture frame" fashion.

in readily available patient-oriented pamphlets.[2,9–11] An enterostomal therapy (ET) nurse is an excellent source of assistance in the custom fitting of these appliances.

Potential Complications

Ostomates may experience both psychologic and physical complications. The pharmacist should be prepared to handle these complications or refer patients to an ET nurse. A thorough explanation before surgery of the type of surgery to be performed, what to expect during the postsurgical recovery period, and the appliances and supplies the patient will use often alleviates the patient's anxiety.

Psychologic Complications

After ostomy surgery, depending on previous mental status and self-confidence, the patient may be psychologically depressed. There may also be fears of not being able to engage in former work, participate in sports, perform sexually, or have children. The pharmacist should reassure the patient that the ability to carry out these activities or functions generally remains unchanged. However, the pharmacist should be aware that most men who have a radical resection of the rectum or bladder are rendered organically impotent. Penile implants or other erection aids could enable a man to regain part or all of this function. If the patient is concerned about impotence, a referral to his urologist would be appropriate. Adverse effects on sexual function also have been reported in women.[12]

The United Ostomy Association, formed in 1962, comprises various ostomy organizations in the United States whose main purpose is to help ostomy patients by giving moral support and supplying information. The names and addresses of those organizations are listed in Appendix 2 at the end of this chapter.

ET is a nursing specialty. Registered nurses with postgraduate education from an accredited school for ET may specialize in ostomy care. A representative listing of ET nurses may be obtained from the Executive Secretary, Wound Ostomy and Continence Nurses Society (WOCN). (See Appendix 2 for address and telephone number.)

Physical Complications

Physical complications of ostomies include stenosis of the stoma, fistula formation, prolapse, retraction, peristomal hernia, and skin irritation. A continuing series of articles concerning physical problems, their assessment, and care has been published in the medical literature.[1,2,13–15]

Stenosis

Stenosis (narrowing) of the stoma is caused by the formation of scar tissue. Excessive scar tissue usually is caused by improper surgical construction, postoperative ischemia, active disease, or alkaline stomatitis or dermatitis. Although dilation of the stoma is often advocated to prevent or palliate this problem, the only cure is revision of the stoma.

Fistula

The formation of an opening, or fistula tract, from inside the body to the skin most often is a manifestation of inflammatory bowel disease. Other causes of this complication are cancer, abscess formation, foreign body retention, radiation, tuberculosis, and trauma. Treatment is with hyperalimentation, surgery, or both.

Prolapse

Prolapse, the telescoping of the bowel through the stoma, frequently results when the opening in the abdominal wall is too large. Women with ileostomies occasionally experience prolapse of the ileostomy during pregnancy. Other causes include inadequate fixation of the bowel to the abdominal wall, poorly developed fascial support, or increased abdominal pressure associated with tumors, coughing, or crying (the latter being of special concern in infants). The prolapse may be reduced by lying on the back and applying continuous pressure against the most distal part of the stoma. Once it is reduced, rigid ring appliances should be avoided because of the risk of strangulation; the appliance may need to be resized. The danger of prolapse is the resultant decrease in blood supply to the bowel outside the abdominal cavity. In some cases, surgical correction may be required.

Retraction

Retraction is the recession of the stoma to a subnormal length. It may be caused by several factors, including active Crohn's disease and weight gain, and may lead to damage of the skin surface. If it is not severe, a convex pouching system may be all that is required. In other cases, treatment is surgical correction.

Peristomal Hernia

Peristomal hernia is the protrusion of the colon or ileum into the subcutaneous layers of the skin around the stoma. Peristomal hernia can be managed by modification of the pouching equipment or technique, modification of clothing, dietary changes, or surgery.

Skin Irritation

The most common causes of skin irration are output excoriation, sensitivity to a product, epithelial hyperplasia, alkaline dermatitis, infection, or Crohn's disease.

Output Excoriation Excoriation, an abrasion of the epidermis by digestive enzymes from output, occurs when an improper pouch is worn, the lumen in the faceplate is too big, or the pouch has leaked and has not been promptly replaced. These problems can allow fecal or urinary output to come in contact with the skin. Fecal output may contain active pancreatic enzymes (especially in the case of an ileostomy) that digest the skin protein. The alkaline nature of the fecal output also is irritating to unprotected skin. Alkaline urine is similarly irritating and causes excoriation. These two conditions are treated differently. After diagnosis and treatment, a skin barrier and pouch may be applied. The pouch should be changed as infrequently as possible to lessen irritation, and treatment should be continued until the skin is clear.

Sensitivity Patch testing of patients with a history of allergy, adhesive tape reaction, eczema, or psoriasis and those with very fair skin can help prevent skin irritation caused by sensitivity to a product. Patch testing can easily be done by the physician or ET nurse and checked by the patient at home.

Hyperplasia Hyperplasia, the overgrowth of hyperplastic skin, occurs when the faceplate opening is too large. In the early stages there is no pain, but later the affected skin cells multiply and cause agonizing pain. The condition resembles a mucosal malignancy. Treatment entails ensuring that the pouch has the correct size opening and that the seal is secure; to this end, sealants, skin barrier powder, or a support device (eg, a belt) may be used. A convex faceplate that is just slightly larger than the stoma is applied, and a snug belt may be added. A mild case of hyperplasia generally resolves in 1 week. Severe cases, although treated the same, may take from 4–6 weeks to heal. Other treatment methods are cauterization and surgical removal.

Alkaline Dermatitis Many patients with urinary diversions have problems with alkaline urine. Although normal urine is not particularly irritating to intact skin, urine that is alkaline may have gross effects on the stoma and skin. It is a major cause of frank blood in the pouch because it renders the stoma extremely friable.

The treatment is to acidify the urine. The patient should avoid alkaline ash foods, especially citrus fruits and juices, which, although originally acidic, are excreted in alkaline form. Ascorbic acid or cranberry juice acidifies the urine.

To minimize the risk of irritation due to alkaline urine, a cloth soaked with a solution of one-third white vinegar to two-thirds water can be applied for 5–10 minutes to the stoma at least once weekly before putting on the appliance. Patients using a two-piece system can apply the solution as often as three to four times daily. The frequency of application is determined by the severity of the case. The vinegar may cause the stoma to blanche, but this is not indicative of damage. Most of the new urinary appliances have an antireflux feature, which keeps the urine from resting on the stoma or exposed skin, thus preventing the development of this condition.

Infection With the possible exception of patients with Crohn's disease, ostomates do not have more frequent infections of the peristomal skin, or other skin, than do nonostomates. However, an infection under the faceplate can be a problem. If the skin is indurated, swollen, and red, it may need incision and draining. At that time, a sample is taken and sent to the lab for culture and sensitivity testing. The appropriate antibiotic can be prescribed topically, systemically, or both. It may be a challenge to devise a way of containing the discharge while leaving the affected area accessible for treatment.

Monilial infection may be a problem in patients who wear appliances continuously. A dark, warm, moist environment provides an area for growth of species of *Candida*. The primary symptom is itching. If the condition is diagnosed early, an application of nystatin powder or 2% miconazole powder is useful. If the infection is allowed to continue unchecked, the skin will become denuded, the faceplate will not stick, and additional skin irritation will result from the output. The antifungal preparation should be used every other day and for 1 week after the skin has become clear.

In treating monilial infections, it is also important to ascertain whether the ostomate is taking antibiotics. Any antibiotic, but especially a broad-spectrum agent, changes the flora of the skin, and the entrenched monilia can become difficult to eradicate. For ostomy patients taking antibiotics, nystatin powder or 2% miconazole powder should be continued for 1 month after the monilial infection is gone.

Excessive Sweating Sweating under the faceplate can decrease wearing time and cause monilial infection. A skin cement and a belt may be necessary to hold the appliance in place. Discomfort from perspiration underneath the collection pouch can be alleviated by purchasing or making a cover or bib to keep the pouch material from touching the skin.

Diarrhea Resulting in Dehydration Ileostomates and ascending colostomates are at risk of severe diarrhea. This can be a result of flu, food poisoning, or other gastrointestinal irritants. The stool becomes very voluminous and watery, and fluid and electrolytes are lost rapidly. Often the only way to replace the loss adequately is by administering intravenous fluids. Patients must be aware of the risk of diarrhea so that they can seek medical treatment before dehydration results.

Diet

Diet does not play an important role in management of the ostomy patient. Most patients can eat a liberal diet, including all the foods eaten before surgery, if the foods are chewed well. However, it is wise to remain on a diet low in fiber for the first 6 weeks after surgery to allow the intestine to heal and swelling to resolve. After that time, a regular diet can be resumed. Urostomates may want to avoid asparagus or other foods that cause odor. Irrigating colostomates should avoid any food that causes them to have loose stools. (This varies with each individual.) Patients with ileostomies are more prone to obstruction from high-roughage foods eaten in large quantities or exclusive of other food; such potentially troublesome foods include popcorn, nuts, corn on the cob, mushrooms, bran products, citrus fruits, coconut, Chinese vegetables, raw celery, and raw carrots. These patients should chew these foods well and eat them in small amounts and with other food.

Because they have no control over gas passage, fecal ostomates may prefer to cut down on gas-forming foods such as beans, vegetables of the cabbage family (onions, broccoli, cauliflower, cabbage), beer, and carbonated drinks. Stool odor can be minimized by reducing the consumption of fish, eggs, asparagus, garlic, beans, turnips, foods in the cabbage family, and some vitamins or medications.

Patients with a urostomy, ileostomy, or ascending colostomy must include an adequate amount of fluid in their diets to prevent the precipitation of crystals or kidney stones in the urine. Absence of the large bowel may not allow the normal absorption of water needed to maintain urinary volume.

TABLE 1 Effects of certain medications on the ostomate

	Colostomate	Ileostomate	Urostomate
Dosage Forms			
Chewable tablets	1	1	1
Enteric-coated tablets	1	3	1
Sustained-release medication	1	3	1
Liquid medication	1	1	1
Gelatin capsules	1	1	1
Compounds			
Alcohol	1	1	1
Antibiotics (poorly absorbed)	1	2,3	1,2
Antidiarrheal agents	1,2	1	1
Calcium-containing antacids	2	2	2
Corticosteroids	1	2	1
Diuretics	1	2	2
Magnesium-containing antacids	2	2	1
Opiates	1,2	1	1
Salicylates	1	1	1
Salt substitutes	1	2	1
Stool softeners	1	2	1
Sulfa drugs	1	1	2
Vitamins	1	2	1

Key:
1 means medication probably has no adverse effects.
2 means medication may cause an increase in adverse effects; patient should be monitored.
3 means medication may be ineffective; patient should be monitored.

Use of Medications

Because part or all of the colon is removed and intestinal transit time may be altered, the ostomate may experience adverse effects from taking prescription or nonprescription medications, or the medications may be ineffective (Table 1).

Coated or sustained-release preparations may pass through the intestinal tract without being absorbed, and the patient may receive a subtherapeutic dose. The ostomate should look for any undissolved drug particles in the pouch. Liquid preparations or preparations that are crushed or chewed before swallowing are best.

The ostomate also must be careful in taking antibiotics, diuretics, and laxatives. Antibiotics may alter the normal flora of the intestinal tract, causing diarrhea or fungal infection of the skin surrounding the stoma. If diarrhea occurs, fluid and electrolyte intake should be increased. Antidiarrheal and antimotility drugs may affect ileal excreta.[16] The physician may prescribe nystatin or miconazole powder to treat fungal overgrowth.

Sulfa drugs should be used with caution. Crystallization in the kidney may occur more often in patients having difficulty with fluid balance. To minimize this problem, fluid intake should be increased and the urine should not be acidified. In ileostomy patients, whose fluid and electrolyte balance is more difficult to maintain, diuretics should be given with care because additional loss of fluid may cause dehydration and electrolyte imbalance.[17] The ileostomate should be monitored for signs of hyponatremia if salt substitutes are prescribed.

Laxatives may be used by colostomy patients, but only under close supervision. Ostomates tend to become obstructed, and the laxative's particular action may cause perforation. If the colostomate is constipated, a stool softener may be recommended. Both prokinetic agents (eg, metoclopramide, cisapride) and antacids may cause problems and should be taken with caution. Products containing calcium may cause calcium stones in the urostomate; products containing magnesium may cause diarrhea in the ileostomate; and aluminum products may cause constipation in the colostomate. To alleviate any anxiety, the patient should be counseled about medications that may discolor the feces. Some of these medications and the discoloration they cause are listed below[18]:

- *Aluminum antacids*: whitish color or speckling;
- *Antibiotics (oral)*: greenish gray;
- *Anticoagulants (excess)*: pink to red to black (bleeding);
- *Bismuth salts*: black;
- *Charcoal*: black;
- *Chlorophyll*: green;
- *Ferrous salts*: black;
- *Heparin*: pink to red to black (bleeding);
- *Indomethacin (Indocin)*: green;
- *Oxphenbutazone (Tandearil)*: pink to red to black (bleeding);
- *Phenazopyridine (Pyridium)*: orange red;
- *Phenolphthalein*: red;
- *Salicylates*: pink to red to black (bleeding);
- *Senna (and other anthraquinone derivatives)*: yellow-green to brown.

Case Studies

Case 17–1

Patient Complaint/History

CG, a 57-year-old male, presents to the pharmacist with a complaint of severe itching of the skin. During questioning of the patient, the pharmacist learns that CG was diagnosed with diverticulitis 10 years ago and had a sigmoid colostomy 2 years ago. The patient noticed severe itching around the stoma a couple of days earlier for which she is applying Benadryl cream. She also noticed very loose, black stools for which she takes Pepto-Bismol. Physical observation of the stoma reveals that it is red and slightly swollen around the face plate. The patient, who wears a close-ended, one-piece, flushable appliance, reports that she is very diligent about replacing the appliance each morning and each night at bedtime.

CG's current medication use includes Biaxin 500 mg q12h for 14 days for a sinus infection (she is on day 6 of therapy); Seldane-D one tablet bid; Tylenol 500 mg q6h prn for pain; Bendadryl cream 2% prn for itching; and Pepto-Bismol 30 mL three to four times a day.

Clinical Considerations/Strategies

The following considerations/strategies are provided to aid the reader in (1) determining whether treatment of the patient's condition with nonprescription medications is warranted, (2) selecting the appropriate nonprescription medication, and (3) developing a patient counseling strategy to ensure optimal therapeutic outcomes:

- Assess the possible cause(s) of the severe itching.
- Assess the possible cause(s) of the diarrhea and black stools.
- Determine the appropriate response to the clinical situation.
- Determine what potential effects the patient's medication regimen (prescription and nonprescription) would have in a person who does not have a colostomy.
- Develop a patient education/counseling strategy that will:
  - Ensure that the patient understands the importance of nonpharmacologic treatment;
  - Ensure that the patient knows when to contact a health care provider.

Case 17–2

Patient Complaint/History

HR, a 32-year-old male, presents to the pharmacist with a complaint of skin irritation around an ileostomy; he says that he has had several bouts of skin irritation in the past 2 months. The patient goes on to reveal that 10 years ago he was diagnosed with Crohn's disease, which was treated with prednisone and sulfasalazine. About 2 years ago, he was hospitalized for an acute exacerbation of the condition. Following a diagnosis of partial obstruction of the small bowel at the terminal ileum, the patient received an ileostomy.

When asked about his appliance and ostomy cleaning regimen, HR explains that he empties his open-ended two-piece appliance four times a day. He also applies a skin paste barrier and skin barrier wafer weekly; he ran out of the custom cut material and has been using a precut wafer for the past 2 weeks. He cleans the stoma with Dial soap once a week at the same time the wafer is changed.

For the past 6 months, HR has been taking the following allergy medications: Beconase AQ two puffs intranasally qAM and qPM; Seldane one tablet qPM; and Seldane-D one tablet qAM. He has no known drug allergies.

Clinical Considerations/Strategies

The following considerations/strategies are provided to aid the reader in (1) determining whether treatment of the patient's condition with nonprescription medications is warranted, (2) selecting the appropriate nonprescription medication, and (3) developing a patient counseling strategy to ensure optimal therapeutic outcomes:

- Assess the appropriateness of the patient's ostomy cleaning regimen.
- Assess the advantages of a two-piece ostomy appliance.
- Assess the need for adding other products to the ostomy cleaning regimen.
- Determine an alternative ostomy cleaning regimen that will help decrease this patient's skin irritation.
- Assess the absorption of the oral medications.
- Develop a patient education/counseling strategy that will:
  - Ensure that the patient understands the importance of a rigorous ostomy cleaning regimen;
  - Ensure that the patient uses the recommended cleaning products properly.

Summary

With proper instructions and equipment, ostomates can lead normal, healthy lives. Pharmacists can help by giving patients information about treatment and ostomy supply services and by referring patients to an ET nurse when appropriate.

References

1. Garvin G. *Nurs Clin North Am*. 1994; 29: 645.
2. Bryant RA. *Cancer Invest*. 1993; 11(5): 565.
3. Benfield BR et al. *Arch Surg*. 1973; 107: 62.
4. Cromar CD. *Dis Colon Rectum*. 1968; 7: 256.
5. Watt R. *Am J Nurs*. 1977; 77: 442.
6. Hensle TW, Ring KS. *Urol Clin North Am*. 1991; 18(4): 701.
7. Cohen Z, Stone R. *Ostomy Manage*. 1980; 2: 4.
8. Sparberg M. *Ileostomy Care*. Springfield, Ill: Charles C. Thomas; 1971: 18.
9. Kuhn JK, Flaherty JM. *J Gerontol Nurs*. 1990; 16(6): 27.
10. Gross L. *Ileostomy: A Guide*. Los Angeles, Calif: United Ostomy Association, Inc; 1974: 28.
11. Gill NN et al. *Instructions for the Care of the Ileostomy Stoma*. Cleveland, Ohio: Cleveland Clinic Foundation; 3.
12. Taylor P. *Nurs Times*. 1994; 90(13): 51.
13. Krasner D. *Am J Nurs*. 1990; 90(40): 46.
14. Anon. *Prof Nurs*. 1993; 9(3): 108.
15. Travers C. *J Enterostomy Ther*. 1980; 7: 8.
16. Kramer P. *Dig Dis*. 1977; 22: 327.
17. Gallagher ND et al. *Gut*. 1962; 3: 219.
18. Strauss S. *Your Prescription and You —A Pharmacy Handbook for Consumers*. 3rd ed. Ambler, Pa: Medical Business Services; 1978.

Appendix 1: Major Manufacturers of Ostomy Products and Accessories

- Austin Medical Products, Inc
  PO Box 1705
  Conway, NH 03818
  800–223–9310
- Bard Patient Care Division
  111 Spring Street
  Murray Hill, NJ 07974
  908–277–8000
  800–526–4930
- Coloplast, Inc
  5610 West Sligh Avenue, Suite 100
  Tampa, FL 33634
  813–886–5634
  800–237–4555
- Convatec
  (A Bristol-Myers Squibb Company)
  PO Box 5254
  Princeton, NJ 08543–5254
  908–359–9200
  800–422–8811
- Cymed, Inc
  1336 "A" Channing Way
  Berkeley, CA 94702
  800–582–0707
- Dansac Ostomy Products Company, Inc
  2920–3000 Wolff Street
  Racine, WI 53404
  414–632–2264
- Ellenberg Associates
  5525 Walter Road
  Oriskany, NY 13424
  315–736–1795
  800–843–8368
- Hollister, Inc
  2000 Hollister Drive
  PO Box 250
  Libertyville, IL 60048
  800–323–4060
  800–942–1141 (Illinois)
  800–263–7400 (Canada)
- Hy-Tape Surgical Products Corporation
  772 McLean Avenue
  Yonkers, NY 10704
  914–237–1234
- Marlen Manufacturing and Development Company
  5150 Richmond Road
  Bedford, OH 44146
  216–292–7060
- Mason Laboratories
  119 Horsham Road
  Horsham, PA 19044
  215–675–6044
- MKM Healthcare Corporation
  1957 Pioneer Avenue, Building H
  Huntingdon Valley, PA 19006
  215–957–1400
- Nu-Hope Labs, Inc
  PO Box 331150
  Pacoima, CA 91333–1150
  818–899–7711
  800–899–5017
- Perry Products
  3803 East Lake Street
  Minneapolis, MN 55406
  612–722–4783
- Rystan Company, Inc
  47 Center Avenue
  Little Falls, NJ 07424–0214
  201–256–3737
- Second Nature
  PO Box 859
  Tallevast, FL 34270–0859
  800–846–5994
- Sender-Care
  PO Box 25–1679
  Los Angeles, CA 90025
  310–280–3220
- Smith & Nephew United, Inc
  11775 Starkey Road
  Largo, FL 34643
  813–392–1261
  800–876–1261
- Sween Corporation
  1940 Commerce Drive
  PO Box 8300
  North Mankato, MN 56002
  507–345–6200
- T.G. Eakin, Ltd
  965 Upper Newtownards Road
  Dundonald, Belfast ST160RL
  North Ireland
  011–44–232–483131
- Torbot Group, Inc
  1185 Jefferson Boulevard
  Warwick, RI 02887
  401–739–2241
- VPI
  PO Box 266
  Spencer, IN 47460
  800–843–4851

Appendix 2: Ostomy Support and Information Organizations

- American Pseudo-Obstruction and Hirschsprung's Disease Society
  PO Box 772
  Medford, MA 02155–0006
  617–395–4255
- Association for Bladder Exstrophy Children
  13823 Shavano Downs
  San Antonio, TX 78230
  210–492–6062
- Better Together Club
  PO Box 7206
  Melville, NY 11747–9210
- Crohn's & Colitis Foundation of America, Inc (CCFA)
  444 Park Avenue South
  New York, NY 10016–7374
  800–343–3637
  212–685–3440 (New York)
- United Ostomy Association (UOA)
  36 Executive Park, Suite 120
  Irvine, CA 92714
  800–826–0826
- Wound Ostomy and Continence Nurses Society (WOCN)
  2755 Bristol Street, Suite 110
  Costa Mesa, CA 92626
  714–476–0268

CHAPTER 18

Diabetes Care Products and Monitoring Devices

Condit F. Steil, R. Keith Campbell, and John R. White, Jr

Questions to ask in patient assessment and counseling

- *Have you ever answered a questionnaire regarding diabetes mellitus?*
- *Is there a history of diabetes in your family? Please describe this history.*
- *Have you been tested for diabetes? If so, what were the results?*
- *If you were diagnosed as having diabetes, what care plan did your caregiver recommend?*
- *Have you seen a dietitian before? What were the dietitian's recommendations?*
- *When did you last review your care plan with your physician, pharmacist, nurse, dietitian, physical therapist?*
- *Describe how you control your diabetes:*
    - *What medications are you taking? How do you use them? Please include all medications, even for problems other than your diabetes. (Are you allergic to any medications, especially sulfa drugs or insulins containing beef and/or pork?)*
    - *If you use insulin, what brand do you use? How do you inject it? What injection sites do you use and how do you rotate them? How do you dispose of your syringes and needles? Will you demonstrate these steps for me? (How do you store your insulin at home and when you travel?)*
    - *Do you test your blood for glucose? If so, what monitoring system do you use? How often do you test? How do you record the results? Will you show me your testing technique?*
    - *Do you test your urine for glucose? For ketones? Please describe your testing procedures. (How do you use the test results to control your diabetes?)*
    - *Describe your diet plan for your diabetes. Do you have trouble following the plan?*
    - *Are you currently using or have you ever used a "fad" diet? If so, describe the diet plan. How did you learn about the plan?*
    - *What exercise guidelines do you follow? Describe your routine exercise habits.*
    - *Do you consume alcoholic beverages? What have you been told about consuming alcohol? What instructions have you received about alcohol and diabetes?*
- *When did you last see an eye specialist?*
- *When did you last see a dentist? What is your visit schedule? Describe how you care for your teeth.*
- *Have you ever seen a podiatrist (foot specialist)? If so, when and how often? Describe how you care for your feet.*
- *What identification do you carry to show you have diabetes?*
- *Are you a member of the American Diabetes Association?*
- *How do you feel about having diabetes? How does your family feel about this? Does your family understand factors that affect control?*
- *Do you have specific questions today about your diabetes care? Is there any problem right now that I can help you with? If so, what is it?*

Approximately 8 million persons with diabetes are being treated in the United States, while approximately 7 million individuals have undiagnosed diabetes (with mild symptoms or none at all).[1] Recent data from the American Diabetes Association show that diabetes is especially prevalent in certain minority populations, including Hispanic Americans, African Americans, American Indians, and Asian Americans.[2] Because the rate of diabetes in these populations is up to two to five times greater than that of Whites, these groups bear a greater burden from the disease's complications.[2] Approximately 50% of the diabetic population is over the age of 55.[1] The overall incidence of diabetes in the US population is about 5%. However, as detection and screening methods are more completely used, increasing numbers of diabetic patients will be identified. Roughly 25% of the population (approximately 50 million people) have diabetes, will develop diabetes, or have a relative with diabetes.

Diabetes is the leading cause of new blindness in individuals between 20 and 74 years of age, and it represents the third leading cause of death by disease in the United States. More than half of all heart attacks are related to diabetes. Diabetic kidney disease is a leading cause of end-stage renal disease. Neurologic complica-

Editor's Note: This chapter is based, in part, on the chapter with the same title that appeared in the 10th edition but was written by John R. White, Jr, and R. Keith Campbell. Portions of the Foot Care section in this chapter are based on material written by Nicholas G. Popovich and Gail D. Newton for the 11th edition version of the chapter "Foot Care Products."

tions, both autonomic and peripheral, occur frequently. Complications of pregnancy due to diabetes are well recognized. More than 55,000 amputations are performed annually owing to diabetes-related complications in the foot and leg. Persons with diabetes are two to three times more likely to suffer from macrovascular disease than their nondiabetic counterparts. Overall, diabetes and its complications are responsible for approximately 8% of hospital admissions.[2,3]

The estimated annual cost of diabetes care in the United States in 1992 was $132 billion, with $85 billion representing direct costs. The remaining $47 billion were indirect costs including lost workdays and sick days.[2] Economic costs are about 13% higher for insulin-dependent patients than for non–insulin-dependent patients.[4] Persons with diabetes spend approximately $2,500 annually for diabetes care products. Frequently, these people have been forgotten by manufacturers of pharmaceuticals, health and beauty aids, food, drinks, and candy, who offer a confusing selection of products that are improperly formulated and/or poorly labeled (ie, lacking adequate patient education and comprehensive instructions essential to optimal self-care). Food labeling revisions have helped to clarify issues involving those products.

The pharmacist has an excellent opportunity to assist the diabetic patient by assessing the patient's ability for self-care, providing education related to self-care measures, monitoring those measures, reinforcing instructions, highlighting warning signs, and verifying that the patient understands the information provided. Additionally, the pharmacist can become a consultant and information source to both the physician and the patient concerning not only the disease but also whatever drugs, devices, and monitoring systems are used in treatment.

Carbohydrate Metabolism

Normal Carbohydrate Metabolism

Under normal conditions, the body maintains a balance among glucose, fatty acids, and ketone bodies in the tissue cells and blood to keep plasma glucose levels within a relatively narrow range and provide adequate glucose to the central nervous system. Insulin, which is stored in pancreatic beta cells, is released in response to an elevated concentration of plasma glucose. An initial, rapid insulin release (first phase) in response to an increase in plasma glucose is followed by a slower, sustained release (second phase), which gradually increases. Insulin, which is needed to facilitate glucose transport into fat and muscle tissues, stimulates glucose uptake and use. It also stimulates the storage of glucose in muscles and the liver as glycogen; synthesis of fatty acids and triglycerides; decreased hepatic glucose output, lipolysis, and production of ketone bodies; and enhanced incorporation of amino acids into proteins. Insulin is then rapidly cleared by the liver, which allows changes in insulin secretion to compensate for fluctuations in blood glucose levels. Together with glucagon, somatostatin, growth hormone, corticosteroids, epinephrine, and other hormones, endogenous insulin maintains blood glucose levels between 50 and 150 mg/100 mL (mg%) at all times. Changes in these hormones or other chemicals—or changes in the response to them—that affect insulin activity (such as those that occur with some drug therapy) can induce hyperglycemia or glucose intolerance, thus producing diabetes. Similar effects in someone with diabetes can worsen that person's glycemic control.

Carbohydrate Metabolism in Diabetes

Type I Diabetes

In Type I diabetes, a gross lack of insulin release in response to increased blood glucose levels after a meal or a snack produces hyperglycemia. To compensate for the failure of insulin to provide glucose to the glucose-deficient tissue, amino acids are converted into glucose by gluconeogenesis and liver glycogen is converted into glucose by glycogenolysis. However, without insulin, the dependent tissues cannot use this glucose either, and the hyperglycemia becomes even more pronounced. These metabolic changes cause a rapid onset of symptoms.

Specifically, the unused glucose produces an increased osmotic load in the kidney, drawing body water with it. This results in the production and excretion of large amounts of urine (polyuria), a loss of fluid, and dehydration. This osmotic diuresis may initially cause dry mouth and can progress to significant hypovolemia, electrolyte loss, and cellular dehydration. A compensatory increase in thirst (polydipsia) occurs. Additionally, since tissue cells also cannot use the circulating blood glucose because of the lack of insulin, the nervous system signals the person to eat (polyphagia), which continues to increase the blood glucose level. Other symptoms resulting from the excess of glucose include weight loss, weakness, and ketonuria.

Insulin is an inhibitor of the enzyme lipoprotein lipase, which mobilizes body fat (lipolysis). An insulin deficiency causes enhanced lipase activity, and fat is converted into free fatty acids. Circulating cholesterol indices tend to be elevated also. In time, this fat metabolism will cause a weight loss. The free fatty acids are further broken down for energy and produce acidic ketone bodies, which can eventually induce metabolic acidosis in the absence of insulin. Fully developed progression of this syndrome can induce a systemic ketoacidosis with deep and labored breathing and air hunger, or Kussmaul's respiration. This is an emergency that can induce coma and death if not treated. Early detection with urine ketone testing can often limit the reaction to a milder form.

Figure 1 shows the clinical manifestations that occur in a patient with untreated Type I diabetes.

With normal levels of blood glucose, no glucose is found in the urine. The blood glucose level at which glucose first appears in the urine is referred to as the renal threshold for glucose. Glucose may be present in the urine when venous blood glucose exceeds 180 mg/100 mL. In persons with diabetes and patients of advanced age, the threshold level for glucose may be higher. This variance in the renal threshold limits the clinical

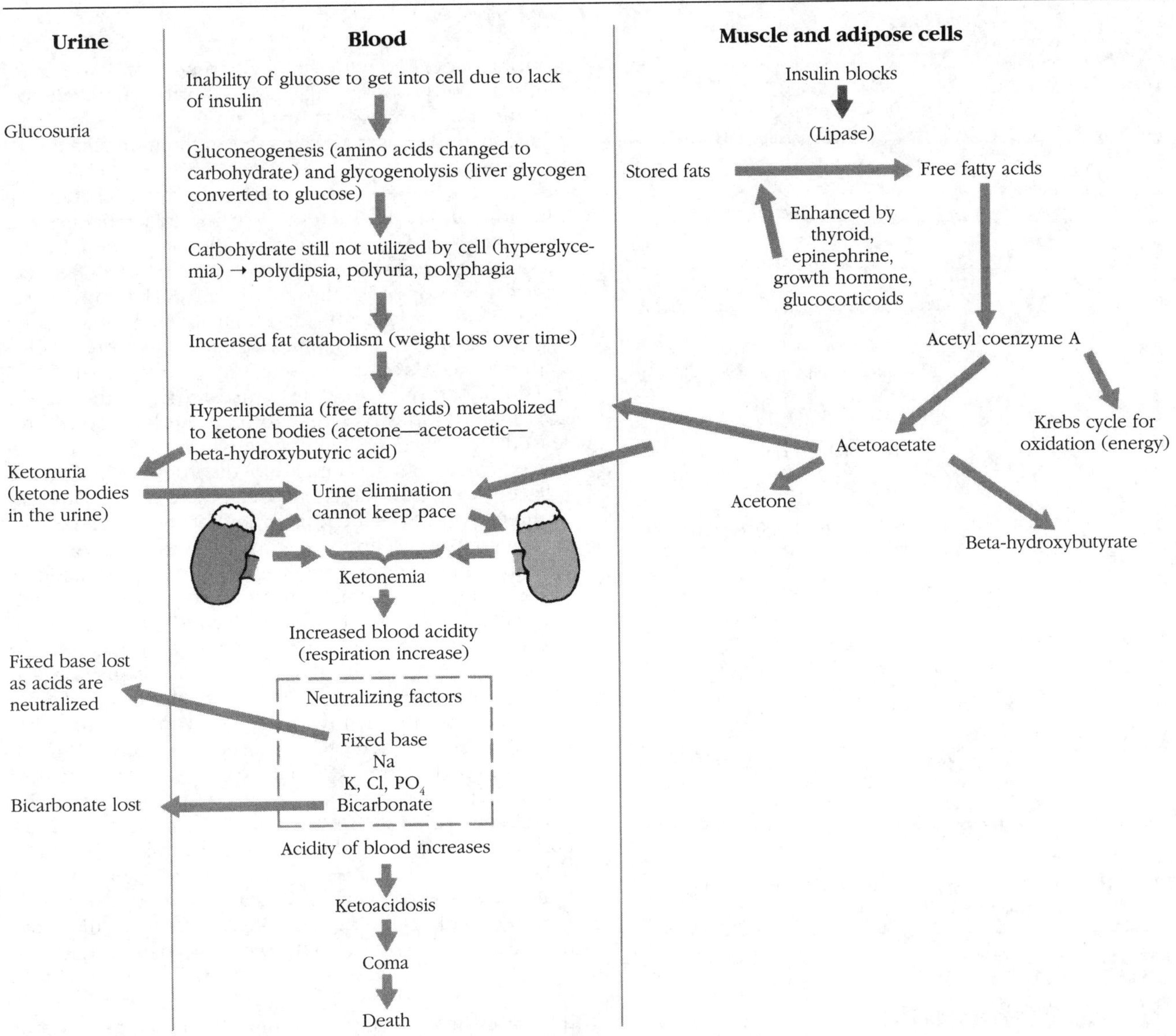

FIGURE 1 Clinical manifestations of Type I insulin-dependent diabetes mellitus.

use of urine glucose testing. For this reason, it is preferable to monitor blood glucose values to determine how well the patient's diabetes is being controlled.

Type II Diabetes

In contrast to Type I diabetes, Type II diabetes is often not accompanied by any symptoms. Instead, it is detected most often when glucose is found in the urine (glucosuria) or when an elevated blood glucose level is found on a routine examination. Figure 2 provides a flow diagram of the pathogenesis of Type II diabetes. Careful study of an older, obese group of patients reveals glucosuria, proteinuria (protein in the urine), postprandial hyperglycemia, microaneurysms, and even retinal exudates.

Nonobese Type II patients may have low, normal, or high blood insulin levels, depending on a number of factors. Obese Type II patients, who are in the majority, usually have normal or elevated blood insulin levels. Glucose is transported into muscle and fat cells, so these patients are not usually ketosis prone and seldom develop ketoacidosis except during periods of significant stress. Because of their high blood glucose levels, they may be prone to a syndrome termed hyperglycemic, hyperosmolar, nonketotic coma. While the acute management of this syndrome is similar to that of ketoacidosis in Type I patients, diagnosis is troublesome because of nonspecific symptoms in the elderly individual.

Increased obesity in Type II patients may cause high levels of insulin in the blood (hyperinsulinemia), resulting in a downregulation or loss of sensitivity of insulin receptors to glucose, which leads to the clinical finding of hyperglycemia. Thus, the controls for normal glucose levels may be "reset." Weight reduction to an ideal body weight will often be accompanied by a return to normal blood glucose levels and a response to alterations.

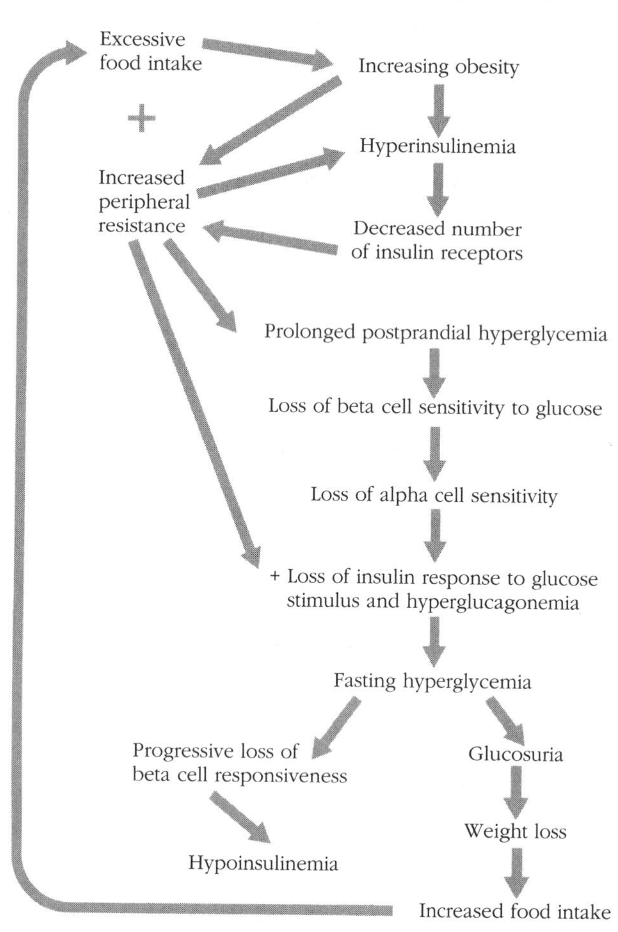

FIGURE 2 Pathogenesis of Type II non–insulin-dependent diabetes mellitus.

Classification of Diabetes Mellitus

Diabetes mellitus is not a single disease but rather a syndrome composed of several specific diseases, all of which are characterized by hyperglycemia and a tendency toward the development of macro- or microvascular disease and neuropathy. This results in shifts in the use of carbohydrates, fats, and proteins for energy. Several types of diabetes have been identified. Table 1 summarizes the current classification system. Table 2 classifies the two major clinical types of diabetes according to their distinguishing features. Currently, a reclassification is under consideration to reflect a recognition of those Type II patients with insulin resistance and those with insulin sensitivity. Approximately 10% of persons with diabetes in the United States are classified as having Type I, or insulin-dependent diabetes mellitus (IDDM); the remaining 90% have Type II, or non–insulin-dependent diabetes mellitus (NIDDM). Approximately 10% of patients with NIDDM are nonobese; the other 90% are obese. Nonobese Type II diabetes often occurs in patients during youth and is inherited in an autosomal dominant pattern. Obese Type II diabetes is more common in adults over the age of 40.

Etiology

Factors associated with the development of diabetes include heredity, obesity, age, stress, hormonal imbalance, vasculitis of the vessels supplying the beta cells of the pancreas, and viruses affecting the autoimmune responses of the body.

Type I diabetes is characterized by an absence of functioning, insulin-secreting pancreatic islet cells. The cells may be affected by factors such as (1) genetic defects in the production of certain macromolecules necessary for proper insulin synthesis, packaging, or release; (2) extrinsic factors that stimulate the loss of insulin synthesis; or (3) the inability of beta cells to recognize endogenous glucose levels or replicate normally.[5] Extrinsic factors may include viruses such as mumps or coxsackie B4, destructive cytotoxins and antibodies released by sensitized lymphocytes, or autodigestion in the course of an inflammatory disorder involving the adjacent exocrine pancreas. Cells have many different antigen types. Specific human leukocyte antigen genes may increase susceptibility to a diabetogenic virus, or certain immune-response genes may predispose patients to a destructive autoimmune response against their own islet cells. In the severe form of Type I diabetes, circulating islet cell antibodies have been detected in as many as 80% of cases in the first few weeks of disease onset.[5,6] Type II patients, like those with severe Type I diabetes, may inherit a response to a viral infection that causes a beta cell defect as a consequence of viral stress.

In Type II patients who have excess insulin and are obese, hyperinsulinism and insulin resistance have been correlated with a decrease in insulin receptors; this decrease is the basic, and commonly reversible, defect in insulin-resistant patients.[7,8] Moreover, studies have shown that the tissues of insulin-resistant, obese patients exhibit reduced insulin binding. Resistance to insulin's action also appears to result from an impairment in the target cells' response to insulin due to a defect in postreceptor binding. In some Type II patients, both a decreased insulin receptor number and a postreceptor defect may exist in combination.[9]

Consequences of Poor Glycemic Control

The basic goals of diabetes therapy largely remained unchanged for several years, with many clinicians assuming that management that approached normalization of blood glucose was beneficial. This changed when the results of a large, multicenter, long-term study investigating the basic premise of tight management were reported in 1993.[10] This study, the Diabetes Control and Complications Trial (DCCT), was conducted in 29 centers in the United States and Canada and involved 1,441 patients with Type I diabetes for more than 7,000 patient years. The study asked two basic questions: "Does tight management prevent the start of diabetes complications?" (primary prevention), and "Does tight management prevent or limit the progression of diabetes complications?" (secondary intervention). Retinopathy assessment was used for assigning patients to the prevention or intervention

TABLE 1 Classification of diabetes and glucose intolerance

Current names	Old names
Clinical Categories	
Type I: Insulin-dependent diabetes mellitus (IDDM)	Juvenile diabetes Juvenile-onset diabetes Ketosis-prone diabetes Growth-onset diabetes Brittle diabetes
Type II: Non–insulin-dependent diabetes mellitus (NIDDM) Type a: nonobese Type b: obese	Adult-onset diabetes Maturity-onset diabetes Ketosis-resistant diabetes Stable diabetes Maturity-onset diabetes of youth
Diabetes mellitus associated with other conditions or syndromes	Secondary diabetes (drug-induced diabetes; impaired glucose tolerance due to other hormonal irregularities)
Impaired glucose tolerance	Asymptomatic diabetes Chemical diabetes Subclinical diabetes Borderline diabetes Latent diabetes
Gestational diabetes	Gestational diabetes
Statistical Risk	
Previous abnormality of glucose tolerance	Latent diabetes Prediabetes
Potential abnormality of glucose tolerance	Potential diabetes Prediabetes

Reprinted with permission from *Diabetes*. 1979; 28 (12): 1039.

cohort. The patients were assigned to an intensive or conventional treatment group, the therapy plans for which are listed in Table 3. The study results, as summarized in Table 4, show that the group receiving intensive treatment achieved better glycemic control. This group showed significant improvement in microvascular and neurologic complication progression, whereas the primary adverse event was a threefold increase in severe hypoglycemia.

The dramatic findings of the study have changed the therapy goals for Type I patient. Additionally, since the cellular changes causing complications in Type II diabetes are similar, the findings have stimulated planning to apply many of the same principles to Type II therapy. Direct application to Type II is difficult, however, because insulin resistance and other disorders may be present, as may be other limiting factors that exist with specific patient characteristics, such as the pediatric individual, the diabetes patient with hypoglycemia unawareness—a condition that, through autonomic neuropathy, renders the person unable to detect hypoglycemia—and the diabetes patient with significant vascular disease. The best news from the DCCT is that when the cohorts were grouped by individuals who achieved similar levels of glycemic improvement and then compared, it was found that *any* improvement in glucose control lowered the complication incidence![10]

All major physiologic systems are adversely affected by chronic hyperglycemia and complications in diabetes (Tables 5 and 6). A number of events have been suggested as possible contributors to these complications. For example, when glucose is consistently elevated, highly reactive glycosylated proteins are formed, which interact to form advanced glycosylation end products, or AGE products.[11,12] These products form covalent bonds with amino groups on other proteins, resulting in cross-linking, accumulation, and thickening in the basement membrane.[12] An investigational drug, aminoguanidine, has demonstrated the ability to inhibit AGE product formation, thereby confirming the usefulness of giving medication to prevent or limit progression of a complication. Data indicate that an angiotensin-converting enzyme (ACE) inhibitor, captopril, limits the progression of diabetic nephropathy.[13] This may be a class effect; other ACE inhibitors appear to have similar action.[14] Another such event

TABLE 2 Distinguishing features of the two major types of diabetes mellitus

	Insulin-dependent Type I (IDDM)	Non–insulin-dependent Type II (NIDDM)
Age of onset	Usually, but not always, during childhood or adolescence	Frequently >35
Type of onset	Abrupt	Usually gradual
Prevalence	0.5%	2–4%
Incidence	<10%	>75%
Family history of diabetes	Frequently negative	Commonly positive
Primary cause	Pancreatic beta cell deficiency	End organ (insulin receptors) unresponsiveness to insulin action
Nutritional status at time of onset	Usually thin with weight loss	Usually obese
Postglucose plasma or serum insulin[a], mcU/mL	Absent or minimal	Normal or elevated
Symptoms	Polydipsia, polyphagia, and polyuria	Maybe none
Hepatomegaly	Rather common	Uncommon
Stability	Blood sugar fluctuates widely in response to small changes in insulin dose, exercise, and infection	Blood sugar fluctuations are less marked
Possible etiologic factors include:		
Inheritance	Associated with specific HLA[b] tissue types, but only 40–50% concordance in twins	95–100% concordance in twins, but not associated with specific HLA[b] tissue types
Autoimmune disease	50–80% circulating islet cell antibodies	Negative; <10% circulating islet cell antibodies
Viral infections	Coxsackie, mumps, influenza	No evidence
Proneness to ketosis	Frequent, especially if treatment program is insufficient in food and/or insulin	Uncommon except in the presence of unusual stress or moderate to severe sepsis
Insulin defect	Defect in secretion; secretion is impaired early in disease; secretion may be totally absent late in disease	Insulin deficiency present in some patients, others are insulin resistant Insulin deficiency—in most patients, insulin secretion fails to keep pace with inordinate demands caused by obesity; this defect may appear initially as a failure to respond to glucose alone, suggesting an impairment in the glucoreceptor of the pancreatic beta cell Insulin resistance—in some patients, there is a defect in tissue responsiveness to insulin and evidence of hyperinsulinemia; in such patients, insulin resistance may be mediated by a decreased number of insulin receptors in target cells Increased hepatic glucose production in response to altered cellular glucose uptake

TABLE 2 *continued*

	Insulin-dependent Type I (IDDM)	Non–insulin-dependent Type II (NIDDM)
Plasma insulin (endogenous)	Negligible to zero	Plasma insulin response may be either adequate but delayed, so that postprandial hypoglycemia may be present when diabetes is discovered, or diminished but not absent
Vascular complications of diabetes and degenerative changes	Infrequent until diabetes has been present for ≈5 years	Frequent
Usual causes of death	Degenerative complications in target organs (eg, renal failure due to diabetic nephropathy)	Accelerated atherosclerosis (eg, myocardial infarct); to lesser extent, microangiopathic changes in target tissues (eg, renal failure)
Diet	Mandatory in all patients	If diet is used fully, hypoglycemic therapy may not be needed
Insulin	Necessary for all patients	Necessary for 20–30% of patients
Oral agents	Rarely efficacious	Often efficacious

[a]Normal response is between 50 and 135 mcU/mL at 60 minutes and less than 100 mcU/mL at 120 minutes after 100 g of oral glucose.
[b]Human leukocyte antigen.

occurs when serum glucose levels are elevated so that glucose is present in high concentrations in non–insulin-dependent tissues, such as the lens of the eye and some neurons. Here, the enzymes normally involved in the polyol pathway metabolize the excess glucose, increasing sorbitol and fructose concentrations. Increased amounts of sorbitol and fructose can be found in the lens and nerves of hyperglycemic diabetic animals, and their accumulation may produce osmotic injury to these cells. When acutely elevated blood glucose levels in persons with diabetes are normalized, previously severe neuropathy symptoms may resolve.[15] Aldose reductase inhibitors hold promise as medications to prevent or reduce the severity of several diabetic complications resulting from excess sorbitol production. Tolrestat (Ayerst) is one such medication currently being evaluated in clinical trials.

Other abnormalities of glycoprotein metabolism have been identified in both Type I and Type II patients and, in some cases, are used clinically. For instance, increased levels of a minor hemoglobin component, hemoglobin A_{1c}, reflect mean blood glucose concentration over a period of about 2 months and are used to assess chronic control of hyperglycemia.

Atherosclerotic lesions in persons with diabetes appear similar to those in persons without diabetes, but they tend to develop earlier, occur more often, and are more severe.[16] Atherosclerosis contributes to the twofold increase in cardiovascular mortality and morbidity that occurs in persons with diabetes. Less clear is what degree of atherosclerosis contributes to the development of microvascular disease.[15] Hyperglycemia causes damage to the intimal cells of the arteries, and this is probably the initial lesion in atherosclerosis. Lower-than-normal levels of plasma high-density lipoprotein (HDL) cholesterol and elevated levels of low-density lipoprotein cholesterol (LDL) may contribute to cholesterol deposition and plaque formation.[16,17] Atherosclerotic lesions produce symptoms in various areas. Persons with diabetes may suffer from occlusive vascular changes in the lower extremities as a result of both atherosclerosis and damage to smaller arteries (microangiopathies). Peripheral lesions, alone or in combination with hemorrheologic factors, may cause increased intermittent claudication and contribute to the development of gangrene. Widespread disease of small vessels is common. Cardiomyopathy, cardiovascular neuropathy, and silent myocardial infarct may also occur in these patients.[16]

Hyperglycemia may impair the phagocytic activity of the body's white blood cells. This effect often makes it difficult for persons with diabetes to eradicate bacterial infections.[18] Because glucose levels in saliva are increased in patients with hyperglycemia, these patients have a higher incidence of dental caries and gum disease. Pharmacists should encourage good oral hygiene and regular dental examinations.

Symptoms of Diabetes

The pharmacist should obtain a careful patient history before attempting an evaluation. The more common symptoms of diabetes (eg, polydipsia, polyphagia, polyuria, fatigue, nocturia [nighttime urination], blurred vision,

TABLE 3 Diabetes Control and Complications Trial (DCCT) treatment parameters

Treatment parameter	Conventional treatment group	Intensive treatment group
Insulin	1 or 2 daily injections	3–4 daily injections or insulin pump
Home monitoring	Daily, blood or urine	Blood monitoring, several tests/day
Diet and exercise	Instruction	Instruction quarterly, refresher monthly
Follow-up examination	Quarterly	Monthly
Care contact	As needed by patient	Weekly by nurse

Reprinted with permission from Diabetes Control and Complications Trial Research Group. The effect of intensive treatment of diabetes on the progression of long-term complications in insulin-dependent diabetes mellitus. *N Engl J Med.* 1993; 328: 977–86.

ketosis, and dry mouth) may be fairly easy to detect. Other symptoms that pharmacists should consider in assessing potential patients and in monitoring diagnosed patients for blood glucose control are discussed below. While nonspecific for diabetes, these symptoms, in combination or with progressive severity, may indicate its development. Pharmacists who detect these symptoms and conditions should refer the patient to a physician.

Weight Loss

Losing weight while consuming regular meals may be an indication of diabetes. In persons with the disease, the pharmacist must evaluate dietary restriction versus loss of blood glucose control as the primary reason for the weight loss. Other conditions associated with weight loss include hyperthyroidism, cancer, and anorexia nervosa.

Recurrent Monilial Infections

Monilial infections, especially fungal infections of the vulva and anus in women, are common in persons with diabetes. Recurrent monilial vaginal infections may be the first indicator of increased blood glucose levels in females. Persons with diabetes may also experience loss of blood glucose control whenever they have infections and may require close monitoring and alterations in their treatment regimen. Chronic skin infections, carbuncles, furuncles, and eczema are also common in patients with this disease. Any recurrent or abnormally slow healing infections should be evaluated by a physician for cause.

Prolonged Wound Healing

Minor cuts and scratches may take approximately twice as long to heal in someone with diabetes. They are also more likely to become infected if not properly treated. All patients at risk of having diabetes, as well as those who do have it, should be instructed in proper wound care. Wounds that do not heal properly or that become infected should be evaluated by a physician.

TABLE 4 Diabetes Control and Complications Trial (DCCT) risk reductions from conventional to intensive cohorts, both primary and secondary interventions

Complication	% reduction
>3-step sustained retinopathy	63
Macular edema	26
Severe nonproliferative or proliferative retinopathy	47
Laser treatment	51
Urinary albumin (>40 mg/24 h)	39
Urinary albumin (>300 mg/24 h)	54
Clinical neuropathy at 5 years	60

Reprinted with permission from Diabetes Control and Complications Trial Research Group. The effect of intensive treatment of diabetes on the progression of long-term complications in insulin-dependent diabetes mellitus. *N Engl J Med.* 1993; 328: 977–86.

Gout

Patients diagnosed with gout have a higher incidence of diabetes than the general population and should be screened for the disease.

TABLE 5 Harmful effects of hyperglycemia (blood glucose ≥150 mg/dL)

Increased capillary basement membrane thickening
Glucose metabolized via polyol pathway, leading to increased levels of sorbitol
Increased plasma viscosity; decreased red blood cell flexibility
Faulty lipid metabolism, leading to higher levels of fat and possibly accelerating atherosclerosis
Abnormally high levels of glycosylated hemoglobin; advanced glycosylated end products
Impairment of phagocytosis and subsequent ability to fight infection
Increased neonatal morbidity and mortality

Updated from Pharmaceutical services for patients with diabetes. *Am Pharm* (module 4). 1986 May; NS26 (5): 7.

Visual Disturbances

Patients who wear glasses may notice that increasingly stronger lenses are required at relatively short time intervals. Ophthalmologists initially identify a large number of persons with diabetes. Cataracts and open-angle glaucoma in older diabetes patients are common. Research suggests that the increased frequency of cataracts seen in these patients may be due to an increased level of sorbitol, which accumulates in certain tissues during hyperglycemia. Cataract formation appears to be associated with the high sugar alcohol concentration in the lens, which produces swelling from an influx of water and the eventual disruption of lens fiber membranes and protein deposits.

Psychologic Changes

Some of the first symptoms of hypoglycemia affecting the nervous system are irritability, nervousness, and anxiety. Generalized fatigue and depression occur more often in persons with diabetes. Frequent emotional flare-ups may signal abnormal biochemistry that may be due to diabetes.

Screening for Diabetes

The pharmacist's role in promoting and supporting diabetes detection programs cannot be overstated. The accessibility and professional competency of the pharmacist provides an excellent opportunity to screen patients for diabetes. Individuals suspected of having the disease can then be referred to a physician for a complete physical examination, history, and laboratory analysis. Patients already known to have diabetes can be monitored by the pharmacist to ensure their understanding of and adherence to the treatment plan. At all times in the process, the pharmacist should be prepared to answer patients' questions concerning diabetes.

If all pharmacists set aside 1 day each month to screen patients for diabetes, they would make substantial headway on detecting the more than 5 million undiagnosed persons with diabetes in the United States. Screening can start with the diabetes survey developed by the American Diabetes Association and shown in Table 7. Adding up the point values of the questions gives a person's relative risk for developing diabetes. Individuals who reveal a high risk for the disease can then be tested by capillary blood glucose (fingerstick). This method of screening is more productive than trying to fingerstick all potential individuals with diabetes. The actual testing itself requires literature, documentation forms, alcohol swabs, lancets, blood test strips, and a glucose meter to test the strip's color changes. The pharmacist should review his or her state's specific laboratory guidelines, the state's application of the federal Clinical Laboratory Improvements Act (CLIA) of 1988, and the blood and body fluid precautions issued by the Occupational Safety and Health Administration (OSHA). Some restrictions as to who may handle blood and blood products may apply via CLIA. Any facility that routinely has the potential for blood and body fluid exposure must comply with OSHA guidelines.

Diagnostic criteria from the American Diabetes Association for nonpregnant adult diabetes mellitus are as follows[19]:

- A random plasma glucose level of at least 200 mg/dL in addition to classic and overt symptoms such as polydipsia, polyphagia, polyuria, and/or weight loss;
- A fasting plasma glucose level of at least 140 mg/dL on at least two separate occasions;
- A fasting plasma glucose level below 140 mg/dL plus at least two oral glucose tolerance tests that yield 2-hour plasma glucose levels of at least 200 mg/dL and one intervening value (at 30, 60, or 90 minutes) of at least 200 mg/dL.

Diagnostic criteria for children and pregnant women are different from those for nonpregnant adults and are also available from the American Diabetes Association.

Treatment

The basic objectives in the treatment of diabetes, in order of importance, are to:

- Relieve and prevent diabetic symptoms;
- Prevent hypoglycemic reactions;
- Maintain blood glucose levels close to euglycemia (between 80 and 150 mg/dL) to prevent or slow progression of chronic complications;
- Achieve and/or maintain optimal weight;
- Promote normal growth and development in children;
- Eliminate or minimize all other cardiovascular risk factors;
- Integrate the patient into health care through intensive education and involvement in self-care, using the premise that the patient must become a primary caregiver.

These objectives can be met only through the combined efforts of the physician, pharmacist, nurse, dietitian, patient, patient's family and/or significant others, and other caregivers.

Key elements in the treatment of diabetes can be easily remembered with the five DEEDS: *D*iet, *E*xercise, *E*ducation, *D*rugs, and *S*elf-monitoring of blood glucose. Caloric planning and increased physical activity are part

TABLE 6 Potential complications of diabetes mellitus and their treatment

Body location	Description	Treatment
Eyes	Retinopathy, cataract formation, glaucoma, and periodic visual disturbances due to microvascular disease and other metabolic complications such as increased sorbitol; leading cause of new blindness	Strict control of blood glucose to avoid need for treatment (eg, laser photocoagulation, vitrectomy)
Mouth	Gingivitis, increased incidence of dental cavities and periodontal disease	Strict control of blood glucose and daily hygiene; see dentist regularly
Reproductive system (pregnancy)	Increased incidence of large babies, stillbirths, miscarriages, neonatal deaths, and congenital defects due to metabolic abnormalities	Strict control of blood glucose before and during pregnancy
Nervous system	Motor, sensory, and autonomic neuropathy leading to impotence, neurogenic bladder, paresthesias, gangrene, altered gastrointestinal motility, and cardiovascular problems	Strict control of blood glucose, daily foot care, surgery, and antidepressants and phenothiazines when indicated
Vascular system	Large vessel disease resulting in atherosclerosis and microvascular disease leading to retinopathy, nephropathy, and decreased peripheral perfusion	Strict control of blood glucose
Skin	Numerous infections and specific lesions such as skin spots, diabetic bullae, lipodystrophies, and necrobiosis lipoidica diabeticorum due to small vessel disease, increased lipids in blood, and pruritus	Strict control of blood glucose, daily hygiene
Kidneys	Diabetic glomerulosclerosis causing nephropathy	Strict control of blood glucose; eventually, diet low in proteins. Prednisone, dialysis, and renal transplantation if necessary. Angiotensin-converting enzyme inhibitors to limit progression.
Reticuloendothelial system (infections)	Cystitis, tuberculosis, skin infections, difficulty in overcoming infections, and moniliasis in diabetic women	Strict control of blood glucose and aggressive anti-infective therapy when indicated

Adapted from Pharmaceutical services for patients with diabetes. *Am Pharm* (module 4). 1986 May; NS26 (5): 8.

of the treatment plan for both types of diabetes. Education is crucial to the patient's understanding of the disease and mastery of the skills needed to achieve glycemic control. Sulfonylureas, metformin, or insulin are used to control hyperglycemia, and nonprescription products—in addition to insulin—formulated especially for use by the person with diabetes are helpful adjuncts. Finally, self-monitoring of blood glucose enables the patient to adjust medication, diet, and exercise carefully to maintain near-normal blood glucose levels.[20]

Insulin Therapy

Although this chapter deals with nonprescription products used in diabetes, the pharmacist must understand the proper use of all drugs used to control the disease. The two groups of prescription drugs traditionally used to treat diabetes—oral sulfonylurea agents and a biguanide, metformin—are discussed in depth in major textbooks on prescription drugs. In September 1995, the FDA approved acarbose, a prescription-only alpha glucosidase inhibitor, for the treatment of Type II diabetes. Acarbose, which will be available on US markets in January 1996, prevents the breakdown of large carbohydrates in the gastrointestinal tract, thus preventing their absorption and thereby lowering blood glucose levels.[21]

Insulin, with the exception of the U-500 preparation, is a nonprescription drug. Pharmacists also need to be familiar with drugs that may affect blood glucose control by themselves or by interacting with sulfonylureas, metformin, or insulin. Further, they should recognize

TABLE 7 Diabetes screening questionnaire

Could you have diabetes and NOT know it?	**Point values[a]**
1. My weight is equal to or above that listed in the chart below.[b]	Yes 5____
2. I am under 65 years of age, and I get little or no exercise during a usual day.	Yes 5____
3. I am between 45 and 64 years of age.	Yes 5____
4. I am 65 years old or older.	Yes 9____
5. I am a woman who has had a baby weighing more than 9 pounds.	Yes 1____
6. I have a sister or brother with diabetes.	Yes 1____
7. I have a parent with diabetes.	Yes 1____
	Total____

Women		Men	
Height (in.) (w/o shoes)	**Weight (lb)[b] (w/o clothing)**	**Height (in.) (w/o shoes)**	**Weight (lb)[b] (w/o clothing)**
57	127	61	146
58	131	62	151
59	134	63	155
60	138	64	158
61	142	65	163
62	146	66	168
63	151	67	174
64	157	68	179
65	162	69	184
66	167	70	190
67	172	71	196
68	176	72	202
69	181	73	208
70	186	74	214
		75	220

[a]A score of 3–5 indicates a low risk for diabetes; a score of >5 indicates a high risk for diabetes. Anyone scoring >5 points should see a physician promptly for evaluation.

[b]Chart lists weights 20% heavier than those recommended for men or women with medium frames.

Adapted with permission from *Diabetes Alert*. Alexandria, Va: American Diabetes Association; 1995.

which drugs can cause or exacerbate peripheral neuropathy, retinopathy, and nephropathy, as well as which drugs can cause hypoglycemia or hyperglycemia (Tables 8–11).

Although insulin is prescribed by a physician, pharmacists are often the health care professionals who are consulted about problems. Because insulin is not a prescription drug in the United States, patient access to the

TABLE 8 Drugs of abuse that impair diabetes management

Alcohol

Impairs judgment

Is metabolized similarly to fat and alters insulin response when taken with carbohydrates

Promotes hypoglycemic attacks

Impairs the manufacture, storage, and release of glycogen

Interacts with other drugs (eg, chlorpropamide)

Can cause precipitous drop in blood glucose in alcoholic persons who have stopped eating

Can increase blood glucose when used with sugar-containing mixers or in "sweet drinks"

Nicotine (smoking)

Is a potent vasoconstrictor

Causes a 1–2°F drop in skin temperature with one cigarette

Significantly alters oral and intravenous glucose tolerance tests

Is a risk factor in etiology of diabetic nephropathy

May decrease subcutaneous absorption of insulin

May increase insulin requirements by as much as 15–20%

Caffeine (coffee, tea, colas)

In large amounts, increases blood glucose levels

Marijuana

Alters time perception, which may affect control

May cause "munchies"

Impairs short-term memory in intoxicated state

Causes a highly dose-related effect, which is dangerous because patient may not know tetrahydrocannabinol content

Yields profound impairment when used with alcohol

With heavy use, impairs glucose tolerance, causing hyperglycemia

Central nervous system stimulants (amphetamines, sympathomimetics, decongestants, anorectics, cocaine, and psychedelics)

Increase blood glucose levels

Increase liver glycogen breakdown, which causes hyperglycemia

Alter time perception, which may affect management steps

May cause anorexia, which increases blood glucose levels

Sedatives and hypnotics

Impair thinking and thus self-control

Opiates (heroin, morphine)

Cause euphoria, which may affect management and increase blood glucose levels

Reprinted from Pharmaceutical services for patients with diabetes. *Am Pharm* (module 4). 1986 May; NS26 (5): 4.

TABLE 9 Drugs that can cause peripheral neuropathies

Antimicrobials	Nitrofurantoin, ethambutol, isoniazid, colistin, streptomycin, metronidazole, amphotericin B
Anticonvulsants	Phenytoin, carbamazepine
Antirheumatics	Indomethacin, colchicine, penicillamine, gold compounds
Cytotoxics	Vincristine, procarbazine, cytarabine, chlorambucil
Cardiovascular drugs[a]	Hydralzine, clofibrate, disopyramide
Miscellaneous agents	Cimetidine, ergotamine, methysergide, amitriptyline, amphetamines

[a]Nitroglycerin can cause postural hypotension in diabetic patients with autonomic neuropathy.

Adapted from Pharmaceutical services for patients with diabetes. *Am Pharm* (module 4). 1986 May; NS26 (5): 5.

TABLE 10 Drugs that can induce nephropathy

Penicillamine, gold salts, nonsteroidal analgesics (large doses over time)

Aminoglycoside antibiotics (neomycin, kanamycin, gentamicin, tobramycin)

Cephaloridine, rifampin, cyclophosphamide, heroin, methotrexate, and methysergide

Adapted from Pharmaceutical services for patients with diabetes. *Am Pharm* (module 4). 1986 May; NS26 (5): 5.

medication is unrestricted. Thus, pharmacists should be knowledgeable about insulin products and the pharmacotherapy of insulin.

Type I patients must be treated with exogenous insulin. Generally, persons who require insulin initially are younger than 30 years of age at diagnosis and are lean, prone to developing ketoacidosis, and markedly hyperglycemic, even in the fasting state. Among Type II patients, insulin is indicated for those who do not respond to diet and exercise therapy alone or to therapy with oral sulfonylureas or metformin, or those who have fasting plasma glucose concentrations of greater than 200 mg/dL. Insulin therapy is also necessary for some Type II patients who are subject to situational stresses such as infection, pregnancy, or surgery. Type II patients must receive intensive education concerning diet and exercise when they start on insulin since increased hunger and a resultant weight gain can be major problems for them.

Patients who are receiving parenteral nutrition, who require large-calorie supplements to meet increased energy needs, or who have drug-induced diabetes are other persons who may require insulin exogenously on a short-term or intermittent basis to maintain normal glucose levels. By combining the appropriate modification of diet, exercise, and variable mixtures of short- and longer-acting insulins with self-monitoring, these patients can achieve acceptable control of blood glucose. Normalization of blood glucose usually requires intensified insulin regimens using multiple daily injections or insulin pumps.

All persons using insulin should be trained to inject themselves. Children with diabetes should probably begin giving themselves their own insulin injections at about

TABLE 11 Drugs that may cause hypoglycemia or hyperglycemia

Hypoglycemia	Hyperglycemia
Acetaminophen	Acetazolamide
Alcohol (acute)	Alcohol (chronic)
Amitriptyline	Amiodarone
Anabolic steroids	Antimicrobial (pentamidine, rifampin, sulfasalazine, nalidixic acid)
Beta blockers	Asparaginase
Biguanides	Beta-agonists
Chloroquine	Caffeine
Clofibrate	Calcium channel blockers
Disopyramide	Chlorpromazine
Fenfluramine	Chlorthalidone
Fluphenazine	Corticosteroids
Guanethidine	Cyclosporine
Haloperidol	Diazoxide
Imipramine	Encainide
Insulin	Estrogens
Lithium	Ethacrynic acid
Monoamine oxidase inhibitors	Fentanyl/Furosemide
Norfloxacin	Indapamide
Pentamidine	Interferon alpha
Perphenazine/Amitriptyline	Lactulose
Phenobarbital	Niacin and nicotinic acid
Prazosin	Oral contraceptives
Propoxyphene	Phenytoin
Quinine	Probenecid
Salicylates in large doses	Sugars (dextrose, fructose, mannitol, sorbitol, sucrose)
Sulfonamide antibiotics	Sympathomimetic amines
Sulfonylurea agents	Thiazide diuretics
Tetrahydrocannabinol	Thyroid preparations
	Tricyclic antidepressants

6–9 years of age. Parents should administer one or two injections each week to stay in practice, to ensure that injection sites are rotated correctly, and to inject in areas that are difficult for the child to reach.[22]

Insulin Preparations

Several insulin products are available in the United States. For ease of discussion, insulins may be categorized based on the species source, type, strength, and purity.

The source from which insulin is derived and its antigenicity can both influence the product's effect on blood glucose control, resistance to insulin, and sensitivity to its actions.[23,24] Commercially available animal-derived insulins are either pure pork or a mixture of beef and pork. Beef insulin has greater antigenicity because it differs in structure from human insulin by three amino acids; pork insulin differs by only one amino acid. Biosynthetic human insulin is now available from two manufacturers in the United States: Eli Lilly and Novo-Nordisk. Each species source of insulin has a distinct time-action profile. Human insulin has a more rapid onset and a shorter duration of action than pork insulin, which has a more rapid onset and a shorter duration of action than beef insulin. Patients switched from one species to another require medical supervision.

Insulins may be divided into three groups according to promptness of action onset, duration (eg, short acting, intermediate acting, or long acting), and intensity of action following subcutaneous (SC) injection. Rapid or short-acting insulin is regular insulin. To increase the duration of action of regular insulin, zinc and protein molecules or zinc alone can be added to bind the insulin. Neutral protamine Hagedorn (NPH) and lente insulin suspensions are intermediate-acting insulins; ultralente insulin suspension is long-acting. NPH is an insulin preparation in which zinc and protamine have been added. Protamine is a fish protein that slows insulin absorption from the site of injection. The lente insulins are produced by adding high levels of zinc to insulin. Two basic crystal types are formed with mixtures of these for specific action defining the lente and ultralente insulins. (Two other insulin preparations, semilente and protamine zinc insulin, were discontinued from US production in 1994.) Fixed-dose mixtures of human insulin at a ratio of 70% NPH to 30% regular and a ratio of 50% NPH to 50% regular are also available. Information concerning the time-action profiles of these insulins is contained in Table 12. Many factors, such as injection site, species source, and ambient temperature, affect the time-action profiles of insulins; thus, the values listed in Table 12 are given in ranges with some degree of variability.

Another factor that can affect the clinical use of insulin preparations is the route of administration. Regular insulin injected intramuscularly (IM) provides faster absorption with a greater initial drop in plasma glucose levels than does injection by the SC route. Regular insulin injected intravenously (IV) produces the highest pharmacologic level of insulin in the least time. Insulin suspensions (eg, NPH, lente, and ultralente) are never administered IM or IV.

Insulin absorption can also be affected by exercise. Leg exercise accelerates absorption from the leg; arm or abdominal injections avoid this response during leg exercise and thus reduce exercise-induced hypoglycemia. A patient whose day includes a hard game of tennis might do well to inject that day's insulin into the abdomen rather than into the arm or leg. Also, if more than 60 U of insulin are injected at one site, there is potential for erratic absorption. Patients receiving large doses of insulin should perhaps split the doses and inject in two different sites, and they should also be monitored closely.

In March 1980, the FDA decertified U-80 insulin, leaving two strengths of insulin—U-40 and U-100—available for diabetic patients. In 1990, the FDA decertified U-40 insulin. Unfortunately, this is the insulin that is usually available in several non–English-speaking countries. Thus, patients traveling abroad need to plan their trip and carry extra insulin and corresponding insulin syringes to prevent problems or errors.[24] U-500 regular insulin is available from Eli Lilly as a prescription-only product for insulin-resistant patients who use more than 100–200 U per injection.

Newer methods of purifying insulin now ensure that all commercially available insulins are highly purified. The average content of common pancreas contaminants proinsulin, arginine insulin, esterified insulin, and glucagon has been decreased, resulting in fewer insulin-sensitivity reactions. All insulin preparations available in the United States contain between 0 and 10 ppm of proinsulin (see product table "Insulin Preparations"). Increased insulin product purity is less antigenic and allows use of lower insulin doses. The ability to manufacture insulin through DNA technology has allowed further improvement. All insulin, including human, clumps

TABLE 12 Insulin time-action profile

Type	Insulin preparation	Onset (h)	Peak activity (h)	Duration of action (h)
Short acting	Regular	0.5–1.0	3–4	6–8
Intermediate acting	NPH	1.0–1.5	6–12	18–24
	Lente	1.0–2.5	8–14	18–24
Long acting	Ultralente	4.0–8.0	12–30	up to 36

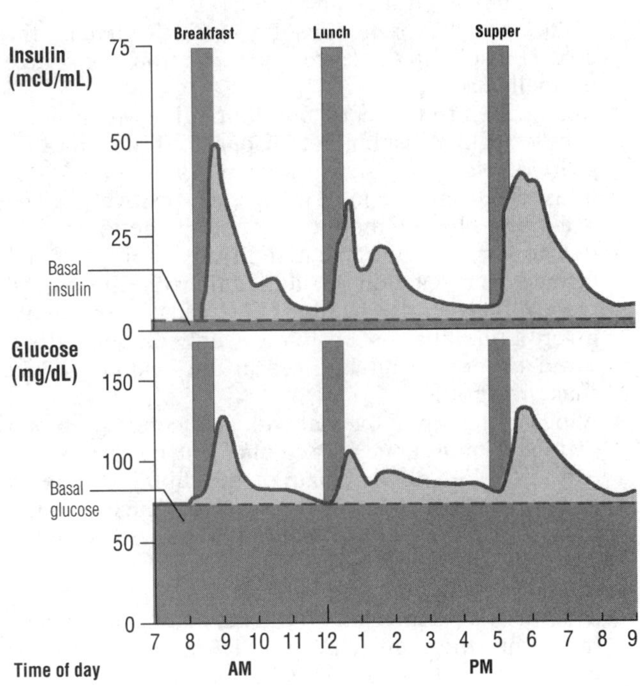

Intensive insulin therapy regimens

	7 AM	11 AM	4–5 PM	Bedtime
1. 2 doses, intermediate	×		×	
2. 2 doses, regular and intermediate	Reg. & intermed.		Reg. & intermed.	
3. 3 doses, regular or regular and intermediate	Reg. & intermed.	Reg.	Reg. & intermed.	
4. 4 doses, regular and long acting	Reg.	Reg.	Reg.	Long acting
5. 3 doses, regular and intermediate, regular only, intermediate only	Reg. & intermed.		Reg.	Intermed.

Note: Many other regimens are used as "intensive" therapy plans. The therapy is individualized to the response of the diabetic patient.

FIGURE 3 Relationship between insulin and glucose. Adapted with permission from *US Pharm.* 1988; 13 (11 suppl): 41.

together in hexamers requiring time in vivo to dissociate and begin its action. By manipulating the structure, researchers have developed monomeric compounds with insulin-like action, which are currently under study. Some of these so-called insulin analogs have very rapid action; others provide extended action.[24]

Insulin Regimens

The insulin regimen is a key element of the overall treatment plan for diabetes. Pharmacists should be familiar with the different types of insulin regimens prescribed by physicians.

Single-injection regimens are not advocated for any newly diagnosed person and provide consistent glycemic control in few patients. By using multiple daily injections or an insulin infusion pump, however, intensified regimens can achieve near-euglycemic blood glucose levels. Although intensively managed patients must monitor their blood glucose multiple—usually four—times daily, these patients are able to maintain their usual activities and may actually increase their lifestyle flexibility. For example, pump patients can more promptly adjust insulin doses to accommodate changes that occur in the activities of daily living. A 19-year-old Type I college scholarship swimmer can adjust her insulin schedule on days of three practices versus only an evening swim meet.

The goal of intensive therapy is to mimic the insulin action of a functioning pancreas. Figure 3 depicts the glucose surges from three daily meals and the resultant insulin release from a pancreas responding to the glucose. Those patients willing to use multiple injections have the option of using various combinations of insulins, depending on the individual's response pattern. Numerous regimens can be devised to fit the patient's needs, lifestyle, etc (Figure 3). For example, regular insulin can be injected before meals, and an intermediate-acting insulin can be injected at bedtime to cover blood glucose levels during the sleeping hours. Another alternative would be to inject long-acting (ultralente) and regular insulin before breakfast, regular insulin before lunch, and regular and ultralente again before dinner.

Insulin Mixtures

As the purity of insulins has improved, the problem of stability in mixing insulins has decreased. Regular insulin may be mixed with NPH insulin in any proportion desired[25]; the resultant combination is stable for approximately 1 month at room temperature and 3 months when refrigerated. Lente insulin binds with regular insulin when the two are mixed, thus decreasing the action of the regular insulin. This reaction occurs within minutes and continues for up to 24 hours. Patients mixing regular and lente insulin should either inject the mixture immediately or allow it to stand for 24 hours and then inject it. Lente and ultralente insulins may be combined with one another in any ratio desired at any time. These mixtures are stable in any proportion for 18 months if refrigerated; however, sterility is not guaranteed. The manufacturers of insulin will also not guarantee the sterility of prefilled syringes produced by the pharmacist or in the home. Home infusion therapy pharmacists are advised to review their policy manuals for appropriate prefilling plans. Patients should be given the smallest possible number of prefilled syringes at any one time. Novo-Nordisk's Velosulin should not be mixed with any lente preparation.

Patients using infusion pumps may use either normal saline or Lilly's Insulin Dilution Fluid to dilute the insulin in the pump. Regular insulin may be mixed in any proportion with normal saline for use in the pump, but the combination should be used within 2–3 hours after mixing because changes in the pH and dilution of the buffer may adversely affect stability. On the other hand, regular insulin may be mixed with Lilly's Insulin Dilution Fluid in any proportion, and it will be stable indefinitely. Because regular insulin may form crystal deposits in the tubing of insulin pumps, Velosulin has added phosphate buffer to help limit or prevent this reaction.

Proper Storage of Insulin

Insulin is a heat-labile protein, so all preparations must be stored carefully to maintain potency and maximum stability. Patients should be instructed repeatedly to inspect their insulin for visible changes in appearance. Color changes may be associated with denaturation of protein and should be interpreted as evidence of potency loss. Regular insulin's potency may decline by as much as 1.5% per month if the insulin is stored at room temperature (59–85°F, 15–29°C), and the rate of potency loss increases as the temperature increases. The lente forms of insulin retain their potency when stored at room temperature for 24 months, but signs of lost potency, such as discoloration and clumping, may occur after 30 months. In one study, NPH at room temperature did not lose potency for up to 36 months. Similarly, many insulins have been shown to be stable in unrefrigerated areas for long periods in a controlled laboratory setting. Thus, patients may keep vials of insulin currently in use out of the refrigerator because the vials contain bacteriostatic agents. However, the insulin should be used within 1–2 months and should be stored away from heaters, radiators, or sunny windows. At 100°F (38°C), all insulins lose a significant amount of potency within 1–2 months, as can be evidenced by clumping, precipitation, or discoloration of the insulin.

The pharmacist should advise patients to keep any extra bottles of insulin in the refrigerator (at 36–46°F, 2–8°C) but not the freezer. The refrigerator door is a good location for storage to keep the insulin from being shifted to the back of the refrigerator, which would increase the risk of its being frozen. Freezing insulin does not necessarily affect potency, but it may cause aggregation, precipitation, and clumping, which can alter the insulin action.[26] When patients are traveling for prolonged periods in warm climates, they can ensure the stability and potency of their insulin by storing it in an insulated container with ice, "blue ice," or some other form of cooling agent or in an insulated carrying case such as Medicool, or by packing it between several layers of clothing in a suitcase. Insulin should never be stored in the glove compartment or trunk of an automobile, or in uninsulated backpacks or cycle bags.

All insulins are produced at a near-neutral pH of 7.4. Regular insulin is a clear solution. If it looks cloudy or has become tinted, it may be contaminated and should not be dispensed or used. All other available insulins are cloudy suspensions that will settle out after standing. If the insulin suspension rapidly settles out, it has been altered and should not be used. Similarly, if it clumps or discolors, if a crystal-like glaze or frost forms on the sides of the vial, or if a white flocculation develops in any of the insulins, the insulin may be contaminated and should not be dispensed or used.

Preparation of Insulin Dose

It is important that patients understand how to mix insulin properly within the syringe. Thus, pharmacists should instruct patients in the following technique:

- Inspect vials for signs of contamination or degradation.
- Wash hands with soap and water.
- Make sure the proper insulin is used—that is, the correct insulin in the correct strength from the source normally used.
- Agitate the insulin gently but thoroughly. All insulins, except regular insulin, are suspensions and must be swirled before they are withdrawn from the vial. New, unused vials may require prolonged, relatively gentle agitation to loosen the sediment on the bottom.
- Before using bottles, wait until any foam that has formed from agitation subsides. Otherwise, gently roll the vial between the palms of the hands or repeatedly invert it until the suspension is evenly distributed. To avoid generating air bubbles in the insulin, do not shake the bottle.
- Wipe off the top of the vial with an alcohol swab or a cotton ball moistened with alcohol, and be sure that no cotton or cloth fibers remain on the rubber stopper.
- Remove a clean syringe from storage. Touch only the hub of the plunger and the barrel of the syringe; avoid touching the hub of the needle.
- Inject into the intermediate-acting insulin vial an amount of air equivalent to the needed insulin dose.
- Inject into the regular insulin vial an amount of air equivalent to the needed insulin dose.
- Invert the vial and syringe and withdraw the appropriate number of units of insulin from the regular insulin vial.
- Repeat the above step with the vial of intermediate-acting insulin.
- When the correct number of units of insulin (without air bubbles) has been measured, withdraw the needle.
- Holding the syringe with the needle upright, draw an air bubble into the syringe, invert the syringe, and roll the bubble through to mix.
- Tap the barrel of the syringe briskly two or three times to remove any tiny air bubbles that may have clung to the barrel.
- Expel the air bubble and recap the needle, or lay the syringe on a flat surface such as a table or shelf with the needle over the edge to avoid contamination.
- Check the administration site and administer the insulin to the patient.

Proper Injection Technique

Pharmacists should also make sure that patients know the correct way to inject insulin. The following procedure is recommended:

- After properly preparing the insulin dose, check the record to confirm where the insulin was injected previously. Injection sites should be rotated (Figure 4).
- Clean the injection site with an alcohol swab or a cotton ball moistened with alcohol.
- Pinch a fold of skin with one hand. With the other hand, hold the syringe like a pencil, place the needle on the skin with the beveled edge up, and push the needle quickly through the fold of skin at a 45–90° angle, depending on the degree of obesity. Before injecting the insulin, draw back slightly on the plunger (aspirate) to be sure a blood vessel has not been penetrated. If blood appears in the syringe barrel, withdraw the needle and repeat the injection in another spot on the body (Figure 5).

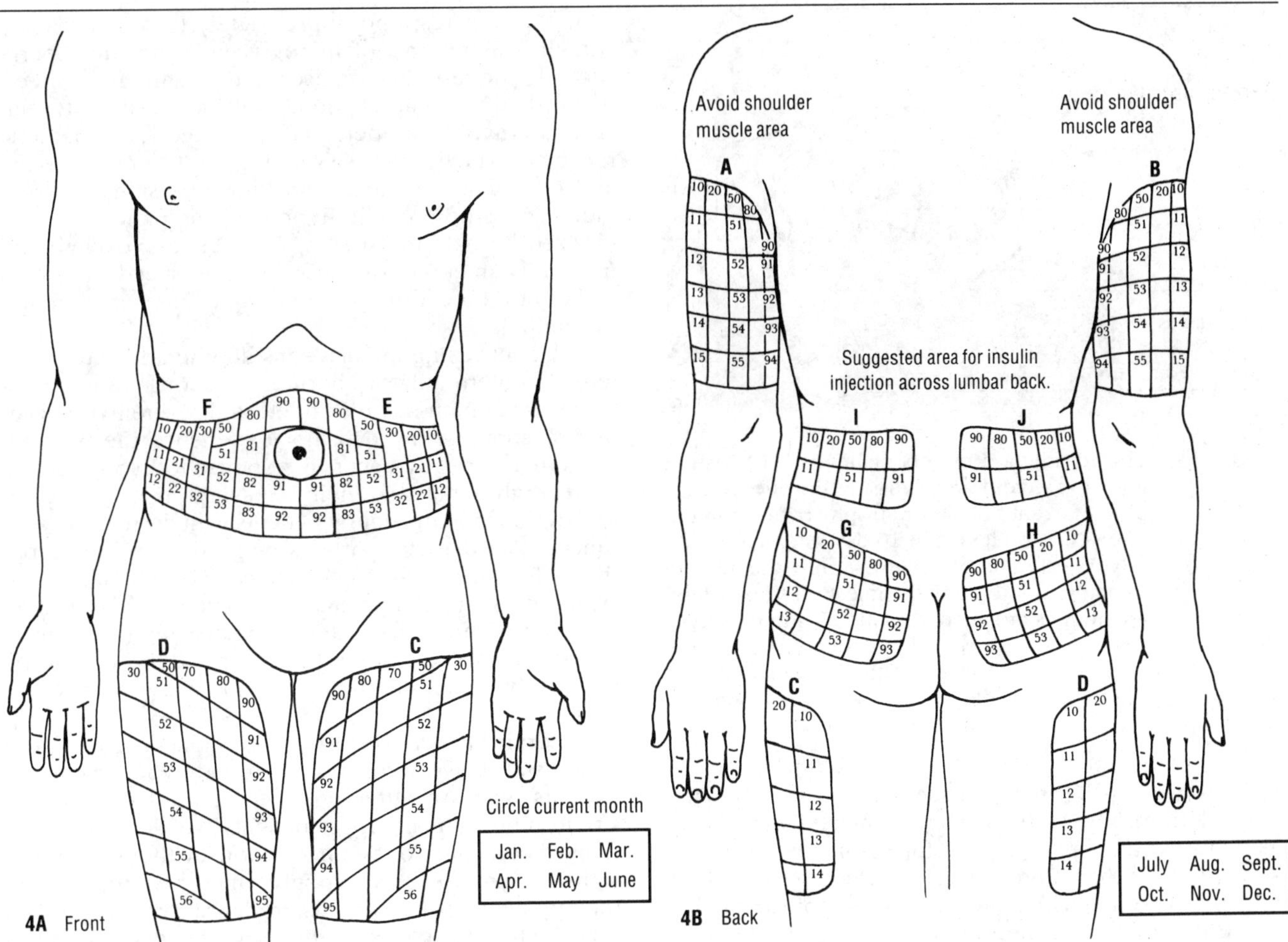

FIGURE 4 Body map of subcutaneous insulin injection sites. This body map, which is for both hospital and home use, is designed to record insulin injection sites systematically. The numbers printed in the squares are mainly for hospital recording of insulin injection sites on each patient's chart; the numbers may be used at home, but a simpler method of recording would be to write the date of each injection in the corresponding square on the map at the time of injection. With continued use, this diagram will facilitate the rotation of insulin injection sites over the entire body and thereby avoid injection too often in a single location. Adapted with permission from *The Body Map*. Birmingham, Ala: Baptist Hospitals Foundation.

- Inject the insulin by pressing the plunger in as far as it will go.
- Withdraw the needle quickly and press on the injection site with the swab or cotton ball moistened with alcohol.
- When injection is completed, dispose of the syringe and needle properly.
- Record the injection site.

Patients should be taught that insulin is to be injected deep into SC tissue. The technique for injection may need to be altered with each individual, depending on the amount of SC fat present. For many, a 60° angle or more with the skin stretched will accomplish the deep SC injection needed (Figure 5). For a thin person, a 45° angle with the skin pinched up may be required to avoid penetrating the muscle. The purpose of pinching the skin is to lift the fat off the muscle and thus avoid IM or IV injection, which may result in a more rapid onset of action and severe hypoglycemia. Properly injected insulin leaves only the needle puncture dot to show the injection site. If insulin leaks through the puncture in the skin, a longer needle should be used, inserted at a right angle to the skin.

Pharmacists should stress to patients the importance of rotating injection sites to limit local irritation, tissue reactions, and lipodystrophy. The site of the injection is one of many factors that can influence the rate at which insulin is absorbed. Injection sites, in decreasing order of degree of absorption, include the abdomen, upper arms (deltoid region), thighs, and hips (Figure 4). Because of variance from one site to another, some clinicians have recommended using all areas of one site (eg, left thigh) before switching sites. Still others have advocated using only the abdomen to eliminate the concern of dose-to-dose variance. Massaging or exercising the injection area, which will increase the rate of absorption from the injection, can affect the patient's glycemic control. Injection into a site where the SC tissue has atrophied or thickened will produce erratic absorption. A patient who is experiencing erratic control might con-

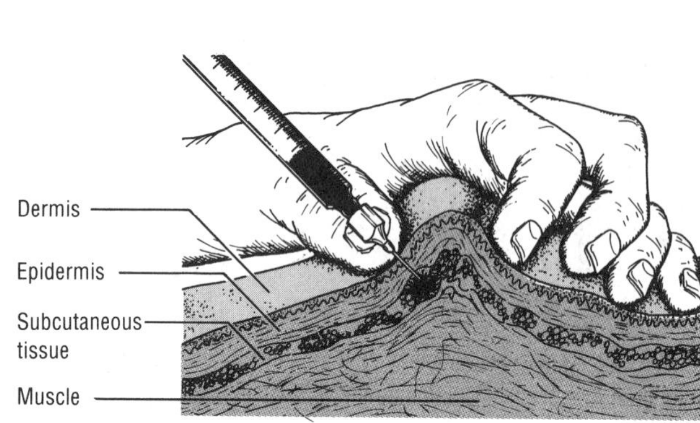

FIGURE 5 Correct method of subcutaneous (SC) insulin injection. Avoid areas already fibrotic or atrophic. Prevent fibrosis or atrophy by injecting in one site at no less than 10-day intervals. Properly injected insulin leaves only the needle puncture dot to show the injection site. Several techniques are good; the one illustrated serves well because the needle penetrates the skin at its thinnest area (dimple) and must enter the SC space. The needle angle should be 45° or more.

sider confining the injection site rotation to a specific area of the body such as the abdomen. Fibrosis and atrophy can be prevented by injection into the same site at no less than 10-day intervals. Deep IM injections will produce a much more rapid onset of action because the absorption rate from the injection site is increased. Fever, exercise, extremely hot weather, or a sauna or Jacuzzi can increase peripheral blood flow, which also speeds insulin absorption. Conversely, cold packs, cold extremities, or a hypothermal blanket may slow the onset of action because the absorption rate is decreased.

The pain and inconvenience of multiple injections may be helped by using the Button Infuser, a flexible catheter inserted SC. Doses of insulin can be injected through the proximal end. Other devices that assist with insertion of the needle into the skin are basically held against the skin and a button is pushed to insert the needle. Patients must learn the proper technique to prevent skin damage.

Adverse Reactions Associated with Insulin Therapy

Adverse reactions to insulin include insulin resistance, insulin allergy, lipodystrophies, and hypoglycemia—the most common complication of insulin therapy.

Hypoglycemia Factors predisposing the patient to hypoglycemia include insufficient food intake (eg, skipping meals, vomiting, diarrhea), excessive exercise, drug interactions, inaccurate measurement of insulin dose, concomitant intake of hypoglycemic drugs, very tight glycemic control, and termination of diabetogenic conditions.

In persons with diabetes, the counterregulatory hormones (glucagon, epinephrine, cortisol, and growth hormone), which serve to protect people from hypoglycemia, may not respond appropriately to hypoglycemic stimuli.[27] Symptoms of hypoglycemia include a parasympathetic response (nausea, hunger, and flatulence), diminished cerebral function (confusion, irritability, agitation, lethargy, and personality changes), sympathetic responses (tachycardia, sweating, and tremor), coma, and convulsions. Ataxia and blurred vision are common. The profile of the hypoglycemic patient is summarized by pale moist skin, nervousness, excitability, irritability, mental confusion, hunger, headache, normal to rapid breathing, and a tongue that may be numb or tingling.

Patients using intensive insulin therapy with an altered counterregulatory hormone response to hypoglycemia are at high risk for undetected severe hypoglycemic reactions. They may not experience the warning signs that normally occur in response to hypoglycemia or hyperglycemia, and their first symptom may be cerebral dysfunction. In elderly patients with decreased nerve function, in diabetic patients with advanced neuropathy, or in patients taking nonselective beta blockers, the symptoms of hypoglycemia are sometimes diminished and may go undetected and untreated until the condition is advanced. Among this group are those with the previously mentioned hypoglycemia unawareness syndrome.

Morning hyperglycemia (Somogyi phenomenon) may be a result of asymptomatic nocturnal hypoglycemia in patients who are otherwise well controlled on intensive insulin regimens. These patients may describe symptoms of confusion or be unconscious without any other signs or symptoms of hypoglycemia, and appropriate therapy may not be administered. Via a reflex survival action to the hypoglycemia, the body releases epinephrine, which releases glucose from the liver—thus, the morning hyperglycemia. Another reaction that can present with a similar morning hyperglycemia is termed the "dawn reaction."[28] While a person is at rest during the night, cortisol and epinephrine are released in preparation for the day ahead. A natural rise in glucose in the early morning hours occurs along with insulin release from the functioning pancreas. If that person has diabetes, the insulin release may not occur, resulting again in morning hyperglycemia. However, it should be noted that the first reaction is due to too much insulin and the second is due to too little insulin. Patients with these symptoms must monitor their blood glucose levels between 2:00 AM and 3:00 AM to determine if the glucose is low (Somogyi phenomenon) or normal/high (dawn reaction).[28] They should record the results along with any changes in their diet and activities, and they should be assisted in interpreting the results and making adjustments in their therapy.

All manifestations of hypoglycemia are relieved rapidly by glucose administration (see product table "Blood Sugar Elevating Products"). Because of the potential danger of insulin reactions progressing to hypoglycemic coma, persons with diabetes should always carry packets or cubes of table sugar, a candy roll, or glucose tablets, and should eat 2 tsp (10 g) or two cubes of sugar, five to six Lifesavers, or two glucose tablets at the onset of mild hypoglycemic symptoms (eg, sweating, hunger, weakness, nausea, dizziness, and mood changes). Alternatively, they may drink at least one-half cup of orange juice, one-third cup of apple juice, or 6–12 oz of any sugar-containing carbonated beverage. If the glucose concentration remains below 60 mg/dL, the treatment may be repeated in 15 minutes and the carbohydrate dose may be increased to 15 g. Candy that contains chocolate is usually not recommended because of a slightly slower carbohydrate absorption rate, the fat content of the chocolate, and the accompanying potential to overshoot or overconsume a proper dose. A snack consisting of one to two cups of milk, a piece of fruit, or cheese and soda crackers is generally enough to treat mild hypoglycemia if mealtime is not imminent.[29] Blood glucose should be monitored frequently to ensure adequate levels and prevent recurrent hypoglycemia.

If symptoms are intermediate (eg, with presenting confusion, poor coordination, headache, and double vision), more aggressive administration of glucose and a sugar load may be required. A glucagon emergency kit containing an ampule of glucagon (1 mg), a syringe of diluent, and clearly illustrated directions should be provided to every Type I patient in case of severe hypoglycemia-associated unconsciousness. Glucagon should be reconstituted with the accompanying solvent. Family members and other patient caregivers and coworkers should be taught to mix and administer glucagon. The usual dose for adults and children weighing more than 20 kg is 1.0 mg administered in a similar manner as insulin; for children weighing less than 20 kg, the usual dose is 0.5 mg. Normally, the patient will regain consciousness within 5–10 minutes and be able to swallow some sweetened water. If there is no response after 5–10 minutes, a second injection may be given. Glucagon injection may cause nausea and vomiting up to 2–4 hours after injection, so care should be taken to prevent aspiration of gastric contents.[29] If the response is still insufficient after the second dose, the patient should be taken to an emergency room or a physician immediately. If response does occur, the physician should be informed of the episode. If a hypoglycemic person is mistakenly thought to be hyperglycemic and given insulin, severe hypoglycemia and subsequent brain damage may result. When there is doubt about whether a patient is hypoglycemic or hyperglycemic, sugar should be given initially until the condition can be accurately evaluated.

Patients who demonstrate a sensitivity to insulin usually develop redness at the injection site. When a patient first begins taking animal-source insulin, such a reaction may be common and may occur over several weeks before gradually subsiding. The reactions may be treated with diphenhydramine chloride (Benadryl) or hydroxyzine. The long-term solution may be changing to human insulin. Newly diagnosed patients requiring insulin are now started routinely on human insulin, and hypersensitivity reactions are very rare.

Insulin Resistance Insulin resistance, a condition in which the patient requires more than 200 U a day of insulin for more than 2 days in the absence of ketoacidosis or acute infection, occurs in about 0.001% of diabetic patients. These patients almost invariably have high titers of insulin-neutralizing immunoglobulin G antibodies and should be switched to human insulin. If this switch does not resolve the problem, glucocorticoids are indicated.

Insulin Lipodystrophy and Allergy Another potential complication of insulin therapy is insulin lipodystrophy. Lipodystrophy occurs in two forms: lipoatrophy (the breakdown of SC fatty tissue, leaving hollowed areas under the skin) and lipohypertrophy (the hyperdevelopment of fatty tissue, causing bulges under the skin). Lipodystrophic changes are usually unattractive and may be difficult for the patient to accept. Lipoatrophy improves in most patients when human insulin is substituted; this is because the condition may be due to an immune response to a more antigenic insulin preparation. Lipohypertrophy is generally seen in patients who use the same sites for repeated insulin injection. The pharmacist should investigate the patient's injection technique and rotation schedule for a solution.

Nondrug Therapy

One objective in controlling diabetes is maintaining normal weight. The pharmacist should stress the importance of proper exercise and diet. Patients who need help adhering to the prescribed exercise program or adjusting their diet should be referred to a physical therapist or dietitian who deals with person with diabetes.

Exercise

Although exercise is now nearly always recommended by physicians as part of the treatment of diabetes, it was rarely considered a vital part of treatment in the past and was seldom prescribed. With the advent of specialized training in exercise physiology and diabetes management, and with the certification of physical therapists as diabetes educators, more physicians are referring patients for individualized exercise training. The physical therapist, who is trained in the physiology of exercise and its effects on glucose levels and overall glycemia control, works with the patient, physician, and dietitian to develop an exercise program tailored to the patient's age, activity level, disability, response of blood glucose levels, and daily glucose variations.[30] This helps ensure long-term adherence and decreases the risk of hypoglycemia (Table 13). The physical therapist can determine the optimal mode and intensity of exercise for the patient's individual lifestyle and diagnosis.

Patients are encouraged to participate in exercise that uses the large muscle groups at submaximal levels (eg, swimming, running, and biking). Activities that require heavy straining, such as weight lifting, are discouraged because of the risk of damage to the smaller optic capillaries. Daily aerobic exercise as prescribed by the physical therapist helps lower blood glucose levels by allowing glucose to penetrate the muscle cells for metabolism without the assistance of insulin. Exercise also improves circulatory function, an important factor in diabetic management; helps achieve and maintain ideal body weight; aids in breathing, digestion, and metabolism; and improves the cardiovascular endurance of the individual.

Effects of exercise on blood glucose levels can vary, however, with the current level of glucose or insulin. Exercise may cause hyperglycemia if there is inadequate insulin available when the patient begins the activity, or it may cause hypoglycemia if the patient's blood glu-

TABLE 13 Guidelines for managing and monitoring diabetes in patients who exercise conscientiously

1. Instruct patients to:
   a. Test blood glucose concentrations before, during, and after exercise.
   b. Prepare for moderate exercise (eg, bicycling or jogging for 30–45 minutes) by decreasing the preceding dose of regular insulin by 30–50%. If glucose concentration is normal or low before exercise, the patient should supplement the diet with a snack containing 10–15 g of carbohydrate.
   c. Avoid increased absorption of regular insulin from exercise by injecting into the abdomen or exercising 30 minutes to 1 hour following injection.
   d. Not exercise if the glucose concentration exceeds 240–300 mg/dL, which indicates severe insulin deficiency and predisposes patients to hyperglycemia secondary to exercise.
   e. Avoid jarring exercise or exercise that involves moving the head below the waist if severe proliferative retinopathy or retinal hemorrhage is present.
2. Use caution in the case of individuals with low glycogen stores (eg, alcoholics, fasting individuals, and patients on diets that are extremely hypocaloric [<800 cal] and low in carbohydrates [<10 g per day]) who may be predisposed to the hypoglycemic effects of exercise.
3. Watch for postexercise hypoglycemia (which can occur 8–15 hours following exercise). Individuals who exercise during the day should increase their carbohydrate intake and test their blood glucose concentration during the night to detect nocturnal hypoglycemia. Patients taking insulin are more susceptible to hypoglycemia than those taking sulfonylureas. Patients with Type II diabetes treated with diet are unlikely to develop hypoglycemia.

Adapted from *Applied Therapeutics: The Clinical Use of Drugs*. Vancouver, Wash: Applied Therapeutics, Inc; 1992: 1697.

cose concentration is normal or low just before exercise and proper precautions are not observed. Consistency with exercise is a key component. Patients should maintain a daily exercise program to complement the insulin dose and avoid extremes in blood glucose levels. Consistent exercise habits are more difficult for the juvenile diabetes patient to maintain, so parents must play an integral role in their child's exercise program.

Patients must be trained to monitor their blood glucose levels before, during, and after exercise and to adjust their diet and insulin injections accordingly (Table 13). Those who monitor their own blood glucose become motivated to exercise because they easily see how exercise contributes to a favorable blood glucose profile. An exercise log may help the patient maintain a regular daily schedule.

The pharmacist should encourage the patient to follow the prescribed exercise plan as part of the total treatment plan, and should be ready to refer a patient who needs information about exercise to an appropriate caregiver. If a problem arises, the pharmacist should check to ensure that the patient is ingesting carbohydrates before exercise, is injecting preexercise insulin at nonexercised sites, is participating in prescribed physical activities at the appropriate time of day with regard to peak insulin activity and food intake, recognizes the symptoms of hypoglycemia, carries a sugar source as well as a glucagon emergency kit, and wears a medical identification necklace or bracelet. Patients may need to be encouraged to tell friends, teachers, or neighbors of their diabetes. If a patient experiences a hypoglycemic event and is unable to self-treat, others must know what is happening so the patient can receive appropriate treatment as swiftly as possible.

Diet

Along with exercise, diet therapy is the cornerstone of diabetes management. This is true for all diabetic patients but especially for those with Type II diabetes. However, diet therapy adherence often is lacking, creating feelings of frustration, pessimism, failure, and anger, which may, in turn, result in worsening patient motivation. Pharmacists can provide positive patient support regarding diet and nutrition, and should reinforce the patient's understanding that consistent adherence to the prescribed diet is key to glycemic control.[31] The pharmacist can also refer the patient to a registered dietitian for more detailed education and training regarding basic nutrition; food selection and preparation; daily food plans; and plans to meet needs during special times, such as on holidays, when traveling, or when eating out.

Factors in Dietary Control Successful diet programs require education, clear goals, motivation, and behavior modification techniques. A team approach to education, counseling, and planning that includes the patient as an integral member should be used. Each patient should be able to discuss the reasons for the diet, set dietary goals, participate actively in developing a meal plan to fit his or her lifestyle, and include foods that are acceptable while meeting nutritional and caloric needs. Failure to consider patient food preferences, ethnic or religious restraints, and lifestyle may contribute to diet therapy failures. The dietitian should review the patient's eating patterns, food exchanges, and variations on meal plans to meet social needs such as parties, eating out, and holidays. Dietary education and counseling is a continual process conducted in an understanding and nonjudgmental manner and includes psychologic, physical, and socioeconomic factors in developing each individual's daily food plan. If the patient has a role in planning and selecting the diet and understands the diet's importance in the overall treatment of diabetes, and if the diet is tailored as much as possible to meet that patient's needs, diet therapy may be more successful.[31]

Recent changes in the American Diabetes Association's nutrition control guidelines have altered somewhat the dietary management of diabetes.[32] Effective diabetes self-management mandates an individualized approach to building a diet plan. The goal of the diet plan for Type I patients is to build a healthy daily nutritional intake into a regimen that allows flexibility in insulin therapy and home monitoring. The goal for Type II patients had been primarily to lose weight, but while this was usually achieved over the short term, long-term success in weight loss was elusive. The emphasis now is on meeting the blood lipid, blood pressure, and blood glucose goals through diet. Healthy food choices to obtain the calories with less saturated fat and protein may be the first step used for the Type II patient.

Limited data indicate some trends for recommending firm protein intake levels. The recommendation is the same as for the general population—about 10–20% of total calories. This is reduced for patients with renal failure. Less than 10% of the total daily intake should come from saturated fats and up to 10% should come from polyunsaturated fats, leaving 60–70% of the total calories coming from carbohydrates and monounsaturated fats. The distribution of calories between these two remaining groups will vary among patients, depending on the assessment and treatment goals. For individuals with near-normal body weight and lipid levels, the recommendation of 30% or less of the calories from total fat could be implemented, leaving 45–60% of the calories from carbohydrates. If obesity and weight loss are the major issues, a reduction in dietary fat can effectively achieve a positive alteration. One may also consider the Step II diet guidelines of the National Cholesterol Education Program, which call for 7% of the total calories from saturated fat, with 200 mg cholesterol daily. Fiber should also be included in the diet plan to assist in regulating the absorption rate of carbohydrates.

The percentage of calories from carbohydrates will vary with the patient's eating habits and treatment goals. Diabetes patients were taught for many years to avoid simple sugars. However, there is little evidence that the assumed rapid absorption and increase in glucose actually occurs when some sugar is part of the basic meal plan. Rather than being concerned about the type of carbohydrate source, one should address the total amount of carbohydrates consumed.

The patient must understand the need for attention to the amount of other nutritive sweeteners (fructose, sorbitol, etc) consumed and their "hidden" nature in foods. The polyols carry the potential for laxative effects. Sodium intake should be watched given the risk link for hypertension. Similar precautions for alcohol consumption apply to persons with diabetes as to the public at large. The risk for hypoglycemia is enhanced when alcohol is consumed on an empty stomach. Even though alcohol has no nutritional value, the calories must be accounted for, and moderation is the key. All patients should monitor their blood glucose at home to see which foods adversely affect their glycemic control.

To help patients modify their eating behaviors, pharmacists should encourage them to keep a diet log similar to the exercise log. In it, patients should record (for 4–10 days) each time they eat, what they eat, how much they eat, and why they eat (eg, social pressure, loneliness, depression, nervousness, time of day, or hunger). This diary can be the cornerstone of an acceptable plan for control with diet. Once eating patterns are defined and understood, modifications can be made and dietary behaviors changed.

Use of Alternative Sweeteners In general, food may be adapted or prepared for the diabetic patient by either restricting the sugar content or altering the sugar content and caloric value. When special foods are being prepared, sucrose should be omitted and other sweetening agents substituted. The term *alternative sweeteners* has replaced the term *artificial sweeteners* because some of the sweeteners used are now derived from natural sources.

The FDA classifies sweeteners as being either nonnutritive or nutritive. The term *nonnutritive* refers to sweeteners without calories, such as saccharin or cyclamates. *Nutritive* refers to sweeteners with calories, such as aspartame, fructose, sorbitol, and mannitol. The use of various sweeteners of both kinds is acceptable in the management of diabetes although the safety of some of these substitutes has been questioned.

Saccharin, which is 400 times as sweet as sucrose, is a common sucrose substitute in the United States. Because it has been implicated in causing malignant tumors in rats consuming exaggerated quantities, the FDA requires a warning on all products containing saccharin. The FDA also requires all retail establishments selling saccharin-containing products to display a warning statement concerning saccharin.

The use of sorbitol and fructose is troublesome because of their significant caloric content and potential to undermine efforts at weight loss and glucose control. Sorbitol, a glucose alcohol that is 60% as sweet as sugar, is absorbed slowly from the gut, converted to glucose, and metabolized. Sorbitol is one of the end products of the polyol pathway of glucose metabolism that results in some of the late complications of diabetes. Although it is generally without side effects, large quantities of sorbitol may produce the aforementioned laxative action via osmotic effects. The amount of sorbitol in foods is not considered to be a risk factor to patients unless very large amounts are consumed. The energy value of sorbitol (4 calories/g) must be counted by patients for whom weight control is necessary. Foods containing sorbitol are often labeled "not for weight control purposes" because they may have more calories than other sweeteners.

Fructose is another sucrose substitute that is found naturally in fruits, honey, and other sources. It, too, is an end product of glucose metabolism by insulin-independent pathways and has some potential for adding to the late complications of diabetes. Patients planning to use fructose as a substitute sweetener should first consult with their physician or dietitian. The quantitative reduction of hyperglycemia that may result from substantial substitution of sorbitol, fructose, and xylitol for glucose and sucrose in the diet should be assessed for long-term effectiveness and safety.

The G. D. Searle Company manufactures aspartame, which is a combination of two naturally occurring amino acids. Aspartame is classified as a nutritive sweetener by the FDA because it technically has calories. However, since the agent is 200 times sweeter than sugar and yields only 0.1 calories/tsp, aspartame is also called a noncaloric sweetener. It is commonly found in diet soft drinks, other drink mixes, candies, and cereals and is available in a crystal form for use. It is heat labile and cannot be used in cooking. Some physicians do not recommend its use in very young children.

The Hoechst Company markets an artificial sweetener, acesulfame potassium, or Sunette, for use in gum and dry food products and for sale in packets and tablets. Sunette is similar to saccharin in that it has no calories, but unlike saccharin, it also has no aftertaste. It differs from aspartame in that it does not lose its potency after heating or long-term storage.

Any patient who ingests an excessive amount of any sweetener requires nutritional counseling and assessment of needs. Limitations on the intake of sweeteners have been established in most cases; however, intake should be individualized, the use of other sweeteners considered, and the overall diet and nutritional adequacy of such products considered.

Pharmacists have a supportive and educational role to play in all phases of diet therapy. They should encourage patients to follow their prescribed diet, discourage prolonged fasting or the use of fad diets to lose weight, and help patients understand the vital importance of diet therapy in the overall treatment plan. Pharmacists can also help patients establish a self-monitoring program that will let them see the effect of food intake on blood glucose control beginning in the initial or survival phase of self-management and continuing throughout the rest of the training and lifestyle adjustment period. Patients should be encouraged to obtain dietitian or physician approval for any change in dietary habits.

Pharmacists should also encourage patients to read the labels of all foods marked "dietetic" because such labeling does not mean "diabetic" and the foods may not be sugarless or even intended for persons with diabetes. New food labeling guidelines from the FDA have clarified many problems regarding the nutritional value of various foods. Some dietetic foods actually have more calories than regular foods. Pharmacists should be familiar with all products that are directed at diet therapy. They should know which ingredients are acceptable for use by the patient, how much fat the product will contribute to the diet, and which products should be avoided. This will assist the patient in selecting the right products for his or her individual situation.

Precautions

Reading the label on all food and drug products is essential to maintaining glycemic control. Patients should develop this habit early to avoid potential adverse effects and complications in managing diabetes (Table 8).

Use of Alcohol and Alcohol-Containing Products

Precautions that apply to the general public regarding the use of alcohol apply to persons with diabetes as well. Alcohol burns like fat; alters insulin response; changes the manufacture, storage, and release of glycogen; and can cause impaired judgment and coordination and a host of other adverse effects. Because avoidance of alcohol is not always possible or desired, patients should be assessed individually to determine if ingesting alcohol to reduce emotional tension, relieve anxiety, or stimulate appetite outweighs the potential adverse effects on blood glucose control. Alcohol consumed as dry wine in moderate quantities (no more than the equivalent of two alcoholic beverages once or twice a week) has been advocated by some diabetologists as part of the therapy.

Either hyper- or hypoglycemia may develop in patients who ingest alcohol. Hypoglycemia is the most common effect, especially when alcohol is consumed on an empty stomach. It is believed to be due to either increased early endogenous insulin response to glucose or inhibition of hepatic gluconeogenesis. Relatively small quantities of alcohol (48 mL of 100 proof) may cause hypoglycemia, but if a patient has adequate amounts of glucose in the blood, the alcohol produces a less significant hypoglycemic effect. Finally, as noted in the American Diabetes Association dietary guidelines, alcohol can play a role in producing neurologic damage, as well as in the neuropathy of diabetes.

Tolbutamide and chlorpropamide have been reported to interact with alcohol, resulting in a disulfiram-like reaction (eg, flushing, headache, nausea, and vomiting). The other oral sulfonylureas (Table 9) are less likely to cause this reaction. The additive hypoglycemic effect of high-level alcohol intake with insulin has produced severe hypoglycemia, resulting in coma, brain damage, and even death. Patients who are well fed and who consume alcoholic beverages may eventually develop hyperglycemia.

Alcohol is one of the most readily oxidizable food substances known, and unlike sugar, it can be metabolized readily without insulin participation. Several studies have shown that diabetic patients who are on diet control alone or in conjunction with insulin or a sulfonylurea can consume up to 2 oz (60 mL) of dry wine daily without any significant alteration in blood glucose values. In fact, there is little evidence to support concern over the consumption of small (temperate) amounts of any alcohol. However, if ethyl alcohol—regardless of source (wine, beer, or distilled spirits)—is consumed in excess, ketosis may occur.

The amount of alcohol contained in a 4-oz glass of wine is equivalent to that in a 1.5-oz shot of distilled beverage or in 12 oz of beer. A typical 4-oz serving of dry table wine contains 90–100 calories with a sugar content generally averaging 400 mg. However, the sugar content in a 2-oz serving of sweet sherry, port, or muscatel may be as high as 6 g. Thus, light beer and dry wine may be better choices because their carbohydrate and caloric contents are lower than those of regular beer or wine.

Alcoholic beverages should always be consumed with food. Four ounces of dry wine could be consumed with the evening meal without difficulty as long as no food is omitted in the Type I diabetes meal plan and there are no other contraindications for use. For individuals with Type II diabetes, alcohol may be substituted for fat exchanges because it is metabolized like fat (1 oz = two fat exchanges). Patients prone to alcohol abuse should be discouraged from using alcohol at any time.

More individualized guidelines for alcohol use in persons with diabetes have been established. Alcohol is generally contraindicated in patients with neuropathies, alcoholism, or proliferative retinopathy; in Type I patients who are prone to hypoglycemia or are pregnant; and in Type II patients who have experienced the chlorpropamide-alcohol flush. Additional guidelines for alcohol use in patients include:

- Discussing the use of alcohol with a physician to ensure that no other contraindications exist;
- Drinking in moderation;
- Eating first and spacing drinks apart;
- Not drinking if overweight or if diabetic control is unstable;
- Avoiding mixes that contain sugar;
- Calculating the alcohol in the diet schedule and decreasing fat intake;
- Considering that alcohol promotes hypoglycemia the "morning after."

Use of Caffeine

The response to caffeine is highly variable among diabetic patients. Caffeine intake may need to be considered in patients who tend toward hyperglycemic episodes at specific times of the day. The caffeine contained in coffee, tea, soft drinks, and other products, if consumed in large amounts, may cause an increase in blood glucose because of increased liver glycogen breakdown. Large amounts of caffeine can also alter the patient's perception of hyperglycemia and affect its management.

Use of Sugar-Containing Products

A list of sucrose-free pharmaceutical preparations is useful so that the pharmacist may suggest a suitable sucrose-free product for patient use. (See Appendix 2, "Sucrose-Free Nonprescription Preparations.") Cough preparations that contain simple syrup may have a clinically significant effect on a brittle insulinopenic diabetic patient. However, the amount of extra sugar ingested to relieve a cough would not be significant in most well-controlled cases of diabetes. To put this in perspective, the difference between a large and small orange could include more sugar than would be found in 2 tsp of most cough syrups. Also, the effect of the illness upon glucose control may be more dramatic.

Use of Sympathomimetic Amines

Ephedrine, pseudoephedrine, phenylpropanolamine, phenylephrine, and epinephrine increase blood glucose and cause increased blood pressure by vasoconstriction. These substances should be used cautiously in persons with diabetes. Sympathomimetic amines do not have as potent an effect on blood glucose as does epinephrine, which can stimulate glycogenolysis. Hyperglycemia, acetonuria, and glycosuria have been reported in three nondiabetic children who received therapeutic oral doses of phenylephrine. The major problem would occur in unstable Type I patients.

Use of Salicylates

Although aspirin products do not bear a warning statement for diabetes patients, they can cause hypoglycemia in these patients, possibly by stimulating general cellular metabolism. In Type I patients, the degree of hypoglycemia resulting from large doses of aspirin (5 or 6 g) could stimulate a hypoglycemic reaction. However, the clinical significance of aspirin is questionable if the patient is monitoring for diabetes control. In addition, aspirin could cause misleading results in urine tests for glucose, but this would be a dose-related phenomenon. False-negative glucose oxidase readings have been associated with daily doses of aspirin of approximately 2.5 g. Similar doses of aspirin can also cause false-positive glucosuria readings when the copper reduction test method is used. Other nonprescription choices for analgesia can pose problems with adverse effects on renal function. Patients should be counseled to limit themselves so they do not develop a habit of using routine doses of these medications.

Use of Vitamins and Minerals

The diet of diabetic patients should meet the standard recommended requirements for vitamins and minerals. There is no evidence that such patients have a unique or special need for specific vitamin or mineral supplementation above the recommended daily allowance unless they are on a very low calorie diet or other special circumstances exist. For example, supplementation of calcium may be necessary for a patient who is pregnant, lactating, or on a calcium-poor diet.

Preventing Complications

The complications of diabetes include microangiopathy, macroangiopathy, dermopathy, retinopathy, neuropathy, nephropathy, and a decreased ability to overcome infections. The results of the DCCT serve as evidence that improved metabolic control is key to slowing the progression of complications, with the ultimate goal of preventing them altogether. Self-monitoring is a vital part of the contemporary therapy plan.

Patients must carefully use products that may affect their diabetes. For instance, the ingestion of large quantities of aspirin or even of ascorbic acid (vitamin C) may influence urine tests and alter glycemic control. Decongestant nasal sprays; asthma, allergy, and hay fever medications containing decongestants; and cold and cough preparations that contain sympathomimetic amines should be used with caution, especially in patients with poorly controlled diabetes, since these agents can directly stimulate blood glucose release. Patients should also avoid medications that contain sugar or alcohol. Antihistamines or other products that produce drowsiness and decrease mental acuity may result in decreased adherence to a therapy plan.

Diabetic patients have a greater incidence of atherosclerosis, which develops earlier in life, progresses at an accelerated rate, and is more extensive than in nondiabetic patients. However, patients considering the use of niacin or nicotinic acid to control or prevent hypercholesterolemia without their physician's knowledge should be warned of the adverse effects of the drug—including its ability to elevate blood glucose—and strongly discouraged from self-medicating.

Patients should be trained in health habits, including general hygiene, foot care, dental care (see Chapter 25, "Oral Health Products"), and eye care (see Chapter 22, "Ophthalmic Products"), to limit or prevent some chronic problems with specific body systems or areas.

General Hygiene

Persons with diabetes are more susceptible to bacterial infection and less able to fight infections, particularly monilial infections, than is the general population. The most easily infected part of the body is the skin. Infections in patients with vascular and neurologic disease may not be detected promptly and heal slowly. Extended periods of hyperglycemia also tend to worsen the skin's wound-healing ability. Minor cuts and scratches should be promptly cleansed thoroughly with soap and water. Any patient with a serious cut, burn, or puncture wound should see a physician immediately.

Daily bathing with thorough drying is recommended; patients should use mild soaps and avoid all harsh chemicals, including caustic powders, iodine-containing preparations, astringents, and any other products that may produce or exacerbate vascular or neurologic complications. Patients should inspect their bodies daily, starting at the top of the head and working down to the feet and toes. They should check for any signs of dry or cracked skin, chafing or irritation, infection, injury, and areas with visible changes from increased pressure by clothing or shoes. Patients should also ensure that any problem areas already identified are being cared for and are healing properly. Any new lesions or old lesions not resolving properly should be brought to the attention of a physician as soon as possible.

Pharmacists should know which products the physicians in their area prefer to use or avoid, and why. This ensures a better working relationship and health care partnership between the pharmacist, the patient, and the physician. The pharmacist should discuss with the patient the appropriate use of nonprescription topical antimicrobial products and should refer the patient to a physician when further medical attention is indicated.

Foot Care

Approximately 25% of persons with diabetes will develop severe foot or leg problems within their lifetime. These individuals are estimated to be 17 times more likely than persons without diabetes to develop gangrene of the extremities; among people 40 years of age and older, gangrene reportedly occurs 50 times more often in diabetic patients. Before the advent of antibiotics, leg amputations were performed on 9 of 10 patients undergoing surgery for gangrene of the foot (see color plates, photograph 1). Even with antibiotics, approximately 50% of major leg amputations (55,000 a year) are performed on patients with diabetes.[2] Yet data further suggest that more than half of these amputations could be prevented through effective diabetes control and patient education about appropriate foot care. These efforts, when coupled with expected advances in microvascular surgical techniques, seem likely to decrease future incidence of amputations among this population group.

Predisposing Factors for Foot Infections

Foot ulcers must be promptly and vigorously treated because they are easily infected, may lead to gangrene, may affect the loss of a limb, and could jeopardize the life of the patient. In the patient who has a foot infection, the risk of limb loss remains substantial for up to 6 months after the infection. Thus, because any constant irritation of the diabetic foot can cause an ulceration within 24 hours if it is not removed, even a small pebble in the shoe for a brief time can have devastating consequences. In addition, calluses may form because of ill-fitting shoes. Ultimately, repeated and unrelieved pressure on the callus site can encourage ischemia and ulceration of the underlying tissue. This situation may go unnoticed until bleeding becomes significant or an odor is noticed from the wound.

Several factors predispose diabetes patients to foot infections.

Angiopathy In time, angiopathies develop in diabetic patients, especially when blood glucose is poorly controlled. *Micro*angiopathies occur in the small-caliber blood vessels of the feet; *macro*angiopathies occur in the larger blood vessels of the foot and leg. These angiopathies contribute to compromised circulation in the foot, thus predisposing diabetic patients to infection of the lower extremities. If feet are exposed to minor trauma or infection, the thick-walled vessels become obliterated more easily.

Peripheral Neuropathy Peripheral neuropathy, which affects one in two patients with long-established disease (ie, greater than 10 years duration), results in decreased perfusion of tissue; increased relative tissue hypoxia; decreased delivery of immune system components to the area; decreased removal of cellular waste; and increased risk of severe ulcerations, gangrene, osteomyelitis, and systemic infections. As peripheral neuropathy can drastically reduce sensitivity of the feet,[33] it becomes almost impossible for the patient to be aware of minor trauma without visual observation. This condition, when combined with decreased blood flow to the foot, can contribute to the development of foot ulcers.

Peripheral Vascular Disease Peripheral vascular disease, which is 20 times more prevalent among persons with diabetes than among the general population, is another mitigating factor in the development of diabetic foot ulcerations. Diabetic patients also develop peripheral vascular disease at an earlier age than does the general population. Arterial insufficiency, which is often in evidence below the knee, results in ischemia. When diabetes is not well controlled, there may also be an increase in LDL cholesterol and a decrease in HDL cholesterol, which nurtures arterial plaque development and may further compromise circulation.

Weakened Immune System If the patient's immune system is weakened (immunocompromised), the body experiences a decreased ability to mobilize leukocytes, decreased phagocytic ability, and decreased oxygen-radical production. Collectively, these factors interfere with the patient's ability to localize and stave off infection. Decompensated peripheral circulation results in reduced clearance of metabolic waste, decreased pH, and greater susceptibility to anaerobic infection. Fungal and bacterial infections are distinct possibilities within the skin and nails of the diabetic foot.

Preventive Foot Care

Daily Inspection The importance of foot hygiene and proper foot care can never be overemphasized. One physician tells his patients, "If you look at your feet every day, they will stay attached to your ankles." This is scary to hear, but it gets the patient's immediate attention. With the aid of a mirror, patients should daily inspect their feet and lower legs (especially between toes and pressure areas) for cuts, blisters, calluses, scratches, cracks, evidence of pressure, changes in color, excessive dryness, and excessive moisture. Some clinicians train family members to perform the daily inspection for patients who cannot easily see their foot skin surface. Feet should also be evaluated by a physician or podiatrist at every clinic or office visit. The potential for this is improved by patients removing their shoes and socks in the examination room, even for a recheck visit.

Proper Hygiene Patients must wash their feet every day with mild soap and lukewarm water, after which the feet should be thoroughly dried, especially between the toes. The patient should not rub too vigorously because this may irritate and break the skin. When the feet have been dried, the patient may rub them thoroughly with a mineral or vegetable oil, lanolin, moisturizing cream, or other appropriate commercial product that does not contain any irritants. The purpose of this is to prevent excessive friction, remove scales of dead skin, and keep the skin soft and moist. Such products should not be applied between the toes, however, because they may promote the development of a bacterial or fungal infection. The pharmacist should assist the patient in product selection to avoid the use of irritants.

While excessively dry skin may crack and fissure, allowing infection to enter, feet that are too soft and moist are more susceptible to skin infections such as athlete's foot. Thus, if feet become too soft and tender, they should be rubbed with alcohol once a week. Alcohol should not be applied too often, however, because of its drying effect.

Care should be taken to avoid dry and brittle toenails. To soften toenails, patients can soak their feet for one-half hour each night in lukewarm water containing 1 tbsp/qt of powdered borax (ie, sodium borate). This can be followed by rubbing vegetable oil or a moisturizing cream around the nails. When the nails become too long, it is often advisable to file them down with an emery board. They should be filed to follow the contour of the toe, but not shorter than the underlying soft tissue of the toe. Care must be taken not to cut the corners of the nails lest an ingrown toenail develop; instead, edges should be filed after cutting to limit the potential for a sharp edge damaging another toe. Some patients may be instructed to have their toenails cared for only by a podiatrist.

Shoes and socks should be changed a couple of times every day, depending on the patient's tendency to retain moisture on the feet and in the shoes. If foot moisture is present, the patient could develop athlete's foot. To prevent this, a prophylactic foot powder can be used on the feet and in the shoes daily.

Prevention of Vasoconstriction To prevent vasoconstriction in lower extremities, patients should massage their feet every day, rubbing upward toward the tips of their toes. If patients have varicose veins, the feet should be massaged gently but the legs should not.

Diabetic patients should also observe usual foot care measures when traveling. It is wise to remove the shoes for a time during prolonged travel. Frostbite is a distinct possibility if travel involves prolonged exposure to the cold. Cold air causes the blood vessels to constrict, thus reducing blood flow to the feet. In the case of poor circulation or cold feet, diabetic patients should keep their feet warm by wearing warm hosiery. However, they should not apply heat in any form (eg, hot water bottles or heating blankets and pads) without a physician's consent. Because there is a sensory deficit, even moderate heat can injure the skin if the circulation is poor. Thus, patients should never step into a bathtub before first checking the temperature with the hands—not feet.

Constricting clothing (eg, elastic hosiery with a tight top band) will also decrease blood flow to the feet and should be avoided by diabetic patients. Similarly, patients should not cross their legs when sitting down because they may compress leg arteries and impair or close off the blood supply to the legs, as well as put pressure on certain nerves. If the weight of the bedclothes is uncomfortable for a patient, it helps to place a pillow under the covers at the foot of the bed. And since components of tobacco can also cause vasoconstriction in the extremities and thus represent an important risk factor in the development of coronary artery disease and peripheral circulation, patients should abstain from using tobacco products.

Recommendations for Footwear The need for properly fitted footwear cannot be overemphasized. Ill-fitting footwear can very easily cause friction and blister formation, particularly in these individuals because of their sensory deficit. Thus, patients should wear soft, professionally fitted leather shoes that are comfortable. Patients who experience neuropathy should be instructed never to walk barefoot inside or outside the home, and especially not in areas where there is a risk of foot trauma (eg, sticker, splinter, or cut). As a preventive measure, they should shake their shoes out after taking them off to remove any foreign objects, and they should also run their hand inside the shoes before putting them on again to ensure that no foreign object is present.

Fashion-conscious women with diabetes pose special problems related to footwear because a comfortable pair of shoes is often not stylish. In any case, the female patient is advised to wear low-heeled shoes of soft leather that correctly fit the shape of the foot. The shoe should have adequate room in the toe box so there is minimal pressure between the toes; it should fit close in the arch and snugly grip the heel. It is important to find a salesperson who is conscientious and knowledgeable and a shoe store that provides good service.

If lower extremity edema is a complicating condition, the patient should purchase shoes at the end of the day. Shoes should then be "broken in"; that is, new shoes should be worn no longer than a half hour the first day, and that time should be increased by an hour each subsequent day.

Pharmacist's Role in Preventive Care The pharmacist can play an active role in preventive foot care by asking persons at risk for diabetic foot ulcers about any neuropathic symptoms, history of claudication or resting pain, history of prior orthopedic foot problems or surgeries, and current or previous smoking habits and alcohol intake. Overweight individuals, especially males, also have a higher risk of foot pathology. Patients with any of the above risk factors should be instructed in the appropriate care of their feet and monitored closely. Pharmacists should also know which foot care products are not recommended for use by persons with diabetes, and they should be available to assist patients in making appropriate decisions as to which products to buy and when to seek additional medical attention. Finally, the pharmacist should be ready with referral choices to help the patient select a diabetologist, general physician, or podiatrist familiar with diabetic foot problems.

Treatment of Foot Conditions

First Aid for Minor Injuries Even with seemingly trivial injuries, proper first-aid treatment is a necessity as the slightest break in the skin could become infected, ulcerated, or gangrenous unless properly treated. Patients should avoid using strong antiseptics (eg, tincture of iodine) to treat infection because these products can irritate and dry the skin. A mild disinfectant might be preferable to use but not without medical supervision. If it is necessary to cover the wound with a gauze bandage, only fine paper tape or cellulose tape (Scotch Tape) should be used to secure the bandage to the skin. Ordinary adhesive tape can make the skin soggy, encourage the growth of microorganisms, and irritate the skin when removed. Any development of redness, blistering, pain, or swelling should be brought to the attention of the physician.

Corns and Calluses Corns and calluses occur as a result of friction, usually from improperly fitting footwear. A common problem for some patients is the development of a callus under the ball of the foot. This can be avoided by wearing shoes that fit well, are not too short, and do not have high heels. Curling and stretching the toes several times during the day also helps to prevent this problem, as does finishing each step on the toes rather than on the ball of the foot.

To remove a bothersome callus or corn, the patient should soak the foot with mild soap in lukewarm water for about 15 minutes. The excess tissue can then be gently rubbed off with a towel, a file, medium sandpaper, or pumice stone. The excess skin should not be torn off, however, and should *never* be allowed to become irritated. Corns and calluses should *not* be cut or trimmed with razor blades or paring knives as this may predispose the patient to an infection, which could have serious and even life-threatening consequences. If the corn or callus is particularly discomforting, a podiatrist should be consulted. The patient should *not* use one of the available nonprescription topical corn or callus removers, whose primary active ingredient is salicylic acid. These can irritate and injure the skin and predispose the patient to harm. Patients should also avoid corn medications, all of which contain keratolytic agents.

Athlete's Foot Athlete's foot in the diabetic patient, which generally begins with peeling and itching around and between the toes, should never be treated with acidic or astringent preparations. Instead, a specific antifungal drug should be used, and the patient should immediately contact a physician or podiatrist. Tinea unguium, a fungal infection of the toenail that is characterized by a brittle and discolored nail bed, should also be treated by a physician or podiatrist.

Foot Ulcers When counseling a patient about a possible foot ulcer, the pharmacist should err on the side of safety and suggest that the patient consult a physician or podiatrist. Depending on the severity of the foot infection, the patient may be treated on an outpatient or an inpatient basis. On an outpatient basis, superficial foot ulcers are treated with topical antibiotic creams or ointments with a simple dressing. If an ulcer shows signs of a local infection, erythema, and swelling, appropriate oral anti-infective therapy may be prescribed. Such therapy should consist of at least 10 days of treatment, subject to change when culture and microorganism susceptibility results become available.

An estimated 20% of all hospitalizations for diabetes are owing to unresolved foot infections, which account for more in-hospital days than any other complication of the disease. Hospitalization may be required when the lesion shows signs of a deep infection, gas is present in the lesion, gangrenous patches are observed, or there are signs of systemic infection. About 70% of foot infections are polymicrobial and may involve between three and five organisms, with *Staphylococcus aureus, Staphylococcus epidermidis*, and *Streptococcus* sp being the most common among those cultured from the lesion. Anaerobes (eg, *Bacteroides* sp, *Peptococcus* sp, and *Clostridium perfringens*), gram-negative aerobes (eg, *Escherichia coli, Proteus* sp, and *Klebsiella* sp), and gram-negative bacilli have also been cultured. Limb-threatening infections dictate aggressive combination parenteral antibiotic therapy; total bed rest; and the incision, drainage, and debridement of the foot ulcer.

Unfortunately, many patients simply do not view their condition as a disease as much as they do a nuisance, so they may minimize the potential consequences of a foot ulcer. If patients do not inspect their feet daily, they might not know an ulcer exists until it is advanced. Further, because their touch sensation might be so minimal, they might not even be aware that foreign objects are present within the ulcer. Tacks and pins are examples of foreign objects podiatrists have removed from diabetic foot ulcers.

An important nondrug measure is to have the patient keep his or her weight off the foot, especially if the foot is swollen or shows signs of a deep infection. As long as the patient keeps walking on it, even for as little as 10 minutes a day, an infected lesion simply may not heal. A wheelchair, cane, or crutches may be used when ambulatory activity is necessary.

Dental Care

Gingivitis and dental caries occur at an increased rate in diabetic patients. Occult abscesses of the teeth are common in hyperglycemic patients and may contribute to poor blood glucose control. Patients should have their teeth checked at least twice each year; they should brush and floss their teeth at least twice daily and should massage their gums with a brush, a Water Pik, or their fingers. Because uncontrolled diabetes seems to predispose patients to the various stages of periodontal disease, they should consult a dentist at the first sign of abnormal conditions of the gums, inform their dentist that they have diabetes, and then discuss appropriate dental care products.

Pharmacists should ensure that patients use sugar- and alcohol-free dental products, know which toothbrush has been recommended, and know how to floss correctly. Patients should be monitored closely for changes in oral health and referred to their dentist when appropriate.

Eye Care

Diabetes is the leading cause of blindness in the United States. The DCCT has demonstrated the positive value of metabolic control on retinopathy. Some cases of blindness can also be avoided or significantly reduced if (1) retinopathy is detected early and the retina is photocoagulated with laser therapy, and (2) glaucoma is detected and treated early. Pharmacists should encourage patients to have their eyes examined at least once each year. Pharmacists can also educate patients concerning the relationship of good vision and good blood glucose control. As mentioned earlier, glucose is metabolized to sorbitol during hyperglycemic episodes. Sorbitol accumulates in the lens as well as in other tissues, resulting in a water influx into the lens and in swelling or precipitation of protein, which may then lead to cataract formation. Drugs with parasympatholytic effects, including anticholinergics, antidepressants, antihistamines, and ganglionic blockers, can alter the pupil and ciliary muscles and result in blurred vision. Patients should be discouraged from using any topical ophthalmic preparations unless such products are recommended or prescribed by their physician, ophthalmologist, or optometrist. Patients who note any change in vision or develop any irritation of the eye should see their doctor immediately.

Product Selection Guidelines

Pharmacists should be able to advise persons with diabetes on the purchase of various diabetes care products and should be able to teach the correct use of any product they have in stock. Several syringe types are available, including those using prefilled and premixed cartridges and insulin pumps that provide high-intensity dosing of insulin without multiple daily injections. Injection aids are available for patients with a fear of needles or with handicaps such as impaired vision. Pharmacists should be aware of any special adapter or product needs associated with the specific aids, as well as of the type and amount of product training available to both them and the patient. There are also many different methods for monitoring blood and urine glucose. Special products have recently been made available for patients who travel or spend a lot of time away from home and carry their insulin with them.

Syringes and Needles

Insulin dosage errors occur when patients use the wrong insulin or syringe, so pharmacists are responsible for ensuring that the patient is purchasing the proper type of equipment. The problems with administering the wrong insulin (source or type) have been discussed previously. Because insulin is administered in units rather than milliliters, syringes are calibrated in units. The calibration of the syringe should correspond to the concentration of the insulin used (eg, U-100 syringes with U-100 insulin).

Two types of syringes are available: glass (reusable) and plastic (disposable). Almost all patients use plastic insulin syringes even though plastic syringes are more expensive than glass ones. The advantages of disposable syringes and needles include ensured sterility and ease of penetration because of thinner metal, a wide bore, and a 25% smaller angle in the needle bevel. The needles are finer (27, 28, and 29 gauge), sharper, and silicone coated for ease of insertion. There is less pain associated with the smaller (28- or 29-gauge) needles, and there is virtually no "dead space"—that is, the measurable space in the needle and at the hub of the needle and syringe that contains drug that is not injected. Dead space is a potential source of error when two different fluids are drawn, measured, and mixed in the same syringe. Needles are available in ½- and ⅝-inch lengths; the longer needle is used for obese patients and when back leakage of insulin occurs.

Disposable U-100 syringes with the capacity of 0.3 cc (30 U) and 0.5 cc (50 U), called low-dose syringes, and those with the capacity of 1.0 cc (100 U) may be used with U-100 insulin only. The low-dose syringes have a smaller-caliber barrel so that the U-100 insulin can be measured in 1-U increments, yielding a more accurate dose. Thus, patients who require less than 30–50 U of U-100 insulin per injection may use the low-dose syringes to measure the dose more accurately. The low-dose syringe barrels are also easier to read. The 1.0 mL syringes, on the other hand, are graduated in 2-U increments. The 1.0 mL syringes resemble the tuberculin syringes but should not be interchanged with them because of differences in labeling.

Several researchers have reported the reuse of insulin syringes. One study revealed that plastic disposable syringes can be reused for at least 3 days with safety and patient satisfaction; another indicated that patients reused syringes for an average of 4 days and that dullness was a major reason for changing to a new syringe.[34] Patients have been reported to place transparent tape over the barrel of the syringe to keep the numbers from rubbing off, refrigerate their syringes between uses, and wipe their needles with alcohol before reusing. There have not been any reports of an increased infection rate at the injection site in these patients, but there are also no large, long-term, well-controlled prospective studies. In general, reuse of disposable plastic syringes is not recommended, although patients who have been following this practice without problems for several years should not be discouraged. Those patients who are not at increased risk for developing infection and who are capable of safely recapping the syringe may be allowed to reuse syringes.[35] Syringes that are to be reused over a few days may be stored at room temperature. It is important to ensure that any patient who reuses a syringe and needle pay close attention to aseptic technique to avoid touch contamination. The needles should probably not be cleaned with alcohol because this removes the silicon coating.

Injection Aids

A variety of products are available for the visually impaired, including "drawing aids" that hold the syringe and vial, align the needle (Holdease, Insulin Needle Guide), and help draw up the insulin (Count-a-dose, Insulgage, Load-Matic, Syringe Support), and that can be used with magnifier devices if necessary. Magnifiers (Insul-eze, Magni-Guide, Tru-Hand) enlarge the calibrations on an insulin syringe to twice their normal size. The syringe usually is inserted or loaded into the magnifier, or has the magnifier attached to the side of the syringe. There are "dose gauges" that allow doses to be dialed in, have audible dose selectors, come in Braille with raised numbers, or have prefilled syringes that are disposable after multiple dose use (see product table "Insulin Syringes and Related Products").

There are also several different types of insulin injection devices or automatic injectors designed for patients who have an aversion to self-injection. These products include insertion aids (Autoject, Automatic Injector, Instaject, Injectomatic), insulin pens (Autopen, Novolin PenFill), jet injectors (Medi-jector EZ, Tender-Touch, Vitajet, Freedom jet), and infusers. An insertion aid is usually a jacket that fits over a filled syringe, is spring-loaded, and guides the needle into the skin. The needle may or may not be visible to the patient, depending on the design of the automatic injector. Some injectors adjust the depth and angle of skin penetration; the size of the injector varies depending on type. The syringe may be prefilled and carried until ready to use. The insulin pens look like writing pens; use disposable cartridges filled with 150 U of human insulin (regular, NPH, or a 30:70 mix); can deliver preset or dial-in doses, depending on the type; and require only one hand for injection. There are also needleless injectors called jet injectors, which allow the insulin to be delivered as a tiny liquid stream that is forced through the skin under pressure. The injected insulin disperses into a very thin spray as it enters the SC tissue. Patients who are using this type of device for the first time may have to adjust the insulin dose because the increased tissue contact may cause the insulin to be absorbed faster than when it is injected with a needle. Patients who do not have enough fat tissue may actually inject insulin into muscle tissue with a jet injector. Jet injector devices cause less lipoatrophy and inflammation than customary needle administration; they also facilitate reaching and rotating the injection sites. As with any device, however, improper use can result in errors of insulin dose. For example, the jet injector must be held firmly against the skin. If the contact is lost, the dose may not be properly administered.

For patients who use the syringe and needle for injection but dislike sticking themselves, a small flexible catheter (the Button Infuser) can be inserted SC, usually in the abdomen, and anchored at the site. It allows the patient to give multiple doses of insulin by simply attaching a syringe to a portal and injecting. The syringe is then disconnected from the SC catheter portal, which is "plugged" until the next dose is administered. The catheter can remain in place for 24–72 hours, and the patient may inject insulin several times a day through the catheter. The Button Infuser is not as complicated as an insulin pump and is often more acceptable to patients requiring multiple daily injections than the individual needle and syringe. The patient must be instructed on how to prepare the site before insertion and how to care for the site while the catheter is in place to prevent infection.

Several other adapter and injector devices are being tested, including a new needle design called the sprinkler needle. This needle has a sealed end hole and 14 small holes in the side walls to allow insulin to be sprinkled into the SC tissue instead of being deposited into a single reservoir. This is supposed to lead to more rapid absorption of the short-acting insulin, thereby allowing patients to inject themselves immediately before eating rather than 30 minutes before eating.

All the devices mentioned above must be used correctly, presenting additional teaching opportunities for the pharmacist. If the patient is not instructed in their proper use, the insulin may be delivered IM or IV, improper doses may be drawn or injected, or only part—or none—of the dose may be injected.

Insulin Infusion Pumps

Intensified insulin therapy to achieve tight control of blood sugar requires either multiple daily injections, as previously discussed, or continuous insulin pump infusion that allows a small (basal infusion) amount of insulin (usually 0.5–1.0 U per hour) to be continuously infused SC and a bolus of insulin to be injected before meals and snacks. The use of portable, battery-driven, open-loop, continuous infusion pumps to administer insulin to some Type I patients has gained support. These pumps, which are referred to as open-loop devices because the regulation of insulin is not automatically controlled by the blood glucose level, do not function like an artificial pancreas. The patient must self-monitor blood glucose at least four times a day and determine how much insulin should be injected and when. Some pumps can be programmed to change basal rates automatically at different times of the day; this allows insulin therapy to be tailored to the patient's lifestyle, prevents early-morning rise in blood sugar, and enables the patient to maintain blood glucose levels that approximate euglycemia.

There are currently two pumps (MiniMed 506, H-Tron V100) available to administer SC insulin. These devices, which are about the size of a credit card and half an inch thick, are basically microcomputers that use rechargeable batteries. They sound an alarm when the battery is running low, the infusion line is occluded, or the insulin reservoir is almost empty. These pumps use a syringe filled with diluted regular insulin and a motorized device that is programmed to push the plunger of the syringe a set distance forward. This forces the insulin through a plastic tube (infusion line) attached to a 27-gauge, ⅝-inch needle or flexible cannula, which is inserted SC and taped in place. The infusion line can be disconnected from the syringe when the patient is swimming, showering, or involved in intimate activities or when the infusion line is occluded. (Buffered insulin such as Velosulin appear to be less likely to precipitate in the insulin pump and cause blockage of insulin flow, although many patients use regular insulin with no reported problems.) Most patients should change the infusion line and cannula sites every 2 days to prevent soreness and infection. When the syringe or reservoir is empty, it must be replaced. Some pumps continue to have "runaway" alarms that sound if a runaway, or high dose, should occur. Most manufacturers say that runaways are so unlikely that such an alarm is not necessary.

The pump is programmed to provide an individualized, continuous basal amount of SC insulin throughout a 24-hour period, and to handle fluctuations in blood glucose when the patient is not eating. Guidelines for adjusting doses to account for food, exercise, and the results of self-monitoring of blood glucose are established when the patient begins using the pump. Before eating, the patient pushes several buttons on the pump to deliver a predetermined bolus amount of insulin to handle what is consumed during the meal.

A number of auxiliary pump devices are also available, including infusion tubing (12–42 inches), batteries and battery rechargers, syringes or reservoirs that fit specific pumps, tape (Micropore, Ensure, Tegaderm, or Op-Site), tape adhesive remover, surgical soap, skin conditioner, diluting fluid for insulin, blood testing supplies, and logbooks. The pharmacist should have a basic plan for training patients in the use of any insulin administration aid products stocked in the pharmacy.

Some problems with pump use are related to the fact that (1) some patients can go into a ketotic phase within a matter of hours, should an interruption of the flow of insulin occur; (2) many patients do not experience the normal symptoms of hypoglycemia; and (3) injection sites must be carefully monitored to prevent infections. Problems at the SC site also include the variability in insulin absorption and local skin reactions.

Blood glucose self-monitoring is essential for pump users, and many studies have shown that various metabolic parameters can be normalized using insulin pumps. The objectives of insulin pump therapy thus include the following:

- Normalization of blood glucose values (80–150 mg/dL);
- Maintenance of blood glucose values under 200 mg/dL;
- Normalization of glycosylated hemoglobin values;
- Prevention or reversal of diabetic complications;
- Maintenance of daily activities;
- Increased lifestyle flexibility (pump patients can more easily adjust to eating, sleeping, and exercise schedules);
- Avoidance of weight gain by maintenance of a well-planned diet;
- Avoidance of infection and complications with pump procedures;
- Achievement of a sense of well-being.

Notice that these goals are very similar to the management goals for all patients with diabetes, with the specific addition of the pump and site care guidelines.

Success in the use of insulin infusion devices is directly correlated with patient characteristics. Patients selected for insulin pump therapy must be highly motivated, capable of being educated, responsible for keeping records, willing and able to follow specific procedures, and willing to perform and log blood tests daily. Not all patients are candidates for insulin pump therapy, however. At present, Type II patients and children with diabetes are not encouraged to use an insulin pump. Patients who are candidates include:

- Pregnant patients;
- Patients with complications;
- Patients with a renal transplant;
- Brittle (difficult to control) patients;
- Motivated Type I patients.

The role of these open-loop systems in delivering insulin to the patients will gain significance in the next few years. Closed-loop systems are also being studied and are in initial clinical trials as an investigational method for insulin delivery. Unlike the open-loop systems, closed-loop systems can monitor serum glucose levels and deliver programmed amounts of insulin in response to a particular level of serum glucose. Such systems include implantable devices and an artificial pancreas. The implantable pumps being tested are primarily constant-rate, vapor-powered Infusaid devices that deliver insulin IV or intraperitoneally. The programmable implantable medication system, which allows remote programming and interrogation by radio telemetry or telephone communication, is also being investigated. There have been several problems with the implantable pumps, including flow stoppage due to tissue blockage and formation of insoluble aggregates of insulin in the pump reservoirs due to prolonged exposure to body heat and movement. The implantable glucose sensors have also produced inconsistent results. An alternative route for insulin delivery is nasal mucosal absorption. Pharmacists should review the literature closely and remain current with new products that are available or in development.

Blood and Urine Testing and Record Keeping

Proper blood or urine testing for glucose and urine ketones, as well as maintenance of adequate records of daily control, is an essential part of the diabetic patient's routine, and especially for that patient who is using insulin and must adjust the daily dose according to test results. Blood glucose testing allows the patient to learn what effect exercise, various foods, various medications, illness, and emotional stress have on blood glucose levels. Thus, it is considered to be the most accurate way for ambulatory patients to determine the level of management needed to control the diabetic condition. It should be remembered that blood glucose levels are approximately 15% lower than whole blood levels reported by laboratories.

As an alternative, urine glucose testing does not indicate the current blood glucose level but gives the patient an idea of what that level has been in the past several hours. Insulin doses should never be adjusted based on urine glucose testing because the test indicates only that there was a blood glucose increase (but not a decrease) in the past hours and that glucose spilled over into the urine when the blood glucose level exceeded the renal threshold.

Testing for urine ketones is advised for all patients who use insulin. The urine should be tested whenever blood glucose levels are greater than 200–250 mg/dL and during periods of illness or stress. The ketone test helps screen for the level of fat breakdown in the patient. Ketones in the urine, combined with elevated blood glucose, are the first indicators of diabetes ketoacidosis. The presence of ketones on two or more consecutive urine tests should be reported to the physician.

Blood Glucose Tests

The ability to achieve and maintain normal blood glucose levels helps prevent or delay the complications of diabetes. Speculation concerning the benefits of tight control is supported by the following DCCT findings:

- The frequent checking of blood glucose at home increases patients' motivation to maintain their blood glucose within normal range and thus to regulate their daily lives.
- The method encourages patients to become more involved in dietary control.
- The availability of more information on diabetic control facilitates proper insulin dosage and allows dosage to be adjusted with confidence.
- Abnormal blood glucose levels are normalized more quickly.

Maintenance of blood glucose control is impossible without measurement, and self-monitoring of blood glucose (SMBG) is the most accurate method a patient can use. It is, in fact, the gold standard for day-to-day assessment of glycemic control in that it can provide the patient immediately with the information needed to make correct decisions concerning therapy changes, which thereby improves the overall control of blood glucose. However, only with proper use and application will it improve glucose control.[36] Thus, the patient must be properly trained in the technique and given specific guidelines for therapy alterations.

Two different consensus development conferences were held in the past decade to evaluate the "state of the art" with monitoring. The first conference, in 1986, stimulated a shift toward more user-friendly blood glucose meters. Meters using the nonwipe method, labeled by many as second-generation meters, were a direct result of this conference. Today, this technology is the standard or most common type of meter in use.

The second consensus conference, in 1993, was held after the FDA completed a study to examine errors made by *all* users of SMBG equipment, including patients, family members, nurses, pharmacists, and other caregivers.[37] This study demonstrated a large need for follow-up training; it recommended that routine users be trained for at least 1 month after the initial training session and receive retraining every 6 months thereafter to review user technique. Many education centers have included this quality component as a part of their patient service. The 1993 conference emphasized the continued need for proper and easy-to-use patient teaching materials. It also validated the place of SMBG in diabetes control, recommending it for all patients who require insulin and for most patients who require drug therapy.

Blood glucose tests can be divided into two types. One type uses only reagent strips; the other type uses reagent strips and a blood glucose meter.

Reagent Strips Reagent strips, which are impregnated with glucose oxidase, can be read visually to obtain a *range* of the blood glucose level. The patient places a drop of blood on the strip and waits 30–60 seconds before wiping or washing the blood off; then, after waiting about a minute longer, the patient compares the color on the strip with the colors on a color meter chart or on the color chart on the side of the bottle containing the strips. If the patient placed the blood properly and waited the correct amount of time, an accurate result can be achieved. There are no known medications that cause false readings while blood glucose is being tested with these strips.

To ensure accuracy, test strips should be stored at room temperature. Also, bottle caps should be replaced immediately and tightly after a strip is removed since most strips will react to moisture. Visually read strips are listed in the product table "Glucose and Ketone Test Products."

Glucose Meters A glucose meter used in conjunction with reagent strips gives the specific blood glucose level rather than a range. There are two types of meters for measuring blood glucose although both kinds are based on (oxidation) glucose oxidase or hexokinase activity (see product table "Blood Glucose Meters"). One type uses a photometric measurement based on a dye-related reaction. As in the above method, the patient places a drop of blood on a reagent strip and blots it; the strip is then inserted into a meter, where it is read photometrically or colorimetrically. The other type measures blood glucose through an electronic charge via a chemical reaction. With this method, the blood on the strip is not blotted but instead remains outside the meter after the strip is inserted, and an electrical impulse is transmitted into the meter for assessment by the system/computer chip. This is the aforementioned nonwipe, or second-generation, meter.

All meters are calibrated and will generally analyze the blood glucose level based on programmed data. Additionally, all meters provide a digital readout of the blood glucose level as well as a visual indicator; some have audio components; several have memories for later recall of recent blood glucose levels; and some can give a printout of the retained data. Many pharmacies have loaded software from the meter company into their computers to allow downloading of data from a meter; this allows the program to print out glucose-level curves to reflect the patient's glucose pattern.

Patients who are selecting a meter can make comparisons based on size, wipe or nonwipe method, timing devices, calibration, accuracy, ease of use, memory/data management and printout features, battery types, need for cleaning, accessories required, audio capabilities, teaching materials or training available, and price. Other variables to assess include the precision of the product; the effect(s), if any, of temperature on accuracy; the effect on the test result of holding the meter at an angle; manufacturer support; and any specific idiosyncrasies of the particular device. The FDA has set specific allowable variances for the meters. However, when blood glucose monitoring equipment is used properly, calibrated frequently, and interpreted correctly, accuracy is ±10%. Finally, the blood glucose monitoring method recommended to the patient must be flexible and capable of being easily incorporated into the patient's daily lifestyle or routine. Patients should be allowed to try several meters before selecting one for home use.

Lancets and Other Test Accessories In addition to these test devices, patients may need blood lancets and lancet holders, alcohol swabs or cotton balls and alcohol, and other accessories. Several lancing devices are available for patient use, so pharmacists are advised to stock various brands to meet individual patient preferences (see product table "Miscellaneous Diabetes Products"). These devices allow for a finger stick with less associated pain. The patient should be instructed to use the sides of the finger, where there are fewer nerve endings than in the middle and thus less pain. The patient should wash hands just before sticking the finger, preferably with warm water to increase blood supply. If this is not possible, alcohol swabs can be used for cleansing, but the patient should ensure that the alcohol has evaporated before sticking the finger since alcohol can alter the test results.

Patient Education in SMBG Because meters are easier to use and support improved glycemic control, SMBG is becoming recommended for all types of patients with diabetes. Cost may be a factor for some patients, but most insurance companies and managed care organizations, under the provisions of major medical plans, will reimburse patients for all or part of the cost of SMBG, including the cost of a meter.

While there are a few patients who are not candidates for self-monitoring, those who should be strongly encouraged to self-test their blood glucose are:

- Patients with abnormal or unstable renal threshold;
- Patients with renal failure;
- Patients whose glycemic control is unstable and insulin dependent;
- Patients with impaired color vision;
- Patients who have trouble with urine testing;
- Patients who have difficulty recognizing true hypoglycemia;
- Patients who are pregnant;
- Patients who are using drug therapy for diabetes control;
- Patients who prefer to self-test their blood glucose.

Proper education in the methods for self-monitoring, in the differences between individual meters, in the importance of multiple daily tests, and in the interpretation and application of test results will encourage more patients to perform SMBG consistently. Pharmacists can become distributors of the blood testing devices and acquire the training needed to ensure that patients using such devices are themselves properly trained. Manufacturers are very helpful in providing education and training materials. Return demonstration by the patient is necessary to ensure patient understanding and to correct any errors as they are observed. Any user error recommendations noted at this time should be incorporated into the patient profile for technique follow-up. The pharmacist should then document the sale and training on the profile and correspond with the patient's primary physician regarding the training session.

Urine Glucose Tests

While blood glucose testing is preferred, urine glucose testing is recommended for patients who cannot or will not monitor their own blood glucose. This includes individuals who refuse to lance themselves, cannot be taught the proper technique, or are otherwise unreliable.

There are two chemical reactions for testing for glucose in the urine: copper reduction tests (Clinitest) and glucose oxidase tests (also called dip-and-read tests). In the qualitative copper reduction tests, cupric sulfate (blue) in the presence of glucose yields cuprous oxide (green to orange). However, this method of testing has a "pass-through phenomenon"; that is, if there is greater than 2% glucose in the urine, the reaction may go past green to orange very quickly and then fade back to brown. Because such a reaction may be erroneously interpreted as less than 2%, the patient must watch the reaction develop. Moreover, copper reduction tests are not specific for glucose but detect the presence of other reducing substances in the urine. Lastly, care must be exercised when using test materials: the tablets and solutions are very caustic, so handling or splashing should be avoided, and because the tablets can also be quite dangerous if accidentally ingested, they must be kept out of the reach of children.

A second qualitative method is based on the enzyme glucose oxidase. Glucose in the urine, in the presence of glucose oxidase, yields gluconic acid and hydrogen peroxide (H_2O_2). In the presence of *o*-toluidine, a color change occurs. The glucose oxidase test is more convenient and less expensive to use than the copper reduction test, but the test strips can be affected by humidity and are not as easily read.

Patients may be taking drugs that can interfere with urine glucose testing methods (Tables 14 and 15) and should be instructed to test their urine using both methods. If the test results differ, there is a strong possibility that a drug is interfering with the test results. Table 16 summarizes the disadvantages of urine glucose testing compared with SMBG.

Patients must consider the accuracy, sensitivity, range, ease of testing and timing, cost, availability of tests, and advantages or disadvantages of multitest versus individual test kits when considering which urine test kit to purchase. And as with the SMBG tests, patients must be specifically trained to use whichever products are selected, and the pharmacist should have the patient demonstrate his or her technique to ensure accuracy and proficiency.

TABLE 15 Substances that interfere with copper-reduction tests to give false-positive results

Ascorbic acid	Levodopa
Aspirin	Metaxalone (Skelaxin) metabolite
Cephalosporins	Methyldopa
Dilute urine	Penicillin
Glucuronic acid conjugates	Probenecid (Benemide)
Homogentisic acid	Reducing sugars
Isoniazid	Salicylates
Lactose in pregnant women	Streptomycin

From *Contemp Pharm Pract.* 1980; 3: 224–5.

Tests for Urinary Ketones

Because ketones in the blood overflow into the urine, urinary ketone levels can be tested to detect whether metabolic changes causing ketoacidosis are occurring. The ketone bodies produced are acetone, acetoacetic acid, and beta-hydroxybutyric acid. The basis for the test is that sodium nitroprusside alkali turns lavender in the presence of acetone or acetoacetic acid.

Acetest reagent tablets are specific for acetoacetic acid and acetone, and will detect 10 mg of acetoacetic acid in 100 mL of serum, plasma, or whole blood. They will not react with beta-hydroxybutyric acid in 100 mL of urine. Acetest can be tested for reliability by using nail polish remover that contains acetone.

TABLE 14 Substances that interfere with glucose oxidase tests

False-positive	
Chloride	Hydrogen peroxide
Glucose hypochlorite	Peroxide
False-negative	
Alcaptonuria	Homogentisic acid
Ascorbic acid	5-Hydroxyindoleacetic acid
Aspirin	5-Hydroxytryptamine
Bilirubin	5-Hydroxytryptophan
Catalase	L-Dopamine
Catechols	Levodopa
Cysteine	Meralluride injection
3,4 Dihydroxy-phenyl-acetic acid	Methyldopa (Aldomet)
	Sodium bisulfate
Epinephrine	Sodium fluoride
Ferrous sulfate (Feosol)	Tetracycline (Tetracyn, Achromycin) with vitamin C
Gentisic acid	Uric acid
Glutathione	

Adapted from *Contemp Pharm Pract.* 1980; 3: 224–5.

Ketostix, Chemstrip K, and other tests will detect 5–10 mg of acetoacetic acid in 100 mL of urine. These tests are easier to perform than Acetest, and no dropper is required. However, the new, improved Ketostix only tests for acetoacetic acid and thus shows a false-negative result if the patient produces acetone or beta-hydroxybutyric acid. It is also difficult to find a substance at home to test the reliability of the Ketostix.

All diabetes patients, particularly those with Type I diabetes, should test for ketones when blood glucose is 240 mg/dL or greater (see product table "Glucose and Ketone Test Products"), and all patients should be counseled on the proper way to test for ketones in the urine.

Factors in Selection of Test Products

Numerous factors should be considered in selecting a product to test the urine or blood of a person with diabetes.

Diabetes Category The type of diabetes a patient has is a major factor in determining which method of SMBG to recommend. Patients who are brittle, or whose blood glucose is very volatile or difficult to control, obviously need to test more often than stable Type II patients.

Patients' Ability and Motivation Willingness to learn and perform the tasks associated with using strips and a glucose meter is also a factor in the selection of home blood glucose tests. Patients who are unable or unwilling to perform the more complex tests should use simpler tests even though such tests may not be as quantitative. Often the health care providers' most important role is to motivate patients to alter their behavior, perhaps by performing SMBG.

Physical Handicaps Manual dexterity plays a role in product selection; Clinitest urine testing and several SMBG systems cannot be manipulated by patients with trembling hands. Patients with poor vision, which is common in

TABLE 16 Disadvantages of urine glucose tests

1. Inability to detect low blood sugar (hypoglycemia)
2. Many possible drug interferences
3. Patient variance with reference to renal threshold for glucose
4. Lack of correlation between urine and blood glucose levels
5. For some patients, difficulty in reading and performing tests
6. More privacy required than blood testing
7. Inability to detect how high blood glucose really is

persons with diabetes, may be unable to see the Clinitest drops or some blood glucose meter readout screens. Problems can occur in performing the tests and interpreting the color changes on the blood or urine glucose monitoring strips. Few visually impaired patients are able to match the strips accurately to the corresponding color chart, especially if lighting is poor; those who perform the color match using single-source direct lighting (eg, a table lamp) are more accurate. Special kits are available for the visually impaired patient, who may also be able to use blood glucose meters that have audio components.

Ketosis-prone patients are advised to test their blood for glucose; those who show elevated levels should also test their urine for ketones. All patients should periodically test their urine for protein as an indication of nephropathy. Protein in the urine can be easily determined by using Albustix, Combistix, Chemstrip 2GP, or Uristix (see product table "Glucose and Ketone Test Products").

The Role of the Pharmacist

The pharmacist should emphasize the importance of testing for and recording urine and blood glucose levels, and can assist the patient in selecting and using any monitoring products. Samples of testing products in the pharmacy's diabetes center can be used to help the patient make the selection. The pharmacist should be ready to instruct the patient in the proper techniques for any in-stock monitoring system and should ask the patient to demonstrate his or her ability to perform the test properly before the instruction session is completed. The patient should be encouraged to keep accurate records of the tests and to return with his or her logbook, which should also contain records of body weight, activities, diet, and medication use, so that the pharmacist can determine how well the diabetes is being controlled. The pharmacist should also discuss drug interferences with each urine monitoring method.[38]

Figures 6 and 7 are patient profile and data collection forms. These forms can be adapted for use in a community pharmacy's computer as the nondrug side of a patient profile after the data have been obtained from the patient. Then the record can be quickly updated with each patient visit. This form of documentation can be invaluable to assess the outcome of pharmacist-based patient teaching.

The pharmacist plays a vital role in helping the patient adhere to the prescribed regimen. Many diabetes educators tend to use the word *adherence* instead of *compliance*. This reflects the need for patients to accept the various components of a potentially complex regimen and adjust their lifestyle to realize the benefits of good control. Because the patient will need to apply the principles of care for a lifetime, the use of adherence indicators seems quite appropriate.[39] This concept is discussed further in the patient education section. The pharmacist can ensure that the patient understands the steps to care and then communicate this to the patient's other health care providers (physician, diabetes educator, etc) via written communication. The pharmacist may also become the "gatekeeper" for access to others in the medical community, maintaining a ready listing of potential referral sources for different diabetes-related needs (podiatrist, dietitian, ophthalmologist, etc).

Identification Tags

All persons with diabetes should wear identification bracelets, necklaces, or tags that can be seen easily and indicate that the person has diabetes and takes medication. Patients should also carry identification cards that contain the person's name, address, and telephone number; the amount and type of medication used; and the name and telephone number of the patient's physician. This identification may be lifesaving if hypoglycemia or ketoacidosis occurs. If a patient becomes unconscious through an accident or a hypoglycemic or hyperglycemic coma, medications that must be taken regularly may be missed. Because a hypoglycemic (insulin) reaction may be confused with drunkenness, there have been reports of hypoglycemic patients being jailed rather than given medical care. Various patient identification systems are listed in the product table "Miscellaneous Diabetes Products."

Recommendations for Travel

Persons with diabetes should always take enough supplies for the entire trip plus 1 week. They should always carry an extra vial of insulin to ensure that they have insulin derived from the same source. Although insulin is not a prescription product, drug abuse issues have altered state-to-state access to syringes, with some states requiring a prescription. And patients traveling abroad should bring an adequate supply of insulin and syringes because the most common type available in most foreign countries is U-40 insulin. They should not travel with prefilled syringes, however, because the syringes may be accidentally jarred and the dose wasted. Patients should also carry one or two glucagon kits and instructions for use.

All patients who travel should carry an identification card and wear an identification bracelet, necklace, or tag that indicates they have diabetes and is written in the

Patient

Name | Home phone ( ) ______

Present address (street, city, zip) | Allergies ______

History

Have you ever answered a questionnaire about diabetes? If "Yes," when?
Have you ever been tested for diabetes? If "Yes," what were the results?
What was recommended for your care?
Is there diabetes in your family? ☐ Yes ☐ No Relationship What type?
When was the last time the nondiabetic members of your family were tested?
How long have you had diabetes?
How do you feel about having diabetes?
Do members of your family understand the conditions and factors that affect control? ☐ Yes ☐ No
Do you belong to a diabetes association? ☐ Yes ☐ No

Physician/Laboratory Test Results

When was your last glucose tolerance test?
At what time was it conducted?
What was your last blood glucose level?

Individual Patient Care Planning

Do you take anything for diabetes? ☐ Yes ☐ No
If "Yes," what?

Do you take insulin? ☐ Yes ☐ No
If "Yes," what kind?

What injection equipment, syringe, injector, etc, do you use?

What do you think has adversely affected the control of your diabetes?

Where do you inject your insulin?
Do you rotate injection sites? ☐ Yes ☐ No
How much do you inject?
How often?

Demonstrate your insulin dose preparation.

How do you carry your insulin with you?
Have you had any infections? ☐ Yes ☐ No
Any other problems?

Diet

Describe your diet plan.

Have you used other diet plans previously? ☐ Yes ☐ No
If "Yes," which one(s)?
Do you use alcohol? ☐ Yes ☐ No
How much?
Are you eating differently? ☐ Yes ☐ No

Exercise

Do you have a regular schedule for exercise? ☐ Yes ☐ No
Type of exercise?
Frequency of exercise?
Are you excercising more or less? ☐ More ☐ Less

Testing

Do you test your urine? ☐ Yes ☐ No If "Yes," how?
Which product? How often?
What do you test for? ☐ Sugar ☐ Ketones ☐ Protein
Do you test your own blood for glucose? ☐ Yes ☐ No If "Yes," how?
Which product? How often?
Show me your test method.

FIGURE 6 Diabetic condition analysis form. Adapted from Pharmaceutical services for patients with diabetes. *Am Pharm* (module 4). 1986 May; NS26 (5): 10, 11.

☐ Insulin-dependent Year of onset ________

☐ Non–insulin-dependent

Patient's name ______________________________

Address ______________________ Tel # ______________ Date of birth ________

Insurance ______________________ Policy/Group # ______________________

Physician ______________________ Tel # ______________________

Dentist ______________________ Tel # ______________________

Ophthalmologist ______________________ Tel # ______________________

Podiatrist ______________________ Tel # ______________________

Dietitian ______________________ Tel # ______________________

Responsible person/emergency ____________ Tel # __________ Relationship to patient ________

HISTORY

Known Allergies/Sensitivities

Causative agent	Occurrence date	Treatment	Outcome
1.			
2.			

Concurrent diseases	Date diagnosed	Treatment
1.		
2.		

ANTIDIABETES THERAPY

Diet: Calories __________ Sweetener __________ Exercise __________ Restriction: y/n

Oral Agent

Agent __________

Date					
Strength					
Frequency					

Insulin

Type __________

Date					
Units					
Frequency					

Type __________

Date					
Units					
Frequency					

Syringe size __________ Needle size __________ Injection aid __________

Monitoring Urine ☐ Ketones ☐ Blood glucose ☐ Correspondence communication follows: y/n

Test or kit __________ __________ __________

FIGURE 7 Diabetic patient record form. From Pharmaceutical services for patients with diabetes. *Am Pharm* (module 4). 1986 May; NS26 (5): 9.

country's dominant language. Many organizations recommend that patients traveling in countries where English is not the dominant language carry the names of English-speaking physicians in each city they will be visiting. Organizations are available that help locate physicians abroad. Patients traveling to foreign countries must be able to communicate their medical needs. Although most metropolitan hotels have English-speaking employees, it is recommended that patients carry cards with some key phrases, such as "I am diabetic," "Please get me a doctor," and "Sugar or orange juice, please," written in the dominant language of the countries to be visited. They should also carry a letter from a physician stating that they have diabetes and noting other major medical problems, current medications by both brand and generic names, and information concerning medical insurance.

Patients who are traveling should control their diets carefully, allow time for physical activity, and carry candy or sugar to combat possible hypoglycemic attacks. Those who are changing time zones should also recognize that changes of 2 hours or more require adjustments of the insulin dose. The diabetic traveler heading west may use this formula to make a one-time/one-day adjustment:

New NPH/lente dose = usual NPH/lente dose × (1 + number of time zones crossed/24).

If the traveler is headed east, the formula is:

New NPH/lente dose = usual NPH/lente dose × (1 – number of time zones crossed/24).

Patients using a mixture of insulins or intensive therapy may not be able to use these formulas and so should monitor their blood glucose more often to ensure control.

Because patients will probably need to monitor their blood glucose more often, owing to changes in diet, activity, and meal schedules, they should also take extra batteries and strips for the glucose meter, a bottle of strips that can be read visually, alcohol wipes, cotton balls, and lancets. Even if patients do not usually monitor their urine for ketones, it is advisable to do so while traveling.

Behavioral and Psychosocial Issues in Diabetes

Despite continuing gains in understanding diabetes, the state of knowledge remains insufficient to prevent the disease, cure it, or provide patients with optimally effective treatment. Thus, there is a need to focus energies on improving the quality of life for patients and their families. This includes finding ways to cope with the psychologic ramifications; noncaloric food that tastes better; lifestyle changes that complement the treatment protocol; and a health team that understands the varied emotional states of the diabetic patient and cares enough to provide honest, helpful, and informed guidance.

Following the diagnosis, patients experience a series of emotions, including depression, fear, anger, and denial. The patient may feel confused and highly anxious about the treatment issues and the daily regimen to be followed. Many patients live with fear because of the serious health implications of the disease. Fear of an early death, apprehension about suffering from diabetic complications, and embarrassment over bizarre behavior during a hypoglycemic reaction may strongly affect a patient's adjustment and decrease good glycemic control. Patients who have suffered a serious insulin reaction often keep their blood glucose high to avoid a repeat episode.

Some patients may try to "beat the odds" or "live each day to the fullest" and not fully adhere to the treatment regimen. They may overindulge themselves and rationalize that having a chocolate shake, for example, will not cause a medical emergency, pain, or any other acute symptom. Then, it is not unusual for them to feel guilty about their lapse. Unfortunately, if the protocol is too stringent, it can cause frustration. Generally, however, bad habits such as overeating are easily formed and difficult to break, leading to chronically poor control.

Living with the fear of complications, when added to the daily demands of a rigorous medical regimen—the need for diet management, rigid meal schedules, blood testing, various daily therapeutic decisions, insulin injections (if required), and alterations in lifestyle—can be stressful, not only for the patient but also for the entire family. While many patients are already subject to powerful, unpredictable mood and behavioral changes caused by metabolic imbalance, the stresses often result in significant emotional disequilibrium and, occasionally, in clinical psychiatric disorders. Impaired self-esteem is common. Denial, anxiety, hostility, and depression also occur and may impair interpersonal relationships at various levels.

These emotions may be partially overcome by empathetic teachers who do not lose sight of the fact that the overall goal for diabetes education is to encourage adherence with the treatment plan and that this goal can only be accomplished when the patient both understands the plan and is motivated to gain control over the disease. To be successful in the treatment program of diabetic patients, each health team member must be sensitive to the patients' emotional concerns. Strong positive encouragement must become the norm from health care providers with regard to the patient's efforts to maintain control and avoid complications. To this end, elimination of a "c" word from the vocabulary of diabetes educators is imperative. The "c" word is cheat, and persons with diabetes do not cheat because their care is not a game. Rather, they make choices just as all individuals do. The health care provider's function is to equip the patient to make those choices wisely.

Most diabetes educators try to provide a phased approach to care, with survival skills initially taught followed by lifestyle changes. The lifestyle segment allows the patient to incorporate an individual treatment plan into his or her life. This is one reason why SMBG is among the most significant advances in diabetes care in the past 40 years. With proper patient education, SMBG allows the patient to monitor blood glucose closely and regulate diet, exercise, and medications.

Acceptance and motivation for controlling diabetes do not occur overnight. In a several-hour or even several-day program of diabetic education, the patient is often exposed to a learning process that includes all components of diabetes care. These programs are usually based on a set of national standards that have been field tested. These standards recommend the inclusion of several health providers in the educational process and mandate proper documentation. A key component of any program is the use of follow-up visits to reenforce portions of the program. Return quality check visits for SMBG can be good opportunities for enhancing the message or clarifying questions of the patient.

Patient Education

Patient education is one of the critical keys to success in controlling diabetes. Some diabetologists insist that the patient know as much about diabetes from the practical management aspect as the physician.

Education, periodic but scheduled and planned re-education, and maintenance of support systems involving friends and family members are essential in fighting the burdens accompanying diabetes. Because diabetes is a particularly difficult disease for children and adolescents, it is especially important that positive steps be taken to help young patients understand their emotions. Diabetes is the only disease in which the young patient and his or her parents are expected to make independent therapeutic decisions based on daily clinical observations. Yet many patients and their families lack an understanding of the disease and mastery of the necessary skills needed to achieve glycemic control. Thus, contracting with appropriate and knowledgeable health care providers to develop plans for specific treatment goals is often very helpful, especially since accessible and well-designed educational programs help maintain motivation for control.

Patients live with their disease 24 hours a day, so it is essential that they understand the condition and know when they are in trouble and need to call for help. Every diabetic patient should know:

- What diabetes is and why treatment is necessary;
- How to test blood for glucose;
- How to test urine for acetone and perhaps sugar;
- How to administer and store insulin and correctly take and store oral medications for control and complication therapy;
- What dose and time is best for administration of oral agents, if appropriate;
- What the symptoms are of uncontrolled diabetes and ketosis;
- What the symptoms are of hypoglycemia;
- What the emergency treatment is for hypoglycemia;
- How to select the proper foods at each meal;
- How to modify treatment for exercise or illness;
- How to care for the feet;
- What precautionary measures to take while traveling;
- How to contact the attending physician, pharmacist, or emergency department;
- When to return for follow-up.

A team approach to patient education is essential. After diagnosing the condition and classifying the patient's type of diabetes, the physician explains the disease and the treatment objectives. The dietitian emphasizes the importance and methods of reaching and maintaining an ideal body weight. The diabetes nurse specialist may train the patient in using syringes and needles, mixing insulins, and injecting insulin SC; the nurse may also give advice on proper personal hygiene, foot care, urine testing techniques, and record keeping. The physical therapist teaches the patient how to incorporate exercise into daily life, develops strategies to avoid the complications of exercise, and instructs the patient in the many benefits related to regular physical exercise.

As the specialty of diabetes education has evolved over the past 2 decades, with it has come the need for recognized experience and ability in the field. Thus, the National Certification Board for Diabetes Education (NCBDE) was developed by the American Association of Diabetes Educators in 1985. The NCBDE is a truly multidisciplinary board with physician, pharmacist, nurse, dietitian, and psychologist/educator membership dictated in its by-laws. Since the fall of 1986, the NCBDE has developed and administered a certification process for diabetes educators, the requirements for which are listed in Table 17.

The pharmacist plays a special role in patient education with regard to mixing, storing, and injecting insulin and monitoring the person's entire drug regimen. In addition, the pharmacist is often called upon to reinforce education and training provided by the physician, nurse, dietitian, and physical therapist. Some practice locations may not be supplied with all of the various practitioners listed, so the pharmacist may become the primary diabetes educator. Diabetes information sources for pharmacists and their patients are listed in Appendix 1. With the aid of this information, pharmacists should be prepared to discuss the following topics with patients:

- The relationship between diet, exercise, and insulin;
- The diabetic diet and prescribed caloric level;
- Products safe to use in weight control;
- The strength, dose, times of administration, and types of insulin;
- Injection sites and proper site rotation;

TABLE 17 Certified diabetes educator requirements

1. Professional education: currently hold a US license as a physician; podiatrist; pharmacist; physician's assistant; nurse; dietitian; registered pharmacy technician; occupational therapist

   OR

   Hold at least a master's level education in the person's chosen health profession
2. Experience: have at least 2,000 hours of direct diabetes patient education, which were obtained within the past 10 years in the United States in an organized education program that has at least a 2-year curriculum
3. Successfully pass the certification examination[a]

[a]Recertification by examination every 5 years.

August 1, 1996

John Jones, MD
Family Practice Clinic
111 Clinic Drive
Suburbia, America

Dear Dr Jones:

This morning we received a prescription for a blood glucose monitoring system from your patient George Sims. We assisted Mr Sims in selecting a meter best suited to his needs, given that he has arthritis, and provided his meter training at 2:30 PM.

Mr Sims and his wife attended the training. In planning the training, we assessed their previous experience with glucose/meter testing and their basic diabetes knowledge. After the monitoring system was selected, we reviewed each part of the system with them and covered the various steps in care for the monitor (calibration, battery replacement, cleaning, etc). A demonstration test was performed using a control solution. After this, Mr Sims demonstrated the proper technique for testing his own blood glucose. He was a bit frustrated with his timing of the test because of his arthritis. I provided some tips for streamlining his technique in obtaining an adequate sample of blood.

Mr and Mrs Sims confirmed what your note states: that Mr Sims is to record the samples and report them for possible dose adjustment. I have scheduled the Sims' 1-month technique check for Friday, September 6, when they will return for prescription refills. At that visit, I will again offer them access to our printout service to download the test results from the meter's memory. We will continue to follow up with Mr Sims and will be happy to provide him and his wife support for interpreting the results.

We appreciate the opportunity to provide diabetes education to Mr and Mrs Sims, and we look forward to working with you and your patients in the future regarding diabetes care. Should you have any questions regarding our programs and information, please contact us at your convenience.

Respectfully submitted,

William Smith, PharmD, CDE

FIGURE 8 Sample letter for communicating care.

- The proper technique for preparing the syringe (withdrawing insulin) and mixing insulin;
- The correct use of insulin syringes and needles, and how to avoid dead space;
- The availability and use of insulin infusion devices;
- Blood and urine testing methods and techniques;
- Urine testing times;
- The proper interpretation of testing results and record keeping;
- The pharmacotherapy of oral hypoglycemic agents;
- The symptoms and appropriate treatment of possible hypoglycemic and hyperglycemic reactions;
- Skin care, foot care, and personal hygiene;
- The treatment of cuts and scratches;
- The use of antihistamines and decongestants;
- The alcohol and sugar content of both prescription and nonprescription drugs;
- Proper identification, including diabetic information cards and MedicAlert jewelry or emblems.

Diabetes Care Center

To emphasize to patients that the pharmacist is truly interested in serving their needs, a clearly identified diabetes section may be established in the pharmacy. This diabetes care center should provide a complete line of diabetic products, including information about available diabetic products and services, nonprescription products that are safe for persons with diabetes to use, and booklets about diabetes. Each brochure should be reviewed for its accuracy, philosophy or approach to care, and reading level (sixth grade or lower). An area may also be established in which patients can practice testing their urine or blood and using syringes properly. Appendix 1 lists several publications that provide information to pharmacists interested in developing a diabetes care center.

Communication

Team effort and coordination are vital in patient education, and communication must be part of that effort. Pharmacists concerned about diabetes control should become involved in their local diabetes association or Juvenile Diabetes Foundation. In addition, they should become familiar with community physicians who treat diabetes and develop a working relationship with them. A consult-type letter, as shown in Figure 8, can be sent to other caregivers following a counseling session; this communication should include all the care provided to the diabetic patient and the level of patient understanding. While this process of documenting the care provided and communicating any relevant information to other health care providers often seems tedious and difficult for the pharmacist to perform, maintenance of patient data is vital to the care of diabetic patients. A system for communication with diabetic patients may also be developed. Using a drug-monitoring checklist or merely a series of questions allows the pharmacist to show concern for the patient and to gather information that may be helpful in monitoring the condition.

Case Studies

Case 18–1

Patient Complaint/History

RB, a 49-year-old male, calls the pharmacy seeking help with his blood glucose meter. Six months earlier, he was diagnosed as having Type II diabetes for which glyburide was prescribed. Four months after the diagnosis, the physician decided that the patient needed insulin injections to control his diabetes. Currently, the patient profile shows that RB uses Novolin 70/30 insulin 32 U qAM and 12 U q4PM. The profile also shows that he purchased his One Touch Profile blood glucose meter and 100 test strips about 5 weeks ago. At the time of the purchase, he was instructed on the proper use of the meter.

The patient, who has been testing his blood glucose three or four times a day, asks, "What could be causing the meter to go bad so quickly?" He notes that 4 days ago, while he was out of town, he bought a new set of test strips. He goes on to explain that the results of the tests performed the past couple of days have appeared erratic and have not reflected how he feels. RB now wants to purchase the type of strips he originally used. He also wants advice on choosing an appropriate cough and cold medication. His cold symptoms, which he describes as a runny nose and raspy cough associated with some chills, began a couple of days ago.

Based on the information provided by the patient, the pharmacist asks him to bring in his meter and the new test strips for evaluation.

Clinical Considerations/Strategies

The following considerations/strategies are provided to aid the reader in (1) determining whether treatment of the patient's condition with nonprescription medications is warranted, (2) selecting the appropriate nonprescription medication, and (3) developing a patient counseling strategy to ensure optimal therapeutic outcomes:

- Assess the patient's current knowledge about and technique for self-monitoring of blood glucose levels.
- Assess the patient's ability to obtain an adequate blood sample for his particular meter.
- Assess the patient's ability to program his meter properly for different test strip lots.
- Assess the patient's interpretation of his blood glucose levels as they relate to control of his diabetes.
- Assess the patient's cold symptoms and recommend a product for symptomatic relief that will not significantly interfere with his glycemic control.
- Describe components of a follow-up education plan that will ensure that diabetic patients understand and adhere to their treatment regimen.
- Develop a plan for continually assessing/reviewing the patient's technique in using his meter.

Case 18–2

Patient Complaint/History

AG, a 56-year-old male whose wife died 3 months ago, has been using insulin for about 2 months to control his Type II diabetes. He also takes Lopressor 50 mg bid and hydrochlorothiazide 25 mg daily to control his blood pressure. During the two and a half years he has had diabetes, the patient has been unable to control his condition adequately; his blood glucose levels are often above 180 mg/dL. His current insulin regimen is two doses of Novolin 70/30 insulin, administered as 34 U qAM and 14 U in the late afternoon (4–5 PM). Now that he is alone, he prefers to eat breakfast at a restaurant close to his work site. His physician has instructed him to inject his morning dose of insulin after driving the 24-mile commute to work and then eat breakfast. His physician also told him that beta blockers could mask signs/symptoms of hypoglycemia.

AG brought the following chart of his blood glucose test results to the pharmacy today for evaluation. Except for the test performed at 10 PM, the results are from preprandial tests.

	6:15 AM	Noon	4 PM	10 PM
Week 1	142	162	118	156
Week 2	149	151	119	161
Week 3	145	139	126	158
Week 4 (current)	214	199	204	221

Although his activities have not changed significantly in the past few weeks, the patient says that he has been feeling sluggish. Further, his medications have not changed in the past month. He asks whether the insulin could be causing the problem; he noticed some white flecks sticking to the inside of the insulin vial.

Clinical Considerations/Strategies

The following considerations/strategies are provided to aid the reader in (1) determining whether treatment of the patient's condition with nonprescription medications is warranted, (2) selecting the appropriate nonprescription medication, and (3) developing a patient counseling strategy to ensure optimal therapeutic outcomes:

- Assess the patient's knowledge of how to detect deterioration of his insulin. Also, assess his technique in inspecting his insulin for signs of clumping, discoloration, frosting, and loss of suspension.
- Assess the patient's injection technique.
- Assess the patient's adherence to the treatment plan (eg, blood glucose monitoring, insulin administration, nutrition, and physical activity).
- Assess the patient's current practices for storing his insulin.
- Discuss with the patient the proper storage technique for insulin vials.
- Develop a plan for instructing diabetic patients on the proper storage and use of insulin.
- Review with the patient the proper use of his antihypertensive medications.

Summary

Diabetes control requires a team effort on the part of the physician, pharmacist, dietitian, nurse, physical therapist, podiatrist, patient, and other caregivers. The pharmacist plays an important role by monitoring patient care, remaining informed about all aspects of the disease, and applying current knowledge to improving patient glycemic control. Patient consultation and follow-up will reinforce the patient's understanding of diabetes and serve to enhance the importance of consistency by the patient in his or her own care. Concerned pharmacists should join their local diabetes associations, consult recent literature, and plan their educational activities to keep their knowledge current.

References

1. Garrelts L. *US Pharm Guide Diabetes Manage.* 1988; 13(11, suppl): 4.
2. *ADA Vital Statistics.* Washington, DC: American Diabetes Association; 1993.
3. Diabetes Care Group, National Institute of Diabetes and Digestive and Kidney Disease. *Diabetes in America.* 2nd ed. NIH Pub No 95–1468. Bethesda, Md: US Department of Health and Human Services; 1995.
4. Foster DW. In: Braunwald E et al, eds. *Harrison's Principles of Internal Medicine.* 11th ed. New York: McGraw-Hill; 1987: 1778–96.
5. Rifkin H, Porte D Jr, eds. *Ellenberg and Rifkin's Diabetes Mellitus: Theory and Practice.* 4th ed. New York: Elsevier Science Publishing; 1990.
6. American Diabetes Association. *The Physician's Guide to Type II Diabetes Mellitus (NIDDM): Diagnosis and Treatment.* New York: American Diabetes Association; 1984: 1–112.
7. Hepp KD. *Diabetologia.* 1977; 13: 177.
8. Gerich JE. *Mayo Clin Proc.* 1986; 61: 787–91.
9. Kolterman OG et al. *J Clin Invest.* 1981; 68: 957.
10. Diabetes Control and Complications Trial Research Group. The effect of intensive treatment of diabetes on the progression of long-term complications in insulin-dependent diabetes mellitus. *N Engl J Med.* 1993; 328: 977–86.
11. Brownlee M. *Diabetes Care.* 1992; 15: 1835–43.
12. Brownlee M et al. *N Engl J Med.* 1988; 319: 1315–21.
13. Lewis EJ et al. *N Engl J Med.* 1993; 328: 1456–62.
14. Sano T et al. *Diabetes Care.* 1994; 17: 420–4.
15. Motlich ME. *Postgrad Med.* 1989; 85: 182.
16. Nathan DM. *N Engl J Med.* 1993; 328: 1676–85.
17. Betteridge DJ. *Br Med Bull.* 1989; 45: 285–311.
18. Rayfield EJ. *Am J Med.* 1982; 72.
19. Standards of medical care, *Diabetes Care.* 1994; 17: 616.
20. American Diabetes Association. Consensus statement. Self-monitoring of blood glucose. *Diabetes Care.* 1994; 17: 76–87.
21. Clissold SP, Edward C. Acarbose. *Drugs.* 1988; 35: 214–43.
22. Skyler JS. *Postgrad Med.* 1987; 81(6): 163–74.
23. Krosnick A. Newer insulin, insulin allergies, and the clinical use of insulins. In: Bergman M, ed. *Principles of Diabetes Management.* New Hyde Park, NY: Medical Examination Publishing Co; 1987: 123–35.
24. Campbell RK. *Pract Diabetes.* 1988 Jan/Feb; 15–7.
25. Brange J et al. *Diabetes Care.* 1990; 13: 923–54.
26. White J, Campbell RK. *Hosp Pharm.* 1991; 26: 12.
27. Peters AL, Davidson MB. *Diabetes Care.* 1986; 9: 180–3.
28. Cryer PE, Gerich JE. *N Engl J Med.* 1985; 313: 232.

29. Stephenson JM, Schernthaner G. *Diabetes Care.* 1989; 12: 245–51.
30. Perragallo-Dittko V, Godley K, Meyer J, eds. *A Core Curriculum for Diabetes Education.* 2nd ed. Chicago, Ill: American Association of Diabetes Educators; 1993.
31. Bogardue C et al. *Diabetes.* 1984; 33: 311–8.
32. Crapo PA. *Clin Diabetes.* 1983; 1: 12–4.
33. Franz MJ et al. *Diabetes Care.* 1994; 17: 490–518.
34. Vinik AI et al. *Diabetes Care.* 1992; 15: 1926–75.
35. Aziz S. *Diabetes Care.* 1984; 7: 118.
36. *Diabetes Care: Clin Pract Rev.* 1991; 14(suppl 2).
37. Nathan DM. Monitoring diabetes mellitus. In: Lebovitz HE. *Educational Therapy for Diabetes Mellitus and Related Disorders.* Alexandria, Va: American Diabetes Association; 1991: 86–91.
38. National Steering Committee for Quality Assurance in Capillary Blood Glucose Monitoring. Proposed strategies for reducing user error in capillary blood glucose monitoring. *Diabetes Care.* 1993; 16: 493–8.
39. Guthrie D, Guthrie R, Hinnen D. *Diabetes Forecast.* 1985; 38(2): 43–5.
40. Funnell MM et al. *Diabetes Educ.* 1991; 17: 37–41.

Appendix 1: Diabetes Information Sources

Information for Pharmacists and Patients

- American Association of Diabetes Educators
  444 North Michigan Avenue
  Suite 1240
  Chicago, IL 60611
  312–644–2233
  Numerous aids in diabetes education, including A Core Curriculum in *Diabetes Education*, 2nd edition.

- American Diabetes Association, Inc
  1660 Duke Street
  Alexandria, VA 22314
  703–549–1500
  Numerous publications on all aspects of diabetes. Monthly magazine for members.

- American Dietetic Association
  216 West Jackson Boulevard
  Suite 800
  Chicago, IL 60606–6995
  312–899–0040
  Numerous publications on diabetes education.

- Becton Dickinson and Company
  Becton Dickinson Consumer Products
  One Becton Drive
  Franklin Lakes, NJ 07417
  201–847–7100
  Pharmacists: numerous diabetes education products.
  Patients: numerous publications on diabetes education and management.

- Boehringer Mannheim Diagnostics
  9115 Hague Road
  Indianapolis, IN 46250
  800–858–8072
  Numerous publications on diabetes education.

- Bristol-Myers Squibb Company
  US Pharmaceutical Division
  PO Box 4500
  Princeton, NJ 08543–4500
  609–897–2000
  Various professional and patient teaching materials.

- Chronomed
  13911 Ridgedale Drive
  Suite 250
  Minnetonka, MN 55305
  800–876–6540
  Numerous publications, including slides and audiocassettes, on diabetes education and management.

- *Diabetes Self-Management*
  Subscription Department
  PO Box 51125
  Boulder, CO 80321–1125
  800–234–0923
  Bimonthly publication.

- Diagnostics Division/Bayer, Inc
PO Box 3115
Elkhart, IN 46515
219–264–8410
Pharmacists: several publications and continuing education programs related to diabetes education. Patients: numerous publications on diabetes management.

- Eli Lilly and Company
Lilly Corporate Center
Indianapolis, IN 46285
317–276–2000
Numerous publications on diabetes management.

- Herc Publishing
PO Box 30090
Lincoln, NE 68503
402–476–2221
Diabetes—Living and Learning, a book for the adult with Type I or Type II diabetes, 1988.
Diabetes—Stuff and More Stuff, a book for children with diabetes and their parents, 1988.

- Hoechst-Roussel Pharmaceuticals, Inc
Medical Information
Route 202–206 North
PO Box 2500
Somerville, NJ 08876–1258
800–445–4774
Numerous publications on diabetes education.

- International Diabetes Center
5000 West 39th Street
Minneapolis, MN 55416
612–927–3393
Numerous publications on diabetes education and management.

- Joslin Diabetes Center
One Joslin Place
Boston, MA 02215
617–732–2400
Numerous publications on diabetes education and management.

- Juvenile Diabetes Foundation
432 Park Avenue South
New York, NY 10016–8013
212–889–7575
Pharmacists: numerous diabetes education products. Patients: numerous publications on diabetes education.

- Lifescan, Inc
A Johnson & Johnson Company
1051 South Milpitas Boulevard
Milpitas, CA 95035
800–227–8862
"Blood Glucose Monitoring: For the Phases of Your Life," published for LifeScan, Inc, by Health Education Technologies.

- MedicAlert Foundation, International
PO Box 1009
Turlock, CA 95381–1009
800–432–5378
MedicAlert Emergency Medical Identification necklace or bracelet engraved with the patient's specific health problem and a wallet card. The patient's medical history is computerized and is available to emergency personnel 24 hours a day via a collect phone call to the MedicAlert Foundation.

- National Institute of Child Health and Human Development
Building 31, Room 2A32
9000 Rockville Pike
Bethesda, MD 20892
301–496–5133
"Understanding Gestational Diabetes: A Practical Guide to a Healthy Pregnancy," D. Thomas-Doberson et al, 1989.

- Novo-Nordisk Pharmaceuticals Inc
100 Overlook Center, Suite 200
Princeton, NJ 08540
800–727–6500
Numerous publications on diabetes education and management.

- Pfizer Inc
235 East 42nd Street
New York, NY 10017
212–573–2323
Pharmacists: numerous diabetes education products. Patients: numerous publications on diabetes education and management.

- *US Pharmacist*
Jobson Publishing Corporation
352 Park Avenue South
New York, NY 10010
212–274–7000
Annual diabetes supplement to *US Pharmacist*.

- The Upjohn Company
7000 Portage Road
Kalamazoo, MI 49001
616–323–4000
Numerous publications on diabetes education.

Additional Suggested Reading

The pharmacist should contact the local diabetes association and diabetes educators association for information to provide diabetic patients about membership and activities.

Appendix 2: Sucrose-Free Nonprescription Preparations

The following sucrose-free preparations were extracted from APhA's nonprescription drug database and grouped by therapeutic category. Because of space limitations and because manufacturers voluntarily designate which of their products are sucrose-free, this list cannot be considered all-inclusive.

Manufacturers freqently change the ingredients in their products; therefore, it is *critical* that patients be instructed to read product labels carefully and not to assume that a product that was once sucrose free has remained free of sucrose. Further, products labeled as "dietetic" or "sugar free" may contain calorigenic sugars such as dextrose, fructose, or sorbitol. Patients with diabetes should check product labels carefully so as to avoid all calorigenic sugars. These patients should also check product labels for alcohol content.

Patients with diabetes who are ill are usually under stress and thus should be instructed to monitor their blood glucose levels more frequently. Although the amount of any calorigenic sugar in a given dose of most medications is not high enough to change a treatment protocol significantly, the following products are less likely to affect blood glucose levels.

Antacid and Antireflux Products

Alka-Seltzer Extra-Strength
Alka-Seltzer Gold
Alka-Seltzer Lemon-Lime
Alka-Seltzer Original
ALternaGEL
Arm & Hammer Pure Baking Soda
Gaviscon ESRF
Gaviscon Liquid
Maalox
Maalox Therapeutic Concentrate

Anthelmintic Products

Pin-X

Antidiarrheal Products

Kaolin Pectin
Lactaid
Pepto-Bismol Maximum Strength
Pepto-Bismol Original Strength

Antiemetic Products

Nauzene

Antiflatulent Products

CharcoCaps
Gas-X Extra Strength
Genasyme
Little Tummys Infant Gas Relief
Maalox Extra Strength Antacid/Anti-Gas

Calcium Products

Calci-Mix
Calciday-667
Calcium Carbonate
Calcium Gluconate
Calcium and Magnesium
Calcium Carbonate
Calcium Complex
Calcium Magnesium
Calcium with Vitamin D
Calcium, Magnesium, and Zinc
Caltrate 600
Caltrate 600 + D
Caltrate Plus
Citracal
Citracal + D
Citracal Liquitabs
Fem Cal
Florical
Liquid Calcium + D
Mag/Cal Mega
Monocal
Nephro-Calci
Os-Cal 250 + D
Os-Cal 500
Oyster Calcium
Oyster Calcium 500 + D
Oyster Shell Calcium
Oyster Shell Calcium with Vitamin D
Oystercal 500
Oystercal-D 250
Parvacal
Super Cal/Mag
Super Calci-Caps

Cold, Cough, and Allergy Products

Benylin Adult Cough Formula
Benylin Multi-Symptom Formula
Clear Cough DM
Clear Cough Night Time
Codimal DM
Diabe-tuss DM
Diabetic Tussin Allergy Relief
Diabetic Tussin Cough Drops, Cherry
Diabetic Tussin Cough Drops, Menthol-Eucalyptus
Diabetic Tussin DM
Diabetic Tussin DM Maximum Strength
Diabetic Tussin EX
Diabetic Tussin, Children's
Dimetapp Allergy, Children's
Fisherman's Friend, Extra Strong, Sugar Free
Fisherman's Friend, Refreshing Mint, Sugar Free
Halls Juniors Sugar Free Cough Drops, Grape or Orange
Halls Mentho-Lyptus Sugar Free Cough Suppressant Drops, Black Cherry
Halls Mentho-Lyptus Sugar Free Cough Suppressant Drops, Citrus Blend
Halls Mentho-Lyptus Sugar Free Cough Suppressant Drops, Mountain Menthol
Hayfebrol
Herbal-Menthol
Luden's Maximum Strength Sugar Free, Cherry
Nasal-D
Propagest
Ricola Sugar Free Herb Throat Drops, Alpine-Mint

Ricola Sugar Free Herb Throat Drops, Cherry- or Lemon-Mint
Ricola Sugar Free Herb Throat Drops, Mountain Herb
Robitussin Sugar Free Cough Drops, Cherry or Peppermint
Safe Tussin 30
Scot-Tussin Allergy Relief Formula
Scot-Tussin DM
Scot-Tussin DM Cough Chasers
Scot-Tussin Expectorant
Scot-Tussin Original
Scot-Tussin Senior
Sinulin
Sudafed Children's Cold & Cough
Sudafed Children's Nasal Decongestant
Sudafed Pediatric Nasal Decongestant
Tricodene Sugar Free

Dentifrice Products

Arm & Hammer PeroxiCare
Dr. Tichenor's Toothpaste
Mentadent Gum Care
Natural White Toothpaste
Natural White Tartar Control Toothpaste
Pearl Drops Whitening Baking Soda Tartar Control
Pearl Drops Whitening Extra Strength
Pearl Drops Whitening Regular Tartar Control
Pearl Drops Whitening Toothpolish, Spearmint
Slimer Toothpaste

Enteral Food Supplement Products

Casec
Criticare HN
Deliver 2.0
DiabetiSource
Impact
Impact 1.5
Impact with Fiber
Isocal
Isocal HN
IsoSource VHN
MCT Oil
Moducal
ReSource Fructose Sweetened/ReSource Diabetic
SandoSource Peptide
Vivonex Pediatric
Vivonex Plus
Vivonex T.E.N.

Gastric Decontaminant Products

CharcoAid
CharcoAid 2000

Histamine II Receptor Antagonists

Tagamet HB
Zantac 75

Infants' and Children's Formula Products

3232A Formula
Enfamil
Enfamil Human Milk Fortifier
Enfamil Next Step
Enfamil Premature Formula
Enfamil Premature Formula with Iron
Enfamil with Iron
Gerber Baby Formula Low Iron
Gerber Baby Formula with Iron
Lactofree
Lofenalac
MSUD Diet
Nutramigen
Pregestimil
ProSobee

Internal Analgesic and Antipyretic Products

Addaprin
Alka-Seltzer Extra-Strength
Alka-Seltzer Lemon-Lime
Alka-Seltzer Original
Aminofen
Aminofen Max
Arthriten
Mobigesic
Motrin IB
PediApap
Supac

Iron Products

Feostat
Fer-In-Sol
Ferro-Sequels
Ferrous Gluconate
Ferrous Sulfate
I.L.X. B_{12} Sugar Free
Iron Plus Vitamin C
Irospan
Niferex
Perfect Iron

Laxative Products

Ceo-Two
FiberCon
Metamucil Original Texture, Effervescent Sugar Free
Purge
Unilax

Menstrual Products

Backaid Pills
Diurex Water Caplet
Lurline PMS

Miscellaneous Mineral Products

Chromium Picolinate
Chromium, Organic
Manganese
Maxi-Minerals
Mega Mineral
Selenium
Selenium, Oceanic
Zinc
Zinc, Elemental

Oral Discomfort Products

Little Teethers Oral Pain Relief
Peroxyl Oral Spot Treatment
Probax

Sore Throat Products

Luden's Maximum Strength Sugar Free, Cherry
Ricola Sugar Free Herb Throat Drops, Alpine-Mint
Ricola Sugar Free Herb Throat Drops, Cherry- or Lemon-Mint
Ricola Sugar Free Herb Throat Drops, Mountain Herb
Vicks Chloraseptic Sore Throat, Cherry Menthol

Vitamin Products

A-D_3-E with Selenium Tablets
Advanced Stress Formula Plus Zinc Tablets
Advanced Stress Formula Tablets (with or without iron)
Akorn Antioxidants Caplets
Antioxidant Formula Softgels
Antioxidant Vitamin & Mineral Formula Softgels
B 100 "1" B Factors Tablets or Timed-Release Tablets
B 100% RDA Complex Tablets
B 150 "11" B Factors Timed-Release Tablets
B 50 "11" B Factors Tablets
B 50 Complex Capsules or Tablets
B Complex Maxi Softgels
B Complex Maxi Tablets
B Complex Tablets
B Complex with C Tablets
B-C Complex Capsules
Beta Carotene Softgels
Brewers Yeast Tablets
Buffered C Tablets
C & E Softgels
C Plus Tablets
C Tablets
C Timed-Release Tablets
C Vitamin Tablets
C Vitamin Timed-Release Tablets
Centrum Tablets
Chelated Calcium Magnesium Tablets
Chelated Calcium Magnesium Zinc Tablets
D-alpha Tocopherol Softgels
Daily Multiple Vitamins & Minerals Tablets
Daily Multiple Vitamins Tablets (with or without iron)
Daily Plus Iron & Calcium Tablets
Daily Vitamins Plus Minerals Tablets
DiabeVite Tablets
Eye-Vites Tablets
Eyetamins Tablets
Fish Liver Oil Softgels
Formula for Life Tablets
Freedavite Tablets
Fruit C Chewable Tablets
Geri-Freeda Tablets
Gerimed Tablets
Herpetrol Tablets
I.L.X. B_{12} Sugar Free Elixir
Jets Chewable Tablets
Kenwood Therapeutic Liquid
Kovitonic Liquid
KPN (Key Prenatal) Tablets
LKV (Liquid Kiddie Vitamins) Drops
Mature Complete Tablets
Maxi-Minerals Tablets
Men's Multi Iron Free Tablets
Multi-Mineral Tablets
Natalins Tablets
Nestabs Tablets
Os-Cal Fortified Tablets
Oxi-Freeda Tablets
Parvlex Tablets
Peridin-C Tablets
Poly-Vi-Sol Vitamin Drops
Pre-Natal Multi Vitamin-Mineral Complex Tablets
Protegra Antioxidant Softgels
Quintabs-M Tablets
Stresstabs High Potency Stress Formula + Iron Tablets
Stresstabs High Potency Stress Formula Plus Zinc Tablets
Stresstabs High Potency Stress Formula Tablets
Sunvite Multi Vitamin-Mineral Formula Tablets
Sunvite Platinum Multi Vitamin-Mineral Formula Tablets
Super A&D_3 Tablets
Super C Tablets
Super Dec B-100 Coated Tablets
Super Multiple 33 with Minerals Tablets
Super Multiple 42 with Beta Carotene Tablets
Super Multiple 50 Tablets
Super Multiple Minus Iron Tablets
Super Quints-50 Tablets
Theragran High Potency Multivitamin Caplets
Theragran Stress Formula High Potency Multivitamin Caplets
Theragran-M High Potency Vitamins with Minerals Caplets
Therapeutic M Multi Vitamins Plus Minerals Tablets
Tri-Vi-Sol Vitamins A,D+C Drops
Tri-Vi-Sol With Iron Vitamin A,D+C Drops
Ultra-Freeda Tablets
Unilife-A Gelcaps
Vitalets Chewable Tablets, Flavored or Unflavored
Vitalize Liquid
Women's One Daily Multiple Vitamin Tablets

CHAPTER 19

Nutritional Products

Loyd V. Allen, Jr

Questions to ask in patient assessment and counseling

- *Why do you think you need a vitamin, mineral, or nutritional supplement?*
- *What are your symptoms? Have they appeared suddenly or gradually?*
- *What is your age and weight?*
- *Do you eat meats, vegetables, dairy products, and grain products every day?*
- *Are you dieting or do you have any type of dietary restrictions?*
- *Do you participate regularly in sports, or do you have a job requiring physical activity?*
- *Do you have any chronic illness (diabetes, peptic ulcer, ulcerative colitis, or epilepsy)?*
- *Are you currently taking any prescription or nonprescription medications?*
- *Are you taking or have you recently taken any vitamins, minerals, or nutritional supplements?*
- *Do you donate blood? How often? When did you last donate blood?*
- *Do you smoke or are you around smokers daily?*
- *Do you drink alcohol? How often and how much?*
- *Are you pregnant?*
- *Do you take oral contraceptives (birth control pills)?*

Vitamins are potent organic compounds (exclusive of protein, carbohydrate, and fat) that are essential in small quantities for the specific body functions of growth, maintenance, and reproduction. Vitamins are classified as fat soluble or water soluble. Because most vitamins (with the exception of vitamin D) cannot be synthesized by the body in sufficient quantities to meet metabolic needs, they must be supplied by food or supplementation. Vitamins are widely consumed by the American public, accounting for annual sales in excess of $3 billion.[1]

In most cases, the typical American diet does not need supplementation. Nutrition experts agree that foods, not supplements, are the preferred source of vitamins and minerals and that most individuals can easily meet their requirements by eating a balanced diet. There is less agreement, however, about the extent to which the US population consumes a balanced diet. There are those who believe that most Americans receive adequate levels of vitamins and minerals from their usual diet; the lack of symptoms of deficiency supports this position. But some segments of society (eg, elderly persons, smokers, nursing home patients, and teenagers) are less likely to consume the recommended dietary allowances (RDAs) of all vitamins and minerals. Primary attention should be directed toward improving the diet; under some circumstances, however, a supplement is appropriate.

The issue of who would benefit from supplements, however, is complex. One of the greatest dangers of food fads, high-potency supplements, and large doses of single vitamins is that they are sometimes used in place of sound medical care. The false hope of superior health or freedom from disease may attract desperate or uninformed individuals who have cancer, heart disease, arthritis, or other serious illnesses and may place them at greater risk because it causes them to delay seeking and receiving appropriate medical attention.

Guidelines for optimum nutrition are provided by two organizations: the Food and Nutrition Board of the National Research Council–National Academy of Sciences and the Food and Drug Administration (FDA).

Recommended Dietary Allowances

RDAs are the levels of daily intake of essential nutrients that, based on scientific knowledge, the Food and Nutrition Board judges to be adequate to meet the known nutrient needs of most healthy persons (Table 1). The RDA is two standard deviations above the minimal daily requirement, which is the minimal amount of a vitamin necessary to prevent deficiency of that vitamin in the US population. RDA values are periodically updated based on new information, and they are set high enough to allow for variations in individual requirements caused by minor illnesses. In the Food and Nutrition Board's recommendations, an "estimated safe and adequate daily dietary intake" of other nutrients for which human requirements are not quantitatively known has also been promulgated (Table 2). These data should be used merely as guidelines for nutritional assessment.

RDAs have certain applications and limitations. Their applications include:

- Evaluating the adequacy of the national food supply;
- Establishing standards for menu planning;
- Establishing nutritional policy for public institutions/organizations and hospitals;
- Evaluating diets in food consumption studies;
- Developing materials for nutritional education;

TABLE 1 Food and Nutrition Board, National Academy of Sciences–National Research Council recommended dietary allowances (RDA),[a] revised 1989

							Fat-soluble vitamins					
Category	Age (y) or condition	Weight[b] (kg)	Weight[b] (lb)	Height[b] (cm)	Height[b] (in)	Protein (g)	Vitamin A (mcg RE)[c]	Vitamin D (mcg)[d]	Vitamin E (mg α–TE)[e]	Vitamin K (mcg)	Vitamin C (mg)	Thiamine (B_1) (mg)
Infants	0.0–0.5	6	13	60	24	13	375	7.5	3	5	30	0.3
	0.5–1.0	9	20	71	28	14	375	10	4	10	35	0.4
Children	1–3	13	29	90	35	16	400	10	6	15	40	0.7
	4–6	20	44	112	44	24	500	10	7	20	45	0.9
	7–10	28	62	132	52	28	700	10	7	30	45	1.0
Males	11–14	45	99	157	62	45	1,000	10	10	45	50	1.3
	15–18	66	145	176	69	59	1,000	10	10	65	60	1.5
	19–24	72	160	177	70	58	1,000	10	10	70	60	1.5
	25–50	79	174	176	70	63	1,000	5	10	80	60	1.5
	51+	77	170	173	68	63	1,000	5	10	80	60	1.2
Females	11–14	46	101	157	62	46	800	10	8	45	50	1.1
	15–18	55	120	163	64	44	800	10	8	55	60	1.1
	19–24	58	128	164	65	46	800	10	8	60	60	1.1
	25–50	63	138	163	64	50	800	5	8	65	60	1.1
	51+	65	143	160	63	50	800	5	8	65	60	1.0
Pregnant						60	800	10	10	65	70	1.5
Lactating	1st 6 months					65	1,300	10	12	65	95	1.6
	2nd 6 months					62	1,200	10	11	65	90	1.6

[a]The allowances, expressed as average daily intakes over time, are intended to provide for individual variations among most normal persons as they live in the United States under usual environmental stresses. Diets should be based on a variety of common foods in order to provide other nutrients for which human requirements have been less well defined.

[b]The use of these figures does not imply that the height-to-weight ratios are ideal.

[c]RE = retinol equivalents. One RE = 1 mcg retinol or 6 mcg beta-carotene. One IU = 0.3 mcg retinol or 0.6 mcg beta-carotene.

- Establishing labeling regulations;
- Setting guidelines for food product formulation.

RDAs have limitations because:

- They are too complex for direct consumer use;
- They do not state ideal or optimal levels of intake;
- The allowances for some categories are based on limited data;
- The data on some nutrients in foods are limited;
- They do not evaluate nutritional status;
- They do not apply to seriously ill or malnourished patients.

Lack of knowledge prevents RDAs from being set for all known nutrients. Further, the application of RDAs to individuals may require adjustment owing to climate, strenuous physical activity, and the presence of a disease state.

The FDA publishes a less comprehensive set of values to be used for labeling purposes. These values, formerly known as the US recommended daily allowances (US RDAs), are included in Table 3. The US RDAs are now called reference daily intakes (RDIs). Other associated terminology includes daily reference values (DRVs) and percent daily value. The nutrition labeling of a dietary supplement of a vitamin or mineral that has an RDI or a DRV is a box with the heading "Nutrition Facts." In addition to information on serving size and servings per container, the label lists all required nutrients that are present in the dietary supplement in quantitative amounts by weight, and the percentage of the RDI or DRV as established and where appropriate. These percentages may be expressed to the nearest whole number except that "less than 1%" may be used in place of "0%" when the material is present in a quantity greater than zero. The percent of daily value is based on RDI values for adults and children 4 years of age or older unless the product is designed for children less than 4 years old, pregnant women, or lactating women. These groups will be specified in a separate column. Pharmacists may find US RDI values useful for patient discussions.

RDAs provided in this chapter are primarily for infants, children, adult men and women, and pregnant and lactating women (Table 1). Resource information is available from several standard textbooks and reference books in nutrition and pharmacy.[2–8] The discussion of product forms is primarily limited to those items available for nonprescription oral administration.

Water-soluble vitamins					Minerals						
Riboflavin (B_2) (mg)	Niacin (B_3) (mg NE)[f]	Pyridoxine (vitamin B_6) (mg)	Folic acid (folate) (mcg)	Cyanocobalamin (vitamin B_{12}) (mcg)	Calcium (mg)	Phosphorus (mg)	Magnesium (mg)	Iron (mg)	Zinc (mg)	Iodine (mcg)	Selenium (mcg)
0.4	5	0.3	25	0.3	400	300	40	6	5	40	10
0.5	6	0.6	35	0.5	600	500	60	10	5	50	15
0.8	9	1.0	50	0.7	800	800	80	10	10	70	20
1.1	12	1.1	75	1.0	800	800	120	10	10	90	20
1.2	13	1.4	100	1.4	800	800	170	10	10	120	30
1.5	17	1.7	150	2.0	1,200	1,200	270	12	15	150	40
1.8	20	2.0	200	2.0	1,200	1,200	400	12	15	150	50
1.7	19	2.0	200	2.0	1,200	1,200	350	10	15	150	70
1.7	19	2.0	200	2.0	800	800	350	10	15	150	70
1.4	15	2.0	200	2.0	800	800	350	10	15	150	70
1.3	15	1.4	150	2.0	1,200	1,200	280	15	12	150	45
1.3	15	1.5	180	2.0	1,200	1,200	300	15	12	150	50
1.3	15	1.6	180	2.0	1,200	1,200	280	15	12	150	55
1.3	15	1.6	180	2.0	800	800	280	15	12	150	55
1.2	13	1.6	180	2.0	800	800	280	10	12	150	55
1.6	17	2.2	400	2.2	1,200	1,200	320	30	15	175	65
1.8	20	2.1	280	2.6	1,200	1,200	355	15	19	200	75
1.7	20	2.1	260	2.6	1,200	1,200	340	15	16	200	75

[d]As cholecalciferol; 10 mcg cholecalciferol = 400 IU of vitamin D.

[e]α-TE = alpha-tocopherol equivalents. 1 mg *d*-alpha-tocopherol = 1 mg α-TE = 1.49 IU.

[f]NE = niacin equivalent, equal to 1 mg of niacin or 60 mg of dietary tryptophan.

Adapted with permission from Food and Nutrition Board, National Research Council–National Academy of Sciences. *Recommended Dietary Allowances.* 10th ed. Washington, DC: National Academy Press; 1989.

Malnutrition

The primary causes of malnutrition include starvation, disease-related factors, eating disorders, alcoholism, and food faddism. Because of pathophysiologic, physiologic, behavioral, or economic situations, certain segments of the population are predisposed to vitamin deficiencies:

- Iatrogenic situations: for example, oral contraceptive and estrogen users, patients on prolonged broad-spectrum antibiotics, or patients on prolonged parenteral nutrition;
- Inadequate dietary intake: for example, alcoholics, the impoverished, the aged, patients on severe calorie-restricted diets or fad diets, or patients with eating disorders;
- Increased metabolic requirements: for example, pregnant or lactating women; women of childbearing age who have regular menstrual blood loss; infants; children undergoing periods of accelerated growth; or patients with major surgery, cancer, severe injury, infection, or trauma;
- Poor absorption: for example, the aged; or patients with such conditions as prolonged diarrhea, severe gastrointestinal (GI) disorders or malignancy, surgical removal of a section of the GI tract, celiac disease, obstructive jaundice, or cystic fibrosis.

Groups in the United States that are most prone to undernourishment include infants, preschoolers, lactating or pregnant women, elderly persons, alcoholics, the homeless, and the impoverished. Epidemiologic surveys have shown that schoolchildren, factory workers, businesspersons, and farmers are less likely to be poorly nourished.

Elderly people have a 34–88% reduction in circulating levels of one or more vitamins. Among those who are homebound, the incidence of vitamin deficiency due to inadequate dietary intake is approximately 10%. The causes of nutritional deficiency in the elderly population may be related to disease, malabsorption, physiologic changes of the GI tract, mastication difficulty, or loss of perception (taste, smell, or sight). Other factors include social isolation, fear for personal safety, lack of knowledge about an adequate diet, poverty, alcoholism, and drug abuse.

Poor nutrition increases the risks of cancer and infection, as well as of complications from surgery and chemotherapy. Wound-healing time and mortality may be increased. The conditions associated with severe mal-

TABLE 2 Estimated safe and adequate daily dietary intakes of selected vitamins and minerals[a]

		Vitamins		Trace elements[b]				
Category	Age (y)	Biotin (mcg)	Panto-thenic acid (mg)	Copper (mg)	Manganese (mg)	Fluoride (mg)	Chromium (mcg)	Molybdenum (mcg)
Infants	0–0.5	10	3	0.4–0.6	0.3–0.6	0.1–0.5	10–40	15–30
	0.5–1	15	3	0.6–0.7	0.6–1.0	0.2–1.0	20–60	20–40
Children and adolescents	1–3	20	3	0.7–1.0	1.0–1.5	0.5–1.5	20–80	25–50
	4–6	25	3–4	1.0–1.5	1.5–2.0	1.0–2.5	30–120	30–75
	7–10	30	4–5	1.0–2.0	2.0–3.0	1.5–2.5	50–200	50–150
	11+	30–100	4–7	1.5–2.5	2.0–5.0	1.5–2.5	50–200	75–250
Adults		30–100	4–7	1.5–3.0	2.0–5.0	1.5–4.0	50–200	75–250

[a]Because there is less information on which to base allowances, these figures are not given in Table 1 and are provided here in the form of ranges of recommended intakes.

[b]Because the toxic levels for many trace elements may be only several times the usual intakes, the upper levels for the trace elements given in the table should not be habitually exceeded.

Adapted with permission from Food and Nutrition Board, National Research Council–National Academy of Sciences. *Recommended Dietary Allowances*. 10th ed. Washington, DC: National Academy Press; 1989: 284.

nutrition include marasmus, kwashiorkor, and mixed malnutrition. Marasmus is caused by inadequate total caloric dietary intake and presents as decreased fat deposits, decreased muscle mass, and cachexia, primarily in infants or children. Kwashiorkor is caused by inadequate dietary intake of protein and is characterized by edema and decreased serum protein levels, including hypoalbuminemia. Mixed malnutrition is caused by inadequate dietary intake of calories and protein and exhibits features of both marasmus and kwashiorkor.

The evolution of vitamin deficiency may include several stages (Table 4).[9]

Nutritional Assessment

Assessment of nutritional status is difficult in the ambulatory environment. Clinical impressions about nutrition are often erroneous because the stages between well-nourished and poorly nourished states are not readily evident. There are guidelines, however, which may help to provide a more objective assessment of a patient's nutritional status. Pharmacists should know which population groups tend to be poorly nourished, should exercise good observational skills, and should know which questions yield helpful information. The more specific the information obtained from the patient, the more helpful the pharmacist can be in determining the need for nutritional supplementation. Questions regarding foods generally not included in the diet and previous treatment of similar symptoms may also be important.

The pharmacist should observe the patient's physical condition but must realize that only severe dietary deficiencies are likely to be reflected physically. A thorough clinical appraisal of nutritional status includes evaluation of growth and development, as determined by the amount of weight loss or gain, body fat (measured by triceps and subscapular skinfold thickness), and somatic protein or muscle mass (measured by midarm muscle circumference, creatinine height index, hair pluckability, and myoderma). The assessment should also include evaluation of fitness, medical and dietary history, and biomedical components such as visceral protein markers (measured by serum albumin, prealbumin, transferrin, retinol levels, skin antigen response, and pitting time), as well as observation of signs consistent with deficiencies.

Although these assessment measures are beyond the scope of routine pharmacy practice, some observations may be made on the status of the patient. For example, a patient's fingernails may indicate malnutrition if they lose their luster and become dark at the upper ends. The texture, amount, and appearance of the hair may indicate the patient's nutritional status. The eyes, particularly the conjunctiva, may indicate vitamin A and iron deficiencies, and the mouth may show stomatitis, glossitis, or hypertrophic or pale gums. The number and general condition of the teeth may reflect the patient's choice of food. Visible goiter, poor skin color and texture, obesity or thinness relative to bone structure, and the presence of edema may also be indications of malnutrition. The pharmacist should be able to recognize overt but nonspecific symptoms of vitamin and mineral deficiencies where prompt physician referral may be crucial.

It is in fact the pharmacist's responsibility to refer patients with a suspected serious illness to a physician. Just as nutritional deficiencies may lead to disease, disease may lead to nutritional deficiencies. Epidemics of vitamin deficiency do not occur in the United States; however, patients may present with one or more deficiencies, which may be very difficult to diagnose. Rarely in the United States do pharmacists encounter patients

TABLE 3 US recommended daily allowances (US RDAs) for labeling purposes

	Unit	Infants	Children under age 4	Adults and children aged 4 or older	Pregnant and lactating women
Vitamin A	IU	1,500	2,500	5,000	8,000
Vitamin D	IU	400	400	400	400
Vitamin E	IU	5	10	30	30
Ascorbic acid	mg	35	40	60	60
Folic acid	mg	0.1	0.2	0.4	0.8
Thiamine	mg	0.5	0.7	1.5	1.7
Riboflavin	mg	0.6	0.8	1.7	2.0
Niacin	mg	8	9	20	20
Pyridoxine	mg	0.4	0.7	2	2.5
Cyanocobalamin	mcg	2	3	6	8
Biotin	mg	0.05	0.15	0.3	0.3
Pantothenic acid	mg	3	5	10	10
Calcium	g	0.6	0.8	1.0	1.3
Phosphorus	g	0.5	0.8	1.0	1.3
Iodine	mcg	45	70	150	150
Iron	mg	15	10	18	18
Magnesium	mg	70	200	400	450
Manganese[a]	mg	0.5	1.0	4.0	4.0
Copper	mg	0.6	1.0	2.0	2.0
Zinc	mg	5	8	15	15
Protein	g	—	20(28)[b]	45(65)[b]	—

[a]Proposed US RDI.
[b]Values in parentheses are US RDIs when the protein efficiency ratio (PER) is less than that of casein; the other values are used when the PER is equal to or greater than that of casein. No claim may be made for a protein with a PER equal to or less than 20% that of casein.

with severe deficiencies resulting in diseases such as scurvy, pellagra, or kwashiorkor. However, milder forms of malnutrition may be seen.

The Pharmacist's Role in Vitamin and Mineral Use

By asking key questions, the pharmacist may detect cultural, physical, environmental, and social conditions that may suggest inadequate vitamin intake. By being familiar with daily RDAs of the various vitamins and minerals, and by knowing which natural food sources provide these RDAs, the pharmacist may be able to educate the patient and improve the diet so that nutritional requirements are met through food. If a supplement is needed, the pharmacist can recommend a product that will provide appropriate levels of the needed vitamins at a reasonable price.

The average American consuming an average diet does not need vitamin supplementation. Although some claim that everyone would benefit from supplements, the general lack of knowledge concerning the risks and benefits of megadose vitamin therapy leads others to argue that vitamin supplements are unnecessary and that megavitamin therapy is even dangerous. The truth probably lies closer to the second claim. Some segments of the population may benefit from supplemental multivitamins, but most others do not. Although there are specific situations in which high doses of specific vitamins have been reported to be of therapeutic benefit, the exaggerated claims of the megavitamin enthusiasts have not been objectively confirmed. Furthermore, prolonged ingestion of vitamins has not been tested for safety; and some vitamins, such as A, D, niacin, and pyridoxine, are known to be toxic in high doses. Thus, patients should be cautioned against initiating high-dose self-medication with vitamins. Chronic ingestion of large doses of any drug, including vitamins, for relief of a relatively mild or self-limiting condition such as the common cold should be discouraged.

The public is constantly being exposed to exaggerated and fraudulent claims concerning vitamin products. The pharmacist can help to expose such claims by keeping up with medical and pharmaceutical literature and not supporting or appearing to support the claims until they are substantiated by reliable clinical studies. Patients inquiring about such claims should be educated about the increased potential risk of the nontraditional use of vitamins; they should be told, for example, about adverse drug reactions that might occur with these products

TABLE 4 Stages in the evolution of a vitamin deficiency

Stages	Effects
Preliminary	Decreased tissue stores, decreased urinary excretion
Biochemical	Reduced enzyme activity, negligible urinary excretion
Physiologic	Malaise, weight loss, insomnia, impaired psychologic functions
Clinical	Increased nonspecific symptoms, appearance of clinical signs
Anatomic	Clear specific symptoms, pathologic tissue changes that may be fatal

when used in alternative doses or in combination with prescription and nonprescription drug products.

Vitamins are used both as dietary supplements and as therapeutic agents to treat deficiencies or other pathologic conditions. As dietary supplements, vitamins are usually dosed at 50–150% of the US RDI. As therapeutic agents, vitamins should be recommended only by physicians according to specific medical indications. Typically, therapeutic doses should not exceed 2–10 times the RDA, depending on the vitamin.

Multivitamin Therapy

Although health authorities agree that a balanced diet and adequate caloric intake obviate the necessity for supplemental vitamins for most individuals, those segments of the population known to be at risk for vitamin deficiencies (see section on Malnutrition) may benefit from special attention to diet or vitamin supplements. The pharmacist should counsel patients on appropriate multivitamin selection. In general, an inexpensive supplemental preparation that supplies close to 100% of the RDA for each vitamin will meet the needs of most patients requiring or desiring supplements (see product table "Vitamin Products"). The need for expensive high-potency vitamins is rare.

"Natural" Vitamins

Frequently, natural vitamin products are supplemented with the synthetic vitamin. For example, because the amount of ascorbic acid that can be acquired from rose hips (the fleshy fruit of a rose) is relatively small, synthetic ascorbic acid is added to prevent too large a tablet size. However, this addition may not be noted on the label, and the price of the partially natural product is often considerably higher than that for the completely synthetic but equally effective product. Patients should be informed that the body cannot distinguish between a vitamin molecule derived from a synthetic source and one derived from a natural source and that synthetic vitamins are therefore absorbed to the same extent as the more expensive natural vitamins.

Fat-Soluble Vitamins

Vitamins A, D, E, and K are the fat-soluble vitamins. They are soluble in lipids and are usually absorbed along with chylomicrons into the lymphatic system of the small intestine, where they pass into the general circulation. Their absorption is facilitated by bile. These vitamins are stored in body tissues, and when excessive quantities or megadoses are ingested, they may be toxic. Deficiencies of these vitamins occur when fat intake is limited or fat absorption is compromised. Drugs that affect lipid absorption, such as cholestyramine (which binds bile acids and thereby hinders lipid emulsification) and mineral oil (which increases fecal elimination of lipids), may precipitate such a deficiency.

Vitamin A

The designation "vitamin A" refers to a group of compounds essential for vision, growth, reproduction, cellular differentiation and proliferation, and integrity of the immune system. There are a number of names and forms of vitamin A, including the retinoids (eg, reti, rl and retinoic acid) and the carotenoids (eg, beta-carotene). The term *retinoid* is also used to refer to this very large group of compounds, some of which are without vitamin A activity. Additionally, more than 500 of the carotenoids, which are precursors of vitamin A, are found naturally, but only about 50 are precursors of retinol. Biochemical changes occur in the retinoids and carotenoids during absorption in the intestine to form active compounds.

More than 90% of the body's supply of vitamin A is stored in the liver, and these reserves are usually sufficient for several months to a year. Infants and young children are more susceptible to vitamin A deficiency because they have not established the necessary reserves.

The primary dietary source of vitamin A is the carotenoids, which are synthesized by plants and converted in the body into vitamin A. Vitamin A is measured in international units (IUs); 1 IU equals 0.3 mcg of retinol, 0.6 mcg of beta-carotene, or 1.2 mcg of other carotenoids. The retinol equivalent (RE) has been recommended by the Food and Nutrition Board as a way to determine the amount of absorption of the carotenoids as well as their degree of conversion to vitamin A in the body. In the RE system, 1 RE equals 1 mcg of retinol, 6 mcg of beta-carotene, and 12 mcg of other carotenoids. This system is appropriate because retinol is assumed to be completely absorbed from the GI tract whereas carotenes are only about one third absorbed. Thus, because only about half of the absorbed beta-carotene is converted to retinol, only one sixth of the intake is actually used. Similarly, because one fourth of the other carotenoids is converted to retinol, only one twelfth of the intake is available. (The carotenoids are split in the intestinal mucosa to form retinaldehyde, which is subsequently reduced to form retinol.)

Vitamin A and carotenoids, which are fat soluble, are found mainly in fatty foods. Good sources are fish, butter, cream, eggs, milk, and organ meats. Carotenoids are the yellow-orange pigments of carrots, squash, and pumpkin; they are also present in many dark, leafy vegetables. However, the color intensity of a vegetable is not a reliable indicator of its vitamin A content.

Indications Vitamin A is essential for normal growth and reproduction, normal skeletal and tooth development, and the proper functioning of most organs of the body, notably the specialized functions involving the conjunctiva, retina, and cornea of the eye. It is thus indicated in the prevention and treatment of symptoms of vitamin A deficiency, such as dry eye (xerophthalmia) and night blindness (nyctalopia). The synthesis of the glycoproteins necessary to maintain normal epithelial cell mucous secretions requires vitamin A, which is also vital to the body's defense against bacterial infections in the upper respiratory system.

Vitamin A deficiency is rare in well-nourished populations and develops slowly because of body stores. It is most common in poorly nourished children under 5 years old. Serum levels usually remain normal until the liver reserve becomes highly depleted. Deficiency occurs when vitamin A plasma levels fall below 10 mcg/dL. (Normal blood levels range from 20 to 80 mcg/dL.) Conditions such as cancer, tuberculosis, pneumonia, chronic nephritis, urinary tract infections, and prostate disease may cause excessive excretion of vitamin A. Conditions in which there is fat malabsorption, such as celiac disease, short gut syndrome, obstructive jaundice, cystic fibrosis, and cirrhosis of the liver, may impair vitamin A absorption. Neomycin or cholestyramine may cause significant malabsorption of vitamin A and other fat-soluble vitamins and may precipitate deficiencies with long-term use. In the United States, vitamin A deficiency occurs more often from diseases of fat malabsorption than from malnutrition.

One of the earliest symptoms of vitamin A deficiency is night blindness, caused by failure of the retina to obtain adequate supplies of retinol for the formation of rhodopsin. If the situation is not reversed, it may be rapidly followed by structural changes in the retina and xerosis (abnormal dryness) of the conjunctiva. Bitot's spots (small patches of bubbles that resemble tiny drops of meringue) may appear on the conjunctiva, which may look dry and opaque, and photophobia (light sensitivity) may occur. If the deficiency continues, xerosis of the cornea occurs, followed by corneal distortion. The loss of continuity of the surface epithelium, with formation of a noninflammatory ulcer and infiltration of the stroma, can lead to softening of the cornea, alteration of the iris, and permanent loss of vision.

Other characteristic clinical findings of a deficiency disorder include increased susceptibility to infection, follicular hyperkeratosis, loss of appetite, impaired taste and smell, impaired equilibrium, and an increase in cerebrospinal fluid pressure. Some of these findings may be masked by concurrent deficiencies of other nutrients. Notable, however, is the drying and hyperkeratinization of the skin, which predisposes patients to infections. The integrity of epithelial tissues depends on vitamin A activity.

One of the most encouraging developments in vitamin research has been the discovery that vitamin A analogs show promise in the prevention and treatment of certain cancers and in the treatment of certain skin disorders. It has long been known that vitamin A deficiency in animals leads to hyperkeratosis and metaplasia (preneoplastic conditions) of epithelial tissues. Systemic administration of high doses of vitamin A may retard the development of these precancerous lesions. Experimental results also suggest that certain systemic retinoids may be useful in treating acne, psoriasis, and other skin conditions characterized by hyperkeratosis. Topical retinoic acid (Retin-A) and systemic isotretinoin (Accutane) are currently used to treat acne vulgaris, although not without side effects.

Dose/RDA The usual requirements for vitamin A are supplied by an adequate diet. The use of supplemental vitamin A would be appropriate in treating vitamin A deficiency and as prophylaxis in at-risk patients during times of increased requirements (eg, infancy, pregnancy, or lactation). Dietary intake of vitamin A should be estimated when determining the dose for administration. Vitamin A is usually administered orally.

The RDA values published by the Food and Nutrition Board express the potency of vitamin A in terms of an RE. Thus, the RDA in adult men and women is 1,000 and 800 mcg RE, respectively. The US RDI still retains the IU as a measure of potency, so the US RDI for adults is 5,000 IU, which is equivalent to 1,000 RE. This is increased to 8,000 IU for pregnant and lactating women, and decreased to 2,500 IU for children under 4 years of age and to 1,500 IU for infants (Table 3). If the pharmacist determines that a vitamin A supplement is appropriate, a nonprescription multiple vitamin that contains no more than the RDA of vitamin A should be recommended. High-dose vitamin A therapy should be undertaken only with close medical supervision. There does not appear to be a special requirement for vitamin A for the elderly. Tables 1, 2, and 3 show the requirements for children; it is interesting to note that individuals are differentiated by sex starting at 11 years of age because that is when differences in lean body mass occur.

Adverse Effects/Drug Interactions Excessive intake of vitamin A may result from overzealous prophylactic vitamin therapy, prolonged self-medication, or increased intake of foods high in vitamin A, such as cod liver oil. Since vitamin A is stored in the body, high doses of it can lead to a toxic syndrome known as hypervitaminosis A. The incidence of hypervitaminosis A is increasing because of publicity regarding the potential application of vitamin A in cancer and skin disorders. Toxicity in the form of bulging fontanelles or hydrocephalus has occurred in infants given doses 10 times the RDA for several weeks. A single dose (2,000,000 IU, or 400,000 RE) may precipitate acute toxicity 4–8 hours after ingestion. Chronic daily ingestion of at least 25,000 IU of vitamin A, a dose readily available to the public, has resulted in toxicity in children. Headache is a predominant symptom, but it may be accompanied by double vision (diplopia), nausea, vomiting, vertigo, hypercalcemia, or drowsiness. Fatigue, malaise, and lethargy are also common symptoms. Abdominal upset, bone and joint pain, throbbing headaches, insomnia, restlessness, night sweats, loss of body hair, brittle nails, abnormal protrusion of the eyeball (exophthalmos), rough and scaly skin, peripheral edema, and mouth fissures may occur as well. Severe constipation, menstrual irregularity, and emotional lability have been reported in some cases. Treatment consists of discontinuing vitamin A supplementation, and the prognosis is good. Beta-carotene does not produce toxicity rapidly because its conversion to vitamin A is slow. However, eating large amounts of carrots daily may result in carotenemia, which can produce a yellow skin hue.

Large doses of vitamin A may increase the hypoprothrombinemic effect of warfarin. Thus, the recommended dose of vitamin A supplements should not be exceeded, and cholestyramine or mineral oil, which may reduce the absorption of vitamin A, should not be used for a prolonged period while using these supplements. Additionally, oral contraceptive use may increase plasma levels of vitamin A, so pregnant women or women of childbearing age who are not using contraception should avoid vitamin A doses above the RDA because of a teratogenic risk.

Vitamin D (Calciferol)

A number of chemicals are associated with vitamin D activity; Table 5 lists the structurally similar chemicals and their metabolites for which vitamin D is a collective name. Cholecalciferol (vitamin D_3) is the natural form of vitamin D. It is synthesized in the skin from endogenous or dietary cholesterol on exposure to UV radiation (sunlight). Ergocalciferol, which differs structurally only slightly from cholecalciferol, is of dietary importance. Ergocalciferol and cholecalciferol are equipotent.

Activation of vitamin D requires both the liver and the kidney. One metabolite, 25-hydroxycholecalciferol, is formed by the liver and then hydroxylated by the kidney to its most active form, 1,25-dihydroxycholecalciferol. This explains why hypocalcemia occurs in patients with renal failure, and why some patients fail to respond even to massive doses of vitamin D_3. Administration of 1,25-dihydroxycholecalciferol (available as calcitriol) to these patients has been successful whereas the 25-hydroxycholecalciferol is sufficient in patients with hepatic failure.

Vitamin D, which has properties of both hormones and vitamins, is necessary for the proper formation of the skeleton and for mineral homeostasis. It is closely involved with parathyroid hormone, phosphate, and calcitonin in the homeostasis of serum calcium.

Milk and milk products are the major source of preformed vitamin D in the United States, given that milk is routinely supplemented with 400 IU of vitamin D per quart. Eggs and animal livers are also rich in vitamin D, and fish, beef, and butter are additional natural sources. Vitamin D is stable, and normal food processing does not appear to alter its activity.

Indications A deficiency of vitamin D may be due to dietary deficiency; GI disorder (hepatobiliary disease, malabsorption, or chronic pancreatitis); acidosis; chronic renal failure; hereditary disorders of vitamin D metabolism; phosphate depletion; renal tubular disorders; poisoning from lead, cadmium, or outdated tetracycline; and prolonged parenteral nutrition without proper vitamin D supplementation.

The signs and symptoms of vitamin D deficiency diseases are reflected as calcium abnormalities, specifically those involved with bone formation. The classic deficiency state is rickets. Vitamin D increases calcium and phosphate absorption from the small intestine, mobilizes calcium from bone, permits normal bone mineralization, improves renal absorption of calcium, and maintains serum calcium and phosphorus levels. As serum calcium and inorganic phosphate decrease, compensatory mechanisms attempt to increase the calcium. Parathyroid hormone secretion increases, possibly leading to secondary hyperparathyroidism. If physiologic mechanisms fail to make the appropriate adjustments in levels of calcium and phosphorus, demineralization of bone will ensue to maintain essential plasma calcium levels. During growth, demineralization leads to a failure of bone matrix mineralization, and in adults, it may lead to severe osteomalacia. The epiphyseal plate may widen because of the failure of calcification combined with weight load on the softened structures during growth. As a result, rickets is manifested by soft bones and deformed joints. The diagnosis is made radiologically by observing the bone deformities. The lack of adequate calcium in muscle tissue results in tetany.

Although the incidence of rickets in the United States is low, the increasing popularity of vegetarian diets has led to rickets in some children who abstain from milk and in infants breast-fed by mothers who do not drink milk, fail to take prenatal vitamins, or otherwise receive inadequate intake of vitamin D. A deficiency of vitamin D may also result in liver disease and myopathy because of decreased muscle phosphate.

Osteomalacia may develop in elderly persons owing to vitamin D deficiency (malabsorption syndromes, inadequate diet or sunlight, gastrectomy, laxative abuse, and pancreatic insufficiency); anticonvulsant, cholestyramine, or glucocorticoid therapy; liver disease; chronic renal failure; hypoparathyroidism; postmenopausal endocrine changes; and/or cadmium and strontium toxicity. In adults, bone fractures may result from the bone loss that accompanies hypocalcemia.

Dose/RDA Most persons obtain the RDA (Tables 1 and 3) of vitamin D from dietary sources and exposure to sunlight. People regularly exposed to sunlight will generally have no dietary requirement for vitamin D. However, a substantial part of the US population is exposed to very little sunlight, especially during the winter.

If a patient asks for a vitamin D supplement and the pharmacist determines that the need is based on poor dietary intake or on indoor confinement, a multivitamin supplement containing no more than 100 IU of vitamin D may be recommended. Liquid preparations that contain vitamin D should be measured carefully, particularly when given to infants. Patients who request therapeutic doses of vitamin D should be referred to a physician; those using a prescription vitamin D product should be encouraged to see their physician regularly.

Vitamin D is included in most multivitamin preparations and is also available alone in various strengths as tablets, capsules, and drops. Two active metabolites, 25-hydroxycholecalciferol (calcifediol) and 1,25-

TABLE 5 Chemicals that have vitamin D activity

Activity ratio	Name	Synonyms	
1	Vitamin D_3	Cholecalciferol	Calciol
2–5	25-Hydroxyvitamin D_3	25-Hydroxycholecalciferol	Calcifediol
10	1,25-Dihydroxyvitamin D_3	1,25-Dihydroxycholecalciferol	Calcitriol
1	Vitamin D_2	Ergocalciferol, Ergocalciol	Ercalciol
2–5	25-Hydroxyvitamin D_2	25-Hydroxyergocalciferol	Ercalcidiol
10	1,25-Dihydroxyvitamin D_2	1,25-Dihydroxyergocalciferol	Ercalcitriol

dihydroxycholecalciferol (calcitriol), are available by prescription for use in patients with hypocalcemia associated with hepatic or renal failure, respectively. The former compound has a longer half-life but is less potent. Dihydrotachysterol, which is available by prescription, is also useful in renal failure because it does not require metabolic activation by the kidneys.

Large daily doses of vitamin D (1,000–4,000 IU) are prescribed for the treatment of rickets. For adults with osteomalacia caused by renal disease, 0.25–1 mcg per day of calcitriol is often prescribed.

Adverse Effects/Drug Interactions Taking five or more times the RDA of vitamin D may lead to adverse effects, including hypercalcemia, hypercalciuria, polyuria, nephrocalcinosis, renal failure, metastatic calcification, and kidney stones. Doses exceeding 400 IU (25 mcg of cholecalciferol) are not advisable. In infants, as little as 1,800 IU of vitamin D per day may inhibit growth.

The more common symptoms of hypervitaminosis D are anorexia, nausea, weakness, weight loss, polyuria, constipation, vague aches, stiffness, soft tissue calcification, nephrocalcinosis, hypertension, anemia, hypercalcemia, acidosis, and irreversible renal failure. If a recent blood test has not been taken to measure serum calcium, a physician should be consulted.

Concurrent drug therapy must be closely monitored because vitamin D may interact with other drugs. Phosphate in chronically used drugs, such as certain laxatives, may lower the calcium level and contribute to a vitamin D deficiency. Patients with such a deficiency because of renal problems should use caution in taking antacids; patients with severe renal problems should be advised to select antacids for the specific ingredients they contain. Aluminum-containing antacids may be chosen because they bind phosphates, and calcium-containing antacids may be used to help increase serum calcium levels. However, magnesium-containing antacids should be avoided because magnesium tends to accumulate to toxic levels in renal disease. Cholestyramine and mineral oil may reduce the amount of vitamin D absorbed, so their prolonged use should also be avoided. Phenytoin or barbiturates may decrease the half-life of vitamin D.

Vitamin E (Tocopherol)

Vitamin E is present in all cell membranes. The term *vitamin E* refers to a series of eight compounds. The tocopherols and the tocotrienols are naturally occurring compounds in plants. Alpha-tocopherol, the most active of these compounds, is used to calculate the vitamin E content of food.

The following equivalents can be used to estimate the total alpha-tocopherol equivalents (α-TEs) of diets containing only natural forms of vitamin E. To use the table below, the number of milligrams of vitamin E in the diet should be multiplied by the number in the factor column. One α-TE equals 1.49 IU.

Item	*Factor*
beta-tocopherol	0.5
gamma-tocopherol	0.1
alpha-tocotrienol	0.3
all-rac-alpha-tocopherol	0.74

Its metabolic roles are not completely understood, but vitamin E functions primarily as an antioxidant in protecting cellular membranes from oxidative damage or destruction. This process may be aided by selenium and ascorbic acid. Vitamin E may also have a more specific coenzyme role in heme biosynthesis, steroid metabolism, and collagen formation.

Foods rich in vitamin E include vegetable oils, margarines (made from plant oils), green vegetables, nuts, wheat germ, and whole grains. Refining grains to produce white flour removes much of the vitamin, and bleaching grains further depletes it. Meats, fruits, and milk contain very little vitamin E.

Indications Vitamin E deficiency is extremely rare but may occur in two population groups: premature, very low birth-weight infants; and patients who do not absorb fat normally, such as children with cystic fibrosis. A deficiency syndrome involving premature infants who were fed a vitamin E-depleted formula has been noted. Symptoms include edema, hemolytic anemia, reticulocytosis, and thrombocytosis, which clears upon supplementation with vitamin E. In adults, the primary signs of vitamin E deficiency are reproductive failure and neurologic abnormalities. Signs or tests include increased hemolysis of red blood cells, creatinuria, and smooth muscle deposits of brown pigment. Evidence for deposition of ceroid (age) pigments, creatinuria, altered erythropoiesis, and myopathy has been found in patients with vitamin E deficiency secondary to steatorrhea. Neurologic abnormalities responsive to supplemental vitamin

E have been reported in some patients with biliary disease and cystic fibrosis. Patients with these conditions should receive vitamin E supplements.

Dose/RDA The average daily diet contains approximately 3–15 mg of vitamin E; therefore, large doses (ie, ≈100 mg per day) are not necessary unless the patient is experiencing malabsorption. Doses of 300–400 mg per day have been prescribed for claudication, angina, and diabetes, with inconclusive results.

Vitamin E requirements may vary in proportion to the amount of polyunsaturated fatty acids in the diet. Although the polyunsaturated fatty acid content of the US diet has increased in recent years, the plant oils responsible for the increase are rich in tocopherol. It has been theorized that, with the increasing oxidant insult to the environment in the form of atmospheric pollutants, the intake of vitamin E should be increased. However, the lack of evidence of deficiency at the present intake supports the current adult RDA of 8–10 mg per day.

Adverse Effects/Drug Interactions Vitamin E is relatively nontoxic. Most adults tolerate 100–1,000 IU daily without adverse effects, but the hazards of long-term, high-dose therapy are unknown. Nevertheless, the enhancement of warfarin anticoagulation has been reported. The pharmacist should caution patients taking oral anticoagulants to avoid vitamin E in large doses. Nor should vitamin E be taken at the same time as iron, as studies with supplementation of infant formulas containing iron and vitamin E show that blood tocopherol levels do not increase.

Vitamin K

Phytonadione (vitamin K_1) was first isolated from alfalfa and is present in many vegetables. Menaquinone (vitamin K_2), which was produced from putrefied fishmeal, is a product of bacterial metabolism, and the colonic bacteria may be able to synthesize about 2 mcg/kg of body weight per day of the vitamin. Menadione (vitamin K_3) is a synthetic compound that is two to three times as potent as the natural vitamin K. There are at least five proteins in the body that depend on vitamin K for hepatic synthesis; these include Factors II (prothrombin), VII, IX, and X of the plasma clotting cascade.

Sources of the vitamin include pork liver and vegetables such as spinach, kale, cabbage, and cauliflower. Food composition tables and product labels may not list vitamin K content because it is not precisely known.

Indications Deficiencies do not readily occur because normal US diets contain 300–500 mcg of vitamin K daily, so there is a low incidence of deficiency among healthy, well-nourished individuals. Moreover, microbiologic flora of the normal gut synthesize enough menaquinones to supply a significant part of the body's requirement for vitamin K. However, because the absorption of vitamin K requires bile in the small intestine, anything that interferes with bile production or secretion may contribute to a vitamin K deficiency. Malabsorption syndromes and bowel resections may decrease vitamin K absorption. Liver disease may also cause symptoms of vitamin K deficiency if hepatic production of the prothrombin clotting factor is decreased. Other potential causes of deficiency include breast-feeding of newborns; regional enteritis; blind loop syndrome; ulcerative colitis; and chronic, broad-spectrum antibiotic therapy. A deficiency may be demonstrated by a prolonged prothrombin time.

Vitamin K deficiencies are almost always associated with severe pathologic conditions in which the patient is receiving intensive medical care. The only evident symptom of a deficiency state—defective blood coagulation with hemorrhage—is also the most common symptom.

Dose/RDA The 1989 RDA values included vitamin K for the first time: 65 mcg per day for adult women and 80 mc per day for adult men. For minor bleeding, 1–5 mg of vitamin K is given daily; for a major hemorrhage, 20 mg is given. The cause of the deficiency and the severity of bleeding will determine whether oral administration is adequate. Vitamin K_1 (phytonadione) is routinely given to neonates at birth (one dose of 1 mg) to prevent hemorrhaging. This is necessary because placental transport of vitamin K is low and the neonate has yet to acquire the intestinal microflora that produce the vitamin.

Only a small number of available nonprescription products contain vitamin K.

Adverse Effects/Drug Interactions Even in large amounts over an extended period, vitamin K does not produce toxic manifestations. However, administration of menadione (but not of phylloquinone) may cause hemolytic anemia, hyperbilirubinemia, and kernicterus in the newborn owing to interaction with sulfhydryl groups.

In addition to agents such as cholestyramine resins and mineral oil, which interfere with the absorption of all fat-soluble vitamins, the oral anticoagulants are antagonists of vitamin K. Although dietary amounts of vitamin K (near the RDA value) do not usually interfere with coumarin anticoagulant activity, an interaction with the 5-mg therapeutic dose of warfarin sodium (Coumadin) may be significant. Conversely, 2.5–25 mg of oral or parenteral vitamin K may be used to counteract an overdose of coumarin anticoagulant.

Long-term, broad-spectrum antibiotic therapy may initiate a vitamin K deficiency by decreasing gut flora; however, this interaction is not usually seen if dietary intake is normal. Vitamins A and E, in large quantities, may interfere with the absorption or metabolism of vitamin K.

Water-Soluble Vitamins

Ascorbic Acid (Vitamin C)

Ascorbic acid is the most easily destroyed of all the vitamins. A relatively simple compound, it is a powerful reducing agent that serves to protect the capillary basement membrane. As a nutrient, ascorbic acid is necessary to form collagen and to serve as a water-soluble antioxidant.

Ascorbic acid, which must be ingested since it is not produced in the body, is necessary for the biosynthesis of hydroxyproline, a precursor of collagen, osteoid, and dentin. It also assists in the absorption of nonheme iron from food by reducing the ferric iron in the stomach and by combining in complex formation with ions that remain solubilized in the alkaline pH of the duodenum.

Ascorbic acid has been promoted for prevention of the common cold and for attenuation of symptoms should a cold occur, but these claims are largely unsupported by well-designed and controlled clinical studies. It has been suggested that a decreased recovery time from cold sores, an increased healing rate of pressure sores, and a decreased incidence of rectal polyps may occur following administration of ascorbic acid. There are conflicting and equivocal data, however, concerning the ability of ascorbic acid to lower cholesterol levels in hypercholesterolemic patients.

Ascorbic acid has been called the "fresh-food" vitamin, and most of the daily intake is derived from the vegetable and fruit groups. Sources relatively high in vitamin C content include green and red peppers, collard greens, broccoli, spinach, tomatoes, potatoes, strawberries, oranges, and other citrus fruits. Meat, fish, poultry, eggs, and dairy products contain some vitamin C, but it is generally absent in grains.

Indications Characteristics of ascorbic acid deficiency include malaise, weakness, capillary hemorrhages and petechiae, hyperkeratotic follicles (corkscrew hairs), swollen hemorrhagic gums, and bone changes. A deficiency may also impair wound healing. A profound dietary deficiency can eventually lead to scurvy, producing widespread capillary hemorrhaging and a weakening of collagenous structures.

Scurvy, the classical deficiency state, is rare in the United States. It develops only when there is chronically inadequate nutritional consumption of ascorbic acid. Infants who are fed artificial formulas without vitamin supplements may develop symptoms of scurvy. In adults, however, scurvy would not occur for 3–5 months after all ascorbic acid consumption was stopped.

Several other uses of ascorbic acid are worthy of mention. For example, ascorbic acid supplementation in institutionalized elderly patients, among whom marginal ascorbic acid deficiencies have been reported, may measurably improve their general health and well-being. Such supplementation may also benefit smokers and women taking oral contraceptives, in whom lower than normal levels of ascorbic acid (and several other vitamins) have been noted. Ascorbic acid can also be used to increase iron absorption because it can form a soluble iron chelate and inhibit the oxidation of ferrous to ferric iron, although this is generally not necessary for patients taking adequate iron supplementation.

Dose/RDA Pharmacists are rarely confronted with overt symptoms of ascorbic acid deficiency. Only 10 mg per day of ascorbic acid prevents scurvy; a normal diet containing fresh fruits and vegetables contains many times this amount. The RDA of ascorbic acid for most adults is 60 mg per day. The apparent average daily intake of vitamin C in the United States is about 77 mg for women and 109 mg for men, although losses during cooking may decrease the actual amount ingested. About 200 mg per day will saturate the body; most of a dose above this level will be excreted.

Most multivitamin supplements contain 60–100 mg of ascorbic acid, an appropriate level to consume if supplements are required. Doses of more than 200 mg are rarely indicated. In patients with a severe vitamin C deficiency, as evidenced by clinical signs of deficiency, 300 mg of ascorbic acid per day is recommended to replenish body stores. Infants who do not have ascorbic acid supplements in their formula should receive 35–50 mg per day; those who are breast-fed by well-nourished mothers will receive a sufficient amount. The Food and Nutrition Board recommends that smokers ingest at least 100 mg of supplemental vitamin C per day to compensate for increased ascorbic acid metabolism and lower levels of ascorbic acid in the body. If a supplement is warranted, a multivitamin product containing 60–100 mg of ascorbic acid may be recommended.

Ascorbic acid tablets should be stored in a sealed container and kept away from heat and moisture to maintain potency. Ascorbic acid and its various salt forms are available in 25- to 1,000-mg regular and chewable tablets, 500- to 1,500-mg timed-release capsules and tablets, 60-mg lozenges, crystal (4 g/tsp), powder (4 g/tsp), solution (100 mg/mL), and syrup (500 mg/5 mL) dose forms, as well as in numerous combination products.

Adverse Effects/Drug Interactions The pharmacist is urged to weigh the relative risks and benefits of ascorbic acid therapy. Short-term use to promote healing or for serious disorders such as rectal polyps may warrant a trial of ascorbic acid with medical supervision. Megadoses, however, may be harmful in certain circumstances, and the expense and potential risks of ingesting large quantities of the vitamin over the long term may be questionable for a seemingly minor beneficial effect on the common cold, a self-limiting condition. While the incidence of toxicity with ascorbic acid is low, ascorbic acid toxicity may increase oxalate excretion, produce nephrolithiasis, and lead to hemolysis in patients deficient in glucose 6-phosphate dehydrogenase.

Urine glucose tests are affected by large quantities of ascorbic acid in the urine: Clinistix urine glucose tests may give false-negative readings whereas Benedict's solutions and Clinitest tablets may give false-positive readings. The pharmacist should instruct the patient on testing procedures to minimize the interaction between tests and ascorbic acid.

Ascorbic acid (0.5–2.0 g every 4 hours) has been used to acidify urine in patients taking methenamine compounds for urinary tract infections. The lower pH of the urine facilitates hydrolysis of methenamine to the antibacterial product, formaldehyde. If sulfonamides are administered simultaneously with ascorbic acid, crystalluria may result because sulfonamide solubility is decreased in the acidified urine. When the urine is acidified, acidic drugs are reabsorbed more readily from the tubules, resulting in higher, more prolonged blood levels. On the other hand, basic drugs such as tricyclic antidepressants and amphetamines may be excreted more rapidly from acidified urine and their effect reduced by ascorbic acid therapy. The clinical significance of the effects of ascorbic acid on the reabsorption and elimination of acidic and basic drugs is controversial because the ascorbic acid–induced decrease in urine pH has been shown to be small. Nevertheless, patients should be monitored if they are on acidic or basic medications eliminated by renal excretion and if they initiate megadose ascorbic acid therapy. Cholestyramine may bind ascorbic acid, reducing not only ascorbic acid absorption but also the bile acid–binding capacity of cholestyramine. Therefore, administration of the two should be separated.

There have been isolated anecdotal reports of oxalate urinary tract stone formation, possible ascorbate-mediated destruction of dietary vitamin B_{12} (cyanocobalamin), and rebound scurvy upon sudden withdrawal of ascorbic acid. This last effect was detected in infants whose mothers took megadoses of vitamin C during pregnancy. Ascorbic acid may increase the serum levels of estrogens and reduce the anticoagulant action of warfarin.

Cyanocobalamin (Vitamin B_{12})

Cyanocobalamin contains a single atom of cobalt and is the most complex vitamin molecule. It is available in the body as methylcobalamin, hydroxycobalamin, and adenosylcobalamin, all designated as "cobalamins." The term *vitamin B_{12}* refers to all cobalamins that have vitamin activity in humans. Cyanocobalamin, the common pharmaceutical form of the vitamin, is one of two commercially available forms and is the most stable; however, it is present in only small amounts in the body.

Vitamin B_{12} is active in all cells, especially those in the bone marrow, the central nervous system (CNS), and the GI tract. It is also involved in fat, protein, and carbohydrate metabolism. A cobalamin coenzyme functions in the synthesis of DNA and in the synthesis and transfer of single-carbon units such as the methyl group in the synthesis of methionine and choline. Vitamin B_{12} participates in methylation reactions and cell division, usually in concert with folic acid. It is necessary for the metabolism of folates; therefore, a folate deficiency may be observed as a feature of vitamin B_{12} deficiency. Vitamin B_{12} is also necessary for the metabolism of lipids, the maintenance of sulfhydryl groups in the reduced state, and the formation of myelin.

Vitamin B_{12} is produced almost exclusively by microorganisms, which accounts for its presence in animal protein (meats, oysters, and clams). It may also be found in small amounts in the root nodules of legumes and in selected vegetables and fruits, again because of the presence of microorganisms.

Indications In healthy individuals who have not restricted their diets, cyanocobalamin levels are maintained by the body. Vitamin B_{12} deficiency may be caused by poor absorption or utilization, or by an increased requirement or excretion of this vitamin. Because vitamin B_{12} is conserved by the body, it requires approximately 3 years for the deficiency to develop. In patients with malabsorption (ileal diseases or resection), the reabsorption phase of the enterohepatic cycle is affected, and the deficiency may occur much earlier.

Because of the general lack of vitamin B_{12} in vegetables, vegetarians who consume no animal products are at risk for developing a vitamin B_{12} deficiency, several cases of which have been reported in infants breastfed by vegetarian mothers. Strict vegetarians should consider taking vitamin B_{12} supplements or adjust their diet to include fermented foods, such as soy sauce, that contain the vitamin.

The symptoms of a vitamin B_{12} deficiency mimic those of a folate deficiency and are manifested in organ systems with rapidly duplicating cells. Thus, one effect of such a deficiency on the hematopoietic system is macrocytic anemia. The GI tract is also affected, with glossitis and epithelial changes occurring along the entire digestive tract. Some people lack the glycoprotein (intrinsic factor) necessary for the gastric absorption of vitamin B_{12}; this results in pernicious anemia. Because vitamin B_{12} is necessary to the maintenance of myelin, deficiency states produce many neurologic symptoms, such as paresthesia (manifested as tingling and numbness in the hands and feet), unsteadiness, poor muscular coordination, mental confusion, agitation, hallucinations, and overt psychosis. Other clinical manifestations of cyanocobalamin deficiency include macrocytic megaloblastic anemia, atrophic gastritis, achlorhydria, neurologic degeneration, and dementia.

The pharmacist should caution patients that an accurate diagnosis of the causes of a suspected anemia is essential in selecting effective treatment. For example, anemia due to a folic acid deficiency should be treated with folic acid, pernicious anemia should be treated with vitamin B_{12}, and iron deficiency anemia should be treated with iron. The use of "shotgun" antianemia preparations containing multiple hematinic factors should be discouraged.

Dose/RDA The RDA for vitamin B_{12} is 2 mcg for adults. Requirements increase to 2.2 mcg during pregnancy and to 2.6 mcg during lactation.

Past treatment of vitamin B_{12} deficiency involved crude liver extracts administered orally or parenterally. Crystalline vitamin B_{12} is now available. Cyanocobalamin is available for oral use as 25-, 50-, 100-, and 250-mcg tablets and as a 400-mcg/0.1-mL unit of nasal gel. Oral forms can be used if the deficiency is nutritionally based; intramuscular or subcutaneous administration is necessary for deficiencies due to malabsorption.

Hydroxycobalamin is a longer-acting form equal in hematopoietic effect to cyanocobalamin. Because it is more extensively bound to proteins at the site of injection and to plasma proteins, renal excretion is slower and the vitamin remains in the body for a longer period.

Adverse Effects/Drug Interactions Excessive doses have not resulted in toxicity, nor has any benefit been reported from nondeficient patients taking large quantities of the vitamin.

Certain drugs such as neomycin may impair absorption of vitamin B_{12}.

Folic Acid (Pteroylglutamic Acid, Folacin)

The term *folacin* is used as a generic term to designate folic acid, pteroylglutamic acid, and other similar-acting compounds. Current guidelines for terminology are that *folate* and *folic acid* are preferred synonyms for *pteroylglutamate* and *pteroylglutamic acid*. Because *folates* can be used in a generic sense referring to the above, the term *folacin* should not be used.

Folates are reduced in vivo to the bioactive form, tetrahydrofolic acid, through a complex process and are involved in the biosynthesis of purine, pyrimidine, serine, methionine, and choline. Folic acid is further biotransformed in the body and is involved in DNA synthesis and maturation and cell production activities. The function of folic acid is closely related to that of vitamin B_{12}. A folic acid deficiency can occur as a consequence of a vitamin B_{12} deficiency.

Folates are present in nearly all natural foods. Primary sources in the diet include liver, lean beef, veal, yeast, leafy vegetables, legumes, some fruits, eggs, and whole-grain cereals. The diet should include some foods that require little cooking, however, because folates are heat labile and the folic acid content of food is subject to destruction depending on how the food is processed. Canning, long exposure to heat, and extensive refining may destroy 50–100% of the naturally occurring folic acid.

Indications The requirements for folic acid are related to the metabolic rate and cell turnover. Thus, increased amounts of folic acid are needed during pregnancy, lactation, and infancy, as well as for infection, hemolytic anemias and blood loss (in which red blood cell production must be increased to replenish blood supply), and hypermetabolic states such as hyperthyroidism. Rheumatoid arthritis may also increase folic acid requirements.

Causes of folic acid deficiency include alcoholism, malabsorption, food faddism, liver disease, and iatrogenic forms associated with the administration of various therapeutic agents.

A deficiency of folic acid results in impaired cell division and protein synthesis. Symptoms of folic acid deficiency are similar to those of vitamin B_{12} deficiency and include sore mouth, diarrhea, and CNS symptoms such as irritability and forgetfulness. The most common laboratory feature of folic acid deficiency is megaloblastic anemia.

Because vitamin B_{12} is essential for the metabolism of folates, a megaloblastic anemia responsive to folic acid administration is a feature of pernicious anemia. Folic acid given without vitamin B_{12} to patients with pernicious anemia will correct the anemia but will have no effect on the more insidious damage to the CNS, symptoms of which include lack of coordination, impaired sense of position, and various behavioral disturbances. Because of the potential for folic acid to mask the signs of pernicious anemia, which is caused by a vitamin B_{12} deficiency, products containing more than 0.8 mg of folic acid per dose are available only by prescription. Pharmacists should refer all patients with suspected anemias for medical consultation.

Dose/RDA The RDA for folic acid is 200 mcg for most adult men and 180 mcg for most adult women, increasing to 400 mcg during pregnancy. Folic acid supplementation starting before pregnancy, if possible, is now recommended to prevent neural tube defects, one of the most common severe congenital malformations.

The oral dose of folic acid for correction of a deficiency is usually 1 mg per day, particularly if the deficiency occurs with conditions that may increase the folate requirement or suppress red blood cell formation (eg, pregnancy, hypermetabolic states, alcoholism, or hemolytic anemia). Doses larger than 1 mg per day are not necessary except in some life-threatening hematologic diseases. Maintenance therapy for deficiencies may be stopped after 1–4 months if the diet contains at least one fresh fruit or vegetable daily. For chronic malabsorption diseases, folic acid treatment may be lifelong and parenteral doses may be required.

Adverse Effects/Drug Interactions Folic acid toxicity is virtually nonexistent because of folic acid's water solubility and rapid excretion. Up to 15 mg have been given daily without toxic effect.

Several drugs taken chronically may increase the need for folic acid. Phenytoin and possibly other related anticonvulsants may inhibit folic acid absorption, leading to megaloblastic anemia. This problem is further complicated by the fact that folic acid supplementation may decrease serum phenytoin levels and complicate seizure control. The pharmacist should note when folic acid is prescribed to patients whose medication records indicate concurrent phenytoin therapy.

Trimethoprim may act as a weak folic acid antagonist in humans. Megaloblastic anemia may be precipitated in patients who possess a relatively low folic acid level at the onset of trimethoprim therapy; however, this problem is rarely seen in most patients using trimethoprim. Pyrimethamine, which is related to trimethoprim, may induce megaloblastic anemia in large doses. The mechanism of pyrimethamine's folic acid antagonism is inhibition of active tetrahydrofolate production. Methotrexate is also a folic acid antagonist, so patients on maintenance regimens for psoriasis or rheumatoid arthritis should be questioned carefully if they request folic acid supplements.

Niacin (Nicotinic Acid)

The physiologically active form of niacin is nicotinamide. Niacin and niacinamide (nicotinic acid amide) are constituents of the coenzymes nicotinamide adenine dinucleotide and nicotinamide adenine dinucleotide phosphate. These coenzymes are electron transfer agents; that is, they accept or donate hydrogen in the aerobic respiration of all body cells. Niacin is unusual as a vitamin in that humans can synthesize it from dietary tryptophan, with about 60 mg of tryptophan being equivalent to 1 mg of niacin. Most individuals receive about 50% of their niacin requirement from tryptophan-containing proteins and the rest as preformed niacin or niacinamide. In therapeutic doses, niacin will lower triglycerides and low-density lipoprotein cholesterol by mechanisms unrelated to its function as an essential micronutrient.

Niacin is present in most foods, including lean meats, fish, liver, cold cereals, whole grains, green vegetables, and legumes.

Indications Clinical findings of niacin deficiency include the three "Ds" of *d*ermatitis, *d*iarrhea, and *d*ementia, often accompanied by neuropathy, glossitis, stomatitis, and proctitis. The classical niacin deficiency state is pellagra. The pellagra syndrome involves dermatitis, diarrhea, dementia, and neurologic changes (eg, mild tremor, depression, and peripheral neuropathy).

Pellagra is rare, occurring most often in alcoholics, poorly nourished elderly persons, and individuals on bizarre diets. It may occur in areas where much corn is eaten because niacin in corn may be bound to undigestible constituents, making it unavailable. The main body systems affected are the CNS, the skin, and the GI tract. Symptoms involving the CNS include peripheral neuropathy, myelopathy, and encephalopathy. Mania may occur. Seizures and coma precede death. Before the cause of CNS manifestations of niacin deficiency was discovered, many psychiatric admissions were occasioned by symptoms of niacin deficiency. Both niacin and niacinamide are effective in treating pellagra.

There is a characteristic rash in niacin-deficient patients. The skin over the face and on pressure points may become thickened or hyperpigmented, or it may appear burned. Secondary infections may occur in such lesions. The entire GI tract is generally affected, with angular fissures around the mouth, atrophy of the epithelium, a beefy-red color of the tongue, and hypertrophy of the papillae. Inflammation of the small intestine may be associated with episodes of occult bleeding and/or diarrhea.

An individual's niacin status can be estimated by measuring the urinary levels of niacin metabolites. Low values together with symptoms point to a diagnosis of pellagra.

Dose/RDA The RDA of niacin is 19 mg for most adult men and 15 mg for most adult women. As previously noted, 1 mg of niacin is equivalent to 60 mg of dietary tryptophan.

Niacin requirements are increased during acute illness; during convalescence after a severe injury, infection, or burns; when either caloric expenditure or dietary caloric intake is substantially increased; or when the patient has a low tryptophan intake (eg, a low-protein diet or a high intake of corn as a staple in the diet).

Treatment of pellagra involves the ingestion of 300–500 mg of niacinamide daily in divided doses. Because other nutritional deficiencies may be present, treatment may include the other B vitamins, vitamin A, and iron.

Niacin has been used in daily dosages of 1 to 2 g three times per day, up to 8 g per day, to treat hypercholesterolemia and hyperlipidemias. Niacin treatment increases beneficial high-density lipoprotein cholesterol and decreases levels of potentially harmful triglycerides, total cholesterol, and low-density lipoprotein cholesterol. In the Coronary Drug Project, niacin treatment correlated with a decrease in nonfatal recurrent myocardial infarct and, upon long-term follow-up, an 11% decrease in mortality from all causes. This beneficial effect was evident 9 years after cessation of both the study and the niacin therapy. Niacin treatment of hyperlipidemias requires close medical supervision for evidence of effectiveness and manifestations of drug-induced toxicity.

Niacin and niacinamide are available as tablets and capsules in strengths ranging from 25 to 500 mg and in both regular and timed-release products. They are also available in elixir form (50 mg/5 mL) as well as in many combination products. Prenatal multivitamins may contain up to 20 mg of niacin.

Adverse Effects/Drug Interactions Niacin toxicity can involve GI symptoms (eg, nausea, vomiting, and diarrhea), hepatotoxicity, skin lesions, tachycardia, hypertension, and flushing. Doses of niacin in excess of 1 g per day may result in flushing and burning sensations. High doses may cause significant and potentially serious adverse effects. Chronic high-dose usage may lead to hyperkeratotic pigmented skin lesions.

Because of the adverse effects on the GI tract, high doses of niacin are contraindicated in patients with gastritis or peptic ulcer disease. Niacin can provoke the release of histamine, so its use in patients with asthma should be undertaken carefully. Niacin may also impair liver function, as evidenced by cholestatic jaundice, and it can disturb glucose tolerance and cause hyperuricemia. If niacin and niacinamide are used in high doses, laboratory parameters suggested by the potential side effects should be followed.

Patients should be forewarned that niacin may cause flushing and a sensation of warmth, especially around the face, neck, and ears. This reaction, which many people experience especially upon initiation of therapy, may be diminished if they take 325 mg of aspirin or 200 mg of ibuprofen 30 minutes before the niacin dose, provided there are no contraindications. Itching or tingling and headache may also occur. All these effects will usually subside or decrease in intensity with continued therapy. If niacin causes GI upset, it should be taken with meals.

Niacinamide does not produce the discomforting flushing associated with therapeutic doses of niacin; however, it also does not have a beneficial lowering effect on plasma lipids.

Pantothenic Acid

Pantothenic acid is a water-soluble vitamin of the B-complex family. Only the dextrorotatory isomer of pantothenic acid has biologic activity; however, pantothenic acid is a precursor of coenzyme A (CoA), a product that is active in many biologic reactions and that plays a primary role in cholesterol, steroid, and fatty acid synthesis. Pantothenic acid is important for acetylation reactions and the formation of citric acid for the Krebs cycle, and it is crucial in the intraneuronal synthesis of acetylcholine. It is also important in gluconeogenesis; the synthesis and degradation of fatty acids; the synthesis of sterols, steroid hormones, and porphyrins; the release of energy from carbohydrates; and acylation reactions.

Pantothenic acid is widely distributed in plant and animal tissues. Sources include meat, liver, milk, eggs, vegetables, cereal grains, and legumes.

Indications Because pantothenic acid is contained in many foods, deficiency states are rare and hard to detect. In malabsorption syndromes, it is difficult to separate pantothenic acid deficiency symptoms from symptoms of other deficiencies. Symptoms of pantothenic acid deficiency include somnolence, fatigue, headache, paresthesia of hands and/or feet followed by hyperreflexia and muscular weakness in the legs, cardiovascular instability, GI complaints, changes in disposition, and increased susceptibility to infections. Administration of pharmacologic doses of pantothenic acid reverses these symptoms and has also been used to eliminate burning feet syndrome.

Dose/RDA The Food and Nutrition Board does not list an RDA value for this vitamin but estimates a safe and adequate daily intake to be 4–7 mg for adults. Pantothenic acid is available as calcium pantothenate in 25-, 100-, 250-, and 500-mg tablets and in multivitamin products.

Adverse Effects/Drug Interactions Pantothenic acid is generally considered nontoxic, even in large doses. Doses as high as 10 g of calcium pantothenate daily have been given to young men for 6 weeks with no toxic symptoms. However, ingestion of more than 20 g has been reported to result in diarrhea and water retention. Dexpanthenol may prolong bleeding time in hemophiliacs and should be used with extreme caution.

Pyridoxine (Vitamin B_6)

Description Pyridoxine serves as a cofactor for more than 60 enzymes, including decarboxylases, synthetases, transaminases, and hydroxylases. It is important in heme production and in the conversion of oxalate to glycine.

This water-soluble vitamin exists in three forms: pyridoxine (vitamin B_6), pyridoxal, and pyridoxamine. Although all three forms are equally effective in nutrition, pyridoxine hydrochloride is the form most often used in vitamin formulations.

Foods rich in pyridoxine include meats, cereals, lentils, nuts, and some fruits and vegetables such as bananas, avocados, and potatoes. Cooking destroys some of the vitamin. The average US diet provides slightly less than the RDA; certain restricted diets may result in low pyridoxine intake. Infant formulas are required to contain pyridoxine hydrochloride.

Indications Causes of pyridoxine deficiency include alcoholism, severe diarrheal syndromes, food faddism, drugs (isoniazid, hydralazine, penicillamine, and cycloserine), malabsorption syndromes, and genetic diseases (cystathioninuria and xanthinuric aciduria).

The symptoms of severe pyridoxine deficiency in infants are convulsive disorders and irritability. Treatment with pyridoxine hydrochloride (2 mg per day for infants) generally brings the electroencephalogram back to normal and resolves clinical symptoms. Symptoms in adults whose diets are deficient in pyridoxine or who have been given a pyridoxine antagonist are difficult to distinguish from symptoms of niacin and riboflavin deficiencies. These symptoms include pellagra-like dermatitis; scaliness around the nose, mouth, and eyes; oral lesions; peripheral neuropathy; and dulling of mentation. Serious deficiency symptoms include convulsions, peripheral neuritis, and sideroblastic anemia.

Dose/RDA The RDA is 2 mg for most adult men and 1.6 mg for most adult women. This requirement is increased to 2.2 mg during pregnancy and to 2.1 mg during lactation.

Treatment of sideroblastic anemia requires 50–200 mg per day of pyridoxine hydrochloride to aid in the production of hemoglobin and erythrocytes. At least five pyridoxine-dependent inborn errors of metabolism have been shown to respond to large doses of pyridoxine. Pyridoxine (100 mg taken three times daily) for at least 11weeks has been reported to relieve paresthesia and pain in the hands of patients with carpal tunnel syndrome, but the value of such therapy has not been clearly and objectively determined. Pyridoxine is available as 25-, 50-, and 100-mg tablets; in 100-mg timed-release tablets; and in combination products.

Adverse Effects/Drug Interactions Pyridoxine may be toxic in high doses. A severe sensory neuropathy, similar to that observed with the deficiency state, has been reported when gram quantities were taken to relieve symptoms of premenstrual syndrome (PMS). Similar symptoms have been reported in women taking doses as small as 50 mg per day for PMS. Recovery occurred upon withdrawal of pyridoxine but was slow.

High daily doses of pyridoxine (200–600 mg) have been shown to inhibit prolactin. Prenatal vitamins, which contain 1–10 mg per dosage unit, do not appear to have a significant antiprolactin effect. Large doses of pyridoxine may also increase the activity of plasma aminotransferase, but the consequences of this effect are unknown.

Several drugs interact with pyridoxine, and it affects the action of several drugs. Isoniazid and cycloserine antagonize pyridoxine; hydralazine may have this effect as well. Perioral numbness resulting from peripheral neuropathy is a clinical manifestation of this antagonism. To overcome the antagonism, 50 mg per day of pyridoxine hydrochloride with isoniazid and as much as 20 mg per day with cycloserine should be used routinely. Another recommended dose is 10 mg of pyridoxine per 100 mg of isoniazid. Psychotic behavior and seizures, both produced by cycloserine, may be prevented with increased pyridoxine intake. Penicillamine may bind with pyridoxine hydrochloride, causing pyridoxine-responsive neurotoxicity. Pyridoxine may reduce the clinical effects of phenobarbital and phenytoin by reducing their serum levels.

Pyridoxine is intimately involved in the metabolism of amino acids, particularly that of tryptophan. Low pyridoxine levels result in the appearance of excess urinary xanthurenic acid, a tryptophan metabolite. In fact, pyridoxine status is assessed by quantitation of urinary xanthurenic acid following administration of a loading dose of tryptophan. Estrogens seem to increase xanthurenic acid production significantly, and women taking oral contraceptives may show laboratory signs of pyridoxine deficiency. Supplementation with daily pyridoxine (2–40 mg) returns the tryptophan metabolic pattern to normal. The pathologic consequences of these events are not known; however, a depressive syndrome occasionally experienced by women taking oral contraceptives has responded to daily pyridoxine supplementation of 20–100 mg. Levels of other vitamins are marginally lower in some oral contraceptive users. Women who take oral contraceptives should consider improving their diet. For some, a multivitamin supplement may be indicated.

Pyridoxine antagonizes the therapeutic action of levodopa (the biologically active form of dopa) by facilitating the transformation of levodopa into dopamine before the former can cross the blood-brain barrier and enter the CNS. The pharmacist should inform patients taking levodopa of the interaction and should advise them to avoid supplemental pyridoxine. On the other hand, pyridoxine may be useful in treating patients who have overdosed on levodopa. Sinemet, the combination product containing levodopa and carbidopa, a peripherally acting dopa decarboxylase inhibitor, does not appear to be affected by the concurrent administration of pyridoxine.

Riboflavin (Vitamin B_2)

Riboflavin occurs in the free state in foods, in combination with phosphates, or with both phosphates and proteins. The free riboflavin is released and absorbed during digestion.

Riboflavin is a constituent of two coenzymes, flavin adenine dinucleotide and flavin mononucleotide. It is involved in numerous oxidation and reduction reactions, including the cytochrome P-450 reductase enzyme system involved in drug metabolism. Cellular growth cannot occur without riboflavin.

Primary sources of riboflavin include meats; poultry; fish; dairy products; enriched and fortified grains, cereals, and bakery products; and green vegetables such as broccoli, turnip greens, asparagus, and spinach.

Indications Riboflavin deficiency, in a pure, uncomplicated form, is probably not encountered alone in patients but rather is accompanied by other nutrient deficiencies that are attributable to an inadequate diet. Early signs of riboflavin deficiency may involve ocular symptoms as the eyes become light sensitive and easily fatigued. Also, blurred vision; itching, watering, sore eyes; and increased capillarization may develop in the cornea with a bloodshot appearance of the eye. Later clinical findings of deficiency include stomatitis, glossitis, seborrheic dermatitis, and magenta tongue. Surveys have revealed lower than anticipated riboflavin levels in women taking oral contraceptives; however, the pathologic consequences are unknown. Marginal riboflavin deficiencies have also been detected in vegetarians and alcoholics.

Dose/RDA The RDA for riboflavin is 1.7 mg for most adult men and 1.3 mg for most adult women. The need for riboflavin appears to increase during periods of increased cell growth, such as during pregnancy and wound healing.

Riboflavin is poorly soluble. If oral absorption is poor, 25 mg of the soluble riboflavin salt may be injected intramuscularly. Riboflavin may also be given intravenously as a component of an injectable multivitamin, but the dose is relatively low (about 10 mg). Riboflavin is available as 25-, 50-, and 100-mg tablets and in various combination products in various strengths.

Adverse Effects/Drug Interactions The use of riboflavin may cause a yellow-orange fluorescence or discoloration of the urine. Patients who report this effect should be reassured that this is normal.

Thiamine (Vitamin B_1)

Thiamine, a water-soluble vitamin, is necessary for several critical functions in carbohydrate metabolism. Its active form, thiamine pyrophosphate (formerly known as cocarboxylase), plays a vital role in the oxidative decarboxylation of pyruvic acid; in the formation of acetyl CoA, which enters the Krebs cycle; and in other important biochemical conversion cycles. Thiamine is also essential in neurologic function. The amount of vitamin that is required increases with increased caloric consumption.

The most familiar natural thiamine source is the hull of rice grains. Other sources are pork, beef, fresh peas, and beans.

Indications Several genetic diseases respond to the administration of thiamine. These fall into the category of vitamin-responsible inborn errors of metabolism and are generally attributable to a defect in the binding of enzyme and cofactor. Large daily doses of vitamins (5–100 mg in the case of thiamine) saturate the enzyme system(s) and usually obviate the pathology. Examples of thiamine-responsive inborn metabolic errors are lactic acidosis due to defective pyruvate carboxylase, branched-chain aminoacidopathy due to defective branched-chain amino acid decarboxylase, and some cases of the Wernicke–Korsakoff syndrome due to defective transketolase. These disorders justify the rational use of megadose thiamine therapy.

The primary causes of thiamine deficiency are generally related to inadequate diet, alcoholism, malabsorption syndromes, prolonged diarrhea, increased use (pregnancy), or food faddism.

Accordingly, thiamine deficiency in the United States is found primarily in alcoholics, in patients with chronic diarrhea, and in patients maintained on a high carbohydrate diet. In fact, among alcoholics, thiamine deficiency is common. Not only is the alcoholic's diet often nutritionally deficient and imbalanced, but alcohol ingestion further impairs thiamine absorption and transport across the intestine and increases the rate of destruction of thiamine diphosphate. High-dose, parenteral thiamine is commonly given to patients who are admitted to hospitals for alcohol detoxification and treatment. A vitamin supplement containing thiamine is often prescribed for the alcoholic patient.

The neurologic signs of thiamine deficiency (Wernicke's encephalopathy) include nystagmus, which occurs when the patient is asked to gaze up and down along a vertical plane or from side to side along a horizontal plane. Damage to the cerebral cortex may occur in patients who survive severe thiamine deficiency, and the deficiency may lead to Korsakoff's psychosis. The symptoms of the psychosis are impaired retentive memory and cognitive function; the patient commonly confabulates when given a piece of information or asked a question. Irreversible neurologic damage and death may ensue if severe thiamine deficiency is left untreated.

A diet consisting chiefly of unenriched white rice and white flour, or situations in which low dietary levels of thiamine are accompanied by the consumption of large amounts of raw fish with thiaminase containing intestinal microbes, may also produce a thiamine deficiency. Individuals subsisting on a diet of 0.2–0.3 mg of thiamine per 1,000 calories (slightly less than the thiamine requirement) may gradually become depleted of thiamine and develop peripheral neuropathy. If the patient has been subsisting on substantially less than 0.2 mg of thiamine per 1,000 calories, the deficiency will be more severe.

Symptoms of thiamine deficiency may become evident in 3 weeks after thiamine intake is stopped. The deficiency causes cardiac dysfunction, possibly accompanied by edema; tachycardia on only minimal exertion; enlarged heart; and electrocardiographic abnormalities. The patient may have pain in the precordial or epigastric areas. Neuromuscular symptoms include paresthesia of the extremities, weakness, and atrophy.

If severe and prolonged, thiamine deficiency may

result in either dry beriberi (evidenced by polyneuropathy, muscle weakness, symmetrical paresthesia, wrist- and/or footdrop, and encephalopathic stages—ie, Korsakoff's and Wernicke's syndromes) or wet beriberi (evidenced by the more common high-output cardiac failure, lactic acidosis-vasodilation, and/or the less common low-output cardiac failure). *Beriberi* literally means "I cannot," stemming from the fact that people affected have difficulty walking. Beriberi may develop in infants whose mothers are on a polished rice diet in regions where thiamine supplements are not used. The symptoms of infantile beriberi are also neurologic. Aphonia, or silent crying, may occur, and the signs of meningitis may be mimicked. Death will ensue if thiamine treatment is not initiated. Today, beriberi caused by nutritional deficiency rarely occurs in developed countries.

Dose/RDA The RDA for most adult men and women is 1.5 mg and 1.1 mg, respectively.

The treatment of beriberi is 25 mg of thiamine two or three times daily for 5 days, followed by a daily dose of 5 mg taken orally. For severe malabsorption, 5 mg daily is given parenterally.

To treat the symptoms of heart failure caused by a thiamine deficiency, 5–10 mg of thiamine is taken three times a day. At this dosage, the failure is rapidly corrected but the neurologic signs correct much more slowly. The daily dose of thiamine for neurologic deficits is 30–100 mg given parenterally for several days or until an oral diet can be started. Thiamine is available as 50-, 100-, 250-, and 500-mg tablets and is included in several strengths in combination products. If it is mixed in a solution, the solution should be acidic because thiamine is labile at an alkaline pH.

Adverse Effects/Drug Interactions The kidney easily clears excessive thiamine intake, and oral doses of 500 mg have been found to be nontoxic. There may be some toxicity from large doses given parenterally, however, with symptoms of itching, tingling, and pain. In rare instances, anaphylactic reactions are possible.

Vitamin-Like Compounds and Pseudovitamins

Bioflavonoids (Vitamin P)

The term *bioflavonoids* has been used to designate flavones and flavonols. The early extract apparently contained several flavonoids, chemically related substances derived from phenol. Because this work was not confirmed, it was recommended that the term *vitamin* be discontinued in this context and the word *bioflavonoids* be used to designate flavonoids with biologic activity.

These flavonoids are widely distributed in plants and are concentrated in the skin, peel, and outer layers of fruits and vegetables. As there is no known bioflavonoid deficiency condition, bioflavonoids have no accepted preventive or therapeutic role in human nutrition.

The average daily dietary intake of flavonoids is approximately 1,000 mg. Consequently, dietary supplementation using 20- to 30-mg tablets would not be significant.

Bioflavonoids are available as capsules and tablets and in combination products (both regular and sustained release) as tablets, capsules, and wafers.

Biotin (Vitamin H)

Biotin, a member of the B-complex group of vitamins, is required for various metabolic functions such as gluconeogenesis, lipogenesis, fatty acid biosynthesis, propionate metabolism, and the catabolism of branched-chain amino acids. There are now up to nine known biotin-dependent enzymes, including six carboxylases, two decarboxylases, and a transcarboxylase; four carboxylases—those for acetyl-CoA, propionyl-CoA, beta-methylglutaconyl-CoA, and pyruvate—occur in human tissues. Biotin plays an important role in fat, amino acid, and carbohydrate metabolism.

Biotin is widely distributed in animal tissue and is thus present in the diet. Sources include liver, egg yolk, cauliflower, salmon, carrots, bananas, soy flour, and yeast. Colonic flora probably contribute to the amount of biotin in the body.

Indications Deficiency states of biotin are rare but have been associated with nausea, vomiting, lassitude, muscle pain, anorexia, anemia, and depression. Dermatitis, a grayish color of the skin, and glossitis may also be among the physical findings, and hypercholesterolemia and cardiac abnormalities may occur.

Biotin deficiency in humans can be caused by the ingestion of a large number of raw egg whites. Raw egg white contains avidin, a protein that binds biotin, thereby preventing its absorption. Biotin deficiency symptoms have also been noted in patients on parenteral nutrition without biotin supplements. In pregnant women, blood biotin levels decrease as gestation progresses.

Individuals undergoing a rapid weight loss program with intense caloric restriction or those with malnutrition may not be obtaining adequate biotin and should receive supplementation.

Dose/RDA Although biotin is known to be necessary for carboxylation reactions in the body, the nutritional requirements for this vitamin are imprecise and no RDA has been determined for it. However, 100–200 mcg per day is generally considered safe and adequate. Biotin has been included in several multivitamin preparations.

Adverse Effects/Drug Interactions Side effects and drug interactions have not been reported with biotin therapy.

L-Carnitine (DL-Carnitine)

Carnitine, a vitamin-like molecule, can be synthesized from lysine and methionine in the liver and kidney; thus, it is considered an essential nutrient but not necessarily a vitamin. A number of actions are attributed to carnitine, including oxidation of fatty acids, promotion of certain organic acid excretions, and enhancement of the rate of oxidative phosphorylation.

L-Carnitine is required to transport long-chain fatty acids in mitochondria, which is prerequisite to their beta oxidation and to maintenance of energy production. Although carnitine is biosynthesized adequately by adults, newborns have a low capacity for carnitine synthesis from lysine and methionine, and they may be further compromised if fed soy formulas or maintained on total parenteral nutrition with no supplemental carnitine.

Dietary sources and synthesis in the liver and kidney satisfy the primary need for carnitine. Food sources include dairy products and meat, especially red meat.

Indications Carnitine deficiency may be evidenced by muscle weakness, cardiomyopathy, abnormal hepatic function, decreased ketogenesis, and hypoglycemia during fasting. Lipids may accumulate between muscle fibers.

Dose/RDA Human carnitine deficiency has been documented, but no RDA has been established. Therapy for carnitine deficiency should include a pharmaceutical supplement and a high-carbohydrate, low-fat diet. L-Carnitine is available as 250-mg capsules, 330-mg tablets, and a liquid containing 100 mg/mL, and it is present in several strengths in various combination products.

Adverse Effects/Drug Interactions L-Carnitine is without appreciable adverse effects in normal adults, and doses of 15 g per day have been well tolerated.

Choline

Choline is contained in most living cells and in foods. It is usually present in the form of phosphatidylcholine, commonly known as lecithin, and in several other phospholipids found in cell membranes. Intestinal mucosal cells and pancreatic secretions contain enzymes capable of splitting phospholipids to release choline. Choline is also found in sphingomyelin and is highly concentrated in nervous tissue.

Choline, a precursor in the biosynthesis of acetylcholine, is an important donator of methyl groups used in the biochemical formation of other substances in vivo. It can be biosynthesized in humans by the donation of methyl groups from methionine to ethanolamine. Further, choline and inositol are considered to be lipotropic agents (ie, agents involved in the mobilization of lipids). They have been used to treat fatty liver and disturbed fat metabolism, but their efficacy has not been established.

Although choline is found in egg yolks, cereal, fish, and meat, it is also synthesized in the body; therefore, it is doubtful that choline is a vitamin. Choline is obtained from the diet as either choline or lecithin.

Indications A deficiency state has not been identified in humans, possibly because choline is readily available in the diet.

Dose/RDA An average diet will furnish 200–600 mg of choline daily. Choline is available as 250-, 300-, 500-, and 650-mg tablets; as a powder; and in combination products in various strengths.

Adverse Effects/Drug Interactions The administration of large doses of lecithin has been associated with sweating, GI distress, vomiting, and diarrhea. Most adults, however, tolerate up to 20 g per day, and some tolerate as much as 30 g per day with no adverse effects.

Essential Fatty Acids (Vitamin F)

The essential fatty acids are involved in the proper development of various biomembranes; they are also important as precursors of prostaglandins, leukotrienes, and various hydroxy fatty acids. The polyunsaturated fatty acids regulate cell permeability to a significant degree because they are constituents of phospholipids. The typical Western diet, with its heavy polyunsaturated fat and oil content, provides ample essential fatty acids.

Linoleic and linolenic acids are essential in human nutrition but do not meet the definition of a vitamin. They are considered macronutrients. Linoleic acid, the 18-carbon fatty acid with two double bonds, cannot be synthesized in the body and must be present in the diet. It is rapidly converted to arachidonic acid, a functioning polyunsaturated fatty acid that is physiologically important. Linolenic acid has some essential fatty acid properties, but its biochemical role is not well defined. It is not a substitute for linoleic acid.

Linoleic acid deficiency symptoms can include scaly skin, hair loss, and impaired wound healing. If the total dietary calories consist of 1–2% linoleic acid, biochemical and clinical evidence for deficiencies do not occur.

Inositol

Inositol is a hexitol found in large amounts in muscle and brain tissues. It is widely distributed in nature and is also synthesized in the body. Inositol seems to be necessary for amino acid transport and for the movement of potassium and sodium, but its value in human nutrition has not been well documented. Like choline, it is considered a lipotropic agent of unproven therapeutic value.

Inositol is a sweet, water-soluble substance occurring in fruits, vegetables, whole grains, meats, and milk. It is present in cells as a phosphatide, and inositol lipids appear to be involved in the calcium-mediated control of cell functions, in cell proliferation, and in the attachment of enzymes to the plasma membrane.

A normal dietary intake is approximately 1 g per day, derived primarily from plant sources. The human requirement has not been established. Inositol is available in 250-, 500-, and 650-mg tablets and in a powder.

Laetrile (Amygdalin, Vitamin B_{17})

Laetrile occurs naturally in almond, apricot, and peach pits and in apple seeds. Consisting of 6% cyanide by weight, it is made up of two parts glucose, one part benzaldehyde, and one part cyanide. When spelled with a capital "L", it refers to a synthetic substance that was never marketed; when spelled with a small "l", it refers to amygdalin, the product marketed by laetrile promoters as a cancer cure, and is a synonym for cyanogenetic glycosides. Many toxic reactions have been reported worldwide with the ingestion of cyanogenetic glycosides; cyanide poisoning has occurred with some laetrile products.

Although it is called vitamin B_{17}, laetrile contains no vitamin activity and has no nutritional or therapeutic value and no approved medical use. Moreover, no physiologic or biochemical abnormalities develop when the diet is deficient in laetrile. Thus, the term *vitamin* B_{17} is erroneous, misleading, and fraudulent, and it should not be used. Use by desperate and uninformed individuals may lead to critical delays in seeking and receiving appropriate medical attention.

Pangamic Acid (Vitamin B_{15})

Pangamic acid is an uncharacterized extract of the Prunus family. The unsupported claim has been that the extract provides immunization against toxic products present in the human or animal system, as well as produces symptomatic relief and immunity to persons afflicted with asthma, eczema, arthritis, neuritis, painful nerve and joint afflictions, and numerous other conditions. Pangamic acid is described as a poorly defined mixture of dimethylglycine and sorbitol. No studies have shown it to have any efficacy in treating any medical disorder. Pangamic acid has been categorized as a pseudovitamin, and it has no nutritional or therapeutic value.

Taurine (Aminoethanesulfonate)

Along with carnitine, choline, and inositol, taurine has been referred to as a vitamin-like compound. It is now considered important enough to be included in human infant formulas, enteral products, and some parenteral nutritional solutions.

A unique chemical aspect of taurine is that it contains a sulfonic acid group that replaces the carboxyl group of what would otherwise be glycine. It is not incorporated into peptides, but it does participate in a few biochemical reactions. Taurine is present in most cells and exhibits a wide range of activity. Some of the physiologic functions that are affected by taurine include retinal photoreceptor activity, bile acid conjugation, white blood cell antioxidant activity, CNS neuromodulation, platelet aggregation, cardiac contractility, sperm motility, growth, and insulin activity.

Taurine, which is important in many metabolic activities, is normally biosynthesized in adequate amounts. Plasma levels of taurine normally range from 50 to 220 mcmol/L, and any excess is excreted in the urine.

Even though it is not known whether taurine is essential for humans, some concern has been expressed about the risk of taurine insufficiency in formula-fed infants—especially those born prematurely—as compared with breast-fed infants. Cow's milk contains lower levels of taurine than does human milk. No RDA is established at this time.

Minerals

Minerals constitute about 4% of body weight. The major mineral content of the skeleton consists of calcium and phosphorus in a ratio of approximately 2:1. Any change of one may be reflected in changes of the other.

Minerals are present in the body in a diverse array of organic compounds such as phosphoproteins, phospholipids, hemoglobin, and thyroxine, as well as in inorganic compounds such as sodium chloride, potassium chloride, calcium, and phosphate; they are also present as free ions. Different body tissues contain different quantities of different elements. For example, bone has a high content of calcium, phosphorus, and magnesium; soft tissue has a higher quantity of potassium. Minerals function as constituents of enzymes, hormones, and vitamins. They are involved in regulating cell membrane permeability, osmotic pressure, and acid-base and water balance.

A well-balanced diet is required to maintain proper mineral balance. Calcium and iron are two elements that may require particular dietary attention from normal individuals. Optimal mineral intake values for humans are still imprecise, and only estimated ranges are available for minerals such as chromium, fluoride, copper, manganese, and molybdenum. These ranges are based on the mineral content of the average diet. Similarly, the possible adverse effects of long-term ingestion of high-dose mineral supplements are unknown, and high doses of one mineral can decrease the bioavailability of other minerals and even of vitamins.

Unlike vitamins, minerals exist in plants in varying amounts, according to the composition of the soil in which the plant is grown. This, in turn, affects the mineral content of local livestock. Mineral intake varies considerably from region to region, although the use of foods delivered from diverse geographic locations tends to minimize intake variations. Marginal deficiencies of minerals have been reported only in certain segments of the population, but the increasing use of highly refined foods, which are low in minerals, may contribute to these deficiencies.

Mineral deficiency is often difficult to evaluate. Hair analysis has received attention in recent years, and its noninvasiveness is advantageous. However, a number of factors, such as distance from the scalp where the sample was obtained, color of the hair, and the use of shampoos, sprays, and conditioners, can adversely influence the accuracy of results. The analysis for zinc and toxic minerals such as arsenic, mercury, and lead has provided interesting results, but accepted normal values have not been established in routine nutritional assessment.

Calcium

The most abundant cation in the body is calcium (about 1,200 g); about 99% of calcium is present in the skeleton and the remaining 1% is present in the extracellular fluid, intracellular structures, and cell membranes. Calcium is a major component of bones and teeth. The calcium content in bone is continuously undergoing a process of resorption and formation. In elderly people, the resorption process predominates over formation, and a decrease in calcium absorption efficiency results in a gradual loss of bone (osteoporosis). This effect can be minimized by ensuring an optimal calcium intake during the formative years to develop optimal bone mass and by promoting weight-bearing exercise.

Calcium is important because it activates a number of enzymes (eg, pancreatic lipase, adenosine triphosphatase, and some proteolytic enzymes), is required for acetylcholine synthesis, increases cell membrane permeability, aids in vitamin B_{12} absorption, regulates muscle contraction and relaxation, and catalyzes several blood-clotting steps. It is also necessary for the functional integrity of many cells, especially those of the neuromuscular and cardiovascular system.

The average blood level of calcium in the body is about 9.0–10.5 mg/dL. There are three forms of calcium in the blood and body fluids; these forms include ionized calcium, calcium complexes with organic acids, and protein-bound calcium.

The small intestine controls calcium absorption. Patients ingesting relatively low amounts of calcium absorb proportionately more, and some patients taking large amounts of calcium excrete more as fecal calcium. Calcium requirements may increase as the consumption of protein increases.

Rich dietary sources of calcium include milk and other dairy products. Teenagers experiencing rapid growth and bone maturation need to consume adequate calcium via dairy products, especially milk, or nutritional supplements in tablet or capsule form. Adults can easily meet calcium RDA levels by incorporating dairy products (especially low-fat and nonfat milk) into their diets. Nonfat milk contains about 300 mg of calcium per 8 oz. As an alternative, calcium supplements are essentially free of adverse effects in daily doses of less than 2 g of calcium.

Dietary factors that increase calcium absorption include certain amino acids such as lysine and arginine, vitamin D, and lactose. Dietary factors that decrease the efficiency of calcium absorption include foods with high phosphate content (eg, unpolished rice, hexaphosphoinositol in bran, and wheat meal) and foods high in oxalate content (eg, cocoa, soybeans, kale, and spinach). Vitamin D deficiency may also reduce the absorption and physiologic effects of calcium.

Indications

Decreased calcium levels may have profound and diverse consequences, including convulsions, tetany, behavioral and personality disorders, mental and growth retardation, and bone deformities, the most common being rickets in children and osteomalacia in adults. Changes that occur in osteomalacia include softening of bones, rheumatic-type pain in the bones of the legs and lower back, general weakness with difficulty walking, and spontaneous fractures.

Common causes of hypocalcemia and associated skeletal disorders are malabsorption syndromes; hypoparathyroidism; vitamin D deficiency; renal failure with impaired activation of vitamin D; long-term anticonvulsant therapy (with increased breakdown of vitamin D); and decreased dietary intake of calcium, particularly during periods of growth, pregnancy, and lactation and among elderly individuals.

Dose/RDA

To maximize bone mass before the inevitable decline that occurs after menopause, the RDA values have been set at 1,200 mg per day for both women and men aged 11–24. The RDA for adults over 24 years of age is 800 mg per day. Some suggest that, for women, about 1,100 mg per day before menopause and 1,500 mg per day after menopause is advantageous; during pregnancy and lactation, 1,200 mg per day is recommended. Weight-bearing exercise is also very important in maintaining bone mass, and any program to decrease the risk for osteoporosis should include regular exercise.

Calcium is available in many salt forms and strengths as tablets (regular, chewable, and effervescent), capsules, powders, and liquids, as well as in combination products (see product table "Calcium Products"). The calcium salts available without a prescription (and the percentage of calcium they contain) are the carbonate (40%), citrate, lactate (21%), gluconate (9%), and phosphate salts (23–39%). Calcium carbonate and calcium phosphate salts are insoluble and should be taken with meals to enhance absorption, which depends on a low pH in the stomach. Patients requiring supplementation who have low levels of gastric hydrochloric acid (achlorhydria) or are on histamine II (H_2) antagonists or omeprazole should probably take a soluble salt (eg, calcium citrate, calcium lactate, or calcium gluconate). Bonemeal (mostly a calcium phosphate matrix) and oyster shell products (calcium carbonate matrix) are insoluble and require an acid pH for absorption. Some products do not disintegrate as well as others, which further limits the amount of calcium available for absorption.

Adverse Effects/Drug Interactions

Calcium in doses greater than 2 g per day can be harmful. Large amounts taken as dietary supplements or antacids can lead to high levels of calcium in the urine and to renal stones; the latter development may result in renal damage. Hypercalcemia, with associated anorexia, nausea, vomiting, constipation, and polyuria, is also possible, particularly in patients taking high-dose vitamin D preparations, even when that intake is independent of calcium supplements. Hypercalcemia can also result in an increased deposition of calcium in soft tissue.

High calcium intake levels may inhibit the absorption of iron, zinc, and other essential minerals. Corticosteriods inhibit calcium absorption from the gut, and their use has been associated with increased bone fractures and osteoporosis. The excessive ingestion of aluminum-containing antacids has been shown to result in negative calcium balances. Several other drugs, including phosphates, calcitonin, sodium sulfate, furosemide, magnesium, cholestyramine, estrogen, and some anticonvulsants, also lower calcium serum levels. Thiazide diuretics, on the other hand, increase serum calcium levels.

Iron

Iron is widely available in the US diet. Iron absorption from the intestinal tract is controlled by the body's need for iron, intestinal lumen conditions, and the food content of the meal. Although iron-deficient persons may absorb about 10–20% of dietary iron, persons with normal iron stores absorb about 5–10%.

Iron plays an important role in oxygen and electron transport. In the body, it is either functional or stored. Functional iron is found in hemoglobin, myoglobin, heme-containing enzymes, and transferrin, the transport form of iron. Stored iron is primarily found in the hemoglobin of red blood cells, which contains 60–70% of total body iron. The rest is stored primarily in the form of ferritin and hemosiderin and is found in the intestinal mucosa, liver, spleen, and bone marrow.

Normally, adult men have iron stores of about 50 mg/kg of body weight; women have about 35 mg/kg of body weight. The normal hemoglobin level in adult men is about 14–17 g/100 mL of blood; in adult women it is 12–14 g/100 mL of blood.

Dietary iron is available in two forms. Heme iron is found in meats and is reasonably well absorbed. Nonheme iron constitutes most of the dietary iron and is poorly absorbed. Therefore, the published values of the iron content of foods are misleading because the amount absorbed depends on the nature of the iron. To gain an accurate assessment of the iron available in a meal, the composition of the meal must be considered in detail. About half of the iron in meats is heme iron, which is about 25% absorbed. The amount of absorbable nonheme iron contributed by vegetables and grains in the diet varies greatly.

The available iron content of foods is calculated by assuming that only 10% of the total iron (heme plus nonheme) is absorbable if no iron deficiency exists. In the iron-deficient state, iron absorption improves so that as much as 20% may be absorbed and used from an average diet. As Americans appear to be moving away from a "red meat" diet, it may be increasingly important to monitor the population for iron status.

Nonheme-ingested iron, which is mostly in the form of ferric hydroxide, is solubilized in gastric juice to ferric chloride, reduced to the ferrous form, and chelated to substances such as ascorbic acid, sugars, and amino acids. Chelates have a low molecular weight and can be solubilized and absorbed before they reach the alkaline medium of the distal small intestine, where precipitation may occur. In intestinal mucosal cells, iron is stored in a protein-bound form as ferritin. As needed, it is released into the plasma, where it is oxidized to the ferric state and bound to a beta globulin to form transferrin. When released at the spleen, liver, bone marrow, intestinal mucosa, and other iron storage sites, the iron is combined with apoferritin to form ferritin or hemosiderin. Iron is used in all cells of the body; however, most of it is incorporated into the hemoglobin of red blood cells. Iron is lost from the body by the sloughing of skin cells and GI mucosal cells; by hemorrhagic loss; by menstruation; and by excretion of urine, sweat, and feces.

Indications

Early symptoms of iron deficiency are vague. Easy fatigability, weakness, and lassitude cannot in themselves be easily related to iron deficiency. Other signs of anemia include pallor, split or "spoon-shaped" nails, sore tongue, angular stomatitis, dyspnea on exertion, palpitation, and a feeling of exhaustion. Coldness and numbness of the extremities may be reported. Small red blood cells and low hemoglobin concentrations (hypochromic, microcytic anemia) characterize iron deficiency.

There are three general stages of iron deficiency:

- Iron depletion, in which iron stores are depleted and associated with plasma ferritin levels below 12 mcg/L;
- Iron-deficient erythropoiesis, in which red cell protoporphyrin levels are elevated but the hemoglobin levels are within the 95% reference range;
- Iron deficiency anemia, in which the total blood hemoglobin levels are below normal levels.

Iron deficiency anemia is a widespread clinical problem and the most common form of anemia in the United States. Although it causes few deaths, it contributes to the poor health and suboptimal performance of many people.

Iron deficiency results from inadequate diet, malabsorption, pregnancy and lactation, or blood loss. Because normal excretion of iron through the urine, feces, and skin is small, iron deficiency caused by poor diet or malabsorption may develop very slowly. This is because iron is stored and conserved (recycled) by the body, and signs may be manifested only after several years.

Despite fortification of flour and educational efforts regarding proper nutrition, iron deficiency remains a problem for certain segments of the population, especially children in poverty and menstruating and pregnant women. Iron supplements are routinely recommended as a component of prenatal care.

The four life periods when iron deficiency is most common are:

- From 6 months to 4 years of age, because of the low iron content in cow's milk;
- During early adolescence, when rapid growth entails an expanding red cell mass and the need for iron in myoglobin;
- During the female reproductive years, owing to menstrual iron losses;
- During and after pregnancy, owing to the expanding blood volume of the mother, the demands of the fetus and placenta, and blood losses during childbirth.

Menstruation normally results in a loss of 60–80 mL of blood per month and about 1.4 mg of iron in addition to that normally lost. The daily amount required for replacement is about 0.7–2.3 mg of absorbed iron. The average US diet contains about 5–7 mg of iron per 1,000 calories, but only about 10% of iron in food is absorbed. If the menstrual blood loss exceeds 60–80 mL, supplemental iron may be desirable because the dietary requirement may be as high as 40 mg/d.

The donation of 500 mL (1 pint or unit) of blood produces a loss of approximately 250 mg of iron. This is not a significant problem in healthy, well-nourished adults with adequate iron stores; however, some blood donors, especially those who donate frequently, may benefit from short-term iron replacement following blood donation.

The differential diagnosis in adults or postmenopausal women should rule out iron deficiency owing to excess blood loss associated with peptic ulcer disease, hemorrhoids, Crohn's disease, esophageal varices, diverticulitis, intestinal parasites, regional enteritis, ulcerative colitis, and cancer.

Chronic use of drugs such as salicylates, nonsteroidal anti-inflammatory drugs, reserpine, corticosteroids, warfarin, ulcerogenic drugs, antiprothrombinemic drugs, or most drugs used to treat neoplasms might indicate drug-induced blood loss. Drug-induced blood loss may occur because of irritating effects on the gastric mucosa or an indirect effect on the GI tract.

The pharmacist may sometimes ascertain the cause of the patient's condition by consulting the medication record. Medications such as aspirin or ibuprofen may not be included on a medication record if they were bought without a prescription. Thus, the pharmacist should routinely question the patient regarding the use of nonprescription drugs. The pharmacist should also ascertain whether the patient's problem is chronic, whether self-treatment has been tried, and whether medical care has been sought or received. Pharmacists should be aware that anemia in patients other than those who are pregnant, lactating, menstruating, or on a restricted diet may be a symptom of a more serious medical disorder, and these individuals should be strongly encouraged to seek medical attention. Such intervention may prevent a more serious problem.

A patient who reports blood loss should be referred to a physician immediately. Abnormal blood loss may be indicated by (1) vomiting blood (coffee-ground vomitus); (2) bright red blood in the stool or black, tarry stools; (3) large clots or an abnormally heavy flow during the menstrual period; or (4) cloudy or pink-red urine (assuming that dyes in drugs that may cause urine discoloration have been ruled out).

Blood loss, particularly through the stool, is not always obvious. Even when abnormal blood loss occurs, the patient may not notice it and the blood loss may not be reported. Periodic testing using home occult blood test kits may be considered for certain high-risk or at-risk patients.

Dose/RDA

The RDA for iron is 10 mg for adult men, 15 mg for adult women, and 30 mg for pregnant women. Most healthy individuals who self-medicate, including menstruating females, will absorb adequate iron from one 325-mg ferrous sulfate tablet per day. In a 325-mg ferrous sulfate tablet, 20% (about 60 mg) is elemental iron. In patients with iron deficiencies, 20% of the elemental iron (12 mg) may be absorbed. Because 36–48 mg of iron daily is enough to support maximum incorporation into red blood cells (0.3 g of hemoglobin per 100 mL of blood) and replace iron stores, the usual therapeutic dose of two to four tablets daily for 3 months is probably reasonable in treating a deficiency. If the patient has an inadequate response after this period, a physician should be consulted. In cases of severe or chronic iron deficiency and when serious medical conditions have been ruled out, continuous low-maintenance doses of three to four tablets daily for approximately 3–6 months should normalize hemoglobin and replace iron stores, provided there is no ongoing bleeding and the diet is adequate.

If iron supplementation is appropriate, the pharmacist may recommend which iron product is best. The choice should be based on how well the iron preparation is absorbed and tolerated, as well as on its price. Because ferrous salts are more efficiently absorbed than ferric salts, an iron product of the ferrous group is usually appropriate. Ferrous sulfate is the standard against which other iron salts (eg, ferrous succinate, ferrous lactate, ferrous fumarate, ferrous glycine sulfate, ferrous glutamate, and ferrous gluconate) are compared. Ferrous citrate, ferrous tartrate, ferrous pyrophosphate, and some ferric salts are not well absorbed (see product table "Iron Products").

Ferrous salts may be given in combination with ascorbic acid. At a ratio of 200 mg of ascorbic acid to 30 mg of elemental iron, the increased amount of iron absorbed validates this practice. Other agents that may help increase absorption include sugars and amino acids. Chemicals that may decrease iron absorption include phosphates in eggs, phytates in cereals, carbonates, oxalates, and tannins.

Iron is available in numerous salt forms as tablets, capsules, liquids, and controlled-release products. It is also available in various strengths in combination products. The enteric-coated and delayed-release products are generally more expensive but may cause fewer symptoms of gastric irritation. Because progressively less iron is absorbed as it moves from the duodenum (the site of maximum absorption) to the ileum of the small intestine, overall iron absorption is decreased by delaying the time of release.

Adverse Effects/Drug Interactions

All iron products tend to irritate the GI mucosa and may produce nausea, abdominal pain, and diarrhea. These adverse effects may be minimized by reducing the dose or giving iron with meals. However, because food may decrease the amount of iron absorbed by as much as 50%, physicians may recommend iron with instructions for between-meal dosing. It is advantageous for absorption if the patient is able to tolerate iron taken in this manner. But if nausea or diarrhea is intolerable, it is usually better to take the iron with food or decrease the number of tablets taken per day than to stop taking iron supplements entirely.

A frequent side effect of iron therapy is constipation. This adverse effect has prompted the formulation of iron products that also contain a stool softener (eg, docusate).

During iron therapy, stools may become black and tarry, usually owing to unabsorbed iron. Black, tarry stools may also indicate GI blood loss and a serious GI problem. Medical referral is indicated if an underlying GI condition is suspected or if there is a history of GI disease. If the stool does not darken somewhat during iron therapy, however, the iron product may not have disintegrated properly or released the iron.

Accidental poisoning with iron occurs most often in children, who are attracted to the sugar-coated, colored tablets. It can also occur from overingestion of chewable multivitamins containing iron. Such poisoning is considered a medical emergency. As few as fifteen 325-mg ferrous sulfate tablets have been lethal to children; however, recovery has followed the ingestion of as many as 70 such tablets. The clinical outcome depends on the speed and adequacy of treatment.

Toxic ingestion of iron may be life-threatening and should be referred to a poison control center or emergency medical facility immediately. Symptoms of acute iron poisoning include pain, vomiting, diarrhea, electrolyte imbalances, and shock. In later stages, cardiovascular collapse may occur, especially if the cause has not been properly recognized and treated as a medical emergency. Treatment of iron toxicity may begin immediately at home by giving ipecac syrup to induce vomiting. (See Chapter 16, "Emetic and Antiemetic Products.")

A more insidious toxicity may occur during prolonged therapy with iron. In the treatment of refractory anemia, oral iron may be excessively absorbed, leading to iron overload. Certain alcoholic patients may also become overloaded with iron because wine contains iron and alcohol increases ferric iron absorption. Patients with chronic liver or pancreatic disease absorb more iron than normal from the gut. Iron overload also may occur if individuals who do not require long-term iron supplementation take iron for prolonged periods. The pharmacist should discourage the chronic use of iron supplements if no clinical evidence indicates its need.

Iron is chelated by many substances. Its interaction with antacids may be clinically significant. The mechanism of this interaction is probably related to the relative alkalinization of the stomach contents by an antacid. The chelate of iron with an antacid is more insoluble in the alkaline medium. Iron appears to chelate with several of the tetracyclines, resulting in decreased tetracycline and iron absorption. If simultaneous administration of an iron salt and a tetracycline is medically necessary, patients should take tetracycline 3 hours after or 2 hours before iron administration. Further, allopurinol should not be given with iron unless recommended by a physician.

Magnesium

Magnesium, which is essential for all living cells, is the second most plentiful cation of the intracellular fluids and the fourth most abundant cation in the body. About 2,000 mEq of magnesium are present in an average 70-kg adult, with about 50% of this in bone, about 45% as an intracellular cation, and 1–5% in the extracellular fluid. Magnesium is required for normal bone structure formation and the proper functioning of more than 300 enzymes, including those involved with adenosine triphosphatase-dependent phosphorylation, protein synthesis, and carbohydrate metabolism. Extracellular magnesium is critical to both the maintenance of nerve and muscle electrical potentials and the transmission of impulses across neuromuscular junctions.

Magnesium tends to mimic calcium in its effects on the CNS and skeletal muscle. Magnesium deficiency blunts the normal response of the parathyroid glands to hypocalcemia. Thus, tetany due to a lack of calcium cannot be corrected with calcium unless the magnesium deficiency is also corrected.

Individuals consuming natural diets should not develop magnesium deficiency because all unprocessed foods contain magnesium, albeit in widely varying amounts. Vegetables are a good source of magnesium; whole seeds such as nuts, legumes, and unmilled grains contain the highest concentrations. Processing, which leads to removal of the germ and outer layers of cereal grains, results in a loss of more than 80% of the magnesium.

Indications

Deficiency states are usually due to GI tract abnormalities, renal dysfunction, general malnutrition, alcoholism, and iatrogenic causes. Additionally, hypomagnesemia may result from diarrhea and steatorrhea, prolonged total parenteral nutrition therapy with magnesium-free solutions, hemodialysis, diabetes mellitus, pancreatitis, diuretic-induced electrolyte imbalance, and primary aldosteronism. Hypomagnesemia may also be associated with hypokalemia and hypocalcemia.

Magnesium deficiencies are rarely noted in the normal adult population because magnesium is present in most foods. Deficiencies have been observed, however, in individuals with alcoholism, diabetes, chronic diarrhea, and renal tubular damage and in patients receiving long-term intravenous feedings without magnesium supplementation. Magnesium deficiency causes apathy, depression, increased CNS stimulation, delirium, and convulsions. Symptoms of hypomagnesemia may include nausea, muscle weakness, irritability, behavioral changes, and myographic changes.

Hypermagnesemia is characterized by muscle weakness, CNS depression, diarrhea, hypotension, and confusion. Excess magnesium intake may also decrease bone decalcification. Because excess magnesium has a direct, depressive effect on skeletal muscle, intravenous magnesium sulfate has been used to prevent the seizures of eclampsia. However, hypermagnesemia can occur with overzealous use of magnesium sulfate (epsom salts) or magnesium hydroxide (milk of magnesia) as a laxative, or even with use of magnesium-containing antacids in patients with severe renal failure.

Dose/RDA

The RDA values of magnesium for men and women over 18 years of age are 350 mg per day and 280 mg per day, respectively. Magnesium is available in numerous strengths and salt forms as tablets, capsules, and liquids and in various combination products.

Adverse Effects/Drug Interactions

No evidence is available to suggest that oral intake of magnesium is harmful to individuals with normal renal function. Hypermagnesemia, if it should occur, may be accompanied by nausea, vomiting, hypotension, bradycardia, cutaneous vasodilatation, electrocardiographic changes, hyperreflexia, and CNS depression. Eventually, respiratory depression, coma, and cardiac arrest may occur. Diarrhea may occur with the oral supplements.

Phosphorus

Phosphorus is present throughout the body. Approximately 85% of the body's store is located in bone. About 1% of body weight, or one fourth of the total mineral content in the body, is phosphorus. Normal plasma levels of inorganic phosphate range between 2.5 and 4.4 mg/dL.

Phosphorus is essential for many metabolic processes. As calcium phosphate, it serves as an integral structural component of the bone matrix and a functional component of phospholipids, carbohydrates, nucleoproteins, and high-energy nucleotides. Accordingly, plasma phosphate levels are under tight biologic control involving parathyroid hormone, calcitonin, and vitamin D. The DNA and RNA structures contain sugar-phosphate linkages. Cell membranes contain phospholipids, which regulate the transport of solutes into and out of the cell. Many metabolic processes depend on phosphorylation. The storage and controlled release of energy—the adenosine diphosphate–adenosine triphosphate system—involves phosphorus compounds. And an important buffer system of the body consists of inorganic phosphates.

There is a reciprocal relationship between calcium and phosphorus. Both minerals are regulated partially by parathyroid hormone. Secretion of parathyroid hormone stimulates an increase in calcium levels through increased bone resorption, gut absorption, and reabsorption in renal tubules. Parathyroid hormone causes a decrease in the resorption of phosphate by the kidney. Thus, when serum calcium is high, serum phosphate is generally low, and vice versa.

Phosphorus is present in nearly all foods, especially protein-rich foods and cereal grains. Milk, meat, poultry, and fish contain about half the dietary phosphorus in the US diet. Other rich sources include seeds, nuts, and eggs.

Indications

Because nearly all foods contain phosphorus, deficiency states do not usually occur unless induced. For example, patients receiving aluminum hydroxide as an antacid for prolonged periods may exhibit weakness, anorexia, malaise, pain, and bone loss. This is because aluminum hydroxide binds phosphorus, making it unavailable for absorption because of the formation of insoluble and poorly absorbed complexes.

In patients with diabetic ketoacidosis, phosphorus deficiency may result from increased tissue catabolism, impaired glucose use and cellular phosphorus uptake, and increased renal excretion of phosphorus caused by metabolic acidosis. The opposite situation, hyperphosphatemia (along with hypocalcemia and hypermagnesemia), may occur with acute renal failure, as renal phosphorus elimination is decreased in the face of continued release of phosphorus from tissues.

Dose/RDA

The RDA for phosphorus is 800 mg for adults over the age of 24, 1,200 mg for those aged 11–24, 800 mg for children aged 1–10, and 1,200 mg for women during pregnancy and lactation. In addition to being used to alleviate the deficiency state, phosphates have been used to increase tissue calcium uptake in osteomalacia and to decrease serum calcium levels in hypercalcemia. Sodium and potassium phosphate salts are available without a prescription for those requiring supplements. Products available include different salt forms and strengths of phosphorus in tablet, capsule, powder, and liquid dose forms, as well as in numerous combination products.

Adverse Effects/Drug Interactions

Side effects and drug interactions have not been commonly reported with phosphorus therapy.

Trace Elements

Trace elements, which are present in minute quantities in plant and animal tissue, are considered essential for numerous physiologic processes. "Ultratrace minerals" have been defined as those elements with an estimated dietary requirement of usually less than 1 mg per day; these include arsenic (E), boron (E), bromine (NE), cadmium (NE), chromium (E), fluorine (NE), lead (NE), lithium (PE), molybdenum (E), nickel (E), selenium (E), silicon (E), tin (NE), and vanadium (PE). The designation "E" represents essential, "PE" means probably essential but further study is required, and "NE" means not essential because the evidence for essentiality is inadequate. Based on the amount of trace elements in the average diet, a range of intake values for those elements thought to be safe and adequate has been published by the Food and Nutrition Board (Table 2) (see product table "Miscellaneous Mineral Products").

Chromium

About 5 mg of chromium is present in the normal adult, and levels decline with age. Higher concentrations occur in the hair, spleen, kidney, and testes; lesser concentrations are present in the heart, pancreas, lungs, and brain.

Chromium functions to maintain normal glucose use. Chromium is a component of glucose tolerance factor, a dietary organic chromium complex that appears to facilitate the glucose usage that is apparently essential for the efficient use of insulin. Fatty acid stimulation and cholesterol synthesis are attributed to chromium, as is the possible role of RNA in protein synthesis.

Significant amounts of chromium are present in liver, fish, whole grains, and milk. There is concern that the increasing consumption of refined foods may lead to a marginal chromium deficiency in the population.

Chromium combined with picolinic acid, a metabolite of tryptophan, forms chromium picolinate, a form of chromium with enhanced bioavailability. Chromium picolinate, in doses of 200 mcg per day, has recently been promoted for lowering cholesterol, producing weight loss, and increasing muscle mass, and as an aid in controlling diabetes. These promotions are based on limited uncontrolled studies and anecdotal reports in the literature, which also report some untoward effects. The above claims should be considered as preliminary and largely unsubstantiated via objective clinical trials.

Indications

Deficiency of trivalent chromium, the chemical form present in diets, is manifested by glucose intolerance, elevated circulating insulin, glycosuria, fasting hyperglycemia, elevated serum cholesterol and triglycerides, neuropathy, and encephalopathy. Impaired glucose tolerance may be a manifestation of chromium deficiency, especially in older persons and protein-calorie malnourished infants.

Low chromium concentrations have been associated with juvenile diabetes and coronary artery disease. However, evaluation of chromium-deficient patients is difficult because of problems associated with total chromium analysis.

Dose/RDA

Chromium intake in the United States is low (about 50 mcg per day) compared with that of other countries. The estimated safe and adequate dietary intake for adults has been set at 50–200 mcg per day. Chromium has a relatively high margin of safety and is available in 1-mg tablets.

Adverse Effects/Drug Interactions

Oral administration of trivalent chromium has not been reported to be toxic. However, the hexavalent forms of chromium can be toxic and carcinogenic. These forms, which are encountered through industrial exposure, may enter the body through inhalation or cutaneous absorption.

Cobalt

Cobalt is an essential component of vitamin B_{12}, but ingested cyanocobalamin is metabolized in vivo to form the B_{12} coenzymes. No deficiency state is reported to exist in humans. No RDA exists for cobalt.

Large doses of cobalt may result in goiter, myxedema, and congestive heart failure. Cardiomyopathy has also been described. Cyanosis and coma may result from accidental ingestion by children.

Copper

Copper ions exist in two states, the cuprous and the cupric (a potent oxidizing agent). Copper is similar to zinc in the complexes it forms with a number of the same chelating agents. Copper is found in virtually all tissues of the body, but concentrations are highest in the liver, brain, heart, and kidney.

Copper is essential for the proper structure and function of the CNS, and it plays a major role in iron metabolism. Ceruloplasmin, one of the copper metalloenzymes, is especially important in the conversion of absorbed ferrous iron to transported ferric iron. Other copper-containing enzymes are cytochrome oxidase, dopamine beta-hydroxylase, and superoxide dismutase.

Food sources for copper include organ meats (especially liver), shellfish, chocolate, whole-grain cereals, legumes, and nuts.

Indications

Copper deficiency is uncommon in humans even though many individuals may have lower than recommended intake. Contemporary diets provide about 0.9 mg per day for women and 1.2 mg per day for men, which is somewhat less than the estimated safe and adequate range of 1.5–3.0 mg per day. Deficiencies have been observed in premature infants; in severely malnourished infants fed milk-based, low-copper diets; and in patients receiving parenteral nutrition with inadequate copper.

One of the prominent features of copper deficiency is impaired iron absorption. This is most likely caused by the loss of activity of the copper metalloenzymes, ferroxidase and ceruloplasmin (a protein-copper complex), which results in hypochromic anemia. In copper-deficient animals, bone cortices are fragile and thin owing to the failure of collagen cross-linking. Spontaneous rupture of major vessels may also be observed in deficiency states.

Wilson's disease is an inborn error of metabolism resulting in failure to eliminate copper. The result is CNS, kidney, and liver damage. Acute symptoms of copper toxicity include nausea, vomiting, diarrhea, hemolysis, convulsions, and GI bleeding. Symptoms respond to treatment with penicillamine.

Dose/RDA

Adults can safely take 2–3 mg of copper per day; 0.7–2.5 mg per day is suggested for children. Copper is available in different salt forms.

Adverse Effects/Drug Interactions

Copper administered orally has an emetic action, with doses in excess of 250 mg of copper sulfate producing vomiting. However, copper salts should not be used for this purpose. Molybdenum, zinc, and cadmium are antagonistic to copper, and large amounts of ascorbic acid impair copper absorption. Oral contraceptives have been shown to increase serum copper at the expense of tissue levels.

Fluorine

Available therapeutic forms of fluorine include sodium fluoride and acidulated phosphate fluoride, both of which are available for oral and topical administration; sodium monofluorophosphate; and stannous fluoride. Sodium fluoride contains about 45% fluoride ion, and stannous fluoride contains about 24% fluoride ion.

Fluoride occurs normally in bones and tooth enamel as a calcium salt. Intake of small amounts has been shown to markedly reduce tooth decay, presumably by making the enamel more resistant to the erosive action of acids produced by bacteria in the oral cavity. Fluoride has also been used in women with osteoporosis at a dose of 50 mg per day. However, this treatment may have adverse effects, so the patient must be carefully monitored.

Fluoride is present in soil and water, but the content varies widely from region to region. Most municipal water supplies are fluoridated to 1 ppm of fluoride, a level that has been shown to be safe and to reduce caries in children by about 50%.

Indications

Fluoride deficiency states in humans, other than potential decay, have not been described.

Dose/RDA

The safe and adequate estimated range for children is 0.5–2.5 mg per day and for adults, 1.5–4.0 mg per day. Fluoride is a normal constituent of the diet, given that it occurs in soils, water supplies, plants, and animals. Fluoride supplements should be routinely administered to children who consume water that is low in fluoride ion, such as well water. Sodium fluoride is available by prescription as oral tablets and solutions, topical solutions, and gels, as well as in combination products. Nonprescription products include topical rinses containing 0.01–0.02% fluoride, such as sodium fluoride.

Adverse Effects/Drug Interactions

Excess fluoride can be toxic. Acute toxicity should not result from the low levels present in drinking water but may result from the administration of excessive doses of fluoride supplements. It has been recommended that sodium fluoride tablets used as dietary supplements be dispensed in containers containing less than 264 mg of sodium fluoride (120 mg of fluoride ion). In unit-dose containers, the limit of 300 mg per package is acceptable.

Because acute toxicity affects the GI system and the CNS, it can be life-threatening. Symptoms include salivation, abdominal pain, nausea, vomiting, diarrhea, dehydration, thirst, urticaria, muscle weakness, tremors, and (rarely) seizures. Because of the calcium-binding effect of fluoride, symptoms of calcium deficiency, including tetany, may be seen. The patient may exhibit mental irritability. Eventually, respiratory and cardiac failure may occur. The dose that causes acute toxicity in adults is approximately 5 g. Death has occurred after ingestion of as little as 2 g in adults, but much larger overdoses have been treated successfully. In children, as little as 0.5 g of sodium fluoride may be fatal. Treatment includes precipitation of the fluoride by using gastric lavage with 0.15% calcium hydroxide solution, administration of intravenous glucose and saline for hydration, and treatment with calcium to prevent tetany.

Chronic fluoride toxicity is manifest as changes in the structure of bones and teeth. Bones become more dense and may be afflicted with disabling disease. Tooth enamel acquires a mottled appearance consisting of white, patchy plaques occurring with pitting brown stains. Prolonged ingestion of water that contains more than 2 ppm of fluoride has resulted in a significant incidence of mottling. Extremely large doses (eg, 20–80 mg per day) have resulted in chalky, brittle bones that tend to fracture easily, a condition known as skeletal fluorosis.

Iodine

The thyroid gland contains about one third of the iodine in the body, stored in the form of a complex glycoprotein, thyroglobulin. The only known function of thyroglobulin is to provide thyroxine and triiodothyronine. These hormones regulate the metabolic rate of cells and therefore influence physical and mental growth, nervous and muscle tissue function, circulatory activity, and the use of nutrients.

Iodine is required to synthesize thyroxine and triiodothyronine and is an essential micronutrient. Although in high concentrations iodine inhibits the release of these hormones, in its absence thyroid hypertrophy occurs, resulting in goiter. However, since iodine is usually present as the iodide in food and water and is sometimes organically bound to amino acids, the consumption of foods from diverse sources and the addition of iodide to table salt have essentially eliminated goiter as a health problem in the United States.

The primary dietary source of iodine is iodized salt, which contains 1 part of sodium or potassium iodide per 10,000 parts (0.01%) of salt. A dose of about 95 mcg of iodine can be obtained from about one fourth of a teaspoon of salt (1.25 g). In the United States, most of the table salt sold is iodized; however, that used in food processing and for institutional use is not. Additional dietary sources of iodine include saltwater fish and shellfish. Seacoast soils produce vegetables with higher iodide content because plants extract iodine from the soil.

Indications

As previously stated, deficiency of iodine can result in goiter.

Dose/RDA

The iodine content of typical diets in the United States has been slowly declining but is still well above the RDA value of 0.15 mg for adults. Iodine supplements are unwarranted for most individuals. Potassium iodide is available as a tablet and solution and is included in various combination products.

Adverse Effects/Drug Interactions

Some individuals are sensitive to iodide or to organic preparations containing iodine. Symptoms of chronic iodide intoxication (iodism) include an unpleasant taste and burning in the mouth or throat, along with soreness of the teeth or gums. Increased salivation, sneezing, irritation of the eyes, and swelling of the eyelids commonly occur.

Manganese

Manganese is required for glucose utilization, synthesis of the mucopolysaccharides of cartilage, biosynthesis of steroids, and the biologic activity of pyruvate carboxylase. Manganese can apparently substitute for magnesium in selected enzymes involved in oxidative phosphorylation.

Manganese is widely available in the diet in vegetables and fruits. Nuts, legumes, and whole-grain cereals are particularly good sources.

Indications

In animals, poor reproductive performance, growth retardation, congenital malformations, abnormal bone and cartilage formation, and impaired glucose tolerance are related to manganese deficiency. Only one case has been reported of human manganese deficiency; symptoms involved the hair and nails, nausea/vomiting, decreased serum phospholipids and triglycerides, and moderate weight loss.

Dose/RDA

Even though manganese is poorly absorbed after oral administration (3%), sufficient quantities are present in the average diet to maintain appropriate levels. A dose or dietary intake of 2–5 mg per day is considered safe and adequate. Manganese is available as different salt forms, primarily as 20- and 50-mg tablets and in various combination products.

Adverse Effects/Drug Interactions

Toxicity is rare for orally administered manganese. It has been observed, however, from inhalation of dust and industrial fumes containing manganese.

There is a possible antagonistic effect between manganese and iron, resulting in less iron absorption. Also, low iron levels may result in enhanced manganese absorption and possible toxicity.

Molybdenum

Molybdenum can readily change its oxidation state and act as an electron transfer agent in oxidation-reduction reactions. It may also function as an enzyme cofactor.

The molybdenum content of food varies, depending on the growth environment. Milk, organ meats, beans, breads, and cereals appear to contribute the most dietary molybdenum.

Indications

Molybdenum is a cofactor for several flavoprotein enzymes and is found in xanthine oxidase. Because xanthine oxidase is involved in the oxidation of xanthine to uric acid, high molybdenum intake has been associated with goutlike symptoms. Parenteral nutrition without molybdenum has resulted in an acquired molybdenum deficiency, which has been treated with ammonium molybdate.

Dose/RDA

It appears that the human molybdenum requirement is low (about 75–250 mcg per day for adults) and is easily furnished by the average diet. A safe and adequate daily dietary intake of 150–500 mcg has been estimated.

Adverse Effects/Drug Interactions

Molybdenum is relatively nontoxic. When consumed in excess, however, it may be antagonistic to copper, resulting in symptoms of copper deficiency.

Nickel

Divalent and trivalent forms of nickel are important in biologic systems. The absorption of nickel may be related to iron, but only a very low percentage is absorbed, most of it being lost in the feces. Nickel is found in highest concentrations in chocolate, nuts, dried beans, peas, and grains.

It has been speculated that nickel is involved in specific metalloenzymes, but its actual activity has not been clearly delineated even though it is essential. Symptoms of a deficiency state have not been documented in humans.

Selenium

Selenium is present in all tissues. Many selenium compounds are analogous to sulfur compounds. Glutathione peroxidase, a selenoenzyme, is important in the destruction of inflammatory hydroperoxides.

Selenium is generally incorporated into organic compounds involving amino acids such as methionine or cysteine. Selenium compounds are about 80% absorbed. The highest concentrations are found in the kidneys and liver; the lowest are in the lungs and brain. The kidney is the primary route of excretion.

Dietary sources of selenium include meat, seafoods, and some cereal grains. Vegetables and fruits contain little of this element. The selenium content of foods depends on the soils in which the plants are grown.

Indications

Selenium is an essential trace element in humans, but deficiencies are not common in the general population. Selenium deficiency has been reported in patients with alcoholic cirrhosis, probably owing to an insufficient diet or the altered metabolism of selenium. It has been rarely reported in patients on long-term parenteral nutrition.

Limited evidence in humans suggests that deficiency results in cardiomyopathy, muscle pain, and abnormal nail beds. Epidemiologic studies suggest that cancer and heart disease may be common in areas of low selenium availability. Keshan disease (a disorder characterized by abnormalities of the myocardium) has been shown to respond to selenium.

Dose/RDA

The RDA for selenium has been set at 70 mcg for adult men and 50–55 mcg for adult women. Selenium is included in some multivitamin and mineral preparations. It is available as 50-mcg tablets and in various strengths in combination products. Doses in excess of 0.2 mg per day are not recommended.

Adverse Effects/Drug Interactions

Toxic effects reported include loss of hair and nails, skin lesions, and CNS and teeth involvement. Selenium toxicity may be evidenced by growth retardation, muscular weakness, infertility, focal hepatic necrosis, dysphagia, dysphonia, bronchopneumonia, and respiratory failure.

Silicon

Little is known about the absorption, distribution, metabolism, and excretion of silicon. It apparently functions in the development and maintenance of connective tissue, and it is required for collagen biosynthesis and for the mineralization process in bone calcification.

Silicon is obtained in diets that consist of primarily foods of plant origin, especially cereal products, root vegetables, and unrefined grains of high fiber content. The role of silicon in human nutrition, if any, is unknown at present.

Indications

Silicon deficiency states in humans have not been described.

Dose/RDA

The daily requirement of silicon has not been established, and the best product form for silicon administration has not been determined.

Adverse Effects/Drug Interactions

When taken orally, silicon is essentially nontoxic. This is evidenced by the administration of silicon-containing magnesium trisilicate, a nonprescription antacid that has been available for more than 40 years without apparent toxic effects, and the ingestion of simethicone, a common antigas ingredient in many nonprescription antacids. The absorption and metabolism of silicon may be altered by fiber, molybdenum, magnesium, and fluoride.

Tin

Tin may be involved in growth and reproductive functions, but evidence of its necessity is lacking. A deficiency state for tin has not been described in humans. Adequate quantities of tin are apparently obtained from the diet.

Vanadium

The most important forms of vanadium in biologic systems are the tetravalent and pentavalent states. The tetravalent form easily complexes with other substances such as transferrin or hemoglobin to stabilize it against oxidation. Vanadium may be involved in functions related to growth and reproduction; however, the evidence of its necessity is not well established.

Vanadium is presumed essential, but a deficiency state has not been confirmed. It is obtained in sufficient quantities in the diet. Shellfish, mushrooms, parsley, and some spices (eg, dill seed and black pepper) are rich in vanadium.

Toxicity can occur through excessive dietary intake. Symptoms include diarrhea, anorexia, depressed growth, and neurotoxicity. Vanadium toxicity may be diminished by administration of ascorbic acid, ethylenediaminetetraacetic acid (EDTA), chromium, protein, ferrous iron, chloride, and possibly aluminum hydroxide.

Zinc

Zinc is an integral part of at least 70 metalloenzymes, including carbonic anhydrase, lactic dehydrogenase, alkaline phosphatase, carboxypeptidase, aminopeptidase, and alcohol dehydrogenase. It is also a cofactor in the synthesis of DNA and RNA, and it is involved in the mobilization of vitamin A from the liver and in the enhancement of follicle-stimulating hormone and luteinizing hormone. It is essential for normal cellular immune functions and for spermatogenesis and normal testicular function, and it is important in the stabilization of membrane structure.

The divalent ion is most commonly found and used in the body. Zinc has a relatively rapid turnover rate, and the body pool appears to be about 2–3 g. Zinc is efficiently regulated in the body.

Most dietary zinc (about 70%) is derived from animal products. Good sources of zinc include oysters; liver; high-protein foods such as beef, lamb, pork, legumes, and peanuts; and whole-grain cereals.

Indications

Although zinc deficiencies are not widespread in the United States, marginally low zinc values have been associated with growth retardation in children, slow wound healing in adults, birth defects, and problems in childbirth. Additional symptoms include loss of appetite, skin changes, and immunologic abnormalities, and may also include delayed sexual maturation, hypogonadism and hypospermia, alopecia, behavioral disturbances, night blindness, and impaired taste and smell.

Malabsorption syndromes, infection, myocardial infarct, major surgery, alcoholism, liver cirrhosis, pregnancy, lactation, and high-fiber diets rich in phytate predispose an individual to a suboptimal zinc status. Zinc depletion is relatively rare but may be seen in patients on long-term parenteral nutrition and patients with GI tract abnormalities such as fistulas and high-output diarrhea.

Zinc deficiencies adversely affect DNA, RNA, carbohydrate, and protein metabolism. Iron supplements decrease zinc absorption just as zinc supplements decrease iron absorption, probably owing to competition for the same transport system. If these minerals are taken with a meal, the adverse interaction is less pronounced. Vegetarian diets, despite their high fiber content, do not result in low plasma zinc levels. In patients with impaired wound healing, zinc supplementation may be marginally beneficial.

Dose/RDA

The RDA for zinc is 15 mg and 12 mg for adult men and women, respectively. The RDA for infants is 5 mg and for children, 10 mg. Typical Western diets supply 10–15 mg of zinc per day. Because zinc is only 10–40% absorbed from the GI tract, ingestion of the 220-mg dose form of zinc sulfate (50 mg of elemental zinc) will supply 5–20 mg of zinc. Treatment of suspected deficiencies usually involves administration of 150 mg of elemental zinc in three divided doses daily. At these dosages, copper deficiency may be induced, so it has been suggested that the zinc dosage be limited to 40 mg per day if therapy with zinc is going to be chronic.

If parenteral nutrition is continued longer than 3–5 days, zinc should be added to the regimen unless otherwise indicated. Patients with large GI losses via fistulas, ostomies, or stool require larger supplemental doses of zinc. Zinc is available in various salt forms as capsules, generally ranging in strength from 1.5 to 50 mg of elemental zinc, and in numerous combination products in various strengths. Chronic ingestion of more than 15 mg per day is not recommended without adequate medical supervision.

Adverse Effects/Drug Interactions

Because the ingestion of 2 g or more of zinc sulfate has resulted in GI irritation and vomiting, zinc can be taken with food. However, dairy and bran products, as well as foods high in calcium, phosphorus, or phytate, may decrease absorption of zinc. Zinc is also toxic, although the emetic effect that occurs after consumption of large amounts may minimize problems with accidental overdose. Reported signs of zinc toxicity in humans include vomiting, dehydration, muscle incoordination, dizziness, and abdominal pain. Copper levels may be decreased by a high intake of zinc, and zinc may decrease tetracycline absorption.

Nutritional Supplements

Supplemental nutritional products should be used as adjuncts to a regular diet and not as substitutes for food. Often, persons who request a nutritional supplement have self-diagnosed their condition. However, although dietary supplements can be obtained without a prescription, they are complex agents with specific indications, and medical assessment should precede their use. The pharmacist should not be reluctant to consult a dietitian or physician concerning nutritional supplementation and should refer patients when necessary.

Patients purchasing a nonprescription dietary supplement should be instructed on its proper use and storage, including dilution and preparation techniques (see product table "Enteral Food Supplement Products"). In addition, the pharmacist should offer to discuss with the patient possible adverse effects such as diarrhea.

Enteral Nutrition

In addition to oral nutritional supplementation, enteral nutrition is being increasingly used for nutritional support in patients who cannot ingest or digest sufficient amounts of food. Advances in products specifically designed for enteral use and the availability of sophisticated formulas, small-bore nasogastric tubes, and constant-infusion delivery systems have lead to a resurgence of interest in enteral nutrition. The increase may also be attributed to the aging population and government cost-containment programs.

Enteral nutrition is defined as the provision of liquid nutrients by tube or by mouth into the GI tract. It is the desired method of feeding patients whose ability to ingest adequate nutrients by mouth is functionally impaired but who have a functional GI tract. The popularity of this mode of feeding has increased significantly in recent years in the hospital, home, and long-term care settings. Its advantages over parenteral feeding include preservation of the structure and function of the GI tract, more efficient use of nutrients, decreased incidence of infections and metabolic complications, and decreased cost. Enteral foods are not diet foods or health food supplements and are not intended for that purpose.

Currently, enteral feeding devices (tubes) are divided into two major categories: those entering the GI tract through the nose (nasogastric or nasoenteral tubes) and those entering through the abdominal wall (gastrostomies, duodenostomies, or jejunostomies). Most tubes are made of either silicone or polyurethane. The nasogastric and nasoenteral tubes are between 30 and 43 in. in length, with diameters from 5 to 16 French. The longer tubes are for nasoduodenal or nasojejunal feeding. The small diameter of these tubes often results in clogging, especially when medications are added to enteral liquids and administered through the tubes. Gastrostomy and jejunostomy tubes are of a larger diameter (16 to 24 French) and do not tend to clog. These tubes also allow quicker and easier administration of medications and feeding preparations. The newer percutaneous endoscopic gastrostomy tubes are increasingly popular because they are easier to place in patients, even on an outpatient basis.

Classification of Enteral Nutrition Products

There are currently more than 100 commercial preparations available for enteral feeding. Some are designed for general nutrition; others are designed for specific metabolic or clinical conditions. In addition to the various vitamins and minerals previously discussed in this chapter, the bulk volume/weight of these supplements consists primarily of proteins, carbohydrates, and lipids (fats, oils). The reader is referred to Chapter 20, "Infant Formula Products," for detailed information on infant nutrition.

Preparations for enteral feeding may be classified according to clinical indications or to composition of the products.

Clinical Indications Method

Using the clinical indications method, enteral feeding products are classified as natural foods, polymeric solutions, monomeric solutions, solutions for specific metabolic needs, modular solutions, and hydration solutions.

Natural foods include blenderized foods either commercially available or prepared at home. Polymeric solutions contain macronutrients in the form of proteins, triglycerides, and carbohydrate polymers. The protein is obtained from casein, lactalbumin, whey, egg white, or a combination of these; the carbohydrate, from glucose polymers such as starch or its hydrolysates; and the fats, from vegetable sources such as corn oil, safflower oil, sunflower oil, or others. Monomeric solutions require less digestion as they contain protein in the form of peptides and/or free amino acids derived from the hydrolysis of casein, whey, and other proteins; carbohydrates are in the form of partially hydrolyzed starch (maltodextrins and glucose oligosaccharides), and the fat is often a mixture of medium and long-chain triglycerides. Monomeric solutions are lactose free and do not contain fiber. Solutions for specific metabolic needs include branched-chain amino acid solutions, essential amino acid solutions, high-fat/low carbohydrate solutions, and immune-modulating solutions. Modular solutions are designed to provide macro- or micronutrients singly or in combination for specialized formulas for both oral and enteral feedings. Hydration solutions are designed primarily to provide fluid and minerals for therapeutic purposes or to prevent dehydration.

Specialty formulations include puddings (Sustacal Pudding), predigested/hydrolyzed formulas (Criticare HN), low-carbohydrate formulas (Pulmocare), high-carbohydrate polymers (Exceed), low-protein formulas (Amin-Aid), isotonic formulas (Osmolite), clear liquid formulas (Citrotein), nutrient-dense products, and modular products (Moducal).

Product Composition Method

Enteral preparations classified according to composition are either supplemental or complete, with general and specialized applications. Supplemental protein-calorie formula products are to be used only as adjuncts to a regular diet because they are not nutritionally complete. Some products (Mull-Soy and Nutramigen) are milk free and can be used by individuals who have a milk allergy and lactose malabsorption. One product (Controlyte) with a low protein and electrolyte content may be appropriate for patients with acute or chronic renal failure.

Complete formulas can be used orally or as tube feedings, and may be used as sole dietary intake (if the patient's electrolytes are monitored) or as supplementation. These products may contain ingredients that make them appropriate for special needs. Several such products (Instant Breakfast, Sustacal, and Meritene) are milk based; others (Compleat-B and Gerber Meat Base Formula) have a mixed-food base. Another type supplies protein in the form of crystalline amino acids or protein hydrolysate, carbohydrate in the form of oligosaccharides or disaccharides, and vitamins and minerals in the form of individual chemicals. These last products are chemically defined diets, also known as "elemental diets"; examples include Vivonex and Jejunal. Some other complete products (Precision LR and Portagen) are only partly chemically defined.

Nearly all elemental diets have low-fat content and contain electrolytes, minerals, trace elements, and water- and fat-soluble vitamins. All chemically based products require little or no digestion, are absorbed over a short distance in the small intestine, and have low residue. These attributes mean that the number and volume of the stools are reduced, making these products appropriate for patients who had ileostomies or colostomies and who wish to decrease fecal output. The low-residue products may also facilitate the care of elderly patients with stool incontinence or patients with brain damage from strokes, congenital defects, or retardation. Because of the ease of absorption and the low fecal residues, these products are often used in postoperative care, in treating GI disease, and in treating neoplastic disease, in which tissue breakdown is extensive.

Administration and Monitoring Guidelines

Supplemental and complete formulas are available in several forms, including powders that must be diluted with water or milk, liquids that must also be diluted, and liquids and puddings that are ready to use. The extent of dilution is based on the amount of nutrients needed and the amount that can be tolerated. Adults will not generally tolerate preparations of more than 25% weight per volume (wt/vol), which generally delivers 1.0 cal/mL. The maximum concentration for infants is 12% wt/vol, which generally delivers 0.5 cal/mL. Infants should generally be started on a concentration of 7–7.5% wt/vol, increasing to 12% over 4–5 days as tolerated. For children over 10 months of age, 15% wt/vol formulas may be initiated, with gradual increases to 25%. Higher concentrations may cause osmotic diarrhea.

If the preparations are taken orally, 100–150 mL should be ingested at one time. Over the course of a day, 2,000 mL of most preparations provide about 2,000 calories. If the patient is tube fed, 40–60 mL of the product per hour may be given initially. Once opened, the container should be kept cold to prevent bacterial growth, and all prepared products remaining after 24 hours should be discarded. Tubing should be rinsed three times a day with water. If diarrhea, nausea, or distention occur, the diet should be withheld for 24 hours and then gradually resumed. For elderly or unconscious persons or for patients who recently had surgery, elevating the head of the bed is advisable during administration to avoid aspiration.

Pharmacists should store supplemental formula products at temperatures under 75°F (23.8°C). Expiration dates should be checked before dispensing.

Patients must be monitored for biochemical abnormalities, electrolyte values, and adequate nutrition and hydration. Urine and blood glucose concentrations can be monitored. Persons with diabetes may require increased insulin doses. Edema may be precipitated or aggravated in patients with protein-calorie malnutrition or cardiac, renal, or hepatic disease because of the relatively high sodium content of the elemental diets. Some commercially available nutritional products (eg, Ensure and Ensure Plus) are a source of vitamin K supplementation, which may interfere with oral anticoagulant therapy. Tube feedings have been shown to interfere with the absorption of phenytoin administered via the tube. This interaction can be avoided by flushing the tube with saline (or water) before and after phenytoin and waiting 15 minutes both before and after the dose is given.

Selected information useful in educating and counseling patients is included in Table 6.

Case Studies

Case 19–1

Patient Complaint/History

JY is the 15-year-old son of a migrant farm family in south Texas. He comes to the pharmacy today seeking help in relieving the recurrence of fatigue; he first experienced the fatigue last summer. At that time he had a busy schedule, working all day and spending time with friends in the evening. His diet consisted mainly of tortillas, pinto beans, rice, and, when available, onions, garlic, and tomatoes. His daily fluid intake included several soft drinks and fruit-flavored beverages; he rarely drank milk.

Subsequently, JY's mother took him to the Migrant Health Care Clinic. A physical examination revealed the following: the patient's height and weight were 5'10" and 135 lb; his temperature (98.8°F [37.1°C]), pulse rate (72 bpm), and blood pressure (115/80 mm Hg) were normal. Based on a hemoglobin level of 9.5 g/dL, the physician prescribed a slow-release iron product and a multivitamin tablet, each to be taken once daily. Over the next several weeks, JY slowly improved; however, about 6 months after the clinic visit, his mother could no longer afford the prescription iron medication and purchased 325-mg ferrous sulfate tablets instead. After JY began taking one ferrous sulfate tablet at bedtime, he developed stomach distress for which he began taking antacids. He continued to take the multivitamin and antacids but stopped taking the ferrous sulfate. He is now experiencing fatigue again.

Clinical Considerations/Strategies

The following considerations/strategies are provided to aid the reader in (1) determining whether treatment of the patient's condition with nonprescription medications is warranted, (2) selecting the appropriate nonprescription medication, and (3) developing a patient counseling strategy to ensure optimal therapeutic outcomes:

- Assess the appropriateness of the physician-prescribed slow-release iron therapy in treating the iron deficiency anemia.
- Assess the appropriateness of the mother replacing the slow-release iron medication with a regimen of ferrous sulfate 325 mg one tablet daily.
- Discuss the possible etiology of the recurrence of fatigue.

TABLE 6 Selected information useful in counseling patients about nutritional supplements

1. Labels on all vitamin or vitamin and mineral preparations should be read carefully before supplements are taken. The contents and the amounts of vitamins and minerals should be compared with those in the RDAs.
2. Doses of vitamins and minerals higher than the RDAs should be taken with caution. All vitamins and minerals have adverse effects that are dose related.
3. High doses of vitamins or minerals may be dangerous and should not be taken indiscriminately. It is best not to exceed the RDA. Label directions should be followed carefully.
4. Vitamins or vitamin and mineral supplements should be taken with meals if their use is associated with GI symptoms. Iron and other supplements may cause less stomach upset if taken with meals.
5. Patients should not self-medicate if they suspect a vitamin deficiency but should instead consult their physician or pharmacist.
6. For proper nutrition, foods from all the basic food groups (meats, fruits and vegetables, dairy products, and grains) should be eaten. Vitamin supplements are not a substitute for a well-balanced diet.
7. Liquid vitamin and mineral supplements may be mixed with food (fruit juice, milk, baby formula, or cereal).
8. Iron supplements or vitamins with iron may turn stool black. This occurrence is not a cause for alarm unless it is associated with other symptoms involving the GI tract.
9. Some vitamin supplements have a special coating and should be swallowed whole. The physician or pharmacist should inform a patient if this is the case.
10. Like any medicine, vitamin and combination vitamin and mineral supplements should be stored out of the reach of children, especially if the product contains iron.
11. Children's vitamins are not candy. Children should be taught that vitamins are drugs, should be respected as drugs and potential poisons, and cannot be taken indiscriminately.
12. Niacin-containing products may cause a flushing sensation, which should decrease in intensity with continued therapy.
13. Riboflavin-containing products may cause a yellow fluorescence in the urine.

- Propose an alternative therapeutic plan for the patient.
- Determine what information about the changes in the prescribed therapeutic regimen should be included in a phone conversation or letter to the patient's physician.
- Develop a patient education/counseling strategy that will:
  - Support/justify the changes in the prescribed therapeutic regimen;
  - Optimize the therapeutic regimen recommended by the pharmacist (ie, dose, time and frequency of administration, warnings/precautions, adverse effects, and drug interactions).

Case 19–2

Patient Complaint/History

JC, a 41-year-old business executive on the fast track, is a confident individual, who says he thrives on his work pressure and many community activities. The 5'11", 190-lb businessman enjoys playing baseball and basketball with his children; he also enjoys hunting and camping. He comes to the pharmacy today to ask about symptoms that occur about an hour after he takes niacin, ascorbic acid, and multivitamin supplements. He says that he becomes very flushed and red-faced; further, his face feels as though "it's on fire."

During his physical checkup performed 2 weeks earlier, JC's temperature (98.6°F [37.0°C]), pulse rate (72 bpm), and electrocardiogram were normal; his blood pressure was 140/90 mm Hg. Laboratory findings showed a hemoglobin level of 15 g/dL; a blood urea nitrogen (BUN) level of 10 mg/dL; a creatinine level of 1.2 mg/dL; a total cholesterol level of 300 mg/dL; a high-density lipoprotein (HDL) cholesterol level of 35 mg/dL; and a triglyceride level of 120 mg/dL.

The patient, who at that time was a heavy smoker and drank six cups of coffee a day, was diagnosed as having borderline hypertension and Type IIa hyperlipoproteinemia. He was advised to stop smoking, reduce his caffeine intake, and increase his participation in sports and outdoor activities. He was also advised to reduce his intake of saturated fat and cholesterol.

JC immediately began to read materials about his condition. After learning that niacin is used to help lower cholesterol levels, he decided to try it. He also decided that his increased participation in sports and outdoor activities warranted his taking a high-potency multivitamin. Last week he purchased 500-mg ascorbic acid tablets (labeled as meeting USP standards), high-potency multivitamin tablets, and long-acting 500-mg niacin tablets at a healthfood store. JC has been taking one tablet of each vitamin in the morning and evening. He now wonders whether his symptoms are related to his change in lifestyle or to the vitamins.

Clinical Considerations/Strategies

The following considerations/strategies are provided to aid the reader in (1) determining whether treatment of the patient's condition with nonprescription medications is warranted, (2) selecting the appropriate nonprescription medication, and (3) developing a patient counseling strategy to ensure optimal therapeutic outcomes:

- Assess the appropriateness of the multivitamin and ascorbic acid therapy.
- Assess the appropriateness of the niacin therapy.
- Discuss with the patient the possibility of seeking medical intervention in the management of his hyperlipoproteinemia.
- Propose alternative products that will meet the patient's actual versus perceived needs.
- Develop a patient education/counseling strategy that will support/justify changes in the patient-selected vitamin therapy.

Summary

Pharmacists can significantly contribute to improving the nutritional status of the population by becoming familiar with these basics of nutrition, observing patients, listening to their requests, and providing general nutritional counseling. Much misinformation is being disseminated, and pharmacists are in a position to dispel myths, downplay exaggerated claims, and provide objective facts on nutritional agents such as vitamins, minerals, and nutritional supplements.

References

1. Ehrlich FJ. Drugstores and nutrition: played right, a winning combination. *Drug Topics.* 1985 Feb; 129: 28–31.
2. Food and Nutrition Board, National Research Council. *Recommended Dietary Allowances.* 10th ed. Washington, DC: National Academy of Sciences; 1989.
3. Shils ME, Olson, JA, Shike M, eds. *Modern Nutrition in Health and Disease.* 8th ed. Philadelphia: Lea and Febiger; 1994.
4. Robinson CH et al. *Normal and Therapeutic Nutrition.* 17th ed. New York: Macmillan; 1990.
5. Goodman AG et al. *The Pharmacological Basis of Therapeutics.* 18th ed. New York: Pergamon Press; 1990.
6. *American Hospital Formulary Service 1992.* Bethesda, Md: American Society of Hospital Pharmacists; 1992.
7. *US Dispensing Information.* 12th ed. Bethesda, Md: US Pharmacopoeial Convention; 1992.
8. Billups NF, Billups SM. *American Drug Index.* 35th ed. St Louis, Mo: JB Lippincott; 1991.
9. Marcus R, Coulston AM. In: Goodman AG et al. *The Pharmacological Basis of Therapeutics.* 18th ed. New York: Pergamon Press; 1990: 1554.

CHAPTER 20

Infant Formula Products

Rosalie Sagraves, Claudia Kamper, and Judi Doerr

Questions to ask in patient assessment and counseling

- *What is your baby's age and weight?*
- *Is your baby under a physician's care?*
- *Are you breast-feeding your baby or is your baby receiving an infant formula?*
- *Is your baby receiving any solid foods, including cereal? If so, is the food fed by spoon or added to bottle feedings?*
- *Does your baby receive other liquids besides breast milk or an infant formula?*
- *Is your baby allergic or sensitive to milk? Does your baby have other dietary restrictions? Does your baby have any chronic health problems?*
- *Are you giving your baby a multivitamin product? Was it recommended by your baby's physician?*
- *Is your baby receiving fluoride supplementation?*
- *Does your baby have diarrhea, constipation, or vomiting?*
- *Does your baby have a fever, a loss of appetite, decreased tearing, decreased salivation, or fewer wet diapers?*
- *Do you understand how your baby's formula should be prepared?*

Breast-feeding is the desired method for feeding infants from birth to at least 4–6 months of age. This is because human milk provides a nutritional source that is physiologically sound and because breast-feeding tends to facilitate a close mother–child relationship.[1] Breast-feeding also decreases the incidence of infant allergy and illness. Women who breast-feed can decrease the amount of time they spend in nutrition preparation, lower the cost of feeding their infants, and decrease their postpartum recovery time.[2–4]

Because some women do not want to breast-feed or are unable to do so, commercially prepared infant formulas are a good alternative in industrially developed nations. Such formulas are less desirable in developing countries, however, where inadequate sanitation, lack of refrigeration, and the inability of illiterate mothers to follow formula preparation instructions increase the risk of infant morbidity and mortality.[4]

Infant Feeding Practice

Infant formulas have evolved to their present quality over the past century. Before the 20th century, most infants not suckled by mothers or wet nurses died during their first year of life. Substitute milk feedings were made possible by discoveries in biology and medicine in the late 19th century, and technical advances in the early 20th century decreased infant mortality and helped to popularize artificial milk feedings. Between 1930 and 1960, evaporated milk was the product used most often for infant formula preparation, but by 1978 fewer than 5% of formula-fed infants received evaporated milk formulas.[5]

In the 1970s, a greater acceptance of breast-feeding resulted in a change in infant feeding patterns in the United States. Between 1971 and 1982, the incidence of breast-feeding at the time of hospital discharge increased from 24.7% to 61.9% (the highest since 1955, when the recording of this information began), and the incidence at age 5–6 months increased from 5.5% to 28.8%.[6–8] However, in 1989 the incidence of breast-feeding at the time of hospital discharge declined to 52.2%, with the incidence at 5–6 months of age being only 18.1%. Declines in breast-feeding occurred in all groups surveyed but were more likely to occur among young African-American women who had less than a high school education; were enrolled in the Special Supplemental Food Program for Women, Infants, and Children (WIC) at the time surveyed; worked outside the home; lived in states other than western states; and had low-birthweight (LBW) infants.[9] It must be noted that many of the women enrolled in WIC at the time of the survey did not do so until after their infants were born. Therefore, these women did not benefit from breast-feeding information offered by the program, which may, in part, account for the lower number of breast-feeding WIC mothers.

The WIC program is intended to give infants a better nutritional start in life. WIC serves one third of all infants in the United States, providing either infant formula or supplemental food for breast-feeding mothers.[10] In 1989, 1.2 million infants were enrolled in the program, and each consumed approximately 28 cans of formula monthly. Some of the cost of the WIC infant feeding program is covered through manufacturers' rebates. Pharmacists can find out more about WIC from local health department employees.

Most women in the United States (77–97%) decide before or early in pregnancy whether they will breast-feed.[11] This decision does not appear to be associated with age but is associated with educational level, social class, race (the incidence being highest among Caucasians and lowest among African Americans), and parity (a higher incidence among first-time mothers).[11] Most women who decide to feed their infants formula do so because they reject breast-feeding even though most acknowledge that human milk is healthier than infant formula. Reasons for rejecting breast-feeding include embarrassment, pain or discomfort, decreased lifestyle freedom, and father's lack of involvement in the breast-feeding process.[11] Formula-feeding, on the other hand, is convenient. Women's attitudes are also influenced by their spouses or significant others, mothers, and friends.

If the goal of Healthy People 2000, proposed by the US Department of Health and Human Services in 1990, is to have 75% of infants breast-fed at birth with 50% receiving some breast milk at age 6 months,[12] women's attitudes about breast-feeding must change. Although education about feeding practices is important after the infant's birth, education of mothers and fathers both before and during early pregnancy is needed to accomplish this goal.[11]

Until that happens, advances in uniformity, convenience, nutritional quality, and safety have established infant formulas as an alternative method for feeding infants.[13] The composition of commercial infant formulas conforms with guidelines based on extensive assessments of infant nutritional needs. Variations among formulas allow for product selection that will meet a specific infant's nutritional requirements. However, these variations produce differences in palatability, digestibility, sources of nutrients, and convenience of administration. The pharmacist, in consultation with the infant's parents and physician, should be able to evaluate indications, advise on the selection of an infant formula, and help ensure its appropriate use.

The pharmacist's role in infant feeding is to be knowledgeable about infant nutritional requirements, commercially prepared infant formulas, differences in formula composition, and specific uses for therapeutic formulas. The pharmacist should also be able to help educate women about breast-feeding and refer women with questions about breast-feeding to organizations such as the La Leche League.

Infant Physiology and Growth

Physiology

The physiology of the infant's gastrointestinal (GI) and renal systems is crucial in infant nutrition. In early infancy, only liquid nutrition is appropriate until the infant can coordinate complex tongue movements and the infant's swallowing reflexes mature. Frequent feedings are necessary because the stomach capacity of a full-term infant (38–42 weeks' gestation and birthweight greater than 2,500 g) is only 20–90 mL at birth but increases rapidly to 90–150 mL by 1 month of age.[14]

Stomach acid and pepsin secretion peak in the newborn infant by day 10, decrease between days 10 and 30, and then gradually increase over the first year of life. A full-term infant can digest most carbohydrates because the intestinal enzymes lactase, sucrase, maltase, isomaltose, and glucoamylase are sufficiently mature at birth.[12] Sucrase, maltase, and isomaltose usually are fully active in preterm infants (gestational age <38 weeks), but lactase activity may be immature. Lactose intolerance is clinically uncommon in full-term infants because of postnatal adaptive responses to ingested carbohydrates. Lactase activity may decline in African-American and Asian children starting at toddler age.[15] Pancreatic amylase activity and glucose transport are low in both full-term and preterm infants at birth and may not fully develop until the child is several years old.[16] Glucose polymers (glucose molecules linked by alpha[1–4] bonds) are used in some formulas for premature infants and infants with special problems, including lactose intolerance. They offer lower osmolality and may be better absorbed than longer-chained carbohydrates.

Newborn infants exhibit low lipase concentrations and slow rates of bile salt synthesis, both of which are important determinants of efficient fat absorption from the small intestine.[16] Breast-fed infants have a compensatory mechanism, bile salt–stimulated lipase, that helps ensure adequate dietary fat intake.[17,18] Long-chain saturated fatty acids (butterfat) are not absorbed as well as unsaturated fatty acids (vegetable oils), but fat absorption improves as the infant matures.

Protein digestion does not differ appreciably between infants and adults, even though infants digest a smaller quantity on an hourly basis.[19] Amino acids produced by protein digestion are absorbed by active transport mechanisms that reach adult levels by 14 weeks of age.[14] Because infants can readily absorb antigenic proteins, they are at an increased risk for developing food allergies later in life.[16]

The renal solute load is composed of soluble waste products that must be eliminated by the kidneys. Such solutes include nitrogenous waste and excess electrolytes and minerals. These are also excreted through the skin (in sweat), lungs (in water vapor), and GI tract. The potential renal solute load (PRSL) is defined as the solute load that is derived from dietary ingestion that would be excreted renally if amino acids from protein digestion were not used for growth or eliminated by nonrenal routes.[20]

The following equation can be used to calculate PRSL for breast milk or various infant formulas:

$$\text{PRSL (mOsm)} = \text{grams of protein}/0.175 + \text{sodium} + \text{chloride} + \text{potassium} + \text{phosphorus},$$

where sodium, chloride, potassium, and phosphorus are expressed in millimoles per unit volume.[13] Renal solute load will be discussed in greater depth in the section Commercial Infant Formulas later in this chapter.

Growth

The human body exhibits standard growth and development patterns. Birthweight is determined primarily by maternal prepregnancy and pregnancy weight and weight changes. The average birthweight for a full-term infant is approximately 3,500 g (about 7½ lb); infants born prematurely may weigh less than 1,500 g (about 4¼ lb).[21]

After birth, a 6–10% weight loss usually occurs, primarily due to fluid loss. Weight gain then generally proceeds at a rate of 20–25 g per day in the first 4 months and 15 g per day in the next 8 months. Most infants can be expected to double their birthweight by 4 months and triple it by 12 months. In the second year of life, weight increase is equal to slightly less than the birthweight. Thereafter, a fairly constant growth rate of about 5 lb per year occurs until 9 or 10 years of age, when growth velocity increases. At adolescence a major growth spurt occurs. Height shows a pattern similar to weight; most infants increase their length by 50% in the first year, 100% in the first 4 years, and 300% by age 13.

Changes in body composition accompany height and weight changes. Most notably, total body water decreases as adipose tissue increases. Total body water accounts for approximately 70% of total body weight at birth and declines to 60% by 1 year of age.[22]

Normal values of weight, height, and growth for infants and children are expressed in terms of percentiles for age; the reference standards most commonly used are those of the National Center for Health Statistics, a compilation of normative data from two major sources, first available in the late 1970s.[23,24] According to these standards (which reflect growth resulting from predominantly formula-feeding), most children fall between the 5th and 95th percentiles in weight, length/height, weight for length, and head circumference. Most children stay within the same percentile as they grow, but spurts and plateaus are common. If growth is not progressing as expected, particularly in the first year of life when the expected growth rate is rapid, the energy and nutrient content of an infant's diet should be evaluated. Studies of healthy, breast-fed infants reveal a slower weight gain in the first 12–18 months of life, although measures of length and head circumference are equivalent to those obtained with formula-feeding.[25] Therefore, it has been suggested that a new reference standard be developed for weight gain of the breast-fed infant.

Growth of the infant born prematurely can be evaluated similarly based on standard intrauterine growth curves.[26,27] Although many disagree with the concept that extrauterine growth should be similar to intrauterine growth, given the many different environmental influences, the goal of nutrition in the premature infant that is promoted most often is to achieve growth rates similar to intrauterine rates.

Nutritional Standards

Acceptable growth is achieved through an adequate intake of energy, protein, carbohydrates, minerals, and vitamins. The Food and Nutrition Board of the National Research Council established recommended dietary allowances (RDAs) designed to meet the needs of most healthy infants. These general guidelines were last revised and published in 1989 (Table 1).[28] Table 2 contains the Food and Drug Administration (FDA) recommendations for nutrition for infants.

Energy requirements vary with age. Total energy expenditure is a combination of basal energy needs, the specific dynamic action of food (the energy required to digest food), and activity and growth. The infant's energy requirement is high in relation to body size but

TABLE 1 Recommended dietary allowances of nutrients for full-term infants

	RDA	
Nutrient	**0–6 mo**	**>6–12 mo**
Energy (kcal/kg/day)	108	98
Protein (g/kg/day)	2.2	1.6
Essential fatty acids		
Linoleic acid (% of kcal)[a]	2.7	2.7
Vitamins		
Vitamin A (mcg)[b]	375	375
Vitamin D (mcg)[c]	7.5	10
Vitamin E (mg)[d]	3	4
Vitamin K (mcg)	5	10
Vitamin C (mg)	30	35
Thiamine (mg)	0.3	0.4
Riboflavin (mg)	0.4	0.5
Vitamin B_6 (mg)	0.3	0.6
Vitamin B_{12} (mcg)	0.3	0.5
Niacin (mg)[e]	5	6
Folate (mcg)	25	35
Pantothenic acid (mg)[f]	2	3
Biotin (mcg)[f]	10	15
Minerals		
Calcium (mg)	400	600
Phosphorus (mg)	300	500
Magnesium (mg)	40	60
Iron (mg)	6	10
Iodine (mcg)	40	50
Zinc (mg)	5	5
Copper (mg)[e]	0.4–0.6	0.6–0.7
Manganese (mg)[f]	0.3–0.6	0.6–1
Fluoride (mg)[f]	0.1–0.5	0.2–1
Chromium (mcg)[f]	10–40	20–60
Selenium (mcg)	10	15
Molybdenum (mcg)[f]	15–30	20–40

[a]No specific recommendations for linolenic acid have been identified by the National Research Council, Food and Drug Administration, or CON/AAP.

[b]Retinol equivalents (REs); 1 RE = 3.33 IU of vitamin A activity from retinol.

[c]Cholecalciferol; 10 mcg of cholecalciferol equals 400 IU of vitamin D.

[d]Alpha-tocopherol equivalents (TEs); 1 mg of delta-alpha-tocopherol = 1 alpha-TE. The activity of alpha-tocopherol is 1.49 IU/mg.

[e]Niacin equivalents (NEs); 1 NE = 1 mg of niacin or 60 mg of dietary tryptophan.

[f]Estimated safe and adequate daily dietary intakes. Because there is less information on which to base allowances, some figures are provided as ranges of recommended intakes.

Reprinted with permission from Food and Nutrition Board, Commission on Life Sciences, National Research Council. *Recommended Dietary Allowances.* 10th ed. Washington, DC: National Academy Press; 1989.

TABLE 2 Nutritional recommendations for full-term infants (per 100 kcal)

Nutrient	FDA regulations Minimum	Maximum
Protein (g)	1.8	4.5
Fat		
(g)	3.3	6.0
(% calories)	30.0	—
Essential fatty acids		
Linoleic acid (g)	0.3	—
Vitamins		
Vitamin A (IU)	250.0	750.0
Vitamin D (IU)	40.0	100.0
Vitamin K (g)	4.0	—
Vitamin E (IU)	0.7	—
Vitamin C (mg)	40.0	—
B_1 (thiamine) (mcg)	40.0	—
B_2 (riboflavin) (mcg)	60.0	—
B_6 (pyridoxine) (mcg)	35.0	—
B_{12} (mcg)	0.15	—
Niacin (mcg)[a]	2.5	—
Folic acid (mcg)	4.0	—
Pantothenic acid (mcg)	300.0	—
Biotin (mcg)[b]	1.5	—
Choline (mg)[b]	7.0	—
Inositol (mg)	4.0	—
Minerals		
Calcium (mg)	60.0	—
Phosphorus (mg)	30.0	—
Magnesium (mg)	6.0	—
Iron (mg)	0.15	3.0
Iodine (mcg)	5.0	7.5
Zinc (mg)	0.5	—
Copper (mcg)	60.0	75.0
Manganese (mcg)	5.0	—
Sodium (mg)	20.0	60.0
Potassium (mg)	80.0	200.0
Chloride (mg)	55.0	150.0

[a]Includes nicotinic acid and niacinamide.

[b]Required only for non–milk-based infant formulas.

Reprinted from *Federal Register*. 1985; 50: 45106.

declines over time. The accepted RDA for infants from birth to 6 months is 108 kcal/kg per day whereas infants 6–12 months of age require a somewhat lower intake of 98 kcal/kg per day; however, there is some disagreement over direct measurements of energy expenditure.[28] One study of children 1.5–4.5 years of age showed direct measurements of total energy expenditure to be 10–12% less than the current recommendations.[29] This has been theorized to be related to a more sedentary lifestyle. No significant differences in energy requirements have been noted between boys and girls younger than 10 years of age.

Components of a Healthy Infant Diet

Fluid

Water is a particularly important component of an infant's diet because water makes up a larger proportion of the infant's body composition than it does of the older person's. Water intake in the first 6 months of life is primarily derived from breast milk or formula. Both contain adequate amounts of water so that the normal, healthy infant should not need supplemental water. From 6 to 12 months of age, when solid foods are introduced, water intake remains high; most children's foods contain 60–70% or more water.[30] Output is predominantly in renal excretion, evaporation from the skin and lungs, and, to a lesser extent, feces. Increases in water loss caused by diarrhea, fever, or unusually rapid breathing, particularly in concert with decreased water intake, may result in significant dehydration and be accompanied by an imbalance of electrolytes. Maintenance water or fluid needs in infancy are estimated to be approximately 100 mL/kg per day for the first 10 kg of body weight plus 50 mL/kg per day for each kilogram between 10 and 20 kg. Additional losses caused by conditions such as diarrhea, fever, and rapid breathing should be offset by fluid intake in excess of maintenance levels.

Carbohydrates

Although there is no RDA for carbohydrates, under normal circumstances an infant can efficiently use 40–50% of total calories from a carbohydrate source.[31] A carbohydrate-free diet is not desirable because such a diet leads to metabolic modifications favoring fatty acid breakdown, tissue protein and cation loss, and dehydration. Fiber intake is of considerable interest because high-fiber diets have been associated with the prevention of diseases such as diverticular disease, colon cancer, and coronary heart disease. The Committee on Nutrition of the American Academy of Pediatrics (CON/AAP) favors adequate fiber intake to ensure regular stool frequency but has not made a specific recommendation.[32]

Lactose is the primary carbohydrate source in human milk and milk-based formulas. It is hydrolyzed by acids and the enzyme lactase to glucose and galactose. Disaccharide hydrolysis may be incomplete in a newborn, and because lactase activity develops late in fetal life, infants born during the seventh or eighth month of gestation may be unable to hydrolyze the same amount of lactose as full-term infants. Therefore, premature infants are relatively lactase deficient and thus are especially prone to lactose intolerance, which may be manifested by diarrhea, abdominal pain or distention, bloating, gas, and cramping.

Secondary lactase deficiency is a temporary reduction in intestinal lactase caused by gastroenteritis or malnutrition. Congenital lactase deficiency is a rare type of milk intolerance in infants that results from an inborn error of metabolism. Because of low levels of lactase in the GI tract, infants with congenital lactase deficiency and LBW infants may be unable to metabolize the quantity of lactose found in breast milk or infant formulas. Formulas with nutrient sources other than cow milk may be used when lactose intolerance or hypersensitivity is suspected.

Protein and Amino Acids

The accepted average RDA for protein is 2.2 g/kg per day from birth to age 6 months and 1.6 g/kg per day from age 6 months to 1 year.[28] Body protein increases by an average of 3.5 g per day in the first 4 months of life and by 3.1 g per day over the next 8 months, representing an overall change in body protein composition from 11% to 15%.[21]

Equally important as the overall protein intake is the amino acid composition of the protein. Amino acids can be classified as essential, nonessential, and conditionally essential. Eight amino acids (isoleucine, leucine, lysine, methionine, phenylalanine, threonine, tryptophan, and valine) are considered essential in adults because the body cannot synthesize them from precursors as it can nonessential amino acids. Conditionally essential amino acids (eg, cysteine, taurine, tyrosine, and histidine) are nonessential ones that become essential because the synthesis process is impaired owing to immaturity or the effects of disease on synthesis or interconversion. Impairment of synthesis may occur in preterm infants with immature enzyme systems.[28]

The National Research Council has accepted estimates of specific amino acid requirements from the World Health Organization and others (Table 3).[28] Despite similar amino acid densities and milk intakes, serum amino acid patterns in formula-fed infants tend to exceed those in infants fed human milk; however, the growth of formula-fed infants is normal.[33] Although the protein content of human milk adjusts to a growing infant's needs, the high protein needs of preterm infants are not completely met by early human milk.[34] Fortification produces reasonable plasma amino acid profiles and helps an infant meet expected intrauterine growth rates.[35–37]

Histidine is found in both human and cow milk in quantities larger than the estimated requirements. Synthesis of this amino acid becomes adequate by 2–3 months of age. Histidine deficiency results in poor nitrogen balance and growth. Supplemental tyrosine and cystine, as well as histidine, may be needed in the first weeks of life for the preterm infant.[28,38]

Taurine is an amino acid found in abundant quantities in breast milk.[39] It serves a major nutritional role as a protector of cell membranes by attenuating toxic substances (eg, oxidants, secondary bile acids, and excess retinoids) and by acting as an osmoregulator.[40] Taurine is not an energy source, nor is it used for protein synthesis. It is considered a conditionally essential nutrient. Taurine deficiency can result in retinal dysfunction, slow development of auditory brain stem–evoked response in preterm infants, and poor fat absorption in preterm infants and in children with cystic fibrosis. These conditions can be improved with taurine supplements. Although disagreement still exists as to the necessity of taurine supplements even in LBW infants, taurine is now added to many infant formulas to provide the same margin of physiologic safety that is provided by human milk.[41]

TABLE 3 Estimated amino acid requirements for infants and young children (mg/kg/day)

Amino acid	Infants (3–4 months old)	Children (≈2 years old)
Histidine	28	—
Isoleucine	70	31
Leucine	161	73
Lysine	103	64
Methionine + cystine	58	27
Phenylalanine + tyrosine	125	69
Threonine	87	37
Tryptophan	17	12.5
Valine	93	38

In evaluating the adequacy of an infant's protein intake, one must consider not only the absolute amount of protein ingested, but also the growth rate of the child, the quantity of nonprotein calories and other nutrients necessary for protein synthesis, and the quality of the protein itself. Some authors have suggested that amino acid and protein requirements are more meaningful when expressed in terms of calories; therefore, requirements or supplementation levels may appear in grams per 100 kcal. In such cases, direct comparisons with RDAs expressed in grams per kilogram of body weight per day are not easily made.

Fat and Essential Fatty Acids

Fat is the most dense source of calories in the diet (9 kcal/g versus 4 kcal/g for protein and carbohydrates). It supplies approximately 40–50% of the energy intake of infants in developed countries.[21] Although there is concern in the adult population about dietary fat intake, the AAP recommends that the current recommendations of the American Heart Association and the National Institutes of Health Consensus Panel on Lowering Blood Cholesterol to Prevent Heart Disease "be followed with moderation" for children. The AAP says that 30–40% of calories from fat "seems sensible for adequate growth and development."[42] The FDA recommends a minimum fat intake of 3.3 g/100 kcal (30% of calories) and a maximum of 6 g/100 kcal (60% of calories).[43]

The diet must contain small amounts of linoleic acid, the polyunsaturated fatty acid (PUFA) that has been proven to be an essential nutrient. Linoleic acid and its derivatives, including arachidonic acid, enable optimum caloric intake and proper skin composition.[44] Linoleic acid deficiency manifests as increased metabolic rate, drying and flaking of the skin, hair loss, and impaired healing of wounds. Manifestations of essential fatty acid deficiency are generally delayed; however, rapid onset may occur in newborns with delayed provision of fat in their diets.[45] Linoleic acid represents the bulk of PUFAs in infant formulas. Generally, an intake of linoleic acid equal to 1–2% of total dietary calories is adequate to prevent biochemical and clinical evidence of deficiency; 4–5% is thought to be optimal.[21] The AAP recommends linoleic acid intakes of 300 mg/100 kcal, or approximately 3% of total calories.[43] Linolenic acid, a PUFA found in plant foods, is thought by some to be essential; however, a specific deficiency state in humans has not been defined. No specific RDAs for fat have been established.

Micronutrients

RDAs for vitamins and minerals, including trace elements, are shown in Table 1. Precise needs are difficult to define and depend on energy, protein, and fat intakes and absorption. Infant formulas are generally supplemented with adequate amounts of vitamins and minerals to meet the needs of full-term infants.

Vitamin A Vitamins A, D, E, and K are classified as fat soluble. Vitamin A and the carotenoids that are vitamin A precursors are essential for vision, growth, and cellular function. Deficiency occurs most often in young children with dietary insufficiencies[28]; however, deficiency in vitamin A and its precursors is uncommon in the United States. Vitamin A activity from food sources is expressed in retinol equivalents (REs); 1 RE is equal to 1 mcg of all-*trans*-retinol, 6 mcg of all-*trans*-beta-carotene, or 12 mcg of other provitamin A carotenoids.[28] Vitamin A needs for rapidly growing infants and children exceed the maintenance levels required by adults; therefore, RDA values change little as the growth rate decreases. Toxicity can occur with acute or chronic ingestion of exceedingly high doses. Sustained daily intakes of 6,000 mcg retinol by infants or young children may cause toxic manifestations such as headache, vomiting, diplopia, alopecia, desquamation, bone abnormalities, liver damage, and dryness of the mucous membranes.[28] The breast milk of well-nourished women in the United States contains adequate amounts of vitamin A and the carotenoids that supply about 10% of total vitamin A activity to prevent deficiencies in infants.[28]

Vitamin D Vitamin D is essential in mineral homeostasis and bone mineralization and is particularly important in infancy. Severe deficiency states in infancy can cause rickets. Adequate amounts of vitamin D can be synthesized with sufficient exposure to sunlight or artificial UV light.[28] Cow milk and infant formulas should be fortified with 400 IU vitamin D per quart.[28] Excessive intake (as little as five times the RDA) in children may result in toxicity with hypercalcemia, hypercalciuria, soft tissue calcium deposition, and irreversible calcium deposition in the kidneys and heart.[28]

Vitamin E Vitamin E serves an important role in muscular and neurologic function. The most potent and common form, alpha-tocopherol, is also an efficient antioxidant. Premature infants and children with fat malabsorption due to cystic fibrosis or other causes are prone to deficiency. Tocopherol levels should be proportional to the oxidants (iron) and oxidizable substrates (PUFAs) in the diet. Most infant formulas are supplemented to provide 0.8 IU/g of PUFAs because cow milk is low in linoleic acid, having only 20–25% as much as human milk.[28] The RDAs of 3 mg per day for infants 0–6 months of age and 4 mg per day for infants older than 6 months should be met in human milk or formula.

Compared with full-term infants, preterm infants are born with disproportionately small body stores of vitamin E and a reduced capacity for intestinal vitamin E absorption.[46] Hemolytic anemia has been reported in preterm infants who received iron-fortified formulas that contain high levels of PUFAs.[47] The additional oxidant activity of iron (≥8 mg/kg) increases the risk for hemolytic anemia in preterm infants who have insufficient tocopherol levels. To avoid hemolytic anemia in preterm infants, the ratio of vitamin E intake to PUFAs (E/PUFAs) should not be less than 0.4 where E/PUFAs is[48]:

$$\frac{\text{vitamin E per unit volume (IU of alpha-tocopherol)}}{\text{PUFAs per unit volume (grams of linoleic and arachidonic acid)}}$$

It has therefore been suggested that up to 17 mg of vitamin E may be required as an oral supplement until 3 months of age.[28]

Vitamin K Vitamin K and vitamin K–active compounds are essential in the formation of prothrombin and other proteins responsible for coagulation of the blood. Vitamin K activity is supplied by dietary sources and intestinal bacteria. Because intestinal flora is limited in the newborn, most hospital-born infants receive vitamin K prophylaxis at birth. Deficiency states are manifested primarily by prolonged clotting times. Milk-based formulas contain enough vitamin K to prevent deficiency. Furthermore, the bacterial flora generated by milk-based formulas in healthy infants contributes to an adequate supply of vitamin K.

Water-soluble vitamins are generally present in both breast milk and formulas in quantities adequate to prevent deficiency states.

Biotin, Choline, and Inositol

Biotin is an integral component of enzyme systems in humans and is considered an essential vitamin. Biotin deficiency in infants younger than 6 months has been reported to be manifested by seborrheic dermatitis, which can be reversed with supplementation.[49] The recommended intake is 10–15 mcg per day.[28] Choline and *myo*-inositol are both components of cell membrane and phospholipids or lipoproteins. The nutritional requirements for choline and inositol are currently unknown.

Minerals

Calcium and Phosphorus Calcium and phosphorus are crucial to the development and maintenance of the human skeleton. In addition, phosphorus is an integral component of many biochemical reactions. Calcium requirements are affected by protein and phosphorus intake because of these nutrients' interactions with the renal tubular reabsorption of calcium. The recommended ratio of calcium to phosphorus is 1.3:1 for infants between birth and 6 months of age and 1.2:1 for infants older than 6 months. A high phosphate intake has been associated with hypocalcemic tetany.[50,51]

Formulas designed for full-term infants are deficient in calcium and phosphorus relative to the needs of LBW or preterm infants. For these infants, additional calcium and phosphorus in special infant formulas are

TABLE 4 Guidelines for the use of vitamin and mineral supplements in healthy infants

	Multivitamin/ multimineral	Vitamin D	Vitamin E[a]	Folate	Iron[b]
Full-term infants					
Breast-fed	0	±	0	0	±
Formula-fed	0	0	0	0	0
Preterm infants					
Breast-fed[c]	+	+	±	±	+
Formula-fed[c]	+	+	±	±	+
Older Infants (>6 mo)					
Normal	0	0	0	0	±
High-risk[d]	+	0	0	0	±

Key:

+ means a supplement is usually indicated; ± means a supplement is possibly or sometimes indicated; 0 means a supplement is not usually indicated.

Vitamin K for newborn infants and fluoride in areas where there is insufficient fluoride in the water are not shown.

[a]Vitamin E should be in a form that is well absorbed by small, preterm infants. If this form of vitamin E is present in formulas, it need not be given separately to formula-fed infants. Infants fed breast milk are less susceptible to vitamin E deficiency.

[b]Iron-fortified formula and/or infant cereal is a more convenient and reliable source of iron than a supplement.

[c]Multivitamin supplements (plus added folate) are needed primarily when calorie intake is below approximately 300 kcal per day or when the infant weigh 2.5 kg; vitamin D should be supplied at least until 6 months of age in breast-fed infants. Iron should be started by 2 months of age.

[d]Multivitamin–multimineral preparations including iron are preferred to supplements containing iron alone.

Adapted from *Pediatrics*. 1980; 66: 1017.

necessary for normal bone growth and mineralization, and breast milk may also need supplementation.[52]

Table 1 contains RDAs for minerals for full-term infants.

Iron Because iron is a component of hemoglobin and several enzymes, it is considered essential. A large portion of iron is found in storage forms in the liver, spleen, and bone marrow. Intestinal absorption is the primary method for regulating iron sufficiency. The FDA recommends that all formulas contain at least the lower level of iron found in human milk (0.3–0.5 mg/L) and that iron be in a bioavailable form.[19,53] Infants are at risk for iron deficiency and should be given formulas supplemented with 1–2 mg/100 kcal of iron, or approximately 6–12 mg/L; most iron-supplemented formulas contain 12 or 13 mg/L. Iron availability may be less in formulas with higher protein concentrations; iron deficiency is more common in infants fed 2.4% protein (3.6 g/100 kcal) than in those fed 1.5% protein (2.3 g/100 kcal) in a milk formula.[53]

Formulas for LBW infants contain less than or equal to 3 mg of iron per liter. Conservative levels of iron are used because iron supplementation in LBW infants up to 2 months of age has been associated with an increased risk of hemolytic anemia owing to iron's interference with vitamin E metabolism. These formulas do not supply enough iron to meet the normal intrauterine accretion rate of iron. The decision to supplement iron in infants fed LBW formulas should be made by the physician.

Zinc, Copper, and Manganese Full-term infants who are entirely breast-fed should meet their zinc requirements (approximately 2 mg per day for an infant 1 month of age) through breast milk and liver stores. Zinc is less bioavailable in formulas; therefore, the RDA for formula-fed infants is 5 mg per day.[28] Less zinc may be absorbed from soy-protein formulas because of the presence of phytate in soy protein.[54] The AAP recommendation for copper in infant formulas is 60 mcg/100 kcal.[28] The requirement for manganese is currently unknown; the provisional recommendations are 0.3–0.6 mg per day for infants 0–6 months old and 0.6–1 mg per day in infants 6 months to 1 year of age.[28]

The Need for Vitamin and Mineral Supplements

There is no evidence that vitamin and mineral supplementation is necessary for formula-fed full-term infants or for normal, breast-fed infants of well-nourished mothers.[55] However, iron and vitamin D supplementation has been recommended for breast-fed full-term infants.[55] In a study supporting iron supplementation at age 4 months and beyond, the iron status in infants exclusively breast-fed for at least 9 months was found to be deficient (as reflected in a 20% higher incidence of anemia and a 28% higher incidence of inadequate iron stores) compared with that in formula-fed infants.[56]

Vitamin and mineral supplementation may be needed for preterm and LBW infants and for infants whose mothers are inadequately nourished. These infants and those with other nutritional deficiencies, malabsorptive and other chronic diseases, rare vitamin dependency conditions, inborn errors of vitamin or mineral metabolism, or deficiencies related to the intake of drugs will need vitamin and mineral supplementation directed by a physician.[55] Table 4 gives guidelines for supplementation.

Breast-Fed Full-Term Infants

Supplementation of vitamin D is recommended for breast-fed infants as a protective measure against the development of rickets.[57,58] However, rickets caused by vitamin D deficiency has been reported in relatively few breast-fed infants in the United States. The vitamin D–fortified foods in the diets of most mothers reduce the risk of vitamin D deficiency. If the mother's diet has been inadequate in vitamin D, supplements of 400 IU of vitamin D per day may be administered.[59] Mothers should be encouraged to maintain a balanced diet and to drink five to six 8-oz glasses of milk a day while breast-feeding. If the mother cannot tolerate milk because of lactose intolerance, products that aid in lactose digestion (eg, Lactaid, Dairy Aid, Lactogest, or Dairy Ease) are available. If she wishes not to drink milk, she should be encouraged to increase her calcium intake from other dietary sources or to supplement her dietary calcium intake with calcium tablets.

Vitamin A deficiency rarely occurs in breast-fed infants; therefore, vitamin A may be omitted from supplements designed to provide vitamin D for infants.

Vitamin B_{12} deficiency has been reported in breast-fed infants of strict vegetarian mothers.[60] This deficiency is also relatively rare in the United States. A malnourished nursing mother and her infant should receive multivitamin supplements containing vitamin B_{12} to prevent megaloblastic anemia.

The concentration of iron in human milk averages about 0.3–0.5 mg/L.[19,53] Iron is well absorbed from human milk (ie, 50% of the iron is absorbed).[61] Breast-fed infants rarely develop iron deficiency anemia before 4–6 months of age because neonatal stores of iron are adequate. After 6 months of age, neonatal stores may be depleted; consequently, in normal, breast-fed full-term infants, the addition of an iron supplement (2 mg/kg per day of ferrous sulfate) may be desirable. An iron supplement is preferable to iron-fortified cereal. Cereal diluted with milk or formula provides about 7 mg of elemental iron per 100-g serving. A 4% absorption of iron from a 50-g serving of cereal yields only 0.14 mg, or 20% of the daily requirement.[7]

The bioavailability of the electrolyte iron powder used to fortify infant cereals has not been studied in human subjects. Because cereals contain potent inhibitors of iron absorption, they are questionable sources of iron. Iron-fortified wet-packed cereal and fruit combinations marketed in jars offer no exposure of the iron sulfate to oxygen until the jar is opened; therefore, oxidative rancidity is not a problem. These products may be better sources of dietary iron supplementation than dry cereals.[7] Products that require reconstitution of dehydrated flakes with water to produce instant baby foods appear to be nutritionally equivalent to the wet-packed foods.[7]

TABLE 5 Supplemental fluoride dosage schedule (mg per day)

Age	Concentration of fluoride in drinking water (ppm)[a]		
	<0.3	0.3–0.7	>0.7
2 wk–2 y	0.25	0	0
2–3 y	0.50	0.25	0
3–16 y[b]	1.00	0.50	0

[a]2.2 mg sodium fluoride contains 1 mg fluoride.

[b]The American Academy of Pediatrics recommends 16 as the termination age. The American Dental Association recommends 13 as the termination age.

Excerpted from *Am J Dis Child.* 1980; 134: 866.

The CON/AAP states that fluoride supplements can be initiated shortly after birth in breast-fed infants if deemed necessary by a physician.[62,63] Since its statement in 1979, the committee has changed its view because infants who are totally breast-fed do not appear to develop caries at a higher rate than bottle-fed infants. Therefore, fluoride supplements may not be necessary if the breast-fed infant lives in an area where the water is fluoridated. If the physician wishes the infant to receive a supplement, Table 5 can be used to determine the proper fluoride supplementation; the level of supplementation should not be sufficient to cause enamel fluorosis. In fluoridated areas where breast-fed infants receive a diet supplemented by additional food and water, fluoride supplementation is not advised because of the risk of mild enamel fluorosis.[63]

Formula-Fed Full-Term Infants

Full-term infants who consume adequate amounts of an iron-fortified commercial milk-based formula do not need vitamin and mineral supplementation in the first 6 months of life.[64] An iron-fortified formula is preferred because of the concern over adequate iron stores for growing infants. Studies have shown that infants fed iron-fortified formulas do not demonstrate a difference in stool consistency, fussiness, colic, or regurgitation compared with infants fed nonfortified formulas.[65,66]

In a 1985 study, infants 7–12 months of age who were fed formula and solid foods had a more balanced intake of nutrients than infants fed cow milk and solid foods.[67] The table foods that were fed to infants on cow milk were high in protein, sodium, and potassium and low in iron and linoleic acid. Thus, the overall diet of infants fed cow milk and supplemental solid foods contained 52% of the RDA for iron.

Vitamin and mineral supplements are not needed for infants older than 6 months of age who receive a diet of formula, mixed feedings, and increased amounts of table food. A multivitamin with minerals may be needed, however, if the infant is at special nutritional risk. If a powdered or concentrated formula is used, fluoride supplements should be administered only if the community's drinking water contains less than 0.3 ppm of fluoride. Ready-to-use formulas are manufactured with defluoridated water and contain less than 0.3 ppm of fluoride. Therefore, if an infant fed ready-to-use formula does not drink water or juice or eat solid foods, the physician may recommend a fluoride supplement.

Preterm Infants

Preterm infants, either breast-fed or formula-fed, need vitamin and mineral supplementation. Their nutrient needs are proportionately greater than those of full-term infants because of their more rapid growth rate, inability to ingest an adequate volume of formula or breast milk, and decreased intestinal absorption.[47,52] Until these infants can consume about 300 kcal per day or until they reach a body weight of 2.5 kg, a multivitamin supplement should be administered to provide the equivalent of the RDAs for full-term infants.

A multivitamin supplement should include vitamin E in a form well absorbed by preterm infants. Because of conflicting data from clinical studies, it may be prudent to monitor vitamin E serum concentrations and to maintain them at 1–3 mg/dL.[68]

Folic acid deficiency has been reported in preterm infants.[69] The instability of folic acid precludes its use in commercial liquid multivitamin and mineral preparations. Folate can be added to a multivitamin preparation to provide the RDA (Table 1). The shelf life of folate is 1 month, and the label should read "shake well."[47]

To minimize the possibility of hemolytic anemia in infants with insufficient vitamin E absorption, iron supplements should be withheld until the preterm infant is several weeks old. Iron is required at a dosage of 2 mg/kg per day starting by at least 2 months of age; this is because iron is transferred from mother to fetus during the third trimester and so the iron stores of preterm infants may become depleted earlier than those of full-term infants. Iron-fortified formulas supply sufficient iron to prevent iron deficiency in preterm infants.[47]

Calcium, phosphorus, and vitamin D supplementation in preterm infant formulas is necessary to ensure adequate bone mineralization and to prevent osteopenia and rickets.[47,52] The prevention of severe bone disease in preterm infants appears to depend on both high oral intakes of calcium and phosphorus and the intake of at least 500 IU of vitamin D per day.[47,52] Therefore, breast-fed preterm infants should receive a special preterm infant formula that contains appropriate amounts of calcium, phosphorus, and vitamin D supplementation.[52] (See Chapter 19, "Nutritional Products.")

Content of Various Milks

Comparison of Human Milk and Whole Cow Milk

Cow milk is the nutrient source for commercially prepared milk-based infant formulas. Both human and cow milk are intricate liquids that contain more than 200 ingredients in the fat- and water-soluble fractions. Estimates of the concentrations of selected nutrients contained in pooled mature human milk and in cow milk are listed in Table 6.

The two types of milk differ significantly in the quantity and availability of nutrients. Differences in milk composition reflect the different needs of the human infant and the calf. Mature human milk is more effective than cow milk in meeting the nutritional requirements of the human infant. Both milks provide similar amounts of water and approximately the same quantity of energy. However, the nutrient sources for energy (ie, calories) are different. Protein supplies approximately 7% of the calories in human milk and 20% of the calories in cow milk. The low protein content of human milk is compensated by its higher protein quality (ie, larger amounts of essential amino acids).[70] The carbohydrate lactose supplies approximately 42% of the calories in human milk and 30% of the calories in cow milk.[19] The percentage of calories provided by fat is approximately 50% in both milks. This percentage is higher than the 30% recommended for children older than 2 years, but there is a well-documented need for a higher dietary fat content for young infants with developing nervous systems.[42,70]

Carbohydrates

The carbohydrate percentage in cow milk is lower than that in human milk, and carbohydrate supplementation is necessary for milk-based formulas. Honey and other unrefined foods are not recommended for carbohydrate supplementation because they may contain spores of *Clostridium botulinum*.[19] Lactose is the carbohydrate source in both cow milk and human milk. Lactose is absorbed into the brush border of the small intestine and is cleaved by the enzyme lactase into galactose and glucose. These sugars are then actively absorbed against concentration gradients.

Protein

Cow milk contains more than three times the ash (mineral residue) and protein normally found in human milk (3.1–3.5 g/100 mL of protein in cow milk versus 1.05 ± 0.2 g/100 mL of protein in human milk).[15,19] This difference reflects the calf's more rapid growth rate and proportionate demand for protein and minerals. Although cow milk administered to human infants is usually diluted with water and carbohydrates, the solute load requiring renal excretion generally remains higher than the load from human milk.

Not only does cow milk contain a higher percentage of protein than human milk, but the protein differs in composition. This difference alters digestibility and can create a milk sensitivity that may induce problems in digesting a milk-based formula or elicit an allergic response to milk protein. Milk proteins are defined broadly as either whey or casein. Mature human milk has an approximate whey-to-casein ratio of 60:40, but colostrum, the initial human milk, has an approximate ratio of 90:10.[15,71] By 8 months postpartum, the whey-to-casein ratio is 50:50.[15] Cow milk, with an approximate whey-to-casein ratio of 20:80, contains six to seven times more casein than does human milk. The whey protein in cow milk contains alpha-lactalbumin, beta-lactoglobulin,

TABLE 6 Composition of mature human milk and cow milk

Composition	Human milk	Cow milk
Water (mL/100 mL)	87.1%	87.2%
Energy (kcaL/100 mL)	69	66
Protein (g/100 mL)	1.05 ± 0.2	3.1–3.5
Casein (% protein)	40%	80%
Whey (% protein)	60%	20%
Alpha-lactalbumin (g/100 mL)	0.2–0.3	0.1
Beta-lactoglobulin (g/100 mL)	—	0.4
Lactoferrin (g/100 mL)	0.1–0.3	trace
Secretory IgA (g/100 mL)	0.08–0.1	trace
Albumin (g/100 mL)	0.05	0.04
Fat (g/100 mL)	3.9 ± 0.4	3.8
Carbohydrate		
Lactose (g/100 mL)	7.2 ± 0.3	4.9
Electrolytes (per liter)		
Calcium (mg)	280 ± 26	1,200
Phosphorus (mg)	140 ± 22	920–940
Calcium/phosphorus ratio	2:1	1.3:1
Sodium (mg)	180 ± 40	506
Potassium (mg)	525 ± 35	1,570
Chloride (mg)	420 ± 60	1,028–1,060
Magnesium (mg)	35 ± 2	120
Sulfur (mg)	140	300
Minerals (per liter)		
Chromium (mcg)	50 ± 5	20
Manganese (mcg)	6 ± 2	20–40
Copper (mcg)	60	110
Zinc (mg)	0.5–1.4	3–5
Iodine (mcg)	110 ± 40	80
Selenium (mcg)	20 ± 5	5–50
Iron (mg)	0.3–0.5	0.5
Vitamins (per liter)		
Vitamin A (IU)	1,898	1,025
Thiamine (mcg)	150	370
Riboflavin (mcg)	380	1,700
Niacin (mcg)	1,700	900
Pyridoxine (mcg)	130	460
Pantothenate (mg)	2.6	3.6
Folic acid (mcg)	85	68
Vitamin B_{12} (mcg)	0.5	4
Vitamin C (mg)	43	17
Vitamin D (IU)	40	14
Vitamin E (mg)	2.3	0.4
Vitamin K (mcg)	2.1	17

Source:
Nutrition in Infancy and Childhood. 5th ed. St Louis: Times Mirror/Mosby College Publishing; 1993: 90.
Williams AF. *Textbook of Paediatric Nutrition.* 3rd ed. London: Churchill Livingstone; 1991: 26-27.
Suskind RM, Lewinter-Suskind L. *Textbook of Pediatric Nutrition.* 2nd ed. New York: Raven Press; 1993: 33–42.

lactoferrin, serum albumin, lysozyme, and immunoglobulins A, G, and M (IgA, IgG, and IgM); human milk contains all of these proteins and immunologic factors except beta-lactoglobulin. Recent evidence supports the fact that the ingestion of cow milk protein may be an environmental stimulus for the destruction of pancreatic cells in children who have a genetic predisposition for diabetes mellitus.[72] The culprit appears to be bovine serum albumin. To date, there is no evidence that this is a problem for the general population.

Whereas whey protein is highly soluble, casein is relatively insoluble and is found in milk as a "tough" curd.[71] The large amount of casein in cow milk mixes with hydrochloric acid in the stomach to produce curds. This action slows the gastric emptying rate and may cause GI distress. Processing cow milk by acidification, boiling, or treatment with enzymes reduces curd tension and makes the milk more digestible. Because of its lower casein content, human milk forms a soft, flocculent, easy-to-digest curd.

Sensitivity to cow milk differs from milk allergy. Sensitivity may be relieved by altering the casein-to-lactalbumin ratio; however, an allergic reaction requires that all animal milk protein be eliminated from the diet. Although heating cow milk may increase its digestibility, it will not alter its antigen activity.

The amino acid content of cow milk is inappropriate for the neonate's immature enzyme systems. The newborn has a limited ability to metabolize phenylalanine to tyrosine; human milk has low concentrations of these amino acids. High concentrations of these amino acids in cow milk have been associated with metabolic abnormalities.[70] Taurine and cysteine are present in higher concentrations in human milk than in cow milk. Cystathionase, an enzyme necessary for the transulfuration of methionine to cysteine, is present in low concentrations in the neonate, which may explain the higher cysteine content of human milk.[15,19]

Fat

Human milk and cow milk have similar total fat contents. Human milk contains 3–4.5% fat that consists of triglycerides (98–99% of total milk fat), phospholipids, and cholesterol. The fat composition of human milk changes during lactation; triglyceride concentrations rise and phospholipid and cholesterol concentrations decrease during the transition from colostrum to mature milk. When human milk is mature, the fat composition remains constant.[18]

Linoleic acid supplies an average of 7% (depending on the maternal diet) of the calories in human milk but only 1% of the calories in cow milk. Most commercially prepared infant formulas contain more than 10% linoleic acid. Essential fatty acids should provide approximately 3% of the total caloric intake.[73] The cholesterol content varies in both milks, from 20 to 47 mg/100 mL in human milk and from 7 to 25 mg/100 mL in cow milk.[19]

The fat found in cow milk differs from that found in human milk in two ways. First, the triglycerides in cow milk contain primarily short- and long-chain fatty acids, whereas human milk fat contains medium-chain but not short-chain fatty acids. In addition, human milk contains primarily PUFAs, and the fat in cow milk (butterfat) consists principally of saturated fatty acids.[19] Commercially prepared milk-based formulas incorporate the highly digestible unsaturated medium-chain triglycerides by replacing butterfat with vegetable oil and special medium-chain triglyceride oils. Recent studies are questioning whether long-chain polyunsaturated fats such as arachidonic acid and docosahexaenoic acid should be added to infant formulas, especially those intended for use in preterm infants. This has been suggested because formula-fed infants exhibit lower plasma and tissue concentrations of long-chain polyunsaturated fats, indicating that they may have a limited capacity for endogenous synthesis from the precursor fatty acids (ie, linoleic and alpha-linolenic).[15,74,75] Additional studies are needed to answer questions in this area.

Both cow milk and human milk contain lipoprotein lipase, but human milk contains additional lipase that contributes significantly to the higher percentage of absorption of human milk fat.[19] However, infants fed milk-based formula can efficiently digest fat from vegetable oil because of gastric enzyme activity.

Minerals and Electrolytes

↑ in cow milk

The mineral content of cow milk is several times greater than that of human milk. Cow milk and human milk differ in absolute and proportionate amounts of calcium and phosphorus. The total calcium and phosphorus content of cow milk is approximately four and seven times that of human milk, respectively. However, cow milk provides less calcium relative to phosphorus than does human milk. In cow milk–based formulas, the total concentration of calcium and phosphorus has been greatly reduced, but the calcium-to-phosphorus ratio imbalance persists and infants receive a relative phosphorus load that occasionally results in neonatal hypocalcemic tetany.[76] Calcium-to-phosphorus ratios are 2:1 in human milk, 1.3:1 in cow milk, and 1.3–1.4:1 in commercially prepared formulas.[76] The effect of differences in the calcium-to-phosphorus ratio on calcium absorption is not clear because of the interrelation of additional factors, such as vitamin D, fat absorption, and active transport.

The iron content of human milk decreases from 0.5 to 0.3 mg/L when the infant is between 2 weeks and 5 months of age. Levels of iron in cow milk remain at 0.5 mg/L throughout the time the calf is being nourished.[19] Because iron in human milk is more bioavailable, an infant should be able to absorb approximately 50% of the iron from human milk (versus only 10% of that from cow milk, 10% of that from unfortified milk-based formula, and 4% of that from iron-fortified formula).[61,77]

The zinc content of human milk is lower than that of cow milk, but it is more bioavailable (approximately 59% versus 42–50%).[78] Zinc binds strongly to casein in cow milk, whereas binding in human milk is minimal.

Cow milk contains more sodium, potassium, and chloride than does human milk. These higher electrolyte and mineral concentrations, when combined with the high protein content of cow milk, result in a smaller margin of safety against hyperosmolar dehydration. The larger renal solute load of cow milk, in combination with higher environmental temperatures or the presence of fever, vomiting, or diarrhea, can place an infant at risk for severe dehydration.

Reduced-Fat Cow Milk

Reduced-fat milks, such as skim milk (0.1% fat) and 2% milk (2% fat), have been used to prevent obesity and atherosclerosis and to provide a "healthy diet."[79,80] However, when the low-fat diet that is recommended for adults is imposed on children younger than 2 years, it puts them at risk for failure to thrive.[79] The CON/AAP does not recommend skim or 2% milks during the first 12 months of life.[64] Most dietitians and other nutrition experts agree that fat restriction is not recommended for young children.[80]

Infants who receive a major percentage of their caloric intake from reduced-fat milks such as skim or 2% milk may receive an exceedingly high protein intake and an inadequate intake of essential fatty acids. The maximum concentration of protein allowed in infant formulas is 4.5 g/100 kcal, but skim milk provides approximately 10 g of protein per 100 kcal and 2% milk provides nearly 7 g of protein per 100 kcal. Thus, a disadvantage of using reduced-fat milks as the only dietary source for infant nutrition is the unbalanced percentage of calories supplied from protein, fat, and carbohydrates.

It is important to recognize that, per unit volume, skim milk has a slightly higher PRSL than does whole cow milk (Table 7). The solute concentration is further increased by water loss during boiling.[64] Reduced-fat milks are not recommended for the treatment of diarrhea because of the possibility of hypertonic dehydration.

Whole Cow Milk

The age at which it is appropriate to introduce unheated whole cow milk into an infant's diet is controversial. Because the concentration and bioavailability of iron in whole cow milk are low, whole cow milk has been associated with iron-deficiency anemia.[64] In the past decade, convincing evidence has accumulated to indicate that iron deficiency impairs psychomotor development and cognitive function in infants. This impairment has been observed even with relatively mild anemia. Through unknown mechanisms, whole cow milk can also cause occult bleeding from the GI tract.[81] Milk-protein intolerance and/or allergy (estimated to affect 0.5–7.5% of the infant population in the first 2 years of life) poses another potential complication for the use of whole cow milk.[81,82]

More research is needed to establish a time frame for the introduction of whole cow milk. In 1976, the CON/AAP recommended that non–breast-fed infants receive an iron-fortified formula during the first 12 months of life. In 1983, the committee reversed its previous recommendation and concluded, "If breast feeding has been completely discontinued and infants are consuming one-third of their calories as supplemental foods consisting of a balanced mixture of cereal, vegetables, fruits, and other foods, whole milk may be introduced."[81,83] When whole cow milk is fed together with solid food, infants receive unnecessarily high intakes of protein and electrolytes, resulting in a high renal solute load.[84] Also, infants fed an infant formula for the first year of life are less likely to develop iron deficiency.[7] The current position of the CON/AAP is that iron-fortified infant formula is the only acceptable alternative to breast milk. Whole cow milk and low-iron formulas are not recommended during the first year of life.[85,86]

Evaporated Milk

Evaporated milk is a sterile, convenient source of cow milk that has standardized concentrations of protein, fat, and carbohydrate. When ingested, evaporated milk produces a smaller, softer curd than that formed from boiled whole milk. Vitamin D is typically added to evaporated milk during processing, but evaporated milk formulas fail to meet recommendations for ascorbic acid, vitamin E for preterm infants, and essential fatty acids.[64,87,88]

Goat Milk

Goat milk is commercially available in powdered and evaporated forms. It contains primarily medium- and short-chain fatty acids and may be more easily digested than cow milk. Unfortified goat milk is deficient in folate and low in iron and vitamin D. The evaporated form of Meyenberg goat milk is supplemented with vitamin D and folic acid. Powdered Meyenberg goat milk is supplemented with folic acid only and is recommended only for infants older than 1 year. Because the powder formulation is not a complete formula for infants, the manufacturer recommends supplementation with vitamins.

TABLE 7 Potential renal solute loads (PRSLs) of selected milks and infant formulas

	PRSL	
	mOsm/L	mOsm/100 kcal
Human milk	93	14
Milk-based formula	135	20
Soy-based formula	177	26
Whole cow milk	308	46
Skim cow milk	326	93
FDA upper limit for PRSL	277	41

Adapted from Ziegler EE, Fomon SJ. Potential renal solute load of infant formulas. *J Nutr.* 1989; 119(suppl): 1785–8.

Breast-Feeding

The initial human breast milk is called colostrum. It is a clear, yellowish fluid that has a high protein content but lower fat and lactose concentrations than are found in mature human milk. It also has high concentrations of various immunologic factors. Within 1 week after delivery, human milk changes in its composition, at which time it is referred to as transitional milk. Approximately 3 weeks later, breast milk is considered mature. Mature breast milk is the standard against which most commercially prepared infant formulas are compared.

During lactation a nursing mother may experience dramatic physiologic changes (eg, increased cardiac output and increased blood flow to the breasts, intestinal tract, and liver). Blood flow to the breasts may be 500 times higher than the volume of milk (600–1,000 mL) produced daily. Maximum milk production occurs in the early morning hours (approximately 6 AM); the lowest production occurs between 6 PM and 10 PM. Thus, milk volume appears to be controlled by diurnal variation.[71] Some medications (eg, vasoconstrictors) reduce blood flow to the breasts and thus decrease milk volume. Similarly, maternal stress and anxiety decrease milk production, as does the return of menses. The latter does this by reducing blood flow to the breasts.[89,90]

Although not bacteriologically sterile, human milk provides certain advantages over cow milk, goat milk, and infant formulas. However, pharmacists should not issue dire warnings to mothers who cannot or do not wish to breast-feed; normal growth and development are possible without human milk.

Benefits of Breast-Feeding

Reported benefits of breast-feeding include protection against infections such as GI illness and respiratory infection. Studies have shown that breast-fed infants have a lower incidence of gastroenteritis, fewer episodes of diarrhea, and infrequent hospitalizations for GI illness.[3] This lower rate has been noted particularly in infants born in nonindustrialized nations. Results of a study from the United Kingdom show a statistically significant reduction in GI illness in infants who were breast-fed for 13 or more weeks, regardless of the introduction of other supplements during this time, compared with infants who were entirely formula-fed.[91] Interestingly, this effect was reported to have been maintained beyond the period of breast-feeding and was associated with a decrease in the rate of hospital admission.

Conflicting results have been reported regarding breast-feeding and a lower rate of respiratory infection. However, respiratory infections in breast-fed infants are likely to be less severe.[3] Overall, the advantages of breast-feeding in lessening respiratory tract infections are most notable in the first 6 months of life.[3] Protective effects of breast-feeding also have been shown to decline in proportion to the degree of supplementation with formula or cow milk.

Although conflicting data have been reported regarding a protective effect of breast-feeding against otitis media, many past studies have lacked methodological strength. A recent, well-designed study supports the advantages of breast-feeding in reducing the incidence of otitis media.[92] In a study group of more than 1,000 infants followed longitudinally, those who were exclusively breast-fed for at least 4 months developed acute otitis media only half as often as those who were not breast-fed at all, and they had 40% fewer episodes than those with supplemented breast-feeding prior to 4 months of age. No additional protective effect was seen against acute otitis media in infants who were exclusively breast-fed for an additional 2 months. Differences in the incidence of recurrent otitis media were also noted, with a cumulative recurrent otitis media rate of 10% for those who were exclusively breast-fed for longer than 6 months compared with 20% for those in other groups.

A review of the literature identifies studies that present conflicting data about other claimed advantages of breast-feeding.[93] Conditions on which conflicting data exist include sudden infant death syndrome, urinary tract infections, bacteremia and meningitis, allergic disease, obesity, anemia, and childhood cancer.

Many questions about the apparent protective effect of breast-feeding remain to be answered. What is the duration of protection after breast-feeding is discontinued? What effect does change in age have on the protective effect? How great is the interactive effect of social and demographic variables? How does the addition of solid foods to the diet of a breast-fed infant influence the protective effect? What consequence does partial formula-feeding have on the protective effect of breast-feeding? Better designed studies are needed to answer these questions and to document the protective effects of breast-feeding against a variety of infections.

Potential Problems with Breast-Feeding

Hyperbilirubinemia

One minor problem associated with human milk is the presence of increased levels of nonesterified fatty acid, caused by abnormal lipolytic activity, in the breast milk of some women.[94] This condition results in the inhibition of uridine diphosphate glucuronyl transferase and leads to a prolonged unconjugated hyperbilirubinemia in infants. Breast-feeding need not be stopped in most cases of breast-milk jaundice[95]; the jaundice subsides even if breast-feeding is continued. If the infant appears in danger from hyperbilirubinemia itself, a temporary pause in breast-feeding for 1–3 days usually reduces the bilirubin to a safe level and can help determine the cause of bilirubin elevation. Formula feeding during this interval appears to increase stool volume and overall bilirubin elimination. Breast-feeding can then be resumed, although slight elevations or rebounds in serum bilirubin are often observed and may persist for several weeks.[96] No detrimental effects have been reported in infants as a result of breast-milk jaundice.

Human Immunodeficiency Virus

Although the risk of transmitting the human immunodeficiency virus (HIV) in breast milk appears to be low, there have been reports of such transmission.[97] Therefore, the Committee on Infectious Diseases of the AAP recommends that women in the United States who are infected with HIV should not breast-feed, nor should they donate breast milk to milk banks.[98] These recommendations may not be appropriate for women in developing countries, where infants may not receive adequate nutrition except from breast milk.[97]

Medications in Breast Milk

Oral Contraceptives It is debatable whether maternal use of an oral contraceptive while breast-feeding significantly affects lactation. Some studies have found decreased milk production, changes in breast milk protein composition, caloric deficits, and decreased weight gain in infants whose mothers used combination (estrogen- and progestogen-containing) oral contraceptives while breast-feeding.[99–102]

Studies that have specifically addressed the maternal use of combination oral contraceptives that contain 30–50 mcg of ethinyl estradiol or 50–100 mcg of mestranol have demonstrated that lactation is not inhibited after the immediate postpartum period. However, the quantity of milk produced and the duration of lactation may be suppressed.[103,104] The use of combination oral contraceptives during lactation has not been clearly related to changes in milk composition. A study on the effects of two combination oral contraceptives and one progestogen-only oral contraceptive reported that milk volume and composition varied even in the absence of steroidal contraception but that changes remained within the normal ranges.[101]

Studies that address the use of progestogen-only oral contraceptives have shown no consistent alteration in breast milk composition, milk production, or lactation duration.[99,103] A study performed by the World Health Organization addressed the effects of a low-estrogen combination oral contraceptive, a progestogen-only oral contraceptive, depot medroxyprogesterone acetate, and a nonhormonal birth control method. Women who used a combination oral contraceptive had decreased milk volume, but their infants grew appropriately.[103]

AAP recommendations state that low-dose combination oral contraceptives or progestogen-only contraceptives are not contraindicated during breast-feeding as long as milk production has been established.[105,106]

Other Medications Health care personnel need to make decisions about the safety of drugs that lactating mothers might pass on to their breast-feeding infants. Anderson's review of drug use during breast-feeding[107] and the textbook *Drugs in Pregnancy and Lactation*[99] are excellent sources of information.

Transfer of Medications to Breast Milk With the exception of water-soluble compounds of low molecular weight (such as ethanol) that gain access to breast milk through water-filled pores, most medications are transferred from maternal blood to breast milk via passive diffusion. This transfer also depends on a variety of other factors. Maternal factors include the dose of medication, the frequency and route of administration, and the pharmacokinetics of the drug. The pharmacokinetics of a particular drug may vary from the immediate postpartum period to a time several weeks after delivery when the physiologic changes of pregnancy wane. Alterations in renal function during pregnancy may affect drug clearance. These functions return to prepregnancy levels with time and thus may affect drug clearance. Blood flow to the breasts increases postpartum. Therefore, drug concentrations in the serum and milk of women several weeks or months postpartum may not be applicable to the early postpartum period. In addition, changes in breast milk composition from the immediate postpartum period through the weaning process may markedly affect drug excretion into breast milk.

Breast factors that affect a drug's ability to cross into breast milk include the quantity of blood flow to the breasts, pH differences between breast milk and maternal plasma, drug ionization, protein binding in breast milk, drug metabolism in breast milk, and possible reabsorption of a drug and/or its metabolites from breast milk into maternal blood.

Drug characteristics that affect passage into breast milk include molecular weight, plasma protein binding, lipid solubility, pK_a, and maternal plasma pH versus breast milk pH. Most drugs can gain access to breast milk based on molecular weight; only drugs with high molecular weights (eg, heparin) are unable to gain access. Typically, a low–molecular weight, un-ionized, basic compound that is lipid soluble and has a low plasma protein binding can easily cross into breast milk. In addition, when a weak base gains access to human milk, a shift in the ratio of un-ionized to ionized drug can occur in the relatively acidic breast milk, and drug trapping results that inhibits passage back into maternal plasma.

Infant factors that must be considered include the infant's sucking pattern, time spent nursing during each feeding, milk volume consumed during feeding, the number of daily feeding periods, GI absorption of the drug by the infant, and the pharmacokinetics of the drug in infants. To determine the theoretical amount of drug that might be ingested by a breast-feeding infant, the reader is referred to the articles by Atkinson and colleagues.[108,109]

To help minimize an infant's intake of a medication via breast milk, the following strategies should be followed when possible:

- A drug should be selected from a class of drugs that is the least likely to be distributed into breast milk.
- A *nonoral* route that minimizes systemic absorption should be selected for maternal medication administration when the option exists (eg, inhaled beta-agonists, topical corticosteroids).
- A drug that can be taken once daily may be recommended.
- When multiple doses are needed, feedings should coincide with trough (ie, predose) rather than peak drug concentrations.
- If there is concern about toxicity to the infant, the infant should be monitored and, if possible, serum or urine drug concentrations should be obtained.
- If the mother needs a short course of a drug that is not recommended during breast-feeding, breast-feeding may be interrupted for four to five half-lives. During this time, the infant should be given previously expressed breast milk or an infant formula, and the woman should pump her breasts to prevent engorgement.
- If the breast-feeding infant is to be weaned soon, the mother could delay beginning a medication if this option is medically acceptable.[110]

Medications listed in Table 8 are contraindicated during breast-feeding, should be used cautiously by nursing women, or require a temporary interruption of breast-feeding.[106,111]

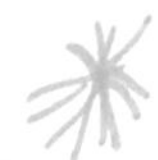

TABLE 8 Medications of concern to breast-feeding women

Medications that are contraindicated in breast-feeding women[a]	
Bromocriptine	Ergotamine
Cimetidine	Gold salts
Cyclophosphamide	Lithium
Cyclosporine	Methotrexate
Doxorubicin	Phenindione
Medications that require cautious use and medical supervision	
Aspirin	Salicylazosulfapyridine
Phenobarbital	
Medications that require temporary stopping of breast-feeding	
Metronidazole	Radiopharmaceuticals

[a]Drugs of abuse (eg, amphetamines, cocaine, heroin, marijuana, nicotine, and phencyclidine) are contraindicated for use during breast-feeding.

Source:

Briggs GG, Freeman RK, Yaffe SJ. *Drugs in Pregnancy and Lactation*. 4th ed. Baltimore: Williams & Wilkins; 1994.

Briggs GG. Drugs in pregnancy and lactation. In: Young YL, Koda-Kimble MA, eds. *Applied Therapeutics: The Clinical Use of Drugs*. 5th ed. Vancouver, Wash: Applied Therapeutics Inc; 1992: 1–33.

Commercial Infant Formulas

Recommendations to standardize the nutrient composition of infant formulas were first published by the CON/AAP in 1967.[112] These recommendations were adopted by the FDA in 1971 and were revised by the AAP in 1976. The FDA published rules concerning the provision of nutrients in infant formulas in 1985.[113]

In 1978, two soy-based formulas were marketed that later were discovered to be deficient in chloride. Some children who received these formulas experienced a hypochloremic metabolic alkalosis, and some failed to grow appropriately. Follow-up studies have shown that these children may be at risk for learning disabilities and language deficits.[114,115] As a result, the US Congress passed an amendment to the Federal Food, Drug, and Cosmetic Act (Infant Formula Act of 1980) that gave the FDA authority to establish quality control, require adequate labeling, and revise nutrient levels.[113,116]

Manufacturers of infant formulas must follow regulations and quality control measures to ensure that infant formulas contain appropriate amounts of nutrients. Suppliers of ingredients used in infant formulas must provide "needed ingredients within rigid tolerance limits of quality" and comply with "good manufacturing practice."[13] Manufacturers may alter a formulation in response to changes in the availability of ingredients or modifications in recommended nutritional allowances, but such changes should not adversely affect the quality or consistency of the formula.[13] An accurate listing of the current ingredients and their quantities for a given formula may be obtained by direct communication with the manufacturer.

Based on an infant receiving 8 oz of infant formula per feeding, the US formula industry produces and sells 3.6 billion 8-oz formula equivalents annually.[117] This is enough formula to feed 4 million infants in the United States for approximately 7 months.[117]

Microbiologic Safety

Guidelines of the Infant Formula Council (a voluntary nonprofit trade association composed of companies that manufacture and market infant formulas) require liquid formulations to be free of all viable pathogens, their spores, and other organisms that may cause product degradation. To ensure that this requirement is met, liquid formulas are usually sterilized by heat treatment and incubated while samples are analyzed. Quality control measures help to ensure the production of a sterile product that is free of microbial effects as long as the container remains intact.[13] Powdered formulas are cultured to ensure that coliforms and other pathogens are absent and that the level of other microorganisms is below the acceptable level set by government standards. The heating required during the final preparation of the infant formula (as indicated on label directions) destroys most microorganisms.[13] If microbiologic contamination occurs, the infant ingesting such a formula could develop diarrhea with subsequent fluid and electrolyte losses.

Physical Characteristics

Infant formulas are emulsions of edible oils in aqueous solutions, but the separation of fat rarely occurs. If separation does occur, the fat can usually be redispersed by shaking the container unless the separation occurred because of a lack of stabilizers or because the formula was stored beyond its shelf life. Liquid infant formulas may contain thickening agents, stabilizers, and emulsifiers to provide uniform consistency and prolong stability.

Protein agglomeration may occur if storage time is excessive. This agglomeration may range from slight, grainy development through increased viscosity and formation of gels to eventual protein precipitation. Agglomeration and separation do not affect the safety or nutritional value of a formula; however, the appearance is a deterrent to its use.

Caloric Density

The RDA for energy is 108 kcal/kg per day for infants from birth to 6 months of age and 98 kcal/kg per day from age 6 months to 1 year.[28] A full-term infant should have no difficulty in consuming enough diluted formula (20 kcal/oz or 67 kcal/100 mL) to meet these caloric needs, but a preterm or LBW (<2,500 g) infant has a higher caloric need and may require as much as 130 kcal/kg per day.[73] An infant recovering from illness or malnutrition also requires more calories.[118] Infant formulas with caloric densities significantly lower or higher than 67 kcal/100 mL are regarded as therapeutic formulas to be used for the management of special clinical conditions and only under medical supervision.

Osmolarity and Osmolality

The osmolarity of an infant formula may be expressed as the concentration of solute per unit of total volume of solution or as the number of milliosmoles of solute per liter of solution (mOsm/L). Osmolarity cannot be measured but must be calculated using the osmolality value for the solution in question.[119] The osmolarity of human milk is approximately 273 mOsm/L. The CON/AAP recommends that formulas for normal infants have osmolarities no higher than 400 mOsm/L; formulas with higher osmolarities should have a warning statement on the label.[120] Hyperosmolar formulas have been implicated in the etiology of necrotizing enterocolitis.[30] However, infant formulas with 67 kcal/100 mL or 80 kcal/100 mL that are routinely used to feed preterm infants have osmolalities less than or equal to 300 mOsm/kg and pose no apparent increased risk of GI mucosal injury.[121]

Osmolality may be expressed as the number of milliosmoles of solute per kilogram of solvent (mOsm/kg). "The osmolality of a formula is directly related to the concentration of molecular or ionic particles in a solution and is inversely proportional to the concentration of water in the formula."[122] The osmolality of human milk is approximately 290 mOsm/kg.[123] Osmolality is related to the carbohydrate and mineral content of the formula. For dilute solutions, there is little difference between osmolality and osmolarity. However, because infant formulas are relatively concentrated solutions, osmolarity may be only 80% of the osmolality.[122] Osmolality is the preferred term for reporting the osmotic activities of infant formulas because osmotic activity is a function of a solute–solvent relationship. Manufacturers report both osmolality and osmolarity.

The relationship between osmolality and caloric density is reasonably linear in formulas with caloric densities of 44–90 kcal/100 mL, the range of caloric concentrations usually fed to infants.[122] If the osmolality of a 67 kcal/100 mL formula is known, that of a formula with a caloric density between 44 and 90 kcal/100 mL can be calculated, assuming a direct proportion between osmolality and caloric density. The osmolality of a formula increases with increasing caloric content.

There is no meaningful difference in the osmolalities of the commonly used ready-to-use formulas that provide 67 kcal/100 mL. The osmolalities of reconstituted concentrated products when diluted to provide 67 kcal/100 mL are not considerably different from the osmolalities of the corresponding ready-to-use products. Directions for diluting concentrated formulas must be followed exactly to prevent harmful hyperosmolar states, such as diarrhea and dehydration. Soy-protein formulas have lower osmolalities than the milk-based formulas because of differences in carbohydrate sources; whereas milk-based formulas usually contain lactose, soy-protein formulas contain sucrose or corn syrup solids.

Renal Solute Load

Renal solute load is related to the protein, electrolyte, and mineral content of an infant formula. It represents the water-soluble substances that must be removed by the kidneys. (See earlier section Infant Physiology and Growth for more information on renal solute load.) Table 7 lists the PRSLs for various milks and infant formulas and provides a comparison with the FDA upper limits for PRSL for infant formulas.[20]

The renal solute load is important because it determines the quantity of water that is excreted by the kidneys. Infants are less able to concentrate their urine than are older children and adults. Most infants can concentrate their urine to between 900 and 1,100 mOsm/kg, but some cannot concentrate to even 900 mOsm/kg. Thus, feeding an infant a formula that is too concentrated may produce a hypertonic urine that may cause dehydration because of increased renal losses. Under normal conditions, infant formulas with 67 kcal/100 mL supply 1.5 mL of water per kilocalorie, an amount that provides adequate water for all losses, including urinary excretion. If an infant has a decreased water intake or an excessive loss, a diet that has a high renal solute load may stress the limited capacity of the infant's renal reabsorptive system. It has been suggested that the upper limit for protein in infant formulas be lowered from 4.5 to 3.2 g/100 kcal, which is the estimated protein requirement for an infant, and that the upper limit for phosphorus be less than 3 mOsm/100 kcal (93 mg/100 kcal). Such changes in two of the primary determinants of PRSL would enable an infant to maintain an adequate water balance and decrease the possibility of hypernatremic dehydration secondary to a high PRSL (ie, ≥39 mOsm/100 kcal).[20]

Effect of Biotechnology on Infant Formula Production

Through the use of genetic coding and the hyperimmunization of pregnant cows with vaccines against various organisms that cause disease in humans (eg, salmonella, listeria), manufacturers may alter cow milk to produce "immune milks" for infant formulas.[117] Cow milk may also be altered via genetic coding to change the concentration of particular nutritional components, such as the casein-to-whey ratio or the type of fat, that currently are different in cow milk and human milk.

Types, Uses, and Selection of Commercial Infant Formulas

Formulas for full-term infants are milk-based or milk-based with added whey protein (whey predominant). These formulas meet the minimum requirements for various nutrients per 100 kcal, as required by the FDA and deemed appropriate by the CON/AAP. Other infant formulas are available for specific needs, but they should be used only on the advice of a physician. (See product table "Infants' and Children's Formula Products" for a comprehensive listing of commercially available formulas for pediatric use.)

Milk-Based Formulas ex) Similac

A milk-based formula is prepared from nonfat cow milk, vegetable oils, and added carbohydrate (lactose). The added carbohydrate is necessary because the ratio of carbohydrate to protein in nonfat milk solids from cow milk is less than is desirable for infant formulas. Protein provides approximately 9% of calories and fat furnishes 48–50% of calories.[121] The most widely used vegetable oils are corn, coconut, safflower, and soy. Replacement of the butterfat with vegetable oils allows for better fat absorption. Vitamins and minerals are added in accordance with the guidelines established by the FDA. Milk-based formulas are available as iron-fortified (approximately 1.8 mg/100 kcal) or low-iron (approximately 0.16 mg/100 kcal) formulas. Similac is an example of a milk-based formula. Although Lactofree is a milk-based formula, it differs from others in this group because it contains corn syrup solids rather than lactose as its carbohydrate source and thus can be used in infants with lactose intolerance.

Milk-Based Formulas with Added Whey Protein ex) Enfamil

When whey is added in proper amounts to nonfat cow milk, the ratio of whey proteins to casein can be altered to approximate that of human milk. The ratio of 60% whey to 40% casein in human milk differs considerably from the ratio in cow milk, in which casein accounts for approximately 80% of the protein and whey for only 20%.[73] Minerals are removed from whey by electrodialysis or ion-exchange processes and then are re-added to the formula to approximate the mineral content of human milk. Formulas containing partially demineralized whey proteins are not nutritionally superior to milk-based formulas. The high nutritional quality and relatively low renal solute load of these formulas are assets in the therapeutic management of ill infants. Enfamil is an example of a whey-predominant formula.

Therapeutic Formulas

Therapeutic infant formulas are used on an individual basis for infants being treated by medical specialists for conditions that require dietary adjustment. Table 9 lists indications for using various therapeutic infant formulas; Table 10 lists formulas for infants who have a variety of metabolic disorders. Therapeutic formulas include soy-protein formulas, casein-based formulas, casein or whey hydrolysate–based formulas, low-sodium formulas, a variety of formulas needed for specific medical problems, and formulas for LBW infants or for specific age groups.

Soy-Protein Formulas added vit K

Soy-protein formulas contain methionine-fortified isolated soy protein.[64] Vegetable oils provide the fat content, and corn syrup solids and/or sucrose supply the carbohydrate in these formulas. Vitamin K is added to provide a concentration of 15 mcg/100 kcal. Other vitamins, taurine, and carnitine (necessary for the optimal

TABLE 9 Indication for the use of therapeutic infant formulas

Problem	Suggested formula	Comments
Allergy or sensitivity to cow milk protein or soy protein	Protein hydrolysate formula (eg, Alimentum, Nutramigen, or Pregestimil)	Protein allergy or sensitivity
Biliary atresia	Portagen	Impaired digestion and absorption of long-chain fats
Carbohydrate intolerance	RCF, 3232A	Formulas are carbohydrate free, and a source of carbohydrate that the patient can tolerate can be added
Cardiac disease	Enfamil, Similac PM 60/40	Whey predominant, low electrolyte content
Celiac disease	Pregestimil or Nutramigen, followed by a soy formula and then a cow milk formula	Advance to more complete formulas as intestinal epithelium returns to normal
Constipation	Routine formula, increase sugar	Mild laxative effect
Cystic fibrosis	Portagen, Pregestimil	Impaired digestion and absorption of long-chain fats
Diarrhea		
Chronic nonspecific	Routine formula or soy formula	Appropriate distribution of calories; impaired digestion of intact protein, long-chain fats, and disaccharides
Intractable	Pregestimil, Alimentum	
Failure to thrive (eg, when intestinal damage is suspected)	Pregestimil, Alimentum	Advance to more complete formulas as intestinal epithelium returns to normal
Gastroesophageal reflux	Routine formula	Thicken with cereal (1 tbsp/oz of formula); also try small, frequent feedings
Hepatitis		
Without liver failure	Routine formula	Impaired digestion and absorption of long-chain fats
With liver failure	Portagen	
Homocystinuria	Low methionine, Analog XMET	Low content of methionine
Lactose intolerance	Soy formula	Impaired digestion and use of lactose
Maple syrup urine disease	MSUD Diet Powder, Analog MSUD	Low content of leucine, isoleucine, and valine
Necrotizing enterocolitis (with resection)	Pregestimil (when oral feeding is resumed)	Impaired digestion
Phenylketonuria	Lofenalac, Analog XP	Low content of phenylalanine
Prematurity	Preterm infant formulas	Whey predominant, easily digestible sources of carbohydrate and fat; appropriate vitamin and mineral content
Renal insufficiency	Similac PM 60/40	Low phosphate content, low renal solute load

Supplemental information extracted from:
Walker WA, Hendricks KM. *Manual of Pediatric Nutrition*. 2nd ed. Philadelphia: BC Decker; 1990: 79.

TABLE 10 Metabolic formulas

Disease	Product
Glutaric aciduria type I	Glutarex-1
Glycogen storage disease type III, IV, V	ProVeMin RCF
Histidinemia	HIST 1 80056-Protein Free Diet Powder
Homocystinuria	3200K-Low Methionine Diet Powder Hominex-1 HOM 1
Hypercalcemia	Calcilo XD
Hyperlysinemia	LYS 1 80056-Protein Free Diet Powder
Hypermethioninemia	Hominex-1
Isovaleric acidemia	I-Valex-1
Maple syrup urine disease	MSUD Diet Powder MSUD 1 Ketonex
Methylmalonic acidemia	80056-Protein Free Diet Powder Propimex-1
Organic acidemia	OS1
Phenylketonuria	Lofenalac Phenex-1 PKU1
Propionic acidemia	80056-Protein Free Diet Powder Propimex-1
Tyrosinemia	3200AB-Low Phe/Tyr Diet Powder Tyromex-1 TYR1
Urea cycle disorders	Cyclinex-1 UCD1 80056-Protein Free Diet Powder

Source:

Pediatric Products Handbook. Evansville, Ind: Mead Johnson Nutritionals; 1993.

Ross Laboratories Product Handbook. Columbus, Ohio: Ross Laboratories; 1992.

oxidation of fatty acids) are also added. Carnitine supplementation of soy-protein formulas is necessary because of carnitine's low concentrations in foods of plant origin compared with foods of animal origin.[124]

Some concerns regarding soy formulas include their high levels of protein and manganese. Absorption of manganese is enhanced in children who are iron deficient. In addition, the phytate content of soy formulas may have a negative effect on vitamin and mineral bioavailability.[125] More studies are needed in this area.

About 15% of infants who are fed formulas receive soy-protein formulas such as Isomil, ProSobee, and Carnation I-Soyalac.[7] These formulas differ in amounts of ingredients, source of carbohydrates, and constituents of the fat source. The fat source in I-Soyalac is soy oil; Isomil contains soy and coconut oils; and ProSobee contains soy, coconut, palm, and sunflower oils.

The carbohydrate source is an important factor in product selection. Isomil contains corn syrup solids and sucrose; I-Soyalac contains only sucrose; ProSobee contains only corn syrup solids. Consequently, infants who are sensitive to corn and corn products and who cannot tolerate a milk-based formula may benefit from a corn-free soy-protein formula. Caution is advised, however, when the type of formulation is selected.

Soy-protein formulas are lactose free and therefore can be used for infants with primary lactase deficiency (eg, galactosemia) and for those with secondary lactose intolerance resulting from enteric infection or other causes of mucosal damage.[64] Resumption of a cow milk formula is generally possible 2–4 weeks after cessation of diarrhea.[118] Soy-protein formulas also provide an alternative nutritional source for infants whose parents are vegetarians and do not wish to use animal protein–based formulas.

RCF (Ross Carbohydrate Free) soy-protein formula does not contain a carbohydrate source. This formula may be used in the dietary management of infants unable to tolerate the type or amount of carbohydrates in cow milk or other infant formulas. A physician may select a carbohydrate source (sucrose, dextrose, fructose, or glucose polymers) that can be added before feeding. RCF is for use only under medical supervision.

Some infants with gastroenteritis develop intolerance to lactose and sucrose because of secondary lactase and sucrase deficiency. Isomil SF and ProSobee contain corn syrup solids (hydrolyzed corn starch, a glucose polymer) as the carbohydrate source and can thus be used in this situation.

Isomil DF is a specific formula for the management of diarrhea. It contains added dietary fiber from soy.

Food allergy occurs in infants because the immature digestive and metabolic processes may not be completely effective in converting dietary proteins into nonantigenic amino acids. The incidence of cow milk allergy in the first 2 years of life is estimated to be 0.5–7.5%.[126] The diagnosis of cow milk allergy is defined as symptomatology involving the respiratory tract, skin, or GI tract that disappears when cow milk is removed from the diet and reappears on two separate challenges when cow milk is given during a symptom-free period. Rechallenge must be done with caution.[127]

Soy-protein formulas are promoted for use in the management of allergy to milk or for infants suspected of having milk allergy. However, the CON/AAP recommends that protein hydrolysate formulas rather than soy-protein formulas be used for infants with documented clinical allergy to cow milk and/or soy protein.[7,124] This recommendation is based on the concern that infants with severe allergy to cow milk—as evidenced by severe diarrhea, vomiting, laryngeal edema, urticaria, or wheezing—have intestinal mucosal damage sufficient to expose them to higher concentrations of foreign protein in soy-protein formulas. Such infants have demonstrated severe allergic manifestations when fed soy-protein formulas.[128,129] However, most infants suspected of having adverse reactions to milk-based formulas have not experienced life-threatening manifestations and appear to tolerate soy-protein formulas, which are less expensive and better tasting, and have been studied more extensively than protein hydrolysate formulas.[7]

For infants with a family history of atopy but who have not shown clinical manifestations of allergy, a soy-protein formula may be used with caution.[124] These infants should be monitored closely for allergy to soy protein.

Soy-protein formulas should not be used for the routine feeding of preterm and LBW infants. In addition, soy-protein formulas are not recommended for infants with cystic fibrosis because these children do not use soy protein adequately, will lose substantial amounts of nitrogen in their stools, and may develop hypoproteinemia or even anasarca. Formula-fed infants with cystic fibrosis appear to do best nutritionally when given an easily used formula that contains predigested protein and medium-chain triglycerides (eg, a casein hydrolysate–based formula).

Casein Hydrolysate–Based Formulas

Casein hydrolysate–based formulas are effective in the nutritional management of infants with a variety of severe GI abnormalities in which intolerance to enteral feeding and the malabsorption of standard forms of protein, fat, and carbohydrate are common. Indications for use include severe or intractable diarrhea, severe food allergies, sensitivity to intact protein, disaccharidase deficiency, intestinal resection, dysfunctional malabsorption, steatorrhea, cystic fibrosis, protein-calorie malabsorption, and severe protein-calorie malnutrition. These formulas are also indicated during a transition from parenteral feeding to a normal diet where lack of enteral stimulation while receiving parenteral nutrition resulted in decreased digestive enzyme activity and nutrient absorptive area.

Use of these formulas for allergy prophylaxis remains controversial. Some studies indicate that prolonged breast-feeding or extended use of hypoallergenic formulas and delayed introduction of solids help prevent allergic disease in infancy, but other studies challenge these findings.[130] To date, the effectiveness of dietary and environmental regimens in the prevention of allergic disease has not been conclusively proven in prospective studies. Infants with documented clinical allergic symptoms to cow milk may benefit from a protein hydrolysate formula because approximately 15–50% of these infants also react to soy protein.[131]

There appear to be few data to support an association between colic and infant formula ingestion.[132] In selected situations, improvement has occurred when cow milk or soy protein was eliminated and a hydrolysate formula was introduced. For this reason, some experts have suggested decreasing cow milk protein and/or soy protein in the diets of infants with moderate to severe colic.[133] However, in the vast majority of infants, symptoms of colic persisted after formula changes. In cases where improvement was noted, it was difficult to attribute the improvement to a formula change.[132,133] Currently, no evidence exists to support the use of hydrolysate formulas for treating colic, restlessness, or irritability.[130] These are common symptoms in infants but they rarely occur as a result of an immune-mediated reaction to cow milk protein.

Extensively hydrolyzed casein protein makes formulas less palatable. However, infants usually accept the feedings satisfactorily. If the formula is rejected when first offered, it may be tried again after a few hours. These products are designed to provide a sole source of nutrition for infants up to 4–6 months of age and to provide a primary source of nutrition through 12 months of age when indicated. Extended use of hydrolysate formulas as a sole source of nutrition in children older than 6 months requires physician monitoring on a case-by-case basis.[134]

Pregestimil, Nutramigen, Alimentum, and 3232A are formulas with enzymatic hydrolysates of casein as the protein source. They contain nonantigenic polypeptides with a molecular weight less than 1,200 daltons[130]; therefore, they can be fed to infants who are sensitive to intact milk protein or other foods. These formulas differ from other formulas in that alpha-amino nitrogen is supplied by enzymatically-hydrolyzed, charcoal-treated casein rather than by whole protein. Casein hydrolysate formulas are supplemented with three amino acids—L-cysteine, L-tyrosine, and L-tryptophan—because the concentrations of these amino acids are reduced during charcoal treatment.

The carbohydrate sources in these formulas vary. Nutramigen contains corn syrup solids and modified corn starch; Pregestimil contains corn syrup solids, modified corn starch, and dextrose; Alimentum contains sucrose and modified tapioca starch; and 3232A contains tapioca starch as a stabilizer and no other source of carbohydrate.

Glucose polymers in corn syrup solids or modified corn starch are particularly useful in infants with malabsorption disorders, who are frequently intolerant to lactose, sucrose, and glucose. Glucose polymers are more easily digested and tolerated by infants whose capacity to handle lactose and sucrose may be impaired.[15,73] In addition, glucose polymers are a low-osmolar form of carbohydrate and contribute little to the total osmolar load. This is an advantage in infants with intestinal disorders who cannot tolerate the osmolar load of disaccharide- or glucose-containing elemental diets.

Medium-chain triglycerides and corn oil are the fat sources found in 3232A. Pregestimil contains the same types of fat and also contains high-oleic safflower oil. Nutramigen contains only corn oil, and Alimentum contains safflower and soy oil (sources of linoleic acid) in addition to medium-chain triglycerides. These triglycerides do not require emulsification with bile and are more easily hydrolyzed than long-chain fats. Shorter-chain fatty acids and medium-chain triglycerides are directly absorbed into the portal system. In addition, medium-chain triglycerides enhance the absorption of long-chain triglycerides. Formulas in which at least 40% of the fat consists of medium-chain triglycerides have been shown to relieve steatorrhea, promote weight gain, and improve calcium absorption in LBW infants.[135–137] Formulas in which at least 80% of the fat consists of medium-chain triglycerides improve the absorption of calcium and magnesium.[73,136,137] A possible adverse effect of medium-chain triglyceride malabsorption due to overfeeding or intestinal mucosal disease is diarrhea.[73]

Pregestimil Pregestimil is an effective nutritional source for infants with massive bowel resection (short-bowel syndrome), severe diarrhea, protein-calorie malnutrition, milk and soy-protein intolerance, transition from intravenous parenteral nutrition, GI immaturity, or cystic fibrosis. Pregestimil is also effective in the intractable diarrhea syndrome of infancy. Pregestimil should not be utilized routinely as a nutrient source for highly stressed LBW infants because of the increased risk of GI complications.[134]

Nutramigen Nutramigen is nutritionally effective for infants with severe diarrhea or GI disturbances and for infants who are allergic or intolerant to intact proteins of cow milk and other foods. In cases of galactosemia, a relatively rare disorder resulting from a deficiency of galactose-*l*-phosphate uridyltransferase or galactokinase, it is necessary to eliminate dietary lactose so that the body may convert glucose to the amount of galactose it requires. Infants with galactosemia may be fed formulas without lactose or sucrose (Nutramigen, Pregestimil, Alimentum, or ProSobee).

Alimentum Alimentum is composed of hydrolyzed casein supplemented with free amino acids and a blend of medium- and long-chain triglycerides. The addition of long-chain triglycerides improves the palatability but increases the allergenic potential for infants with cow milk allergy.[138] Alimentum contains two carbohydrates (sucrose and modified tapioca starch) in lower concentrations than are found in other hydrolysate formulas. These carbohydrates are digested and absorbed by separate mechanisms (principally glucoamylase and sucrase-alpha-dextrinase). This formula can be utilized for infants with protein sensitivity, pancreatic insufficiency (eg, that caused by cystic fibrosis), or intractable diarrhea.

3232A The fat source in 3232A, a monosaccharide- and disaccharide-free formula base, is 87% medium-chain triglycerides and 13% corn oil. Tapioca starch is used as a stabilizer and is the only carbohydrate in the formula base. The physician selects the carbohydrate source (eg, sucrose, dextrose, fructose, or glucose polymers). The formula base is iron fortified and contains all essential vitamins and minerals. It can be used for infants with disaccharidase deficiencies, impaired glucose transport, or intractable diarrhea.

Amino Acid–Based Formula

Occasionally there are infants who are intolerant to even hydrolyzed casein and require an amino acid–containing formula.[15] Neocate Powder contains 100% free amino acids, as well as 35% medium-chain and 65% long-chain triglycerides. Carbohydrate sources are maltodextrin, sucrose, and corn syrup solids. Neocate Powder contains 1 kcal/mL and is available in orange or pineapple flavors.[15]

Sodium Caseinate Formula

Portagen is a sodium caseinate formula. It contains corn syrup solids and sucrose as its carbohydrate sources. Medium-chain triglycerides account for 87% of its fat. It also contains higher concentrations of both lipid- and water-soluble vitamins than are found in casein hydrolysate formulas. Higher concentrations of medium-chain triglycerides and vitamins in Portagen compensate for their impaired digestion or absorption from conventional foods. Portagen has been effective in feeding infants with pancreatic insufficiency (eg, that caused by cystic fibrosis), bile acid deficiency, intestinal resection, lymphatic anomalies, and celiac disease. It can be used on a physician's recommendation as the sole dietary source for both infants and older children, or as a beverage to be consumed with each meal.

Whey Hydrolysate–Based Formulas

Casein hydrolysate formulas have been used for many years for infants with defects in protein digestion and adverse reactions to intact cow milk protein. Recently, heat-treated whey protein has been used as the protein source in an infant formula (Carnation Good Start) for similar purposes. Enzymatic hydrolysates of whey contain some peptides with molecular weights greater than 2,000; these can increase the antigenicity of the product.[130] Anaphylactic-type reactions have been reported in patients with severe milk allergy who received hydrolysate formulas.[139] Therefore, whey hydrolysate–based formulas should not be used in infants with documented IgE-mediated allergy to cow milk protein.[126] The effectiveness of whey hydrolysate formula in infants who have GI intolerance to cow milk but are not allergic to it suggests that whey hydrolysate formula may be an acceptable alternative to milk-based and soy-protein formulas. This product is promoted as having a pleasant taste, smell, and appearance, and it may be better accepted than casein-hydrolysate formulas, which mothers and infants find noticeably different from milk-based and soy-protein formulas in appearance and taste.

Metabolic Formulas

Infants with inherited metabolic disorders require specific formulas tailored to their particular conditions. Table 10 lists various metabolic diseases and formulas available to treat them.

Low Birthweight and Preterm Formulas

Because of their increased caloric needs and decreased ability to consume an adequate volume of formula, LBW infants (weight <2,500 g) and preterm infants (gestational age <38 weeks, but especially <34 weeks) may need formulas that offer a higher caloric concentration for growth. For very low birthweight (VLBW) infants, human milk is insufficient in protein, phosphorus, and calcium.[140] The nutritional goal for preterm infants is to achieve postnatal growth that approximates the in utero growth of a normal fetus at the same postconceptional age. No commercially available formula is completely satisfactory for LBW or VLBW infants; however, improvements in special formulas permit individualization of dietary regimens for these infants. Examples of special formulas that may be beneficial are Enfamil Premature Formula, Similac Special Care, and Similac PM 60/40.

TABLE 11 Dilution of concentrated liquid infant formulas[a]

Desired caloric concentration (kcal/oz)	Amount of liquid formula concentrate (oz)	Amount of water to add (oz)
10	1	3
20	1	1
24	3	2
26–27	3	1.5
28–29	5	2

[a]Commercial infant formula concentrates that contain 40 kcal per fluid ounce before dilution with water.

Adapted from Walker WA, Hendricks KM. *Manual of Pediatric Nutrition*. 2nd ed. St. Louis: Mosby; 1990: 86.

These formulas share common features, such as whey-predominant proteins; carbohydrate mixtures of lactose, corn syrup solids, and glucose polymers; and fat mixtures containing combinations of medium- and long-chain triglycerides. They may differ in electrolyte, vitamin, mineral, and caloric content. Each formula has been shown to be associated with adequate growth and metabolic stability in preterm infants. An isotonic osmolality (approximately 300 mOsm/kg of water) is maintained at a dilution of 24 kcal/oz or 80 kcal/100 mL.[121]

Preterm and LBW infants are especially susceptible to iron deficiency anemia because they have lower iron stores. Without supplemental iron, body stores of iron in these infants will be depleted by 2 months of age, in contrast to depletion at 4–6 months of age in full-term infants.[28] Therefore, supplementation of elemental iron at 2 mg/kg per day of iron is recommended by the CON/AAP for infants older than 2 months.[28] Iron supplementation before 2 months of age must be accompanied by ample vitamin E and PUFA additions to the diet to reduce the possibility of hemolytic anemia from vitamin E deficiency. A formula without iron is preferable for VLBW infants in the first 2–4 postnatal weeks to prevent decreased vitamin E serum concentrations.[141]

A new product has been developed for premature infants for continued catch-up growth after hospital discharge. Similac Neocare has more calories (22 kcal/oz), protein, vitamins, and minerals than standard formulas but contains less than in preterm formulas. It also contains 25% medium-chain triglyceride oil.

Human Milk Fortifiers

Whether human milk provides optimal nutrition for VLBW infants is a controversial issue. Mothers who deliver preterm produce milk that is higher in protein, sodium, potassium, and possibly other nutrients than the milk of mothers who deliver at term. However, it is thought that these nutrients gradually decline to levels found in mature milk at 4–8 weeks postdelivery.

Most of the mineral content for an infant's development is delivered through the placenta during the last 2 months of gestation. During the third trimester, the fetus receives 125–150 mg per day of calcium and 65–80 mg per day of phosphorus, which are primarily deposited in bone. Human milk, preterm or mature, cannot supply the amount of calcium and phosphorus needed to prevent osteopenia of prematurity.[142]

Commercial products have been developed to enhance the nutrient content of human milk. Enfamil Human Milk Fortifier is a powder that can add nutrients to human milk without displacing volume, thereby allowing for a higher intake of human milk. Similac Natural Care is a liquid that may be given alternately with human milk or mixed in various ratios with human milk. Both products are made from cow milk with a whey-to-casein ratio of 60:40 and a carbohydrate mixture of lactose and glucose polymers. Enfamil Human Milk Fortifier contains little fat and Similac Natural Care contains a mixture of medium- and long-chain triglycerides. Studies support adequate weight gain and nutrient retention in infants when either human milk with fortifier or preterm commercial formulas are ingested.[142–144]

Concentrated Formulas

A child with special nutritional needs that exceed normal requirements may be given concentrated formula under medical supervision. Such ready-to-use formulas made from cow milk are available in concentrations of 24 kcal/oz and some are available in concentrations of 27 kcal/oz. Various concentrations can be prepared from liquid concentrates or powdered products by varying the amount of water added (Tables 11 and 12). When concentrated formulas are used, the resulting increase in protein and electrolytes and decrease in fluid require careful monitoring of the infant's fluid intake and output, weight, serum electrolytes, blood urea nitrogen, and urine specific gravity and osmolality.[118]

Modular components are available as an alternative to formula concentration. Carbohydrates can be added in liquid or powdered form. Protein powder is available, but it should be used with caution because its use may increase the renal solute load. Fat may be added as medium-chain triglycerides (MCT Oil) for infants with fat malabsorption or intolerance. Microlipid, made from safflower oil, is also available as an emulsion that mixes well with formula.

Follow-up Formulas

"Follow-up" or "follow-on" formulas such as Enfamil Next Step and Carnation Follow Up are designed for infants 4–12 months of age. The CON/AAP, however, has stated that these formulas offer no nutritional advantage. Standard formulas are appropriate for infants up to 12 months of age.[15,145]

Formula for Children Aged 1–10 Years

PediaSure, PediaSure with fiber, and Kindercal are nutritionally complete, isotonic, lactose-free enteral formulas designed for young children who cannot tolerate a normal diet or eat solid food. They have a pleasant

TABLE 12 Dilution of concentrated powdered infant formulas[a]

Desired caloric concentration (kcal/oz)	Amount of powdered formula concentrate (tbsp)[b]	Amount of water to add (oz)
10	1	4
20	1	2
24	3	5
28	7	10

[a]Powdered infant formulas that contain 40 kcal per level, packed tablespoonful before dilution. Because the powder displaces water and makes the volume larger and the formula more dilute, water should be added to the powder to equal the volume expected if a large volume of formula is to be prepared.

[b]1 tbsp = 1 scoop.

Adapted from Walker WA, Hendricks KM. *Manual of Pediatric Nutrition*. 2nd ed. St Louis: Mosby; 1990: 86.

taste and can be used as supplements to increase caloric intake. They contain adequate amounts of calcium, phosphorus, iron, and vitamin D for this age group; the amounts contained in adult nutritional enteral products are typically inadequate for children aged 1–10 years.

Several therapeutic formulas have also been developed for this age group. Peptamen Junior, a peptide-based elemental formula, and Vivonex Pediatric and Neocate One+, both amino acid–based elemental formulas, are now available.

Potential Problems with Infant Formulas

Diarrhea

Infants are particularly susceptible to dehydration because of their high metabolic rate and ratio of surface area to weight and height. Fluid volume depletion by diarrhea may quickly (within 24 hours) produce severe dehydration with fluid and electrolyte imbalances, shock, and possible death. A common cause of diarrhea is the improper dilution of a concentrated liquid or powdered formula.

If diarrhea is a problem, the pharmacist should ascertain the severity and duration of the diarrhea, frequency of stools, and method of preparing the infant formula. If the diarrhea is serious (many more stools per day than normal) or has continued for 48 hours, or if the infant is clinically ill (with fever, lethargy, anorexia, irritability, dry mucous membranes, decreased urine output, or weight loss), the infant should be referred to a physician. (See Chapter 13, "Antidiarrheal Products.")

Mild diarrhea of short duration may resolve without medical measures, but the infant should be observed closely. Although improper digestion of the infant's formula may initiate diarrhea, continuation of the formula while diarrhea persists may yield only marginal nutrient absorption. A temporary (24-hour) discontinuation of usual dietary intake may be helpful. Oral electrolyte replacement solutions (eg, Pedialyte, Infalyte) may be used cautiously for short-term management of fluid and electrolyte loss. However, these solutions should not be used when parenteral rehydration is required, nor should they be used to provide adequate nutrition. A solution such as Pedialyte should not replace infant formula for the baby after diarrhea has ceased. A nutritionally adequate formula should be resumed under a physician's direction. (See Chapter 13, "Antidiarrheal Products.")

There are various recommendations for resuming formula. Formula may be resumed at half strength for 24 hours and then increased to full strength over a 48-hour period. If diarrhea resumes when the formula is reintroduced, a lactose-free formula such as one of the soy-protein formulas may be used at half strength for 24 hours or resumed at full strength; then full-strength soy-protein formula may be used for 1–3 weeks (depending on the severity of the diarrhea); finally, a milk-based formula may be resumed.[14]

Other Gastrointestinal Problems

Adverse effects of formula on an infant's GI tract range from mechanical obstruction (inspissated milk curds), diarrhea, and dehydration from a hyperosmolar formula to hypersensitivity from specific milk protein. Intolerance to cow milk is associated most often with an inability to digest lactose or milk proteins. It is estimated that approximately 15% of infants in the United States are fed soy-protein formulas because of concerns about cow milk allergy or sensitivity.[7]

Hyperosmolar formulas may adversely affect LBW infants during the early neonatal period and may be a potential cause of necrotizing enterocolitis.[30] Appropriately prepared formulas for LBW infants (20–24 kcal/oz) are isotonic, with osmolalities less than or equal to 300 mOsm/kg; other infant formulas in concentrations of 20–24 kcal/oz have osmolalities less than or equal to 400 mOsm/kg.[121]

Tooth Decay

Baby bottle tooth decay can occur in children who bottle-feed beyond the typical weaning period and is especially prevalent in children who sleep with their bottles after 1 year of age. Caries are seen in children younger than 2 years and may involve the maxillary incisors, maxillary and mandibular first molars, or maxillary and mandibular canines.[146]

Nutritional Deficiencies

Generally, infant formulas have proven to be nutritionally adequate and safe. A number of past nutritional deficiencies associated with infant formulas have been corrected with appropriate supplementation procedures and technological advances in processing infant formulas. Some deficiencies that have occurred include:

- Vitamin K deficiency in infants who were fed certain soy or non–milk-based formulas[55,147,148];
- Vitamin E deficiency and hemolytic anemia in LBW infants who received iron-fortified formulas with high concentrations of PUFAs[47];
- Thiamine deficiency in infants fed soy-protein formulas low in thiamine[149];

- Convulsions in infants who received pyridoxine-deficient formulas[150];
- Goiters in infants who were fed soy-protein formulas that were not supplemented with iodine[151];
- Metabolic alkalosis in infants fed soy-protein formulas that contained low concentrations of chloride.[152] Some children who received these formulas failed to grow appropriately. These children may be at an increased risk for learning disabilities and deficits in language skills.[114,115]

Another potential problem is vitamin D over- or undersupplementation of infant formulas and fortified milk. Researchers who measured the vitamin D content of five brands of infant formulas (10 samples) determined that none of the samples had vitamin D concentrations within 20% of the labeled content.[153] None contained less than the amount of vitamin D stated on the label, but 70% of the samples contained more than 200% of the labeled amount. One formula contained 419% of the labeled vitamin D content. This study also found inconsistency in the vitamin D content of fortified milk: 26 of 42 milk samples (62%) contained less than 80% of the labeled amount of vitamin D. In skim milk samples, 3 of 14 (21%) samples contained no detectable vitamin D. The authors concluded that better monitoring of vitamin D fortification is needed.

A more recent problem occurred in VLBW infants who developed rickets while receiving a soy-protein formula. This condition was caused by poor absorption of the calcium, phosphorus, and vitamin D contained in the formula.[154,155]

Recently there has been concern about possible aluminum contamination of infant formulas, especially if such formulas are ingested by infants who have immature or impaired renal function. Infants fed soy formulas have been shown to have serum aluminum concentrations similar to those found in breast-fed infants, who have lower aluminum intakes. However, serum concentrations may not accurately reflect the body aluminum load because aluminum may be deposited in tissue as well as in the blood.

The highest concentrations of aluminum (455–2,346 mcg/L) have been reported in soy-based formulas.[156] Human milk typically contains less than 5–45 mcg of aluminum per liter, and cow milk–based formulas have concentrations of 14–565 mcg/L. Formulas containing plant proteins, such as soy, appear to have higher aluminum concentrations because plants receive high aluminum concentrations from soil. The CON/AAP has stated that daily elemental aluminum doses in infants and children with underlying renal disease should not exceed 30,000 mcg/kg. The Joint Expert Committee on Food Additives of the Food and Agricultural Organization of the United Nations has set the maximum weekly aluminum intake for infants, children, and adults at 7,000 mcg/kg.[156]

Formula Preparation

The preparation of infant formula requires careful technique. For all formulas, including special dilutions of therapeutic formulas and other modified formulas, the directions on the product container should be followed closely. If bottles with disposable plastic liners are used, the formula should not be mixed in the liner but should be prepared before the formula is poured into the liner; the measurements on the bottle are only approximate.

Infant formulas are available in three types: liquid ready-to-use, liquid concentrate, and powdered concentrate. Ready-to-use formulas do not require the addition of water and, as the name implies, are ready for use. Concentrated liquid and powdered formulations require the addition of water. Mixing equal amounts of water and concentrated liquid formula (eg, 4 oz water to 4 oz formula) provides the desired 20 kcal/oz or 67 kcal/100 mL formula (Table 11). Most powdered formulas require the addition of 1 packed level measure (1 tbsp) of powder for every 2 oz of water to obtain a concentration of 20 kcal/oz (Table 12).[19,157]

McJunkin and colleagues reported that 11% of formulas (133 samples) provided and classified by mothers as either ready-to-use or concentrates were either hypoconcentrated (6%) or hyperconcentrated (5%).[158] Haschke et al stated that 11–21% of formulas prepared from powdered concentrates by 88 women were hyperosmolar because of improper reconstitution.[159] Failure to properly dilute a concentrated formula can result in a hypertonic solution, precipitating diarrhea and dehydration. In extreme cases, the ingestion of overly concentrated formula has produced renal failure, disseminated intravascular coagulation, gangrene of the legs, and coma resulting from hypernatremic dehydration and metabolic acidosis.[19,160]

Overdiluting infant formulas or substituting water for milk may lead to water intoxication, which may result in irritability, hyponatremia, coma, or brain damage.[19] Such a situation may occur when a parent or caregiver misunderstands the instructions for preparing a concentrated formula, dilutes a ready-to-use formula, or tries to make a formula last longer by diluting it further.[19]

Because infants are susceptible to infection, various methods (eg, the aseptic method and the terminal heating method; Table 13) have been recommended for infant formula preparation.[157] The AAP's Committee on the Fetus and the Newborn does not recommend using unsterilized equipment and hot tap water to prepare formula but does recommend that some method of sterilization be used.[161]

Although the AAP does not recommend it, some parents use the clean technique for formula preparation.[19] In this method, one bottle is prepared for each feeding. The person preparing the formula washes his or her hands carefully. Then all equipment for formula preparation (including cans of concentrated formula, bottles, and nipples) is washed thoroughly with detergent and hot water. The formula is then prepared, the opened can of concentrated formula is refrigerated, and the prepared formula is heated. Formula remaining in the bottle after feeding should be discarded. Studies have shown that the clean method of formula preparation is as safe as terminal sterilization if the water supply used for formula preparation is safe (ie, if municipal water is available). If well water is used, it should be boiled for approximately 5 minutes before formula preparation.[162–164] If tap water is used for formula preparation, the water should be run for at least 2 minutes to clear any lead

TABLE 13 Methods for infant formula preparation

Aseptic sterilization

When this method for infant formula preparation is selected, bottles and other equipment (eg, glass measuring cup, spoons, nipples, rings, and disks) are sterilized separately from the formula.[a]

- Wash hands before preparing formula and again if interrupted.
- Place all equipment in a deep pan or sterilizer, cover all equipment with tap water, and boil for 20 minutes.
- Remove all items from the pan or sterilizer with tongs and place on a clean towel. Place the bottles and nipples on the towel with their open ends facing down.

For concentrated liquid or powdered formula:

- While the equipment is being cleaned, boil water for the formula preparation in a clean pan or teakettle for at least 5 minutes.
- Remove the boiled water from the stove and allow it to cool almost to room temperature with the lid left in place.

For concentrated liquid formula:

- Wash the top of the formula can with hot water and detergent, rinse in hot running water, and dry. Shake the can, open it with a clean punch-type can opener, and mix appropriate amounts of concentrated liquid and sterilized water (according to instructions on the product label). All measurements should be made with a measuring cup for accuracy.
- Pour formula into the sterilized bottles. Place nipples, rings, and disks on the bottles.
- Tightly cover any unused formula and store in the refrigerator. It should be used within 48 hours.

For concentrated powdered formula:

- Wash the top of the can with hot water and detergent, rinse in hot running water, and dry. Open the can and mix appropriate amounts of powder and sterilized water (according to instructions on the product label). All measurements should be made with a measuring cup for accuracy.
- Pour formula into the sterilized bottles. Place nipples, rings, and disks on the bottles.
- Tightly cover any unused formula and store in the refrigerator. It should be used within 48 hours.
- Cover the can containing any remaining powder with its plastic top. Store in a cool, dry place for up to 1 month.

For ready-to-use formula:

- Wash the top of the can with hot water and detergent, rinse in hot running water, and dry. Shake the can and open it with a clean punch type can opener. Add the amount of formula needed per feeding to a sterilized bottle. *Do not add water.* Place nipple and ring on the bottle.
- Tightly cover any formula remaining in the can. Store in the refrigerator for up to 48 hours.

For all types of formula:

- Warm the bottle to the desired temperature and shake well before feeding. After feeding, discard any formula left in the bottle and rinse the bottle and nipple in cool water immediately.

Terminal heating method

This method is for the preparation of infant formula from concentrated liquid formula only.

- Wash hands before preparing formula and again if interrupted.
- Wash all needed equipment (eg, glass measuring cup, spoon, bottles, nipples, rings, and disks) with hot water and detergent. Rinse well with hot running water.
- Wash the top of the formula can with hot water and detergent, rinse in hot running water, and dry. Shake the can and open it with a clean punch-type can opener.
- Measure the needed amount of concentrated formula and the correct amount of water in a glass measuring cup (according to instructions on the formula label). Mix well; pour the formula into clean bottles; and attach nipples, disks, and rings. Apply rings loosely.
- Place filled bottles on a rack in a deep pan or sterilizer that contains approximately 3 in. of water. Heat water to boiling and allow it to boil gently for 25 minutes while covered. Remove the pan from the stove.
- After the sides of the pan have cooled enough to be touched comfortably, remove the bottles. Tighten the nipple rings and store bottles in the refrigerator until needed. Use bottles within 48 hours.
- Warm the bottle to the desired temperature and shake well before feeding. After feeding, discard any formula left in the bottle and rinse the bottle and nipple in cool water immediately.

[a]If disposable bottle liners are used, only the nipples, rings, and screw tops of bottle need to be sterilized. The bottle liners are sterilized by the manufacturer.

Source:

How to Prepare Your Baby's Infant Formula. Evansville, Ind: Mead Johnson Nutritionals; 1991.

Feeding Baby: A Guide for New Parents. Evansville, Ind: Mead Johnson Nutritionals; 1994.

that might have accumulated in the pipes to decrease an infant's exposure to lead.[164]

The heating of infant formulas, warming of breast milk, or thawing of frozen breast milk in a microwave oven is a questionable practice. Some of the hazards associated with the use of microwave ovens are scald injuries and palatal burns in infants and exploding containers. Glass bottles get much hotter than plastic bottles, and the temperature of the milk may be uneven.[165] It also appears that microwaving can have detrimental effects on the anti-infective factors found in breast milk. When breast milk was microwaved at temperatures of 162°–208° F (72°–98° C), marked decreases in anti-infective factors (eg, total IgA, specific secretory IgA, and lysozymes) occurred; significant decreases in IgA specific for *Escherichia coli* serotype 06 and lysozymes were noted even at temperatures between 68° and 77° F (20° and 25° C).[166] Sigman-Grant and colleagues reported that the microwave heating of infant formula did not adversely affect riboflavin or vitamin C, ingredients in infant formula that are typically monitored to determine if formula degradation has occurred.[167] They also stated that microwave heating could be as safe as heating infant formula with a commercial bottle warmer if a few principles were followed. They made the following recommendations for microwaving infant formula[167]:

- Heat only *refrigerated* formula, 4 oz or more at one time.
- Make sure the formula bottle is uncovered to allow heat to escape during microwaving.
- Make sure the formula bottle is standing upright in the microwave oven.
- Heat on full power for no more than 30 seconds for 4 oz of formula; 45 seconds for 8 oz of formula.
- After heating, replace the nipple assembly and invert the bottle 10 times.
- Test the formula's temperature before feeding. This can be done by testing a few drops of formula on your tongue or on the top part of your hand. The formula should be cool to the touch; if it is warm to your touch, it is too warm to feed to an infant.

Ready-to-use formula in bottles requires no preparation. Bottles can be stored at room temperature and the formula does not need to be warmed before feeding. The protective cap must be removed and a sterile nipple screwed onto the bottle before feeding. The bottle should be shaken to allow for adequate formula mixing. After feeding, the bottle and any unused formula should be discarded.[157] Ready-to-use formula in cans also needs no preparation. The top of the can should be washed with soap and hot water, shaken to allow for formula mixing, and then opened with a clean punch-type opener. Formula is then added to one bottle for a single feeding or to the bottles needed for a full day's feeding. If the latter is done, the bottles should be covered and refrigerated until needed. Formula remaining in the can may be covered and stored in the refrigerator for as long as 48 hours.

Formulas have specific instructions for preparation and most formulas have symbols on the cans of concentrated formula, ready-to-use formula, and powders that can be used as guidelines in formula preparation. Formula containers should be checked for expiration dates and dents. Parents should store unopened formula where it will not be subjected to extreme temperature changes.[157]

Frequency of Feedings

The frequency of feeding for a newborn infant will vary from every 2 hours to every 4 hours. Smaller infants usually require more frequent feedings because they have lower stomach capacities and shorter stomach emptying times. Breast-fed infants desire more frequent feedings than do bottle-fed infants. Infants usually lengthen the interval between feedings to 4 hours by the time they are 3–4 weeks old. Typically, infants begin to stop nighttime feedings by the age of 3–6 weeks.[87] Average numbers of daily feedings for infants of different ages are shown in Table 14.

By the end of the first week of life, full-term infants increase the volume of their feedings from 30 mL to between 80 and 90 mL. The amount of formula offered to a bottle-fed infant should be consistent with the RDA for energy based on age and weight. The infant should be fed on demand and should not be forced to take more formula than is desired at any one feeding. If the infant finishes a bottle and still seems hungry, another bottle should be offered. An infant who is no longer losing weight by 7 days of age and who is gaining weight by 2 weeks of age appears to be receiving an appropriate amount of formula.[87] Thereafter, growth curves (weight, height, and head circumference) are used to determine whether an infant is growing appropriately. Table 15 lists typical quantities of feedings by age.

Product Selection Guidelines

For healthy full-term infants without the need for a therapeutic formula, a milk-based formula or milk-based formula with added whey protein is indicated. When recommending a type of formula, the pharmacist should consider the method of preparation, the parents' ability

TABLE 14 Number of daily feedings, according to age

Age	Average number of daily feedings
Birth–1 wk	6–9
1 wk–1 mo	6–8
1–3 mo	5–6
3–4 mo	4–5
4–8 mo	3–4
8–12 mo	3

Adapted from Barness LA. Nutrition and nutritional disorders: nutritional requirements. In: Behrman RE, ed. *Nelson Textbook of Pediatrics*. 14th ed. Philadelphia: WB Saunders; 1992: 105–30.

TABLE 15 Quantity of milk ingested per feeding, according to age

Age	Average quantity of milk per feeding (oz)
Birth–2 wk	2–3
3 wk–2 mo	4–5
2–3 mo	5–6
3–4 mo	6–7
5–12 mo	7–8

Adapted from Barness LA. Nutrition and nutritional disorders: nutritional requirements. In: Behrman RE, ed. *Nelson Textbook of Pediatrics*. 14th ed. Philadelphia: WB Saunders; 1992: 105–30.

to follow directions, the parents' attitudes and preferences, and the sanitary conditions and refrigeration facilities available.

For many parents, cost may be a critical factor in selecting an infant formula. Concentrated liquids and powdered formula preparations are less expensive than ready-to-use products. Convenience is also a consideration. The preparation of powdered and concentrated liquid formulas requires more manipulative functions and more attention to aseptic technique. The formula selected should be one that is well tolerated by the infant, convenient for the parents to prepare, and priced to fit the family's budget.

Case Studies

Case 20–1

Patient Complaint/History

A mother presents to the pharmacist with JJ, her 2-month-old infant son who has a 2-day history of frequent spitting up; irritability; and frequent loose, watery stools. The mother is purchasing acetaminophen for the infant's mild fever. She asks for advice on changing infant formulas because JJ is "not tolerating his formula."

In discussing the infant's symptomatology, the pharmacist determines that the infant weighs 13 lb and that the mother administers saline nose drops and uses a nasal aspirator prior to the infant's feedings if he has mild to moderate congestion. There is no family history of food allergy or formula intolerance.

Clinical Considerations/Strategies

The following considerations/strategies are provided to aid the reader in (1) determining whether treatment of the patient's condition with nonprescription medications is warranted, (2) selecting the appropriate nonprescription medication, and (3) developing a patient counseling strategy to ensure optimal therapeutic outcomes:

- Determine what additional questions the pharmacist should ask to give the mother appropriate advice and why these questions are relevant to this case.
- If the infant's pediatrician thinks that the symptoms are related to a sequelae of a self-limiting viral gastroenteritis, determine what strategies to consider in resuming formula feedings after resolution of the symptoms with clear liquids appropriate for the infant's age (eg, Pedialyte, an oral electrolyte solution).
- If specialized strategies are used in resuming formula feedings, determine at what point to make the transition to the infant's usual formula.
- Develop a patient education/counseling strategy that will instruct the mother on techniques and precautions to use in preparing a powder formulation of the infant's usual formula.

Case 20–2

Patient Complaint/History

EA, the 30-year-old mother of a 2-day-old infant, presents a prescription for a postpartum analgesic (acetaminophen/hydrocodone); she also asks for refills of her prescription oral contraceptive and albuterol inhaler. The mother reveals that she is breast-feeding and requests information about her medications and the advisability of breast-feeding while taking them. EA's patient profile shows that mild asthma is her only chronic health concern; the dosage shown for the albuterol inhaler is two puffs qid prn for wheezing. The prescription oral contraceptive, ethinyl estradiol 35 mcg/norethindrone 0.5 mg, was last filled 16 months ago. After confirming the information on her profile, the patient reports that her physician has advised her to continue taking one prenatal vitamin tablet daily.

Clinical Considerations/Strategies

The following considerations/strategies are provided to aid the reader in (1) determining whether treatment of the patient's condition with nonprescription medications is warranted, (2) selecting the appropriate nonprescription medication, and (3) developing a patient counseling strategy to ensure optimal therapeutic outcomes:

- Assess the advisability of the patient breast-feeding while taking either of the medications shown on her profile as well as any new medications.
- Consider alternative nonprescription or nondrug alternatives to opioid-containing analgesics in controlling mild postpartum pain.
- Develop a patient education/counseling strategy that will optimize the efficacy of the patient's medications while minimizing the infant's exposure to them during breast-feeding.

References

1. Garza C, Hopkinson J. Physiology of lactation. In: Tsang RC, Nichols BL, eds. *Nutrition during Infancy*. St Louis: CV Mosby; 1988: 20–32.
2. Lawrence RA. Breastfeeding and medical disease. *Med Clin North Am*. 1989; 73: 583–603.

3. Cunningham AS, Jelliffe DB, Jelliffe EF. Breast-feeding and health in the 1980s: a global epidemiological review. *J Pediatr.* 1991; 118: 659–66.

4. Jason J. Breast-feeding in 1991. *N Engl J Med.* 1991; 325: 1036–8. Editorial.

5. Cone TE Jr. Infant feeding redux. *Pediatrics.* 1990; 86: 473–4.

6. Martinez GA, Krieger FW. 1984 milk-feeding patterns in the US. *Pediatrics.* 1985; 76: 1004–8.

7. Fomon SJ. Reflections on infant feeding in the 1970s and 1980s. *Am J Clin Nutr.* 1987; 46(suppl 1): 171–82.

8. Hoekelman RA. Highs and lows in breast-feeding rates. *Pediatr Ann.* 1992; 21: 615–7.

9. Ryan AS et al. Recent declines in breast-feeding in the US, 1984 through 1989. *Pediatrics.* 1991; 88: 719–27.

10. Batten S, Hirschman J, Thomas D. Impact of the Special Supplemental Food Program on infants. *J Pediatr.* 1990; 117(suppl): S101–9.

11. Losch M et al. Impact of attitudes on maternal decisions regarding infant feeding. *J Pediatr.* 1995; 126: 507–13.

12. Public Health Service. *Healthy People 2000: National Health Promotion and Disease Prevention Objectives—Full Report, with Commentary.* DHHS Pub No PHS 90-50212. Washington, DC: US Department of Health and Human Services; 1990

13. Hansen JW et al. Human milk substitutes. In: Tsang RC, Nichols BL, eds. *Nutrition during Infancy.* St Louis: CV Mosby; 1988: 378–98.

14. Jones EG. In: Kelts DG, Jones EG, eds. *Manual of Pediatric Nutrition.* Boston: Little, Brown; 1984: 17–34.

15. Redel CA, Shulman RJ. Controversies in the composition of infant formulas. *Pediatr Clin North Am.* 1994; 41: 909–24.

16. Hamilton JR. Gastrointestinal tract: normal digestive tract phenomena. In: Behrman RE, ed. *Nelson Textbook of Pediatrics.* 14th ed. Philadelphia: WB Saunders; 1992: 935–40.

17. Watkins JB. Lipid digestion and absorption. *Pediatrics.* 1985; 75(suppl): 151–6.

18. Hamosh M et al. Lipids in milk and the first steps in their digestion. *Pediatrics.* 1985; 75(suppl): 146–50.

19. Pipes PL. Infant feeding and nutrition. In: Pipes PL, ed. *Nutrition in Infancy and Childhood.* 5th ed. St Louis: Times Mirror/Mosby College Publishing; 1993: 87–120.

20. Ziegler EE, Fomon SJ. Potential renal solute load of infant formulas. *J Nutr.* 1989; 119(suppl): 1785–8.

21. Pipes PL. Nutrition: growth and development. In: Pipes PL, ed. *Nutrition in Infancy and Childhood.* 5th ed. St Louis: Times Mirror/Mosby College Publishing; 1993: 1–29.

22. Fomon SJ et al. Body composition of reference children from birth to age 10 years. *Am J Clin Nutr.* 1982; 35: 1169–75.

23. Hamil PV et al. Physical growth: National Center for Health Statistics percentiles. *Am J Clin Nutr.* 1979; 32: 607–29.

24. National Center for Health Statistics. NCHS growth curves for children, birth–18 years, 1977. *Vital and Health Statistics: Data from the National Health Survey; 165.* Series 11. DHEW Pub No DHS 78–1650 (PHS). Hyattsville, Md: US Department of Health, Education, and Welfare, Public Health Service; Nov 1977.

25. Dewer KG et al. Growth of breast-fed and formula-fed infants from 0 to 18 months: the DARLING study. *Pediatrics.* 1992; 89(6): 1035–41.

26. Lubchenco LO et al. Intrauterine growth as estimated from live born birth-weight data at 24 to 42 weeks of gestation. *Pediatrics.* 1963; 32: 793–800.

27. Lubchenco LO, Hansman C, Boyd E. Intrauterine growth in length and head circumference as estimated from live births at gestational ages from 26 to 42 weeks. *Pediatrics.* 1966; 37: 403–8.

28. Food and Nutrition Board, Commission on Life Sciences, National Research Council. *Recommended Dietary Allowances.* 10th ed. Washington, DC: National Academy Press; 1989.

29. Davies PSW, Gregory J, White A. Energy expenditure in children aged 1.5 to 4.5 years: a comparison with current recommendations for energy intake. *Eur J Clin Nutr.* 1995; 49: 360–4.

30. Kliegman RM, Behrman RE. The fetus and neonatal infant: the digestive system. In: Behrman RE, ed. *Nelson Textbook of Pediatrics.* 14th ed. Philadelphia: WB Saunders; 1992: 474–81.

31. Pipes PL. Nutrient needs of infants and children. In: Pipes PL, ed. *Nutrition in Infancy and Childhood.* 5th ed. St Louis: Times Mirror/Mosby College Publishing; 1993: 29–57.

32. Committee on Nutrition, American Academy of Pediatrics. Plant fiber intake in the pediatric diet. *Pediatrics.* 1981; 67: 572–5.

33. Picone TA et al. Growth, serum biochemistries, and amino acids of term infants fed formulas with amino acid and protein concentrations similar to human milk. *J Pediatr Gastroenterol Nutr.* 1989; 9: 351–60.

34. Sanchez-Pozo A et al. Changes in the protein fractions of human milk during lactation. *Ann Nutr Metab.* 1986; 30: 15–20.

35. Polberger SKT, Axelsson IE, Raiha NCR. Amino acid concentrations in plasma and urine in very low birthweight infants fed protein-unenriched or human milk protein-enriched human milk. *Pediatrics.* 1990; 86: 909–15.

36. Boehm G et al. Protein quality of human milk fortifier in low birth weight infants: effects on growth and plasma amino acid profiles. *Eur J Pediatr.* 1993; 152: 1036–9.

37. Itabashi K et al. Fortified preterm human milk for very low birth weight infants. *Early Hum Dev.* 1992; 29: 339–43.

38. Gaull G, Sturman JA, Raiha NCR. Development of mammalian sulfur metabolism: absence of cystathionase in human fetal tissues. *Pediatr Res.* 1972; 6: 538–47.

39. Rassin DK, Sturman JA, Gaull GE. Taurine and other free amino acids in milk of man and other mammals. *Early Hum Dev.* 1978; 2: 1–13.

40. Gaull GE. Taurine in pediatric nutrition: review and update. *Pediatrics.* 1989; 83: 433–42.

41. Michalk DV et al. The development of heart and brain function in low-birth-weight infants fed with taurine-supplemented formula. *Adv Exp Med Biol.* 1987; 217: 139–45.

42. Committee on Nutrition, American Academy of Pediatrics. Prudent life-style for children: dietary fat and cholesterol. *Pediatrics.* 1986; 78: 521–5.

43. Committee on Nutrition, American Academy of Pediatrics. Commentary on breast-feeding and infant formulas, including proposed standards for formulas. *Pediatrics.* 1976; 57: 278–85.

44. Schlenk H. Odd numbered and new essential fatty acids. *Federal Proc.* 1972; 31: 1430–5.

45. Friedman ZA et al. Rapid onset of essential fatty acid deficiency in the newborn. *Pediatrics.* 1976; 58: 640–9.

46. Gross S, Melhorn DK. Vitamin E, red cell lipids and red cell stability in prematurity. *Ann N Y Acad Sci.* 1972; 203: 141–62.

47. Committee on Nutrition, American Academy of Pediatrics. Nutritional needs of low-birth-weight infants. *Pediatrics.* 1977; 60: 519–30.

48. Dicks-Bushnell MW, Davis KC. Vitamin E content of infant formulas and cereals. *Am J Clin Nutr.* 1967; 20: 262–9.

49. Bonjour JP. Biotin in human nutrition. *Ann N Y Acad Sci.* 1985; 447: 97–104.

50. Committee on Nutrition, American Academy of Pediatrics. Calcium requirements in infancy and childhood. *Pediatrics.* 1978; 62: 826–34.

51. Mizrahi A, London RD, Gribetz D. Neonatal hypocalcemia—its causes and treatment. *N Engl J Med.* 1968; 278: 1163–5.

52. Committee on Nutrition, American Academy of Pediatrics. Nutritional needs of low-birth-weight infants. *Pediatrics.* 1985; 75: 976–86.

53. Dallman PR. Iron, vitamin E, and folate in the preterm infant. *J Pediatr.* 1974; 85: 742–52.

54. Prasad AS, Oberleas D. Zinc deficiency in man. *Lancet.* 1974; 1: 463–4.

55. Committee on Nutrition, American Academy of Pediatrics.

Vitamin and mineral supplement needs in normal children in the United States. *Pediatrics.* 1980; 66: 1015–21.

56. Calvo EB, Galindo AC, Aspres NB. Iron status in exclusively breast-fed infants. *Pediatrics.* 1992; 90: 375–9.
57. O'Connor P. Vitamin D–deficiency rickets in two breast-fed infants who were not receiving vitamin D supplementation. *Clin Pediatr.* 1971; 16: 361–3.
58. Fomon SJ et al. Recommendations for feeding normal infants. *Pediatrics.* 1979; 63: 52–9.
59. Bachrach S, Fisher J, Parks JS. An outbreak of vitamin D deficiency rickets in a susceptible population. *Pediatrics.* 1979; 64: 871–7.
60. Higginbottom MC, Sweetman L, Nyhan WL. A syndrome of methylmalonic aciduria, homocystinuria, megaloblastic anemia and neurologic abnormalities in a vitamin B_{12}–deficient breast-fed infant of a strict vegetarian. *N Engl J Med.* 1978; 299: 317–23.
61. Saarinen UM, Siimes MA, Dallman PR. Iron absorption in infants: high bioavailability of breast milk iron as indicated by the extrinsic tag method of iron absorption and by the concentration of serum ferritin. *J Pediatr.* 1977; 91: 36–9.
62. Committee on Nutrition, American Academy of Pediatrics. Fluoride supplementation: revised dosage schedule. *Pediatrics.* 1979; 63: 150–2.
63. Committee on Nutrition, American Academy of Pediatrics. Fluoride supplementation. *Pediatrics.* 1986; 77: 758–61.
64. Committee on Nutrition, American Academy of Pediatrics. Formula feeding of infants. In: Forbes GB, Woodruff CW, eds. *Pediatric Nutrition Handbook.* Elk Grove Village, Ill: American Academy of Pediatrics; 1985: 16–27.
65. Oski FA. Iron-fortified formulas and gastrointestinal symptoms in infants: a controlled study. *Pediatrics.* 1980; 66: 168–70.
66. Nelson SE et al. Lack of adverse reactions to iron-fortified formula. *Pediatrics.* 1988; 81: 360–4.
67. Montalto MB, Benson JD, Martinez GA. Nutrient intakes of formula-fed infants and infants fed cow milk. *Pediatrics.* 1985; 75: 343–51.
68. Hittner HM et al. Retrolental fibroplasia: efficacy of vitamin E in a double-blind clinical study of preterm infants. *N Engl J Med.* 1981; 305: 1365–71.
69. Stevens D et al. Folic acid supplementation in low birthweight infants. *Pediatrics.* 1979; 64: 333–5.
70. Benkov KJ, LeLeiko NS. A rational approach to infant formulas. *Pediatr Ann.* 1987; 16: 225–6, 228, 230.
71. Raiha NC. Nutritional proteins in milk and the protein requirement of normal infants. *Pediatrics.* 1985; 75(suppl): 136–41.
72. Sheard NF. Cow's milk, diabetes, and infant feeding. *Nutr Rev.* 1993; 51: 79–81.
73. Klish WJ. Special infant formulas. *Pediatr Rev.* 1990; 12: 55–62.
74. Giovannini M, Agostoni C, Riva E. Fat needs of term infants and fat content of milk formulae. *Acta Paediatr.* 1994; 402(suppl): 59–62.
75. Decsi T, Koletzko B. Polyunsaturated fatty acids in infant nutrition. *Acta Paediatr.* 1994; 395(suppl): 31–7.
76. Greer FR. Calcium, phosphorus, and magnesium: How much is too much for infant formulas? *J Nutr.* 1989; 119(suppl): 1846–51.
77. Chierici R, Gamboni C, Bigi V. Milk formulae for the normal infant. III: lipids and trace elements. *Acta Paediatr.* 1994; 402(suppl): 50–6.
78. Milner JA. Trace minerals in the nutrition of children. *J Pediatr.* 1990; 117(suppl): S147–55.
79. Pugliese MT. Parental health beliefs as a cause of nonorganic failure to thrive. *Pediatrics.* 1987; 80: 175–82.
80. Taras HL. Early childhood diet: recommendations of pediatric health care providers. *J Am Diet Assoc.* 1988; 88: 1417–21.
81. Oski FA. Whole cow milk feeding between 6 and 12 months of age? Go back to 1976. *Pediatr Rev.* 1990; 12: 187–9.
82. Woodruff CW. Milk intolerances. *Nutr Rev.* 1976; 34: 33–7.
83. Committee on Nutrition, American Academy of Pediatrics. The use of whole cow's milk in infancy. *Pediatrics.* 1983; 72: 253–5.
84. Ziegler EE. Milk and formulas for older infants. *J Pediatr.* 1990; 117(suppl): S76–9.
85. Committee on Nutrition, American Academy of Pediatrics. The use of whole cow's milk in infancy. *Pediatrics.* 1992; 89: 1105–9.
86. Sullivan PB. Cows' milk induced intestinal bleeding in infancy. *Arch Dis Child.* 1993; 68: 240–5.
87. Barness LA. Nutrition and nutritional disorders: nutritional requirements. In: Behrman RE, ed. *Nelson Textbook of Pediatrics.* 14th ed. Philadelphia: WB Saunders; 1992: 105–30.
88. Committee on Nutrition, American Academy of Pediatrics. Supplemental foods for infants. In: Forbes GB, Woodruff CW, eds. *Pediatric Nutrition Handbook.* 2nd ed. Elk Grove Village, Ill: American Academy of Pediatrics; 1985: 28–36.
89. Wilson JT. *Drugs in Breast Milk.* Sydney, Australia: ADIS Press; 1981.
90. Kirksey A, Groziak SM. Maternal drug use: evaluation of risks to breast-fed infants. *World Rev Nutr Diet.* 1984; 43: 60–79.
91. Forsyth JS. Is it worthwhile breast-feeding? *Eur J Clin Nutr.* 1992; 46(suppl 1): S19–S25.
92. Duncan B et al. Exclusive breast-feeding for at least 4 months protects against otitis media. *Pediatrics.* 1993; 91: 867–72.
93. Kovar MG et al. Review of the epidemiologic evidence for an association between infant feeding and infant health. *Pediatrics.* 1984; 74(suppl): 615–38.
94. Poland RL, Schultz GE, Garg G. High milk lipase activity associated with breast milk jaundice. *Pediatr Res.* 1980; 14: 1328–31.
95. Poland RL. Breast-milk jaundice. *J Pediatr.* 1981; 99: 86–8. Editorial.
96. Hopkinson JM, Garza C. Management of breastfeeding. In: Tsang RC, Nichols BL, eds. *Nutrition during Infancy.* St Louis: CV Mosby; 1988: 298–313.
97. Ruff AJ et al. Breast-feeding and maternal–infant transmission of human immunodeficiency virus type 1. *J Pediatr.* 1992; 121: 325–7.
98. Committee on Infectious Diseases, American Academy of Pediatrics. Summaries of infectious diseases: AIDS and HIV infections. In: Peter G et al, eds. *Report of the Committee on Infectious Diseases.* 22nd ed. Elk Grove Village, Ill: American Academy of Pediatrics; 1991: 115–31.
99. Briggs GG, Freeman RK, Yaffe SJ. *Drugs in Pregnancy and Lactation.* 4th ed. Baltimore: Williams & Wilkins; 1994.
100. Miller GH, Hughes LR. Lactation and genital involution effects of a new low-dose oral contraceptive on breast-feeding mothers and their infants. *Obstet Gynecol.* 1970; 35: 44–50.
101. Lonnerdal B, Forsum E, Hambraeus L. Effect of oral contraceptives on composition and volume of breast milk. *Am J Clin Nutr.* 1980; 33: 816–24.
102. Hull VJ. The effects of hormonal contraceptives on lactation: current findings, methodological considerations, and future priorities. *Stud Fam Plann.* 1981; 12: 134–55.
103. World Health Organization Task Force on Oral Contraceptives. Effects of hormonal contraceptives on breast milk composition and infant growth. *Stud Fam Plann.* 1988; 19: 361–9.
104. Koetsawang S. The effects of contraceptive methods on the quality and quantity of breast milk. *Int J Gynaecol Obstet.* 1987; 25(suppl): 115–27.
105. Committee on Drugs, American Academy of Pediatrics. Breast-feeding and contraception. *Pediatrics.* 1981; 68: 138–40.
106. Committee on Drugs, American Academy of Pediatrics. Transfer of drugs and other chemicals into human milk. *Pediatrics.* 1989; 84: 924–36.
107. Anderson PO. Drug use during breast-feeding. *Clin Pharm.* 1991; 10: 594–624.

108. Atkinson HC, Begg EJ. Prediction of drug distribution into human milk from physicochemical characteristics. *Clin Pharmacokinet.* 1990; 18: 151–67.

109. Atkinson HC, Begg EJ, Darlow BA. Drugs in human milk. Clinical pharmacokinetic considerations. *Clin Pharmacokinet.* 1988; 14: 217–40.

110. Sagraves R. Drugs in breast milk. In: Kuhn RJ, Piecoro JJ Jr, Shannon MC, eds. *Pediatric Pharmacotherapy.* Lexington, Ky: University of Kentucky; 1991. Module 28.

111. Briggs GG. Drugs in pregnancy and lactation. In: Young YL, Koda-Kimble MA, eds. *Applied Therapeutics: The Clinical Use of Drugs.* 5th ed. Vancouver, Wash: Applied Therapeutics Inc; 1992: 1–33.

112. Committee on Nutrition, American Academy of Pediatrics. Proposed changes in Food and Drug Administration regulations concerning formula products and vitamin–mineral dietary supplements for infants. *Pediatrics.* 1967; 40: 916–22.

113. Food and Drug Administration. Nutrient requirements for infant formulas. *Federal Register.* 1985; 50: 45106–8.

114. Silver LB et al. Learning disabilities as a probable consequence of using a chloride-deficient infant formula. *J Pediatr.* 1989; 115: 97–9.

115. Malloy MH et al. Hypochloremic metabolic alkalosis from ingestion of a chloride-deficient infant formula: outcome 9–10 years later. *Pediatrics.* 1991; 87: 811–22.

116. Food and Drug Administration. Infant formula: labeling requirements. *Federal Register.* 1985; 50: 1833–40.

117. Filer LJ. A glimpse into the future of infant nutrition. *Pediatr Ann.* 1992; 21: 633–6, 639.

118. Chicago and Suburban Dietetics Association. Nutritional care of the high risk infant. In: *Manual of Clinical Dietetics.* Chicago: American Dietetics Association; 1988: 115–37.

119. Santeiro ML, Sagraves R, Allen LV Jr. Osmolality of small-volume iv admixtures for pediatric patients [published erratum *Am J Hosp Pharm.* 1990; 47: 1978]. *Am J Hosp Pharm.* 1990; 47: 1359–64.

120. Anderson TA, Fomon SJ, Filer LJ. Carbohydrate tolerance studies with 3-day-old infants. *J Lab Clin Med.* 1972; 79: 31–7.

121. *Comparison of Feeding of Infants and Young Children in the Hospital.* Columbus, Ohio: Ross Laboratories; 1990.

122. Tomarelli RM. Osmolality, osmolarity, and renal solute load of infant formulas. *J Pediatr.* 1976; 88: 454–6.

123. Lifschitz CH. Carbohydrate needs in preterm and term newborn infants. In: Tsang RC, Nichols BL, eds. *Nutrition during Infancy.* St Louis: CV Mosby; 1988: 122–32.

124. Committee on Nutrition, American Academy of Pediatrics. Soy-protein formulas: recommendations for use in infant feeding. *Pediatrics.* 1983; 72: 359–63.

125. Lonnerdal B. Nutritional aspects of soy formula. *Acta Paediatr.* 1994;(suppl 402): 105–8.

126. Merritt RJ et al. Whey protein hydrolysate formula for infants with gastrointestinal intolerance to cow milk and soy protein in infant formulas. *J Pediatr Gastroenterol Nutr.* 1990; 11: 78–82.

127. Gerrand JW et al. Cow milk allergy: prevalence and manifestations in an unselected series of newborns. *Acta Paediatr Scand.* 1973; 234(suppl): 1–21.

128. Goel K et al. Monosaccharide intolerance and soy-protein hypersensitivity in an infant with diarrhea. *J Pediatr.* 1978; 93: 617–9.

129. Powell GK. Milk- and soy-induced enterocolitis of infancy: clinical features and standardization of challenge. *J Pediatr.* 1978; 93: 553–60.

130. Committee on Nutrition, American Academy of Pediatrics. Hypoallergenic infant formulas. *Pediatrics.* 1989; 83: 1068–9.

131. Sampson HA. Safety of casein hydrolysate formula in children with cow milk allergy. *J Pediatr.* 1991; 118(suppl): 520–5.

132. Barr RG et al. Feeding and temperament as determinants of early infant crying/fussing behavior. *Pediatrics.* 1989; 84: 514–21.

133. Lothe L, Lindberg T. Cow's milk whey protein elicits symptoms of infantile colic in colicky formula-fed infants: a double-blind crossover study [published erratum *Pediatrics.* 1989; 84: 17]. *Pediatrics.* 1989; 83: 262–6.

134. *Pediatric Products Handbook.* Evansville, Ind: Mead Johnson Nutritionals; 1993.

135. Andrews BF, Lorch V. Improved fat and CA absorption in LBW infants fed a medium chain triglyceride containing formula. *Pediatr Res.* 1974; 8: 378. Abstract.

136. Tantibhedhyangkul P, Hashim SA. Medium-chain triglyceride feeding in premature infants: effects on calcium and magnesium absorption. *Pediatrics.* 1978; 61: 537–45.

137. Tantibhedhyangkul P, Hashim SA. Medium-chain triglyceride feeding in premature infants: effects on fat and nitrogen absorption. *Pediatrics.* 1975; 55: 359–70.

138. Businco L, Cantani A, Longhi MA. Severe anaphylactic reactions following cow's milk protein hydrolysates (CMPHs) ingestion. *Pediatr Res.* 1987; 22: 222. Abstract

139. Businco L et al. Anaphylactic reactions to a cow's milk whey protein hydrolysate (Alfa-Ré, Nestlé) in infants with cow milk allergy. *Ann Allergy.* 1989; 62: 333–5.

140. Forbes GB. Is human milk the best food for low birthweight babies? *Pediatr Res.* 1978; 12: 434.

141. Dallman PR. Upper limits of iron in infant formulas. *J Nutr.* 1989; 119(suppl): 1852–4.

142. Thompson M, McClead RE. Human milk fortifiers. *J Pediatr Perinatal Nutr.* 1987; 1(Fall/Winter): 65–75.

143. Ehrenkranz RA, Gettner PA, Nelli CM. Nutrition balance studies in premature infants fed premature formula or fortified preterm human milk. *J Pediatr Gastroenterol Nutr.* 1989; 8: 58–67.

144. Kashyap S et al. Growth, nutrient retention, and metabolic response of low-birth-weight infants fed supplemented and unsupplemented preterm human milk. *Am J Clin Nutr.* 1990; 52: 254–62.

145. Committee on Nutrition, American Academy of Pediatrics. Follow-up or weaning formulas. *Pediatrics.* 1989; 83: 1067.

146. Johnsen D, Nowjack-Raymer R. Baby bottle tooth decay (BBTD): issues, assessment, and an opportunity for the nutritionist. *J Am Diet Assoc.* 1989; 89: 2–6.

147. Moss MH. Hypoprothrombinemic bleeding in a young infant: association with a soy protein formula. *Am J Dis Child.* 1969; 117: 540–2.

148. Goldman HI, Amadio P. Vitamin K deficiency after the newborn period. *Pediatrics.* 1969; 44: 745–9.

149. Cochrane WA, Collins-Williams C, Donohue WL. Superior hemorrhagic polioencephalitis (Wernicke's disease) occurring in an infant—probably due to thiamine deficiency from use of a soy bean product. *Pediatrics.* 1961; 28: 771–7.

150. Molony CJ, Parmelee AH. Convulsions in young infants as a result of pyridoxine (vitamin B_6) deficiency. *JAMA.* 1954; 154: 405–6.

151. Hydovitz JD. Occurrence of goiter in an infant on a soy diet. *N Engl J Med.* 1960; 262: 351–3.

152. Roy S III, Arant BS Jr. Alkalosis from chloride-deficient Neo-Mull-Soy. *N Engl J Med.* 1979; 301: 615. Letter.

153. Holick MF et al. The vitamin D content of fortified milk and infant formula. *N Engl J Med.* 1982; 326: 1178–81.

154. Kulkarni PB et al. Rickets in very low-birth-weight infants. *J Pediatr.* 1980; 96: 249–52.

155. Finberg L. One milk for all—not ever likely and certainly not yet. *J Pediatr.* 1980; 96: 240–1. Editorial.

156. Litov RE et al. Plasma aluminum measurements in term infants fed human milk or a soy-based infant formula. *Pediatrics.* 1989; 84: 1105–7.

157. *How to Prepare Your Baby's Infant Formula.* Evansville, Ind: Mead Johnson Nutritionals; 1991.

158. McJunkin JE, Bithoney WG, McCormick MC. Errors in formula concentration in an outpatient population. *J Pediatr.* 1987; 111: 848–50.

159. Haschke F, Pietschnig B, Vanura H. Infant formulas improperly prepared from powdered cow milk. *J Pediatr.* 1988; 113: 163. Letter.

160. Owen GM et al. A study of nutritional status of preschool children in the United States, 1968–1970. *Pediatrics.* 1974; 53(suppl): 597–646.

161. Committee on the Fetus and the Newborn, American Academy of Pediatrics. Sterilization of milk-mixtures for infants. *Pediatrics.* 1961; 28: 674–5.

162. Hughes RB et al. Outcome of teaching clean vs terminal methods of formula preparation. *Pediatr Nurs.* 1987; 13: 275–6.

163. Gerber MA, Berliner BC, Karolus JJ. Sterilization of infant formula. *Clin Pediatr.* 1983; 22: 344–9.

164. Howard CR, Weitzman M. Breast or bottle: practical aspects of infant nutrition in the first 6 months. *Pediatr Ann.* 1992; 21: 619–21, 625–7, 630–1.

165. Nemethy M, Clore ER. Microwave heating of infant formula and breast milk. *J Pediatr Health Care.* 1990; 4: 131–5.

166. Quan R et al. Effects of microwave radiation on anti-infective factors in human milk. *Pediatrics.* 1992; 89: 667–9.

167. Sigman-Grant M, Bush F, Anantheswaran R. Microwave heating of infant formula: a dilemma resolved. *Pediatrics.* 1992; 90: 412–5.

CHAPTER 21

Weight Control Products

Paul L. Doering

Questions to ask in patient assessment and counseling

- *What is your age, height, and weight?*
- *Why are you trying to lose weight?*
- *How long have you had a weight problem?*
- *How many pounds overweight do you think you are?*
- *Is there a family history of obesity? Do either of your parents have a weight problem?*
- *Do you eat a nutritionally sound diet? How much do you know about nutrition?*
- *Have you consulted a physician about your desire to lose weight?*
- *Are you or have you been on a diet to help you lose weight?*
- *What weight loss preparations have you used previously? How did they work?*
- *Do you have a regular exercise program? Does your physician recommend that you exercise?*
- *Are you being treated for any chronic disease such as hypertension, angina, diabetes, or a thyroid condition?*
- *What medications, both prescription and nonprescription, are you currently taking?*

A health paradox exists in America today: many people who do not need to lose weight are trying to do so, and most who do need to lose weight are not succeeding. Why are so many people trying to modify the way they look? Many seek to improve their self-images. These people may or may not be overweight or have physical or emotional health problems caused by their weight; in fact, some are of normal or even low weight. Some persons are severely overweight by current medical standards and attempt to lose weight to reduce their risk for weight-related health problems. Other people attempt weight reduction to improve their own perception of their health.

Every period of history has had its own standards of physical beauty. Each culture develops different notions about the proper size, shape, and decoration of the body. Between 1959 and 1978, the body weight and measurements of contestants in the Miss America Pageant decreased significantly.[1] But even though this theoretical "perfect" woman has become leaner in the past 20 years, the average American woman has actually become heavier.

The media can have a profound effect on the health practices of Americans. Viewers of popular television shows see and hear of the health successes of stars and average people alike and thus become motivated and enthusiastic to begin their own quest for renewed health and beauty. When a popular talk show hostess announced on a November 1988 show that she had lost 67 pounds by using Optifast, a very low calorie diet (VLCD) formula (described in the Weight Loss Methods section), the product's manufacturer reportedly received 1 million telephone inquires from people interested in using the formula diet to lose weight.[2]

In December 1988, the *Journal of Consulting and Clinical Psychology* published a report by a well-respected group of obesity researchers describing the long-term effectiveness of their obesity treatments, including, a VLCD.[3] The disappointing results from this study showed that the large initial weight losses (mean of 31 lb) were poorly maintained: after 1 year, patients had regained two thirds of their weight back. Three years after treatment, the average subject was back to within 5 lb of his or her original weight. The two alternative treatments in the study, behavioral therapy and the combination of behavioral therapy and a VLCD, fared no better.

Overall, obese persons experience a lower quality of life.[4] Federal health authorities have thus targeted a reduction in the prevalence of overweight as a national health objective to be achieved by the year 2000.[5] Pharmacists who understand the problems of obesity and can communicate the health risks associated with overweight can help motivate patients to set realistic, attainable weight loss goals for themselves and avoid being victims of diet fads or scams.

Body Fat and Obesity

Obesity can be defined as an excessive accumulation of body fat to the extent that it is thought to impair health. When the percentage of body fat equals or exceeds 30% of total weight in women or 25% in men, an individual is considered obese. Severe obesity is characterized by a body fat content that exceeds 40% in women or 35% in men.

The fat distribution after puberty is characteristically different in men and women. Women tend to store

Editor's Note: This chapter is based, in part, on the chapter with the same title that appeared in the 10th edition but was written by Glenn D. Appelt.

TABLE 1 Metropolitan height and weight tables for men and women according to frame, ages 25–29

Men				Women			
	Weight in (lb)[b]				Weight (lb)[b]		
Height (in.)[a]	Small frame	Medium frame	Large frame	Height (in.)[a]	Small frame	Medium frame	Large frame
62	128–134	131–141	138–150	58	102–111	109–121	118–131
63	130–136	133–143	140–153	59	103–113	111–123	120–134
64	132–138	135–145	142–156	60	104–115	113–126	122–137
65	134–140	137–148	144–160	61	106–118	115–129	125–140
66	136–142	139–151	146–164	62	108–121	118–132	128–143
67	138–145	142–154	149–168	63	111–124	121–135	131–147
68	140–148	145–157	152–172	64	114–127	124–138	134–151
69	142–151	148–160	155–176	65	117–130	127–141	137–155
70	144–154	151–163	158–180	66	120–133	130–144	140–159
71	146–157	154–166	161–184	67	123–136	133–147	143–163
72	149–160	157–170	164–188	68	126–139	136–150	146–167
73	152–164	160–174	168–192	69	129–142	139–153	149–170
74	155–168	164–178	172–197	70	132–145	142–156	152–173
75	158–172	167–182	176–202	71	135–148	145–159	155–176
76	162–176	171–187	181–207	72	138–151	148–162	158–179

[a]Shoes with 1-in. heels.

[b]Indoor clothing weighing 5 lb for men and 3 lb for women.

Source of basic data: Society of Actuaries and Association of Life Insurance Medical Directors of America. *Build Study, 1979.* New York: Metropolitan Life Insurance Company; 1983.

fat in the breasts, hips, and thighs (gynecoid distribution) whereas men tend to accumulate fat in the abdomen (android distribution). However, some women have a relatively central (or android) fat distribution whereas some men exhibit a predominantly peripheral (or gynecoid) fat distribution. An android fat distribution may be more strongly associated with atherosclerosis, diabetes mellitus, and gouty arthritis than a similar amount of fat in a gynecoid distribution.

Methods of Determining Obesity

When is a person considered "overweight"? What level of overweight is associated with adverse health risks? When should a person decide to lose weight? The answers to these questions may not be as clear as once thought. Some patients will seek the help of a dietitian or nutritionist before deciding on when and how to diet, while others will seek the pharmacist's guidance in determining their weight status. It is important to understand some key points relative to the measurement of weight and body fat, the expression of "normal" or "ideal" weight, and the limitations in using the latter term.

Measuring Body Fat

Unfortunately, aside from postmortem analyses of cadavers, there are no truly direct ways to measure body fat. However, close estimates of percentage of body fat can be made indirectly through an assessment of body density. Because fat and fat-free mass have different specific densities, a comparison of a person's weight under water versus out of water allows a determination of the proportion of body weight that is fat. This underwater weighing method currently is considered the "gold standard" for assessing body fat. However, it is a cumbersome procedure that is not always practical for routine clinical purposes.

An easier way to assess body fat is by measuring skinfold thickness, but this approach can suffer from problems related to the reliability of its measurement. Newer methods, such as x-ray densitometry and bioelectrical impedance, have been developed for assessing body fat but have not found their way into clinical practice. Ultrasound has been used to estimate body fat; however, using calibrated fiberglass tape to take circumference measurements of certain body parts may provide a better estimation. The waist-to-thigh ratio has been reported to be an appropriate index for upper and central body fat distribution, especially in women.

TABLE 2 Body weights corresponding to height and body mass index[a]

	Body mass index (kg/m²)													
	19	**20**	**21**	**22**	**23**	**24**	**25**	**26**	**27**	**28**	**29**	**30**	**35**	**40**
Height (in.)	Body weight (lb)													
58	91	96	100	105	110	115	119	124	129	134	138	143	167	191
59	94	99	104	109	114	119	124	128	133	138	143	148	173	198
60	97	102	107	112	118	123	128	133	138	143	148	153	179	204
61	100	106	111	116	122	127	132	137	143	148	153	158	185	211
62	104	109	115	120	126	131	136	142	147	153	158	164	191	218
63	107	113	118	124	130	135	141	146	152	158	163	169	197	225
64	110	116	122	128	134	140	145	151	157	163	169	174	204	232
65	114	120	126	132	138	144	150	156	162	168	174	180	210	240
66	118	124	130	136	142	148	155	161	167	173	179	186	216	247
67	121	127	134	140	146	153	159	166	172	178	185	191	223	255
68	125	131	138	144	151	158	164	171	177	184	190	197	230	262
69	128	135	142	149	155	162	169	176	182	189	196	203	236	270
70	132	139	146	153	160	167	172	181	188	195	202	207	243	278
71	136	143	150	157	165	172	179	186	193	200	208	215	250	286
72	140	147	154	162	169	177	184	191	199	206	213	221	258	294
73	144	151	159	166	174	182	189	197	204	212	219	227	265	302
74	148	155	163	171	179	186	194	202	210	218	225	233	272	311
75	152	160	168	176	184	192	200	208	216	224	232	240	279	319
76	156	164	172	180	189	197	205	213	221	230	238	246	287	328

[a]To use the table, find the appropriate height in the left-hand column; then move across the row to a given weight. The number at the top of the column is the body mass index for the height and weight.

Reprinted with permission from NIH Technology Assessment Conference Panel. Methods for voluntary weight loss and control. *Ann Intern Med.* 1993; 119(7 pt 2): 764–70.

Because of the difficulties inherent in measuring body fat, relative weight has become the most popular and convenient indicator of obesity. Relative weight is calculated by dividing a person's actual weight by the ideal weight for his or her height and sex (Table 1). A relative weight of 1.20 or greater (ie, 20% or more over ideal weight) is used as an operational definition of obesity.[6]

Problems occur when using relative weight or percentage overweight as an indicator of obesity. First, a person may be overweight without being obese. The increased weight may reflect increased muscle mass rather than fat, as is often seen in weight lifters or other athletes. Second, the point of overweight at which increased risk for disease occurs is not clear. The cutoff point of 20% overweight is an arbitrary rather than precise point above which a pathologic state may be seen. Third, as discussed in the next section, the concept of ideal weight, as used in professional and lay literature, is based on information derived from samples that were not representative of the US population.

Determining Ideal Weight

The most popular weight tables developed over the years have been those published by the Metropolitan Life Insurance Company; the 1983 Metropolitan Life Table is in use today (Table 1). Until the 1983 table was published, selection of the appropriate body frame was left to the judgment of the person or the physician. The 1983 table used elbow breadth for men and women at different weight ranges to identify the three frame categories.

The current Metropolitan Life Insurance table was developed based on findings from the 1979 Build Study (conducted by the Society or Actuaries and Association of Life Insurance Medical Directors of America).[7] Weights of individuals associated with the lowest mortality were derived from 4.2 million life insurance policies issued between 1950 and 1971. The study included a disproportionately larger number of men, Caucasians, and individuals from middle and upper socioeconomic strata, and it omitted people over age 59. The so-called ideal weights used to compile the 1983 tables may therefore require adjustment for age, as they are too liberal for young adults and too restrictive for persons in their 50s and 60s.[7] In fact, they accurately reflect the life insurance experience only for those persons about 40–45 years of age.

Calculating Body Mass Index

The 1985 National Institutes of Health Consensus Development Conference on obesity[6] recommended that body mass index (BMI) be used as an appropriate measure of the tendency toward obesity. In this capacity, BMI offers several advantages over relative weight. It is derived by dividing weight in kilograms by the square of height in meters. For persons of average height, one BMI unit is equivalent to approximately 3.1 kg (6.8 lb) in men and 2.6 kg (5.8 lb) in women. The 1985 conference concluded that, in young persons, a BMI greater than 27 increases the risk for morbidity and death. Table 2 presents body weight by height and in correspondence with selected BMI values. The table can be used to gauge an individual's approximate BMI value quickly without making an exact calculation.

Prevalence of Obesity

Previous national estimates of overweight in the United States were based on data from the second National Health and Nutrition Examination Survey (NHANES II) of 1976–1980. Since then, a new estimate for the prevalence of overweight for the entire adult population and for sex, age, and racial/ethnic groups has been published from phase 1 (1988–1991) of the third NHANES study (NHANES III). This estimate shows some disturbing trends.[8]

In NHANES III, BMI was used as a measure of weight for height. Overweight was defined as a BMI value of greater than or equal to 27.8 for men and 27.3 for women. These are the sex-specific 85th percentile values for BMI for men and women aged 20 through 29 years from NHANES II. These values represent approximately 124% of desirable weight for men and 120% of desirable weight for women, desirable weight being defined as the midpoint of the range of weights for a medium frame from the 1983 Metropolitan Life tables (Table 1), after appropriate adjustment for clothing and shoes.

Results of NHANES III indicate that, overall, approximately one third (33.4%) of all adults in the United States are overweight. The prevalence of overweight varies by race/ethnicity, sex, and age. For men, the prevalence is highest among Mexican/Americans (35.5%). For women, there are larger differences among racial/ethnic groups, ranging from 32.9% for non-Hispanic Caucasian women to 46.7% for Mexican-American women and 48.6% for non-Hispanic African-American women. These estimates indicate that nearly half of all adult non-Hispanic African-American and Mexican-American women in the United States are overweight.

Comparison of the 1988–1991 data for adults aged 20 through 74 years with data from earlier surveys indicates dramatic increases in the prevalence of overweight. During the period covered by the previous surveys, the estimated prevalence of overweight for these adults increased slightly both overall and within race/sex groups. However, between NHANES II (1976–1980) and NHANES III phase 1 (1988–1991), there was a much larger increase, especially among Caucasian and African-American adults both overall and for each 10-year increment of age. The increase was largest for Caucasian men and women, ranging from 8 to 9%, and was somewhat less for African-American men and women.

Between NHANES II and NHANES III phase 1, the mean weight of adults aged 20 through 74 years increased by approximately 3.6 kg. Based on 1990 population estimates of the civilian noninstitutionalized population from the US Census Bureau, 58 million US adults (26 million men and 32 million women) are currently overweight. The increase in the prevalence of overweight suggests that the national health status objective that was set to reduce overweight to a prevalence of no more than 20% by the year 2000[5] may not be met. Indeed, the trend appears to be moving away from rather than toward this objective.

Adolescent overweight is also increasing in prevalence. Among the 1490 study participants between the ages of 12 and 19 years for whom complete height and weight data were collected in NHANES III, the prevalence of overweight was 21%, an increase of 6% over that reported in NHANES II. As with adults, this trend is disturbing, and it may be attributed to the decrease in physical exercise undertaken by today's youth. These data also show a move in the wrong direction from the health objective for the year 2000 to achieve a prevalence of overweight among adolescents not to exceed 15%.

Etiology of Obesity

Simply put, excess weight gain in our population is determined by an imbalance between caloric intake and energy expenditure. The physiologic controls of caloric intake have been difficult to define. However, it is well known that the human body aggressively responds to underweight with an enhanced hunger and a decreased metabolic rate, yet it counteracts the accumulation of excess weight poorly. This may derive from the age-old struggle for survival, with the primary risks to the species historically being death due to famine rather than the danger of excess food.

Caloric Intake and Fat Distribution

Most obesity is associated with overeating, particularly of carbohydrates or fats. The calories ingested beyond those necessary for normal energy requirements usually are deposited and stored as fat. To avoid obesity, individuals must decide how much and what type of food to consume.

Daily caloric allowances for persons with moderate physical activity may vary with age and sex. As a general rule, an intake of 3,500 Cal (kcal) over expenditure will produce a weight gain of approximately 0.454 kg (1 lb) whereas an expenditure of 3,500 Cal over intake will result in a 0.454-kg (1-lb) loss of body fat. Daily caloric allowances for average men (weight = 70 kg or 154 lb;

height = 1.78 m or 5 feet 10 inches) in a temperate climate range from 3,200 Cal at 25 years of age to 2,550 Cal at 65 years of age. Corresponding figures for average women (weight = 58 kg or 128 lb; height = 1.63 m or 5 feet 4 inches) are 2,300 and 1,800 Cal at ages 25 and 65, respectively. The daily caloric requirement for women increases slightly during pregnancy (by 300 Cal) and significantly during lactation (by 500 Cal for one child and 1,000 Cal for twins).

Why people take in more calories than they need may be related to physiologic, genetic, social and environmental, or psychologic factors, or to an interrelationship of two or more of these factors.

Physiologic Factors

Lack of Appetite Control The hypothalamus of the brain contains centers that are involved in the food ingestion process: studies of the rat hypothalamus show a "satiety center" and an "appetite center." Destroying the satiety center leads to marked overeating with subsequent obesity; obliterating the appetite center results in emaciation. These results indicate that impulses from the satiety center may inhibit feedback of the appetite center after food is ingested. The glucostatic hypothesis of appetite regulation states that hunger is related to the degree to which glucose is used by cells called glucostats. When glucose use by glucostats in the satiety center is low, the inhibitory effect on the appetite center is reduced, favoring eating behavior. Conversely, when glucose use is high, the appetite center is inhibited and the desire for food intake is reduced.

The hypothalamus contains a high concentration of noradrenergic terminals. A discrete fiber system that supplies the hypothalamus with most of its norepinephrine-secreting terminals is called the ventral noradrenergic bundle. Food-induced enhancement of sympathetic activity is modulated by the ventral noradrenergic bundle; in animals with lesions of this region, food intake increased significantly. It has been suggested that the ventral noradrenergic bundle normally mediates satiety and may serve as a substrate for amphetamine-induced appetite suppression. Destroying the noradrenergic terminals in the hypothalamus or damaging the ventral noradrenergic bundle results in obesity in animals.

Visual and chemical food-related stimuli are interpreted in the cerebral cortex, the area of the central nervous system (CNS) that is involved in accepting or rejecting the sight, aroma, or taste of food. An obese person may respond differently to the appearance, taste, or smell of food than a person of normal weight. Endogenous opioids increase food intake in animals, and naloxone (an opioid antagonist) decreases food intake in animals and in obese humans. Opiate receptors, which exist in the taste pathways, are believed to modulate human taste. Thus, an emerging hypothesis suggests that an endogenous opioid system is involved in human gustatory perceptions. Research involving the trigeminal nerve, a pathway relaying sensory input from the oral cavity to the hypothalamus, supports this system's possible role in food intake. The trigeminal circuit is a system of oral touch, and the excessive nibbling common to obese individuals may be caused by their greater sensitivity to this stimulus.

Thermogenesis Theory Some researchers believe that thin and obese people differ in the degree of thermogenesis that occurs after food ingestion. Overeating in nonobese subjects causes increased heat production, which tends to dissipate the excess calories. In obese subjects, the dissipation of thermal energy may be less pronounced, resulting in fat storage. Animal models of obesity have indicated a defective thermogenic component, but the evidence for this metabolic defect in human obesity is largely circumstantial. A subnormal thermogenic response to food has been reported in the obese and the postobese. Although these studies may be criticized on the grounds that reductions in diet-induced thermogenesis (DIT) may not be a cause but rather a result of the obesity and/or the metabolic adaptation to a low caloric intake, the concept of defective DIT in the etiology of obesity remains provocative.

The thermogenesis theory was expanded to include a specialized form of fat tissue (brown fat), which participates in thermogenesis. The exact role of brown fat is unclear, but it appears to favor increased triglyceride hydrolysis. Animal studies have indicated that sympathetic denervation of brown fat results in an increase in body fat in lean animals and an increase in norepinephrine turnover in brown fat during elevated DIT. The ability of norepinephrine to stimulate activity of brown adipose tissue further implicates the sympathetic branch of the autonomic nervous system in obesity. Several reports present evidence that, in humans, the thermogenic response to food plays an important role in the relationship of the sympathetic nervous system to brown fat.

Enzyme Activity A biochemical basis for obesity involving sodium-potassium adenosine triphosphatase (ATPase) has been suggested. This enzyme facilitates the sodium-potassium pump process in body cells, which could result in caloric expenditure. Red blood cells in obese people were noted to have lower levels of sodium-potassium ATPase as compared with those in individuals of normal weight. Individuals with reduced sodium-potassium ATPase activity burn fewer calories and thus may be more likely to store fat than those individuals with normal enzyme activity.

Excessive Fat Cells Another hypothesis suggests that the presence of excessive fat cells in infancy may predispose an individual to obesity later in life. Obese patients not only have larger than normal fat cells but also have an increased number of these cells. Apparently, as people lose weight on a low-calorie diet (LCD), the size of each fat cell decreases but their total number remains the same; when these people return to increased weight levels, their fat cells regain their original size. Obesity in children may result from the addition of new fat cells whereas "adult onset obesity" may represent an expansion of fat cells already present. Previous experiments suggest that the earlier the onset of obesity, the greater the number of fat cells. After the age of 20, obesity is caused almost exclusively by the expansion of existent cells. Accordingly, an overweight child or adolescent may be more susceptible to obesity as an adult.

Other Physiologic Factors The correlation of a primitive "hibernation response" with human obesity has been proposed. Adaptive reactions that prepare the body for an impending shortage may be predominant in the obese individual. Although humans do not hibernate, an "endomorphic system" may be present to initiate the overeating typical of most obese persons. It is suggested that this "hunger reaction" may be initiated by the beta-endorphins.

The connection that exists between metabolism and sleep may be related to obesity. Obesity has been correlated with the frequency of ultraradian brain rhythms (rapid eye movement [REM] and non-REM sleep). This observation lends credence to the proposal that the amount of sleep decreases in obese people when they lose weight whereas sleep time increases when anorectic patients gain weight.

Endocrine disorders, such as hypothyroidism or Cushing's syndrome, are apparently rarely involved in causing obesity per se. Obesity may result from an anatomic or biochemical lesion in the brain's feeding centers; however, this hypothesis has not been proven in humans.

Genetic Factors

Genetics plays a prominent role in obesity. A child who has one obese parent has a 40% chance of being obese; if both parents are obese, the child's chance of obesity increases to 80%. Twinning studies demonstrate a 0.86 concordance for obesity.[9] These data suggest a direct genetic component, as evidenced by the extraordinarily high prevalence of obesity in Native Americans and Pima Indians, and although this component has not been absolutely proven in human obesity, it has been indicated in animal studies. In experimental animals, genetic transmission of obesity is associated with modified organ size and composition. Human data also suggest fundamental relationships between body build and obesity. Studies reveal that obese women differ from nonobese women in morphologic characteristics other than the degree of adiposity. Specifically, obese women are more endomorphic than nonobese women: Their abdomen mass overshadows their thoracic bulk, all their regions are notably soft and round, and their hands and feet are relatively small.

Social and Environmental Factors

Obesity may result from environmental influences such as the widespread advertising of food products. Occupational, economic, sociocultural, and lifestyle factors may also be considered in the broad environmental sense. Obesity is seven times more common among women of low socioeconomic status than among those of higher status, a trend that is similar although less marked in men. The mental health indices of obese subjects in the low socioeconomic group reflect immaturity, rigidity, and suspiciousness compared with those of normal weight individuals in the same group; a defect in impulse control may be suggested by the immaturity rating. The prevalence of obesity in lower socioeconomic classes is first noted in early adulthood. Suggestive relationships between ethnic and religious factors and obesity have also been noted for both sexes.

In today's society, people have numerous labor-saving devices, both at work and at play. Moreover, leisure-time activities often involve passive entertainment such as watching television or playing computer games rather than active sports. A sedentary way of life and a lack of exercise contribute to the problem of obesity.

Psychologic Factors

Obesity has a psychogenic component in the vast majority of cases. Although the psychologic aspect of caloric excess is usually exemplified by compulsive overeating replacing other gratifications, other factors are also involved. Decreased physical activity often coexists with mental depression and may play a role in obesity. Depression may not be an incidental occurrence in obese people but rather one of the main reasons for the obesity.

Consequences of Obesity

Health Risks

Studies have shown a significant association between morbidity, early mortality, and obesity. The health care costs to this country of the morbidity related to obesity were estimated at $39 billion in 1986.[10]

Cardiovascular Disease Cardiovascular diseases (eg, hypertension, myocardial infarct, heart failure, and coronary artery disease) and cerebrovascular diseases (eg, stroke) are associated with obesity. There is evidence that sustained hypertension is more common in overweight people. In the Framingham Heart Study, nonsmoking men whose body weights were more than 10% above the ideal weight had 30-year mortality rates that were 3.9 times higher than those of men of desirable weight.[11] Therefore, persons at high risk for hypertension, such as those with a family history of youthful obesity, should consider controlling their weight and reducing their salt intake.

Diabetes Mellitus The relationship between obesity and diabetes mellitus is well documented. (See Chapter 18, "Diabetes Care Products and Monitoring Devices.") An early study revealed that 85% of patients over 40 years of age who developed diabetes mellitus were overweight. Glucose intolerance commonly occurs with obesity, and relative insulin resistance is noted in obese subjects although insulin production may be normal or high. Obesity that persists over long periods is generally associated with partial exhaustion of the beta cells and a resultant hypoinsulinemia. The hyperinsulinemia that occurs in obesity of shorter duration is related to increased body fat. Weight reduction leads to improved glucose tolerance in obese persons with diabetes and to reduced hyperinsulinemia in obese persons both with and without diabetes. It may also decrease or eliminate the severity of diabetes mellitus and the need for insulin or oral sulfonylureas.

Skin Disorders Certain skin disorders, including candidiasis, tinea infections, furunculosis, pruritus vulvae, and trophic ulcerations, occur more often in obese individuals. These conditions have also been associated with diabetes mellitus, which may explain their particularly high incidence in obese persons. Entrapment of moisture in skinfolds, which produces a better culture medium for some microorganisms, is certainly a contributing factor.

Cancer In postmenopausal women, obesity appears to be positively related to the risk of both breast and endometrial cancer. Obesity is also associated with increased estrogen production, which is proportionately more significant in postmenopausal women because the ovaries no longer contribute to production of estrogen. The peripheral aromatization of androstenedione (a major adrenal hormone) to estrone via the aromatase reaction in adipose tissue is the principal source of estrogen in postmenopausal women; an increased rate of this reaction has been reported in obese women. Excess estrogen production predisposes women to the development of breast and endometrial neoplasms.

Hyperlipidemia Obesity-associated hyperlipidemia may be related to cholesterol gallstone formation because the level of cholesterol is characteristically elevated in obesity. The positive effects and associated health benefits of weight reduction on lipoprotein levels are well documented.

Respiratory Problems Excessive obesity may contribute to respiratory distress, impaired gas exchange, and pulmonary embolism. Obesity alters pulmonary function, resulting in reduced lung volume, hypercapnia, and pulmonary hypertension. Charles Dickens' description of Joe, the fat boy in *The Pickwick Papers*, as obese and somnolent may be the first account of this condition in literature; the pickwickian syndrome describes a person who is obese, exhibits narcoleptic behavior, and has an excessive appetite.

Other Health Risks Although obesity is generally caused by overeating, it may mask malnutrition. Often the obese individual overconsumes carbohydrates and fats while omitting other nutrients such as protein, vitamins, and minerals from the diet.

Obesity may predispose individuals to the development of gout, may aggravate degenerative joint disease (osteoarthritis) in weight-bearing joints (eg, knees and ankles), may produce or aggravate lower back pain, and may be associated with menstrual irregularities.

Data on the health effects of repeated weight gains and losses, or weight cycling, are also inconclusive. Weight cycling appears to affect energy metabolism and may result in the faster regaining of weight, but the contention that weight cycling has long-term negative effects on psychologic and physical health needs confirmation.

Social and Economic Consequences

Obesity may create a psychologic burden and lead to low self-esteem. Dexterity, coordination, and mobility may be impaired, which can have serious implications in a job situation. Among very obese individuals, weight loss has been followed by greater functional status, reduced work absenteeism, less pain, and greater social interaction.

Studies have shown a striking inverse relationship between obesity and socioeconomic status in the developed world, especially among women. Gortmaker et al studied the relationship between overweight (BMI above the 95th percentile for age and sex) and educational attainment, marital status, household income, and self-esteem in 10,039 randomly selected individuals aged 16–24 years in 1981.[12] To assess the social consequences of obesity, the investigators compared disability from obesity with that associated with other forms of chronic illness. The prevalence of overweight was 3.4% in men and 3.9% in women (5.8% in African-American women versus 2.5% in non-Hispanic Caucasians). A follow-up study 7 years later indicated that the overweight women were less educated (0.3 fewer years of school), were less likely to be married (20%), had lower household incomes ($6,710 less), and had 10% higher rates of poverty than women who had not been overweight, independent of baseline socioeconomic status and aptitude test scores. Similar trends were found among the men.

The US Equal Opportunity Commission, responding to complaints of widespread discrimination against obese persons, has now declared obesity a protected category under the federal Americans with Disabilities Act.[12] It has been said that obesity causes chronic health problems that influence job status, yet subjects with chronic health problems who were not obese did not suffer from the same low attainments. In a 1993 letter in *JAMA*, Robert Yaes wrote, "Certainly, at a time when it is fashionable to claim that alcoholism and drug abuse are illnesses whose treatment should be covered by health insurance, it is inconsistent to blame fat people for their own condition."[13]

TABLE 3 Study of weight loss efforts in adolescents

	Female (%)	Male (%)
Self-perception		
Too fat	34	15
Too thin	7	16
Weight loss effort		
Trying to lose	44	15
Trying to gain	26	15
Trying to maintain	7	26
Doing nothing	23	44
Weight loss method used (past/present)		
Exercise	80	44
Diet pills	21	5
Vomiting	14	4

Information extracted from Serdula MK et al. Weight control practices of US adolescents and adults. *Ann Int Med.* 1993; 119(7pt2): 667–71.

Weight Loss Methods

Data from four recent federal surveys of health practices indicate that 33–40% of adult women and 20–24%

of men are currently trying to lose weight, with an additional 28% of each group trying to maintain their weight. Among women and men trying to lose weight, the reported time on a weight loss regimen in the past year averaged 6.4 and 5.8 months, respectively, and the number of attempts to lose weight in the past 2 years averaged 2.5 and 2.0, respectively.

Data about weight loss efforts among adolescents in the United States have been reported in at least two studies: (1) The Youth Risk Behavior Surveillance System, which collected data from a representative sample of US high school students in 1990,[14] and (2) the Behavioral Risk Factor Surveillance System, which collected data from adults in 38 states and the District of Columbia in 1989.[15] These studies used data derived from a self-administered questionnaire that inquired about weight loss practices during the previous 7 days. The results of these studies are shown in Table 3.

A variety of methods, alone or in combination, are used to accomplish weight loss. Different approaches are successful for different people. Below is a short discussion of common weight loss methods.

Dietary Change

Dietary change is the most commonly used weight loss strategy. Methods range from caloric restriction to changes in dietary proportions of fat, protein, and carbohydrate or use of macronutrient substitutes. Appropriate dietary programs can have positive health effects on factors other than weight loss. Short-term success for some of these methods has been documented, but information on their long-term effectiveness and safety for up to 5 years is limited. Weight loss at the end of relatively short-term programs can exceed 10% of initial body weight; however, there is a strong tendency to regain the weight—as much as two thirds of it within 1 year after completing the program and almost all of it after 5 years. Importantly, however, a small percentage of participants do maintain their weight loss over more extended periods. The duration of most dietary change programs appears to be from several weeks to a few months. Dropout rates can be as high as 80% and seem to vary considerably.

Caloric Restriction

Two levels of caloric restriction are commonly used. The low-calorie diet (LCD) of about 1,000–1,500 kcal per day may involve a structured commercial program with formulated and calorically defined food products or with guidelines for selecting conventional foods. The very-low calorie diet (VLCD) at 800 or fewer calories per day is conducted under physician supervision and monitoring and should be restricted to severely overweight persons.

VLCDs and fasting are associated with a variety of short-term adverse effects. Patients often report fatigue, hair loss, dizziness, and other symptoms, but these appear to be transitory. The increased risk for gallstones and acute gallbladder disease during severe caloric restriction is more serious.

Total fasting or semistarvation is sometimes proposed as a means of weight reduction in severely obese persons. However, starvation, either total or partial, depletes the body of some lean tissue (protein) and essential electrolytes in addition to fat. The ketosis and ketoacidosis that result from a fasting state represent a significant metabolic alteration. If total fasting is used to treat obesity, hospitalization and intensive medical supervision are recommended to deal effectively with the alteration of physiologic functions.

Altered Proportions of Food Groups

High-protein, low-carbohydrate diets of 800–1,000 Cal (kcal) per day are often used in weight reduction programs. Low-carbohydrate diets have been advocated on the premise that individuals may eat as much as they desire as long as no carbohydrates are ingested. However, fat from food may be deposited as fat in the body, and proteins may be converted into fat. The excess fat metabolized may result in an increased production of ketones to the degree that ketosis, acidosis, and dehydration may occur.

Some low-carbohydrate diets recommend the inclusion of large quantities of fat. But although a high-fat diet may suppress fat synthesis, it does not prevent fat deposition. Additionally, a high-fat diet can cause the elevation of serum lipids. And while a carbohydrate-free, high-fat diet does bring about an immediate weight reduction owing to water loss (dehydration), it does not significantly affect adiposity. The "drinking-man's diet" adds alcohol to this regimen, which tends to add more calories and the increased liability of fat deposition. A high-meat (protein and fat), no-carbohydrate diet presents an extra burden to the kidneys because of the resultant increase in urea load. In addition, an increase in the uric acid levels in this diet may precipitate gouty arthritis in susceptible persons.

A low-protein, low-fat rice diet, which was advocated several years ago, is unbalanced and could lead to ill health. A diet containing kelp, vinegar, lecithin, and vitamin B_6 has been proposed. Excess kelp, which contains high amounts of iodine, may decrease thyroid function by negative feedback mechanisms. The other ingredients in this diet do not have any established value in weight reduction. The weight loss in this diet is due to the low caloric intake rather than to the use of these specific additives.

The extent of injuries and deaths caused by the use of extremely low calorie protein diets is unclear. The complaints reported to the Food and Drug Administration (FDA) often include nausea, vomiting, diarrhea (from liquid preparations), constipation (from dry preparations), faintness, muscle cramps, weakness or fatigue, irritability, cold intolerance, decreased libido, amenorrhea, hair loss, dry skin, cardiac arrhythmias, recurrence of gout, dehydration, and hypokalemia. Studies oriented toward geographic incidence, concurrent pathology, age, and other factors need careful scrutiny. The possibility of drug-food interactions with these diets also exists. Patients taking prescription medicines such as diuretics, antihypertensives, hypoglycemic agents, insulin, adrenergics, high doses of corticosteroids, thyroid preparations other than those used in replacement therapy, and lithium should not use the liquid protein diet.

The patient's age should also be taken into consideration because elderly obese persons may be more susceptible to cardiovascular stress, diabetes, and gout. Thus, the pharmacist should warn the patient not to undertake this type of diet without proper medical supervision.

A low-calorie, balanced diet containing no less than 12–14% protein, no more than 30% fat (preferably unsaturated), and the remainder composed of complex carbohydrates (low sucrose) is recommended over unbalanced diets of questionable value that are also potentially dangerous.

Contraindications to Unsupervised Dieting

Weight loss is indicated for persons with current health problems that can be lessened by weight loss (such as sleep apnea, hypertension, or non-insulin-dependent diabetes mellitus). However, unsupervised weight loss is contraindicated for severely overweight persons, pregnant or lactating women, children, persons over age 65, and those with medical conditions that make such an undertaking dangerous. For persons at high medical risk, a properly trained physician should be involved in a multidisciplinary approach to care throughout the weight loss process. Diets of 800 or fewer calories per day should not be undertaken without medical supervision and monitoring because of attendant health risks.

For those within the height/weight range who are not obese but desire to lose weight for other reasons, such as improved appearance or sense of well-being, the decision to lose weight should take into account the difficulty of the task as well as the potential adverse physical and psychologic effects of weight loss regimens. These effects include the risk of poor nutrition, the possible development of eating disorders, the effects of weight cycling, and the sometimes serious psychologic consequences of repeated failed attempts at weight loss.

TABLE 4 Caloric expenditure rates

Activity (1 h)	Calories expended
Bicycling (6 mph)	240
Bicycling (12 mph)	410
Cross-country skiing	700
Jogging (5.5 mph)	740
Jogging (7 mph)	920
Jumping rope	720
Running in place	650
Swimming (50 yd/min)	500
Tennis (singles)	400
Walking (2 mph)	240
Walking (3 mph)	320
Walking (4.5 mph)	440

Exercise

The amount of weight loss that can be achieved by exercise programs alone—usually from 4 to 7 lb—is more limited than the amount that can be obtained by caloric restriction. Table 4 lists the calories expended during 1 hour of various types of exercise. This amount is usually in addition to that lost through caloric restriction. Unfortunately, data indicate that the percentage of adults who exercise or play sports regularly decreased between 1985 and 1990 among African-American, Hispanic, lower-income, and unemployed persons.[16]

Behavioral Modification

Behavioral modification involves (1) identifying eating or related lifestyle behaviors to be modified, (2) setting specific behavioral goals, (3) modifying determinants of the behavior to be changed, and (4) reinforcing the desired behavior. Behavioral modification can be undertaken through group or individual sessions, under the guidance of professional or lay personnel, and alone or in conjunction with other approaches.

When used alone, the typical program takes about 18 weeks and can generate a 1–1.5 lb/wk weight loss. Typically about one third of this weight will be regained at the end of 1 year and most will be regained by 5 years after completion of the program.

Surgical Intervention

In refractory cases of severe obesity that pose a serious health threat, intestinal bypass operations have been performed. This procedure is probably the most hazardous and debatable measure used to treat extreme obesity, and it has led to alternative, perhaps safer, procedures such as gastric partitioning. Liposuction and other cosmetic surgical procedures are also used in some cases of obesity.

Drug Therapy

Drug therapy combined with some degree of caloric restriction can produce weight loss that is equivalent to that obtained with VLCDs alone over comparable periods. Renewed research interest in appetite suppressant drugs has led to some promising discoveries. The ideal appetite suppressant should have the following characteristics[17]:

- It should be safe and acceptable for long-term administration, as established by data documenting 6 months of efficacy and 2 years of safety.
- It should produce a dose-related reduction in body fat.
- It should spare body protein and other body tissues.

- It should be free of significant side effects and abuse potential.

Unfortunately, drugs available to date have not met these stringent criteria.

Dextroamphetamine

Introduced in the 1930s, dextroamphetamine was originally developed as a treatment for narcolepsy but was subsequently and serendipitously found to produce weight loss by reducing appetite. This initiated a new era of pharmaceutical therapy for obesity. Amphetamines, however, suffer from the serious disadvantage of having a substantial abuse potential. In an extensive review of more than 200 studies of the effectiveness of amphetamine-like drugs in the early 1970s, 90% of the studies showed more weight loss in the active drug group than in those subjects using placebo.[18] The drug-related weight loss, however, was small and variable. Of greatest concern is the apparent loss of effectiveness after a few short weeks of therapy. Although amphetamines are still labeled for short-term use as appetite suppressants, their use in weight loss programs has diminished greatly. Some states prohibit the prescribing of amphetamines and other related agents for diet purposes.

Fenfluramine

Fenfluramine, which resembles the amphetamines chemically but not pharmacologically, has advanced the understanding of appetite and its control. This drug acts to partially inhibit the reuptake of serotonin and to release serotonin from nerve endings. The increased serotonin in the neuronal cleft is believed to reduce food intake. The D-isomer of fenfluramine is available in Europe and, at the time of this writing, has been recommended for approval in the United States. This drug and the understanding of appetite control that has resulted from its research hold promise as advancements to the pharmacologic control of appetite when fenfluramine is approved in the United States.

Fenfluramine-Phentermine

This combination drug is being prescribed by large numbers of practitioners around the country, owing in part to widespread media attention given the research with these drugs. Phentermine inhibits reuptake of norepinephrine and has a stimulating effect while fenfluramine, through its effects on serotonin, may cause sleepiness. The combined mechanism seems to prevent the development of tolerance seen with phentermine alone. This combination was tried as an adjunct to behavioral, nutritional, and exercise counseling in a 34-week double-blind trial involving 121 obese patients weighing between 130% and 180% of ideal body weight. After 7 months, the average weight loss with 15 mg of phentermine and 60 mg of fenfluramine was 14.3 kg (31.5 lb), compared with 4.6 kg (10.1 lb) with placebo. In both groups, weight loss tended to level off after 18 weeks; beyond that period, the patients on placebo began to gain back the weight they had lost while active drug patients did not. After the double-blind study period, some patients remained on the medication at least intermittently for more than 2 years. Of the 121 patients who started the study, 112 completed 34 weeks and 51 completed 190 weeks. Four years after the start of the trial, only 3 of the patients still under surveillance weighed less than 120% of ideal body weight.[19]

Fluoxetine

Currently marketed as an antidepressant, fluoxetine inhibits serotonin uptake. Some patients taking this and other selective serotonin-reuptake inhibitors have lost weight. Several studies of 5- to 6-months' duration have shown significantly greater weight loss with fluoxetine than with placebo, especially when the drug is combined with behavioral modification or nutritional counseling.[20,21] Longer studies will help determine if weight loss will continue beyond this short period. At present, however, fluoxetine is not indicated for weight loss.

Drugs that interfere with food absorption, such as lipase inhibitors (eg, tetrahydrolipstatin or Orlisatat), and some that accelerate caloric loss, such as selective beta-adrenergic agonists, have been under study for several years. While preliminary data on the efficacy of these approaches are encouraging, if and when these drugs will be marketed is uncertain at this time.

Phenylpropanolamine

Drug treatment of obesity is of limited value because the only satisfactory means of long-term weight control is lifestyle change incorporating caloric reduction and increased physical activity. In 1992, the FDA issued a final rule establishing that 111 active ingredients in over-the-counter (OTC) weight control products are not generally recognized as safe and effective.[22] These products are listed in Table 5. The final monograph on OTC weight control products includes only phenylpropanolamine (PPA) and benzocaine as Category I drugs (see product table "Appetite Suppressant Products").

Mechanism of Action Anorexiants of the amphetamine class suppress appetite and reduce body weight by activating beta-adrenergic and/or dopaminergic receptors within the perifornical hypothalamus. Although PPA is often considered to be a member of the amphetamine class of anorexiants, it is an atypical adrenergic anorexiant.[23] Unlike amphetamine, PPA microinjected into the perifornical hypothalamus does not suppress feeding. Moreover, PPA-induced anorexia is not reversed by the dopamine antagonist haloperidol. Instead, the anorexic action of PPA may result, in part, from its interaction with $alpha_1$-adrenergic receptors within the paraventricular medial hypothalamus.

Some researchers think that anorexiants act primarily by lowering the body's metabolic set point and only secondarily by suppressing appetite.[24] This theory is supported largely by anecdotal reports of the rapid regaining of body weight after cessation of appetite suppressants in contrast to the relative stability of weight loss achieved without medication.

PPA is a sympathomimetic agent related chemically and pharmacologically to ephedrine. PPA stimulates both alpha- and beta-receptors and also acts indirectly by releasing norepinephrine from peripheral nerve endings. PPA exerts predominant peripheral adrenergic effects and weak central stimulant actions. In the past, controversy has existed as to PPA's effectiveness as an anorexigenic agent. Early studies indicate its usefulness in

TABLE 5 Ingredients determined by the FDA to be not generally recognized as safe and effective

Alcohol	Ferric ammonium citrate	Papain
Alfalfa	Ferric pyrophosphate	Papaya enzymes
Alginic acid	Ferrous fumarate	Pepsin
Anise oil	Ferrous gluconate	Phenacetin
Arginine	Ferrous sulfate (iron)	Phenylalanine
Ascorbic acid	Flax seed	Phosphorous
Bearberry	Folic acid	Phytolacca
Biotin	Fructose	Pineapple enzymes
Bone marrow, red	Guar gum	Plantago seed
Buchu	Histidine	Potassium citrate
Buchu, potassium extract	Hydrastis canadensis	Pyridoxine hydrochloride (vitamin B_6)
Caffeine	Inositol	Riboflavin
Caffeine citrate	Iodine	Rice polishings
Calcium	Isoleucine	Saccharin
Calcium carbonate	Juniper, potassium extract	Sea minerals
Calcium caseinate	Karaya gum	Sesame seed
Calcium lactate	Kelp	Sodium
Calcium pantothenate	Lactose	Sodium bicarbonate
Carboxymethylcellulose sodium	Lecithin	Sodium caseinate
Carrageenan	Leucine	Sodium chloride (salt)
Cholecalciferol	Liver concentrate	Soybean protein
Choline	Lysine	Soy meal
Chondrus	Lysine hydrochloride	Sucrose
Citric acid	Magnesium	Thiamine hydrochloride (vitamin B_1)
Cnicus benedictus	Magnesium oxide	Thiamine mononitrate (vitamin B_1 mononitrate)
Copper	Malt	Threonine
Copper gluconate	Maltodextrin	Tricalcium phosphate
Corn oil	Manganese citrate	Tryptophan
Corn silk, potassium extract	Mannitol	Tyrosine
Corn syrup	Methionine	Uva ursi, potassium extract
Cupric sulfate	Methylcellulose	Valine
Cyanocobalamin (vitamin B_{12})	Mono- and diglycerides	Vegetable
Cystine	Niacinamide	Vitamin A
Dextrose	Organic vegetables	
Docusate sodium	Pancreatin	
Ergocalciferol	Pantothenic acid	

Source: *Federal Register*. 1991 Aug; 56 (153): 37797.

diminishing food intake in animals, and a qualitative difference between the anorexigenic activities of PPA and amphetamines has been reported.[25] The weight-reducing action of PPA may reflect a combined effect on both food intake[26,27] and brown adipose tissue thermogenesis.[28]

In a physician-managed weight reduction program that included behavioral modification, mild caloric restriction, and exercise, subjects taking PPA lost significantly more weight (6.1 kg) than subjects taking placebo (4.3 kg).[29] And a 14-week study that evaluated the anorectic activity of 75-mg daily doses of PPA in 102 overweight subjects found PPA to be associated with significant weight loss as early as week 6 of the study and to be a superior anorexiant compared with placebo.[30] Studies evaluating the safety and efficacy of nonprescription anorexiants beyond 12–14 weeks are lacking. Long-term maintenance of weight loss remains the ultimate goal.

Dosage In 1982, the FDA Advisory Review Panel on Over-the-Counter Miscellaneous Internal Drug Products found PPA to be generally safe and effective for short-term weight control.[31] The FDA permits a PPA dose of up to 37.5 mg in immediate-release products and of up to 75 mg in sustained-release products. The maximum daily dose is set at 75 mg.[31]

Adverse Effects Side effects such as nervousness, restlessness, insomnia, dizziness, perspiration, anxiety, headache, nausea, and an excessive increase in blood pressure may occur with PPA, especially if the recommended dose is exceeded. Cardiovascular adverse reactions, including hypertensive episodes and stroke, have been reported following both excessive and recommended doses of products containing PPA alone or in combination with other drugs.[32] Hypertension has been cited as the most likely cause of PPA-associated intracranial hemorrhage.[33] Intracerebral hemorrhage and cerebral vasculitis have been associated with prolonged PPA use and with use at doses in excess of those recommended in package labeling.[34,35] Vascular etiology involving multiple focal areas of arterial narrowing and segmental vascular injury has been implicated in lobar subcortical and subarachnoid hemorrhages.[34] Various cardiac rhythm disturbances, myocardial infarct, and atrioventricular blockage have also been attributed to PPA.[36–40] Acute renal failure, sometimes associated with rhabdomyolysis, has been reported after PPA ingestion.[41–44]

Hypertensive reactions in previously normotensive individuals have been reported with exaggerated single oral doses of 85 mg PPA in an immediate-release product form.[45,46] Similarly, a double-blind study in young normotensive adults revealed that significant elevations in blood pressure may occur after a single dose of PPA.[47] There is evidence that the immediate-release product in these studies was a different isomer, (+)norpseudoephedrine, than the racemic form, (±)norephedrine, which is available in the United States.[48] Thus, it has been suggested that hypertensive effects are more likely to occur when PPA is in the immediate-release form than when it is in a sustained-release preparation.[49]

However, a review of prospective clinical trials indicated that PPA is an appropriately marketed nonprescription drug with an acceptable margin of safety.[50] Controlled clinical studies have demonstrated an absence of significant side effects or hypertensive activity with PPA in either obese patients[51] or healthy, nonobese subjects.[52,53] A study of obese normotensive patients[54] demonstrated the absence of significant pressor effects with a 75-mg sustained-release PPA product form, even when combined with caffeine. Other reports[55–57] document the absence of significant pressor effects with PPA in recommended nonprescription doses. Finally, the safety and efficacy of PPA at therapeutic doses was noted in a pilot study conducted with a population of adult patients with stable, controlled hypertension.[58]

CNS stimulation as evidenced by PPA-associated convulsive seizures has been noted,[59] as have been psychiatric adverse effects attributed to PPA.[60] Mental disturbances have been described in considerable detail, and the possibility of PPA-associated psychotic episodes clearly exists.[61,62] Amphetamine-like reactions to PPA have been reported from emergency room records over a 6-month period. All adverse CNS effects, which included respiratory stimulation, tremor, restlessness, increased motor activity, agitation, and hallucinations,[63] occurred within 1–2 hours after ingestion of PPA in combination with caffeine. Pharmacists should advise patients of the possible CNS adverse effects of PPA. However, although some clinicians believe PPA poses a danger to the public and should be regarded as a drug with potential for abuse,[64] a recent study provides evidence that PPA administered at recommended doses does not produce the euphoriant or stimulant subjective effects that characterize drugs of abuse.[65]

Although the FDA Advisory Review Panel on Over-the-Counter Cold, Allergy, Bronchodilator, and Antiasthmatic Drug Products did not review anorexiants as such, it concluded that the incidence of side effects with oral PPA is low at recommended doses.[66] Additionally, an analysis of 70 cases of accidental or deliberate overdose with PPA or PPA with caffeine revealed that symptoms such as nausea or vomiting, nervousness, headache, tachycardia, or dizziness occurred in adults only if the amount ingested exceeded the manufacturer's recommended dosage.[67]

Because PPA is an adrenergic substance, it may elevate blood glucose levels and produce cardiac stimulation. For these and other reasons, the labels on products containing PPA warn that individuals with diabetes mellitus, heart disease, hypertension, or thyroid disease should seek medical advice before taking this drug.

Drug Interactions A severe hypertensive episode was reported when indomethacin was taken with an 86-mg immediate-release form of PPA,[68,69] and psychotic reactions have been described with 50 mg of PPA consumed in combination with isopropamide and phenyltoloxamine.[70] PPA has also been implicated in drug-drug interactions with monoamine oxidase inhibitors,[71] and severe hypertensive episodes may be more likely when patients who are already taking monoamine oxidase inhibitors ingest preparations containing PPA in an immediate- rather than a sustained-release form.

Among other drug-drug interactions, PPA was found to cause various adverse effects when ingested concurrently with aspirin and acetaminophen (nausea, vomiting, headaches, weakness, malaise, and severe muscle tenderness; brown-colored urine; and acute interstitial nephritis)[72,73]; with thioridazine (fatal ventricular arrhythmia)[74]; with methyldopa or oxyprenolol (severe hypertension)[75]; and with fluphenazine treatment in conjunction with PPA overdose (catatonia).[76]

Evidence suggests a pharmacokinetic interaction of PPA with caffeine. Coadministration of a sustained-release PPA preparation and a sustained-release caffeine preparation increased plasma caffeine concentration fourfold and the concentration-time curve approximately threefold in human volunteers.[77] In another reported interaction, an additive increase in blood pressure occurred.[78] In a study of the effects of five drug preparations (75 mg PPA, 150 mg PPA, 75 mg PPA plus 400 mg caffeine, 400 mg caffeine, and placebo) in 16 resting, normotensive subjects, significant blood pressure increases occurred over several hours following the 150-mg dose of PPA and the 75-mg dose of PPA plus 400 mg caffeine but occurred less often after ingestion of 75 mg PPA alone and 400 mg caffeine alone.[79] PPA-induced hypertension has been treated with nifedipine[80] and propranolol.[81]

There is one report of a positive phentolamine test for pheochromocytoma in PPA-induced hypertension,[82] and a pseudopheochromocytoma syndrome has been described following PPA use.[83]

The reports of adverse reactions with PPA and PPA-containing combinations should be interpreted within the total context of use. Many of these reports involve only one case or report of multiple drug ingestion and are, in a sense, anecdotal in nature. Factors such as hypersensitivity, dosage and product forms ingested, concurrent pathology, and the presence of other drugs should be established before the use of PPA is discounted.[84] In fact, some of the very drugs implicated as causing drug-drug interactions are marketed as combination products (eg, cold remedies combining PPA and aspirin) without substantial risk of adverse effects.

Benzocaine

Benzocaine was first incorporated into a weight control preparation in 1958.[85] A preparation containing benzocaine and methylcellulose in chewing gum wafers was tried for 10 weeks in 50 patients who were 5.5–46 kg overweight. Results showed that 90% of the subjects lost weight. However, the study did not use a placebo control group, and the weight loss could have been caused by benzocaine, methylcellulose, or the diet alone. The benzocaine dose was small, and any marked degree of numbness in the oral cavity was questionable. It is conceivable that subtle effects on taste sensitivity or taste modification may occur, and perceived analgesia or numbness is not necessary for appetite suppressant activity.

When the two nonprescription anorectic drugs, PPA and benzocaine and their combination, were compared in a 30-patient study, benzocaine produced less weight loss than PPA ($P < .05$). Weight loss with PPA was not enhanced by combination with benzocaine.

Constant snacking is characteristic of the "oral syndrome" in many obese persons. A nontraditional appetite control plan using benzocaine, glucose, caffeine, and vitamins in a hard candy form was tried. The subjects ingested the candies when they wanted a snack and before and after meals; this approach kept the patients orally active while elevating their blood glucose levels. The influence of benzocaine was considered an essential component of the significant weight reduction in the study group.

Because capsules or tablets containing benzocaine are designed to be swallowed, the drug does not come in contact with the oral cavity. Thus, any appetite suppression would depend on an effect on the gastrointestinal mucosa. However, no conclusive clinical data support such an activity. The FDA Advisory Review Panel on Over-the-Counter Miscellaneous Internal Drug Products classified benzocaine as generally effective for short-term weight control. This panel also determined that a dose of 3–15 mg for use in gum, lozenges, or candy just prior to food consumption was generally safe and effective for weight control. However, the director of the FDA Monograph Review Staff does not agree with the advisory panel's assessment and has advised manufacturers of benzocaine-containing products of the FDA's intent to classify this agent as an ineffective weight loss product.[86] Citing serious design flaws in the clinical trials of oral benzocaine's efficacy, the FDA advised the manufacturers that additional data from properly conducted, well-designed studies is required to provide evidence that benzocaine alone provides a statistically significant weight loss when compared with placebo. In response to this advisory letter, most of the manufacturers have already removed benzocaine from their weight loss products.

Clinical Considerations

Obesity is a subject of intense study. Many factors affect metabolic equilibrium. Excessive eating (caloric intake) is the major cause of obesity, and caloric restriction is the cornerstone of any weight control program. Appetite control is only part of the answer, however, and use of pharmacologic agents tends to treat only the short-term manifestations. Where poor nutrition or psychologic factors contribute to overeating, self-therapy groups often help in treating the cause. Caloric expenditure by physical activity can promote maintenance of a nonobese state in the motivated individual. The rates at which various physical activities expend calories are presented in Table 4. When one considers that basal metabolism over a typical 24-hour period consumes approximately 1,000 Cal/m^2 body surface area (the average body surface area being 1.73 m^2), it is easy to see how significant exercise can be in accelerating weight loss.

The resistance of overweight conditions to treatment argues strongly for the need for pediatricians and family practitioners to emphasize preventive efforts beginning in childhood and continuing into adolescence and young adulthood. Guidelines were recently published to assist health care personnel in the identification of persons aged 10 through 24 years who are at risk for overweight.[87]

Dietary Food Supplements

Low-Calorie Balanced Foods

The "canned diet" products are considered substitutes for the usual diet. One product typical of this group supplies 70 g of protein per day, an amount the manufacturer states "is the recommended daily dietary allowance of protein for normal adults." It also contains 20 g of fat and 110 g of carbohydrate in a daily ration for a total daily caloric intake of 900 Cal. Powder, granule, and liquid forms are available; these products are also formulated as cookies and soups.

These dietary products are low in sodium. Weight loss in the first 2 weeks is probably caused, in part, by water loss from the tissues. It is questionable, whether a weight loss over a short period is significant with regard to the effective long-term treatment of obesity.

The pharmacist should be aware that products that substitute 900 Cal daily for the usual diet are usually effective in reducing weight. Moreover, it appears that any diet of 900 Cal that supplies adequate protein and lowers carbohydrate and fat intake should enable an obese patient to lose weight. Some manufacturers recommend that these products be used as substitutes for several meals a day, allowing the dieter to eat a "reasonable" regular meal at the other times.

There are many different dietary products available in supermarkets, department stores, and other retail outlets. Some companies have developed complete lines of low-calorie products to be used as calorie substitutes. The Slim-Fast line is heavily advertised and can be very helpful to the dieter who can follow the diet plan enclosed in the package.

Convenience and palatability of marketed products have been improved in the last few years. Premixed liquids and easily dispersible powders have replaced older powder formulations, which required a blender to prepare the final mixture. Now, nutritional bars and other forms of calorie-substitute products are available to add variety. When used properly, Slim-Fast and other products like it can serve an important function for the person trying to lose weight.

Artificial Sweeteners

Saccharin

Saccharin, a sucrose substitute, is about 400 times more potent than sucrose as a sweetener, and it provides no calories. Although it produces a bitter taste in some individuals, it is the most popular artificial sweetener, especially since the nonregulated use of cyclamates was prohibited. Saccharin may have considerable importance in reducing caloric intake in some individuals. For instance, if it is used instead of one heaping teaspoonful of sugar to sweeten a cup of coffee, 33 Cal are removed from the diet.

In 1972, after bladder tumors were discovered in rats fed very large doses of saccharin in utero and throughout life, the FDA removed saccharin from the list of food additives generally recognized as safe. Saccharin is currently permitted in products labeled specifically as diet foods or beverages. Human epidemiologic studies have not revealed a clear-cut relationship between saccharin consumption and urinary bladder carcinoma. However, saccharin may accumulate in fetal tissues and therefore should not be used during pregnancy.

Aspartame

Aspartame is a synthetic dipeptide that is about 180 times as sweet as sugar. The FDA has determined that it too is safe as a food additive. However, individuals with phenylketonuria or patients who should avoid protein foods must be alerted to the fact that it contains phenylalanine. Thus, products containing aspartame must carry the warning: "Phenylketonurics: Contains Phenylalanine." In addition, directions not to use aspartame in cooking or baking (because the compound loses its sweetness) are required on table products containing aspartame.

Other Sweeteners

Fructose, sorbitol, and xylitol may be used as alternatives to saccharin, but these sweeteners contain calories and should not be viewed as "sugar-free" diet items. Fructose and xylitol are sweeter than sucrose, and xylitol is less calorigenic and more expensive. Apparently, neither sorbitol nor xylitol causes tooth decay, and some products containing xylitol have a more pleasant taste. However, some evidence implicates xylitol in the development of urinary tract abnormalities, kidney stones, and tumors in laboratory animals. Further tests are under way to evaluate this possibility. The ingestion of sufficient amounts of dietetic candies containing sorbitol may result in an osmotic diarrhea in small children.

Several naturally occurring compounds show promise as substitutes for sucrose. Monellin, thaumatin, and miraculin are proteins from plant sources and are currently being investigated as possible sucrose substitutes.

Fat Substitutes

These substitutes mimic the "mouth-feel" of fat but contain fewer calories. For example, Simplesse, a blend of egg white and/or milk protein whipped to a creamlike consistency, is a frozen dessert that contains less than 1 g of fat per serving. Oatrim is a cholesterol-free fat substance designed to replace the fat in meats, cheeses, baked goods, and frozen desserts. Olestra looks and tastes like fat but is not absorbed by the body; because it is heat resistant, it can be used for cooking and frying.

Nutrient Supplements

Vitamins and minerals are present in some nonprescription weight control products. If a dieting patient is not receiving adequate quantities of vitamins and minerals in the diet regimen chosen, the administration of vitamins and minerals is warranted. Although recommended daily allowances for vitamins and minerals are present in any well-balanced LCD, to be on the safe side a pharmacist might want to recommend a once-daily vitamin tablet to guard against inadequate intake. (See Chapter 19, "Nutritional Products.")

Dosage Forms

Nonprescription products for obesity control are available as liquids, powders, granules, tablets, capsules, sustained-release capsules, wafers, cookies, soups, chewing gum, and candy preparations. If wafers, chewing gum, or candy cubes are substituted for high-calorie desserts or snacks, the candylike nature of the dosage form may offer patients a psychologic aid that is not found when a standard tablet or capsule is used. Ingesting large quantities of diet candy would, of course, contribute significantly to caloric intake.

Commercial Weight Loss Programs and Products

Weight Loss Programs

More than 1 million people participate in weight loss groups each week. The typical member of a commercial program is a woman between 30 and 50 years of age who weighs 150–176 lb. People who stay in programs achieve modest weight losses (4.8–15.6 lb during the first 12 weeks and 7–13.2 lb more during the next 12 weeks), but fewer than 20% of participants stay in programs long enough to lose an appreciable amount of weight.[16]

In one study of commercial weight loss programs, men lost significantly more weight than women, members between ages 21 and 51 were slightly more successful than those on either side of that range, and those who worked outside the home fared better than those who did not.[88] In another study, encouragement from the leaders and inclusion in a group were the most important factors in successful weight loss.[89] About one third of self-help group members tend to reach long-term goals.[16]

Many weight loss programs include 1,000- to 1,500-Cal per day diets in which projected weight loss averages 1 or 2 lb/wk. The member usually follows a carefully controlled menu plan. In some cases, the participant is required to purchase specially packaged meals available only from the company, and most often these purchases are not reimbursable through health insurance. The costs for these programs vary considerably, ranging from $250 to $1,000 or more.

Leading Weight Control Programs

There are many commercial weight loss programs in the United States; some are large franchise operations while others are local operations. Rosenblatt reports on a few of the larger programs operating in the United States.[90]

TOPS Take Off Pounds Sensibly (TOPS) is patterned after Alcoholics Anonymous. This program, founded in 1948, is one of the oldest major weight control clubs. The program has five components: medical research; medical supervision of members' diets; group therapy; competition among members, with special recognition given to those who lose the most weight; and instruction in behavioral modification. In one study, 28% of all members lost more than 20 lb.[91] Over time, weight loss at TOPS compares favorably with that at other commercial and medical group programs.

Weight Watchers Established in 1961, Weight Watchers is one of the largest commercial weight loss programs, with franchises found throughout the country. The program charges a moderate fee to join as well as a weekly fee. Members must attend and weigh in at least once a week; if meetings are missed, the member must pay a "penalty" fee.

Weight Watchers has a four-part approach: an eating plan that includes some sample menus, an optional exercise plan, a self-discovery plan, and a group support program. More than 7,000 members lost an average of 1.6 lb/wk. In a 15-month follow-up of 721 members, 50% were within 5% or less of their goal. Weight losses in this program are comparable to those of groups treated in general practice or outpatient hospital clinics. In one study, 50% of participants dropped out within 6 weeks and 70% dropped out within 12 weeks.[92]

Diet Center Diet Center, a franchise organization, began in 1970. The weight reduction phase involves daily supervision and behavioral modification classes once or twice a week. Women are placed on a 915-Cal diet and men, on a 1,000-Cal diet; both are given a special supplement of soy protein, fructose, dextrose, and vitamin B complex.

In one survey, the average weight loss in the Diet Center program was 3.1 lb/wk.[93] When evaluated 1 year after completion of the program, 79% of enrollees were within 10 lb, 64% were within 5 lb, and 52% were at their ideal weight; the average weight loss was 39 lb.

Nutri/System Nutri/System is based on eating special portion-controlled and nutritionally balanced foods purchased from Nutri/System at additional cost. The diet, which contains 800-1,000 Cal per day and a daily vitamin and mineral supplement, is prepared and portioned in advance so that little choice is left to the client.

This program made claims that its clients can lose up to 1 lb a day and that more than 80% maintain the weight loss. Clients are refunded 50% of their money by staying with the program for 1 year and 25% by staying for 6 months.

Overeaters Anonymous Overeaters Anonymous is a voluntary, nonprofit, self-supporting fellowship started in 1960. The program is founded on the belief that compulsive eating is an illness that cannot be cured but can be arrested.

Members meet weekly to solve their common problem of overeating but do not use weigh-ins as a motivational tool. Special diets are neither advocated nor discussed. Rather, a 12-step program patterned after that of Alcoholics Anonymous is used to motivate members to change their eating habits and lifestyle.

Overeaters Anonymous estimates that 25% of its members reach normal weight and that 22% maintain that weight for just over 2 years. In another survey by the fellowship, the average member was found to have lost 31.4 lb, and participants reported many medical and psychologic improvements.[93]

Optifast Optifast is a brand name for a powdered product distributed by physicians as part of a protein-sparing modified fast (PSMF) diet. The manufacturer sets guidelines for the product's use and provides training for the physician and staff. The cost to clients varies in different locations but averages about $2,800 for 9 months. The program is designed for people who (1) are 30–100%, or at least 50 lb over their ideal weight, and (2) have a medical problem that necessitates weight loss.

A 2- to 4-week period of a LCD is followed by 12 weeks of a supplemented fast consisting of 420 Cal per day for women and 800 Cal per day for men.

Advertising Practices of Programs

Commercial weight loss programs can be very successful for the right patient under the right circumstances. The government, however, is concerned about the advertising practices of certain programs. In September 1993, the Federal Trade Commission (FTC) charged that five of the nation's largest commercial diet program companies have misled consumers by making unsubstantiated weight loss claims and using deceptive testimonials. The FTC alleged that none of the five firms could substantiate that its customers are typically successful in reaching their weight loss goals or in maintaining those goals over the long term. The FTC also alleged that four of the companies made unsubstantiated claims that their customers maintained weight loss permanently. Pharmacists are urged to help their patients evaluate the promotional claims of these and all other weight loss plans before paying for them.

Selecting a Weight Loss Method/Program

In evaluating a weight loss method or program, one should not be distracted by anecdotal "success" stories or advertising claims. Information about program success that should be obtained (ideally from independent sources) includes[16]:

- The percentage of all beginning participants who complete the program;

- The percentage of those completing the program who achieve various degrees of weight loss;
- The proportion of weight loss that is maintained at 1, 3, and 5 years;
- The percentage of participants who experienced adverse medical or psychologic effects and the kind and severity of those effects;
- The relative mix of diet, exercise, and behavioral modifications;
- The amount and kind of counseling: individual and closed groups (in which membership does not change except by attrition) are both more successful than open groups (in which members may come and go);
- The nature of available multidisciplinary expertise (including medical, nutritional, psychologic, physiologic, and exercise);
- The training provided for relapse prevention to deal with high-risk emotional and social situations;
- The nature and duration of the maintenance phase;
- The flexibility of food choices and suitability of food types;
- The manner in which weight goals are set, whether unilaterally or cooperatively with the director of the weight loss program.

In formal programs, continued regular contact with a supervising professional may be necessary to maintain weight loss. In any case, new eating behaviors must be learned and adopted, which can be difficult. Such behaviors include modifying the quantity and kinds of food, and possibly developing a different attitude toward eating and toward oneself.

Even though a caloric deficit must be achieved, the diet must provide all essential nutrients. A regular exercise regimen, which could be as simple as walking, is essential both to better health and to maintenance of long-term weight loss.

Methods whose primary goal is short-term rapid or unsupervised weight loss, or that rely on diet aids such as drinks, prepackaged foods, or pharmacologic agents but do not include education in and eventual transition to a lasting pattern of healthful eating and activity, have never been shown to lead to long-term success.[16]

Weight Loss Products/Diets

A succession of fad diet products has come and gone over the years. The "half-life" of such fads is usually only a couple of years, each giving way to the next fad to come along or falling victim to FDA regulation. Some examples of previously popular, nutritionally based diets that proved to be ineffective include:

- *Beverly Hills Diet*: The premise of this diet, which consisted of 90% carbohydrates, 6% protein, and 4% fat, was that most enzymes cannot work simultaneously and so cancel one another out, (ie, "when you mix proteins and carbs, the carbs will usually be trapped in your stomach...")
- *False Mayo Diet*: The premise of this diet was that grapefruit has certain enzymes that "subtract calories" by acting as catalysts and enhancing the fat-burning process. Dieters could eat as much as they wanted of even fatty foods.
- *Twenty-first Century Diet*: This diet restricted food consumption to goose and quail eggs for breakfast and three green peppers for dinner.
- *Other unbalanced diets*: Other diets that proved to be ineffective include the (1) Immune Power Diet, (2) Fit for Life Diet, (3) Living Healthy Diet, (4) It's Not Your Fault You Are Fat Diet, (5) Atkin's Diet, and (6) Stillman's Diet.

The electronic age has opened new avenues for the marketing of weight control products, including those products of questionable safety and efficacy. Pharmacists need to know that their patients have instant access to a vast array of (mis)information about weight loss products via the Internet. Questionable products being promoted range from herbal appetite control mixtures to a PSMF powder. Further, the FDA has issued warnings about potentially dangerous diet products.

Potentially Dangerous Diet Products

Botanical weight loss products are very popular today. Their proponents point to the long history of their use and the fact that they are made up of "natural" ingredients as evidence of safety and efficacy. Recently, the FDA issued a warning about the use of certain botanical weight loss products after receiving reports of adverse effects associated with their use.

Botanical Products with Stimulant Effects The FDA is particularly concerned about products containing multiple pharmacologically related ingredients, including ma huang (*Ephedra sinica* or Chinese ephedra, a botanical source of ephedrine, pseudoephedrine, and nor-pseudoephedrine), guarana or kola nut (sources of caffeine), white willow (salicin source), and chromium. These products are often touted for their reported stimulant effects and their ability to enhance metabolism with subsequent weight loss (so-called fat burners). As their use has increased, however, the FDA has received an increasing number of reports of adverse reactions associated with them. Reactions vary from the milder adverse effects known to be associated with sympathomimetic stimulants (eg, nervousness, dizziness, tremor, alterations in blood pressure or heart rate, headache, and gastrointestinal distress) to chest pain, myocardial infarct, hepatitis, stroke, seizures, psychosis, and death. These adverse reactions have been reported in both young, otherwise healthy individuals and in persons with confounding or complicating conditions such as hypertension. In addition, a stimulant "overdose" syndrome has been reported in children and teenagers who have used these products.[94]

Capwell[95] reported the case of a 45-year-old man who developed ephedrine-induced mania from an herbal diet supplement containing ma huang. Upon discovering the use of the herbal capsule, the physician advised the patient to discontinue its use and prescribed a sedative, which was discontinued 1 week later. The patient had no evidence of mood instability after 1 year of follow-up.

Cal-Ban 3000 Another dangerous diet product is Cal-Ban 3000, diet tablets and capsules that were extensively advertised on television and in magazines a few years ago. Cal-Ban's main ingredient is guar gum, a complex sugar that swells when it becomes wet and can create a sense of fullness when ingested. After receiving reports from health professionals of at least 17 people who experienced esophageal obstruction after ingesting Cal-Ban tablets, the FDA ordered that the distribution of Cal-Ban be halted because it may cause esophageal, gastric, and intestinal obstruction and because promotional materials for the product make unproven claims.

Weight Loss Teas Weight loss products often marketed as "dieter's or slimming teas" contain a variety of strong botanical laxatives (*Cassia* species [senna], cascara sagrada [botanical name *Rhamnus purshiana*]) and diuretics. Adverse reactions reported to the FDA as being associated with these products are characteristic of those seen in laxative abuse syndromes and include severe electrolyte imbalances leading to cardiac arrhythmia and death.

Pharmacists are reminded that the above products are not classified as drugs by the FDA and hence do not undergo extensive premarket review of their safety or effectiveness. There is no good dosing information or monitoring advice available, and there are no standards for potency and purity of ingredients. When patients inquire about such products, the pharmacist should very carefully review the patient's current prescription and nonprescription drug history. Whenever taking a drug history for any purpose, the pharmacist should ask about the use of botanicals and any other unproven "nutritional" products and should discourage their use by anyone with significant diseases superimposed on obesity.

Products/Diets of Questionable Safety/Efficacy

Protein-Sparing Modified Fast Diet Promotional information on the Internet describes a particular brand of PSMF diet as a "fast weight loss regimen" consisting of five servings of a powder spaced 2-3 hours apart. Each serving contains only 120 Cal for a net daily caloric intake of 600 Cal. This is an extremely restricted caloric intake, which should never be used without medical supervision. Yet, anyone with a credit card can order the product for almost $30.00 per can (a can may last up to 1 week).

A discussion of the PSMF diet in a November 1978 issue of *JAMA* concluded that the diet "should be considered investigational; informed consent is desirable. Unlike balanced deficit dieting, the PSMFD is a potent clinical tool that has definite risks and indications and contraindications for clinical use similar to other efficacious clinical procedures."[96]

Lipotrophic Substances Another weight loss system sold on the Internet is a combination of "amino acids, minerals, lipotrophic factors, unsaturated fatty acids, and vitamins designed to enhance the weight loss process." Lipotrophics are further defined as "substances which may liquify or homogenize fats," a description that conjures up a mental picture of fat melting away.

Citrin Still one other weight loss system proposes use of a product called citrin, an extract of *Garcinia combogia*, which is a fruit used in India and China as a spice. Promoters go on to say that this fruit is rich in hydroxycitric acid and that the acid has the following effects:

- Inhibits fat and cholesterol accumulation by slowing down the enzyme process that produces fat in the cells;
- Enhances caloric burning through a thermogenic process;
- Controls the appetite by interfering with pertinent signals sent to the brain by the glucoreceptors in the liver;
- Reduces appetite and subsequently food intake because "the brain sends fewer and less intense appetite signals."

As with other diet products, the capsules of this diet program are accompanied by a sensible plan with easy-to-follow recommendations. If weight loss is achieved with this product, it is likely attributable to the decreased caloric intake in the plan rather than to the product itself.

Cleanse, Build, and Burn Pack A "natural health and nutrition shop" advertising on the Internet is promoting a group of products called the Cleanse, Build, and Burn Pack. The Cleanse products are high-fiber substances and laxative ingredients whose purpose is to eliminate wastes more often so that there is less time for excess calories to be absorbed. The Burn phase contains a product with Chinese ephedra, kelp, dandelion root, parruva brava, capsicum, and chromium; this product is touted to "stimulate burning of fat, increase metabolism, control appetite, and feel more energy." The Build phase consists of a meal replacement shake with carbohydrates, vitamins, minerals, and L-carnitine. The cost of this system is about $150.00 for a month's supply.

USAI Diet Another diet involves a company called United States of America, Incorporated (USAI), which is based in Dallas. This company claims as members of its scientific advisory board some prominent scientists, many of whom have received generous research "grants" from USAI. In 1986, the multi-level marketing program had first-year sales of $150 million; annual sales in 1989 were estimated at $1 billion. Consumer costs to use the USAI nutritional plan were estimated at $135 per month.

The USAI program consists of several different products that contain a total of 36 ingredients, each claimed as a "must" for nutritional enrichment. A fiber energy bar is said to provide a complete nutritious meal or a wholesome snack; the "secret formula" of this bar is not being released to the American consumer. The Formula Plus product is a marine lipid concentrate rich in omega-3 fatty acids and in eicosapentaenoic and docosahexaenoic acids. The Calorie Control Formula is claimed to be a scientific and technical breakthrough, yet the formula is similar to that of other popular, low-calorie liquid diets. It is claimed to be effective if used with the Master Formula. However, the specific analysis of the additional 26 ingredients is not released to the consumer.

Questions of safety arise over the use of unusual ingredients such as roasted dahlia root powder, yucca powder, yucca fiber, bee root powder, and allium sativum extract. The safety of a daily consumption of 900 mg of fish oils, especially for an extended time, is also not known.

Spirulina One of the earliest weight loss fads involved the substance spirulina. The popularity of spirulina, boosted by an article in the *National Enquirer* hailing this substance as a diet breakthrough, led to sales by mail order firms, health food stores, and pharmacies. The *Enquirer's* article claimed that phenylalanine, an amino acid found in spirulina, "acts on the brain's appetite center to switch off your hunger pangs, so you can eat less . . . and lose weight." However, a 1979 FDA advisory panel on OTC drugs reviewed this substance and found no reliable scientific data to demonstrate that it is a safe and effective appetite suppressant.

Spirulina, considered a food or food supplement, is sold in many health food stores as a dark green powder or pill. It is one of about 1,500 known species of blue-green algae that grow in brackish ponds and lakes in mild and hot climates throughout the world. Pure spirulina is a source of protein and contains various vitamins and minerals. Although the active ingredient is extremely cheap, finished products were selling for exorbitant prices and the public was clamoring to try spirulina when it was first being touted as a "miracle." Some promoters sold spirulina as a single-entity product while others sold it mixed with herbs, vitamins, minerals, and other ingredients.

As a food, spirulina is being marketed legally as long as it is labeled accurately, contains no contaminated or adulterated substances, and bears no specific health claims. There is little, if any, evidence that spirulina is effective at suppressing appetite. However, some distributors soon began promoting it through word-of-mouth representations, pamphlets, and other written materials as a safe, quick way to lose weight, maintain health, and rejuvenate the body. In 1981, the FDA sent a mailgram to health professionals and others advising consumers who want to lose weight not to rely on these products but instead to consult with a physician, dietitian, or other health specialist.

Starch Blockers In the early 1980s one of the most popular diet fads was the starch blockers. Over a 2-year span, 200 products were estimated to have poured onto the market and an estimated 1 million tablets were being consumed daily before the FDA ordered their marketing discontinued. Although the presence of amylase inhibitors (their more scientific classification) in certain cereals and beans was reported in the 1940s, no attention was paid to the possible pharmacologic effects of such agents until the mid-1970s, when researchers purified and characterized the amylase inhibitor in the kidney bean and named it phaseolamine. Because of the inhibitor's ability to bind human salivary and pancreatic amylases in vitro, it had been proposed that phaseolamine, when taken orally, can block the digestion of starch in meals and thus be an effective agent in weight control.

Rats fed diets containing the inhibitor have been reported to excrete more fecal starch and gain less weight than control rats. From this early research, manufacturers began to market products for human weight loss, claiming that each starch-blocker tablet would produce enough antiamylase activity to block the digestion and absorption of 100 g (400 kcal) of starch. Thus, people who enjoy eating bread, spaghetti, and potatoes but who still want to lose weight were urged in advertisements to take starch blockers with their meals. Indeed, eaters were instructed to "titrate" their dose of the starch blocker to the amount of the starchy food they wished to eat.

Despite the commercial success of starch blockers, there is no convincing scientific evidence that these preparations actually inhibit the absorption of the starch calories in human beings. Many unpublished studies claiming miraculous results were mentioned in promotional materials, but when controlled experiments were conducted using 1-day calorie balance techniques, no increase in fecal calorie excretion was demonstrated. In one study, fecal calorie output was not higher after ingestion of three starch-blocker tablets than after ingestion of placebo. It is likely that, even though starch blockers block amylase activity in vitro, the human pancreas probably secretes many more times the amount of amylase after meals than is needed for hydrolysis of the ingested starch. Thus, the effects of the starch blocker are probably overwhelmed by the amount of amylase available in the gut.

Concerned about the lack of effectiveness and safety of these products, the FDA declared them to be drugs and not foods, and because there was no approved new drug application on file for these agents, their manufacture and distribution was halted in July of 1982. Even then, reports surfaced that patients had stockpiled the product while the FDA had been deliberating their ban.

Glucomannan Glucomannan is a hydrophilic hemicellulose extracted from the tubers of *Amorphophallus konjac* (Koch), a large cultivated herb used as a food source in Indonesia and Japan. It is composed of glucose and mannose linked through beta-glucoside bonds. Human digestive enzymes do not break down polysaccharides of this type. These compounds were heavily promoted as therapy for patients with diabetes mellitus, hyperlipidemias, and obesity. Only glucomannan's claimed effects on obesity are considered here.

Use of glucomannan as a diet aid is based on its ability to absorb water in the stomach, creating bulk and a feeling of fullness. Glucomannan absorbs about 60 times its weight in water, but like other bulk-forming agents, it has not produced dramatic effects when used in dieters. One controlled trial demonstrated diminished hunger intensity and an increased number of patient-days in which hunger was recorded by diary.[97] However, details of this trial were not adequate to allow critical review of the research.

The action of bulk-producing agents in producing feelings of satiety is poorly demonstrated and transient at best. When a barium marker was added to bulk-forming diet tablets, radiographic studies demonstrated that 30 minutes following ingestion only trace amounts of material remained in the stomach and the mass had advanced well into the small bowel.[98] Thus, taking glucomannan capsules 30–60 minutes prior to a meal, as directed on most weight loss products, is unlikely to cause the claimed sensation of fullness.

Weight loss claims were plentiful for these products, but in 1982 the FDA stated that manufacturers of glucomannan had supplied insufficient data to substantiate claims of effectiveness. In one controlled trial that evaluated the use of glucomannan as a weight loss product, 20 obese subjects (group mean = 54.5% above ideal body weight) took two 500-mg capsules of purified glucomannan or two 500-mg starch capsules with 8 oz of water 1 hour before breakfast, lunch, and dinner.[99] Participants knew they were involved in an assessment of the supplement's effectiveness as a diet aid. Although they were further advised not to alter their usual eating or exercise patterns, no determination of the patients' before- or during-study diet was made. After 8 weeks, subjects given glucomannan had lost an average of 2.5 kg (5.5 lb) compared with an average gain of 0.7 kg (1.5 lb) in the placebo group.

Side effects of glucomannan were usually minor. Diarrhea occurred in a small percentage of individuals given these products. Use of glucomannan has all but disappeared from the US market.

Chromium As this chapter is being written, chromium is the one of the hottest dietary supplements promoted for weight loss. It is also used in the treatment of diabetes, as an ergogenic aid to increase strength and endurance, and for various other purposes. It is marketed either as a single-entity product (in oral or sublingual dosage forms) or in combination with a host of other ingredients.

Chromium is considered a cofactor in the maintenance of normal lipid and carbohydrate metabolism. It is part of the glucose tolerance factor (GTF), which was first isolated from brewers' yeast. The GTF contains one chromium atom in complex with single molecules of glycine, cysteine, and glutamic acid and two molecules of nicotinic acid. The chromium atom is considered the active constituent of GTF. Picolinic acid, a metabolite of tryptophan, forms stable complexes with transitional metal ions such as chromium, which results in an improved bioavailability of the metal ion.

Chromium has also been shown to be essential for the efficient use of glucose in man and animals.[100] It potentiates glucose uptake by cells, oxidation of glucose to carbon dioxide, and incorporation of glucose into fatty acids and cholesterol. A decrease in insulin binding and in the number of insulin receptors has been reported in the absence of adequate amounts of chromium.

The recommended daily allowance for chromium is 50–200 mcg; at present, however, it is very difficult to get a valid assessment of human chromium balance. No toxicity has been reported from the oral administration of trivalent chromium salts (chromium picolinate is Cr^{+++}). In contrast, the hexavalent chromium compounds can be quite toxic orally. The median lethal dose of trivalent chromium by intravenous injection into rats varied between 10 and 30 mg/kg of body weight. Signs of toxicity from intravenous chromium chloride include nausea, vomiting, convulsions, and coma.

Chromium likely plays an important role in maintaining normal glucose and lipid metabolism; however, research defining its precise role is still under way. Although the medical literature contains numerous anecdotal and case reports describing the beneficial effects of GTF on glucose tolerance in diabetic patients, there are few well-designed, controlled clinical trials evaluating those effects. There is even less evidence to support the use of chromium in weight loss programs as its usefulness in this regard has only been extrapolated from its apparent role in regulating glucose metabolism. Until such time as well-controlled clinical trials of chromium as a weight loss ingredient are completed, pharmacists should advise patients to avoid this compound. Although it is probably safe, it is certainly not the miracle substance it is purported to be.

The Pharmacist's Role in Weight Counseling

Although the role of nonprescription appetite suppressants is limited, the pharmacist is in a key position to help people who wish to lose weight. The typical patient who requests a nonprescription weight loss product may not be well informed about weight-related issues, including basic physiology and human nutrition. Many have incorrect notions, reinforced by the media and the popular press, about methods of weight loss and their effectiveness, and they often have inflated expectations about the latest diet method being touted. The well-informed pharmacist can offer the following assistance:

- Answer questions about weight loss methods and products;
- Help the patient set realistic weight loss goals;
- Counsel the patient on the proper use of drugs and supplements;
- Refer the patient to a dietitian for evaluation and diet management;
- Help monitor the patient for adverse events that may occur during therapy.

Increased attention is being given to the problem of obesity and to the drugs that treat it, and safer and more effective diet drugs will likely become available in the next few years. Thus, it is important for the pharmacist to stay abreast of developments in the field of obesity research. Combinations of currently marketed drugs (eg, phentermine and fenfluramine) are being promoted as the latest "breakthrough" in the treatment of obesity. Time will tell if these combination products and other drugs in development are effective. Until that time, pharmacists can help their patients spot fraudulent weight loss schemes while recommending legitimate alternatives.

Some people, especially adolescent girls, attempt weight loss when, in fact, they are already at their normal weight. By carefully monitoring the purchases of nonprescription weight loss products, the pharmacist can spot the beginnings of an eating disorder and take the necessary steps to get help for the person. Much of the information in this chapter may not apply directly to nonprescription weight loss products but instead is provided as background information necessary for helping with diet information in a broader sense.

Recognizing Diet Fads

One of the biggest challenges for the pharmacist is answering questions about diets seen on television, read about in newspapers or magazines, or heard about from a neighbor. Among patients in whom disappointment and frustration with failed diet methods abound, "hope springs eternal." Otherwise rational people are attracted to the latest fad diets or products. This attraction is strengthened by anecdotal evidence, personal endorsements from famous celebrities, and the urging of close friends or relatives who have tried a new diet and have been able to lose several pounds quickly. Patients fall victim to seemingly plausible but scientifically invalid concepts, such as the ability of a particular food or chemical to help the body break down fat, increase metabolism, or prevent absorption.

These products are sold legally because there is little government regulation of the diet supplement industry. Most diet plans are sold as food products, not as drugs, and thus are not subject to the same burden of proof of safety and efficacy required for drugs. Rarely has the FDA been able to take action against a diet manufacturer. However, since the FTC has authority over the promotional and business practices of the diet industry, it has, on a case-by-case basis, imposed sanctions on programs making false or deceptive claims about their products.

Commercial "nutrition" organizations have also proliferated. Some of these entities offer memberships and titles, such as nutritional consultant or nutritional counselor, for various fees. According to a 1990 article in the *American Journal of Gastroenterology*, most of these organizations promote vitamins, minerals, and other supplements through advertising, seminars, brochures, and other channels.[101] Some of these organizations are listed here in the event that patients might ask about them:

- American Association of Nutrition Consultants;
- American College of Advancement Medicine;
- International Academy of Biomagnetic Medicine;
- International Academy of Nutrition and Preventative Medicine;
- International Health Institute;
- International Institute of Natural Health Sciences;
- National Accreditation Association;
- National Health Federation;
- National Medicine Council;
- National Nutritional Foods Association;
- Nutritional Research Foundation;
- The Council for Responsible Nutrition.

There are hundreds of "miracle" diets on which a receptive and gullible public wastes money. Even well-educated and sophisticated patients succumb to pervasive psychologic and social factors as well as to the "commonsense notion of health" (which ensures the success of fad diets). Rather than sell products of unproven efficacy or safety, the pharmacist can help patients evaluate promotional literature before they invest large sums in products that, at best, are worthless and, at worst, could cause them harm. Accordingly, the pharmacist should advise patients to be wary of programs that:

- Make exaggerated health claims for particular nutrients or nutrient combinations;
- Make unsubstantiated and false claims;
- Invent their own nonsensical "physiology" to impress the consumer;
- Use "hooks" or gimmicks;
- Offer unorthodox treatments or diagnostic methods;
- Promise quick results for little effort by using "breakthrough formulas";
- Use anecdotal data, testimonials, one-sided radio/television talk show propaganda and infomercials, or unpublished or unscientific data;
- Preach their version of "good nutrition" and blame a "conspiracy" involving organized medicine for criticizing their "discovery."

Product Selection Guidelines

As a health care professional, the pharmacist should emphasize the importance of a rational, low-calorie, balanced diet and proper exercise to correct caloric imbalance, as well as of individual effort in maintaining a diet management program. The patient may be referred to a support group.

In recommending a nonprescription product for weight control, the pharmacist should stress that weight cannot be reduced without a concerted effort to change one's eating and exercise lifestyle and to maintain the new behavior long term. The patient should be made aware of the caloric value of various food types. The pharmacist should inquire about previous diet control regimens the patient has attempted so that other nonprescription diet management adjuncts may be considered. However, a nonprescription obesity control product should be considered only as an adjunct to a planned weight reduction program. Vitamins sometimes are added to such products on the assumption that dieting individuals may not have an adequate vitamin intake. This practice may be justified in individual cases but should not be applied to all patients. The pharmacist may also participate in monitoring the patient's weight reduction efforts.

Case Studies

Case 21–1

Patient Complaint/History

RM, a 47-year-old female who is 5'2" tall and weighs 182 lb, comes to the pharmacy counter to ask about a "miracle" diet product. RM often comes in and questions pharmacy staff about a new diet plan or product that she has read about. The latest product of interest purportedly allows its users to eat all they want without gaining weight. The patient remembers only that the product contains chromium.

Clinical Considerations/Strategies

The following considerations/strategies are provided to aid the reader in (1) determining whether treatment of the patient's condition with nonprescription medications is warranted, (2) selecting the appropriate nonprescription medication, and (3) developing a patient counseling strategy to ensure optimal therapeutic outcomes:

- Assess the patient's understanding of and expectations from medications or dietary products in producing weight loss versus traditional methods of weight loss, such as modifying eating habits, restricting high-calorie foods and snacks, decreasing consumption of high-fat foods, and exercising.
- Using typical weight standards, determine whether the patient is overweight. If she is, apprise her of the health benefits of losing the extra weight.
- Find out the patient's weight loss goals.
- Assess the patient's past attempts at losing weight: determine which methods, if any, worked well; find out if the patient has a regular exercise program.
- Determine whether the patient has any chronic or acute illnesses and whether she is currently taking any prescription and/or nonprescription medications. If so, determine whether she has consulted a physician about her desire to lose weight.
- Assess the patient's understanding of the role diet and nutrition play in any weight loss program. If necessary, discuss the need for balancing caloric intake with caloric expenditure; be prepared to refer the patient to a nutritionist or diet counselor.
- Determine whether the patient has a support group that will encourage her to adhere to a diet and maintain a weight loss.
- Assess the medical evidence that taking chromium is a pharmacologically and therapeutically sound approach to weight loss: determine whether reliable, objective published literature based on controlled clinical trials is available to support the safety and efficacy of such products.
- Assess whether an alternative weight-loss regimen is more appropriate.

Case 21–2

Patient Complaint/History

PM, a 15-year-old local high school student, and her mother approach the pharmacy counter late one afternoon. The mother wants to ask the pharmacist, whom she considers her "neighborhood health expert," about the Dexatrim caplets she found in her daughter's backpack. PM says that she takes the diet product "to get rid of this ugly fat." The mother wants to know whether the product is addictive or otherwise harmful. According to her mother, PM, who is 5'6" tall and weighs 128 lb, is in good health except for seasonal allergies associated with certain blooming plants.

The package label identifies the diet product as Dexatrim Caffeine-Free Caplets; each caplet contains 75 mg of phenylpropanolamine in a sustained-release dosage form. PM reveals that she is also currently taking Dimetapp Allergy tablets "every so often"; the allergy medication was recommended by her pediatrician.

Clinical Considerations/Strategies

The following considerations/strategies are provided to aid the reader in (1) determining whether treatment of the patient's condition with nonprescription medications is warranted, (2) selecting the appropriate nonprescription medication, and (3) developing a patient counseling strategy to ensure optimal therapeutic outcomes:

- Ask the teenager why she thinks she needs to lose weight.
- Assess the teenager's self-image and try to determine whether an underlying psychologic problem or other factors are behind the desire to lose weight. Be prepared to make appropriate referrals.
- Determine the teenager's goals or desired effects from using the appetite suppressant (eg, weight loss or stimulant effects).
- Try to determine whether an underlying eating disorder is associated with the desire to lose weight.
- Determine whether the teenager is eating a nutritionally balanced diet and whether she has tried to lose weight by modifying her intake of high-caloric and/or high-fat foods.
- Explain to the teenager and her mother the proper role of nonprescription products in weight-loss programs as well as the limitations of such adjunctive products.
- Determine whether the teenager is experiencing adverse effects consistent with CNS stimulant toxicity (eg, jitteriness, irritability, insomnia, dizziness).
- Explain to the teenager and her mother the potential consequences of duplicating the intake of phenylpropanolamine, which is an active ingredient in the allergy medication and the appetite suppressant.
- Explain to the teenager and her mother the potential consequences of taking a nonprescription product without fully understanding the potential risks and benefits of the product.
- Find out whether other girls at the patient's school are taking weight loss products; if so, find out what products they are taking.

Summary

A patient should recognize that a successful weight reduction program includes reduced caloric intake, increased physical activity, and possibly a pharmacologic aid such as a nonprescription product, and that the effectiveness of such a program depends largely on the patient's motivation, education, and acceptance of a regimen necessary to achieve long-term weight control. The role of the pharmacist is to supply pertinent and accurate information regarding methods of weight loss and their relative merits. The pharmacist should be able to advise on the health risk of overweight and encourage the dieter during the difficult days ahead. The pharmacist should also help people avoid being victimized by fraudulent products and methods.

References

1. Garner DM et al. Cultural expectations of thinness in women. *Psychol Rep.* 1980; 47: 483–91.
2. Foreyt JP. The addictive disorders. In: Franks CM et al, eds. *Review of Behavior Therapy: Theory and Practice.* Vol 12. New York: Guilford Press; 1990: 178–224.

3. Wadden TA et al. Three year follow-up of the treatment of obesity by very low calorie diet, behavior therapy, and their combination. *J Consult Clin Psychol.* 1988; 56: 925–8.
4. Rodin J. Cultural and psychosocial determinants of weight concerns. *Ann Intern Med.* 1993; 119(7 pt 2): 643-5.
5. Public Health Service. *Healthy People 2000: National Health Promotion and Disease Prevention Objectives.* DHHS Pub No. PHS 90–50212. Washington, DC: US Department of Health and Human Services; 1990.
6. Health implications of obesity. National Institutes of Health Consensus Development Conference. 11–13 February 1985. *Ann Intern Med.* 1985; 103: 977–1077.
7. 1983 Metropolitan Height and Weight Tables. In: *Stat Bull Metropolitan Life Insurance Co.* 1984; 64: 2–9.
8. Kuczmarski RJ et al. Increasing prevalence of overweight among US adults: the National Health and Nutrition Examination Surveys, 1960–1991. *JAMA.* 1994; 272: 205–11.
9. Stunkard AJ et al. A twin study of human obesity. *JAMA.* 1986; 256: 51–4.
10. Colditz GA. Economic costs of obesity. *Am J Clin Nutr.* 1992; 55: 503S–7S.
11. Kannel WB et al. The relationship of adiposity to blood pressure and development of hypertension. The Framingham Heart Study. *Ann Intern Med.* 1967; 67: 48–59.
12. Gortmaker SL et al. Social and economic consequences of overweight in adolescence and young adulthood. *N Engl J Med.* 1993; 329: 1008–12.
13. Yaes RJ. Futility and avoidance: medical professionals in the treatment of obesity. *JAMA.* 1993; 270: 1423. Letter.
14. Kolbe LJ. An epidemiological surveillance system to monitor the prevalence of youth behaviors that most affect health. *Health Educ Q.* 1990; 21: 44-8.
15. Remington PL et al. Design, characteristics, and usefulness of state based behavioral risk factor surveillance, 1981–1987. *Public Health Rep.* 1988; 103: 366–75.
16. NIH Technology Assessment Conference Panel. Methods for voluntary weight loss and control. *Ann Intern Med.* 1993; 119(7 pt 2): 764–70.
17. Bray GA. Use and abuse of appetite-suppressant drugs in the treatment of obesity. *Ann Intern Med.* 1993: 119(7 pt 2): 707–13.
18. Scoville, BA. Review of amphetamine like drugs by the Food and Drug Administration: Clincial data and value judgement. In: Bray GA, ed. Obesity in Perspective. DHEW Pub No. NIH 75-708. Washington, DC: National Institutes of Health; 1975: 441–3.
19. Weintraub M. Long-term weight control: the National Heart, Lung, and Blood Institute funded multimodal intervention study. *Clin Pharmacol Ther.* 1992; 51: 581–5
20. Goldstein DJ eta la. Fluoxetine: a randomized clinical trial in the treatment of obesity. *Int J Obes Relat Metab Disord.* 1994; 18: 129.
21. Gray DS et al. A randomized double-blind clinical trial of fluoxetine in obese diabetics. *Int J Obes Relat Metab Disord.* 1992; 16(suppl 4): S67–72.
22. *Federal Register.* 1991 Aug; 56: 37792–9.
23. Wellman PJ. Overview of adrenergic anorectic agents. *Am J Clin Nutr.* 1992 Jan; 55(1 suppl): 193S–8S.
24. Stunkard AJ. In: Garattini S, Somani R, eds. *Anorectic Agents: Mechanisms of Action and Tolerance.* New York: Raven Press; 1981: 191–210.
25. Wellman PJ. The pharmacology of the anorexic effect of phenylpropanolamine. *Drugs Exp Clin Res.* 1990; 16(9): 487–95.
26. Hoebel BG et al. Appetite suppression by phenylpropanolamine in humans. *Obes Bariatr Med.* 1975; 4: 192.
27. Hoebel BG et al. Body weight decreased in humans by phenylpropanolamine taken before meals. *Obes Bariatr Med.* 1975; 4: 200.
28. Wellman PJ. Weight loss induced by chronic phenylpropanolamine: anorexia and brown adipose tissue thermogenesis. *Pharmacol Biochem Behav.* 1986 Mar; 24: 605–11.
29. Weintraub M et al. Phenylpropanolamine OROS (Acutrim) vs placebo in combination with caloric restriction and physician-managed behavior modification. *Clin Pharmacol Ther.* 1986 May; 39: 501–9.
30. Greenway F. A double-blind evaluation of the anorectic activity of phenylpropanolamine versus placebo. *Clin Ther.* 1989 Sep-Oct; 11: 584–9.
31. *Federal Register.* 1982; 47: 8466.
32. Lake CR et al. Adverse drug effects attributed to phenylpropanolamine: a review of 142 case reports. *Am J Med.* 1990; 89: 195–208.
33. Fallis RJ, Fisher M. Cerebral vasculitis and hemorrhage associated with phenylpropanolamine. *Neurology.* 1985; 35: 405–7.
34. Maertens P et al. Intracranial hemorrhage and cerebral angiopathic changes in a suicidal phenylpropanolamine poisoning. *South Med J.* 1987 Dec; 80: 1584–6.
35. Glick R et al. Phenylpropanolamine: an over-the-counter drug causing central nervous system vasculitis and intracerebral hemorrhage. Case report and review. *Neurosurgery.* 1987; 20: 969–74.
36. Clark JE, Simon WA. Cardiac arrhythmias after phenylpropanolamine ingestion. *Drug Intell Clin Pharm.* 1983; 17: 737–8.
37. Pentel P et al. Myocardial injury after phenylpropanolamine ingestion. *Br Heart J.* 1982; 47: 51–4.
38. Weesner KM et al. Cardiac arrhythmias in an adolescent following ingestion of an over-the-counter stimulant. *Clin Pediatr.* 1982; 21: 700–1.
39. Woo OF et al. Atrioventricular conduction block caused by phenylpropanolamine. *JAMA.* 1985; 253: 2646–7.
40. Burton BT et al. Atrioventricular block following overdose of decongestant cold medication. *J Emerg Med.* 1985; 2: 415–9.
41. Bennett W. Hazards of the appetite suppressant phenylpropanolamine. *Lancet.* 1979; 2: 42-3. Letter.
42. Swenson RD et al. Acute renal failure and rhabdomyolysis after ingestion of phenylpropanolamine-containing diet pills. *JAMA.* 1982; 248: 1216.
43. Rumpf KW et al. Rhabdomyolysis after ingestion of an appetite suppressant. *JAMA.* 1983; 250: 2112.
44. Duffy WB et al. Acute renal failure due to phenylpropanolamine. *South Med J.* 1981; 74: 1548.
45. Frewin DB, Leonello P, Frewin M. Hypertension after ingestion of Trimolets. *Med J Aust.* 1978; 2: 497–8.
46. Horowitz JD et al. Hypertension and postural hypotension induced by phenylpropanolamine (Trimolets). *Med J Aust.* 1979; 1: 175–6.
47. Horowitz JD et al. Hypertensive responses induced by phenylpropanolamine in anorectic and decongestant preparations. *Lancet.* 1980; 1: 8159, 60-1.
48. Morgan JP. In: Morgan JP, ed. *Phenylpropanolamine.* Fort Lee, NJ: Burgess; 1986: 13–25.
49. Cuthbert MF. Anorectic and decongestant preparations containing phenylpropanolamine. *Lancet.* 1980; 1: 367.
50. Morgan JP, Funderburk FR. Phenylpropanolamine and blood pressure: a review of prospective studies. *Am J Clin Nutr.* 1992 Jan; 55(1 suppl): 206S–10S.
51. Noble RE. Phenylpropanolamine and blood pressure. *Lancet.* 1980; 1: 1419.
52. Silverman HI et al. Lack of side effects from orally administered phenylpropanolamine and phenylpropanolamine with caffeine: a controlled three-phase study. *Curr Ther Res.* 1980; 28: 185.
53. Saltzman MB, Dolan MM, Doyne N. Comparison of effects of two regimens of phenylpropanolamine on blood pressure and plasma levels in normal subjects under steady-state conditions. *Drug Intell Clin Pharm.* 1983; 17: 746–50.

54. Noble R. A controlled clinical trial of the cardiovascular and psychological effects of phenylpropanolamine and caffeine. *Drug Intell Clin Pharm.* 1988; 22: 296–9.
55. Goodman RP et al. The effect of phenylpropanolamine on ambulatory pressure. *Clin Pharmacol Ther.* 1986; 40(2): 144–7.
56. Liebson I et al. Phenylpropanolamine: effects on subjective and cardiovascular variables at recommended over-the-counter dose levels. *J Clin Pharmacol.* 1987; 27: 685–93.
57. Klesges RC et al. The effects of phenylpropanolamine on dietary intake, physical activity, and body weight after smoking cessation. *Clin Pharmacol Ther.* 1990 Jun; 47: 747–54.
58. Bradley MH, Raines J. The effects of phenylpropanolamine hydrochloride in overweight patients with controlled stable hypertension. *Curr Ther Res.* 1989 Jul; 46(1): 74–84.
59. Deocampo PD. Convulsive seizures due to phenylpropanolamine. *Med Soc N J.* 1979; 76: 591–2.
60. Lake CR, Masson EB, Quirk RS. Psychiatric side effects attributed to phenylpropanolamine. *Pharmacopsychiatry.* 1988; 21(4): 171–81.
61. Norvenius G et al. Phenylpropanolamine and mental disturbances. *Lancet.* 1979; 2: 1367–8.
62. Scavullo BC, Dementi B. Psychotic reactions following the naive ingestion of an anorectic, phenylpropanolamine, in psychiatric patients. *J Am Coll Toxicol.* 1986; 5: 577–81.
63. Dietz AJ. Amphetamine-like reactions to phenylpropanolamine. *JAMA.* 1981; 245: 601–2.
64. Blum A. Phenylpropanolamine: an over-the-counter amphetamine? *JAMA.* 1981; 245: 1346–7. Editorial.
65. Morgan JP et al. Subjective profile of phenylpropanolamine: absence of stimulant euphorigenic effects at recommended dose levels. *J Clin Psychopharmacol.* 1989 Feb; 9: 33–8.
66. Summary Minutes of the FDA OTC Panel on Cold, Cough, Allergy, Bronchodilator, and Antihistamine Drug Products. Washington, DC: Food and Drug Administration; 1973 June.
67. Ekins BR, Spoerke DG. An estimation of the toxicity of nonprescription diet aids from seventy exposure cases. *Vet Hum Toxicol.* 1983; 25: 81–5.
68. Lee KY et al. Severe hypertension after ingestion of an appetite suppressant (phenylpropanolamine) with indomethacin. *Lancet.* 1979; 1: 1110–1.
69. Lee KY et al. Severe hypertension after administration of phenylpropanolamine. *Med J Aust.* 1979; 1: 525-6. Letter.
70. Kane FJ, Green BQ. Psychotic episodes associated with the use of common proprietary decongestants. *Am J Psychiatry.* 1966; 123: 484–7.
71. Smookler S, Bermundez AJ. Hypertensive crisis resulting from an MAO inhibitor and an over-the-counter appetite suppressant. *Ann Emerg Med.* 1982; 11: 482–4.
72. Yu PH. Inhibition of monoamine oxidase activity by phenylpropanolamine, an anorectic agent. *Res Commun Chem Pathol Pharmacol.* 1986; 51: 163–71.
73. Bennett WM. Hazards of appetite suppressant phenylpropanolamine. *Lancet.* 1979; 2: 8132.
74. Chouinard G et al. Death attributed to ventricular arrhythmia induced by thioridazine in combination with a single Contact C capsule. *Can Med Assoc J.* 1978; 119: 729–30.
75. McLaren EH. Severe hypertension produced by interaction of phenylpropanolamine with methyldopa and oxyprenolol. *Br Med J.* 1976; 2: 283–4.
76. Castellani S. Catatonia associated with phenylpropanolamine overdose and fluphenazine treatment: case report. *J Clin Psychiatry.* 1985; 46(7): 288.
77. Lake CR et al. Phenylpropanolamine increases plasma caffeine levels. *Clin Pharmacol Ther.* 1990; 47: 675–85.
78. Brown NJ, Ryder D, Branch RA. A pharmacodynamic interaction between caffeine and phenylpropanolamine. *Clin Pharmacol Ther.* 1991; 50: 363–71.
79. Lake CR et al. Transient hypertension after two phenylpropanolamine diet aids and the effects of caffeine: a placebo-controlled follow-up study. *Am J Med.* 1989; 86: 427-32.
80. Gibson RG et al. Nifedipine therapy of phenylpropanolamine-induced hypertension. *Am Heart J.* 1987; 113: 406–7.
81. Pentel PR, Asinger RW, Benowitz NL. Propranolol antagonism of phenylpropanolamine-induced hypertension. *Clin Pharmacol Ther.* 1985 May; 37: 488–94.
82. Duvernoy EC. Positive phentolamine test in hypertension induced by a nasal decongestant. *N Engl J Med.* 1969; 280: 877.
83. Hyans JS et al. Pseudopheochromocytoma and cardiac arrest associated with phenylpropanolamine. *JAMA.* 1985; 253: 1609–10.
84. Appelt GD. The safety of phenylpropanolamine. *J Clin Psychopharmacol.* 1983; 3: 322–3.
85. Plotz M. Obesity. *Med Times.* 1958; 86: 860–3.
86. Gilbertson WE. Benzocaine's Status as an OTC Active Ingredient. Rockville, Md: Food and Drug Administration; Apr 7, 1993 [FDA advisory letter].
87. Himes JH, Dietz WH. Guidelines for overweight in adolescent preventive services: recommendations from an expert committee. *Am J Clin Nutr.* 1994; 59: 307–16.
88. Stuart RB. Self-help group approach to self-managment. In: Stuart RD, ed. *Behavioral Self-Management: Strategies, Techniques, and Outcomes.* New York: Brunner/Mazel; 1977: 278.
89. Ashwell M, Garrow JS. A survey of three slimming and weight control organizations in the UK. *Nutrition.* 1975; 29: 347–56.
90. Rosenblatt E. Weight-loss programs. *Postgrad Med.* 1988; 137-48.
91. Stunkard AJ. Studies on TOPS: a self-help group for obesity. In: Bray GA, ed. Obesity in Perspective. DHEW Pub No. NIH 75–708. Washington, DC: National Institutes of Health; 1975: 387–91.
92. Stunkard AJ. The current status of treatment for obesity in adults. In: Stunkard AJ, Stellar E, eds. *Eating and Its Disorders.* New York: Raven Press; 1984: 157–73.
93. Rosenblatt E. Weight loss programs. *Postgrad Med.* 1988; 86(6): 137–42, 148.
94. *FDA Medical Bulletin.* 1994 Sep; 24: 3.
95. Capwell RR. Ephedrine-induced mania from an herbal diet supplement. *Am J Psychiatry.* 1995; 152: 647.
96. Bistrian BR. State of the art. *JAMA.* 1978; 240: 2299–302.
97. Shearer RS. Effects of bulk producing tablets on hunger intensity in dieting patients. *Curr Ther Res.* 1976; 19: 433–41.
98. Drenck EJ. Bulk producers. *JAMA.* 1975; 234–71.
99. Walsh DE et al. Effect of glucomannan on obese patients: a clinical study. *Int J Obes.* 1984; 8: 289–93.
100. Robinson CH, Lawler MR. Normal and Therapeutic Nutrition. 16th ed. New York: Alan R. Liss; 1980.
101. Mogadam M. Nutritional fads. *Am J Gastroenterol.* 1990; 85: 510–5.

CHAPTER 22

Ophthalmic Products

Mark W. Swanson and Jimmy D. Bartlett

Questions to ask in patient assessment and counseling

- *Is your vision blurred?*
- *Do your eyes hurt? Is the pain sharp or dull? Is it constant or intermittent?*
- *Do your eyes itch or sting?*
- *How long have these symptoms been present? What were you doing when you noticed them? Have you had a similar problem before?*
- *Have you recently used a nonprescription eye product? Which one(s) did you use? For what symptoms?*
- *Have you recently been in an accident or injured your head in any way?*
- *What is the nature of your work?*
- *Have you been working outside or in an environment that would cause your eyes to water, itch, or burn?*
- *Have your eyes been exposed recently to irritants such as smog, chemicals, or sun glare? Have you recently applied any pesticides or fertilizers?*
- *Do you have any other eye problems (double vision, redness, scratchy feeling, discharge, or twitch)?*
- *Do you have a chronic disease such as diabetes, glaucoma, or hypertension?*
- *Have you recently had a head cold or sinus problem?*
- *Are you currently taking any prescription or nonprescription medications?*
- *Do you have any allergies? If so, to what are you allergic?*
- *Do you wear contact lenses? Are they hard or soft lenses?*
- *What contact lens products do you use?*
- *Do you use eye cosmetics? Have you changed brands of eye makeup or used a friend's eye makeup?*
- *Do you use hair spray or spray deodorants?*

Many common conditions causing ocular discomfort are minor and self-limiting. In some instances, however, relatively minor symptoms may be associated with severe, potentially blinding conditions. Pharmacists should be well versed in eye anatomy and physiology and in common ocular conditions to provide the best possible guidance to patients who seek assistance in choosing between self-treatment or professional medical care.

Eye Anatomy and Physiology

External Eye

The external location and exposure of the eye make it susceptible to environmental and microbiologic contamination. However, the eye has many natural defense mechanisms to protect it against such contamination. The eyelids are one of the major protective elements (Figure 1).

The eyelids are a multilayer tissue covered externally by the skin and internally by a thin, mucocutaneous epithelial layer, the palpebral conjunctiva. The intermediate portion of the eyelid contains glandular tissue and muscles for lid closure and opening. There are five main types of glandular tissue found within the eyelid: the meibomian glands, the glands of Zeis and Moll, and the accessory glands of Krause and Wolfring.[1] The meibomian, Zeis, and Moll glands are sebaceous in nature and are found near the cilia (eyelashes). The glands of Krause and Wolfring are lacrimal glands found deep within the palpebral conjunctiva near the junction of the eyelid and globe. Their secretion constitutes the bulk of nonstimulated tears.

The eyelids serve primarily to protect the front surface of the eye. Through neural reflex mechanisms, the lids are physically able to block many foreign contaminants from reaching the ocular surface. The lashes also collect debris before it encounters the eye. The second principal function of the eyelids is to spread the tears produced by the glandular tissue. The eyelids close in a zipperlike manner from the outer to the inner margin, thereby forcing the flow of tears toward the nose, where drainage canals are located in the upper and lower eyelids. The drainage canals converge, forming the lacrimal sac between the inner eyelid and nose. The lacrimal sac is drained by a canal opening just below the inferior turbinate of the nasal cavity. The lacrimal drainage system is lined by a highly vascularized epithelium, and absorption into the systemic circulation along this pathway gives rise to potential systemic effects of topically administered eye medications.[1]

Editor's Note: This chapter is based, in part, on the chapter with the same title that appeared in the 10th edition but was written by Jimmy D. Bartlett and Mark W. Swanson.

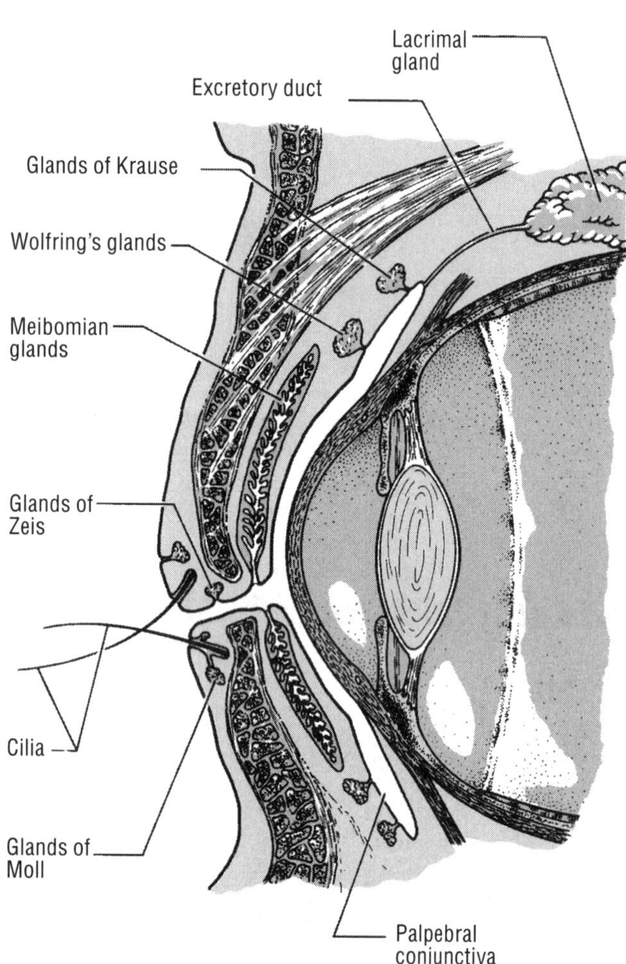

FIGURE 1 Cross-sectional anatomy of the eyelid.

The tear layer functions to keep the ocular surface lubricated, provides a mechanism for removing debris that touches the ocular surface, and has a potent antimicrobial action provided by specific enzymes and a number of immunoglobulins, notably IgA. The tear layer is a trilayer film. The outer surface is a thin lipid layer produced by the meibomian, Zeis, and Moll glands of the lids. The lipid layer complex prevents evaporation and maintains the optical properties of the tear layer. Even with the beneficial effect of the lipid layer, however, as much as 25% of total tear volume is lost to evaporation.[2] The middle, and largest, layer of the tear film is aqueous and is produced by the accessory lacrimal glands of Krause and Wolfring. This layer is largely responsible for the wetting properties of the tear film. The inner layer of the tear film is mucinous and is produced by goblet cells found within the conjunctiva. The mucinous layer allows the aqueous and lipid layers to maintain constant adhesion across the cornea and conjunctiva. Abnormalities within any one of these three layers can result in ocular discomfort.

The tears are produced at a rate of 1–2 mcL/min, with a turnover of approximately 16% total volume per minute.[2,3] An ambient tear volume of approximately 7–10 mcL is found on the ocular surface at any point in time.[2] During episodes of ocular irritation, reflex tearing is stimulated by the lacrimal gland found underneath the outer portion of the upper eyelid, and tear production increases to more than 300% of the nonstimulated production rate.[4]

The visible external portion of the eye is composed of the cornea and sclera (Figure 2). The sclera is a tough, collagenous layer that gives the eye rigidity and encases the internal eye structures. The visible sclera is covered by two epithelial layers, the episclera and the bulbar conjunctiva. The bulbar conjunctiva is contiguous with the palpebral conjunctiva at the junction between the eyelid and the ocular surface (the fornix). The episcleral and bulbar conjunctival layers contain the vascular and lymphatic systems of the anterior eye surface and are the source of visible eye redness during ocular irritation or inflammation. The sclera, episclera, and bulbar conjunctiva join the cornea in a transitional zone (the limbus).

The cornea is an aspherical, avascular tissue that is the principal refractive element of the eye. Approximately 12 mm wide and 0.5 mm thick,[1] it consists of five distinct layers: the epithelium, Bowman's layer, the stroma, Descemet's membrane, and the endothelium. The epithelium and endothelium maintain corneal hydration, Bowman's and Descemet's layers serve barrier and protective functions, and the stroma provides the cornea with its clarity.

The unique anatomic structure of the cornea affects drug absorption. The corneal epithelium is lipophilic and facilitates the passage of fat-soluble drugs. The corneal stroma is hydrophilic and allows the passage of water-soluble drugs. Therefore, optimum penetration of a drug through the cornea depends on biphasic solubility. Damage to the corneal epithelium may markedly change drug absorption rates. Comparative studies with intact and compromised epithelium have shown that drug penetration into the aqueous layer may be increased by as much as threefold in corneas with compromised epithelium.[5] Corneal epithelium can be compromised by trauma, routine contact lens wear, topical ophthalmic anesthetics, and thermal or UV light exposure.

Reflex tearing occurs immediately upon the instillation of a drug into the eye, diluting the drug's concentration. It has been shown that solutions as hypertonic as 2.5% sodium chloride are diluted to the concentration of tears (0.9–0.95%) within 1–2 minutes.[2] The difficulty for drugs to penetrate through the cornea, combined with their rapid removal through the tear system and their dilution by reflex tearing, can hinder efforts to maintain therapeutic drug concentrations in the eye. Studies have shown that as much as 90% of an instilled dose administered to the eye may be lost.[6]

Internal Eye

Directly behind the cornea is the anterior chamber, a cavity filled with aqueous humor (Figure 2). The aqueous functions to maintain the normal internal eye pressure and provides nutritional support for the cornea and crystalline lens. It is produced at a constant rate by the epithelium of the ciliary body and is drained from the

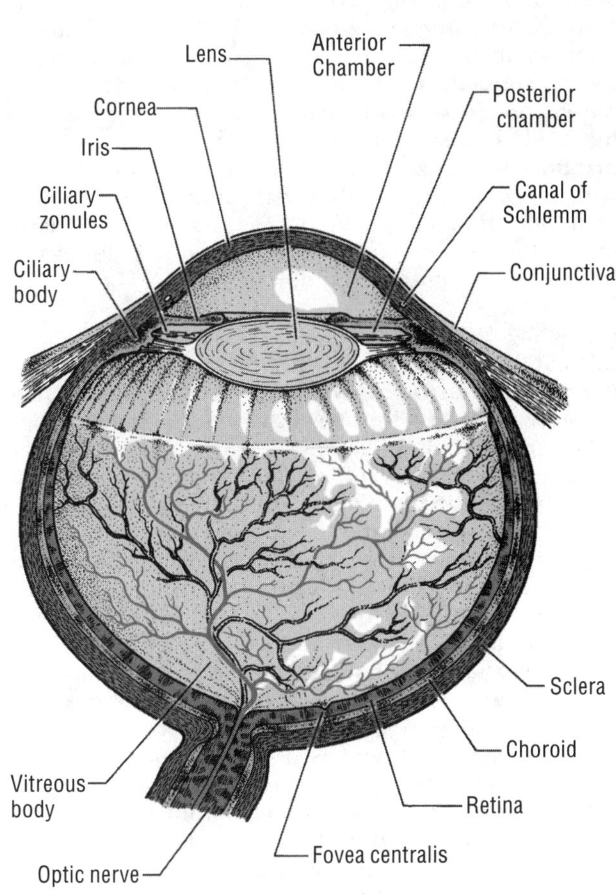

FIGURE 2 Major anatomic features of the eye.

anterior chamber via the trabecular meshwork found at the junction between the iris and the back surface of the cornea. During episodes of internal eye inflammation, the aqueous becomes filled with white blood cells and protein released by the ciliary body. Large amounts of inflammatory cells may block the drainage system, causing the internal eye pressure to rise. Similarly, during episodes of angle-closure glaucoma, the trabecular meshwork is physically blocked by the iris, with a resultant increase in intraocular pressure.

The iris is the visible colored portion of the eye. It functions in much the same way as an aperture on a camera to regulate light striking the retina. The central opening in the iris is the pupil. The pupillary diameter is controlled by two opposing muscles within the iris, the sphincter and the dilator. As the names imply, the sphincter decreases the pupil diameter whereas the dilator increases it. The sphincter is controlled by the parasympathetic nervous system, and the dilator is controlled by the sympathetic nervous system. Both topical and systemic drugs may affect the tonus of these muscles, thereby altering the pupil diameter. Prostaglandins released by the iris during episodes of inflammation may also affect the sphincter muscle, resulting in constriction of the pupil. This constriction may help distinguish simple external irritation from more severe internal inflammation.

Directly behind the pupillary aperture is the crystalline lens, an avascular, biconvex structure that alters its shape to focus light on the retina. The focusing is a response to the viewing of a near object and is referred to as accommodation. With normal aging, the lens becomes less able to focus light, and at some point the individual must rely on optical devices to focus near objects on the retina. Presbyopia, or lack of near focusing ability, commonly begins to manifest itself at ages 40–45. Focusing of the lens is directly controlled by the ciliary body.

The ciliary body is bordered anteriorly by the iris and is continuous posteriorly with the choroid. The ciliary body is composed of the ciliary muscle and the ciliary epithelium. The lens is connected to the ciliary body by the ciliary zonules, threadlike protein fibrils attached to the lens surface. The ciliary muscle is largely controlled by the parasympathetic nervous system. During accommodation, the ciliary muscle constricts, releasing tension on the ciliary zonules and allowing the lens to change shape. During episodes of ocular inflammation, the ciliary muscle may begin to spasm, resulting in fluctuating vision and pain. For this reason, inhibition of the ciliary muscle (cycloplegia) using anticholinergic agents is a frequent treatment during internal ocular inflammation.

Behind the lens lies the vitreous body. It comprises about 80% of the total eye volume and is filled with vitreous humor, a gellike, fluid collagen matrix that helps maintain eye volume. Posteriorly, the vitreous humor abuts the retina, a multilayer neural tissue that begins the visual pathway. Light is initially captured by the rods and cones of the retina in a complex photochemical process. Ultimately, the photic message is transmitted by the optic nerve and visual pathways to the posterior cerebral cortex, where the visual information is decoded. The retina adheres relatively loosely to the retinal pigment epithelium beneath it. Trauma may cause the retina to separate from the pigment epithelium, resulting in retinal detachment. A number of inflammatory conditions of the retina can occur, and most have prominent symptoms. Some, however, have relatively mild symptoms mimicking common irritative conditions.

Common Ocular Disorders

Ocular inflammation and irritation can be caused by many conditions, some of which can be treated safely and effectively with nonprescription ophthalmic products. These products are used primarily to relieve minor symptoms of burning, stinging, itching, and watering. The Food and Drug Administration (FDA) has suggested that self-medication may be indicated for tear insufficiency, corneal edema, and external inflammation or irritation.[7] Self-medication also may be effective in managing hordeolum (stye), blepharitis, and conjunctivitis.[8] Referral for medical care is mandatory for embedded foreign bodies, uveitis, flash burns, chemical burns, tear duct infection, and corneal ulcers.

The FDA has recommended that consumers not self-treat ophthalmic conditions for longer than 72 hours without consulting a doctor.[7] It refers specifically to self-

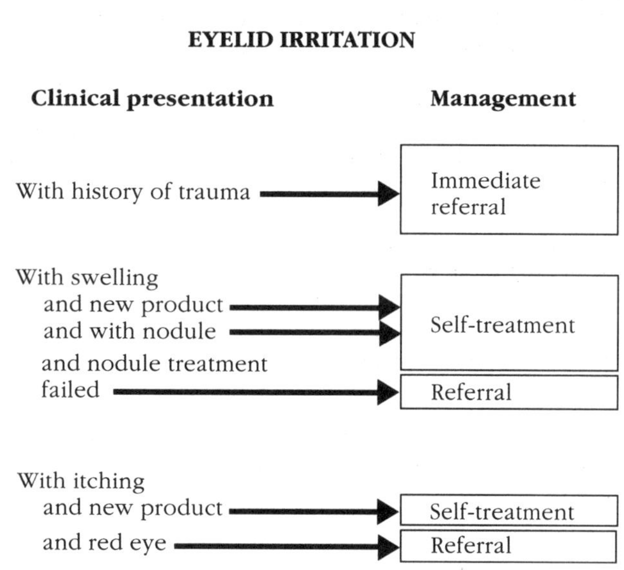

FIGURE 3 Decision-making algorithm for management of patients with eyelid irritation.

treatment with ophthalmic lubricants and decongestant (vasoconstrictor) products. The pharmacist should advise patients of this general rule on duration of use when recommending nonprescription ophthalmic products. Care should be taken when counseling patients because many seemingly harmless ocular conditions can prove to be devastating. Figures 3 and 4 provide general algorithms that may be used in the decision-making process when managing eyelid irritation and red eye. It must be emphasized that if the etiology is not clearly due to simple external irritation, referral to an optometrist or ophthalmologist is strongly encouraged.

Eyelid Disorders

Blunt Trauma

Because the eyelids are a highly vascular tissue, blunt trauma can easily rupture blood vessels and cause bleeding into the eyelid tissue space, resulting in swelling and ocular discomfort. Under most circumstances, blunt trauma does not result in internal damage and treatment is largely supportive, entailing cold compresses and oral nonprescription analgesics as needed. However, all individuals with blunt trauma should be evaluated by an ophthalmologist or optometrist as soon as possible after the event. In addition to the visible external damage, blunt trauma can result in internal eye bleeding, secondary glaucoma, and retinal detachment.

Blepharitis

Blepharitis is an extremely common inflammatory condition of the eyelid margins. It is almost always due to *Staphylococcus epidermidis, Staphylococcus aureus,* seborrheic dermatitis, or a mixture of these conditions.[9] Red, scaly, thickened eyelids, often with loss of the eyelashes, are typical of blepharitis. Itching and burning are the most common accompanying complaints. All forms of blepharitis tend to be chronic, and individuals are often aware of their diagnosis. Treatment may include topical antibiotics or nonprescription lid hygiene preparations. Lid scrubs with baby shampoo are also effective. Lid scrubs consist of cleansing along the eyelid margin with gauze pads or cotton applicators soaked with prepackaged solution, baby shampoo, or topical antibiotic ointment. The chronic nature of blepharitis makes the use of careful lid hygiene preferable to the long-term use of topical antibiotics.

Lice Infestation

Infestation of the eyelids with the organisms *Phthirius pubis* (crab louse) or *Pediculus humanus capitis* (head louse) may cause symptoms similar to blepharitis. These organisms are also responsible for sexually transmitted lice infestation. Children are rarely affected by the crab louse but are commonly affected by the head louse. Adults with eyelid infestation will often be aware of the involvement of other body areas. Pediculicides (eg, RID, Nix, and A-200) are useful for treating noneyelid areas but should not be used around the eye because they could cause severe hypersensitivity reactions. A bland ophthalmic ointment (eg, petrolatum) used for 10 days is also effective because it suffocates the louse and deprives its eggs of adequate oxygen. A 0.25% physostigmine ointment is effective, but the side effects due to its powerful anticholinesterase activity are not well tolerated. Pharmacists should also carefully instruct patients about the need to take hygienic measures, such as washing clothing and bedding that may contain unhatched eggs.

Contact Dermatitis

Swelling, scaling, or redness of the eyelid along with profuse itching are common with contact dermatitis. A change in makeup or soap, or exposure to some foreign substance is usually the cause. The equal involvement of each eyelid suggests allergy because both eyes are often exposed. Questioning the patient about new products used (eg, eyeliner and eye shadow) quickly identifies the offending substance, removal of which is the best treatment. Swelling of the eyelid can be marked in some cases, and nonprescription oral antihistamines along with cold compresses will help reduce the inflammation and itching.

Hordeolum

Hordeolum is an inflammation of either the meibomian gland (internal hordeolum) or the glands of Zeis and Moll (external hordeolum). A palpable, tender nodule is always present. Swelling of the eyelid, almost to the point of closure, can occur with a severe internal hordeolum. The cause is invariably one of the staphylococcal species associated with blepharitis. Hordeola typically respond well to hot compresses applied three to four times daily for 5–10 minutes at each session. Clearing usually occurs within 1 week. Although external hordeola may be treated with a topical antibiotic, internal hordeola do not respond well to such treatment and are best treated with a course of oral antibiotics. In recalcitrant cases, surgical drainage may be required.

A chalazion, which is a sterile granuloma, is very similar in appearance to an internal hordeolum. However, chalazia are not tender to gentle touching whereas hordeola are typically quite tender. Hot compresses applied the same as for treatment of hordeola are usually sufficient to drain chalazia. Recalcitrant chalazia may require an intralesional steroid injection or surgical excision. Recurrences of chalazion and hordeolum may be reduced by the periodic use of lid scrubs.

Ocular Surface Disorders

Foreign Substance Contact

Despite the protective effect of the lids, foreign substances often contact the ocular surface. The immediate response of the eye is watering. If reflex tearing does not remove the foreign substance, the eye may need to be flushed. Lint, dust, and similar materials can usually be removed by rinsing the eye with sterile saline or specific eyewash preparations (irrigants). Foreign particles trapped between the upper lid and the bulbar conjunctiva can be particularly difficult to flush and may need to be removed by an optometrist or ophthalmologist. Metallic foreign bodies are often not removed by self-irrigation and can cause abrasion, scarring, and chronic red eye if not removed. Moreover, when such particles contact the eye as a result of high-speed grinding or activities that entail metal striking metal, intraocular penetration is possible. Thus, immediate medical referral is indicated.

Abrasions

Contact with foreign matter can also cause abrasions of the cornea and conjunctiva. These injuries result in partial or total loss of the epithelium and are especially painful if the cornea is involved. Scratches by fingernails and metallic foreign bodies are a common source of this type of injury. Self-treatment is not recommended owing to the risk of bacteria or fungi contaminating and infecting the eye.

Chemical Exposure

Chemical exposure by splash injury, a solid chemical, or fumes can be a serious problem and should be considered a medical emergency. The initial treatment should include flushing the eye with sterile saline for at least 10 minutes. If saline is not available, water may be used. Because the lids and ocular surface are particularly sensitive to alkali damage, severe scarring can occur. This type of injury should be referred immediately to an emergency facility.

Thermal Damage

Thermal damage may range from minor to severe. One common form of thermal damage occurs from exposure to UV radiation during snow skiing without protective goggles. This form of irritation is typically minor and usually responds well to artificial tear solutions or ointments. If such treatment does not provide relief within 24 hours, medical referral is indicated. More severe forms

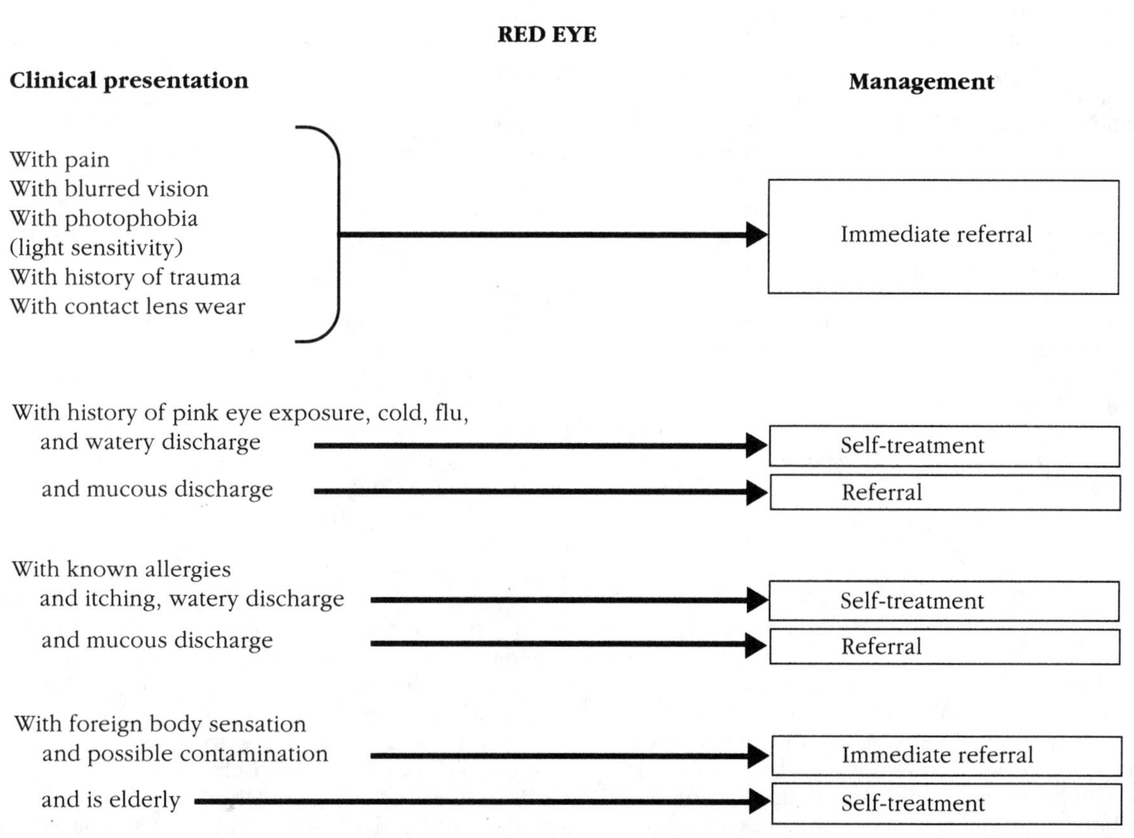

FIGURE 4 Decision-making algorithm for management of patients with red eye(s).

of thermal injury, however, may occur from welder's arc. These injuries may require a visit to the optometrist or ophthalmologist to provide definitive care, including eye patching.

Conjunctivitis

Conjunctivitis is the term given to inflammation of the bulbar conjunctiva. Four general types of conjunctivitis are commonly seen: viral, allergic, bacterial, and chlamydial.

Viral Conjunctivitis Viral conjunctivitis is probably the most common form. A recent cold, sore throat, or exposure to someone with pinkeye (acute contagious conjunctivitis) is a common precursor of this condition. Individuals with viral conjunctivitis will usually have a "pink eye" with a copious amount of watery discharge. Symptoms include nondescript ocular discomfort and mild to moderate foreign body sensation; vision may occasionally be blurred. Low-grade fever may be present, and swollen preauricular or submandibular lymph nodes may be found. Viral conjunctivitis is usually self-limiting, with symptoms resolving over 1–3 weeks. Treatment is aimed at relief of the major symptoms using artificial tear preparations and ocular decongestants. Because certain forms of viral conjunctivitis can be extremely contagious, counseling should include warnings about washing hands, not sharing towels, and properly disposing of tissues used to blot the eye.

Allergic Conjunctivitis Allergic conjunctivitis is characterized by a red eye with watery discharge. The hallmark symptom accompanying ocular allergy is itching. Vision is usually not impaired but may be blurred owing to excessive tearing. The list of antigens that can cause ocular allergy is virtually endless, but the most common allergens include pollen of various types, animal dander, and topical eye preparations. Persons with ocular allergy will often report seasonal allergic rhinitis as well. Questioning the patient about exposure to an allergen may help identify the offending substance. Removal or avoidance of the cause is the best treatment, but ocular decongestants, ocular decongestant antihistamine preparations, nonprescription oral antihistamines, and cold compresses will help relieve symptoms.

Bacterial Conjunctivitis Bacterial conjunctivitis can be caused by a number of organisms, including *S aureus, S epidermidis, Streptococcus pneumoniae,* and *Haemophilus influenzae.*[9] This condition is characterized by a red eye with purulent discharge. The most common complaint is of general eye discomfort along with the key symptom of the eyelids sticking together on awakening. Bacterial conjunctivitis is typically self-limiting within 2 weeks, but topical antibiotics can clear the infection more quickly.

Chlamydial Conjunctivitis A fourth type of conjunctivitis is caused by chlamydial infection. In the United States, this is a sexually transmitted disease and thus is often seen in the sexually active population. Chlamydial conjunctivitis may have many signs and symptoms in common with both viral and bacterial conjunctivitis, and it is often initially misdiagnosed. Misdiagnosis can be a serious problem because afflicted individuals often harbor other sexually transmitted diseases. Women with chlamydial urethritis are at risk of pelvic inflammatory disease. Because of the pitfalls in separating chlamydial infection from self-limiting viral and bacterial conjunctivitis, self-treatment should be discouraged if symptoms and signs are vague.

Keratitis

Keratitis is the inflammation of the cornea. It may accompany any of the forms of conjunctivitis or exist as a separate entity. Individuals with keratitis, which is potentially a vision-threatening problem, will generally have signs of conjunctivitis accompanied by one or more additional symptoms, including blurred vision, photophobia, and pain. Individuals with red eye and signs of keratitis need to be evaluated as soon as possible by an optometrist or ophthalmologist. This is especially true for patients who wear contact lenses who are contemplating self-treatment of red eye. Corneal ulceration and loss of the eye are more likely among those who wear contact lenses than among those who do not. Contact lens wearers who sleep in lenses overnight are particularly at greatest risk of corneal ulceration.[10] *Pseudomonas aeruginosa,* the most common cause of corneal ulcer among contact lens wearers, produces a collagenase that can destroy the cornea within 24 hours.[11]

Corneal Edema

Corneal edema may occur from a variety of conditions, including overwear of contact lenses, surgical damage to the cornea, and inherited corneal dystrophies. The edematous area of the cornea is often confined to the epithelium. Because fluid accumulation distorts the optical properties of the cornea, halos or starbursts around lights, with or without reduced vision, are a hallmark symptom of corneal edema. Once the initial diagnosis is established, hypertonic saline in solution or ointment form, usually in 2% and 5% concentrations, can be used to dehydrate the cornea. Pharmacists should forewarn individuals using a 5% solution that profound stinging may occur on instillation.

Dry Eye

Dry eye is among the most common disorders affecting the anterior eye. This condition is characterized by a white or mildly red eye; a sandy, gritty feeling or complaint of something in the eye is common. Contrary to what the name suggests, dry eye is often accompanied by excess tearing. Abnormalities in the tear layer cause less than optimal lubrication of the ocular surface. This leads to the production of more inadequate tears, and a vicious cycle is set up. Dry eye is most often associated with the aging process, but it can also be caused by lid defects; loss of lid tissue turgor; Sjögren's syndrome; Bell's palsy; a variety of collagen diseases, including rheumatoid arthritis; and systemic medications. Antihistamines, anticholinergics or drugs with anticholinergic properties (eg, antihistamines and antidepressants), diuretics, and beta blockers are some of the more common pharmacologic causes of dry eye.

Treatment of dry eye is the instillation of nonprescription artificial tears and lubricants. The products are similar, but the buffering agents, preservatives, pH, and other formulation factors may vary. Preparations without preservatives have been shown to have a greater beneficial effect on the ocular surface than do those with preservatives.[12] Both drop and ointment preparations are available. Because all ointments tend to blur vision for some time after instillation and have longer contact time with the eye, their preferred usage is at bedtime; drops are generally recommended for use during the day. Vitamin A preparations are also available for treatment of dry eye. Although these have generally been shown to be no more effective than artificial tear preparations in the treatment of routine dry eye, they may be of greatest benefit in treating severe dry eye associated with glandular tissue destruction.[13] The most severe cases of dry eye may be treated with ocular inserts or sodium hyaluronate, or by occlusion of the lacrimal drainage system to increase the available tear pool.

Internal Eye Conditions

Uveitis

Uveitis is the general term for inflammation of the uveal tract (iris, ciliary body, or choroid). This disorder is divided into anterior, posterior, and panuveal (ie, affecting both anterior and posterior) types. Anterior uveitis is also known as iritis, whereas posterior uveitis is synonymous with vitritis. In these conditions, white blood cells are found within the anterior chamber or vitreous body. Uveitis can be caused by a number of conditions, including trauma and systemic inflammatory disease, but in many individuals it is idiopathic. Persons with uveitis can have symptoms very similar to those of viral conjunctivitis or keratitis, with pain, blurred vision, and photophobia commonly reported. The eye is usually mildly to markedly red with reflex tearing. The absence of contact with infected individuals may help determine whether the cause is simple viral conjunctivitis. Untreated uveitis can cause secondary glaucoma, destruction of the iris, and in some cases blindness. Treatment involves topical, depot, or systemic oral steroids, depending on the underlying cause. Because of the severe consequences of untreated or improperly treated uveitis, care must be taken in recommending self-treatment.

Angle-Closure Glaucoma

Narrow-angle or angle-closure glaucoma may present as a red, painful eye. Symptoms associated with angle closure occur as a result of obstruction of the trabecular meshwork and the aqueous draining system. The angle-closure attack may be precipitated by dilation of the pupil with mydriatics; the attack often occurs as the pupil is returning to its normal state several hours after the mydriatic has been instilled. The most common symptoms are brow-ache or headache, often accompanied by nausea and vomiting; these symptoms are typically severe enough to cause the individual to visit an eye doctor. Due to the potentially vision-threatening nature of angle-closure glaucoma, individuals complaining about headache or eye pain occurring after an eye examination that involved pupillary dilation should be referred immediately to their eye doctor.

Ophthalmic Drug Formulations

Ophthalmic medications available without a prescription are necessarily formulated to reduce the stinging and other side effects common with many prescribed ophthalmic drugs. The pH, buffers, tonicity adjusters, and preservative systems must be carefully controlled to produce a product that is comfortable to use and will therefore encourage compliance with the self-medication process. Ophthalmic products that sting, burn, or otherwise irritate ocular tissues will, of course, be poorly tolerated by the patient who self-treats. Among the inactive ingredients of nonprescription ophthalmic products, the drug vehicle and preservative systems are the most important, and the pharmacist must have adequate knowledge of these components to assist the patient in selecting the appropriate ophthalmic product. In addition, various other ingredients are often included as excipients.

Vehicles

An ophthalmic vehicle is an agent other than the active drug that is added to a formulation to enhance drug action by providing increased viscosity. Although aqueous solutions can be used, the vehicles listed in Table 1 are more viscous and thus retard drainage of the active ingredient from the eye; this increases the retention time of the active drug and enhances bioavailability at the external ocular tissues. These polymers are generally of high molecular weight, and some of the molecules can even bind at the corneal surface to increase drug retention and stabilize the tear film. Among the most commonly used vehicles for ophthalmic solutions are povidone, polyvinyl alcohol (PVA), hydroxypropyl methylcellulose (HPMC), and poloxamer 407. Ointments are also used as vehicles for ophthalmic drugs.

Polyvinyl Alcohol

PVA is a water-soluble viscosity enhancer commonly used in a concentration of 1.4%.[14] This vehicle is generally nonirritating to the eye, and documentation has shown that it actually facilitates healing of abraded corneal epithelium.[15]

TABLE 1 Selected ophthalmic vehicles
Carboxymethylcellulose (CMC) sodium
Dextran 70
Gelatin
Glycerin
Hydroxyethylcellulose (HEC)
Hydroxypropyl methylcellulose (HPMC)
Methylcellulose
Poloxamer 407
Polyethylene glycol
Polyvinyl alcohol (PVA)
Povidone
Propylene glycol

Hydroxypropyl methylcellulose

Like PVA, the viscosity enhancer HPMC is available in several molecular weights and in formulations with different substitutions. These polymers are often called "substituted cellulose ethers." When used as ophthalmic lubricants, these vehicles enhance tear film stability. HPMC (0.5%) has been documented to exhibit twice the ocular retention time of 1.4% PVA.[16]

Povidone

Povidone is not bound to membrane surfaces and thus does not provide long-lasting viscosity enhancement beyond its normal residence time in the tears. Its viscosity does not change until near pH 1.0, when it doubles. Thus, there is no appreciable ionic character to the povidone molecule at pharmaceutical or physiologic pH values. Consolute binding, however, can cause a change in the size of the polymer molecule, influencing the viscosity and other properties of the solution.

Poloxamer 407

The first polyionic vehicle to be evaluated in the eye was poloxamer 407, a vehicle with a hydrophobic nucleus, hydrophilic end groups, and surfactant properties. Polyionic vehicles such as poloxamer 407 are unique in their ability to produce an artificial microenvironment in the tear film, which can greatly enhance the bioavailability of certain drugs used in the eye.[17]

Ointments

Ophthalmic ointments represent a special type of vehicle produced by mixing white petrolatum and mineral oil with or without a water-miscible agent such as lanolin. The mineral oil is added to the petrolatum to allow the vehicle to melt at body temperature, and the lanolin is added to absorb water. This allows for water and water-soluble drugs to be retained in the delivery system. Commercial ophthalmic ointments are generally derivatives of a hydrocarbon mixture of 60% petrolatum (USP) and 40% mineral oil (USP), which is a semisolid at room temperature but which melts at body temperature. In general, ointments are well tolerated by the ocular tissues.

The primary clinical purpose for an ophthalmic ointment is to increase the ocular contact time of the instilled product. The ocular contact time of an ointment vehicle is about twice as long in the blinking eye and four times as long in the nonblinking or patched eye as that of a saline vehicle. Nonmedicated ophthalmic ointments are often used for self-medication in treating dry eye syndromes. Patients should be informed, however, that their use may cause temporary blurred vision because ointments coat the eye.

Preservatives

Preservatives are incorporated into ophthalmic products designed for multidose use. These components are intended to destroy or limit multiplication of microorganisms inadvertently introduced into the product. Commonly used preservatives in commercial ophthalmic products are listed in Table 2.

TABLE 2 Preservatives commonly used in ophthalmic products

- Benzalkonium chloride (BAK)
- Benzethonium chloride
- Cetylpyridinium chloride
- Chlorhexidine
- Chlorobutanol
- Disodium ethylenediaminetetraacetic acid (EDTA)
- Methylparaben
- Phenylethyl alcohol
- Phenylmercuric acetate
- Phenylmercuric nitrate
- Propylparaben
- Sodium benzoate
- Sodium propionate
- Sorbic acid
- Thimerosal

Preservatives currently available for ophthalmic use are of two distinct types. One group, the surfactants, are molecules that disrupt the plasma membrane and are usually bactericidal. The other group includes the metals mercury and iodine, their derivatives, and alcohols. These compounds are considered bacteriostatic if they only inhibit growth, or bactericidal if they destroy the ability of bacteria to reproduce.

Quaternary Surfactants

The quaternary surfactants, benzalkonium chloride (BAK) and benzethonium chloride, are preferred by many manufacturers because of their stability, excellent antimicrobial activity, and long shelf life. Unfortunately, these agents have toxic effects on both the tear film and the corneal epithelium.[18] A single drop of 0.01% BAK can break the superficial lipid layer of the tear film into numerous oil droplets. This preservative can reduce the tear film breakup time and thus may represent a poor choice for an antimicrobial preservative in artificial tear products.[19] The inclusion of BAK in artificial tear formulations does not provide protection to corneal epithelium or promote a stable oily tear surface.

Chlorhexidine

Chlorhexidine is useful as an antimicrobial agent in the same range of concentrations as BAK, yet it is used at lower concentrations in commercial ophthalmic formulations. Because it does not alter corneal permeability to the same extent as does BAK, chlorhexidine is not as toxic to the eye.

Other Preservatives

Thimerosal Of the mercurial preservatives, thimerosal is less likely to degrade into toxic mercury than either phenylmercuric acetate or phenylmercuric nitrate. Compared with BAK, which undermines tear film stability, thimerosal has no known effects on the tear film. An important clinical point, however, is that some patients develop contact blepharitis or conjunctivitis after several weeks of exposure to thimerosal and must therefore discontinue use of products containing this preservative. Moreover, products containing thimerosal are rapidly disappearing from the commercial marketplace because this preservative induces contact allergy.

Chlorobutanol Chlorobutanol is less effective than BAK as an antimicrobial preservative and, indeed, tends to disappear from bottles during prolonged storage.[14] Compared with thimerosal, however, chlorobutanol does not appear to produce allergic reactions associated with prolonged use.

Methylparaben and Propylparaben During the past decade, methylparaben and propylparaben have been introduced into some ophthalmic medications, especially artificial tears and nonmedicated ointments. However, these preservatives are unstable at high pH and can sometimes induce allergic reactions.

Ethylenediaminetetraacetic Acid Ethylenediaminetetraacetic acid (EDTA) is a chelating agent that preferentially binds and sequesters divalent cations. The role of EDTA in preservative systems is to assist the action of thimerosal, BAK, and other agents. As with those other preservatives, EDTA can sometimes induce contact allergies.[20]

Excipients

Useful excipients are antioxidants, wetting agents, buffers, and tonicity adjusters. Antioxidants prevent or delay deterioration of products exposed to oxygen in the air, and wetting agents reduce surface tension, allowing the drug solution to spread more easily over the ocular surface. Buffers help to maintain ophthalmic products in the range of pH 6.0–8.0, thus promoting ocular comfort upon instillation. Tonicity adjusters allow the medication to be isotonic with the physiologic tear film. Products in the sodium chloride equivalence range of 0.9% ± 0.2% are considered isotonic and will help reduce ocular irritation and tissue damage. Solutions in the tonicity range of 0.6–1.8% are usually comfortable when placed on the human eye.

Major Categories of Nonprescription Ophthalmic Products

Numerous nonprescription ophthalmic products for treating minor ocular irritations are commercially available for self-administration by the patient under minimal or no supervision. Such products are also adequate for treating certain clinical conditions that have been diagnosed by health practitioners. The pharmacist must actively assist patients in selecting the appropriate product that will enhance compliance, minimize or avoid side effects, and reduce the attendant costs of therapy. Nearly all ophthalmic conditions amenable to nonprescription therapy can be treated by using the appropriate product chosen from the following categories of medications.

Lubricants

Many advances have been made in understanding the mechanisms involved in tear film formation, but the role of tears in maintaining a normal conjunctival and corneal surface is still not completely understood. The availability of synthetic chemicals suitable for topical application to the eye has resulted in the development of various solutions to help alleviate dryness of the ocular surface. The use of water-soluble polymer solutions and bland, nonmedicated ointments remains the primary therapy for the dry eye. Because almost all these products are available without a prescription, the pharmacist has a primary responsibility to assist and counsel the patient regarding their selection and proper use. Although a benefit of ophthalmic lubricant therapy is to increase the viscosity of existing tears, it must be emphasized that high viscosity alone does not necessarily provide relief for all dry eye conditions. Consequently, other, less viscous hydrophilic substances are now included as the primary polymeric ingredients of many artificial tear formulations.

Artificial Tear Solutions (Demulcents)

Lubricants formulated as solutions consist of preservatives, inorganic electrolytes to achieve tonicity and maintain pH, and water-soluble polymeric systems. These solutions are usually administered three to four times daily (Table 3), but depending on the patient's clinical needs and response to therapy, they may be given as often as hourly or only occasionally.

Cellulose Ethers The substituted cellulose ethers are commonly incorporated into many artificial tear solutions. These ethers include HPMC, hydroxyethylcellulose (HEC), hydroxypropylcellulose (HPC), methylcellulose, and carboxymethylcellulose. These solutions are colorless and vary in viscosity (see product table "Artifical Tear Products").

Methylcellulose is usually used in a concentration of 0.25–1.0%. At a concentration above 2%, the methylcellulose solution becomes sufficiently viscous to be classified as an ointment. Most contemporary artificial tear solutions incorporate other substituted cellulose ethers, especially HEC and HPC. Solutions of these polymers are usually less viscous than—but have emollient properties equal or superior to—those of methylcellulose. These ethers can also be combined with other polymers for use as artificial tears. Perhaps the most important property of the cellulose ethers in artificial tear formulations is that they stabilize the tear film and prevent tear evaporation, both of which are beneficial effects for patients with dry eye.[21] These effects generally occur without irritation or toxicity to the ocular tissues. Thus, their relative lack of toxicity, their viscous properties, and their beneficial effects on the tear film have made cellulose ethers extremely useful components of artificial tear preparations.

Polyvinyl Alcohol PVA is another commonly used viscosity enhancer for artificial tear preparations. This polymer is usually used in a 1.4% concentration and is considerably less viscous than methylcellulose. Like the cellulose ethers, PVA also enhances stability of the tear

TABLE 3 Procedure for self-administration of eyedrops

1. Wash hands thoroughly.
2. Tilt head backward.
3. Gently grasp lower outer eyelid below lashes and pull eyelid away from eye to create a pouch.
4. Place dropper over eye by looking directly at it.
5. Just before applying a single drop, look upward.
6. After applying the drop, look downward for several seconds.
7. Release the eyelid slowly.
8. Close eyes gently for 1–2 minutes. Minimize blinking or squeezing the eyelid.
9. With a finger, put gentle pressure over the opening of the tear duct at the inner corner of the eye.
10. Blot excessive solution from around the eye.

film without causing ocular irritation or toxicity. Although PVA is compatible with many commonly used drugs and preservatives, certain compounds, including sodium bicarbonate; sodium borate; and the sulfates of sodium, potassium, and zinc, can thicken or gel solutions that contain it. For example, sodium borate, found in some extraocular irrigants, may react with contact lens wetting solutions containing PVA.[22] Thus, it is important to be cautious when clinically using solutions containing PVA with solutions containing any of these other agents.

Povidone PVP has surface-active properties similar to those of the cellulose ethers. This compound is thought to form a hydrophilic layer on the corneal surface, mimicking natural conjunctival mucin. This "mucomimetic" property has firmly established the role of PVP as an artificial tear formulation. Because PVP promotes wetting of the ocular surface, both mucin- and aqueous-deficient dry eyes seem to benefit.

Retinol Solution Vitamin A deficiency can affect many epithelial-lined organs, including the eye; therefore, the topical administration of retinol, the alcohol form of vitamin A, has been advocated for treating various dry eye disorders. Unfortunately, few controlled clinical trials have been conducted to substantiate the usefulness of retinol solution in dry eye syndromes. Some preliminary studies claim possible benefits for patients with conjunctival hyperemia, superior limbic keratitis, superficial punctate keratitis, and giant papillary conjunctivitis. Many patients may respond favorably to solutions that contain vitamin A because those solutions have emollient qualities. Until more definitive data become available, however, the specific benefits of topically applied vitamin A solution for treating dry eyes will remain speculative. Retinol is available in nonprescription formulations, usually containing 5,000 IU of vitamin A and polysorbate 80.

Preservative-Free Formulations In recent years, artificial tear preparations have been introduced in preservative-free formulations. This is beneficial for patients who are sensitive to preservatives such as BAK and thimerosal. Nonpreserved artificial tear preparations are now available in a variety of unit-dose dispensers, and some of these products are formulated to provide electrolyte support to the damaged surface epithelium of the eye. For example, Refresh Plus and Celluvisc are designed in lower and higher viscosity vehicles, respectively, to provide nutritional support to the ocular surface of patients with moderate to severe dry eye syndromes.[23] In general, however, nonpreserved formulations have the disadvantage of increased cost compared with preserved artificial tear solutions, and they can become easily contaminated by the patient during use. Thus, strict hygienic procedures for self-administration must be followed, and any unused solution should be properly discarded after 12 hours of use.

Clinical results and patient acceptance remain the final criteria for determining efficacy in the treatment of patients with dry eyes. It must be emphasized that no single formulation has yet been identified that will universally improve clinical signs and symptoms while maintaining patient comfort and acceptance.[22]

Prosthesis Lubricant/Cleanser Finally, a sterile, buffered isotonic solution containing 0.25% tyloxapol and 0.02% BAK is available specifically for cleaning and lubricating artificial eyes. Tyloxapol is a detergent surfactant that liquefies solid matter on the prosthesis, and BAK aids tyloxapol in wetting the artificial eye. This solution is used in the same manner as ordinary artificial tears. With the artificial eye in place, one or two drops of solution should be applied three or four times daily. In addition, the solution can be used as a cleaner to remove oily or mucous deposits; in this case, the artificial eye is then rubbed between the fingers and rinsed with tap water prior to insertion.

Nonmedicated Ointments (Emollients)

The principal advantage of nonmedicated (bland) ointments is their enhanced retention time in the eye, which appears to enhance the integrity of the tear film. Thus, both mucin- and aqueous-deficient eyes can benefit from the application of lubricating ointments.

Ointment formulations are usually administered twice daily (Table 4), but depending on the patient's clinical needs and therapeutic response, they may be administered as often as every few hours or only occasionally as needed. Many patients prefer to instill the ointment at bedtime to keep the eyes moist during sleep and to improve morning symptoms of dry eye.

Because of the viscosity of the melted ointment base in the tear film, many patients complain of blurred vision during ointment therapy. This problem can usually be resolved by decreasing the amount of ointment instilled or by administering it at bedtime. Counseling on the blurring of vision with ointments should be a rou-

TABLE 4 Procedure for self-administration of eye ointments

1. Wash hands thoroughly.
2. Tilt head backward.
3. Gently grasp lower outer eyelid below lashes and pull eyelid away from eye.
4. Place ointment tube over eye by looking directly at it.
5. With a sweeping motion, place 1/4- to 1/2-inch of ointment inside the lower eyelid by gently squeezing the tube.
6. Release the eyelid slowly.
7. Close eyes gently for 1–2 minutes.
8. Blot excessive ointment from around the eye.
9. Vision may be temporarily blurred. Avoid activities requiring good visual ability until vision clears.

tine component of dispensing. Although ointment preparations are generally nonirritating, preservatives can be toxic to ocular tissues. Some patients develop hypersensitivity reactions, which prompt them to discontinue therapy. Alternatively, symptoms associated with preserved ointment products can often be eliminated by changing to nonpreserved formulations; this is especially true for patients who require long-term treatment for dry eye. As a rule, it is better to recommend nonmedicated ointments without preservatives for the treatment of dry eye to overcome potential problems that might occur with the use of preserved products.

Decongestants

Four decongestants are available in nonprescription strength for topical application to the eye: phenylephrine, naphazoline, tetrahydrozoline, and oxymetazoline (see product table "Opthalmic Decongestant Products").

Phenylephrine

Phenylephrine, which acts primarily on alpha-adrenergic receptors of the ophthalmic vasculature, is commercially available in concentrations ranging from 0.12 to 10%. However, only the 0.12% or 0.125% concentration is available without a prescription. Higher concentrations are generally reserved for the short-term dilation needed for eye examinations. To prolong shelf life, sodium bisulfite, an antioxidant, is often added to the phenylephrine vehicle. Expiration dates should be strictly enforced because loss of pharmacologic activity may occur without visible changes in solution color.

The low concentrations of phenylephrine used in nonprescription topical decongestants may dilate the pupil if enough of it penetrates the corneal epithelium. This is not uncommon in persons who wear contact lenses who may instill the medication following lens wear. Because a patient can use phenylephrine indiscriminately to quiet an irritated eye, the drug can induce pupillary dilation and precipitate angle-closure glaucoma in eyes predisposed with narrow anterior chamber angles. This adverse effect is more likely if the cornea is damaged or diseased, allowing increased corneal drug penetration. Thus, patients should be cautioned against instilling this and other ophthalmic decongestants too often, and should be encouraged to seek professional eye care if offending ophthalmic signs or symptoms do not resolve within 72 hours.

The most important and common side effect following chronic use of phenylephrine for ocular decongestion is rebound congestion of the conjunctiva, in which the conjunctival vessels become progressively more dilated with continued use of the drug. This phenomenon can create a vicious cycle in which phenylephrine is instilled to quiet an inflamed conjunctiva, which becomes progressively more inflamed with repeated instillation of the medication. Patients with apparent rebound effect should be referred for professional eye care for differential diagnosis and management.

Systemic adverse effects are extremely rare following the topical instillation of nonprescription phenylephrine for ocular decongestion. Although not reported in the literature, certain drug-drug interactions involving low concentrations of phenylephrine are theoretically possible. The pressor effects of phenylephrine may be enhanced in patients taking atropine, tricyclic antidepressants and monoamine oxidase inhibitors, reserpine, guanethidine, or methyldopa. The drug should therefore be used cautiously by patients with cardiovascular disease or diabetes, or by patients taking the concomitant medications listed above. Because of these possible adverse reactions, phenylephrine and other ocular decongestants should not be used as ocular irrigants.

Imidazoles

Like phenylephrine, the imidazoles have greater alpha- than beta-receptor activity and are therefore clinically useful in constricting conjunctival vessels. Moreover, these drugs have only minimal effect on underlying vessels of the episclera and sclera.

Naphazoline Naphazoline has been documented to be effective in constricting conjunctival vessels as well as in reducing tearing and pain associated with superficial ocular inflammation.[24] However, patients with lightly pigmented irides (eg, blue eyes or green eyes) appear to be more sensitive to the mydriatic effects of naphazoline.

Tetrahydrozoline Satisfactory results have similarly been obtained with tetrahydrozoline in most patients with allergic or chronic conjunctivitis, and the beneficial effects can last from 1 to 4 hours. Unlike phenylephrine or naphazoline, tetrahydrozoline does not appear to alter pupil size. However, certain patients may experience mild, transient stinging immediately following instillation of the drops.

Oxymetazoline Oxymetazoline has been evaluated as a topical agent for treatment of allergic and noninfectious conjunctivitis. Topical treatment will improve most symptoms associated with allergic or noninfectious conjunctivitis, including burning, itching, tearing, and foreign body sensation. The clinical effects of oxymetazoline can last up to 4–6 hours. Oxymetazoline (0.025%) appears to be relatively free of both ocular and systemic side effects.

Comparison of Decongestants

It is difficult to reach definitive conclusions regarding clinical comparisons of the available nonprescription ocular decongestants. Although most of the tested preparations produce blanching of conjunctival vessels, 0.02% naphazoline seems to produce greater blanching when compared with other nonprescription decongestants containing 0.05% tetrahydrozoline or 0.12% phenylephrine.[25] Investigators have observed no significant differences in conjunctival blanching with preparations containing naphazoline in concentrations of 0.02%, 0.05%, or 0.1%.[25] Thus, 0.02% naphazoline is an excellent choice for nonprescription therapy of mild to moderate conjunctivitis that is of environmental or noninfectious origin.

The imidazoles generally do not induce ocular or systemic side effects. However, patients should be cautioned that their liberal or indiscriminate use can lead to excessive systemic absorption and the possibility of cardiovascular side effects. Moreover, some patients may experience epithelial xerosis (abnormal dryness) occurring with prolonged topical instillation of local decongestants. Because rebound congestion appears to be less likely following topical ocular use of naphazoline or tetrahydrozoline, these agents should generally be recommended over phenylephrine or oxymetazoline. And because it has superior documented efficacy and produces a relative lack of side effects, 0.02% naphazoline can be recommended with confidence as an ocular decongestant of choice.[26]

Antihistamines

Two nonprescription antihistamines are available for topical ophthalmic use: pheniramine maleate and antazoline phosphate. Pheniramine is a member of the alkylamine group of antihistaminic drugs while antazoline is classified as an ethylenediamine.[27] Both drugs act as specific H_1 receptor antagonists. They do, however, differ somewhat in their pharmacologic actions, both systemically and on the ocular surface. Antazoline has been shown to have some anesthetic properties, but these are insufficient to produce clinical effects when antazoline is used topically.[28] Pheniramine has been shown to have little effect on intraocular pressure whereas antazoline can slightly increase it.[28] This effect during typical usage is not significant.

The topical antihistamines are indicated for the rapid relief of symptoms associated with seasonal or atopic conjunctivitis. Although they are effective individually, all nonprescription preparations contain the decongestant agent naphazoline. The use of a decongestant with the topical antihistamines has been shown to be more effective than the use of either agent singly.[24,29] Most preparations containing the pheniramine-naphazoline combination (Naphcon-A, AK-Con-A, Opcon-A) are formulated with 0.3% pheniramine and 0.025% naphazoline, while the antazoline-naphazoline product (Vasocon-A) is formulated with a higher concentration of naphazoline, 0.05% (see product table "Ophthlamic Decongestant Products"). Recommended dosage for all the products is one or two drops applied to each eye three or four times daily. The FDA has classified the topical antihistamines in the less than effective category primarily because clinical trial data on effectiveness is lacking.

Severe side effects (death, thrombocytopenia, allergic pneumonitis) that may be associated with systemic antihistamine use have not been reported with topical ophthalmic preparations.[30–34] Burning, stinging, and discomfort on instillation are the most common side effects. Although both pheniramine and antazoline may produce stinging, pheniramine may be somewhat more comfortable.[35] There are no absolute contraindications to the use of the topical antihistamines other than sensitivity to one of the components. These drugs do have anticholinergic properties and may cause mydriasis. The mydriatic effect is most commonly seen in persons with light-colored irides or persons with compromised corneas, such as contact lens wearers.[36] In susceptible persons, mydriasis could lead to angle-closure glaucoma. These drugs are contraindicated in persons with a known risk of angle-closure glaucoma.

Irrigants

Extraocular irrigating solutions, or irrigants, are used to cleanse ocular tissues while maintaining their moisture; these solutions must be physiologically balanced with respect to pH and osmolality. Because the tissues with which they come in contact obtain nutrients elsewhere, the role of irrigants is primarily to clear away unwanted materials or debris from the ocular surface. Extraocular irrigants are used only on a short-term basis. All the ophthalmic irrigating solutions are available without a prescription and therefore can be used by patients and practitioners alike (see product table "Miscellaneous Ophthalmic Products").

In the ophthalmic practitioner's office, these solutions come in handy after certain clinical procedures, and they are often used to wash away mucus or purulent exudates from the eye. They are also administered in the hospital to clean out eyes between changes of ocular dressings. When used for these routine purposes, ocular irrigants should not be applied with contact lenses in place because the solutions tend to cause contact lens irritation by reducing the mucin component of the tear film or, in the case of rigid gas-permeable lenses, by reducing the hydrophilicity of the lens surface.[37] Furthermore, absorption of the preservatives BAK or phenylmercuric acetate by soft lenses can have a deleterious effect on the corneal epithelium. Although irrigating solutions may be used to wash out the eyes after contact lens wear, they have no particular value as contact lens wetting, cleansing, or cushioning solutions.

One of the most useful applications of extraocular irrigants is in ocular lavage following chemical injuries to the eye. Penetrating chemicals, such as alkalis, must be washed out immediately. Although the ideal irrigating solution for this purpose is physiologic saline, water may be the only available, practical substance, and it can be recommended when no commercial ocular irrigant is handy. In the particular case of alkali burns to the ocular surface, however, lavage with extraocular irrigants may be inadequate to prevent or minimize ocular damage. In emergency situations involving alkali or acid burns, prompt professional evaluation and treatment by an ophthalmologist or optometrist are strongly encouraged.

In cases in which the patient experiences continuous eye pain, changes in vision, or continued redness or irritation of the eye, or in which the ocular condition persists or worsens, evaluation by an eye care professional should similarly be strongly encouraged. Extraocular irrigants should not be used for open wounds in or near the eyes. As previously discussed, ocular irrigants should not be used in conjunction with contact lens wetting solutions or with other eye care products containing PVA. Commercial irrigating products that use an eyecup should generally be avoided because of difficulties in cleaning the eyecup, with the resultant risk of bacterial or fungal contamination.

Hyperosmotics

Topically applied hyperosmotic formulations are intended to increase the tonicity of the tear film, thereby promoting movement of fluid from the cornea. When applied to the eye, these agents withdraw water from the cornea to the more highly osmotic tear film, which, in turn, is eliminated through the normal tear flow mechanisms. Many patients with mild to moderate corneal epithelial edema may experience improved subjective comfort and vision following appropriate use of these medications. Of the topical ophthalmic hyperosmotic agents that are commercially available, only sodium chloride can be obtained without a prescription in both solution and ointment formulations (see product table "Miscellaneous Ophthalmic Products").

For clinical use, sodium chloride is available in 2% and 5% solution as well as in 5% ointment. In general, the 5% concentration in ointment form is the most effective in reducing corneal edema and improving vision. However, since application of 5% sodium chloride tends to produce symptoms of stinging and burning, patients often prefer the 2% concentration for long-term therapy. Usually one or two drops of the solution are instilled every 3–4 hours (Table 3). The ointment formulation, however, requires less frequent instillation and is usually reserved for use at bedtime to minimize symptoms of blurred vision (Table 4). Because vision associated with edematous corneas is often worse on arising, several instillations of the solution during the first few waking hours may be helpful. Hypertonic saline is nontoxic to the external ocular tissues, and allergic reactions are rare.

Perhaps the most important contraindication to topical hyperosmotic sodium chloride is its use to clear edematous corneas with traumatized epithelium. The intact corneal epithelium exhibits only limited permeability to inorganic ions; therefore, an absent or compromised corneal epithelium will promote increased corneal penetration of the hyperosmotic and thereby reduce the osmotic effect. Consequently, the management of corneal edema associated with traumatized epithelium requires the use of organic hyperosmotic agents that are available only on prescription.[38] Patients whose history or physical appearance suggests a damaged corneal epithelium should be referred for immediate professional eye care.

Antiseptics

Several nonprescription agents are commercially available to reduce the bacterial population on the ocular surface, including the eyelid margins. Although the efficacy of most of these agents is largely unsubstantiated, they may be recommended for patients with only minor conjunctival or eyelid inflammation that is possibly associated with an infectious organism. Of the available agents, only yellow mercuric oxide has received adequate scientific attention to document its effectiveness for some minor ocular infections. Yellow mercuric oxide is, however, no longer commercially available. The others (silver protein, boric acid, and zinc sulfate) have not been adequately studied clinically for use in most ocular surface infections. The "Ophthalmic Decongestant Products" table lists some products that also contain an antiseptic.

Silver Protein

Silver protein is indicated for treatment of ocular infections and for preoperative use in ocular surgery. At low doses, this agent has antimicrobial activity against both gram-positive and gram-negative organisms. When instilled prior to surgery, silver protein stains and coagulates mucus; all stained material should then be removed before operating to reduce the incidence of postoperative infection. For preoperative use, two or three drops are instilled into the eye and then rinsed with sterile irrigating solution. For treatment of mild ocular infections, several drops of silver protein are generally instilled every 3–4 hours for several days. Frequent topical application to the eye for prolonged periods should be avoided, however, because it can result in permanent discoloration of the eyelid skin or conjunctiva, a condition known as argyria. Silver protein is incompatible with topically applied sodium sulfacetamide preparations.[39]

Boric Acid

Boric acid is indicated for the treatment of irritated or inflamed eyelids. Available in 5% or 10% ointment formulations, boric acid should generally be applied in a small quantity to the inner surface of the lower eyelid once or twice daily. If ocular irritation persists or increases, the patient should receive medical attention.

Zinc Sulfate

Zinc sulfate is a mild astringent for temporary relief of minor ocular irritation. It is generally used in a dosage of one to two drops up to four times daily. Zinc salts have also been used for infections caused by *Moraxella*. The application of 0.25% zinc sulfate solution, although effective against the bacteria, is not as effective as prescription antibacterial therapy.

Eyelid Scrubs

Although there are many forms of blepharitis, the mainstay of therapy is generally careful eyelid hygiene. The patient can easily accomplish this at home by using hot compresses for 15–20 minutes, two to four times daily. Each application should be followed by lid scrubs using a mild detergent cleanser compatible with ocular tissues (Table 5). These lid scrub procedures are usually effective and well tolerated.

Although baby shampoo is often used for this purpose, recent experience has shown other commercially available cleansers to be as effective with potentially less ocular stinging, burning, and toxicity.[40] Commercial lid scrub products are intended for the removal of oils, debris, or desquamated skin associated with the inflamed eyelid (see product table "Miscellaneous Ophthlamic Products"). The lid scrubs can also be used for hygienic eyelid cleansing in people who wear contact lenses. These products are designed to be used full strength on eyelid tissues and must not be instilled directly into the eyes. The most effective application technique is to close the eyes and gently scrub the eyelids and eyelashes using side-to-side strokes. The solution should be rinsed thoroughly, and the applications should generally be repeated twice daily. Some of the commercial products are packaged with gauze pads, which provide an abrasive action to augment the cleansing properties of the detergent solution. Eyelid scrubs using commercially available detergents are most effective in patients with noninfectious blepharitis. Thus, if the patient's signs or symptoms fail to improve, the patient should be referred for professional ocular examinations and treatment with appropriate antibacterial agents.

Multivitamins

Deficiencies of vitamin A and zinc have been associated with certain adverse ocular effects. Beyond replacement of documented nutritional deficiencies, which occur rarely in the United States, treatment or prevention of ophthalmic diseases using vitamins and/or minerals is not clearly established.

In recent years, investigations have explored the prophylactic use of vitamins A, C, and E as well as zinc to guard against the degenerative ophthalmic changes that appear to be associated with the aging process. The primary mechanisms of action offered to explain the theoretical efficacy of such therapy include antioxidation and free radical scavenging. Several products are now commercially available for the prevention and treatment of macular degeneration, but considerably more data will be required before these products can be generally recommended.[41]

TABLE 5 Procedure for eyelid scrubs

1. Wash hands thoroughly.
2. Apply three to four drops of baby shampoo or eyelid cleanser to cotton-tipped applicator or gauze pad.
3. Close one eye and clean the upper eyelid and eyelashes using side-to-side strokes, being careful not to touch eyeball with applicator or fingers.
4. Open eye, look up, and clean lower eyelid and eyelashes using side-to-side strokes.
5. Repeat the procedures on other eye using a clean applicator or gauze pad.
6. Rinse eyelids and eyelashes with clean, warm water.

Patient Counseling

The pharmacist has an important responsibility in guiding patients to appropriate nonprescription ocular therapy. Both the safety and effectiveness of ophthalmic products can be enhanced by paying strict attention to drug selection, contraindications, and appropriate dosage schedules and administration technique. Careful consideration of the patient's medical history, including concomitant medication use, will often minimize the risk of adverse reactions. Appropriate dosing procedures are important to ensure maximum effectiveness of the self-administered medications.

Patient History

A careful history not only alerts the pharmacist to possible adverse drug reactions, but also may assist the pharmacist to select the best product for the patient's ocular condition. Among the most important issues to be investigated in the patient's history is concomitant medications.

Drug Interactions/Allergies

Drug interactions can play a significant role in potentiating or impairing drug effects and may even exacerbate any potential adverse reaction. For example, topically applied phenylephrine may heighten the pressor effects of certain prescription drugs.[26]

Inquiry regarding a history of drug allergies is essential. Hypersensitivity to thimerosal and other mercurial compounds is not uncommon among those who wear contact lenses, and topically applied ophthalmic medications containing mercurial preservatives, especially when used long term, can lead to allergic reactions.

Coexisting Medical Conditions

Patients with systemic hypertension, arteriosclerosis, and other cardiovascular diseases may be at risk when topically applied ocular decongestants such as phenylephrine or the imidazoles are used. Adverse cardiovascular events are also possible when these agents are used in patients with hyperthyroidism.[26]

Although most topically administered drugs can be used safely during pregnancy, it is prudent to limit topical ophthalmic dosing in pregnant women. Artificial tears can be used without limit, but agents with ingredients that affect the autonomic nervous system, such as ocular decongestants, should be used sparingly during pregnancy.

Medical Referral

The pharmacist should carefully consider the nature and extent of ocular involvement. Because a definitive ocular diagnosis requires professional examination by an ophthalmologist or optometrist, it is difficult to give precise guidelines on when the pharmacist should refer patients who are not responding to nonprescription therapy. As a general rule, however, patients who fail to respond within 72 hours should be referred for medical evaluation, especially if they are not currently under the care of an ophthalmic practitioner. It is important for patients with acute ocular disease to receive a prompt definitive diagnosis, including baseline visual acuity, before the appropriateness of nonprescription therapy is considered. Some acute conditions, presenting with or without ocular pain or blurred vision, can be appropriately treated with nonprescription agents, but a recent diagnosis from the ophthalmic practitioner can give the pharmacist additional reassurance and confidence in recommending such treatment.

On the other hand, many patients with chronic ocular conditions, especially dry eye, may fail to respond to initial nonprescription therapy with artificial tears or other lubricants. In many of these cases, the most appropriate strategy is to change to a different lubricant, especially one with a different polymer or preservative system. Then, if there is still no response, the patient should be strongly encouraged to seek professional assessment and care from an ophthalmic practitioner. Although the cost-effectiveness of ophthalmic care can be greatly improved through the use of nonprescription agents, severe visual impairment, including blindness, can be a serious clinical and medicolegal complication if referral for definitive diagnosis and treatment is delayed.

Self-Administration of Ophthalmic Medications

Proper drug instillation technique is critical if the target tissue (the eye) is to receive the maximum benefit from the medication. The following general guidelines should help promote the safe and effective use of nonprescription ophthalmic products, and should help the pharmacist decide whether the patient should be referred for professional ophthalmic care.[42,43]

- Nonprescription ophthalmic products should be used only in situations in which vision is not threatened, and they should generally not be used for longer than 72 hours without medical referral if the condition being treated persists or worsens.
- Nonprescription ocular medications should not be recommended to patients who have demonstrated an allergy to any of the active ingredients, preservatives, or other excipients in the product.
- Patients who are already using a prescription ophthalmic product should use nonprescription products only after consulting with an ophthalmic practitioner or pharmacist.
- Patients with a history of narrow anterior chamber angles or narrow-angle glaucoma should not use topical ocular decongestants because of the risk of angle-closure glaucoma.
- The lowest concentration and conservative dosage frequencies should be used, and overdosage should be avoided.
- Drug application should be conservative in patients with hyperemic conjunctiva because of the potential for increased systemic drug absorption and the risk of adverse effects.
- Patients should be reminded to use all medications only as directed. There is generally no additional benefit from receiving more than the intended amount of the drug.
- If multiple drop therapy is indicated, the best interval between drops is at least 5 minutes. This helps to ensure that the first drop is not flushed away by the second, or that the second drop is not diluted by the first.
- If both drop and ointment therapy are indicated, the drop should be applied at least 10 minutes before the ointment so that the ointment does not become a barrier to tear film or corneal penetration of the drop.
- Patients should wipe excessive solution or ointment from the eyelids and lashes after instillation.
- Because ointments may blur the patient's vision during the waking hours, they should be used with caution if visual acuity is critical; otherwise, bedtime instillation is most appropriate.
- Use of eyecups should be discouraged because of potential bacterial, fungal, or viral contamination.
- Ophthalmic medications should not be used beyond their expiration dates. Eyedrop bottles should be replaced or discarded 30 days after the sterility safety seal is opened because the manufacturer's expiration date does not apply once the seal is broken.
- Patients should store all medications out of children's reach.
- The pharmacist should recognize adverse drug reactions, including the clinical signs of drug toxicity or allergy.

Ophthalmic solutions and ointments, as well as eyelid scrubs, are often misused. The pharmacist should help ensure maximum safety and effectiveness of these agents by carefully instructing patients in the proper self-administration procedures. Appropriate patient education and counseling must accompany dispensation of any ophthalmic product. Tables 3, 4, and 5 summarize the step-by-step procedures in using these agents.

Case Studies

Case 22–1

Patient Complaint/History

LY, a 67-year-old female, presents to the pharmacist with complaints of redness, burning, and watering of both eyes; she is not experiencing itching of the eyes or any discharge other than the watering. The symptoms, which are more severe when the patient arises in the morning, have been present for several years; however, they have recently become worse. Physical observation of the patient reveals red and teary eyes.

LY's current medical problems include osteoarthritis, mild osteoporosis, and hypertension. She also has recurrent sinus infections associated with seasonal allergic rhinitis. Her current medications include Monopril 20 mg one tablet daily; Premarin 1.25 mg one tablet daily for 21 days, off for 7 days; Os-Cal 500 one tablet daily; and Advil 200 mg two tablets prn for joint pain, headache, or vague functional aches and pain. A few days earlier, the patient selected the following nonprescription products to manage the current symptoms: Refresh PM, Lacrilube Ophthalmic Ointment, and Visine.

Clinical Considerations/Strategies

The following considerations/strategies are provided to aid the reader in (1) determining whether treatment of the patient's condition with nonprescription medications is warranted, (2) selecting the appropriate nonprescription medication, and (3) developing a patient counseling strategy to ensure optimal therapeutic outcomes:

- Determine whether the patient has used eye drops or ointment to manage previous similar eye conditions. If so, determine whether the medications were effective.
- Assess the need for an artificial tear solution.
- Assess the need for applying a lubricating ointment at bedtime.
- Assess the need for preserved versus nonpreserved solutions.
- Assess the cost versus benefit ratio of the selected product(s).
- Develop a patient education/counseling strategy that will:
  - Address appropriate products and their usage for dry eye therapy;
  - Instruct the patient to apply the ointment only at bedtime and provide appropriate instructions for its application;
  - Explain the limited effectiveness of ophthalmic decongestants for the symptoms (ie, discourage their use);
  - Explain the chronic nature of the condition;
  - Advise the patient of the need for professional eye care if the symptoms persist.

Case 22–2

Patient Complaint/History

CJ, a 37-year-old male, presents to the pharmacist after being told by his eyecare professional to treat a "scabies" infestation of his eyelids by scrubbing the eyelids and then applying an ointment to them. The patient complains of itching and burning of his eyelids. When questioned about the presence of other symptoms, the patient admits that he also has itching of the scalp and genitals. Physical observation reveals reddened eyelid margins.

To treat the scabies infestation, CJ's eyecare professional prescribed doxycycline 250 mg qid po for 30 days. The patient selected the following nonprescription products for additional treatment of his condition: Lacrilube Ophthalmic Ointment, Eye-Scrub solution, and 1% Nix cream rinse.

Clinical Considerations/Strategies

The following considerations/strategies are provided to aid the reader in (1) determining whether treatment of the patient's condition with nonprescription medications is warranted, (2) selecting the appropriate nonprescription medication, and (3) developing a patient counseling strategy to ensure optimal therapeutic outcomes:

- Assess whether the patient has had this condition before. If so, find out whether he used the described nonprescription medication regimen to treat the previous occurrence(s).
- Assess the appropriateness of the patient-selected ophthalmic products.
- Assess the need to treat the condition with the prescribed and patient-selected products.
- Assess the appropriateness of the patient-selected nonophthalmic product.
- Assess the need for additional nonophthalmic products.
- Develop a patient education/counseling plan that will:
  - Explain the potential toxicity of nonophthalmic products when used on or around the eye;
  - Indicate the appropriate duration of treatment for each product;
  - Explain strategies to prevent spread of the scabies infestation;
  - Explain appropriate use and possible reuse of the nonophthalmic products;
  - Explain the proper application of ophthalmic ointments and use of eyelid scrub solutions.

Summary

The pharmacist is strategically positioned in the community to treat patients with ophthalmic pathology or to recommend self-management with one or more nonprescription drugs. Several such pharmaceuticals are available to manage the symptoms of minor acute or chronic conditions of the eye and eyelid. By understanding the pathophysiology of certain ocular conditions and knowing how to assess patients who present with such conditions, a pharmacist should be able to optimize the safe, appropriate, effective, and economical use of nonprescription drugs in the management of various conditions of the eye and eyelid.

References

1. Warwick R. *Anatomy of the Eye and Orbit.* 7th ed. Philadelphia: WB Saunders; 1975: 195–219.
2. Milder B. The lacrimal apparatus. In: Moses RA, Hart WM, eds. *Adler's Physiology of the Eye.* 8th ed. St Louis, Mo: CV Mosby; 1987: 15–35.

3. Mishima S et al. Determination of tear volume and tear flow. *Invest Ophthalmol.* 1966; 3: 264–76.
4. Jordan A, Baum J. Basic tear flow. Does it exist? *Ophthalmology.* 1980; 9: 920–30.
5. Pfister RR, Burstein N. The effects of ophthalmic drugs, vehicles, and preservatives on corneal epithelium; a scanning electron microscope study. *Invest Ophthalmol.* 1976; 15: 246–59.
6. Harris LS, Galin MA. Dose response analysis of pilocarpine-induced ocular hypotension. *Arch Ophthalmol.* 1970; 1: 605–8.
7. Ophthalmic drug products for over-the-counter human use; final monograph. *Federal Register.* 1988; 53(43).
8. Ophthalmic drug products for over-the-counter human use; establishment of a monograph; proposed rulemaking. *Federal Register.* 1980; 45(89): 30002–50.
9. Jones DB, Liesegang TJ, Robinson NM. Laboratory diagnosis of ocular infections. Paper presented at Washington, DC: American Society for Microbiology; 1981.
10. Alfonso E et al. Ulcerative keratitis associated with contact lens wear. *Am J Ophthalmol.* 1986; 101: 429–33.
11. Cohen EJ et al. Corneal ulcers associated with contact lenses including experience with disposable lenses. *CLAO J.* 1991; 1: 173–6.
12. Lopez-Bernal D, Ubels JL. Quantitative evaluation of the corneal epithelial barrier effect: effect of artificial tears and preservatives. *Curr Eye Res.* 1991; 7: 645–66.
13. Schilling H et al. Treatment of dry eye with vitamin A acid: an impression cytology controlled study. *Fortschr Ophthalmol.* 1989; 5: 530–4.
14. Mullen W, Sheppard W, Leibowitz J. Ophthalmic preservatives and vehicles. *Surv Ophthalmol.* 1973; 17: 469–83.
15. Sabiston DW. The dry eye. *Trans Ophthalmol Soc N Z.* 1969; 21: 96–100.
16. Linn ML, Jones LT. Rate of lacrimal excretion of ophthalmic vehicles. *Am J Ophthalmol.* 1968; 65: 76–8.
17. Burstein NL. Ophthalmic drug formulations. In: Bartlett JD, Jaanus SD, eds. *Clinical Ocular Pharmacology.* Boston: Butterworth-Heinemann; 1995: 21–45.
18. Burstein NL. Preservative cytotoxic threshold for benzalkonium chloride and chlorhexidine digluconate in cat and rabbit corneas. *Invest Ophthalmol Vis Sci.* 1980; 19: 308–13.
19. Wilson WS, Duncan AJ, Jay JL. Effect of benzalkonium chloride on the stability of the precorneal tear film in rabbit and man. *Br J Ophthalmol.* 1975; 59: 667–9.
20. Mondino BJ, Salamon SM, Zaidman GW. Allergic and toxic reactions in soft contact lens wearers. *Surv Ophthalmol.* 1982; 26: 337–44.
21. Norn MS. Desiccation of the precorneal film: I. corneal wetting time. *Acta Ophthalmol.* 1969; 47: 865–80.
22. Jaanus SD. Lubricants and other preparations for ocular surface disease. In: Bartlett JD, Jaanus SD, eds. *Clinical Ocular Pharmacology.* Boston: Butterworth-Heinemann; 1995: 355–67.
23. Grene B et al. A clinical study comparing the efficacy of two ophthalmic lubricating solutions using impression cytology. *Invest Ophthalmol Vis Sci.* 1990; 31(suppl): 529.
24. Miller J, Wolf EM. Antazoline phosphate and naphazoline hydrochloride, singly and in combination for the treatment of allergic conjunctivitis—a controlled double-blind clinical trial. *Ann Allergy.* 1975; 35: 81–6.
25. Abelson MB, Yamamoto GK, Allansmith MR. Effects of ocular decongestants. *Arch Ophthalmol.* 1980; 98: 856–8.
26. Jaanus SD, Pagano VT, Bartlett JD. Drugs affecting the autonomic nervous system. In: Bartlett JD, Jaanus SD, eds. *Clinical Ocular Pharmacology.* Boston: Butterworth-Heinemann; 1989: 69–148.
27. Jaanus SD, Hegeman SL, Swanson MW. Antiallergy drugs and decongestants. In: Bartlett JD, Jaanus SD, eds. *Clinical Ocular Pharmacology.* Boston: Butterworth-Heineman Publishers; 1995: 337–53.
28. Krupin T et al. The effect of H_1 blocking antihistamines on intraocular pressure in rabbits. *Ophthalmology.* 1980; 87: 1167–72.
29. Abelson MB, Allansmith MR, Freidlaender MH. Effects of topically applied ocular decongestant and antihistamine. *Am J Ophthalmol.* 1980; 90: 254–7.
30. Petrusewicz J, Kalizan R. Blood platelet adrenoreceptor: aggregatory and antiaggregatory activity of imidazole drugs. *Pharmacology.* 1986; 33: 249–55.
31. Pahissa A et al. Antazoline induced allergic pneumonitis. *Br Med J.* 1979; 2: 1328.
32. Bengtsson U et al. Antazoline induced immune hemolytic anemia, hemoglobulinuria, and acute renal failure. *Acta Med Scand.* 1975; 198: 223–7.
33. Neilsen JL, Dahl R, Kissmeyer-Neilsen F. Immune thrombocytopenia due to antazoline. *Allergy.* 1981; 36: 517–9.
34. Ogbuihi S, Audick W, Bohn G. Sudden infant death—fatal intoxication with pheniramine. *Z Rechtsmed.* 1990; 103: 221–5.
35. Berdy GJ et al. Allergic conjunctivitis—a survey of new antihistamines. *J Ocul Pharmacol.* 1991; 7: 313–24.
36. Gelmi C, Occuzzi R. Mydriatic effect of ocular decongestants studied by pupillography. *Ophthalmologica.* 1994; 208: 243–6.
37. Hales RH. *Contact Lenses: A Clinical Approach to Fitting.* Baltimore: Williams & Wilkins; 1978: 32–50.
38. Lamberts DW. Topical hyperosmotic agents and secretory stimulants. *Int Ophthalmol Clin.* 1980; 20: 163–9.
39. Kastl PR, Ali Z, Mather F. Placebo-controlled, double-blind evaluation of the efficacy and safety of yellow mercuric oxide in suppression of eyelid infections. *Ann Ophthalmol.* 1987; 19: 376–9.
40. Polack FM, Goodman DF. Experience with a new detergent lid scrub in the management of chronic blepharitis. *Arch Ophthalmol.* 1988; 106: 719–20.
41. Sperduto RD, Ferris FL, Kurinij N. Do we have a nutritional treatment for age-related cataract or macular degeneration? *Arch Ophthalmol.* 1990; 108: 1403–5.
42. Bartlett JD, Cullen AP. Clinical administration of ocular drugs. In: Bartlett JD, Jaanus SD, eds. *Clinical Ocular Pharmacology.* Boston: Butterworth Publishers; 1989: 29–66.
43. Bartlett JD. Dosage forms and routes of administration. In: Bartlett JD et al, eds. *Ophthalmic Drug Facts.* St Louis, Mo: Facts and Comparisons; 1992: 1–7.

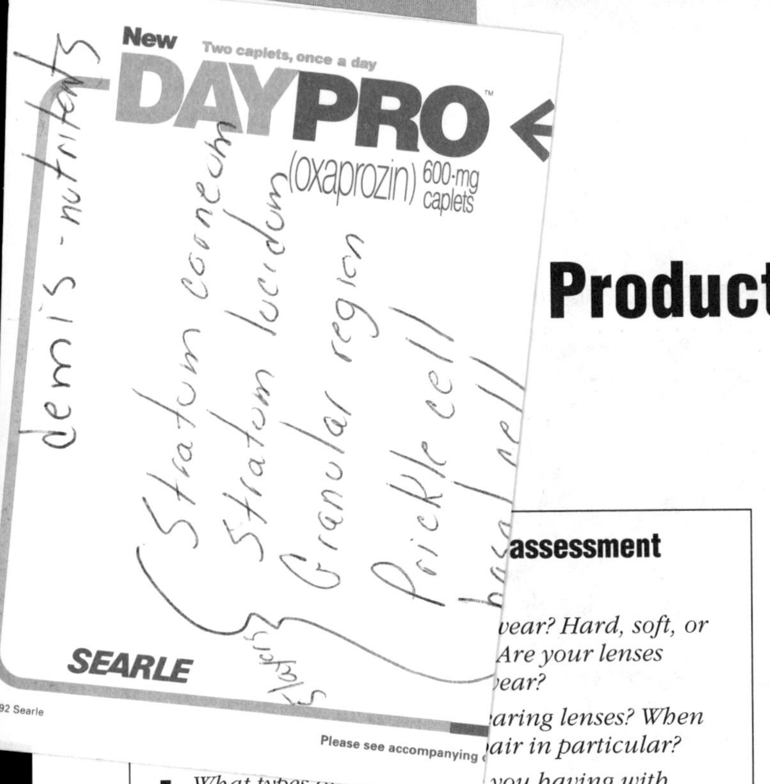

Products

assessment

- ...ear? Hard, soft, or ... Are your lenses ... ear?
- ...aring lenses? When ... air in particular?
- What types of pro... you having with your lenses? Are they related to eye irritation or to changes in vision? When did the problems start?
- *How many hours per day do you wear your lenses before problems start? Do you remove your lenses during the day?*
- *When did you last see your optometrist or ophthalmologist?*
- *How do you take care of your lenses?*
- *Have you recently changed brands of any of your solutions?*
- *How often do you change your storage solutions?*
- *How often do you clean or replace your storage container? Does it need to be replaced?*
- *Have you become pregnant or begun using oral contraceptives since you were prescribed lenses?*
- *What nonprescription and prescription medications are you now taking?*
- *Do you have any allergies?*

Annual sales of contact lens care products exceed $400 million in pharmacies and $900 million overall, and are growing faster than any other category of nonprescription items. With the introduction of soft contact lenses in the 1970s, the greatly enhanced comfort of lenses has led to a significant expansion of the contact lens market. Similarly, developments with rigid gas-permeable (RGP) hard lenses provide the comfort of soft lenses and the enhanced optical qualities of hard lenses. Extended-wear lenses, toric lenses for astigmatism, tinted lenses, bifocal contact lenses, and disposable lenses have also greatly expanded the potential patient population. It is estimated that, by the year 2000, the number of persons wearing contact lenses (contacts) will be the same as the number using eyeglasses.

Figure 1 illustrates the current demographic characteristics of contact lens wearers. Although much of the motivation to wear contacts may be cosmetic, properly fitted lenses can provide significant vision advantages over spectacles. Of the 25 million Americans currently wearing contacts, nearly 90% use the lenses to correct the vision of an otherwise healthy eye. Contact lenses reduce size distortion and prismatic effects and improve peripheral vision. Elimination of spectacle fogging, dirt accumulation, and frame distraction may also be a significant advantage to many users. Most soft contact lens wearers state that their lenses are more comfortable than eyeglasses.

However, it has been well established that contacts, even when expertly fitted, somewhat alter ocular tissues and change the corneal metabolism. These effects make it imperative that both the user and the health professional understand the proper care, maintenance, and safe use of these products. Failure to do so can greatly increase the chance of corneal infection, corneal ulcers, and other ocular conditions that may result in permanent eye damage. Fortunately, however, most side effects of contact lens use are reversible if attended to promptly.

More than 200 nonprescription contact lens care products are available, and consumers are likely to be overwhelmed by the variety. Except for the prescriber, pharmacists are the most qualified to counsel contact lens wearers as to which products to choose.[1] Product selection depends on the products' compatibility with each other as well as with the specific contact lens. It is therefore the pharmacist's responsibility to understand this area of professional practice and provide effective, up-to-date information when consulting with the contact lens wearer.

Characteristics of Contact Lenses

Contact lenses are often broadly classified into three distinct groups based on their chemical makeup and physical properties (Table 1). Lenses that are relatively inflexible, do not appreciably absorb water (<10%), and retain their shape when removed from the eye are commonly called rigid lenses. Rigid lenses that are made of polymethylmethacrylate (PMMA) are not permeable to oxygen and are often called hard lenses. Rigid lenses that are made of less inflexible polymers are permeable to oxygen and are called rigid gas-permeable, or RGP lenses. Hard lenses are seldom now prescribed initially but may be replaced for individuals who were successful with them before the advent of RGP lenses. Contact lenses that are moderately to highly flexible, absorb a high percentage of water (>10%), and conform to the

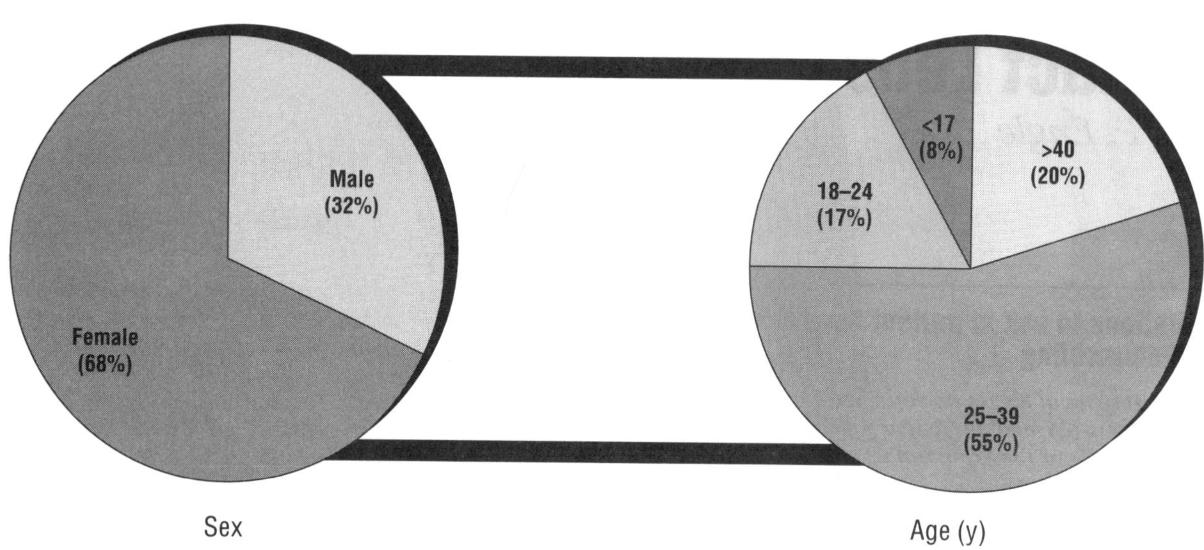

FIGURE 1 Demographics of contact lens wearers.

shape of a supporting structure are commonly called soft lenses. But although the overwhelming majority of contact lenses fall into these three categories, there are a few that do not. These few may be called flexible nonhydrogel lenses.

Subgroups of contacts are extended-wear lenses and disposable lenses. Extended-wear lenses can be either soft or, occasionally, RGP lenses that are designed to be worn for an extended time before removal. Disposable lenses are designed to be worn for 1–14 days and then thrown away.

Contact lenses are manufactured from polymers that vary widely in their chemical and physical properties. Each material has physical and surface characteristics that correlate to the specific problems the patient may encounter.[2]

Physical characteristics of contact lenses include dimensional stability, physical breakage, and polymer stability. Generally, hard lenses are dimensionally stable and tend to hold their parameters with little change. Soft lenses, however, are much less stable physically; water content, to a large extent, will dictate their physical strength. RGP lenses generally have a high degree of dimensional stability. As they dehydrate, however, curvature of the plastic surfaces may alter slightly.

The characteristics of the different contact lenses account for most of the problems that patients will encounter. Unfortunately, many patients do not know which type of lens they are wearing. This underscores the importance of the pharmacist establishing an excellent relationship with contact lens practitioners in the area.

To maintain a healthy cornea, an adequate amount of oxygen is needed. The more oxygen that passes through the contact lens, the more adequately corneal metabolism can be maintained. *Oxygen permeability* describes the ability of a specific material to permit the passage of oxygen. Oxygen permeability is expressed as the *Dk* value of the material, where *D* is the diffusion coefficient and *k* is the solubility coefficient. The higher the *Dk* value, the higher the oxygen permeability. The *Dk/L* value, in which *L* corresponds to the thickness of the material, is a measure of *oxygen transmissibility* (ie, the amount of oxygen that can be transmitted through a contact lens of specific thickness) and is thus the value to which most practitioners and manufacturers refer. Because the lens thickness will vary depending on the power of the lens, many manufacturers will report the *Dk/L* value for a lens with a −3.00D prescription. For example, a lens that corrects a large myopia (minus lens) will be thinner in the center than a lens that corrects hyperopia (plus lens), which will be thicker in the center than on the periphery.

The minimal oxygen transmission values needed to prevent corneal edema in most patients have been extensively debated. For a daily-wear soft lens, the *Dk/L* value ([cm mL O_2]/[sec mL mm Hg]) should be at least 24.1 × 10–9; for extended-wear soft lenses, the *Dk/L* value should be 34.3 × 10–9. This limits overnight corneal swelling to approximately 8% and provides for adequate daytime deswelling to occur.[3] Paradoxically, RGP lenses now have a greater oxygen capability than do soft lenses but, owing to a "tear fluid pumping" mechanism, do not require the oxygen transmissibility to be as high.

Oxygen transmission primarily depends on the water content of the soft lens. The higher the water content, the more oxygen is transmitted through the lens. However, as water content increases, durability decreases, and the lens must be made thicker, which hinders oxygen permeability. Thus, a thick lens with a high water content may transmit the same amount of oxygen as a thin lens with a lower water content.[4] Another problem is that, as water content increases, the lenses tend to attract tear deposits such as lipids, proteins, and polysaccharides. Further, and especially if large pores or many pores are present, lenses with a high water content tend to be more susceptible to the growth of bacteria and fungi on the surface than lenses with a lower water content.[5]

TABLE 1 Comparisons of contact lens characteristics

	Coventional hard lenses	Soft contact lenses	Rigid gas-permeable hard lenses
Lens characteristics			
Rigidity	+++	0	+++
Durability	+++	+	++
Oxygen transmission	0	+	+++
Chemical adsorption	0	+++	0
Optical quality			
Visual acuity	+++	+	+++
Correction of astigmatism	Yes	Toric	Yes
Photophobia	+++	+	++
Spectacle blur	+++	0	++
Convenience			
Comfort	+	+++	++
Adaptation period	Weeks	Days	Days
Extended wear	No	Yes	Yes
Intermittent wear	No	Yes	No

Key:
+ indicates the degree to which the characteristic is present.
0 means the characteristic is not present.

Types of Contact Lenses

The majority of contact lens–wearing patients (85%) are fitted with soft (hydrophilic) lenses.[6] Of these, 47% are daily-wear conventional soft lenses and 38% are disposable or planned replacement lenses. Rigid (primarily RGP) lenses are prescribed for 15% of patients; extended-wear lenses (soft or RGP) are worn by another 15%. By 1996, it is estimated that 74% of patients wearing contacts will be wearing some type of disposable or planned replacement lenses.[7]

Hard Lenses

Hard contact lenses were the first lenses to be used in the United States. Hard lenses are polymerized products of esters of acrylic acid or methacrylic acid. The most common plastic found in hard lenses is PMMA, which is known commercially as Lucite or Plexiglas.

PMMA is not significantly permeable to oxygen; therefore, for the cornea to remain healthy, the lens must be able to slide and rock over the corneal surface in response to a blink so that oxygenation can occur. As the hard lens moves, a layer of tears forms under it and is continually recirculated by the sliding and rocking motion. This process provides oxygen-saturated tears to the corneal surface and is commonly referred to as the tear fluid pumping phenomenon. To allow this movement over the eye, hard lenses are made relatively small in diameter (8.0–9.5 mm) and thus may pop out of the wearer's eye.

Another phenomenon associated primarily with hard lenses is spectacle blur. A hard lens, while in place on the cornea, alters the surface topography of the eye and creates hypoxic edema. As a result, the patient may not see well with glasses immediately after removing the lens. Generally, spectacle blur abates in 20–30 minutes.

Contact lenses made of PMMA are hydrophobic and PMMA is now rarely used for new contact lens fittings because of its negligible permeability to oxygen. However, PMMA possesses many characteristics that make it ideal for a corrective lens in contact with the ocular surface:

- Lenses are very light because of a specific gravity of 1.18–1.20.
- The refractive index, 1.49–1.50, is similar to that of glass spectacle lenses.
- Lenses allow a light transmission of 90–92%.
- Lenses are not affected by weak alkalis or weak acids.
- The plastic does not cause sensitivity reactions when placed on the cornea.

The hardness of these lenses is less than that of glass but is more than that of RGP or soft lenses. Thus, reasonable care must be exercised with hard lenses to avoid scratching or chipping them. Inadequate care or neglect of hard lenses may lead to corneal problems or wearer discomfort, but the lens will still maintain its optical qualities.

In rigid lenses, a small colored dot marker or an etch mark on one lens identifies it as being for the right eye. This marker, located at the outer periphery of the lens, is not perceived by the wearer when the lens is on the cornea.

RGP Lenses

The new generation of RGP lenses combines the optical qualities of PMMA and the oxygen permeability of soft lenses. Generally, RGP lenses can deliver two to three times more oxygen to the cornea than soft lenses of the same thickness. Although, to maintain rigidity (important for the correction of astigmatism and the fit of the lenses), RGP lenses are generally thicker than soft lenses, most recent RGP lenses still transmit much more oxygen to the cornea than do soft lenses while covering only the central 75% of the cornea. RGP lenses, unlike soft lenses, also exchange up to 20% of the postlens tear volume per blink.

RGP lenses have been investigated for extended-wear use, and some have been approved for 1–7 days of extended wear. The use of extended-wear lenses is somewhat controversial as these lenses have been implicated in causing corneal ulcers (eruptions on the corneal surface), which in rare instances can lead to partial or complete blindness.

RGP lenses are available in several materials. One type of lens is made of cellulose acetate butyrate (CAB). CAB lenses transmit more oxygen than PMMA lenses but much less oxygen than other RGP lenses. CAB also has several disadvantages, including its relative ease of surface scratching and its tendency to warp. CAB lenses are only occasionally used because they are more wettable than other RGP lenses.

Another type of lens is composed of silicone acrylates that combine silicone with methyl methacrylate and methacrylic acid and/or hydroxyethyl methacrylate (HEMA) in varying amounts. This material is relatively stable and fairly inflexible. A disadvantage of most silicone acrylates when compared with PMMA and CAB, however, is a decrease in surface wettability owing to the relatively higher hydrophobicity of silicone. In addition, silicone acrylate lenses tend to have a negative surface charge, which attracts lysozyme and other deposits that have a positive charge. Examples of this type of lens include Polycon II and Paraperm O_2.

Silicone resin contact lenses had been available for many years but experienced limited market success and consumer popularity. Pure silicone lenses are uncomfortable because of silicone's extreme hydrophobicity. These lenses are also lipophilic, making their surfaces susceptible to lipid deposits. Their use as a rigid lens has been discontinued, but their elastomeric flexible counterparts still enjoy a niche among pediatric cases.

Fluorine may also be a component of RGP lenses. This may be in the form of fluorosilicone acrylate or fluoropolymer lenses. Fluorine increases the oxygen permeability of the lens. Fluorinated lenses have the advantages of increasing oxygen transmissibility, decreasing tear deposits owing to less surface reactivity, and reducing problems with lipophilicity. Their disadvantages are that they tend to have greater mass, which may change the way RGP lenses fit, and they tend not to be highly wettable. An example of this type of lens is the Boston Equalens.

Alkyl styrene copolymers, another type of RGP lens, are moderately oxygen permeable and lighter than other RGP lens materials. However, these lenses are brittle, have poor wettability, and lack surface stability.[8] They also have low density and a relatively high refractive index. Although these lenses are seldom prescribed, Novalens is an example.

Of the many RGP materials available, the silicone acrylates and the fluorosilicone acrylates are the most commonly used.[9] Table 2 lists examples of RGP contact lenses currently available in the United States.

Soft Lenses

The main chemical difference between the hydrophobic rigid lens and the hydrophilic soft lens is that the soft lens contains hydroxyl or hydroxyl and lactam groups, which allow it to absorb and hold water. Table 3 classifies the different types of soft contact lenses into four groups according to water content and ionic charge based on 1986 Food and Drug Administration (FDA) recommendations. Soft lenses are composed of hydrophilic groups including hydroxyl, amide, lactam, and carboxyl, with small amounts of cross-linking agents that form a hydrophilic gel (hydrogel) network. The degree of cross-linking determines lens hydrophilicity and water content. Greater cross-linking means that fewer hydrophilic groups are available to interact with water, which in turn produces a less flexible, less hydrated lens than those originally available.

Ionic lenses have a negative surface charge, which tends to attract more protein deposits than nonionic lenses; soaking ionic lenses in sorbate-preserved saline will yellow the lenses prematurely. Nonionic lenses are electrically neutral and tend to be less reactive with the tear film, resulting in a more deposit-resistant lens. High-water lenses (>50%), which tend to attract tear film deposits into their matrix, usually cannot withstand daily heat disinfection. If soaked in enzymes for a prolonged period, these lenses may also cause sensitivity reactions.

The water content of soft lenses has gradually increased since they were introduced. Increasing the water content improves the oxygen permeability of a material. However, permeability also depends on lens thickness. Highly hydrated lenses are more comfortable but are also more fragile. Because these lenses must therefore be thicker to offset their fragility, the two factors often cancel each other out regarding oxygen transmissibility. Lowering the water content produces a more durable and longer-lasting lens. The water content of a HEMA-type (2-hydroxyethyl methacrylate) material can vary between 5 and 90%, but a theoretical ideal value might be 75–78%, which matches the hydration of the corneal stroma. However, reducing the percentage of water in a soft HEMA lens also reduces the thickness of the hydrated lens, thereby improving the wearer's comfort. Thus, the optimum water content actually appears to be between 55% to 65%, given the thicknesses at which these materials can be reliably worn. Many lens wearers find they cannot tolerate lenses with a thickness above

TABLE 2 Examples of rigid gas-permeable contact lenses

Brand name	Manufacturer	Composition
Boston II	Polymer Technology	Silicone acrylate
Boston RXD	Polymer Technology	Fluorosilicone acrylate
Polycon II	Sola/Barnes Hind	Silicone acrylate
Paraperm 0_2	Paragon Vision Sciences	Silicone acrylate
Bifocal lenses		
Novalens Perception	Ocutec	Alkyl styrene copolymer
Tangent Streak	Fused Kontacts	Fluorosilicate acrylic
Extended-wear (1–7 days) or daily wear RGP lenses		
Boston Equalens	Polymer Technology	Fluorosilicone acrylate
Fluoroperm 92	Paragon Vision Sciences	Fluorosilicone acrylate
Paraperm EW	Paragon Vision Sciences	Silicone acrylate
Polycon HDK	Pilkington Barnes Hind	Silicone acrylate

0.4 mm because of lid discomfort. For those who cannot tolerate regular soft lenses, several ultrathin soft lenses are available with a thickness as low as 0.04 mm.

Soft lenses in the nonhydrated (dry) state are rigid and extremely brittle and should not be handled by the wearer. When hydrated, the lenses expand as water is absorbed into the gel matrix. These lenses are most comfortable when they are larger than the diameter of the cornea, have thin edges, and undergo just enough movement on the eye to ensure lubrication of the ocular surface under the lens.

Types of Soft Lenses

The increased oxygen permeability and reduced eyelid interaction of soft contact lenses enable certain lenses to be broken in more quickly and worn continuously. Table 4 lists examples of the various kinds of soft contact lenses approved for wear in the United States.

Extended-Wear Lenses Soft extended-wear lenses were originally intended to be worn for weeks. However, as with RGP extended-wear lenses, problems with contamination, infection, and ulceration suggest that they should not be worn for more than 7 days.[10] Recent evidence strongly supports removing them overnight, at least once per week, to reduce the risk of ulcerative keratitis.[11,12]

Disposable and Planned Replacement Lenses Disposable lenses represent the fastest-growing segment of the soft lens market. Depending upon the lens, there are several approved wearing schedules. Some lenses are worn for 1 day and then discarded; others are worn daily for up to 2 weeks and then discarded; and still others can be worn as extended-wear lenses for up to 2 weeks, with the patient wearing them for 6 nights and then removing them for 1 night. Planned replacement lenses are discarded and replaced usually after 1 to 3 months of wear, depending on how quickly the lenses build up deposits and on how well the patient complies with lens care. Planned replacement lenses and disposable lenses other than the daily disposables are cared for similarly to other soft contact lenses except that an enzymatic cleaner is generally not necessary.

Among the advantages of daily disposables are that each lens is sterile prior to removal from its package for immediate insertion into the eye; that no cleaning regimen is necessary since the lens is just thrown out after wear; that deposit formation is minimal; and that lens-related problems such as giant papillary conjunctivitis or allergic reactions to lens care solutions occur less often. However, at a cost of $1.70 to $2 per day for daily disposable lenses to correct both eyes, they are not yet affordable for some patients.

Specialty Lenses Some soft contacts are classified as specialty lenses. These include toric, bifocal, and tinted lenses. Toric soft lenses have been developed specifically to correct astigmatic (improper focusing owing to an irregularly shaped

TABLE 3 Soft contact lens classification

Group I: low water, nonionic	Group III: low water, ionic
Polymacon	Bufilcon A (45%)
Hefilcon A and B	Etafilcon (43%)
Tefilcon	Phemfilcon A (38%)
Tetrafilcon A	
Group II: high water, nonionic	**Group IV: high water, ionic**
Lidofilicon A and B	Bufilcon A (55%)
Surfilcon	Perfilcon
Netrafilcon A	Phemfilcon A (55%)
	Etafilcon A (58%)

TABLE 4 Examples of soft contact lenses

Brand name	Manufacturer	% water/saline	Group[a]
Daily-wear soft lenses			
AO Soft	CIBA Vision	42.5	I
Cibasoft	CIBA Vision	37.5	I
DuraSoft	Wesley-Jessen	38.0	III
Hydrocurve II	Sola/Barnes-Hind	55.0	III
Sof-Form 67	Salvatori Ophthalmics	67.0	II
Soflens	Bausch & Lomb	38.6	I
Softcon	CIBA Vision	55.0	IV
Extended-wear soft lenses			
Cibathin	CIBA Vision	37.5	I
DuraSoft 3	Wesley-Jessen	55.0	IV
Permaflex Natural	CooperVision	74.0	II
Permalens	CooperVision	71.0	IV
Softmate I	Sola/Barnes-Hind	45.0	III
Softmate II	Sola/Barnes-Hind	55.0	IV
Disposable soft lenses			
1 Day Acuvue	Vistakon	58.0	IV
New Vues	CIBA Vision	55.0	II
SeeQuence	Bausch & Lomb	38.0	I
Soft toric lenses			
Hydrocurve II Toric	Sola/Barnes-Hind	45.0	III
Optima Toric	Bausch & Lomb	45.0	I
Spectrum Toric	CIBA Vision	55.0	IV
Soft bifocal lenses			
Bi-Soft	CIBA Vision	37.5	I
Hydrocurve II	Sola/Barnes-Hind	45.0	III
PA1	Bausch & Lomb	38.6	I
Soft daily-wear tinted lenses			
Hydron Zero4 Sof Blue (soft blue visibility tint)	Allergan Optical	38.0	I
Illusions (deep blue, deep green, gray, soft blue, soft green, soft amber)	CIBA Vision	37.5	I
Soft extended-wear tinted lenses			
Durasoft 3 colors (sapphire blue, baby blue, emerald green, jade green, aqua, hazel, misty gray, violet)	Wesley-Jessen	55.0	IV
Freshlook colors (disposable) (blue, green, hazel, violet)	Wesley-Jessen	55.0	IV

[a]Group I: low water, nonionic.
Group II: high water, nonionic.
Group III: low water, ionic.
Group IV: high water, ionic.

cornea) visual conditions. Traditional soft lenses do not correct astigmatism because they conform to the corneal surface rather than retain their original shape, as do rigid lenses. Toric soft lenses are fabricated with both spherical and cylindrical optical corrections and remain on axis because of design features such as weighting on the bottom edge of the lens. Spherical soft lenses can be fitted to eyes with an upper limit of astigmatism of about 1.00 diopters (a unit of refracting power used as a quantitative measure of the abnormal refraction of light at surfaces such as the cornea). However, this figure is highly dependent on the criticality and motivation of the patient.

Bifocal lenses, which can be weighted in a fashion similar to that of toric lenses, are prescribed to correct presbyopia (ocular changes due to age).

Tinted lenses are available to facilitate handling and for cosmetic purposes (to change eye color) as well as for corrective uses. Three types of tinted lenses are available: translucent, opaque, and UV-absorbing lenses. Translucent lenses can be tinted in varying degrees, from light/number 1 intensity to facilitate handling and increase the visibility of the lens, to medium/number 2 and dark/number 3 intensities to enhance eye color. Translucent lenses work best on light eye colors. Opaque lenses cover the iris and hide its natural color; they can completely change the apparent eye color, even in individuals with dark brown eyes. These lenses may also be used as a prosthetic to mask corneal scarring or to cover an amblyopic (lazy) eye. Finally some tinted lenses have UV-absorbing material incorporated into them. These lenses are used in aphakic patients or to help protect any patient from the harmful effects of UV radiation.

Advantages of Soft Lenses

Soft lenses are easier to remove and are considerably more comfortable than rigid lenses. This effect is most apparent during the initial break-in period. Photophobia is not likely to occur with soft lenses, and glare is significantly reduced. As with rigid lenses, however, flare around the periphery may be noticed at night, particularly in individuals who have large pupils. This flare is caused by refractive light entering the eye through the edge margin of the contact lens.

Soft lens wearers can change more easily from their lenses to eyeglasses after a period of wear. The typical soft lens wearer does not usually experience the spectacle blur common among hard lens wearers and even occasionally experienced among RGP wearers.

Soft lenses are less likely than rigid lenses to trap dust particles, eyelashes, or other foreign material under the lens. They are also less likely to become dislodged or fall out. Therefore, soft lenses are often better suited for occasional wear and sports, including contact sports.

Disadvantages of Soft Lenses

Although many people prefer the comfort of soft lenses, not all soft lens wearers can achieve excellent visual acuity. The hydration of the lens may change either in or out of the eye, particularly with extreme temperatures and low relative humidity; this change can decrease the quality of the visual image. Because a soft lens conforms in large part to the corneal shape, it is difficult to project the degree of vision improvement before the lens is actually placed on the eye. Further, because soft lenses cannot be as precisely tailored to the specific requirements of an individual cornea, the fitting process is less exact than it is with rigid lenses. As a result, the overall quality of vision with soft contact lenses does not usually equal that of a properly fitted pair of rigid lenses. Fortunately, these differences are often small and should not concern many wearers.

Unlike rigid lenses, soft lenses can absorb chemical compounds from topically administered ophthalmic products.[13] As previously discussed, ocular irritation may result, and the lens may be damaged. With the exception of a few specially formulated rewetting solutions, no solution should be instilled into the eye with the soft lens in place. If a drug solution is instilled into the eye prior to lens insertion, the wearer must wait until the solution has cleared from the precorneal (conjunctival) pocket—about 5 minutes. In some instances, the prescriber may prefer that the lenses be worn while a prescription medication is being instilled so that they may serve as a reservoir for the drug. If no instructions accompany an ophthalmic prescription for a soft lens wearer, the prescribing practitioner should be contacted. This is also true for a nonprescription ophthalmic product not specifically designed for use with contact lenses. When topical ophthalmic ointments, gels, or suspensions are being used, the lenses should not be worn at all.

Unlike rigid lenses, soft lenses cannot be easily marked to identify which is for the left and right eyes. A soft lens wearer who is uncertain of the identity of the lenses may have to see the vision specialist.

Soft lenses generally cost more than hard lenses. Although the initial cost of acquiring soft lenses has decreased, the overall cost is greater because they must be replaced more often owing to changes in the refractory requirements of the eye. Soft lenses are also more costly because they are less durable than hard ones and require more cleaning and disinfecting products.

The care given to contact lenses varies considerably with each wearer. Soft lenses rapidly degenerate to useless pieces of plastic if they are neglected. When used with a fastidious care and cleaning program, however, daily wear soft lenses can have an average life of 12–18 months compared with 18–36 months for similarly used RGP lenses.

Use of Contact Lenses

Indications

Therapeutic Necessity

The decision to wear contact lenses rather than eyeglasses is sometimes based on therapeutic necessity. For example, with keratoconus, a gradual protrusion of the central cornea, satisfactory vision is usually unattainable with ordinary eyeglasses but can be obtained with rigid contact lenses.[14] Other examples of therapeutic necessity are lenses used as collagen shields and soft contact lenses saturated with antibiotic agents.

Aphakia results when the crystalline lens of the eye is removed because of an opacified lens or cataract and an intraocular lens is not implanted. Aphakic individuals characteristically see better with contact lenses than with spectacles. Extended-wear contacts are particularly beneficial for such patients because their poor vision makes it difficult for them to insert and remove lenses.

Visual aberrations caused by corneal scarring are also often better corrected with rigid contact lenses. Whereas eyeglasses simply correct refractive error by changing the focus of light incident on the cornea, the proximity of the rigid contact lens actually masks irregularities in the corneal topography. Prosthetic lenses may also make corneal scarring cosmetically unnoticeable.

Refractive Exam

Other indications for the use of contacts include refractive errors such as myopia (nearsightedness), hyperopia (farsightedness), astigmatism, and presbyopia.

Astigmatism occurs when there is unequal curvature of the refractive surfaces of the eye, resulting in a fuzzy image. RGP lenses, hard lenses, and toric soft lenses, to a lesser extent, can be used to correct an astigmatism.

Presbyopia (old vision) is a condition caused by aging, in which the crystalline lens cannot properly focus on near objects. More than 50% of visually corrected patients are presbyopic. Contact lenses have not been overly successful for these patients; because vision correction is needed for both near and far, two optical corrections are required in each bifocal contact lens. For most bifocal contact lenses to be successful, the patient should be highly motivated and should not be in an occupation with rigorous visual demands.[15,16]

To correct presbyopia with spectacles, bifocal or trifocal lenses (often called multifocal lenses) are needed. If properly selected and indoctrinated, patients trying bifocal contacts can be successful 60–70% of the time. Monovision is one method of presbyopic contact lens correction that has been successful in some cases: the dominant eye is fitted with a lens for far vision; the other eye, with a lens that corrects for close-up objects and reading. In most individuals, the eyes will adjust in a relatively short time; reading will be done with the nondominant eye, and distant objects will be noted with the dominant one.

Other Benefits

Perhaps the main reason for choosing contact lenses is the perceived improvement in personal appearance. Other strongly influencing factors include no obstruction of vision from eyeglass frames, greater clarity in peripheral vision, no fogging of lenses caused by sudden temperature changes, and more freedom of motion during vigorous activity (eg, sports). A number of factors, such as increased sensitivity to light and improved quality of the retinal image, contribute to the subjective perception of vision improvement by the contact lens wearer. With eyeglasses, the myopic individual sees a smaller than normal image and the hyperopic individual sees a larger than normal image. With contacts, both myopic and hyperopic individuals see objects in nearly their true sizes; for highly myopic persons, the image size increase with contact lenses is significant and decidedly beneficial.

Contraindications

Some individuals who require vision correction cannot or should not wear contact lenses. Contraindications are often based on lifestyle as well as on medical history.

Occupational Hazards

Occupational conditions that may prohibit the wearing of contact lenses include exposure to wind, glare, molten metals, irritants, dust and particulate matter, tobacco smoke, chemicals, and chemical fumes.[17] Certain chemical fumes have been suggested as being particularly hazardous because of the potential concentration of irritants under a hard lens or inside a soft lens. The lens theoretically prolongs contact of such substances with the cornea and can lead to corneal toxicity. However, these theoretical occupational contraindications have not been proven.

Medical Conditions

Contact lenses should not be used for cosmetic reasons if a patient has active pathologic intraocular or corneal conditions. Medical reasons that contraindicate contact lens wear include chronic conjunctivitis; blepharitis; recurrent viral, bacterial, or fungal infections; and poor blink rate or incomplete blink. Insufficient tear production, a deficiency or excess of mucin, excessive lipid production, or excessively dry environments may also preclude successful contact lens use. So, too, may dry spots on the cornea, often found in postmenopausal women. These spots, possibly caused by the absence of the precorneal film, are often identified with lacrimal insufficiency. Diabetic patients are often advised against extended-wear contact lenses because of retarded healing processes and the tendency toward prolonged corneal abrasion with such use. This precaution is probably unnecessary for daily wear of lenses unless problems occur. Chronic common colds or allergic conditions such as hay fever and asthma may also make lens wear extremely uncomfortable or impossible.

Contact lenses should be used with caution by patients with epilepsy or severe arthritis. The corneal topography may be altered by pregnancy or the use of oral contraceptives. The fluid-retaining properties of estrogen may lead to edema of the cornea and eyelids as well as to decreased tear production.

Contact lenses can be used with care by elderly persons; care is needed because of possible lacrimal insufficiency and loose lid tissues, which create a sagging conjunctival cul-de-sac and therefore make lens retention difficult. Individuals with arthritis may lack the dexterity needed to insert lenses. Lens wearers moving from a low to a high altitude may encounter hypoxia or metabolic deficiency, resulting in irritation and corneal abrasions.

During the period needed for adapting to rigid contact lenses, the eyelids may become hyperemic; this condition may lead to blepharitis, especially in the upper lid. Short pseudoblinks, by new wearers of hard lenses, may irritate the conjunctiva of the upper eyelid. Chin elevation and squinting may result from the patient's efforts to minimize the irritation.

Precautions

Contact lenses generally can match or exceed the vision obtained with spectacles. However, depending on the type of lens, there are situations in which vision may become worse.[18] Some patients wearing lenses with high water content may experience hazy vision around the edges of objects. In some cases, patients wearing hard lenses experience nighttime ghosting, which occurs when the patient's pupil dilates enough to see the edges of the lens. This can sometimes be corrected with larger-diameter lenses. Other patients complain of spiderweb vision, usually at night; this can be due to crazing, the development of fine cracks, usually in RGP lenses.

Potential Transmission of Viral Infections

The human immunodeficiency virus (HIV) has been isolated from the tears of infected individuals as well as from the contact lenses worn by infected individuals. This seemingly becomes an issue in the case of trial contact lenses, which may be reused by different patients in the lens fitter's office. Generally, these lenses are not dispensed to a patient except as a loaner lens (ie, to a patient waiting for new replacement lenses). Even in this scenario, after the lenses have been used in any patient, they are disinfected with heat or chemicals before being dispensed to another patient. Studies have shown that heat and the routinely available hydrogen peroxide products are effective in inactivating the HIV virus. The FDA also requires that all contact lens regimens kill herpes simplex, another enveloped virus. There have been no reported cases of HIV transmission via a contact lens fitting.[19]

Adverse Effects of Drugs

Topical Drugs Many undesired effects have been reported when a patient who wears contact lenses ingests or topically applies certain drugs (Table 5). The pharmacist must understand the problems these medications may cause. In general, patients should be counseled not to place any ophthalmic solution, suspension, gel, or ointment into the eye when contact lenses are in place. The only exceptions to this rule are products specifically formulated to be used with contact lenses, such as rewetting drops, or those products that an eye care practitioner has specifically recommended for use with contact lenses.

Topical administration of ophthalmic drugs may have physiologic consequences or may modify pharmacologic responses to drugs. The use of solutions that may be considered benign, such as artificial tears, may reduce tear breakup time and alter the distribution of the mucoid, aqueous, and lipid components of tears, perhaps causing initial discomfort upon instillation of the drops.[13] The pharmacologic effect of a topically administered drug while soft lenses are in place may be exaggerated: the soft lens may absorb the drug and either release it over time, thus creating a sustained-release dosage form, or bind it tightly so that none of it is released into the eye. Further, the presence of any kind of contact lens may increase the amount of time the medication is in contact with the eye. Finally, some increased drug absorption may occur secondary to a compromised corneal epithelium that is present during contact lens wear.[13]

TABLE 5 Drug–contact lens interactions

Changes in tear film and/or production	
Tear volume decreased	
Anticholinergic agents	Timolol (topical)
Antihistamines	Tricyclic antidepressants
Diuretics	
Tear volume increased	
Cholinergic agents	Reserpine
Changes in lens color (primarily soft lenses)	
Diagnostic dyes (ie, fluorescein)	Phenothiazines
	Phenolphthalein
Epinephrine (topical)	Phenylephrine
Fluorescein (topical)	Rifampin
Nicotine	Sulfasalazine
Nitrofurantoin	Tetracycline
Phenazopyridine	Tetrahydrozoline (topical)
Changes in tonicity	
Pilocarpine (8%)	Sodium sulfacetamide (10%)
Lid/corneal edema	
Chlorthalidone	Oral contraceptives
Clomiphene	Primidone
Ocular inflammation/irritation	
Gold salts	Salicylates
Isotretinoin	
Changes in refractivity (ie, induction of myopia)	
Acetazolamide	Sulfamethoxazole
Sulfadiazine	Sulfisoxazole
Sulfamethizole	
Miscellaneous	
Digoxin (increased glare)	
Ribavirin (cloudy lenses)	
Topical ciprofloxacin/Prednisolone acetate (precipitate)	
Hypnotics/Sedatives/Muscle relaxants (decreased blink rate)	

Adapted with permission from Engle JP. Contact lens care. *Am Druggist.* 1990 Jan; 201: 54–65.

There are some cases in which patients will be treated with topical ophthalmic medications while wearing contact lenses. For example, such medications are used in conjunction with disposable soft contact lenses as an alternative to bandage contact lenses in the treatment of persistent epithelial corneal defects. Yet there have been some case reports of an opaque precipitate noted in patients using SeeQuence disposable contact lenses when treated with topical ciprofloxacin and topical prednisolone acetate concurrently.[20] When studied in the laboratory, neither drug alone produced precipitates in the contact lens; white crystalline deposits were noted only when the two topical agents were used in combination. In another study, it was noted that the combination of topical gentamicin and methylprednisolone produced precipitates.[21] Thus, if a patient who wears contact lenses is treated with a topical antibiotic and steroid combination, the eye care practitioner must carefully monitor for deposits in the lenses. If deposits are noted, the lenses should be removed and replaced with a new pair.

Additionally, the preservatives, vehicles, tonicity factors, and pH of the solution to be instilled into the eye could alter the lenses. For instance, instillation of hypertonic solutions such as sodium sulfacetamide 10% or pilocarpine 8% may cause soft lens dehydration and lens disfigurement. Topical medications with an acidic pH promote lens dehydration and steepening; alkaline medications promote hydration and flattening.[22] Topical suspensions may lead to lens intolerance because particulate matter build up and cause discomfort. Gel and oil formulations may alter the surface relationship between the contact lens and the cornea.[13] Finally, the active ingredient of certain topical products (eg, epinephrine) may discolor lenses.

Airborne Drugs Some drugs that are present in indoor air may damage lenses. For example, some nurses who care for patients receiving ribavirin have reportedly experienced cloudy lenses after repeated exposure to the drug.[23,24] Similarly, contact lens wearers who are exposed to a large amount of cigarette smoke may discover a brown discoloration and nicotine deposits on their lenses. This is especially true for those who smoke and have nicotine-stained fingers.[25]

Systemic Drugs Some systemic medications are secreted into tears and may interact with (primarily soft) contact lenses through this mechanism. For example, rifampin will stain the lenses and tears orange. Drugs such as gold salts are secreted into the tears and may cause ocular irritation. Others drugs may affect tear production, the refractive properties of the eye, the shape of the cornea, or the actual lens (Table 5).[26]

Use of Cosmetics

Patients who wear contact lenses should choose—and use—cosmetics with care.[27] Individuals should insert lenses before applying makeup and should avoid touching the lens with eyeliner or mascara. Cosmetics, moisturizers, and makeup removers with an aqueous base should be used because oil-based products may cause blurred vision and irritation if they are deposited on the lens. Cream eye shadows are preferable to powder shadows. Water-resistant as opposed to waterproof mascara (which requires an oil-based remover) should be applied only to the very tips of the lashes. Eyeliners should never be applied inside the eyelid margin as the liner can clog glands in the eyelid and contaminate the contact lens. Any aerosol products, in particular, must be used with caution: irritation may occur if some of the spray particles are trapped in the tear layer beneath the lens, and some sprays may actually damage the lens. One way to avoid a problem is to insert the lenses, go to another room, cover the eyes with a cloth, use the spray, and then leave the area with the eyes still closed.

Nail polish, hand creams, and perfumes should also be applied only after the lenses have been inserted. Nail polish and remover can destroy a lens. Men often contaminate their lenses with hair preparations and spray deodorants; they should take special care to clean their hands thoroughly before handling their contacts. Soaps containing cold cream or deodorants should be avoided because they can leave a film on the fingers after rinsing. This residue is readily transferred to a lens and can cause blurred vision. Moreover, if the lens comes in contact with residual petrolatum-based lotion on the patient's fingers, the lens' surface can be modified. This modification cannot be detected by inspection; it will be noted, however, once the lens is worn. Approximately 20–30 minutes after insertion of the lens, the surface-wetting properties of the lens are disrupted.[28]

Corneal Hypoxia and Edema

An adequate supply of oxygen exists only if the cornea is continuously bathed with oxygenated tears.[29] During blinking, metabolic by-products from the surface epithelium are flushed from under the contact lenses, and oxygen is brought in as the lenses move toward and away from the cornea. Even when properly fitted, however, both rigid and soft lenses can produce a progressive hypoxia of the cornea while the lenses are in place, especially in persons who have low blink frequency or incomplete blinks.

One major effect of this hypoxia is edema of the corneal tissues. It has been demonstrated that corneal thickness is increased to a greater extent by hard (PMMA) lenses. After approximately 16 hours of continuous wear, hard and, to a lesser extent, soft lenses cause the glycogen content of the cornea to fall to a level that is accompanied by significant edema. Symptoms associated with corneal edema include photophobia, rainbows around a light, sensations of hotness, grittiness and itchiness, fogging of vision, and blurred vision. Although it is not usually necessary, a patient experiencing corneal edema from overuse of contact lenses can be treated with one to two drops of sodium chloride (2 or 5%) every 3–4 hours after the lenses have been removed. The patient should be counseled that transient stinging or burning may occur upon instillation of the drops. Further, the patient should be counseled not to overuse the lenses.

Another effect of corneal hypoxia is neovascularization. The development of new vessels is potentially irreversible. Routine follow-up visits to the lens care specialist are important for monitoring for this effect of contact lens wear.

Corneal Abrasions

Corneal abrasions are surface defects in the epithelial layer of the cornea. Causes of these abrasions range from poorly fitted lenses or simple overwear to scratches caused by the entrapment of foreign bodies under the lens. The cornea is sensitive to abrasion, so reflex lid closure (blepharospasm), tearing, and rubbing the affected eye are immediate. However, rubbing the eye must be avoided because it can cause more extensive damage while the lens remains in the eye.

Fortunately, the pain associated with corneal abrasion is usually of greater magnitude than the damage. The epithelium regenerates quickly: most minor epithelial defects (ie, those that are 22 mm in diameter or less) generally heal within 12–24 hours. The lens should be left out for 2 days to a week. The wearer may then proceed using a modified break-in schedule suggested by the vision specialist. More extensive abrasions require the attention of an eye care specialist.

Symptoms of Lens Problems

Lens wearers may initially encounter various problems in adapting to lenses, particularly RGP ones; even long-time wearers occasionally experience difficulty. Many of these problems arise from different causative factors, and identifying and solving a specific problem may require a trained vision specialist. The following list provides a perspective for counseling a lens wearer who seeks advice. Most of this information is particularly applicable to rigid lens wear.

- *Deep aching of eye:* This pain persists even after the lens is removed, and it may be caused by poorly fitted lenses. The eye care practitioner must be consulted.
- *Blurred vision:* This effect may be produced by improper refractive power, lenses switched right for left, lenses placed on the eye inside out, tear film buildup, cosmetic film buildup, corneal edema, or use of oral contraceptives.
- *Excessive tearing:* Tearing is normal when lenses are first worn; however, tearing may also be caused by poorly fitted lenses or chipped, rough edges on the lenses.
- *Fogging:* Misty or smoky vision can be caused by corneal edema, overwearing of contact lenses, coatings or deposits on lens surfaces, or poor wetting of the lens while on the eye.
- *Flare:* Point sources of light having a sunburst or streaming quality can be caused by inadequate optic zone size or decentration of a poorly fitting lens.
- *Itching:* This may be caused by allergic conjunctivitis and may be treated with short-term use of topical steroids.
- *Lens falling out of eye:* Poorly fitted lenses could be the cause. However, even properly fitted rigid lenses may occasionally slide off the cornea or be blinked out of the eye.
- *Inability to wear lenses in the morning:* This may be caused by corneal edema or mild conjunctivitis. Most likely, however, the patient's eyes dry out overnight owing to incomplete eyelid closure.
- *Pain after removal of lens:* This effect is usually caused by corneal abrasion. The presence of the lens anesthetizes the cornea owing to hypoxia; sensation returns after 4–6 hours and pain develops.
- *Sudden pain in the eye:* A foreign body or chipped or folded lens may be the problem.
- *Squinting:* This effect is caused by excessive lens movement or a poorly fitted lens. The wearer squints to center the optical portion of the lens over the pupil.

Lens Care Products and Procedures

Contact Lens Solutions

Formulation Considerations

The manufacturing and marketing of contact lenses are regulated by the ophthalmic devices division of the FDA. Even though contact lens solutions are not considered drug products, formulation considerations still apply. Contact lens wearers should use only lens care products that have been approved by the FDA for use with their specific contact lens.

The basic considerations for a well-formulated contact lens solution include pH, viscosity, isotonicity with tears, stability, sterility, and provision for maintenance of sterility (bactericidal action). The pH range of comfort is not well defined because while normal tear pH is 7.4, tear pH varies among individuals. It is best to have a weakly buffered solution that can readily adjust to any tear pH, given that highly buffered solutions can cause significant discomfort, even ocular damage, when instilled. However, as with therapeutic ophthalmic solutions, stability of the solution components takes precedence over comfort. For this reason, many contact lens solutions are formulated with pH values above or below 7.4. These systems are weakly buffered and are usually well tolerated by the eye.

Routine daily use of any contact lens solution allows the potential for bacterial contamination. Depending on specific lens care procedures, a single container may last for a month or more. The solution must therefore contain a bactericidal agent that is both effective over the long term and nonirritating with daily use in the eye. Few preservatives fulfill these criteria. Commonly used agents are benzalkonium chloride, thimerosal, and sorbic acid products, all of which can cause irritation, depending on concentration and patient sensitivity.

Solutions from different manufacturers should not be mixed because a precipitate may result. For instance, a product containing alkaline borate buffers forms a gummy, gel-like precipitate on lenses if mixed with a wetting solution containing polyvinyl alcohol. Further, solutions containing cationic preservative, such as chlorhexidine, polyquaternium-1 (Polyquad), or polyaminopropyl biguanide (Dymed), should not be mixed with solutions containing an anionic preservative such as sorbic acid because this, too, will cause a precipitate.[30]

Preservatives

Benzalkonium Chloride Benzalkonium chloride is a surface-active agent and germicide that is effective against a variety of gram-positive and gram-negative bacteria. In sufficient concentration, it is also effective against perhaps the most worrisome bacterial ocular pathogen, *Pseudomonas aeruginosa*. However, several properties of benzalkonium chloride require that care be exercised with respect to its concentration in a hard lens solution. High concentrations of benzalkonium chloride cause ocular damage, either directly by instillation into the eye or indirectly by adsorption onto the lens.[31] The maximum tolerable concentration is reportedly about 0.03% (1:3,000), with solutions of 0.02% having been shown to be tolerated up to several times a day. However, most solutions for direct instillation into the eye contain concentrations between 0.004 and 0.01%.[31]

Some persons using a solution preserved with benzalkonium chloride develop ocular irritation because the surfactant builds up on their soft lenses. Switching to a solution with a lower benzalkonium chloride concentration may alleviate this, but change to a solution with a different preservative or cleaning agent may be required. Benzalkonium chloride should not be used concurrently with soft contact lenses because the agent is adsorbed onto the matrix of the lens, and severe toxicity may result from its sustained release from the lens.

Thimerosal Thimerosal, or sodium ethylmercurithiosalicylate, was introduced as an alternative to benzalkonium chloride, with which it is incompatible. Like benzalkonium chloride, it acts by interfering with cell metabolism, glycolysis, and respiration. It is effective against *P aeruginosa* but is slow to act because it depends on sustained release of mercurial ions that penetrate the bacterial cell. Like other mercurials, thimerosal may also cause sensitization in a large proportion of individuals after repeated application. The reaction can be delayed and may take months to occur.

In general, thimerosal does not pose a significant problem except when used with soft contact lenses. Thimerosal may bind to debris in soft lenses and remain in contact with the eye for as long as the lens is in place. Moreover, the concentration of the preservative carried to the eye via soft lenses appears to cause a significant incidence of irritation. Thus, most practitioners have discouraged its use in soft lens care products because of the high incidence of sensitivity in the patient. On the other hand, thimerosal is rapidly cleared from the tear fluid when instilled with RGP lenses and therefore is less likely to be problematic for these patients.

Sorbic Acid or Potassium Sorbate Sorbic acid was once very popular as a preservative. Less irritating than mercurials, it is the preservative ingredient often included in products labeled "thimerosal free" or "for sensitive eyes." However, it reportedly may increase age-associated yellowing of some lenses, particularly those containing a methacrylic acid.[32] In addition, sorbic acid's maximum antimicrobial activity is at a pH that is too low to be of optimum value for use on the eye.

Chlorhexidine Chlorhexidine can irritate the eyes, and its degradation products may produce a yellow-to-green coloration.[33] It can be precipitated by borates, phosphates, and carbonates. At the concentration in which it is used in soft lens solutions, chlorhexidine is less effective against several yeasts and fungi than is optimal. There are also problems associated with its use in RGP lens soaking or conditioning solutions, which generally contain high–molecular weight wetting agents that may impair its disinfecting action. Chlorhexidine-containing solutions that appear greenish should not be used because the color change indicates decomposition of the product.[33]

Sodium Salts of EDTA Sodium salts of ethylenediaminetetraacetic acid (EDTA) are often used in lens solutions because EDTA disrupts the integrity of bacterial cell walls and, in so doing, enhances the action of other preservatives. It also complexes with other substances, such as metallic ions, that might reduce benzalkonium chloride activity; by complexation, calcium deposits on lenses may be prevented. EDTA is often used in contact lens solutions that contain another chemical agent as their primary preservative. Solutions of EDTA cannot be claimed to be preservative free, even if there is no other primary preservative. Addition of EDTA to nonpreserved saline solutions will increase their shelf life after opening.

Polyquaternium-1 Polyquaternium-1 is a quaternary ammonium lens care preservative shown to be effective against certain bacteria, fungi, and yeast. Few toxicity or sensitivity problems have been noted with this preservative thus far. When first introduced to the market, formulations containing Polyquad were not compatible with lenses that had a high water content since the methacrylic acid component of the lens had the ability to adsorb the preservative in toxic levels. However, recent formulations do not seem to have this problem.

Polyaminopropyl Biguanide Polyaminopropyl biguanide is a cationic polymeric biguanide effective against certain bacteria and yeast although its activity against *Acanthamoeba* and fungi does not appear to be optimal. Some solutions were formerly preserved with chlorhexidine, and there were reports of contamination of the solution with *Serratia marcescens*, which is able to feed on the high molecular weight wetting agents. However, no significant adverse effects to polyaminopropyl biguanide have been reported in lens wearers. One manufacturer of RGP solutions uses higher concentrations of this preservative than are found in soft lens solutions; this is necessary because the RGP solutions contain high molecular weight wetting agents, which decrease the effectiveness of the preservative. The higher concentrations do not seem to cause toxicity to the wearer because RGP lenses do not adsorb the preservatives to the degree that soft lenses do.

Care of Hard Lenses

Lens care products help to minimize the stress on the eye from hard contacts. These products aid the wearer, providing comfort and safety (see product table "Hard Lens Products").

Hard lens care involves three important steps: cleaning, soaking, and wetting (Figure 2). For optimal lens care, all three steps should be performed each time the lenses are removed from the eye.

Cleaning Solutions

Normal tears are composed of secretions from many specialized glands lining the lacrimal apparatus, conjunctiva, and lids. Many components are somewhat hydrophobic and tend to adhere to the surface of a hard lens during normal daily wear. This residue, primarily

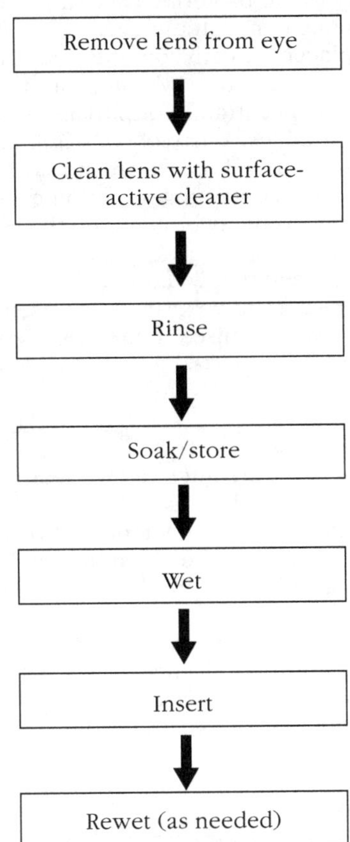

FIGURE 2 Hard contact lens care.

proteinaceous debris and oils, acts as a growth medium for bacteria. If it is not routinely removed by daily cleaning, it may harden to form coatings or tenacious deposits that create an irregular surface on the lens. This residue will eventually irritate the eyelids and corneal epithelium, and may progress to infection or other pathology. Decreased visual acuity and lens wear time are likely consequences of a cloudy lens or allergenic reactions to the residue.

Typical cleaning solutions contain nonionic or amphoteric surfactants that emulsify oils and aid in solubilizing other debris. Proteins and lipids are soluble in highly alkaline media, but a high pH can cause lens decomposition. Weak alkaline solutions may be helpful in dislodging deposits from the lens in conjunction with the surface tension-lowering properties of the surfactants.

Lenses should be thoroughly rinsed after cleaning because residual cleaning agents may lead to ocular irritation. Lenses should never be wiped dry with tissue because this can cause surface scratches. Also, homemade cleaning solutions, such as mixtures of baking soda with distilled water or cleaning solution, should not be used; they may scratch the lens and may not be easily rinsed off.[34] Similarly, dishwashing detergent, lighter fluid, toothpaste, or other cleaners not formulated for contact lens use may accumulate on the lens and cause damage or ocular irritation.

There are four basic techniques for cleaning rigid lenses.

Friction Rubbing A contact lens cleaning solution or gel is applied to both surfaces of the lens. The lens is then rubbed between the thumb and forefinger or between the forefinger and palm of the opposite hand for about 20 seconds. Friction rubbing is the most common cleaning method and it is effective, but it may result in scratched and warped lenses if rubbing is too vigorous.

Spray Cleaning The lenses are placed into a perforated holder and held under a stream of running water from an ordinary faucet. The pressure of the water flow dislodges debris that has been loosened by overnight soaking in the storage case.

Hydraulic Cleaning The lenses are placed into separate baskets in a plastic container that has a rotating cap (ie, Hydra-Mat II). The cap, which is connected to the baskets, is rotated for 20–30 seconds to provide a high level of turbulence. The unit is filled with a special cleaning solution to assist in the removal of deposits.

Ultrasonic Cleaning The lenses are placed in a water bath through which ultrasound waves are passed. These specialized cleaning units have not been shown to be superior in cleaning contact lenses, and their cost is high.

Soaking Solutions

A soaking solution is used to store hard contact lenses whenever they are removed from the eyes. The solution maintains the lens in a constant state of hydration for maximum comfort and visual acuity. It also aids in removing deposits that accumulate on the lens during wear.

A rigid lens absorbs between 1 and 3% moisture by weight. Upon exposure to air, the lens dehydrates; it subsequently rehydrates when it comes in contact with a soaking solution or the lacrimal fluid. Placing a dehydrated lens into the eye causes discomfort as the lens absorbs tears from the precorneal area. In addition, a dehydrated lens is flatter than a hydrated lens; this factor causes problems with both comfort and visual acuity.

If lenses are allowed to dry out during overnight storage, accumulated deposits are more difficult to remove by normal cleaning. Storage in a soaking solution reduces the likelihood of deposits forming.

To maintain sterility, storage solutions use essentially the same preservatives as wetting solutions. The main difference is that the concentration can be somewhat higher in a soaking solution because the solution is rinsed from the lens before insertion. However, preservative levels are carefully selected because higher levels do not necessarily give increased effectiveness and may lead to impaired wetting or corneal irritation because of the adsorption of preservatives onto the lens.

Wetting Solutions

The functions of an ideal wetting solution are:

- To convert the hydrophobic lens surface to a hydrophilic surface by means of a uniform film that does not easily wash away;
- To increase comfort by providing cushioning and lubrication between the corneal surface and the inner

surface of the lens, and between the lens and the inner surface of the eyelid;
- To place a viscous coating on the lens to protect it from oil on the fingers during insertion;
- To stabilize the lens on the fingertip to ease insertion, particularly for individuals with poor manual dexterity or unsteady hands.

If the lens is thoroughly cleaned before insertion, lacrimal fluid can adequately wet the lens. Indeed, the wetting action of popular wetting solutions is sometimes not significantly better than that of saline. Further, patients whose tears are capable of wetting a lens almost immediately upon insertion often do not use these solutions.

The basic wetting solution comprises components from four main categories:

- Cushioning agents, such as viscosity-inducing additives (usually cellulose gum derivatives such as methylcellulose or hydroxypropyl methylcellulose);
- Wetting agents, such as polyvinyl alcohol or other surfactants;
- Preservatives, such as benzalkonium chloride, thimerosal, polyquaternium-1, sorbic acid, and polyaminopropyl biguanide;
- Buffering agents and salts added to adjust the pH and tonicity.

The cushioning effect of a wetting solution is achieved by hydrophilic polymers that lubricate the interface between the lens and the surfaces of the cornea and eyelid. Cellulose gum derivatives are often used. Although compounds such as methylcellulose possess a degree of surfactant activity, they do not promote uniform wetting of a rigid lens. For this reason, polyvinyl alcohol is also used often to decrease surface tension.

The concentration of the cushioning polymer in wetting solutions affects both eye comfort and the quality of vision immediately following insertion. In some individuals, a concentration that is too low causes discomfort after only a short time. In other wearers, a high polymer concentration results in blurred vision because the viscous solution mixes poorly with tears. Overspill of solution onto the lids and eyelashes causes crusting as the solution dries; this crusty residue can be a source of foreign material falling into the eye. Saliva should never be used to wet contact lenses because it can lead to infection by *Acanthamoeba, P aeruginosa,* or other pathogens.

Multifunctional Products

Initially, manufacturers recommended three different solutions for the cleaning, soaking, and wetting of hard contact lenses. However, there has been a trend toward using combination solutions for these functions: some single solutions claim to be effective for all three procedures.

The major problem with an all-purpose solution is that ingredients required in its formulation perform different and somewhat incompatible functions. For example, high concentrations of benzalkonium chloride are necessary to kill bacteria in soaking solutions; however, these same concentrations can cause ocular irritation when placed directly on the eye with a contact lens. If lenses are stored overnight in a solution containing a high concentration of polymers for cushioning and wetting, the lenses may become gummy and cause discomfort. Similarly, if lenses are stored overnight in a cleaning solution containing an anionic surfactant, the detergent may eventually build up on the lens and cause irritation.

No single agent that will optimally perform all three basic functions currently exists. The present all-purpose solutions are compromises. They are marginally effective but cannot be expected to perform as well as separate solutions.

Rewetting Solutions

Rewetting solutions are intended to clean and rewet the contact lens while the lens is in the eye. These solutions depend on the use of surfactants to loosen deposits; removal is assisted by the natural cleaning action of blinking. An agent used to promote this action is polyoxyl 40 stearate. Although these products function well to recondition the lens, the cornea benefits more if the lens is actually removed, cleaned, and rewetted. Removing the lens for even a brief time allows the cornea to be resurfaced with a new proteinaceous or mucinaceous layer.

Other Products

Other ophthalmic products are available to the hard lens wearer for occasional use. Some, such as artificial tears and ocular decongestants, are not recommended for use with the lenses in place. Because of their emollient and lubricating effect, artificial tears can be used to soothe the eye. Ocular decongestants reduce mild conjunctival hyperemia associated with prolonged lens wear. However, these topical decongestants can induce conjunctival hypoxia, which may harm the patient.[35] Thus, routine use of these products should be avoided. If symptoms requiring their use persist, a visit to a vision specialist is advised.

Product Selection Guidelines

The variety of lens care solutions available to hard lens wearers poses a selection problem. The availability of single- and multiple-function products within the same product line can further frustrate and confuse some wearers. Thus, product selection is an area in which pharmacists can perform a much needed role as a consultant. Unfortunately, information at hand is not always sufficient to provide a complete foundation for patient consultation. One factor that could help determine which products to recommend is the adequacy of the labeling. Product labeling is often incomplete or limited to general information; the specific agents and concentrations of preservatives are usually listed adequately, but concentrations of cushioning and lubricating polymers are often absent; and other ingredients are often listed simply as cleaning agents or buffers, making alternate selections a random process. A surfactant cleaner, a soaking solution, a wetting solution, and a rewetting solution should be recommended.

Insertion and Removal

Wearers of hard contact lenses should be instructed in the proper procedures for inserting and removing their lenses as follows: After washing hands, remove the lens from the lens storage case, rinse it with fresh conditioning/soaking solution, and inspect it for cleanliness and signs of damage (cracks or chips). If a wetting or conditioning solution is being used, place a few drops on the lens. Place the lens on the top of the index finger. Place the middle finger of the same hand on the lower lid and pull it down. With the other hand, use a finger to lift the upper lid and then place the lens on the eye. Release the lids and blink. Check vision immediately to ascertain that the lens is in the proper position. If the lens is not placed correctly after three to four blinks (blurry vision), it may be off center, on the wrong eye, or dirty. Instill one to three drops of rewetting or reconditioning drops into the eye. If there is no improvement, remove the lens, place several drops of wetting/conditioning solution onto both surfaces, and reinsert. Repeat this procedure with the other lens.

Before removing the lens, fill the storage cases with soaking/conditioning solution. Remove the top from the cleaning solution. Place a hand (or a towel) under the eye. Two methods are appropriate for removing the lens from the eye:

- *Two-finger method:* Place the tip of the forefinger of one hand on the middle of the eyelid by the lashes. Place the forefinger of the other hand on the middle lower lid margin. Push the lids inward and then together. The lens should pop out. If it only becomes decentered onto the white part of the eye, recenter and try again.
- *Temporal pull/blink method:* Place an index finger on the temporal edge of the lower and upper lids. Widen the eyelids a little, initially. Stretch the skin outward and slightly upward without allowing the lid to slide over the lens. Blink briskly. The lens will pop out because of the pressure of the eyelids at the top and bottom of the lens. Blinking facilitates removal after the lids have been tightened around the lens.

Care of RGP Lenses

Procedures

The diversity and variation in materials used in RGP lenses preclude generalizations. Lens wearers should be advised by their eye care professionals about the products and regimens recommended for their particular lenses. The labeling on contact lens products also indicates the lenses for which they are approved (see product table "Rigid Gas-Permeable Lens Products").

The care of an RGP lens is similar to that of a hard contact lens (Figure 3). The first step, after removing the lens from the eye, is to clean the lens. After cleaning, the lens is soaked in a soaking or conditioning solution. The lens may be wetted and then reinserted into the eye. Rewetting or reconditioning drops may be used while the lens is on the eye. With some lenses, once weekly enzymes are also recommended.

Some RGP lenses have a high silicone content and thus have decreased surface wettability. As previously noted, the lens surface tends to have a negative charge, which promotes the binding of positively charged tear constituents. Cleaners that are designed for conventional hard or RGP lenses may not be effective in removing the more tenacious deposits. Other cleaners that are formulated for this type of lens (ie, Boston Advance Cleaner) contain silica gel, which acts to mechanically break the adhesive bonds that have formed between the lens and the deposits. However, these cleaners have also been associated with hairline scratches on the RGP lens.[36]

It is important to counsel the patient to rinse the lens carefully and not apply too much pressure when cleaning. RGP lenses tend to coat on the concave surface rather than on the convex surface, as is the case with hard lenses. Care should be taken to clean both surfaces of the lens thoroughly, even though the concave surface may be harder to reach. The lenses should be cleaned in the palm of the hand to decrease the risk of chipping an edge, which may occur when the lens is cleaned between the fingers.[36]

Because high-silicone lenses have decreased surface wettability, conditioning solutions are generally used instead of soaking solutions to aid the formation of a cushioning tear layer. A conditioning solution is essentially a specially formulated wetting solution. The conditioner system enhances wettability of the lens, increases comfort, and disinfects the lens. The lenses must be soaked at least 4 hours in this solution before they are reinserted into the eyes. It is important to counsel the patient that the Boston Advance Conditioning solution must be discarded 90 days after opening. There is a space on the label to record the date that the product is opened.

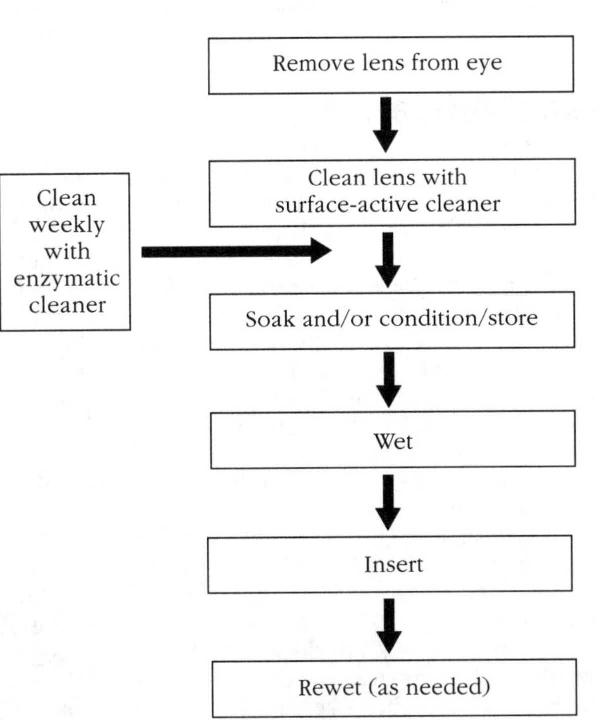

FIGURE 3 Gas-permeable lens care.

Reconditioning/rewetting drops may also be used while the lens is on the eye to rewet the lens as necessary. Boston Rewetting Drops must be discarded 60 days after opening. Heat disinfection cannot be used with RGP lenses.

As the silicone content of RGP lenses increases, so does the amount of protein adherence. Silicone acrylate lenses have an active surface that promotes the binding of tear constituents. Protein deposits on the lens will decrease the oxygen permeability, and the patient may experience discomfort.[37] Lenses of this type should be cleaned with an enzymatic product once weekly. Failure to comply with this cleaning step may result in the need for professional polishing or replacement of the lens.

Products containing chlorhexidine gluconate should not be used with silicone or styrene lenses because this agent will make the lens surface more difficult to wet and may also cause surface clouding. Fluorosilicone acrylate lenses should not be disinfected with hydrogen peroxide or cleaned more than one time with MiraFlow. Cracking, changes in parameters, and brittleness have been noted when this type of lens is cleaned repeatedly with MiraFlow.

Product Selection Guidelines

The appropriate lens care regimen for RGP lenses must be compatible with the particular lens. Lens wearers should be advised against substituting other products for those specifically recommended by their eye care professional. Patients wearing RGP lenses should be advised to purchase a surface-active cleaning product, an enzymatic product, and a conditioning or soaking solution, depending on the type of lens worn. A rewetting or reconditioning product should also be recommended.

Insertion and Removal

Wearers of RGP lenses should be counseled to follow the insertion and removal procedures for hard lenses.

Care of Soft Lenses

Conventional hard lens solutions should never be used with soft lenses because absorption of the ingredients can damage the lenses (see product table "Soft Lens Products"). Because soft lenses contain a high percentage of water, they are most prone to bacterial contamination. Lens disinfection is crucial to prevent ocular infection and damage to the lens material by bacteria and fungi. Wearers of soft hydrophilic contact lenses should also be particularly cautious in exposing their lenses to chemicals. These chemicals, many of which penetrate and bind with the lens material, can come from cosmetics, environmental pollutants, and ophthalmic and systemic products.

The basic regimen of care for soft lenses is different from that for hard lenses (Figure 4). All steps must be completed to avoid ocular complications. The only exception is with daily-wear disposable soft contact lenses; because these lenses are disposed of within 2 weeks, enzymatic cleaners are usually not necessary. Disposable lenses should, however, be cleaned and disinfected after each wearing until disposal. Products such as Opti-One are multipurpose solutions (for cleaning and disinfecting) formulated specifically for contact lenses that have a replacement schedule of 2 weeks or less.

Cleaning Products

A troublesome aspect of soft lens wear is the accumulation of deposits on the lens.[38] The nature of these deposits varies, but generally they consist of proteins and lipids from the wearer's lacrimal secretions. Deposits are a greater problem with the more highly hydrated lenses, but the rate at which these deposits accumulate depends on the lens and the tears. Some wearers experience little difficulty and wear soft lenses for long periods without significant buildup; others may show deposits in as little as 2 or 3 days. Whatever the cause or accumulation rate, the result is an uncomfortable lens of poor optical quality.

Soft contact lenses require two cleaning steps to rid them of debris. Cleaning with a surface-active cleaner must be done daily or, in the case of extended-wear lenses, each time they are removed from the eyes. Cleaning with an enzymatic cleaner should be done weekly or biweekly and can be done more often if necessary.

Surface-Active Cleaners A common method of cleaning soft lenses uses surface-active materials and friction rubbing. Several drops of a cleaning product are placed onto the lens surface, and the lens is gently rubbed between the thumb and forefinger. Another method is to place the lens in the palm of the hand and rub gently with a fingertip. With both methods, care must be used to avoid cutting the soft lens with a fingernail or scratching the lens surfaces with grit or dirt on the hands. Soft lens cleaning solutions generally contain a nonionic detergent, a wetting agent, a chelating agent, buffers, preservatives, and, in some cases, polymeric cleaning beads. Friction cleaning usually takes about 20–30 seconds, and then the cleaner must be thoroughly rinsed from the lens. Rinsing is an essential part of soft lens care; it should be carried out using a sterile isotonic buffered solution. Tap water should *never* be used with soft contact lenses because it is not isotonic and it contains harmful pathogens.

Enzymatic Cleaners Although the surface-active cleaners generally are quite effective in removing lipid deposits, they are less successful in removing tenacious protein debris. Enzymatic cleaners are an additional cleaning aid that can help solve this problem. These enzymes hydrolyze polypeptide bonds of protein and dissolve the protein deposits. For the enzyme solution to work properly, however, the lens must be cleaned with a surface-active cleaner first; enzymes are ineffective in the presence of debris covering or mixed with protein.

Generally, enzymatic cleaners are used in the following manner. The enzyme tablet (papain, pancreatin, or subtilisin) is placed in a solution recommended by the manufacturer, and the lens is allowed to soak from as briefly as 15 minutes (high-water lenses) to as long as overnight (low-water lenses). The enzymatic cleaner is then thoroughly rinsed from the lens to prevent eye irritation. With most enzymatic products (the exception being certain subtilisin products), the lens then must be disinfected to complete the cleaning procedure. It is usually sufficient to use enzyme cleaning as a once-a-

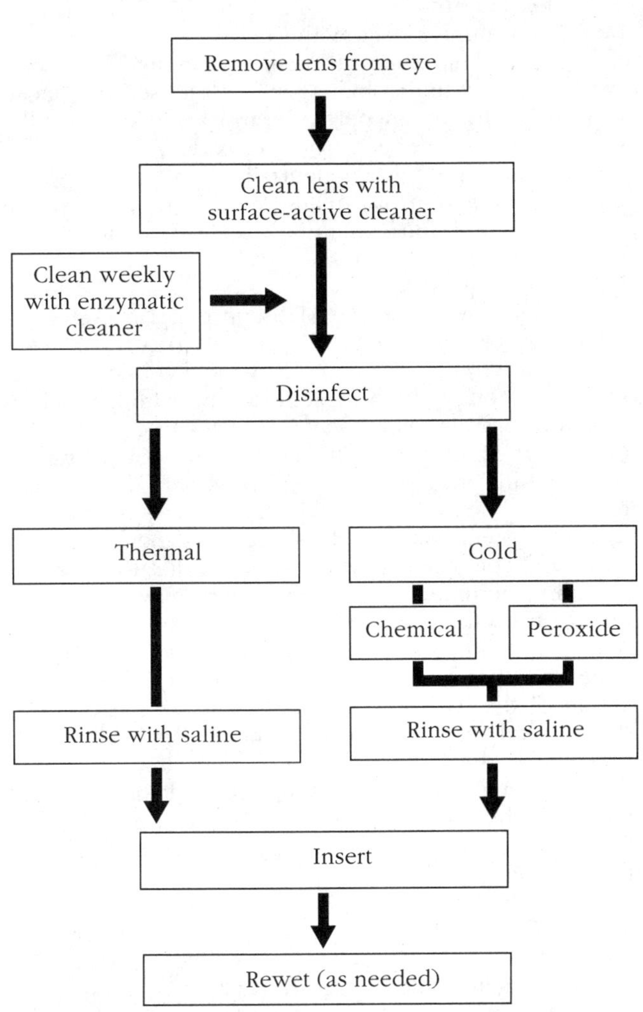

FIGURE 4 Soft contact lens care.

week supplement to daily cleaning with surface-active chemicals. Some enzymatic regimens have been developed to be used simultaneously with thermal and chemical disinfection.

Table 6 shows some of the differences between various enzymatic products. Of particular note are the products that allow the patient to combine the enzymatic cleaning and disinfection steps. These products are dissolved in the hydrogen peroxide used for disinfection or in the saline that will be heated in the disinfection step. This decreases the number of steps necessary for lens care and may increase compliance.

Disinfecting Methods

The FDA recommends disinfecting soft contact lenses before each reinsertion. Disinfection occurs after cleaning the lens. Two methods of disinfection are currently approved: thermal and chemical. Studies have shown that microorganisms do not actually enter the matrix of soft lenses but that surface contamination could lead to ocular infection.[39] Both disinfecting methods are reliable for most ocular pathogens. Chemical disinfection with hydrogen peroxide has increased in popularity with certain types of lenses over thermal and earlier chemical disinfectants because of decreased ocular allergenicity and toxicity.

Thermal Disinfection The basic method of thermal disinfection involves placing the cleaned lenses into separate compartments of a storage case filled with saline. The case is then placed into a heating unit, and the temperature is increased to a specific level for a prescribed time. Originally, the lenses were disinfected by raising the temperature to the boiling point for about 20 minutes. Units that use a lower temperature (about 176°F [80°C]) for a longer time are now available. The FDA requirement is at least 176°F (80°C) for at least 10 minutes. This process is as effective as boiling for most organisms, and it prolongs lens life. The procedure is usually done at night.

TABLE 6 Enzymatic cleaners

	Allergan Enzymatic	Opti-Zyme	Opti-Free Enzymatic	ReNu Effervescent	ReNu Thermal	Ultrazyme
Has an odor	Yes	No	No	No	No	No
Requires disinfection as a separate step	Yes	Yes	No	Yes	No	No
Is effective with a short soak	Yes	Yes	Yes	Yes	Yes	Yes
Can be used concurrently with heat disinfection	No	No	No	No	Yes	No
Can be used concurrently with hydrogen peroxide disinfection	No	No	No	No	No	Yes

Adapted with permission from Engle JP. Contact lens care. *AM Druggist*. 1990 Jan; 201: 54–65.

For situations in which it is not possible to use a heat disinfection unit, the patient may place the tightly closed lens case containing the lenses and saline in a pot of boiling water for at least 10 minutes (15 minutes if at an altitude above 7,000 feet). The water must not boil away. The pot with the water and lenses should then be removed from the heat and allowed to cool for 30 minutes. The patient should resume use of the heat disinfection unit as soon as possible.

Thermal disinfection has several advantages. It can be done with a preservative-free solution and is therefore less likely to cause eye irritation. Additionally, it kills microbial contamination better than any other method. Thermal disinfection is the only approved contact lens disinfection method known to be effective against cysts of *Acanthamoeba*, and it is generally more effective against chemically resistant microorganisms such as fungi and bacillus species. It also kills organisms on and surrounding the contact lens case, further preventing potential contaminants from entering the lenses.

Thermal disinfection also has several drawbacks. Lenses with a high water content cannot withstand daily heating. Some individuals find the method cumbersome and less convenient than chemical disinfection. There is also a high initial cost for equipment, although long-term costs of chemical disinfectant solutions may offset this. The user must take care to remove proteinaceous and other debris by cleaning the lenses first. Lens cases used with thermal units, and the units themselves, should be routinely inspected for damage, cracks, or leaks and replaced at the earliest sign of a problem.

Chemical Disinfection In chemical disinfection, the lenses are stored for a prescribed period of time in a solution containing bactericidal agents that are compatible with soft lens materials. There are two basic chemical disinfection methods available in the United States. The first method is based on the original chemical disinfecting solutions, which consisted of antimicrobial preservatives of sufficient concentration in storage solutions primarily composed of saline. These initial disinfecting solutions contained chlorhexidine and thimerosal, both of which induce sensitivity reactions in many soft lens wearers. These solutions no longer contain thimerosal, but several still contain chlorhexidine. Patients are less sensitive to chlorhexidine and apparently can tolerate it better than thimerosal. To avoid sensitivity reactions, solutions with several new disinfecting preservatives are currently being marketed for soft contact lens care. These preservatives are sorbic acid, polyquaternium-1, and polyaminopropyl biguanide, touted to be much less toxic or allergenic than their predecessors. However, these agents may also be less effective, especially against fungi and protozoans.

Patients should soak their lenses in the disinfecting solution for a minimum of 4 hours. The lenses may be stored for longer periods in these solutions; however, if they are stored longer than 3 days, the patient should clean and disinfect them with fresh solution for at least 4 hours prior to inserting the lenses into the eyes.

An exception to the minimum 4 hours soaking time is Quick Care, which is used to clean and disinfect soft lenses in only 5 minutes. The patient first rubs a hypertonic starting solution containing isopropyl alcohol and surfactants onto the lens to clean and disinfect the lens. The lenses are then soaked in a finishing solution after being thoroughly rinsed with saline.

The second chemical method uses hydrogen peroxide as the antimicrobial agent. Soft lenses are placed in purified hydrogen peroxide and are disinfected by the liberation of oxygen from peroxide. Following disinfection, the peroxide is neutralized to trace levels by the catalytic action of a platinum disc, by soaking the lenses in a solution containing catalase, sodium pyruvate, or sodium thiosulfite, or by—least desirably—dilution techniques.

Patients who use the platinum disc (ie, AO Sept) for neutralization should be counseled to replace the disc after 100 uses or 3 months, whichever comes first. Failure to comply with these instructions may result in disc failure, and the patient may sustain a peroxide burn on the cornea. Moreover, although the catalytic disc systems only require one step, that step takes 6 hours for disinfection and neutralization, which decreases the flexibility of the system. Suboptimal disinfection is another concern with AO Sept. The catalytic disc will neutralize the surrounding peroxide quickly, and there may not be adequate time for disinfection. Another disadvantage is that, depending on the design of the case, bacteria beneath the disc may be protected from the disinfecting action of the hydrogen peroxide.[40] Once the catalytic disc neutralizes the peroxide, a nonpreserved solution remains. If the lenses are left in the case for several days, bacterial contamination may occur. Patients should not store their lenses in neutralized AO Sept for more than 24 hours unless they disinfect the lenses again prior to insertion.

Most hydrogen peroxide systems that require two steps for disinfection and neutralization work in only 20–30 minutes. The patient may use these products in the morning just before insertion. For most patients, one of the products that use a neutralizing solution is appropriate. These products require only 20–30 minutes to use; the neutralizing step is easy; and if the neutralizing agent contains a preservative, there is less chance that the resultant solution will become contaminated.

Table 7 outlines the differences among the various peroxide products.

One potential disadvantage of hydrogen peroxide disinfection is that patients may insert the lens directly from the peroxide solution without neutralization. A peroxide-soaked lens placed on the eye will cause great pain, photophobia, redness, and, perhaps, corneal epithelial damage. If this occurs, the patient should immediately remove the lens from the eye and flush the eye with sterile saline solution. The pain should subside within a few hours. If it does not, the patient should consult an eye or vision care specialist. If the patient has any doubt as to whether the peroxide was neutralized, the entire disinfection cycle should be started over again to avoid the risk of inserting a peroxide-soaked lens without a neutralizing step.

There are two hydrogen peroxide products that help the patient avoid the possibility of forgetting to do the neutralization step. With one product, UltraCare, the user adds a delayed-release neutralizing tablet at the beginning of the disinfection cycle. This tablet contains cyanocobalamin, which turns the solution pink, thus reminding the user that the tablet has been added. There

TABLE 7 Differences in peroxide products

	Neutralizing dilution agent	Flexibility		Potential risks
		Overnight	Morning	
AO Sept	Platinum disc	Yes	No	Disc failure[a]
Consept	Chemical solution	Yes	Yes	None
Lensept	Chemical solution	Yes	Yes	None
Mirasept[b]	Chemical solution/tablets	Yes	Yes	None
Oxysept	Chemical solution/tablets	Yes	Yes	None
UltraCare	Delayed-release chemical tablets	Yes	No	None
Pure-Sept	Saline (osmotic extraction)	Yes	Yes	Possible irritation from leftover peroxide
Quik-Sept	Saline (osmotic extraction)	Yes	Yes	Possible irritation from leftover peroxide

[a] Disc wears out and must be replaced every 3 months or after 100 uses.

[b] Mirasept neutralizing solution (multiuse bottles) must be discarded 4 months after opening.

Adapted with permission from Engle JP. Contact lens care. *Am Druggist.* 1990 Jan; 201: 54–65.

are no additional steps to remember as disinfection and neutralization will occur at the appropriate time intervals. Another advantage of UltraCare is that the lenses are exposed to the disinfecting effects of hydrogen peroxide for 2 hours, the time necessary for optimal activity against *Acanthamoeba*. Patients using UltraCare should be counseled as follows:

- This product requires a minimum of 2 hours to complete disinfection and neutralization of the peroxide.
- The neutralizing tablet should not be crushed or used if there are cracks in the coating; the tablet will start neutralizing the peroxide before adequate disinfection occurs.
- MiraFlow or Pliagel, which are used for surface-active cleaning, can leave a film on the lenses and lens cup if not carefully rinsed off the lens. This may result in foaming and overflow of the peroxide/neutralizer solution.[41] If this occurs, lenses should be rinsed more carefully or another surface-active cleaner should be used.
- Before lenses are removed from the eye, the lens container should be filled with fresh UltraCare disinfection solution, the cap tightened, and the cup turned upside down so that the solution bathes the upper portion of the cup and the top. The cup is left in this position until the patient is ready to disinfect the lenses.
- Ultracare should not be used with Illusions opaquely tinted soft contact lenses. Lens damage may result.
- If the lenses are not going to be worn for awhile, they can be stored unopened in the neutralized solution; however, they should be disinfected once weekly and just before wear.

Another product that helps the patient avoid the risk of peroxide burns is AO Sept. Since the platinum disc is always present in the lens case, the need for the patient to remember to do a separate neutralization step is eliminated. Neutralization of the peroxide automatically occurs as long as the disc is in the case and has been replaced on an appropriate schedule.

Soaking lenses in the peroxide solution longer than the manufacturer recommends is another potential problem for patients using hydrogen peroxide systems. Exceeding the recommended time is not a good practice because it may take longer to neutralize the peroxide.

Using household hydrogen peroxide solutions to disinfect soft lenses may discolor the lenses. Contaminants and other chemicals within such solutions cause the discoloration. Further, the pH of topical hydrogen peroxide is too low for use with contact lenses.[42]

The following points should be discussed with patients who are using hydrogen peroxide disinfecting systems:

- Neutralizers from different peroxide systems should never be mixed. Some ingredients in different neutralizers may interact, forming a precipitate. Incomplete neutralization may also occur. The lenses may be ruined.
- A neutralizing solution should never be placed in a case with a catalytic disc. An unwanted chemical reaction may occur, or a gummy residue may form on the disc.
- If using MiraSept neutralizing solution, the bottle must be discarded 4 months after opening.

- Catalase-based neutralizers should not be used with Illusions opaquely tinted soft contact lenses. Lens damage may result.
- Lenses should not be soaked in the peroxide solution for longer than the recommended time; otherwise, it may take longer to neutralize the peroxide.
- Household hydrogen peroxide solutions should not be used to disinfect soft lenses because the lenses may become discolored. Also, the pH of these solutions is too low for such use.[42]
- The lens cup that comes with a product should be used. Lens cases/cups should not be switched between products.

Saline Solutions

The hydrophilic soft contact lens must be maintained in a constant state of hydration. Furthermore, the hydrated lens must be isotonic with tears because changes in tonicity can alter the conformation and optical properties of the lens. Isotonic normal saline is the basic solution used for rinsing, thermally disinfecting, and storing soft contact lenses.

Prepared saline is available in either preserved or preservative-free forms. Because thimerosal and chlorhexidine can cause sensitivity reactions or irritation in a great many patients, sorbic acid–preserved products are commonly promoted for sensitive eyes and appear to be acceptable to most wearers. Salines preserved with Polyquad and Dymed are also available for patients who are sensitive to other preservatives.

Several preservative-free salines are also available. Preservative-free buffered saline is available in unit-of-use containers (which should be used and discarded once opened) and in several sizes of multiuse bottles (which must be discarded 14–30 days after opening, depending on the product formulation). Nonpreserved salines are also available as aerosol sprays.

Some nonpreserved saline products contain EDTA, which prevents deposits of calcium and other divalent ions on the surface of the lens. EDTA, although not a preservative, will inhibit the growth of certain bacteria, thus extending the shelf life of the product. Nonpreserved, nonaerosol saline generally has a shelf life of 15 days once opened. When EDTA is added to the product, that shelf life may be extended to 30 days.

Patients should avoid using other forms of saline such as intravenous normal saline or saline squirts because these products are usually too acidic for use with soft contact lenses.

Some persons prepare their own preservative-free saline using salt tablets and USP purified water. The use of salt tablets is inexpensive, but the clear superiority of commercial salines argues strongly against it. The use of homemade saline from salt tablets and the application of improper lens care are the greatest predisposing factors to acanthamoeba keratitis, a rare but vision-threatening eye disease, and to many anterior eye infections contracted by hydrophilic lens wearers.[43] The FDA no longer condones the use of salt tablets, and neither should a concerned pharmacist.

Acanthamoeba, of which there are 15 species, is an opportunistic protozoan. Usually nonpathogenic, *Acanthamoeba* has been isolated from airborne dust, soils, surface water, tap water, and even distilled water. In unfavorable environments, it forms a very resistant cyst that can survive many antimicrobial agents, even though its vegetative form (trophozoite) may be susceptible. Viable cysts have been found in swimming pools and hot tubs that are adequately chlorinated to kill trophozoites.

Most victims of acanthamoeba keratitis have used improper lens hygiene, gone swimming without removing their contact lenses, used nonsterile saline solution made from salt tablets and distilled water, or used tap water in the maintenance of their soft contact lenses. Because they are very resistant, *Acanthamoeba* cysts often can survive attempts to eradicate them antimicrobially from the eye. Multiple antibiotic regimens have been applied with variable or poor therapeutic response. Many cases of acanthamoeba keratitis are severe enough to require keratoplasty, a partial or complete cornea transplant, in an attempt to save the eye. Unfortunately, the persistent presence of cysts gives this eye infection a poor prognosis, which, in many cases, ultimately leads to enucleation—the partial or total removal of the affected eye. As a diagnosis of the keratitis has become more definitive and awareness of the disease has become more acute, the apparent incidence of acanthamoeba keratitis has risen from 11 cases reported between 1973 and 1983, to 24 cases reported between mid-1985 and February 1986. More than 200 cases were diagnosed through the first quarter of 1989.

Rewetting Solutions

Accessory solutions for use with soft lenses permit lubricating and rewetting (and, in some cases, cleaning) of the lens in the eye. These solutions typically contain a low concentration of a nonionic surfactant to promote cleaning and a polymer to lubricate the lens surface, along with buffering agents. These solutions are particularly useful to patients with highly hydrated lenses, such as the extended-wear type. Exposure of lenses to wind and high temperature causes some dehydration, even of the lens in the eye. The resulting discomfort can sometimes be relieved by one or two drops of rewetting solution. To minimize contaminations, the tip of the applicator bottle should not touch the eye, eyelid, or any other surface. The pharmacist should be aware of the preservative content of these products. Some are available without thimerosal and may be less sensitizing to patients with preservative allergies.

Product Selection Guidelines

Many problems associated with soft lens wear arise from the way people handle their lenses; unsatisfactory results may stem from improper procedures rather than from inadequate products.[44] In one investigation, only 26% of contact lens wearers fully complied with care instructions, and the occurrence of signs and symptoms of potential wearing problems was directly correlated with noncompliance. Specific questions about the care and maintenance regimen used by a wearer can often bring these problems to light.

Surface-Active Cleaners Some surface-active cleaners have a lower viscosity and may be easier to rinse off the lens (eg, Bausch & Lomb Sensitive Eyes Daily Cleaner). These products are good choices for patients who have difficulty completely rinsing the cleaner off their lens.

In addition to surfactants, some products (eg, Opti-Clean II) contain mild abrasives that aid in the removal of lens deposits. Patients who have difficulty removing deposits from their lenses will benefit from this type of cleaner. These products should be shaken before use. Some patients may have difficulty in rinsing these cleaners off their lens. Care should be taken to be sure that no residue from the cleaning solution remains on the lens prior to insertion.

Finally, one surfactant cleaner (MiraFlow) contains isopropyl alcohol. This product is useful for patients who discover heavy lipid deposits on their lenses.

Enzymatic Cleaners Enzymatic cleaners can be recommended based on the disinfection system the patient uses. If the patient uses thermal disinfection, ReNu Thermal is a good choice because it eliminates the need to perform the enzymatic cleaning and disinfection steps separately. An exception to this is a patient who wears crofilcon A soft lenses (eg, CSI, CSI-T, or AZTECH); the plastic in these lenses has been found to stiffen when used with ReNu Thermal enzymatic cleaner. If the patient uses a hydrogen peroxide cleaning system, Ultrazyme is a good choice. This product can be placed in the peroxide solution, thus cleaning and disinfecting at the same time. If the patient uses Opti-Free disinfecting solution, Opti-Free Enzymatic Cleaner would be a good choice as it can be placed directly in the Opti-Free solution during the disinfection cycle. If the patient uses another chemical disinfection system, the comparisons between products become very idiosyncratic unless the patient has an allergy to one of the components.

Disinfecting Methods When counseling a patient about the best disinfection method to use, the pharmacist should ask what type of lenses the patient wears. If the patient wears low-water lenses, heat disinfection or UltraCare (2-hour exposure to hydrogen peroxide) is best because they are the only methods that eradicate *Acanthamoeba*. If a patient wears high-water lenses or is not sure what type of lenses he or she has, a hydrogen peroxide system or a second-generation chemical system (ie, Opti-Free or ReNu) can be recommended.

Soft lens wearers may freely switch from thermal to chemical disinfection methods, but the switch from chemical to thermal may present problems. If lenses that have been chemically disinfected are not completely free from all traces of the chemicals, they can be damaged by heating. Prolonged soaking in several changes of saline is recommended to clean the lenses before using a heating unit.

Product Incompatibility Several incompatibilities may occur when mixing soft lens products. Most manufacturers test for compatibility within their own product lines; however, compatibility with other manufacturers' products is usually not determined. Generally, chemical disinfecting solutions should not be interchanged or used concurrently. If a patient mixes a disinfecting solution containing chlorhexidine and thimerosal (ie, Flex-care) with a product containing a quaternary ammonium compound (ie, Allergan Hydrocare), a toxic keratopathy known as mixed solution syndrome may occur. Patients should be counseled not to switch from a chlorhexidine-containing chemical disinfection system to a hydrogen peroxide system unless they procure new lenses. A fine black precipitate may form on the lenses if chlorhexidine is still present in the lens matrix. Other chemical disinfection system residue on soft lenses may cause the lens to turn pink, yellow, brown, black, or purple if the lens is exposed to a hydrogen peroxide system. Barnes Hind Daily Cleaner should not be mixed with a cleaner containing poloxamer 407 (ie, Mirasoft) because cloudy precipitates may form on the lens.[30]

Insertion and Removal

When inserting soft lenses, the wearer should carefully follow these steps:

- Wash the hands with noncosmetic soap and rinse thoroughly; dry the hands with a lint-free towel.
- Remove the lens for the right eye from its storage container. Rinse it with saline solution to dilute any preservatives left from disinfection.
- Place the lens on the top of a finger and examine it to be sure it is not inside out. This can be done by using the "taco test." Gently fold the lens at the apex (not the edges) between the thumb and forefinger. The edges should look like a taco shell with the edges pointed inward. If the edges roll out, the lens is inverted and must be reversed.
- Examine the lens for cleanliness. If necessary, clean it and rinse again with saline.
- Insert the lens on the right eye.
- Repeat the process for the left eye.
- Before removing the lenses, wash hands with a noncosmetic soap; rinse the hands thoroughly and dry them with a lint-free towel.
- Using the right middle finger, pull down the lower lid of the right eye. Touch the right index finger to the lens and slide the lens off the cornea. Using the index finger and thumb, grasp the lens and remove it.
- Repeat the procedure for the left eye.

Patient Counseling

Although contacts are usually safe, lens wearers can experience a variety of problems. Many lens care–related problems are minor and can be easily solved by the knowledgeable pharmacist. Others require ocular inspection and should be referred to the prescriber. A few problems are serious and may be vision threatening. In these cases, the pharmacist must certainly refer the patient to an appropriate specialist.

General Instruction for Lens Wearers

Pharmacists should ask patients wearing contact lenses the questions at the beginning of this chapter; the answers will give the pharmacist a sense of the urgency and a general sense of the etiology of the problem, and will help the pharmacist determine whether the problem is related to noncompliance with care regimens or to drug–lens interactions. The pharmacist should then ask specific questions related to the type of lens the patient is currently wearing. Only then can the pharmacist give appropriate counseling information.

The following are general instructions the pharmacist can give patients for successful contact lens wear.

- The hands should be washed with noncosmetic soap and thoroughly rinsed before contact lenses are touched.
- Oily cosmetics should be avoided while lenses are being worn. Bath oils or soaps with a bath oil or cream base may leave an oil film on the hands that will be transferred to the lenses.
- When lenses are being handled over a sink, the drain should be covered or closed to prevent the loss of a lens.
- Lenses should be checked to be sure that they are not scratched, chipped, or torn; that there are no foreign particles on them; and that they are clean and thoroughly rinsed of cleaner. Lens warpage and discoloration may also cause discomfort.
- Contact lenses are individually fitted to correct the refractive error of each eye. To avoid mixing up the lenses, it is helpful always to work with the same lens first. Hard lenses may be marked or etched with a dot in the periphery to avoid confusion.
- If the lenses are not comfortable after insertion or if vision is blurred, the patient should check to be sure that they are not on the wrong eyes or on inside out.
- Aerosol cosmetics and deodorants damage the lens and should be applied either before lens insertion or with eyes closed until the air is clear of spray particles.
- Lenses should not be inserted in red or irritated eyes. If the eyes become irritated while lenses are being worn, the lenses should be removed until the irritation subsides. Should irritation or redness not subside, an eye care practitioner should be consulted.
- Except for extended-wear lenses, and then only by prescription, contact lenses must not be worn while sleeping.
- Lenses should not be worn while sitting under a hair dryer if excessive dryness of the eyes results. The same caution applies to overhead fans and air ducts.
- When cleaning the lens, the wearer should rub it in a back-and-forth rather than a circular direction.
- The second lens should be cleaned as thoroughly as the first. Some patients have "left lens syndrome," in which the left lens has more deposits than the right lens because the right lens is often removed first and cleaned more thoroughly.
- The eyes should be protected when lenses are worn outside on windy days because soot and other particles may become trapped under the lens and scratch the cornea.
- Contact lenses do not preclude the use of eye protection in industry, sports, or any other occupation or hobby that has the potential for eye damage.
- Contact lenses should always be stored in a proper lens case when not in use.
- Contact lens solutions should never be reused.
- Soaking solutions in lens cases should be replaced after each use. Lenses must never be stored in tap water.
- Contact lenses should be cleaned only with agents specifically made for that purpose.
- Each type of lens should be cared for only with commercially manufactured products made specifically for that type of lens.
- Contact lens care products from different manufacturers may not be chemically compatible with each other and should not be mixed unless they are identified as compatible by a lens care specialist.
- Care products should be discarded if the labeled expiration date has passed.
- Contact lenses should generally not be worn in swimming pools, hot tubs, ocean waters, or other natural bodies of water unless there is external eye protection such as goggles.
- To prevent contamination, dropper tips or the tips of lens care product containers should not be touched.
- Contact lenses and contact lens care products should be kept out of the reach of children.
- Saliva should never be used to wet contact lenses. This practice can result in eye infections.
- If an eye infection is suspected, the attention of an eye care practitioner should be sought immediately.
- Only ophthalmic solutions specifically formulated for contact lens use should be used in the eye while wearing lenses.
- All instructions for care should be carefully followed.

Specific Instructions for Lens Wear

Hard Lenses

Pharmacists should ask hard lens wearers the following additional questions:

- Do you soak your lenses when they are not in use? Lenses should not be stored dry.
- How often do you clean your lenses? Patients should clean their lenses every time they remove them from their eyes.
- What lens care products do you use? Do you use a combination-type solution, which may not provide optimal lens care?
- Do you inspect your lenses regularly for chips and scratches?

The following special instructions will help ensure successful hard contact lens wear.

- The eyes should not be rubbed while lenses are in place.
- Contact lenses should not be rinsed with very hot or very cold water because temperature extremes may warp the lenses.
- Lenses should be cleaned before storage.
- Wearers should not get oils or lanolin on the lens.

RGP Lenses

Pharmacists should ask RGP lens wearers the following additional questions:

- What brand of RGP lenses do you wear?
- Do you routinely use enzymatic cleaners? How often? What do you use to dissolve the enzymatic tablet?

- Do you clean your lenses immediately upon removal from the eye?
- Do you routinely use a soaking/conditioning solution formulated for your type of RGP lenses?

The following special instructions will help ensure successful RGP lens wear:

- Patients should be sure to apply cleaner to and clean both sides of the lens.
- When cleaning the lens, patients should not apply too much pressure. If debris is still present, a cotton swab can be soaked in the surfactant cleaner and used to clean the lens.
- If tap water is used to rinse the cleaner off the lens (not recommended), the lens should be disinfected before being placed in the eye.[45]
- Heat disinfection should not be used with RGP lenses.

Soft Lenses

Pharmacists should ask soft lens wearers the following additional questions:

- What type of soft lenses do you wear (ie, brand, high- or low-water content, ionic or nonionic)?
- Do you clean your lenses before disinfection?
- What method of disinfection do you use?
- How often do you disinfect your lenses?
- Do you use commercial saline solutions or do you mix your own? How often do you replace your solution?
- Do you use any cosmetics that are applied to the eye area? How do you apply these products?
- Do you routinely use enzymatic cleaners? How often? How do you dilute the enzymatic tablet?
- Are your lenses extended-wear lenses? How long do you wear them?

The following special instructions will help ensure successful soft contact lens wear:

- Soft contact lenses must be thoroughly cleaned before chemical or especially thermal disinfection.
- Chemical disinfectants must be completely rinsed off before the lens is placed in the eye.
- Hydrogen peroxide disinfectants must be completely neutralized before the lens is placed in the eye.
- Enzyme cleaner tablets should be discarded if any discoloration has appeared.
- Soft lenses must be handled with care because they are very fragile and can easily be torn.
- Soft contact lenses should be removed before instillation of any ophthalmic preparation that is not specifically intended for concurrent use with soft contact lenses. The wearer should wait at least 20–30 minutes before reinserting the lenses unless directed otherwise by an eye care specialist. Lenses should not be worn at all when a topical ophthalmic ointment is being used.
- Soft contact lenses should not be worn in the presence of irritating fumes or chemicals.
- Extended-wear soft lenses should not be worn continuously for more than 7 days without complete cleaning and disinfection.
- Disposable soft contact lenses should be used strictly in accordance with manufacturer's guidelines and under the supervision of an eye care practitioner.

Extended-Wear Lenses

Extended-wear lenses can be either RGP or soft. The following instructions should be given to patients wearing extended-wear lenses[17]:

- Each morning, look carefully at your eyes. Is there unusual, persistent redness? (Some redness is normal upon wakening; it should abate within 45 minutes.) Is there any unusual discharge? Pain? If any of the above are present, remove the lens and call your lens care practitioner.
- Can you see well with your lenses? (Some hazy vision is normal upon awakening because of corneal hypoxia, which develops overnight.) Application of a few drops of rewetting agent may improve the hydration of the lens and help resolve the hypoxia. If it does not, remove the lenses, clean them, and reinsert. If your vision still has not improved within an hour, remove your lenses and call your lens care practitioner.
- Female patients should remove mascara before sleeping because mascara can flake off during sleep and become trapped underneath the lens.[46]
- If your lenses appear to be lost upon awakening, check your eyes to see if the lenses were displaced. Soft lenses can fold over on themselves and get lodged underneath the top or bottom eyelid.

Storage Case

Choice of a lens storage case is important. The case should have left and right clearly identified on the caps and in the lens wells. There should be ridges or flutes in the lens wells so that the RGP lens does not adhere to the case, an occurrence that is common in smooth cases and can cause warpage of the lens or inversion upon removal.

As important as lens care is the proper care and cleaning of the contact lens storage case. A storage case should be able to hold at least 2.5 mL of the storage solution.[47] This minimizes the chance that the soaking solution will be overwhelmed by an inoculum of bacteria. The lens case should be cleaned thoroughly and replaced at least every 3 months.[48] Routine cleaning entails air drying the case between periods of use and scrubbing it weekly. Air drying should be done daily as it discourages biofilm formation. Some manufacturers recommend cleaning the case twice weekly using a few drops of lens cleaner and hot water.[49] If the case can withstand boiling (such as those cases made of polycarbonate or noryl plastic), it can be boiled in a pot of water for 10 minutes weekly.[50] It should be examined for cracks and replaced periodically. Lens cases can be contaminated with a biofilm that will attract pathogens and increase the risk of infection.

Value-Added Pharmacy Services

The continued growth of contact lens use for both cosmetic and therapeutic reasons further increases the need for pharmacists to keep up to date with all aspects of lens products, lens materials, and care and maintenance programs. This is especially true for the pharmacist who dispenses replacement contact lenses (where allowed by law).

When maintaining a patient medication profile, pharmacists should note that the person wears contact lenses and include specific information regarding the patient's sensitivities to ingredients in lens care products. Concurrent use of any systemic drug that could affect tear flow or the refractive properties of the eyes or could discolor lenses should be considered when counseling a lens wearer about health care. Particular attention should be given to the possible effects of ophthalmic medications on contact lenses. This is a service that many patients do not currently receive.

To further enhance this service, the pharmacist should develop a relationship with contact lens prescribers in the area. A questionnaire could be sent to these practitioners asking which lenses they commonly prescribe and which lens care systems they prefer. It could ask if the practitioner fits bifocal, toric, extended-wear, or disposable lenses. After the questionnaire is returned, the pharmacist could call the practitioner and either discuss it on the telephone or make an appointment to discuss the responses in person. The pharmacist could develop a brochure and ask the practitioners to distribute it among their patients. The pharmacist could also ask the practitioners for a supply of business cards to facilitate referrals not only of appropriate lens patients for problems they may be having but also of patients who currently wear glasses and are interested in trying contact lenses. Eye care practitioners will be more likely to refer patients to a particular pharmacy if the pharmacist has a personal relationship with them. The pharmacy should have in stock the products most commonly used by the practitioners in the area.

Because of the wide variety of lens care products, stock should be carefully selected to provide a complete care program for most wearers. The contact lens department should be 24–28 linear feet in size and contain 95–100 SKUs (ie, sizes and quantities in which products are available).[51] Use of Plan-O-Grams—blueprints that show the ideal arrangement of products within a given section—will help to reduce inventory cost. Monthly sales should be approximately $1,100.[51] Generally, more than three quarters of the contact lens department should be devoted to soft lens products; the remainder should include hard and RGP lens products.[51] Items such as heating units, lens cases, and replacement catalytic discs should also be included in the department. When choosing a product line, pharmacists should consider stocking all products in the line to properly serve contact lens wearers.

The pharmacist can communicate his or her expertise to patients and encourage patients to ask questions by posting a sign in the contact lens product department that states, "The pharmacist on duty will be happy to answer your questions about contact lenses and lens care products." Educational literature about contact lenses and lens care can be displayed. The pharmacist who provides information, products, and services to the contact lens patient will be assured of consumer loyalty.

Case Studies

Case 23–1

Patient Complaint/History

CS, a 28-year-old female, presents to the pharmacy with complaints of eye discomfort associated with soft contact lenses. Questioning of the patient reveals that she began wearing soft contact lenses, and this particular pair of lenses, 2 months ago; she is unsure of the brand name of the lenses. CS did not experience discomfort when she first began wearing the lenses; however, over the past 2–3 weeks she began to notice discomfort and some irritation that occurred only when she wore the lenses. She does not complain of other symptoms such as discharge from the eye. Her last visit to the lens prescriber was 2 months ago when she received the soft lenses.

The patient's lens care regimen includes cleaning the lenses with Bausch & Lomb Sensitive Eyes Daily Cleaner each time she removes them. She then soaks the lenses in Ultracare with a neutralization tablet (hydrogen peroxide disinfection system) for 2 hours. Further, she always uses fresh solutions and cleans her storage container once a week according to the manufacturer's recommendations. Although CS does wear a water-based cream eye shadow and water-resistant mascara (but no eyeliner), she inserts her lenses before she applies any cosmetics. She also washes her hands with a noncosmetic soap before inserting the lenses.

Questions about the patient's medical history reveal no history of ocular problems, no known allergies, no current use of prescription medications (including oral contraceptives), and no past or present history of pregnancy; her family history is noncontributory. Her use of nonprescription medications includes acetaminophen for occasional headaches and diphenhydramine taken about three times a month for insomnia. The patient does not smoke; she drinks five to six beers a week.

Clinical Considerations/Strategies

The following considerations/strategies are provided to aid the reader in (1) determining whether treatment of the patient's condition with nonprescription medications is warranted, (2) selecting the appropriate nonprescription medication, and (3) developing a patient counseling strategy to ensure optimal therapeutic outcomes:

- Assess the contact lens care regimen. Call the lens prescriber to determine the appropriate care regimen and to discuss suggested changes in the care regimen.
- Assess the patient's history of lens wear along with symptomatology and allergy history.
- Develop a patient education/counseling strategy that will:
  - Design a lens care regimen that is optimal for compliance and ease of use;

- □ Justify changes in the care regimen;
- □ Optimize proper use of new product(s) added to the regimen;
- □ Educate the patient about contact lens wear and symptoms of lens problems;
- □ Educate the patient about possible medication-lens interactions;
- □ Reinforce proper usage of cosmetics when wearing contact lenses.

Case 23–2

Patient Complaint/History

ED, a 36-year-old male who began wearing soft contact lenses 1 week ago, comes to the pharmacy seeking information about the proper care of his lenses. He had worn hard contact lenses for the prior 10 years. He says that his lens prescriber told him to clean the soft lenses with Opti-Clean II each time he removes them; however, he cannot remember the rest of the care regimen. He also complains of difficulty in removing all of the cleaner from the lens surface.

Questioning of the patient reveals that he is wearing AO Soft lenses and that, when he first started wearing the lenses, his eyes felt "dry." Over the past few days, he noticed that the lenses also felt "gritty" when he inserted them. He experiences these sensations only when wearing the lenses; he has not experienced other symptoms such as discharge from the eye.

ED's lens care regimen includes cleaning the lenses with Opti-Clean II each time he removes them and then soaking them in aerosolized saline. He has used the same saline solution for the past week and has not added fresh saline solution. He also has not cleaned his storage container since purchasing it.

Although questions about the patient's medical history reveal no history of prior ocular problems, a history of hayfever and sensitivity to thimerosal is revealed; his family history is noncontributory. In addition to contact lens products, ED's medication use includes hydrochlorothiazide 25 mg once daily and nonprescription chlorpheniramine 4 mg q6h prn. He smokes one pack of cigarettes a day and is a social drinker.

Clinical Considerations/Strategies

The following considerations/strategies are provided to aid the reader in (1) determining whether treatment of the patient's condition with nonprescription medications is warranted, (2) selecting the appropriate nonprescription medication, and (3) developing a patient counseling strategy to ensure optimal therapeutic outcomes:

- Assess the contact lens care regimen. Call the lens prescriber to determine an appropriate care regimen and to discuss suggested changes in the regimen.
- Assess the patient's history of lens wear along with symptomatology, allergy history, and medication history.
- Develop a patient education/counseling strategy that will:
  - □ Design a lens care regimen that is optimal for compliance and ease of use;
  - □ Justify changes in the care regimen;
  - □ Optimize proper use of new product(s) added to the regimen;
  - □ Reinforce proper principles of lens care (eg, never reusing solutions, cleaning lens storage cases frequently);
  - □ Educate the patient about contact lens wear, symptoms of lens problems, and drug-lens interactions;
  - □ Encourage the patient to quit smoking.

References

1. MacKeen DL. Contact lens solutions. *Am Pharm.* 1986 Oct; NS26: 691–6.
2. Feldman GL. Contact lens materials. *Int Ophthalmol Clin.* 1981 Summer; 21: 155–62.
3. Holden BA, Mertz GW. Critical oxygen levels to avoid corneal edema for daily and extended wear contact lenses. *Invest Ophthalmol Vis Sci.* 1984; 25: 1161–7.
4. Hayworth NA, Asbell PA. Therapeutic contact lenses. *CLAO J.* 1990 Apr; 16: 137–42.
5. Yamaguchi T et al. Fungus growth on soft contact lenses with different water contents. *CLAO J.* 1984; 10: 166–71.
6. Levy B. Current trends in contact lens care. *Ophthalmol Clin North Am.* 1993; 6: 531–41.
7. Barr J. 1993: the year of both innovation and frustration. *Contact Lens Spectrum.* 1994; 29(1): 19–24.
8. Lembach RG. Rigid gas permeable contact lenses. *CLAO J.* 1990 Apr; 16: 129–34.
9. Callender MG. Contact lenses and care systems. *Pharm Pract.* 1990 Mar; 6: 26–45.
10. Weinstock FJ, Zucker JL. Extended-wear cosmetic contact lenses. *Int Ophthalmol Clin.* 1991 Spring; 31: 25–33.
11. Schein OD et al. The relative risk of ulcerative keratitis among users of daily-wear and extended-wear soft contact lenses. *N Engl J Med.* 1989 Sep; 321: 773–8.
12. Kershner RM. Infectious corneal ulcerations with over-extended wear of disposable contact lenses. *JAMA.* 1989 Jun; 261: 3549–50.
13. Krezanoski JZ. Topical medications. *Int Ophthalmol Clin.* 1981 Summer; 21: 173–6.
14. Lembach RG. Keratoconus. *Int Ophthalmol Clin.* 1991 Spring; 31: 71–82.
15. Stein HA. Contact lenses in the management of presbyopia. *Int Ophthamol Clin.* 1991 Spring; 31: 61–70.
16. Stein HA. The management of presbyopia with contact lenses: a review. *CLAO J.* 1990 Jan; 16: 33–8.
17. Freeman MI. Patient selection. *Int Ophthalmol Clin.* 1991 Spring; 31: 1–12.
18. Kastl PR. Is the quality of vision with contact lenses adequate? Not in all instances. *Cornea.* 1990; 9(suppl 1): S20–2.
19. Pepose JS. Contact lens disinfection to prevent transmission of viral disease. *CLAO J.* 1988 Jul; 14: 165–8.
20. Macsai MS et al. Deposition of ciprofloxacin, prednisolone phosphate, and prednisolone acetate in SeeQuence disposable contact lenses. *CLAO J.* 1993 Jul; 19: 166–8.
21. Lee BL et al. The solubility of antibiotic and corticosteroid combinations. *Am J Ophthalmol.* 1992; 114: 212–5.
22. Plotnik RD, Mannis MJ, Schwab IR. Therapeutic contact lenses. *Int Ophthalmol Clin.* 1991 Spring; 31: 35–52.
23. Diamond SA, Dupuis LL. Contact lens damage due to ribavirin exposure. *DICP, Ann Pharmacother.* 1989 May; 23: 428–9.
24. Rodriguez WJ et al. Environmental exposure of primary care personnel to ribavirin aerosol when supervising treatment of infants with respiratory syncytial virus infections. *Antimicrob Agents Chemother.* 1987 Jul; 31: 1143–6.

25. Broich J, Weiss L, Rapp J. Isolation and identification of biologically active contaminants from soft contact lenses. *Invest Ophthalmol Vis Sci.* 1980; 19: 1328–35.
26. Miller D. Systemic medications. *Int Ophthalmol Clin.* 1981 Summer; 21: 177–83.
27. Koetting RA. Cosmetics. *Int Ophthalmol Clin.* 1981 Summer; 21: 185–93.
28. Mandell RB, Respicio SG. Efficacy of contaminant removal by RGP lens cleaners. *Contact Lens Spectrum.* 1988 Jun; 3: 57–60.
29. White PF, Miller D. Corneal edema. *Int Ophthalmol Clin.* 1981 Summer; 21: 3–12.
30. Rakow PL. Mixing contact lens solutions. *J Ophthalmic Nurs Technol.* 1989; 8(2): 67–8.
31. Eriksen S, Dabezies OH. Preservatives. In: Dabezies OH, ed. *Contact Lenses, The CLAO Guide to Basic Science and Clinical Practice.* 2nd ed. Boston: Little, Brown and Co; 1992: 28.1–8.
32. Lowther G, Shannon BJ, Weisbarth R, eds. Contact lens care products and their use. In: *The Pharmacist's Guide to Contact Lenses and Lens Care.* Atlanta: CIBA Vision; 1988: 27–36.
33. Tripathi RC, Tripathi BJ. Lens spoilage. In: Dabezies OH, ed. *Contact Lenses, The CLAO Guide to Basic Science and Clinical Practice.* 2nd ed. Boston: Little, Brown and Co; 1992: 45.1–33.
34. Diefenbach CB, Seibert CK, Davis LJ. Analysis of two home remedy contact lens cleaners. *J Am Optom Assoc.* 1988; 59(7): 518–21.
35. Butrus SI, Abelson MB. Contact lenses and the allergic patient. *Int Ophthalmol Clin.* 1986 Spring; 26: 73–81.
36. Terry R, Schnider C, Holden BA. Rigid gas permeable lenses and patient management. *CLAO J.* 1989 Oct; 14: 305–9.
37. Mobley CL. Letter. *Contact Lens Forum.* 1989 Apr; 14(suppl 4): 13–4.
38. Stenson S. Soft contact lens deposits. *JAMA.* 1987 May; 257: 2823.
39. Tripathi BJ, Tripathi RC, Rhee JM. Adherence of bacteria to soft contact lenses. In: Dabezies OH, ed. *Contact Lenses, The CLAO Guide to Basic Science and Clinical Practice.* 2nd ed. Boston: Little, Brown and Co; 1992: 42.1–17.
40. Morgan JP. Problems associated with current care systems for contact lens. Paper presented at Las Vegas: CLAO annual meeting; January 1990.
41. Wittman G. Personal communication of data on file at company. Irvine, Calif: Allergan, Inc; January 17, 1995.
42. Harris MG. Practical considerations in the use of hydrogen peroxide disinfection systems. *CLAO J.* 1990 Jan; 16(suppl 1): S53–60.
43. Fiscella RG. New eye infection: difficult to detect, easier to prevent. *US Pharm.* 1989 Apr; 14: 75–81.
44. Lowther G, Shannon BJ, Weisbarth R, eds. The importance of compliance. In: *The Pharmacist's Guide to Contact Lenses and Lens Care.* Atlanta: CIBA Vision; 1988: 23–5.
45. Campbell RC, Caroline PJ. RGPs and tap water. *Contact Lens Forum.* 1990 Jul; 15: 64.
46. Key JE, Bennett ES. Rigid gas-permeable extended wear contact lenses. In: Kastl PR, ed. *Contact Lenses, The CLAO Guide to Basic Science and Clinical Practice.* 3rd ed. Dubuque, Iowa: Kendall/Hunt Publishing; 1995; II: 51–74.
47. Krezanoski JZ, Dabezies OH. Hard lens hygiene. In: Dabezies OH, ed. *Contact Lenses, The CLAO Guide to Basic Science and Clinical Practice.* 2nd ed. Boston: Little, Brown and Co; 1992: 31.1–7.
48. Driebe WT. Contact lens cleaning and disinfection. In: Kastl PR, ed. *Contact Lenses, The CLAO Guide to Basic Science and Clinical Practice.* 3rd ed. Dubuque, Iowa: Kendall/Hunt Publishing; 1995; II: 237–62.
49. *Boston Equalens Patient Care Guide.* Polymer Technology Corporation; 1987.
50. Callender MG. Contact lens care systems: part 1. hard and gas permeable lenses. *Pharm Pract.* 1990 Mar; 6: 26–31.
51. Hamacher DP. Contact lens solutions. *NARD J.* 1992 Mar; 114: 55–6.

CHAPTER 24

Otic Products

Keith O. Miller

Questions to ask in patient assessment and counseling

Earache

- *Do you have an earache? How long have you had it?*
- *Is the pain sharp and localized or dull and generalized?*
- *Is the pain constant or made worse by pulling on the ears or chewing?*
- *Do you have or have you recently had a cold or the flu?*
- *Do you have a fever?*
- *Have you been swimming during the past few days?*
- *Have you attempted to clear your ears recently to remove earwax? If so, what method did you use?*
- *Are your ear canals dry and flaky or wet and sticky?*
- *Have you had similar symptoms in the past? If so, how long ago?*
- *What, if anything, have you already done to treat your earache?*
- *Do you wear dentures or have any dental problems?*
- *What is your occupation?*

Hearing Loss

- *When did you notice that your hearing is not as good as it used to be?*
- *Do you have a cold or the flu?*
- *Have you been swimming during the past few days?*
- *Are your eardrums damaged from a prior illness or injury?*
- *Have you been traveling in an airplane recently or been in any places where the air pressure has changed suddenly (eg, fast elevators)?*
- *Does anyone else in your family have a hearing loss?*
- *Do any of your relatives wear a hearing aid?*
- *Would you be interested in taking a 5-minute hearing test for your own information only?*
- *Are you taking any prescription medications, even for other medical problems?*
- *Have you been hospitalized recently? If so, why?*

Tinnitus

- *Are the abnormal sounds you are sensing continuous or intermittent?*
- *Are you taking aspirin or any prescription or nonprescription medications? If so, what doses are you consuming?*

Discharge

- *Could you describe the appearance and the amount of discharge from your ear(s)?*
- *Was your ear itchy before the discharge appeared?*
- *Did you have any ear pain after the discharge appeared? Before the discharge started?*
- *Have you taken oral analgesics (eg, aspirin) or pain-relieving eardrops, or have you tried to rinse out the ear?*
- *Do you have diabetes or any other medical condition?*
- *Do you have a problem with dandruff?*

Disorders of the ear are very common and usually cause discomfort. Patients often complain of earache, impacted ear, running ear, cold in the ear, itching in the ear, or a combination of these symptoms. Ear disorders may be caused by a disease of the auricle (most external portion of the ear), external ear canal (external auditory meatus), or middle ear, or by a disease in another area of the head and neck. A traumatic or pathologic condition of the tongue, mandibles, oropharynx, tonsils, or paranasal sinuses may cause referred pain to the ear and may appear to the patient as an earache. These conditions are often caused by an underlying disease process that requires accurate diagnosis and treatment by a physician. In such cases, self-treatment may be unwise.

Home remedies and nonprescription drugs are usually restricted to self-limited disorders that are related only to the external ear. In such cases, self-treatment may be used effectively to aid the normal body defenses and to improve the integrity of the skin that lines the auricle and external auditory canal. However, self-treatment should be reserved for minor conditions.

Before recommending any nonprescription product to persons with ear disorders, the pharmacist should recognize the symptoms of the various disorders and their corresponding pathophysiology. This information will permit an accurate evaluation of the problem and assist the pharmacist in recommending treatment plans.

Anatomy and Physiology of the Ear

The external ear is composed of the auricle (pinna) and the external auditory canal (Figure 1). The auricle is the external appendage of cartilage (elastic type); it is covered by a thin layer of normal skin that is highly vascularized except for the lobule, which is composed primarily of fatty tissue. The skin covering the ear is thinner than skin elsewhere on the body because it lacks a protective layer of fat. The absence of this subcutaneous tissue makes the auricular skin subject to frostbite despite the rich supply of superficial blood vessels.[1,2] The auricle, which is oval, flattened, and irregular, is considered an extension of the cartilaginous ear canal. The cartilaginous projection anterior to the external opening of the ear (not shown in Figure 1) is called the tragus.

A thin tissue layer called the perichondrium covers both the cartilaginous auricle and the outer cartilaginous half of the external auditory canal.[1] The periosteum, a specialized connective tissue, covers the inner bony half of the external auditory canal.[1] The external auditory canal is tubular, forming a channel that permits sound waves to pass to the tympanic membrane (eardrum) and protects the tympanic membrane from injury. In adults, the external auditory canal is approximately 24 mm long.[2] Both the auricle and the external auditory canal show much individual variation in size and shape. The ear canal is the only epidermal-lined cul-de-sac in the body.

The auricular skin is continuous and lines the entire ear canal and the outer covering of the tympanic membrane.[1] The skin covering the cartilaginous portion of the canal, which is thicker than the skin covering the bony portion, contains hair follicles, large sebaceous glands that open either to the skin surface or into the hair follicle lumen, and ceruminous glands.[2] Hair appears to serve a protective function, with its ability to trap foreign bodies in a waxy network. No hair follicles or glands are found in the bony inner half of the external auditory canal.

Cerumen (earwax) is derived from the watery secretions of the apocrine glands (which mature and become functional at puberty) and the oily secretions of the sebaceous glands.[1] Collectively, these glands are referred to as ceruminous glands. Ceruminous glands are functional throughout life; however, older individuals may have fewer of them because the glands atrophy. Cerumen turns brown when it mixes with desquamated epithelial cells and dust particles. Cerumen lubricates the skin and traps foreign material entering the external auditory canal, thus providing a protective barrier.[2] Semisolid cerumen is expelled unnoticed by epithelial migration. This migration involves movement of epithelial cells across the surface of the tympanic membrane and the epithelial lining of the external auditory canal to the outside during the processes of chewing and talking.[2] The skin of the normal external auditory canal is water-resistant with a pH between 5.0 and 7.2, which helps prevent pathologic bacterial growth.[1,3,4]

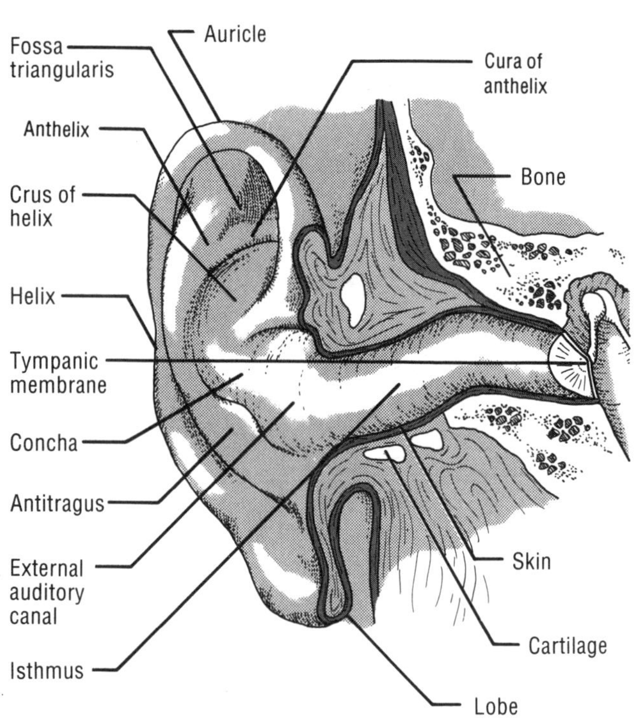

FIGURE 1 Anatomy of the auricle and external ear.

The tympanic membrane is pearly gray, egg shaped, semitransparent, about 0.1 mm thick, and 8–9 mm wide.[2] The outer epithelial layer is continuous with the epidermis of the external auditory canal; the middle layer is tough, fibrous tissue; and the innermost layer is a mucous membrane continuous with the tympanic cavity lining.[3] In adults, the membrane forms approximately a 45-degree angle with the external canal floor; it is almost horizontal in infants. It protects the middle ear from foreign material and also functions in transmitting airborne sound waves into the middle ear. Anatomically, the tympanic membrane is part of the external auditory canal (Figure 1); functionally, however, it is considered part of the middle ear (tympanic cavity).

Etiology of Ear Conditions

Hairs in the outer half of the canal, the size of the ear canal and its isthmus, and cerumen act as natural defensive barriers of the normal ear canal, collectively preventing the introduction of foreign material that may

TABLE 1 Symptoms of selected otic disorders

	Boil	Otomycosis	Bacterial external otitis	Nonsuppurative otitis media	Impacted cerumen	Suppurative otitis media
Pain[a]	Often	Possibly	Often	Rarely	Rarely	Usually
Hearing deficit	Rarely	Possibly	Possibly	Possibly	Often	Usually
Purulent discharge	Rarely	Rarely	Often	Rarely	Rarely	Occasionally and indicative of perforation
Bilateral symptoms	Rarely	Rarely	Possibly	Often	Rarely	Occasionally
Appropriateness of self-medication	Auricle only	Never	Never	Never	Never	Never

[a]Pain is increased with chewing, traction on the auricle, and pressure on the tragus except in otitis media, where pain may be knifelike and steady.

cause injury or infection. The integrity of the skin layers and the acid pH of the canal also provide natural protection against infection.

Predisposing factors often lead to the breakdown of these natural defense barriers. An inherited narrowed ear canal, a malformation of the mandible, or excessive hair growth in the canal may impair the normal cleansing process and decrease the efficiency of epithelial migration. In addition, hyperactive ceruminous glands may cause excessive wax to accumulate and become impacted. African Americans tend to have shorter and straighter ear canals, and thus they develop external otitis less often than non-African Americans.[5]

Certain conditions and activities also contribute to the breakdown of natural defensive barriers of the normal ear canal. Intensely warm, humid climates, along with sweating and exposure to water (swimming and bathing during the summer months), have been implicated. Increased exposure to moisture may result in tissue maceration that breaks down the protective barrier of the skin and alters skin pH. Collectively, these factors predispose the ear canal to infection.[1,4] A positive correlation exists between the amount of water exposure in the ear canal and the incidence of external otitis.[5]

Ear disorders may also be due to various trauma-induced causes. Improperly cleaned or poorly fitted earplugs may cause trauma or maceration of the skin in the ear canal. Poorly fitted hearing aids or ear molds of hearing aids may be another source of trauma-induced injury.[4]

The removal of cerumen or the lack of natural protection provided by its presence may increase the predisposition for bacterial or fungal infection in the ear canal. Using an instrument, a cotton-tipped applicator, or other device to clean ears is likely to push the earwax deeper into the ear canal, causing it to become tightly impacted and increasing the difficulty of subsequent removal. This cleaning process also often causes trauma to the skin covering the ear canal, further predisposing the ear to infection.

After the protective layer of the skin of the ear canal has been compromised, a preinflammatory stage occurs in which the patient tends to scratch the ear involuntarily or rub the auricle in response to an itch. These actions further abrade the skin, causing deep fissures in the epidermis of the cartilaginous portion of the ear canal. An inflammatory reaction follows this fissure formation, as evidenced by edema, pain, swelling, and redness of the affected area. This large area thus becomes a good culture site for bacteria or fungi, making subsequent infection likely.

Neurodermatitis is a condition that is presumably caused by chronic rubbing, scratching, or cleaning the ear in response to a vague itch or feeling of fullness that sometimes occurs. The itch sensation may also be characteristic of superficial fungal infection, contact dermatitis, or eczema.[1,6] Some individuals produce a scant amount of cerumen and may be subject to itching, maceration, and subsequent infection.[3]

Common Problems of the Ear

Many disorders of the external ear are minor and easily resolved. However, the pharmacist should keep in mind that pain associated with minor disorders can be significant. Some untreated ear problems can result in hearing loss. The pharmacist can assist the patient by assessing the symptoms (Table 1), discussing the proper course of action (self-treatment or referral to a physician), and recommending a nonprescription product, when appropriate.

Disorders of the Auricle

Disorders associated with the auricle, the external part of the ear, are generally minor and self-limiting. They

TABLE 2 Interpretation of physical findings associated with disorders of the external ear

Physical findings	Probable appearance	Physiologic basis	Example
Enlarged lymph node	Swollen, tender to touch, pre- and postauricular	Inflammation of lymph node; spread of infection outside the ear	Mastoiditis, otitis media
Tophus	Hard, pale node on helix, chalklike dust upon rupture	Urate crystals	Gout
Sebaceous cyst	Swollen, erythematous postauricle lesion in the skin of the ear	Inflammation of sweat gland	Skin infection
Cerumen	Red-orange pastelike discharge	Normal secretion of wax	Normal finding
Blood	Red-blue discharge	Ruptured blood vessel	External otitis
Serous fluid	Clear discharge	Blocked eustachian tube	Chronic (purulent) otitis media
Pus	Yellowish discharge	Acute inflammation	Acute suppurative otitis media

Adapted with permission from Longe RL, Calvert JC. *Drug Intell Clin Pharm*. 1977; 11: 660.

often involve lacerations, boils, and dermatitis. Table 2 provides examples of some common physical findings related to disorders of the external ear.

Trauma

Lacerations, including scrapes and cuts involving only the skin of the auricle, usually heal spontaneously. Wounds that do not heal normally should be checked by a physician, as should deep wounds that may involve injury to the cartilage. Injury to the auricle that does not perforate the subperichondrium may cause subcutaneous bleeding and produce a hematoma. A hematoma may require aspiration or incision by a physician because it may obliterate normal auricular contours and often results in inflammation and perichondritis (cauliflower ear). The swelling can also cause local pruritus and pain upon touch.

Boils

Boils (furuncles) are usually localized infections of the hair follicles. In a high percentage of cases in young adults, no specific causative or predisposing factor can be established. Poor body hygiene may contribute to the development of boils. The etiologic organism of a boil is usually a *Staphylococcus* species.[2]

A boil often involves the anterior portion of the external auditory canal. It usually begins as a red papule and develops into a round or conical superficial pustule with a core of pus and erythema around the base. The lesion gradually enlarges, becomes firm, and then generally softens and opens within 2 weeks, discharging the purulent contents. Because the skin is very taut, even minimal swelling may cause severe pain.

Boils are usually self-limiting; however, they may be severe, autoinoculable, and multiple. Deeper lesions may lead to perichondritis.

Perichondritis

Perichondritis is an inflammation involving the perichondrium (the fibrous connective tissue surrounding the auricular cartilage) usually following a poorly treated or untreated burn, injury, hematoma, or local infection. Its onset is characterized by a sensation of heat and stiffness of the auricle with pronounced pain. As the condition worsens, an exudate forms and the auricle becomes dark red, swollen, and shiny, with uniform thickening caused by edema and inflammation. The lesions are usually confined to the cartilaginous tissue of the auricle and external canal, but some patients may experience generalized fever and malaise.

Perichondritis often results in severe auricular deformity, and atresia (a pathologic closure) of the external auditory canal may occur. A patient suspected of having perichondritis should be seen by a physician.

Dermatitis of the Ear

Inflammation of the skin may result from an abrasion of the auricle; if untreated, a dermal infection may develop. Inflammatory conditions such as seborrhea, psoriasis, and contact dermatitis (eg, poison ivy and poison oak) may also affect the skin of the auricle and the external ear canal. Contact dermatitis may be caused by an allergic response to jewelry, cosmetics, detergents, or topical drug applications of antihistamines or antibiotics (dermatitis medicamentosa).[3,7,8] Dermatitis lesions may spread from ear molds. Methyl methacrylate, a component of ear molds, has been reported to be an offender.[9]

Dry, scaly skin associated with an itchy ear canal suggests the presence of seborrheic dermatitis, especially in the presence of severe dandruff and other signs of seborrhea.[1] Symptoms of dermatitis of the ear usually include itching and local redness followed by vesication, weeping, and erythema. The lesions, which form scales and yellow crusts on the skin,[3,6] may spread to adjacent unaffected areas. Excessive scratching may cause the lesions to become infected. Topical drugs should be used cautiously in treating dermatitis because their potential allergenicity could exacerbate the condition. Because seborrheic dermatitis of the ear is usually associated with dandruff, treatment of the scalp with dandruff-control shampoos is recommended. Cases that are difficult to control should be referred to a physician.

Itching or Pruritus of the Ear

Itching commonly begins as an annoying itch-scratch cycle that results in trauma, infection, epidermal barrier destruction, and inflammation of the affected areas following repeated scratching. Ear scratching may be a compulsive nervous habit.[1] Careful observation to determine the cause of itching is often helpful before any attempt is made to provide symptomatic relief.

An itchy ear canal is a common symptom that may mask the preinflammatory stages of acute external otitis. Itching can be related to dryness but may be a complaint when no abnormalities or lesions actually exist.[4] For patients with chronic external otitis, the chief complaint is itching[2] caused by dry ears that may lack sufficient cerumen, a circumstance that is more common in older individuals owing to atrophy of cerumen glands.[4] Itching may also be caused by infections, allergic seborrheic dermatitis, eczema of the skin around the ears, psoriasis, contact dermatitis, superficial fungal infection, or neurodermatitis.[1]

Aural Drainage

Excess water and fluids in the external auditory canal may cause a feeling of fullness in the ear. Fluid can be removed by having the patient tilt the head to one side with the affected ear down. This position allows the excess fluid to drain out of the ear by gravity. To permit direct visual examination of the tympanic membrane, it may be necessary to straighten the canal by applying traction to the auricle in an upward and backward direction.

Any patient with a discharge or drainage from the ear should be referred to a physician for proper diagnosis and treatment. The drainage or discharge may be blood, watery fluid (serum), or purulent or mucoid material. Head trauma may cause leakage of cerebrospinal fluid into the ear. Infection of the external ear canal may produce a watery discharge. A ruptured tympanic membrane usually produces a serosanguineous fluid. Any trauma of the ear canal may cause bleeding; and, if infected, the ear may exude a purulent fluid from which the causative organisms may be cultured and appropriate antibiotics chosen.

Self-treatment of ear disorders is inappropriate whenever drainage, pain, or dizziness are present; whenever an infection is suspected; whenever there is known injury in or perforation of the eardrum; or within 6 weeks following otic surgery.[10,11]

Disorders of the External Auditory Canal

Boils

Symptoms induced by boils include pain at the infected site, which is usually exacerbated by chewing. The ear canal may be partially occluded by swelling, but hearing is impaired only if the opening is completely occluded. Edema and pain over the mastoid bone directly behind the auricle may occur. Traction of the auricle or the tragus is very painful. Patients with boils in the external auditory canal should be referred to a physician because unresolved conditions may lead to more generalized infections.

Otomycosis

Otomycosis, an external fungal infection of the ear, is more common in warmer, tropical, or semitropical climates than in mild, temperate zones. Species of *Aspergillus* and *Candida* are the most common causative agents.[1,2] *Aspergillus niger* forms characteristic black growth in the canal.[2] Antibiotic treatment of a bacterial ear infection with resultant suppression of normal bacterial flora, immunosuppression (drugs, disease), and diabetes mellitus may predispose an individual to a fungal external ear infection.

A superficial mycotic infection of the external auditory canal is characterized by pruritus accompanied by a feeling of fullness and pressure in the ear. Intense itching is the primary complaint of patients with otomycosis.[2] Pain, if present, may increase with chewing and with traction on the pinna and tragus. The fungus leads to an accumulation of epithelial debris, exudate, and cerumen. In the acute state, the fungal infection may obstruct the external auditory canal, and hearing may be impaired.

Depending on the nature of the fungus, the color of the accumulated mass may vary. The skin that lines the external auditory canal and the tympanic membrane may become beefy red and scaly. A musty-smelling discharge may be present.[3] The skin may be eroded or ulcerated with the fungus filaments.

Otomycosis is particularly serious in diabetic patients because of the microangiopathy and associated cutaneous manifestations common to diabetes mellitus. Mycotic ear infections in diabetic patients should be treated promptly.

Keratosis Obturans

Keratosis obturans is a rare condition with an unclear etiology.[1] Wax accumulates in the deeper parts of the external auditory canal and, with adjacent epithelial cells, leads to an obstruction that exerts pressure on the surrounding tissue. The condition is probably related to faulty migration of squamous epithelial cells from the surface of the tympanic membrane. Pain may be present owing to erosion of the epithelial tissue surrounding the tympanic membrane.[1] The infection may form abscesses in the subcutaneous tissue or mastoid bone.

Pain in the ear and decreased hearing are common symptoms. A discharge and tinnitus may also occur. Mechanical removal of the obstruction is necessary but often difficult and should be performed by a physician—preferably an ear, nose, and throat specialist. Patients should not attempt to remove the obstruction themselves.

Impacted Cerumen

The accumulation of cerumen in the external auditory canal may be caused by (1) overactive ceruminous glands; (2) a tortuous or small canal or an abnormal narrowing of the canal, which may not permit normal migration of the cerumen to the outside; or (3) the secretion of abnormal cerumen, which may be drier or softer than normal cerumen and may interfere with the normal epithelial migration process. Individuals who get water in their ears while swimming or showering sometimes will experience a sudden loss of hearing in one ear. This may be caused by the increased bulk of the earwax or by water trapped behind the wax.[2] Cerumen is often packed deeper into the external auditory canal by repeated attempts to remove it with cotton-tipped devices and other instruments; ordinarily there is no pain unless the ear is secondarily infected.[2] There is usually no cerumen in the inner half of the canal unless it has been pushed there. In elderly persons, cerumen is often admixed with long hairs in the canal, forming a matted obstruction in the canal and preventing the natural removal of cerumen.

Foreign Objects in the Ear

Young children often insert small items into the ear canal; such items include candy, pretzel sticks, pencil erasers, toy stuffing, beans, peas, marbles, pebbles, beads, or metal nuts unscrewed from toys.[12] An object lodged in the ear canal will usually cause a hearing deficiency, pain, or pressure in the ear during chewing. An exudate may form because of secondary bacterial infection. Vegetable seeds (eg, dried beans or dried peas) lodged in the external auditory canal swell when moistened during bathing or swimming and become wedged in the bony portion of the canal, causing severe pain. Furthermore, if an obstruction of the external auditory canal is not removed promptly, acute bacterial otitis may result. Insects enter the canal and cause stress by beating their wings and crawling. In such a case, olive oil (sweet oil) drops or mineral oil may be used to suffocate the insect and stop the movement.

Foreign objects lodged in the ear canal may not always cause symptoms and may be found only during a routine physical examination. Mechanical removal should be performed only by a physician because unskilled attempts at removal often damage the skin surrounding the external auditory canal or lodge the objects deeper into the ear canal.

External Otitis

External otitis (inflammation of the skin lining the external auditory canal, often due to infection) is one of the most common diseases of the ear. It is also very painful and annoying. The external auditory canal is considered a blind cul-de-sac lined with skin. It is dark, warm, and well suited for collecting moisture. Prolonged exposure to moisture tends to disrupt the continuity of the epithelial cells, causing skin maceration and fissures that provide a fertile environment for bacterial growth. It also tends to raise the pH above the normal range of 5–7,[12] which improves the growth environment for bacteria and fungi. Factors contributing to susceptibility to external otitis are race, age, climate, and occupation.[9] The most common causative organisms of external otitis include species of *Pseudomonas, Staphylococcus, Bacillus,* and *Proteus*. Fungi may be the causative organisms in some cases.[2]

A bacterial infection of the external auditory canal leads to inflammation and epidermal destruction of the tympanic membrane. The infection may progress through the fibrous layer of the tympanic membrane, perforating the membrane and spreading the infection into the middle ear; this results in intense pain and discomfort. External otitis caused by bacterial infection, like otomycosis, is particularly difficult to control in individuals who have diabetes.[1,13]

There is very little subcutaneous tissue between the skin that is tightly bound to the perichondrium on the cartilaginous portion and the periosteum on the bony portion of the external auditory canal. When there is swelling, the lack of space available for expansion increases skin tension. Thus, the inflammation that causes edema provokes severe pain that is disproportionate to any visible swelling. As the inflammation increases, pain may increase significantly during chewing.

Symptoms often develop following attempts to clean the ear with cotton swabs, hairpins, matchsticks, pencils, fingers, or other objects. Symptoms may also be caused by foreign debris or scratching of the ear to relieve itching. This may traumatize and damage the horny skin layer, forming an opening that allows invasion by microorganisms. Because a normal, healthy, external auditory canal is impervious to potentially pathologic organisms, skin integrity generally must be interrupted before an organism can produce an infection.

Swimmer's Ear Another type of trauma-induced external otitis is called swimmer's ear, or desquamative external otitis. Heat, humidity, and moisture cause the stratum corneum of the skin to swell, which may block the follicular glands. Introduction of extraneous moisture or water during swimming or bathing increases the maceration of the skin lining the ear canal and sets up a condition favorable for bacterial growth.[3] The accumulation of water in the tympanic recess may contribute to the tissue maceration, possibly predisposing the ear canal to infection. Attempts to clear the canal of water with objects that can abrade or lacerate the skin lining may result in infection. Also, cerumen accumulated in the external auditory canal absorbs water and expands, and the trapped water provides a medium for bacterial growth. Within a few hours to 1 day following exposure to excess moisture, symptoms of itching, pain, and possible draining from the ear may occur, with swelling causing partial occlusion.

Often the initial symptoms include itching in the ear followed by a feeling of wetness in the ear canal and discomfort leading to pain. The amount of wetness may vary from minimal to frank discharge. The discharge is often cream colored or yellow. A hearing loss, if present, may be caused by epithelial debris mixed with purulent discharge, which causes blockage.

Acute External Otitis Symptoms of acute external otitis are related to the severity of the pathologic conditions. There is usually mild or moderate pain, which becomes more pronounced by pulling upward on the auricle or pressing on the tragus. A discharge may be present. Hearing loss may occur if the ear canal is obstructed by swelling and edema, debris, or a cerumen plug.

TABLE 3 Physical findings associated with selected conditions of the middle ear

Physical findings	Probable appearance	Interpretation
Perforation	Dark, thin, oval discoloration	Rupture of the eardrum
Acute purulent otitis media	Yellowish pus behind eardrum; bulging, hyperemic membrane; light reflex absent	Acute infection of the middle ear
Chronic serous otitis media	Amberlike fluid behind eardrum; observable fluid level with air bubbles; retraction of handle of malleus	Blockage of eustachian tube

Reprinted with permission from Longe RL, Calvert JC. *Drug Intell Clin Pharm*. 1977; 11: 661.

Allergic External Otitis/Dermatitis of the External Auditory Canal In allergic external otitis and dermatitis of the external auditory canal caused by seborrhea, a common symptom is itching, burning, or stinging of the lesions. Often the complaints seem excessive compared with the visible signs.

Chronic External Otitis Chronic external otitis is usually caused by the persistence of predisposing factors. Many cases are of fungal origin and occur in individuals whose ear canals are exposed to excessive moisture.[6] The most common symptom is itching, which prompts patients to attempt to scratch the ear canal for relief. However, scratching can break the skin,[10] thereby allowing the entry of the pathogen(s).

Chronic cases, especially those with symptoms of severe pain, lymphadenopathy, discharge, possible hearing loss, and fever, should be referred to a physician. Tender lymph nodes may be felt anterior to the tragus, behind the ear, or in the upper neck just below the pinna. Progressive symptoms of disease processes involving the external ear canal or auricle should be treated by a physician.

Malignant External Otitis Malignant external otitis is the most progressive form of otitis. It occurs most often in elderly patients and in patients with chronic lymphocytic leukemia, granulocytopenia, or poorly controlled diabetes mellitus.[14,15] In these patients, the ear becomes inflamed and may involve the temporal bone area. The most common complaints are severe, persistent pain and swelling. Clinical findings include persistent aural drainage, severe tenderness, and swelling in the region of the ear and mastoid bone. The tragus is always tender to touch and the auricle is tender to traction.

Disorders of the Middle Ear

Disorders of the middle ear should not be treated with nonprescription otic products. Although some symptoms of middle ear disorders are the same as those of external ear disorders, others are not (Table 3). All bacterial infections of the middle ear should be promptly evaluated and treated by a physician. The usual treatment is systemic antibiotic therapy. A brief review of the common conditions involving the middle ear will aid the pharmacist in evaluating symptoms.

Otitis Media

Otitis media is an inflammatory condition of the middle ear that occurs most often during childhood. Conditions that interfere with eustachian tube function, such as upper respiratory tract infection, allergy, adenoid lymphadenopathy, and cleft palate, predispose individuals to otitis media.[1] Blockage of the eustachian tube allows oxygen in the middle ear cleft to be absorbed. This produces a relative negative pressure or vacuum that results in a transudation (movement) of fluid into the middle ear cleft. Generally, symptoms of eustachian tube blockage are mild intermittent pain, mild hearing loss, and fullness in the ear. If infection is absent, the color of the tympanic membrane, when retracted, is pearly gray. Inflation of the eustachian tube by Valsalva's maneuver (blowing against pressure) or by swallowing may help send air up the eustachian tube. The tube should not be inflated when the nasopharynx is infected because of the danger of spreading the infection into the middle ear.

Children often experience repeated episodes of eustachian tube obstruction, which are caused by masses of adenoids that become edematous and block the eustachian tube opening, resulting in otitis media. Adenoidectomy usually prevents future occurrence. In adults, recurrent otitis media may be caused by nasopharyngeal tumors.

Nose blowing and sneezing against occluded nostrils may worsen the condition and therefore should be avoided.[16,17] If the serous fluid in the middle ear cavity remains sterile, the condition is called serous otitis media and is most often of viral origin; if the fluid is infected by bacteria, the condition is generally called purulent or suppurative otitis media.

Serous Otitis Media Symptoms of serous otitis media include a sensation of fullness in the ear accompanied by hearing loss.[4] The condition worsens as fluid accumulates and fills the middle ear cleft. The sensation of fullness is associated with voice resonance, a congested feeling in the ears, a hollow sound, or a popping or cracking noise in the ears during swallowing or yawning. These symptoms are usually not present in external otitis.

Purulent (Suppurative) Otitis Media The most common symptoms in the acute phase of purulent otitis media are pain, hearing loss, fever as high as 104°F (40°C), and feeling ill. As noted by one author, "the strategic location of middle cleft and mastoid cells separated from the sigmoid sinus and meninges by a mere thin shell makes every infection of the middle ear capable of intracranial infection."[1] The severity of symptoms increases as the condition worsens. The pressure of fluids in the middle ear causes an outward tension on the tympanic membrane, which is innervated by sensory nerves. The rapid production of fluid and tension in a short period of time causes acute pain, which is described as sharp, knifelike, and steady. The pain usually does not worsen with mastication or with traction applied to the auricle or tragus. Excessive nose blowing, especially against occluded nostril(s), may force additional purulent mucus into the eustachian tube and worsen the condition. Nonprescription eardrops or prescription antibiotic drops do *not* help to resolve acute otitis media while the tympanic membrane is intact. The use of nonprescription otic drugs to treat any form of otitis media is not recommended.

Chronic Otitis Media

Chronic serous otitis media occurs most often in small children. It may be caused by inadequate treatment of previous episodes of otitis media or by recurrent upper respiratory tract infections associated with eustachian tube dysfunction.[3] Often, long-standing fluid becomes more and more viscous, which accounts for the term *glue ear*.[3]

The most common symptom is impaired hearing, but the onset is insidious. Children may have no acute symptoms,[3] and pain is usually absent. Frequently, parents may note that the child has become inattentive and disobedient, and the child's school performance may decline. Diagnosis requires visual inspection of the tympanic membrane, which appears yellow or orange, lusterless, and less flexible. The membrane is not perforated but often appears to be retracted.

Treatment may involve evacuation of the fluid by aspiration through an incision in the tympanic membrane (myringotomy) and implantation of temporary, pressure-equalizing tubes.[3]

Tympanic Membrane Perforation

The most common causes of traumatic perforation of the tympanic membrane are water sports, such as diving or waterskiing.[3] Any corrosive agent introduced into the ear canal may also perforate the tympanic membrane. Other causes of perforation include blows to the head with a cupped hand, foreign objects entering the ear canal with excessive force, and forceful irrigation of the ear canal. At the moment of injury the pain is severe, but it decreases rapidly. Hearing acuity usually diminishes quickly, and if the condition is untreated, it may lead to otitis media. Other complications may include tinnitus, nausea, and vertigo (disequilibrium). Any patient suspected of having an acute perforated tympanic membrane should be referred to a physician for examination.

Barotrauma (Acute Aero-Otitis Media)

Barotrauma occurs during a quick descent from high altitude.[6] The eustachian tube fails to ventilate, resulting in a negative pressure in the middle ear. This negative pressure causes a suction and forces the tympanic membrane to retract, causing pain. Barotrauma may occur in individuals who fly with an upper respiratory tract infection or with any condition associated with impaired eustachian tube ventilation. For such patients, pretreatment with antihistamines or decongestants may help to avoid serious symptoms during air travel. Treatment of acute episodes consists of oral decongestants, antihistamines, and autoinflation of the eustachian tube (Valsalva's maneuver).[1,18] Swallowing or blowing against pressure may assist in sending air up the eustachian tube, thereby helping to equalize the pressure on both sides of the tympanic membrane.

Hearing Disorders

Obstructive Hearing Loss

Accumulated cerumen is a common cause of hearing loss, especially in persons with overactive cerumen glands. The accumulated cerumen causes an obstruction and produces a feeling of fullness or diminished hearing. Hearing impairment may occur when cerumen occludes the canal, impairing the transmission of sound waves to the tympanic membrane. After the patient swims or bathes, water can be trapped in the ear canal behind the cerumen. The trapped water is absorbed by the cerumen, causing expansion of the cerumen to worsen occlusion and thus causing an acute hearing deficit. As discussed previously, temporary hearing impairment may also result from excessive edema, which, in combination with accumulated cerumen and debris, may occlude the canal. Impacted cerumen can be removed only by direct manipulation; the procedure should not be attempted by the patient or untrained persons.

Tinnitus

Tinnitus is defined as alien noise in the ear, which is subjective and audible only to the patient. It is described as sounding like steam escaping from a small pipe, ringing, roaring, pulsating, chirping (crickets), or humming. Tinnitus can be very annoying and may be constant or intermittent. The intensity of the disturbance varies from patient to patient, and patients' reactions may vary from minor distraction to severe mental depression.

Tinnitus can arise from a variety of causes involving the inner ear. It may be the result of blockage of the ear canal or of the eustachian tube and middle ear cavity, which is easily corrected following proper diagnosis. Tinnitus, which may be the first and only sign of a hearing disorder,[2] may be associated with hearing loss, exposure to high noise level, or acoustic trauma, or it may be a symptom of drug toxicity or systemic disease.[17] (Vertigo also may be of toxic origin, the result of intracranial or neurologic diseases, infection, hyperventilation, or severe ceruminal impaction.[19])

External otitis, serous otitis media, acute otitis media, and chronic otitis media seldom produce tinnitus as the sole or predominate complaint. Sometimes, when there are no other signs or symptoms, the cause of tinnitus can only be suspected.

Patients with tinnitus caused by such drugs as salicylates (arthritis patients), quinidine (heart patients), and quinine (malaria patients or patients using quinine to relieve leg cramps) usually will notice a decrease in the intensity of the tinnitus following discontinuation of the offending medication. Any patient who experiences tinnitus should receive a medical examination and evaluation. Nonprescription eardrops are not effective and are not recommended for the treatment of tinnitus.

Patient Assessment

To choose appropriately between recommending patient self-treatment and physician referral, as well as to make the proper product selection and to instruct the patient appropriately, the pharmacist must be able to assess the nature and severity of the patient's otic condition by evaluating overt signs and symptoms (Table 1). The most common complaints may include one or more of the following: localized pain, itchiness in the ear canal, a feeling of fullness, hearing loss, lymphadenopathy, fever, and malaise. The patient should always be referred to a physician if the symptoms include severe pain, lymphadenopathy, discharge from ear, possible hearing deficit, or fever.

The pharmacist should have the patient describe the symptoms and should ask whether the patient has experienced similar symptoms previously and, if so, when and how they were treated. Evaluation of the patient's present health status must also be based on information in the medical and drug history records, as well as on information concerning predisposing factors or conditions that may influence the patient's response to self-treatment, such as seborrheic dermatitis, psoriasis, eczema, allergies, and contact dermatitis, or the presence of chronic diseases that may impair healing, such as diabetes mellitus.

The skin of patients with diabetes mellitus is more prone to infection (bacterial and fungal), especially when the diabetes is poorly controlled. Infections in diabetic patients tend to resolve more slowly and to recur more often. The increased predisposition to infection of the ear canal may be related to impairment of the skin's integrity and abnormalities in immunologic responses. Ear infections, especially external otitis, are difficult to treat in diabetic patients. Rigid control of both diabetes and predisposing factors cannot be overemphasized.

Having assessed the severity of the otic disorder and recognized any potential or actual complications associated with the condition, the pharmacist may either provide appropriate nonprescription medication with instructions for proper use or refer the patient to a physician. Appropriately selected nonprescription drug products can be relied upon to provide a suitable therapeutic response in certain conditions. Adults with recurrent otitis who respond poorly to treatment should be examined by a physician. Health professionals (pharmacists, physicians, and nurses) properly trained to visualize the tympanic membrane and ear canal with a suitable otoscope and properly instructed in aural hygiene may, in most cases, perform irrigation safely with an ear syringe or a forced water spray.

Ear Pain

Pain in the ear, commonly identified by the patient as an earache, may be caused by various disorders. Careful inspection by trained personnel with proper instrumentation is often necessary to determine the etiology of the pain. External otitis, foreign material or cerumen packed against the tympanic membrane, and acute otitis media with its possible complications (eg, mastoiditis or abscesses) are all common causes. Pain may be referred to the ear from the sinuses, nasopharynx, tongue, hypopharynx, larynx, or temporomandibular joint. Loose-fitting dentures may also induce frank ear pain. In all such cases, the source of the pain should be determined and proper medical diagnosis should be made.

Pressure on the pinna or the tragus increases pain in external otitis,[4] although patients with otitis media rarely report increased pain in such cases. Chewing may also cause increased pain in patients with either external otitis or otitis media.

Before suggesting self-treatment of an external ear disorder, the pharmacist should rule out an earache caused by otitis media secondary to an upper respiratory tract infection. A history of pressure in, or referred pain to, the ear may be caused by a pathologic condition in the area around the ear. Recent injury or trauma to the head or neck regions may also cause referred pain to the ear. Trauma to the ear canal is to be avoided at all times.

Boils

The signs and symptoms of a boil in the ear canal include localized, burning pain that increases when the patient chews, when traction is applied to the auricle, and when the tragus is pressed medially. A red, inflamed, raised lesion can be seen in the ear canal. The skin around the affected area is intact, provided the patient has not attempted to scratch the boil. The patient's subjective hearing is also usually intact. If lymphadenopathy, fever, malaise, or severe pain is present, the patient should be referred to a physician for treatment.

Foreign Objects

The signs and symptoms typically produced by a foreign object in the external ear usually include a feeling of fullness with hearing loss from the affected ear. Pain may be present and may increase with chewing, traction on the auricle, and pressure applied to the tragus. Lymphadenopathy, fever, or malaise do not occur acutely but may develop later, and there may be a foul-smelling discharge from the affected ear. Collectively, these characteristics indicate a secondary ear infection that is typically of bacterial or fungal origin. All patients with foreign objects in the ear, with or without secondary infection, should be evaluated and treated by a physician as promptly as possible.

TABLE 4 Differential assessment of acute external otitis and acute otitis media

	Acute external otitis	Acute otitis media
Season	Summer	Winter
Movement of tragus painful	Yes	No
Ear canal	Swollen	Normal
Eardrum	Normal (or red)	Perforated or bulging
Discharge	Yes	Yes, but through a perforation
Nodes	Frequent	Less frequent
Fever	Yes	Yes
Hearing	Normal or decreased	Always decreased

Adapted with permission from DeWeese D et al. *Otolaryngology—Head and Neck Surgery*. 7th ed. St Louis: CV Mosby; 1988: 398.

External Otitis

The only means by which bacterial or fungal external otitis may be confirmed is by microbiologic culture. However, a culture is not always practical or necessary. Pain and swelling localized in the ear canal are usually the motivating symptoms that cause the patient to seek professional help (Table 4). A bacterial infection may be characterized by increased pain with chewing, traction applied to the auricle, and pressure applied medially on the tragus, as well as by a foul-smelling, mucopurulent discharge. Lymphadenopathy, a feeling of fullness, and fever and associated malaise may be additional characteristics of infection. Otoscopic examination may reveal a swollen, inflamed ear canal and an inflamed tympanic membrane. Patients with external otitis should be referred to a physician for thorough evaluation and treatment of the ear canal.

Hearing Loss

Hearing loss is a complaint that should be evaluated and diagnosed by a physician or audiologist. A 5-minute hearing test is sometimes useful to assess some patients with a suspected hearing deficit; it is not intended to be a test in sound discrimination (Table 5). Acute hearing loss without pain may be experienced and identified during an examination of the ear canal.

Patients with impacted cerumen without secondary complications may be treated safely with nonprescription cerumen-softening agents. Patients with hearing loss without pain, and whose tympanic membrane is visible and not obstructed, should be evaluated and treated by a physician. Such decreased hearing may be due to a perforated tympanic membrane. Usually the patient with this injury has experienced a sharp pain of short duration at the time of the injury. Treatment of a perforated tympanic membrane may include repair and medical therapy to prevent infection in the middle ear.

Otomycosis

Patients with otomycosis usually complain of itching and a feeling of fullness in the affected ear. The most common initial symptom of fungal external otitis is pruritus as opposed to the deep-seated pain and tenderness typically seen with predominately bacterial infections. Initially, the ear canal may reveal mild erythema and edema only. An established infection shows tender, red, and edematous tissue.[1] A colorless discharge may or may not be present. Pain is usually not present but may occur in severe cases. The pain increases with chewing, traction on the auricle, and pressure applied medially on the tragus. Systemic disturbances usually occur only in severe cases, which are often due to secondary bacterial infections with obstruction of the ear canal.

Otitis Media

The only conclusive means of diagnosing otitis media is via a complete patient history and physical examination using a pneumatic otoscope. Otitis media, which is most often caused by eustachian tube dysfunction, is common in children. Patients may be asymptomatic or may complain of occasional fullness and a cracking or hollow sound in the ears. There may be earache and fever, especially in children. The effect is usually bilateral.

TABLE 5 Five-minute hearing test

	Almost always	Half the time	Occasionally	Never
1. I have a problem hearing over the telephone.				
2. I have trouble following the conversation when two or more people are talking at the same time.				
3. People complain that I turn the television volume too high.				
4. I have to strain to understand conversations.				
5. I miss hearing some common sounds like the phone or doorbell ringing.				
6. I have trouble hearing conversations in a noisy background such as a party.				
7. I get confused about where sounds come from.				
8. I misunderstand some words in a sentence and need to ask people to repeat themselves.				
9. I especially have trouble understanding the speech of women and children.				
10. I have worked in noisy environments (on assembly lines, with jackhammers, around jet engines, etc).				
11. Many people I talk to seem to mumble (or do not speak clearly).				
12. People get annoyed because I misunderstand what they say.				
13. I misunderstand what others are saying and make inappropriate responses.				
14. I avoid social activities because I cannot hear well and feel I will reply improperly.				
To be answered by a family member or friend: 15. Do you think this person has a hearing loss?				

Mark the column that best describes the frequency with which you experience each situation or feeling. To calculate your score, give yourself 3 points for every time you checked "almost always," 2 for every "half the time," 1 for every "occasionally," and 0 for every "never." If you have a blood relative who has a hearing loss, add another 3 points. Total your points.

Scoring:
0 to 5: Your hearing is fine. No action required.
6 to 9: Suggest you see an ear, nose, and throat (ENT) physician.
10 and above: Strongly recommend you see an ENT physician.

Reprinted with permission from the American Academy of Otolaryngology—Head and Neck Surgery, Inc, Alexandria, Va.

On examination, pneumatic otoscopic findings are specific and demonstrate a bulging, poorly resilient tympanic membrane resulting from the pus and exudate that accumulate behind the tympanic membrane. The symptoms are often consistent with the severity of the disorder. Pain is often dull and throbbing at first; then it rapidly becomes sharp, knifelike, and agonizing. The symptoms often follow an upper respiratory tract infection and may include chills, fever, and malaise. A bloody, purulent, foul-smelling discharge flows from the infected ear only after tympanic membrane perforation, at which time the patient experiences sudden relief from pain.

Patients with symptoms of either fever, malaise, or lymphadenopathy associated with any ear disorder should be thoroughly evaluated by a physician.

Treatment

Normally, the skin that lines the external auditory canal provides adequate protection against bacterial or fungal infection. Cerumen provides a continual, self-cleaning process that removes particulate matter and debris from the external auditory canal. An infection of the auricle or external auditory canal is a skin infection and should be treated as such.

Surgical intervention may be necessary for deep cuts, bruises, or abrasions of the ear. Severe infections often require both systemic and local antibiotics. Progressive symptoms of otic disease should be evaluated and treated only under a physician's supervision.

External Ear Disorders

Boils

Small boils may be treated by good hygiene combined with topical compresses. Self-treatment may be instituted by applying hot compresses of saline solution to the affected area, followed by an antibiotic ointment. A soft cotton applicator is useful for applying a topical drug over and around the boil. An antibiotic ointment may be used in the absence of known or suspected sensitivity. The lesion usually is self-limiting and clears after several days of frequent applications of heat and ointment. Boils that do not respond rapidly to topical therapy should be examined by a physician. Resistant lesions require incision and drainage by a physician. Recurrent boils may require systemic antibiotic therapy.

External Otitis

Treatment of external otitis typically includes antibiotic and hydrocortisone drops applied in the ear canal. When cellulitis and lymphadenopathy are present, oral antibiotics are effective. Trauma to the ear should be avoided. The ear canals should be kept clean and dry at all times.

A 5% aluminum acetate solution (Burow's solution) may be used as an astringent to obtain rapid resolution of eczematous or weeping skin.[1,2] Soaking with warm water, saline, or aluminum acetate solution is often useful in the treatment of crusting and edema involving the auricle and surrounding tissue.[15]

Cleansing the ear with a soft rubber bulb ear syringe may be uncomfortable but should never be painful. Severe, knifelike pain occurs if the tympanic membrane is ruptured, and it may be followed by intense vertigo. If frank pain does occur, irrigation must be stopped at once.

Cleansing repeatedly with saline or water at body temperature helps to clear debris from the ear canal. The irrigation solution should always be at body temperature; if it is too cold, the patient may experience vertigo.[4] A bulb ear syringe may be appropriate for cleansing purposes; however, proper technique is very important. The water column should be superior against the canal wall so that the returning stream can push the debris (cerumen) from behind.[3] Patients with otomycosis and those with impacted mycotic debris should have their ears cleaned and treated by a physician. The use of a forced water spray (eg, Water Pik) should be reserved for health professionals trained in aural hygiene.

External otitis should always be treated promptly to prevent spread to the mastoid bone or middle ear cavity. Severe cases may result in permanent hearing loss.

Pharmacologic Agents

Although some nonprescription topical otic products have been recommended in the past to prevent swimmer's ear and dry water-clogged ears, a Food and Drug Administration (FDA) final ruling issued in February 1995 said that insufficient data exist to establish the safety and effectiveness of acetic acid, isopropyl alcohol, anhydrous glycerin, or any other nonprescription otic ingredients for these uses.[20] The ruling went on to say that any ingredient labeled, represented, or promoted for these uses is considered nonmonograph and is misbranded.[20] Some of these ingredients, however, are used in the treatment of external otitis (see product table, "Otic Products").

Because most bacteria or fungi do not thrive in acidic environments, an important feature of any otic solution is that the pH is acidic.[2] In mild cases of external otitis, topical treatment is all that is necessary.[2] Following careful cleansing, an acidified soothing liquid (ie, dilute acetic acid in alcohol) placed in the ear canal is suitable and even preferred, except for diabetic patients and for unusually severe cases of external otitis. In severe cases, these solutions may be used to flush debris from the ear canal to improve the effectiveness of topical antibacterial otic drops.[1]

All nonprescription otic preparations may be contraindicated in individuals who are susceptible to local irritation and hypersensitivity. Patients should be advised to discontinue using the medication if rash, local redness, or other adverse symptoms occur.

Acetic Acid Solutions

Acetic acid solution in the form of household vinegar has been used successfully for many years to treat mild forms of external otitis.[1,21] Its application reduces redness, inflammation, and edema, thereby relieving the signs and symptoms of external otitis. It is recommended for treatment of swimmer's ear. Acetic acid is well tolerated and nonsensitizing, and it does not induce resistant organisms. However, it does have an unpleasant vinegar-like odor, and it can be very painful if applied to the middle ear through a tympanoplasty tube or a perforation. If it does irritate or if sensitivity develops, use should be discontinued.[22]

Acetic acid has bactericidal and fungicidal properties when used properly, particularly against *Pseudomonas* sp, *Candida* sp, and *Aspergillus* sp. An environmental pH of 7.2–7.6 appears to be optimal for bacterial growth in the ear. This was confirmed in a study of 42 otitis cases in which pus cells and bacteria were observed in a pH range of 6.5–7.2.[23] Concentrations of 2–3% acetic acid provide effective and dependable treatment for mild forms of otitis by lowering the pH of the ear canal; however, solutions of less than 1% lack bactericidal properties. The recommended treatment is four drops of dilute acetic acid 2–3% placed into the ear canal four times daily. This will provide an environmental pH of less than 3.[23]

A suitable concentration of acetic acid can be made easily and inexpensively in the pharmacy from white distilled household vinegar, which is usually 5% acetic acid. A 50:50 mixture of distilled household vinegar with either water, propylene glycol, glycerin, or rubbing alcohol (70% isopropyl or 70% ethyl alcohol) will provide a 2.5% acetic acid solution.[22] Because propylene glycol is viscous, mixing it with vinegar will increase the contact time of acetic acid with the epithelium. Anhydrous glycerin, alone or mixed with vinegar, will help to remove water from the ear. Alcohol alone or mixed with vinegar has anti-infective properties and provides a drying effect.[6] Decreasing the alcohol concentration may lessen the burning sensation as well as the drying effect, whereas increasing the alcohol concentration will increase the drying effect.

Patients can be treated at home with dilute acetic acid solution using eight drops of white vinegar diluted to 10 mL with 10% isopropyl alcohol or aluminum acetate solution.[1] The solution should be applied as two to four drops into the ear using the following technique[1,24]:

- Tilt head downward, affected ear up.
- If there is *no* possibility that there is a hole in the eardrum, carefully squeeze a medicine dropper full of the solution into the ear canal.
- With one hand, move the ear back and forth to move the solution all the way into the ear.
- Tilt the head to the other, affected side to let the solution out, gently tapping the unaffected side.
- Repeat the procedure in the opposite ear.

Aluminum Acetate Solution (Burow's Solution)

External otitis or local itching of the external ear caused by external ear dermatitis may be treated with an astringent such as 1:10 or 1:40 aluminum acetate solution.[2,3,25] One tablet or one packet dissolved in 500 mL of water yields a concentration of 1:40. Aluminum acetate solution is used widely for conditions involving the external ear. Its major value is its acidity, which restores the normal antibacterial pH of the ear canal.

Applied locally as protein precipitants, astringents dry the affected area by reducing the secretory function of the skin glands.[25] Contraction and wrinkling of the affected tissue may be seen; astringents also toughen the skin to help prevent reinfection. When applied properly, aluminum acetate may be used to treat bacterial infections or otomycosis.

When the ear canal is swollen, weeping, and inflamed, an aluminum acetate solution is helpful, given its anti-inflammatory, antipruritic, astringent, and limited antibacterial properties.[25] Aluminum acetate solution may also be used to treat the edema and crusting associated with acute moist ear canals, for which the abundant desquamative debris that forms requires special cleansing.[3]

A wet compress may be used with a gauze dressing on the auricle.[15] Drops may be instilled into the canal. The usual dosage of aluminum acetate solution is four to six drops every 4–6 hours until itching or burning subsides. Aluminum acetate solution is suitable for children and adults. Used properly, it is nonsensitizing and well tolerated.[26] Adverse reactions are rare.

Antipyrine

The FDA has concluded that antipyrine is neither safe nor effective for nonprescription use as a topical otic analgesic and anesthetic, and that it should be used only under the advice and supervision of a physician.[27]

Benzocaine

The utility of benzocaine or other local anesthetics for local analgesia in the ear is not clear. The FDA has concluded that evidence is lacking to classify benzocaine as either safe or effective for nonprescription use as a topical analgesic, and it has suggested that benzocaine is ineffective topically as an analgesic and/or anesthetic on the tissue of the tympanic membrane and ear canal.[10,27] Hypersensitivity to benzocaine is considered a general contraindication to its topical use in the ear or elsewhere on the skin.

Boric Acid

Boric acid is an ingredient in some ear preparations. It is a weak, local anti-infective and is nonirritating to intact skin in a dilute solution of 1–5%. Alcohol-boric acid solutions show improved bactericidal action over alcohol alone (either 99% isopropyl or 70% ethyl alcohol) because the addition of boric acid increases the acidity of the preparation, which, when applied topically, increases the acidity of the skin. Because of its toxicity, boric acid should be used with caution, particularly in children and on open wounds where the potential for systemic absorption is high.[25]

Camphor

The safety and effectiveness of camphor as an ingredient in nonprescription eardrops have not been substantiated.

Cerumen-Softening Agents

Cerumen-softening and cerumenolytic agents only soften and loosen the cerumen. These agents do not readily remove cerumen. Patients can remove minor amounts of excessive ear wax by rinsing the ear canal with an ear syringe. However, hardened or impacted earwax should be removed by a physician. If ear pain is present, the patient should be referred to a physician.

Carbamide Peroxide The antibacterial properties of carbamide peroxide (urea hydrogen peroxide) are owing to the release of nascent oxygen, the primary value of which is in cleansing wounds. The effervescence caused by oxygen release mechanically removes debris from inaccessible regions. In otic preparations, the effervescence assists in disintegrating wax accumulations. Carbamide (urea) helps debride the tissue. These actions soften residue in the ear. Removal of the softened cerumen may be assisted by warm water irrigation.

The FDA has determined that 6.5% carbamide peroxide formulated in an anhydrous glycerin vehicle is safe and effective for occasional nonprescription use as an aid to soften, loosen, and remove excessive earwax.[11] The FDA recommends usage twice each day for up to 4 days if needed, or as directed by a physician. Five drops of the solution should be instilled into the affected ear and allowed to remain at least 15 minutes; this is done by either tilting the head (affected ear up) or inserting a small amount of cotton into the canal opening. The applicator tip should not enter the ear canal. Wax remaining after treatment may be removed by gently flushing the ear with warm water, using a soft rubber ear syringe. The process may be repeated a second time if necessary. Failure to obtain relief after 4 days of treatment could indicate a more serious condition, and a physician should be consulted. This process is not recommended for children under 12 years of age.

Unless it is under physician supervision, carbamide peroxide should not be used if there is ear drainage, pain, or dizziness; if there is known injury or perforation of the eardrum; or if ear surgery has been performed within the past 6 weeks. This treatment should be discontinued whenever irritation or rash appears. It is not recommended for treating pain of raw inflamed tissue, swimmer's ear, or itching of the ear canal.

Other Cerumen-Softening Products The occasional instillation of olive oil, mineral oil, glycerin, diluted hydrogen peroxide solution, or propylene glycol in the ear can also soften the cerumen and promote the normal process of removal.

The patient may rinse the ear canal every few days with a mixture of 20–30% alcohol and water or aluminum acetate solution to help prevent cerumen buildup. If the tympanic membrane is perforated or is not known to be intact, these cerumen-softening products should be used only under a physician's supervision. If perforation of the tympanic membrane is not suspected, a 1:1 solution of warm water and hydrogen peroxide can be used to flush the ear canal.[1] Patients can be instructed to use cerumen-softening agents for 3–4 days, at which time the cerumen should be softened enough to be easily removed by rinsing with an ear syringe.[2] The overuse of undiluted 3% hydrogen peroxide and the indiscriminate or chronic use of aqueous hydrogen peroxide (1:1) instilled into the ear canal are not recommended because maceration of the skin may predispose to infection.

Chloroform

The safety and effectiveness of chloroform as an ingredient in nonprescription topical ear products have not been established.

Glycerin

Glycerin may be used as a solvent or an emollient; it may also be used as a humectant because of its hygroscopic properties. Glycerin is widely used as a vehicle in many otic preparations (prescription and nonprescription). It is safe and nonsensitizing when applied to open wounds or abraded skin.

Dehydrated glycerin contains no less than 98.5% glycerin; glycerin (USP) contains no less than 95% glycerin (it may contain a maximum of 5% water).[25,29] Anhydrous glycerin may be prepared by heating glycerin (USP) at 302°F (150°C) for 2 hours to drive off moisture.[11] Because of glycerin's hygroscopic properties, patients should be advised not to rinse the applicator because this will dilute the glycerin and reduce its effectiveness.

Ichthammol

Ichthammol is a weak antiseptic and irritant with emollient properties. Its primary activity is as an emollient rather than an antiseptic. Ichthammol ointment (10%) is used for treating local inflammation associated with minor boils or abscesses. The safety and effectiveness of ichthammol in treating disorders of the ear have not been established.

Menthol

The safety and effectiveness of menthol as a nonprescription ingredient in eardrops have not been substantiated.

Olive Oil (Sweet Oil)

Olive oil is used as an emollient and topical lubricant.[25] It may be instilled into the ear canal to alleviate itching and burning. It is also helpful for softening earwax.[13] If an insect becomes trapped in the ear canal, olive oil can be instilled to smother the insect.

Phenol in Glycerin

Phenol (5–10%) in glycerin has been used to treat pain caused by ear disorders. Its use is no longer recommended, however, because it poses inherent dangers of necrosis and perforation of the tympanic membrane.

Propylene Glycol

Propylene glycol is a solvent that has preservative and humectant properties. Used in both prescription and nonprescription otic preparations, propylene glycol is a clear, colorless, nonirritating, viscous liquid. It is useful as a vehicle because it is hygroscopic and its viscosity increases contact time with tissues of the external auditory canal.[3] Adding acetic acid to propylene glycol increases the solution's acidity, enhancing its anti-infective properties.[3] If used over a long period of time, propylene glycol may cause allergic dermatitis in susceptible individuals.[2,8]

Thymol

Thymol, a phenolic compound obtained from thyme oil, has a more agreeable odor than phenol. It has been used traditionally in topical preparations for its aromatic properties. It has antibacterial and antifungal properties in a concentration of 1%[21]; in the presence of large amounts of proteins, however, its antibacterial activity is greatly reduced. The clinical effectiveness of thymol for treating ear disorders has not been well studied and objectively determined. The value of thymol in managing any disorder of the external ear is unsubstantiated.

Other Medications

Nonprescription drug products used for palliative treatment of ear disorders should include selective products useful for treating skin disorders. For example, when applied to the skin, salicylic acid acts as an irritant; continuous application may cause dermatitis.[26] Thus, the use of salicylic acid in topical preparations applied to the ear is considered inadvisable unless recommended by a physician.

Topical antibiotic ointments, either with single or multiple antibiotics, are adequate for treating minor lesions of the auricle. They should be used only in the absence of known or suspected hypersensitivity. Antibiotics do not readily penetrate boils or abscesses; therefore, incision and drainage may be required.

Patient Counseling

Cleansing procedures and self-treatment for treating ear disorders should not be delegated to patients unless they understand proper techniques of drug administration and use. Patients must be evaluated for their ability to understand the hazards of inappropriate self-treatment. The pharmacist with proper skill in aural visualization and irrigation procedures can usually make these judgments.

Patients should be instructed on the use of nonprescription drugs for the ear consistent with any other drug product dispensed by the pharmacist. They should also fully understand the proper use of medicine droppers for administering eardrops into the ear and of ear syringes for irrigating the ear. Water to irrigate the ear canal should be sterile or sterilized by boiling to prevent contamination.[28] Eardrops should be warmed to body temperature by holding the medication container in the palm of the hand or placing it into a vessel of warm water for a few minutes before administration. Heated eardrops should never be applied to the ear canal because they are likely to damage the ear. Also, excessive heat may damage the ingredients in the eardrop. Eardrops may be applied as often as four times daily. The involved ear should be tilted up for at least 2 minutes following the placement of two to four eardrops to permit effective contact of the medication.

A cotton wick may be inserted gently into the ear canal to help the medication maintain contact with the affected area in the ear canal. Gently pulling the auricle backward may allow medication to reach a greater depth in the ear canal. Cotton wicks, however, usually require insertion with appropriate instruments and should be used only by trained personnel.

Patients should be advised that symptoms usually begin to subside within 1–2 days if self-treatment is appropriate. If symptoms persist or if an adverse reaction to the medication occurs, the patient should consult a physician immediately.

Case Studies

Case 24–1

Patient Complaint/History

RA, a 27-year-old male, presents a request for refill of his wife's prenatal vitamins. During conversation with the pharmacist, he reveals that his ears have been bothering him for several weeks and requests eardrops for "itching" ears. To relieve the itching, he had on several occasions scratched his ear canals with toothpicks, hair pins, or cotton swabs. His symptoms now include a burning sensation in the left ear plus itching in both ears; however, no unusual ear discharge, pain, or subjective change in hearing acuity is present. Further, no previous history of ear injury exists. The patient admits that he may scratch his ears more often when he is "under a lot of pressure."

RA is in good general health and currently takes no prescription medications. He takes nonprescription antihistamines and decongestants as needed to relieve symptoms associated with allergic reactions to hay, grass, ragweed, and pine pollen; he also takes nonprescription antitussives, antacids, and other nonprescription medications as needed.

RA smokes a pipe and is a social drinker.

Clinical Consideration/Strategies

The following considerations/strategies are provided to aid the reader in (1) determining whether treatment of the patient's condition with nonprescription medications is warranted, (2) selecting the appropriate nonprescription medication, and (3) developing a patient counseling strategy to ensure optimal therapeutic outcomes:

- Assess the patient's practice of "scratching" the ear canal and advise accordingly.
- Advise the patient of techniques for proper otic hygiene and the dangers associated with inappropriate procedures for cleaning the ears.
- Assess whether the current condition warrants medical referral or a regimen of one or more nonprescription medications.
- Recommend one or more products that are astringent and mildly acidic in nature.
- Recommend a therapy regimen (eg, medication(s), dose, frequency of administration, and duration of therapy).
- Review techniques for proper administration of otic solutions/suspensions.
- Recommend follow-up procedures as well as a course of action to take if current symptoms persist and/or worsen or if new symptoms develop.

Case Study 24–2

Patient Complaint/History

JD, a 64-year-old cattle rancher, presents to the pharmacy with complaints of a "feeling of fullness" and slight pain in his right ear as well as difficulty in hearing. He reports no other complaints. JD requests a nonprescription medication to relieve his present symptoms. His past history of compliance with the pharmacist's advice and suggested treatment regimens has been good.

JD's current prescription medications include phenytoin 100 mg tid; benzapril 10 mg QAM; hydrochlorothiazide 25 mg QAM; aspirin 325 mg QAM; and doxepin 25 mg hs. He is also currently taking the following nonprescription medications: Humulin 70/30 insulin taken before breakfast and before the evening meal (dose is dependent on the results of self-monitored blood glucose levels); docusate calcium 240 mg QAM; one multivitamin tablet QAM; and vitamin E 400 IU QAM. JD has no history of allergies.

Clinical Consideration/Strategies

The following considerations/strategies are provided to aid the reader in (1) determining whether treatment of the patient's condition with nonprescription medications is warranted, (2) selecting the appropriate nonprescription medication, and (3) developing a patient counseling strategy to ensure optimal therapeutic outcomes:

- Assess the patient's overall health status and determine what etiologic risk factors may exist that could predispose to external otitis, excessive accumulation of cerumen, or other complications of the external auditory canal.
- Assess whether the current condition warrants medical referral or a regimen with one or more nonprescription medications or devices.
- Select an appropriate treatment regimen based on the family practitioner's diagnosis of impaction and excessive accumulation of cerumen in both ears.
- If a ceruminolytic medication is to be used, recommend appropriate medication(s), dose, frequency of administration, and duration of therapy.
- If irrigation of the external auditory canal(s) is warranted, recommend at what point this process should occur after the ceruminolytic therapy has begun.
- Explain the proper irrigation of the external auditory canal (eg, technique, frequency, and duration of therapy).
- Recommend a course of action to take if current symptoms persist and/or worsen or if new symptoms develop.
- Advise the patient of techniques for proper otic hygiene to initiate once the current condition is resolved, the potential consequences of inappropriate otic hygiene, and procedures for preventing recurrence of cerumen accumulation and impaction.

Summary

Otic disorders affect both young and old people, and visible signs are not always proportional to the degree of pain suffered. Nonprescription products are available to treat disorders of both the auricle and the external auditory canal. Disorders involving the middle ear should not be treated with nonprescription drug products.

By assessing the complaint and reviewing the patient's history, the pharmacist should be able to judge whether symptoms may be self-treated or referral to a physician is indicated. Health professionals trained in otic procedures may examine the tympanic membrane with an otoscope and irrigate the ear canal gently with a syringe or a forced water spray. This procedure should be performed only if the tympanic membrane is known to be intact and there are no underlying disorders as determined by a recent physician examination.

Objects such as hairpins, pencils, matchsticks, cotton swabs, or other sharp instruments should never touch the external auditory canal, and objects smaller than a finger draped with a clean washcloth should never enter the external auditory canal. The warning "Never clean the ear with anything smaller than the elbow" may be good advice.[2] Good personal hygiene, especially of facial and neck areas, should be maintained at all times. Dandruff and dirty hair can be controlled with appropriate shampoos and washing. A skin infection must not be neglected because it may be transferred very easily to uninfected areas.

Many nonprescription otic products have been shown to be safe and effective. The pharmacist should advise the patient to consult a physician if symptoms do not subside within 1 or 2 days after treatment is initiated or if adverse reactions occur.

References

1. Paparella MM, Shumick DA. *Otolaryngology*. 3rd ed. Philadelphia: WB Saunders; 1991: 23, 26, 595, 1077, 1228–30, 1246, 1259, 1293.
2. DeWeese D et al. *Otolaryngology—Head and Neck Surgery*. 8th ed. St Louis: CV Mosby; 1994: 353, 357, 403–7, 409, 410, 437, 489.
3. Austin DF. Diseases of the external ear. In: Ballenger JJ et al, eds. *Diseases of Nose, Throat, Ear, Head, and Neck*. 14th ed. Philadelphia: Lea & Febiger; 1991: 925, 1069, 1075–6, 1106, 1117, 1179, 1229.
4. Meyerhoff WL, Rice DH. *Otolaryngology and Head and Neck Surgery*. Philadelphia: WB Saunders; 1992: 16, 18–9, 48, 157, 293, 353–4, 356, 1072, 1077, 1106, 1109–11.
5. *Federal Register*. 1977; 42: 63559.
6. Senturia BH et al. *Diseases of the External Ear, An Otologic-Dermatology Manual*. 2nd ed. New York: Grune and Stratton; 1980: 79–80.
7. Rutka J, Alberti P. *Toxic and Drug Induced Disorders in Otolaryngology*. The Otolaryngology Clinics of North America; 1984: 761–74.
8. Booth J. In: Kerr A, ed. *Scott-Brown's Otolaryngology*. 5th ed. London: Butterworth's & Co; 1987: 55–6, 164.
9. Meding B, Ringdahl A. *Ear Hear*. 1992; 13: 122–4.
10. *Federal Register*. 1982; 47: 30014, 30018.
11. *Federal Register*. 1986; 51: 28656–61.
12. Bordely J et al. *Ear, Nose, and Throat Disorders in Children*. New York: Raven Press; 1986: 56–7, 61, 89.
13. Cohn A. *Arch Otolaryngol*. 1974; 99: 138.
14. Corcoran JG, Atline SG. Infectious diseases in the geriatric patient: symposium on geriatric otolaryngology. *Otolaryngol Clin North Am*. 1982 May; 15(2): 425.
15. Lucente FE. In: English GM, ed. *Otolaryngology—Diseases of the Ear and Hearing*. Vol 1. Philadelphia: Harper & Row; 1983: 1–2.
16. Bossi J, Jackman J. *Drug Intell Clin Pharm*. 1977; 11: 665.
17. Smyth GDL. In: English GM, ed. *Chronic Otitis in Otolaryngology*. Philadelphia: Harper & Row; 1976: 2.

18. Lee KJ. *Differential Diagnosis, Otolaryngology*. New York: Arco; 1978: 91, 94, 115.
19. Wood RP, Northern FL. *Manual of Otolaryngology*. Baltimore: Williams & Wilkins; 1979: 39, 42.
20. Topical drug products for over-the-counter human use; products for the prevention of swimmer's ear and for the drying of water-clogged ears; final rule. *Federal Register*. 1995 Feb; 60(31): 8916–20.
21. Ochs I. *Arch Otolaryngol*. 1950; 52: 935–7.
22. *AMA Drug Evaluations Annual*. Chicago: American Medical Association; 1992: 1128, 1480.
23. Goffin F. *N Engl J Med*. 1963; 268: 287–9.
24. Goldstein JC. What to advise patients on swimmer's ear. *Wellcome Trends Pharm*. 1989 Aug; 9.
25. *Remington's Pharmaceutical Sciences*. 18th ed. Easton, Pa: Mack; 1990: 761, 1310, 1316, 1318.
26. Wade A, Reynolds JE. *Martindale, The Extra Pharmacopoeia*. 27th ed. London: Pharmaceutical Press; 1979: 212, 272.
27. *Federal Register*. 1977; 42: 63564.
28. *USP DI*. 21st ed. Rockville, Md: US Pharmacopoeial Convention; 1992: 158, 768.

CHAPTER 25

Oral Health Products

Arlene A. Flynn

Questions to ask in patient assessment and counseling

General Assessment

- *What are your symptoms?*
- *How long have you had this dental problem?*
- *Have you seen a dentist about the problem? When?*
- *What remedies have you tried? How did you use them? How long did you use them? Did they work?*
- *Have you had this problem before?*

Mouth Pain

- *Where is the pain?*
- *Is the pain severe? Is there swelling in the area?*
- *Is the pain continuous and throbbing, or does it come and go?*
- *Is the pain triggered or made worse by hot or cold substances or by chewing?*
- *Have you found anything that makes the pain go away? If so, what?*
- *Do you feel ill?*
- *Do you have a cold, sinus infection, or ear infection?*
- *Do you have a fever?*
- *Are there any prior events such as trauma associated with the pain?*
- *Are there any other symptoms associated with the pain?*

Mouth Irritation or Discomfort

- *Where is the area of irritation or lesion? Is it visible? What color is it?*
- *Is the discomfort continuous?*
- *Is the discomfort aggravated by eating or drinking?*
- *Is there a discharge from the lesion?*
- *Do your gums bleed when you brush your teeth?*
- *Do you have a bad taste in your mouth?*
- *Do you have bad breath continuously?*
- *Are any of your teeth loose?*
- *Do you wear dentures? Are they loose?*
- *Do your dentures cause sore spots?*

General State of Oral Health

- *How do you brush your teeth or clean your dentures? How often?*
- *Do you use dental floss? How often?*
- *How often do you see your dentist for checkups?*
- *Do you use supplemental fluoride in any form (eg, rinse or tablet)?*

Additional Patient-Specific Factors

- *Do you suffer from any chronic medical illness (eg, diabetes mellitus, rheumatic heart disease, asthma, seizure disorder, or high blood pressure)?*
- *What prescription and nonprescription medications are you currently taking?*
- *Do you have a pacemaker?*
- *Have you had joint replacement surgery?*
- *Do you smoke or use any tobacco product (including smokeless tobacco products)?*
- *Do you have any food or drug allergies? If so, what are they?*

Dental diseases are among the most prevalent chronic diseases in our society. Pertinent statistics include the following:

- Fifty percent of the population needs dental treatment.
- Only 55% of the adult population visit a dentist during a year.
- Of all 17-year-olds, 84% have experienced tooth decay.
- The average adult has 23 decayed or filled tooth surfaces.
- Each year, dental diseases cause 6.73 million days of disability that result in confinement to bed.
- Nearly 80% of all Americans have some degree of periodontal disease.
- Forty-one percent of older Americans have lost all their natural teeth.
- Oral cancer accounts for 4% of all cancers.[1]

Since the 1970s, the incidence of dental caries has declined significantly in school-age children in this country. The National Institute of Dental Research reports that

49.9% of all US children aged 5–17 in 1990 had no episodes of dental caries in their permanent teeth, as compared with 36.6% in 1980 and 28% in 1970.[1] Nevertheless, dental caries remains a public health problem, and the importance of prevention should not be ignored. In addition, root caries, an age-related problem that affects the root surfaces of adult teeth exposed by gingival recession, is becoming increasingly significant as adults retain greater numbers of teeth later in life and the number of older people in the population increases. Finally, periodontal disease, the prevalence and severity of which is related primarily to oral health care, remains the principal cause of tooth loss in adults over 35 years of age.[2] Yet this common and significant public health problem can be prevented or controlled.

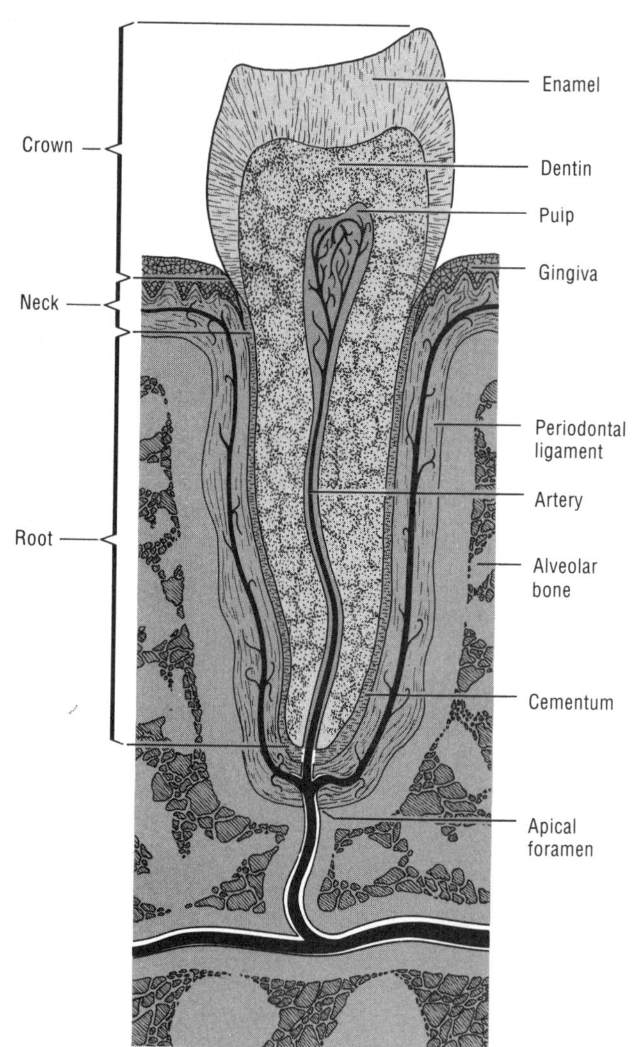

FIGURE 1 Anatomy of the tooth.

Dental Anatomy and Physiology

The teeth and supporting structures are necessary for normal mastication and articulation and for aesthetic appearance. The primary dentition first appears at approximately 6 months of age with the eruption of the mandibular (lower jaw) central incisors; it is usually complete with the eruption of the upper second molars at approximately 24 months. There are 20 deciduous teeth, 10 in each arch. Generally, the permanent dentition first appears with the eruption of the mandibular first molar behind the deciduous second molar at approximately 6 years, and it continues in a regular pattern, replacing shedding deciduous teeth. The last permanent teeth to erupt are the third molars (wisdom teeth), which may appear between 17 and 21 years of age.

Anatomically, the teeth are grossly viewed as having two parts, the roots and the crown (Figure 1). The roots are normally below the gingival (gum) line or margin and are essential for support and attachment of the tooth to the surrounding tissues. The crown is above the gingival margin and is responsible for mastication. The teeth comprise four basic components: enamel, dentin, pulp, and cementum.

Enamel is composed of very hard, crystalline calcium salts (hydroxyapatite). It protects the underlying tooth structure and covers the crown of the tooth to the cementoenamel junction, enabling the crown to withstand the wear of mastication. Dentin, which is softer, lies beneath the enamel and makes up the largest part of the tooth structure. Its tubules enable transport of nutrients from the dental pulp. Dentin protects the dental pulp from mechanical, thermal, and chemical irritation.

The pulp occupies the pulp chamber and is continuous with the tissues surrounding the tooth by means of the apical foramen, an opening at the apex of the root. The pulp consists primarily of vascular and neural tissues. The only type of nerve endings in the pulp are free nerve endings; thus, any type of stimulus to the pulp is interpreted as pain.

The periodontium comprises the tissues that support the teeth, including the cementum, the periodontal ligament, the encompassing alveolar bone, and the gingiva. The bonelike cementum is softer than dentin and covers the root of the tooth, extending apically from the cementoenamel junction. Its major function is to attach the tooth to the periodontal ligament via periodontal fibers. The periodontal ligament is connective tissue that attaches the tooth to the surrounding alveolar bone and gingival tissue. The four functions of the periodontal ligament are supportive, formative, sensory, and nutritive. The alveolar bone forms the sockets of the teeth. Alveolar bone is thin and spongy, and it attaches to the principal fibers of the periodontal ligament as well as to the gingiva. The gingiva is the soft tissue surrounding the teeth. It is normally pink and keratinized, and it is attached to the cementum by the gingival group of periodontal ligament fibers.

The mucosa covering the pharyngeal region, soft palate, floor of the mouth, vestibule (between the alveolar ridge and cheek), and cheeks is normally more pinkish-red than the gingiva. This is because the outer surface of the mucosa, which is stratified squamous epithelium, does not have a keratinized stratum corneum outer layer as do the gingiva and hard palate.

The tongue functions in mastication, swallowing, taste, and speech. Its dorsal or upper surface is usually irregular and rough in appearance. Taste buds are usually small, oval-shaped organs of flat epithelial cells surrounding a small opening (taste pore).

The major salivary glands are the parotid, submandibular, and sublingual salivary glands. They are responsible for secreting saliva, which is an alkaline, slightly viscous, clear secretion that contains enzymes (lysozymes and ptyalin), albumin, epithelial mucin (a mucopolysaccharide), immune globulin, leukocytes, and minerals. Normal salivary gland function promotes good oral health in several ways. Saliva components clear carbohydrates and microorganisms from the oral cavity. Saliva also reduces the acid concentration formed by carbohydrate fermentation, and it buffers the pH fall caused by acid production. Its mineral components have a protective role in the demineralization and remineralization process of tooth enamel.

Patient Assessment and Counseling

The oral health care market has grown an average of 6.1% per year since 1986. An analysis of 1994 retail sales for five categories of oral health care products (toothpaste, dental accessories, mouthrinses [mouthwashes], denture products, and oral hygiene) indicated overall sales at approximately $3.5 billion. Drugstore sales for these categories totaled about $1 billion (29%) and accounted for 54% of all sales in the oral hygiene category, an 8.2% increase over 1993; drugstore sales in the remaining four categories showed a slight drop of about 3% on average.[3] Nonprescription products are widely available in the pharmacy for both the prevention and treatment of oral disease or discomfort. Therefore, a pharmacist may be the first health care professional to evaluate and counsel a patient with oral health care needs. On the basis of thorough patient assessment, the pharmacist can inform and advise the patient regarding self-care or the need for professional referral. Questions the pharmacist should ask the patient presenting with a dental problem (see list of questions at beginning of this chapter) relate to several factors:

- The clinical manifestation of the particular problem (eg, pain);
- The patient's general state of oral health;
- Possible etiology;
- Patient-specific factors (eg, history of chronic disease, prescription medications, allergies, and previous dental care);
- Lifestyle risks;
- Product selection.

It is important for the pharmacist to assess each complaint to determine whether the problem (1) is a recurring one, (2) is likely to resolve with self-treatment using nonprescription products, (3) could lead to progressive and potentially serious consequences, or (4) presents a dental emergency requiring immediate professional care.

It is also important for the pharmacist to determine if the patient is currently under a dentist's care and is experiencing a problem related to a recent dental procedure. A recurrent problem (eg, swelling, drainage, chronic pain) may signal a condition that warrants referral to a dentist. Previous self-treatment with nonprescription oral products needs to be evaluated for possible misuse, abuse, or inappropriate response.

Counseling a patient about nonprescription medication should include more than merely explaining that a product is preventive, curative, or palliative. The patient should be informed about how to use the product properly, how long to use it, what to expect from it, what precautions to take with its use, and what to do if it is ineffective. It is equally important for the pharmacist to tell the patient which nonprescription medications should not be used and why. The patient should realize that nonprescription drugs should improve the condition being treated. If their use results in no change, worsens the condition, or causes another problem, the drugs should be discontinued and the patient should see a dentist or other physician.

Assessment of Clinical Manifestations

Pain

Pain can accompany many common oral problems. Different features of pain indicate different underlying problems. Tooth pain triggered or worsened by stimuli such as heat, cold, or pressure upon biting often indicates a pulpal response to deep carious lesions or a cracked or broken tooth. Continuous tooth pain may indicate pulpal infection and necrosis, an abscess, or serious periodontal disease. Fever, malaise, and swelling may indicate an oral abscess; a patient who exhibits these symptoms should be referred to a dentist for immediate professional care.

Mouth Irritation or Discomfort

Continuous irritation, soreness, or pain that is associated with the soft tissues of the mouth and is more severe upon eating or drinking is a common symptom of canker sores and acute atrophic candidiasis. Pain along the gingival ridge under a denture prosthesis suggests ill-fitting dentures, denture stomatitis, or possible candidiasis. The color, shape, and location of various oral anomalies help in assessment. Recurrent oral sores on nonkeratinized oral mucosa (eg, canker sores), recurrent vesicular sores on the skin bordering the lip (eg, cold sores and fever blisters), and inflammation under seldom-cleaned dentures (eg, denture stomatitis) are examples of location-specific lesions that can help define oral problems (see product table "Oral Discomfort Products"). Some examples of pathologic color changes include the white plaques of candidiasis, the erythema (redness) associated with the margins of canker and cold sores, and the gingival erythema associated with periodontitis. Halitosis may result from poor oral hygiene, acute necrotizing ulcerative gingivitis (trench mouth), periodontal disease, or dentopyogenic infections, and it merits inquiry and possible referral.

Assessment of Patient-Specific Factors

If available, the patient's medication profile should be reviewed. This history, which should include prescription and nonprescription drug use, may suggest to the pharmacist potentially serious dental or medical complications, such as endocarditis secondary to an oral abscess in a patient with rheumatic heart disease. Patients who have undergone surgery for placement of a pacemaker or prosthetic joint may be at high risk for bacterial endocarditis. Use of oral irrigating devices may be contraindicated in these groups because of the possibility of bacteremia.[1] The pharmacist should also be alert to predisposing factors or conditions that might result in oral pathology. Signs and symptoms of oral candidiasis (eg, white plaques with a milk curd appearance, erythematous tissue, angular cheilitis) might be observed in the presence of a disease (eg, leukemia, autoimmunodeficiency syndrome, or cancer) or with some treatment regimens. Patients treated with an antihistamine with high anticholinergic activity that dries the mouth, an orally inhaled steroid that decreases the immune response in the mouth, a broad-spectrum antibiotic that results in overgrowth of nonsusceptible organisms, or therapy (eg, cancer chemotherapy) that produces an immune deficiency disorder may be at risk.

Assessment of General Oral Health

Poor oral hygiene or infrequent dental care can greatly increase the likelihood of dental caries, infection, periodontal disease, ill-fitting or broken dentures, and other oral health problems. Patients sometimes notice bleeding gingiva, the presence of plaque and calculus on teeth, and loose teeth during brushing and flossing. Such symptoms should prompt the pharmacist to refer the patient to a dentist for evaluation.

Assessment of Lifestyle Risks

Alcohol Consumption

Adverse effects of alcohol consumption on oral health include xerostomia (dry mouth) and increased risk for development of oral cancer.

Use of Tobacco Products

Use of tobacco products, both smoked and smokeless, has been associated with oral cancer, sinusitis, discoloration of the teeth, halitosis, xerostomia, periodontal disease, dental calculus, and other hard and soft tissue damage in the oral region.[1] Smoking accounts for about 30% of all cancer deaths, and about 390,000 premature, smoking-related deaths in the United States occur annually. If diagnosed early enough, however, many precancerous changes in the oral cavity can be reversed with the cessation of smoking or tobacco use.[1]

It is estimated that at least 10 million Americans, about 30% of whom are under 21 years of age, use smokeless tobacco. Use among teenage boys continues to increase. Epidemiologic and clinical case studies provide evidence of an increased risk of oral cancer among smokeless tobacco users, particularly those who regularly use snuff. Although the adverse effects associated with snuff use have been more fully documented than those associated with the use of other such products, the carcinogenic potential of all smokeless tobacco products is recognized.[4]

Evidence also supports an association of smokeless tobacco use with gingival inflammation and recession; increased dental caries (because these products contain sugar, which is kept in contact with the teeth); cervical erosion of the teeth; and oral leukoplakia, a precancerous oral lesion of which 3–6% of cases progress to become squamous cell carcinoma.[5]

Any patient who complains of persistent mouth irritation and who uses tobacco products of any type should be advised to visit a dentist for evaluation and to seek help in stopping tobacco use. A National Cancer Institute program promotes the use of the "four A's," which pharmacists can adopt in counseling their patients:

- *Ask* patients about their smoking behaviors.
- *Advise* all smokers to quit.
- *Assist* patients in stopping.
- *Arrange* for supportive follow-up.[1]

Pharmacists might also seriously consider providing a smoke-free environment and eliminating the sale of tobacco products in the pharmacy.

Chewing Ice Cubes

Chewing ice cubes can cause tooth enamel to develop cracks because of pressure, shearing force, and the expansion and contraction caused by temperature changes. These tiny cracks provide surfaces for plaque and stain to accumulate.

Common Oral Problems

The following sections discuss common oral problems, disease, and health concerns that pharmacists may encounter. Each section presents etiology and pathophysiology; suggestions for preventive care; and guidelines for treatment, product selection, and patient counseling as appropriate.

Plaque and Calculus Buildup

Etiology and Pathophysiology

Plaque is commonly recognized as the source of microbes that cause caries and periodontal disease; thus, plaque buildup is related to the incidence of oral disease.[6] Plaque is thought to start with the formation of acquired pellicle on a clean tooth surface. Pellicle appears to be a thin, acellular, glycoprotein-mucoprotein coating that adheres to the enamel within minutes after a tooth is cleaned. Its source is thought to be saliva. The pellicle seems to serve as an attachment for cariogenic bacteria that produce, along with acids, long-chain polymers such as dextrans and levans that adhere to the pellicle and tooth surface. The resulting sticky adherent mass is called dental plaque. It is soft and readily disrupted by toothbrushing or flossing.

After meals, food residue may be incorporated into plaque by bacterial degradation. Left undisturbed, plaque thickens and bacteria proliferate. Plaque growth begins in protected cracks and fissures and along the gingival margin.[7] If not removed within 24 hours, dental plaque begins to calcify by calcium salt precipitation from the saliva and forms calculus, or tartar. This hardened, adherent deposit is removable only by professional dental cleaning.[7]

Calculus is generally considered to be a substrate on which additional plaque can develop, and it is not regarded as the primary causative oral accumulation in periodontal disease.[7] However, most periodontists agree that supra- (above) and subgingival (below the gingival margin) calculus can promote the progression of periodontal disease in several ways. Both can promote the retention of new bacterial plaque accumulation in contact with sensitive tissue sites, and both can interfere with local self-cleaning processes and patient plaque removal. Subgingival calculus also may intensify the inflammatory process. Thorough removal of subgingival calculus in periodontal therapy is an important step in delaying the reestablishment of periodontal pathogens and the resolution of inflammation.[8,9]

Plaque Removal

The best way to ensure healthy teeth and gingival tissues is to remove plaque buildup by brushing at least twice daily and flossing at least once a day. Toothbrushing removes plaque from the lingual (tongue) side, buccal (cheek) side, and occlusal (biting) surfaces of the teeth. Plaque found between the teeth (interproximal surfaces) can be removed efficiently only with dental floss and other interdental cleaning aids (eg, interproximal brush, dental tape, or tapered picks). Effective plaque removal will help prevent both dental caries and periodontal disease by removing disease-causing bacteria and preventing their growth. Eating fibrous foods such as celery, apples, or carrots does not prevent plaque accumulation or aid in its removal.[10]

Chemical management of plaque and calculus can enhance mechanical removal either by acting directly on the plaque bacteria or by disrupting components of plaque to aid its removal during routine oral hygiene. The use of chemical agents in plaque removal may be particularly appropriate for selected patients who may be either unable to brush and floss effectively or inhibited from doing so. Physically or mentally handicapped individuals (who may not be able to master the manual techniques necessary) and orthodontia patients or those with fixed prostheses may benefit from the addition of antiplaque agents to their oral hygiene regimen.

Products for Plaque Removal

In 1990, the Food and Drug Administration (FDA) issued a call for data on oral health care products that make antiplaque and related claims.[11] This call was the initial step in developing the final segment of the rulemaking for over-the-counter (OTC) oral health care drug products, which will address antiplaque and related claims. Because plaque reduction or removal is intended to prevent disease (ie, gingivitis, caries, and periodontal disease), the FDA considers plaque removal and reduction claims to be drug claims.[11]

Two classes of oral health care products have made antiplaque claims. These classes include those products that rely on the mechanical action of abrasives to remove plaque, and those that claim to reduce or remove plaque by chemical or antimicrobial activity. These products are available in multiple forms (eg, dentifrices, gargles, and mouthwashes). Manufacturers of products bearing antiplaque and related claims (eg, for the reduction or prevention of plaque, tartar, calculus, or gingivitis) and containing active ingredients that have been marketed for such indications—and that meet conditions of FDA rules governing eligibility for review—may submit supporting safety and effectiveness data to the OTC drug review for consideration.[11] At the time of this publication, no final rule has been issued. However, the FDA has received a substantial amount of information, and the Plaque Subcommittee of the FDA Dental Products Panel is engaged in continuing discussions to develop guidelines for determining the safety and effectiveness of antiplaque products. That panel will advise the FDA Commissioner on the promulgation of a monograph establishing conditions under which oral antiseptic drugs for antiplaque and antiplaque-related use are generally recognized as safe and effective.[12]

Products for plaque removal may have cosmetic and/or therapeutic activity. Those that contain therapeutic ingredients specific to caries prevention (eg, fluoride) or hypersensitivity are discussed in the following sections Dentifrices and Mouthrinses (Mouthwashes).

American Dental Association Product Evaluation Programs For 35 years, the American Dental Association (ADA) seal program has been the consumer's guide to dental product safety and efficacy. The ADA evaluates the safety and efficacy of dental products used by dental professionals and the public through the evaluation programs of the Council on Dental Therapeutics (CDT) and the Council on Dental Materials, Instruments, and Equipment (CDMIE). Manufacturers voluntarily submit their products for detailed analysis of safety and efficacy. Moreover, product labels and promotional material must comply with ADA standards. Dental products are evaluated based on data regarding their safety and effectiveness for their intended use,[13] and those products that carry ADA seals or statements have scientifically earned their recognition.

The CDT evaluates the safety and efficacy of nonprescription and prescription therapeutic drugs used in the diagnosis, treatment, or prevention of dental disease. Council acceptance is valid for 3 years. Historically, the CDMIE maintained three evaluation programs (for acceptance, certification, and recognition), which differed in the mechanisms used. However, the recognition program for products not currently covered by a formal acceptance or certification program was terminated June 30, 1992. It is intended that certification program specifications or acceptance program guidelines will be developed for the product categories formerly in the recognition program so that the previously recognized products can be assimilated into the other programs.

Toothbrushes and Similar Devices The toothbrush is the most universally accepted device available for removing dental plaque and maintaining good oral hygiene. Toothbrush sales at retail are estimated in the $500 million range. Manual toothbrushes vary in size, shape, texture, and design, with new product designs proliferating rapidly. Dentists recommend toothbrushes based on the individual patient's manual dexterity, oral anatomy, and periodontal health. The toothbrush should be of a size and shape to allow the patient to reach every tooth in the mouth. Many dentists and dental hygienists prefer soft, rounded, multitufted nylon bristle brushes. This is because nylon bristles are more durable and easier to clean than natural bristles and because soft, rounded bristle tips are more effective in removing plaque below the gingival margin and on proximal tooth surfaces. Unfortunately, toothbrush firmness is not standardized; toothbrushes designated as soft, medium, or hard may not be comparable across manufacturers. Innovations in head shapes and bristle configurations continue to be introduced. The Dentrust toothbrush has earned the ADA seal and features a three-sided head with bristles that cup the teeth, surrounding them at a 45-degree angle. It also features ridges on the back of the head that can be used to clean the tongue. The Colgate Total design also carries the ADA seal and features bristles of three different lengths (angled outer bristles with both long and short inner bristles) to improve cleaning contact with tooth and gumline surfaces.

Characteristics considered desirable in selecting a toothbrush include:

- A relatively small brush head for easy access;
- A multitufted, dense, straight-trimmed brushing surface;
- Soft, resilient, nylon filaments with rounded ends.[14,15]

The handle size and shape of a toothbrush should allow the individual to maneuver the brush easily while maintaining a firm grasp. Most toothbrushes marketed in the United States have a flat handle design. Many modifications that may improve contact between the bristles and some less accessible tooth surfaces, such as angle bends or flexible areas in the handle, have been introduced.

The proper frequency and method of brushing will vary from patient to patient, depending on individual factors. After a clinical evaluation, the dentist or dental hygienist will recommend a method, time, and frequency for toothbrushing. Thoroughness of plaque removal without gingival trauma is more important than method. Patients should brush thoroughly at least twice a day, taking time to clean all tooth surfaces systematically. A gentle scrubbing motion with the bristle tips at a 45-degree angle against the gumline is indicated because the tips of the brush do the cleaning. Excessive force should be avoided because it may result in bristle damage, cervical abrasion, irritation of delicate gingival tissue, and gingival recession with associated hypersensitivity. Gentle brushing of the upper surface of the tongue is recommended to reduce debris, plaque, and bacteria.

As to how often the patient should buy a new toothbrush, there is no definite answer although 3 months has been suggested as a guide for toothbrush life expectancy. Marketing data suggest that consumers on average replace their toothbrushes only 1.7 times per year.[16] There are two major reasons for replacing toothbrushes frequently: wear and bacterial accumulation. Different methods of brushing cause bristles to wear differently. Worn, bent, or matted bristles do not remove plaque effectively. Thus, patients should replace toothbrushes at the first sign of bristle wear rather than after a set period of use, and ideally they should rotate two or three toothbrushes to allow each to dry completely between use, thereby decreasing bristle wear and matting. An innovation in the toothbrush product line is the Oral-B Indicator. This brush has a band of center bristles colored with a dye that fades with wear as a visual reminder to replace the brush.

Toothbrushes have been found to be a receptacle for bacteria. One study has reported that it takes just 17–35 days to accumulate a heavy buildup of bacteria on a toothbrush.[17] Patients with infectious diseases of the oral tissues (eg, gingival or periodontal disease) should change brushes every 2 weeks, and it is advisable to replace a toothbrush following a respiratory infection to prevent reinfection.[17] Patients should be advised to rinse their toothbrushes thoroughly after each use to dislodge food debris and dilute sugar residue, both of which may serve as media for bacterial growth.

Manual toothbrushes had been covered by the ADA recognition program but are in the process of being assimilated into the acceptance program. More than 100 brands of manual toothbrushes representing more than 50 manufacturers had participated in the recognition program at the time it was terminated.[18]

Standard electric toothbrushes mimic the motion of hand brushing. Although they have not consistently proven superior to properly manipulated manual toothbrushes, electric toothbrushes may benefit patients who are handicapped, who lack manual dexterity, who require someone else to clean their teeth, or who wear orthodontic appliances. Models such as the Water Pik may offer an advantage for some handicapped individuals because the brushing action can be started by either depressing a button or simply applying pressure to the toothbrush bristles. These devices may also be useful for young children when parents do the brushing and for patients who may be motivated by the novelty of a powered toothbrush to increase the frequency and efficiency of their oral hygiene.[19,20] It has been suggested that "level of instruction, motivation, cost, ease of use and maintenance will determine long-term acceptance by patients."[15]

Electric toothbrushes, which are available from numerous manufacturers, use essentially three brush-head motions to clean (ie, back and forth, up and down, and a combination pattern). Best results can be expected if a patient uses a brush carrying the ADA seal of acceptance and follows the specific directions of a dental professional. ADA criteria for acceptance are based primarily on safety concerns. Advertising may mention plaque reduction but may not claim improvement of any existing oral disease.[1] Comparative studies to date have yielded mixed results and modest differences. Variations in study design and specific patient factors or situations have influenced interpretation. Positive results (ie, significant reductions in dental plaque accumulation) depend to some extent on proper use of the device, implicating the need for patient education.[21]

Besides the familiar electric toothbrush, other types of powered rotary devices for plaque removal have been marketed and evaluated. Because conventional dentifrices may clog these devices, a dentifrice specifically formulated for use with the device (eg, Interplak toothpaste) and/or a fluoride rinse is advised. The Rota-dent comes with three interchangeable brush heads or tips shaped like interproximal brushes, and it rotates in a fashion similar to instruments used during a professional cleaning.[1] Clinical trials comparing the Rota-dent with conventional manual plaque-removal devices show the Rota-dent to be well accepted by users, generally superior to manual toothbrushes alone in removing plaque, and equivalent to manual toothbrushing when combined with a comprehensive oral hygiene program that includes instruction in the use of dental floss, toothpicks, interspace brushes, and disclosing agents.[21,22]

The Interplak Home Plaque Removal Instrument has a brush head with 10 tufts of bristles arranged in two rows positioned to follow the gumline. Each tuft spins independently in the opposite direction of adjacent tufts at the rate of 4,200 rpm. If used properly, the Interplak is more effective than manual brushing in eliminating plaque for most patients.[23] In addition, patients with orthodontic bands may find this device beneficial.

A new addition to this category is a dental hygiene device using high-frequency sound vibrations to remove plaque. The Sonex ultrasonic toothbrush is safe for use with any toothpaste.

Selected ADA-accepted powered oral hygiene devices include the Braun/Oral-B Plaque Remover, Interplak, Home Plaque Removal Instrument, Oralgiene, Plaque Control 2000, Braun Power Toothbrush, Panasonic Power Floss and Brush, Plak Trac, Sunbeam Automatic Toothbrush and Automatic Angle Toothbrush, Rota-dent, and Stimu-gum.[13]

Oral Irrigating Devices Oral irrigators work by directing a high-pressure stream of water through a nozzle to the tooth surfaces. Studies have shown that these devices can remove only a minimal amount of plaque from tooth surfaces.[20,24] Thus, oral irrigators cannot be viewed as substitutes for a toothbrush, dental floss, or other plaque-removal devices but should be considered as adjuncts in maintaining oral hygiene.[20] The ADA views these devices as potentially useful for "removing loose debris from those areas that cannot be cleaned with the toothbrush such as around orthodontic bands and fixed bridges."[20] A multicenter study of periodontitis patients receiving supportive periodontal treatment (maintenance phase) determined that adjunctive daily water irrigation provided meaningful clinical outcomes.[25] Oral irrigators have also been valuable as vehicles for administering chemotherapeutic agents that inhibit microbial growth in inaccessible regions of the mouth.[26] Yet the ADA cautions that patients with advanced periodontal disease should use these devices only under professional supervision as it is possible for transient bacteremia to occur after manipulative procedures with the oral irrigator.[20] Oral irrigation devices should also be considered contraindicated in patients pre-disposed to bacterial endocarditis.

Two types of oral irrigation devices are available: pulsating (intermittent low- and high-water pressure) and steady-stream (constant water pressure). In general, steady-stream types are less expensive than pulsating models; however, neither type has shown superior ability to remove debris or plaque. Oral irrigators should be operated with warm or tepid water within recommended water pressure levels. Operating these devices parallel to the long axis of the teeth may traumatize soft tissue or impact food within a periodontal pocket.

The ADA has evaluated and given its seal of acceptance to several brands of irrigating devices, including Dento Spray, Hydro Pik, Interjet Gingival Care Instrument, Sunpak Aqua Floss Oral Irrigator, and Water Pik Oral Irrigator.[13]

Dental Floss Plaque accumulation in the interdental spaces contributes to proximal caries and periodontal pocketing. Interdental plaque removal has been reported to reduce gingival inflammation and prevent periodontal disease and dental caries.[20] Dental flossing is the most widely recommended method of removing dental plaque from proximal tooth surfaces not adequately cleaned by toothbrushing alone.[20] Besides removing plaque and debris interproximally, proper flossing also polishes the tooth surfaces, massages interdental papillae, and reduces gingival inflammation.

Floss is a multifilament nylon yarn that is available in waxed or unwaxed form and in varying widths, from thin thread to thick tape. New introductions in product lines feature flosses impregnated or coated with additives such as baking soda and fluoride. Also, several manufacturers are marketing floss made of materials with superior antishredding properties (eg, Glide and Colgate Precision). The low-friction fibers are especially helpful for patients with tight contacts between teeth. Because no particular product has proven superior, patient factors such as tightness of tooth contacts, tooth roughness, manual dexterity, and personal preference should be considered in product selection.[27] Similarly, clinical studies show no difference between waxed and unwaxed floss in terms of plaque removal and prevention of gingivitis,[28,29] and concern about a residual wax film deposited on tooth surfaces when using waxed floss is not supported by available evidence.[30]

Proper flossing technique requires some finger dexterity and practice. If done improperly, flossing can injure gingival tissue and cause cervical wear on proximal root surfaces.[1] Patients should be instructed to use approximately 18 in. of floss and wrap most of it around a middle finger. The remaining floss should be wound around the same finger of the opposite hand. About an inch of floss should be held between the thumbs and forefingers. The patient should not snap the floss between the teeth but should use a gentle, sawing motion to guide the floss to the gumline. When the gumline is reached, the floss should be curved into a C-shape against one tooth and gently slid into the space between the gum and tooth until there is resistance. The patient should hold the floss tightly against the tooth and gently scrape the side of the tooth while moving the floss away from the gums. Next, the patient should curve the floss around the adjoining tooth and repeat the procedure.

Waxed floss may pass interproximally between tight-fitting teeth without shredding easier than unwaxed floss. If contacts at the crowns of teeth are too tight to force floss interdentally, floss threaders can be used to pass floss between the teeth and around fixed bridges. Floss threaders, which are available in reusable and disposable forms, are usually thin plastic loops or soft plastic, needle-like appliances; in either case, the device should have one or two forks rigid enough to keep floss taut and a mounting mechanism that allows quick rethreading of floss.[27] Floss threaders should be used cautiously so as not to physically traumatize the gingiva. One manufacturer offers special precut floss with a stiff floss threader at the end (Oral-B Super Floss). Floss holders may promote compliance among some people and are recommended for patients lacking manual dexterity and for caregivers assisting handicapped or hospitalized patients. The ADA has recognized nearly 100 brands of dental floss and tape as safe and effective.[13]

Specialty Aids Cleaning devices that adapt to irregular tooth surfaces better than dental floss does are recommended for interproximal cleaning of teeth with large interdental spaces, such as is found in patients with periodontal disease.[27] Specialty brushes and aids are available to remove plaque from hard-to-clean areas (eg, spaces around a fixed bridge or orthodontic bands) and dentures. The most common aids are tapered triangular wooden toothpicks (Stim-U-Dent), holders for round toothpicks (Perio-aid), miniature bottle brushes (Py-Co-Prox or Proxabrush), rubber stimulator tips, denture brushes, and denture clasp brushes.

Conflicting findings are reported for plaque-removal efficacy among these interproximal cleaning devices. Differences in methodology and patient populations prevent generalizations while individual patient motivation and dexterity may influence results.[31] One study reported no difference in plaque-removal efficacy when comparing dental floss, an interdental brush, and a rubber tip stimulator used in addition to a toothbrush.[32] All three devices improved plaque removal in patients who brushed normally. Another study, which used a group of patients previously treated for periodontal disease, found the interdental brush superior to dental floss in removing plaque from large, open, interproximal spaces.[31] Patient oral anatomy, the presence of periodontal disease, the size of the interproximal spaces, and patient dexterity should all be considered when choosing an interdental cleaning aid.

Disclosing Agents Disclosing agents are used at home by the patient for self-evaluation of plaque removal and in the dental office when the dentist is instructing the patient in proper cleaning technique. Disclosing agents contain a vegetable dye (eg, erythrosine or FD&C Red No. 3), which stains dental plaque so that the patient can easily see it. This enables patients to evaluate their oral hygiene efforts and detect areas they missed, where more thorough brushing and flossing is indicated. The dye stains plaque but not tooth enamel, gingiva, or restorations, and it is easily rinsed away because it is soluble in water. (See color plates, photograph 2.)

Disclosing agents are available for home use as either a solution or a chewable tablet. These agents are not intended for daily or continuous long-term use; they should be used intermittently as a plaque indicator to monitor cleaning technique. Chewable tablets may be preferred for normal home use because they are individually wrapped in unit-of-use doses, thereby eliminating any problems with spilling that might occur with the liquids. The tablets are chewed, swished around the mouth, and then expectorated. Because they are sweet, usually containing mannitol or sorbitol, and brightly colored, the tablets may be mistaken for candy.[33] Thus, these products should be kept out of the reach of children, and use by children should be supervised. Solutions may be preferred in some cases because they can be applied with a cotton-tipped applicator to a handicapped patient's or child's dentition by another person, and they can be diluted with water. Disclosing products should be expectorated completely and not swallowed; the mouth should be rinsed with water and the water should also be expectorated.

Dentifrices Dentifrices are used with a toothbrush for cleaning accessible tooth surfaces. Use of a dentifrice enhances removal of dental plaque and stain, resulting in a decreased incidence of dental caries and gum disease, reduced mouth odors, and enhanced personal appearance.[7]

Dentifrices are available as powders, pastes, or gels (see product table "Dentifrice Products"). The powder forms commonly contain abrasive and flavoring agents and sometimes a surfactant (foaming agent). Dentifrice powders are either moistened to form a slurry and applied with a dry brush or used dry with a brush moistened with water. The powder is more abrasive when used dry. The anticaries tentative final monograph classified fluoride powdered forms as Category III, stating that powders were found to be imperfect as vehicles for therapeutic agents (ie, fluoride).[34] Monograph status for powdered dentifrices containing sodium fluoride with the abrasive sodium bicarbonate is supported by data submitted since the tentative final monograph was published in 1988 and will be published in the forthcoming final monograph.[35] The gels and pastes commonly contain an abrasive, a surfactant, a humectant (moistening agent), a binder/thickener, flavoring agents, a sweetener, and, commonly, a therapeutic agent, such as fluoride for anticaries activity or potassium nitrate for treating hypersensitivity.

Dentifrice abrasives are pharmacologically inactive and insoluble compounds. Common abrasives include silicates, dicalcium phosphate, alumina trihydrate, calcium pyrophosphate, calcium carbonate, and sodium metaphosphate.[7] Although dentifrices vary in their degree of abrasiveness, this is an essential property for removal of stained pellicle from teeth.[7,36] The ideal abrasive would maximally aid in cleaning and minimally cause damage to tooth surfaces. Unfortunately, because of the variance in patient brushing techniques and oral conditions, the ideal dentifrice abrasive does not exist. Although dentifrice abrasives do not pose a risk to dental enamel, the softer material of exposed root surfaces (cementum) and dentin can be damaged by toothbrushing action and excessive abrasiveness, which may lead to tooth hypersensitivity.[7]

Unless advised otherwise by their dentists, patients—especially those with periodontal disease, significant gum recession, and exposed root surfaces—should choose the least abrasive dentifrice that effectively removes stained pellicle. Low-abrasive dentifrices, which make up the great majority of dentifrice formulations currently marketed in the United States,[7] usually have a low concentration (10–25%) of silica abrasives, whereas high-abrasive dentifrices typically have higher concentrations (40–50%) of the inorganic calcium or aluminum salts listed above. Baking soda, a mild abrasive, is found in a number of dentifrices (eg, Colgate Baking Soda, Arm & Hammer Dental Care, etc). Although safe to use, toothpastes with baking soda have not been shown to be better at cleaning teeth than toothpastes without. Baking soda is water soluble, and even at higher concentrations, its polishing action is limited.[37,38]

Surfactants are incorporated into most dentifrices because their detergent action aids in removing debris. The most frequently used surfactants are sodium lauryl sulfate and sodium dodecyl benzenesulfonate.[7] There is no evidence that surfactants in dentifrices possess anticaries activity or reduce periodontal disease, and they are considered inactive ingredients by the FDA.[39]

Humectants and binding agents are used in paste and gel dentifrices. The humectant (most commonly sorbitol or glycerin) provides a vehicle for other dentifrice components, prevents the preparation from drying out, and provides microbial resistance. The binder/thickener system, which commonly uses gums and silicas,[7] determines dentifrice texture, dispersibility, and appearance. Selection of the binder/thickener is determined by its compatibility with other components of the dentifrice formulation in producing the desired qualities.

Flavoring and sweetening agents are added to these preparations to make them more appealing. Sweeteners include sorbitol, glycerin, xylitol, saccharin, sodium saccharin, and aspartame. Flavoring agents, which are selected to provide a refreshing aftertaste, include essential oils and other flavorings (eg, spearmint, wintergreen, and cinnamon).[7]

The most common therapeutic agent added to dentifrices is fluoride for its anticaries activity. Other therapeutic agents (eg, potassium nitrate) are also added to treat hypersensitive dentin.

Chemical agents to control plaque and help prevent or reduce calculus formation have received much attention as additives to dentifrices and mouthrinses. Desirable characteristics for antiplaque agents include:

- Selective antibacterial activity and/or interference with the rate of accumulation or metabolism of supragingival plaque;
- Substantivity (sustained retention of the agent in the mouth);
- Compatibility with dentifrice ingredients;
- Lack of undesirable side effects for the user;
- Noninterference with the natural ecology of the normal oral microflora.[40,41]

Several dentifrice manufacturers make claims of antiplaque or tartar control effectiveness. Agents with antiplaque potential for inclusion in dentifrices include plant extracts (sanguinarine), metal salts (zinc and stannous), phenolic compounds (triclosan), and essential oils (thymol and eucalyptol).[40–42] The antibacterial triclosan is used in toothpastes marketed abroad. In a review of clinical studies on sanguinarine-containing dentifrices, however, only one in five trials reported a significant antiplaque effect.[43] Combinations of ingredients (eg, triclosan and zinc citrate) have been shown to reduce plaque accumulation significantly and to be more effective at lower concentrations than either agent alone at higher concentrations.[40,42] There are few clinical data to support inclusion of enzymes (eg, dextranases and oxidases) for antiplaque purposes, and quaternary ammonium compounds are incompatible with most conventional toothpaste ingredients.[42]

However, no dentifrice is currently accepted by the ADA as efficacious in the antiplaque/antigingivitis therapeutic category, and patients should not forgo the benefits of fluoride in favor of chemical antiplaque ingredients. Manufacturers of dentifrices with therapeutic potential for gingivitis and supragingival dental plaque control may voluntarily submit data to the ADA for evaluation. To gain the ADA seal for this therapeutic effect, the product must fulfill very stringent ADA guidelines.[44] Certain fluoride dentifrices for which antiplaque claims are made bear the ADA seal of approval for their anticaries effect only. The CDT requires that accepted fluoride dentifrices that contain peroxide, baking soda, or a combination of the two include a statement on package labeling and advertising that indicates that peroxide and baking soda, alone or in combination, have not been shown to have a therapeutic effect on periodontal diseases.[45]

A number of fluoride dentifrices containing anticalculus or tartar-control compounds are currently being marketed. Although plaque, not supragingival calculus, is the primary etiologic factor in marginal periodontal disease, the reduction of calculus formation is still a goal of oral hygiene.[7,46] The ingredients incorporated to prevent or retard new calculus formation are zinc chloride, zinc citrate, and soluble pyrophosphates, which act to inhibit crystal growth. Placebo-controlled clinical studies have reported efficacy; findings have shown significant reduction in calculus occurrence and severity.[46,47] Patients who form heavy calculus between dental visits may consider using a fluoride dentifrice with added tartar-control ingredients instead of a plain fluoride dentifrice. A patient's appearance may benefit from a lessening of visible supragingival calculus buildup, and reports indicate that professional dental cleaning may be easier because the calculus that does form is less adherent.[48]

The ADA regards inhibition of supragingival calculus as a nontherapeutic use and therefore does not evaluate anticalculus claims. However, all advertising claims made for accepted products are reviewed for accuracy. The ADA has directed that the following additional statement appear on all package and container labeling for accepted fluoride dentifrice products with calculus-control activity: "[Product name] has been shown to reduce the formation of tartar above the gumline, but has not been shown to have a therapeutic effect on periodontal diseases."[48]

Use of tartar-control toothpastes has been related to a type of contact dermatitis in the perioral region.[49] The addition of pyrophosphate compounds to these products increases alkalinity and requires increased concentrations of other components, such as flavorings and surfactants for solubilizing. It is hypothesized that the pyrophosphates, either alone or in combination with the higher concentrations of inactive ingredients, are implicated as the cause of irritant contact dermatitis. Patients experiencing such a reaction should be advised to discontinue the tartar-control dentifrice and switch to a non–tartar-control fluoride product. The skin eruption has been shown to resolve by decreasing or eliminating exposure.[49]

Cosmetic dentifrices make no therapeutic claims and are usually chosen by patients because of taste, whitening ability, or antistain properties. Some dentifrices claiming to remove stubborn coffee or tobacco stains may contain higher concentrations of abrasives. High-abrasive formulations are not advised for long-term use or for use by patients with exposed root surfaces. Plain baking soda, which is a mild abrasive, or toothpastes containing baking soda have limited polishing and stain removal capacity. Other products may contain a pigment (eg, titanium dioxide) that produces a temporary brightening effect. Rembrandt Whitening Toothpaste contains a chemical complex of aluminum oxide, a citrate salt, and papain. Whitening dentifrices containing oxygenating agents depend on debriding action to remove stained pellicle. Recent market entries combine baking soda and peroxide with fluoride (eg, Arm & Hammer Peroxicare, Mentadent, Triplex).

Popular gel dentifrices are flavored and disperse rapidly in the mouth. Manufacturers of gel dentifrices have advertised that children brush longer and more thoroughly because of the gel's consistency, translucence, dispersibility, and flavor. This claim has not been substantiated, but many dentifrices marketed for children are of the gel type. The children's products usually have fruit flavors rather than the breath-freshening minty or cinnamon flavors that adults prefer.

Mouthrinses (Mouthwashes) Mouthrinse and dentifrice formulations are very similar. Like dentifrices, mouthrinses may be cosmetic or therapeutic (see product table "Oral Hygiene Products"). Both may contain surfactant(s), humectant(s), flavor, coloring, water, and therapeutic ingredient(s). A mouthrinse approximates a diluted liquid dentifrice containing ethanol and no abrasive. Alcohol adds bite and freshness, enhances flavor, solubilizes other ingredients, and contributes to the cleansing action and antibacterial activity. Flavor contributes to pleasant taste and breath freshening. Surfactants are foaming agents that aid in removal of debris. Other ingredients may include astringents, demulcents (soothing agents), antibacterial agents, and fluoride.[7] New additions to the mouthrinse category include dry formulations that contain ingestible surfactants rather than alcohol (Spritz) and a nonaerosol gel formulation (Morgan & Berry Breath Gel).

Mouthrinses can be classified by appearance, alcohol content, and active ingredients. In general, mouthrinses are minty (green or blue) or spicy (red), medicinal or alcoholic, and they contain various miscellaneous ingredients, such as glycerin, a topical protectant that tastes sweet and is soothing to oral mucosa; benzoic acid, an antimicrobial agent; and zinc chloride/citrate, an astringent that neutralizes odoriferous sulfur compounds produced in the oral cavity. Cosmetic mouthrinses freshen the breath and clean some debris. The most popular cosmetic mouthrinses are phenolic (medicinal) and mint flavored. To have some degree of oral malodor (eg, morning breath) is normal in a healthy individual. This is because reduced activity of tongue, cheeks, and salivary flow enhance bacterial activity and production of odoriferous sulfur compounds.[7] Thus, products that are intended to eliminate or suppress mouth odor of local origin in healthy persons with healthy mouths are considered by the FDA Advisory Review Panel on Over-the-Counter Oral Health Care Products to be cosmetics unless they contain antimicrobial or other therapeutic agents,[50] and the ADA acceptance program does not evaluate mouthrinses labeled and advertised only as cosmetic agents. An important consideration is the potential for breath-freshening mouthrinses to disguise and delay treatment of pathologic conditions that may contribute to lingering oral malodor (eg, periodontal disease, purulent oral infections, and respiratory infections). The ADA suggests that "if marked breath odor persists after proper toothbrushing, the cause should be investigated" and not masked with mouthrinse.[20]

The alcohol content in mouthrinses ranges from zero to 27%; most popular adult mouthrinses contain between 14% and 27%.[51] This issue has drawn attention for two reasons. Ingestion of alcohol-containing products poses a danger for children, who may be attracted by bright colors and pleasant flavors, and there is a potential association between the use of mouthrinses containing alcohol and an increased risk of oral cancer.

Toxicity data concerning children's ingestion of ethanol-containing mouthrinse demonstrate that the amount of ethanol in available mouthrinse preparations is sufficient to cause serious illness and injury to children.[51] Acute alcoholic intoxication and death resulting from high-dose ingestion is possible.[1] Clearly, these products should be kept out of the reach of children. Responding to concern over the potential danger to children, the Consumer Products Safety Commission issued a final rule in January 1995[51] requiring child-resistant packaging for mouthrinses with 3 g or more of absolute ethanol per package—the amount that is present in a small quantity (approximately 2.6 oz) of mouthrinse with 5% ethanol. "For the purposes of this final rule, the term *mouthwash* includes liquid products that are variously called mouthwashes, mouthrinses, oral antiseptics, gargles, fluoride rinses, anti-plaque rinses, and breath fresheners. It does not include throat sprays or aerosol breath fresheners."[51]

The Dental Products Panel continues to consider the use of alcohol in oral health care products. The FDA Plaque Subcommittee has recommended that the alcohol content of mouthrinse products be clearly stated on the principal display panel and that epidemiologic studies on mouthrinse use by nonsmokers and nonalcohol drinkers are needed to further investigate a possible connection between the use of alcohol-containing mouthrinse and oral cancer.[52] These preliminary recommendations were accepted by the Dental Products Panel in December 1994 and will be considered in the panel's final report.

Alcohol-free formulations in the various mouthrinse categories, such as Clear Choice and Rembrandt Breath Refreshing Rinse, are entering the market. In the nonprescription fluoride rinse category, Act Fluoride Anti-Cavity Rinse is now alcohol free as well.

Over the last decade, nonprescription mouthrinses promoted for antiplaque or tartar-control activity have proliferated. Ingredients added to mouthrinses for plaque control include plant extracts (sanguinarine); aromatic oils (thymol, eucalyptol, menthol, and methyl salicylate), which are antibacterial and have some local anesthetic activity; and agents with antimicrobial activity such as quaternary ammonium compounds. Of the latter, cetylpyridinium chloride is a cationic surfactant capable of bactericidal activity although it does not penetrate plaque well, and domiphen bromide is a bactericidal agent similar to cetylpyridinium. Another ingredient, phenol, is a local anesthetic, antiseptic, and bactericidal agent that penetrates plaque better than either cetylpyridinium or domiphen.

Regarding products for chemotherapeutic control

of plaque and gingivitis, the ADA acceptance program invites manufacturers to submit data voluntarily.[44] Listerine was the first mouthrinse to be accepted by the ADA as a nonprescription antiplaque/antigingivitis mouthrinse; its mechanism of action involves bacterial cell wall destruction, bacterial enzymatic inhibition, and extraction of bacterial lipopolysaccharides.[53] The ADA has authorized use of the following label statement:

> Listerine has been shown to help prevent and reduce supragingival plaque accumulation and gingivitis when used in a conscientiously applied program of oral hygiene and regular professional care. It has not been shown to have a therapeutic effect on periodontitis.[54]

The ADA has since accepted Cool Mint Listerine and an increasing number of private-label antiseptic mouthrinses in the antiplaque/antigingivitis category of accepted therapeutic products.[13]

The quaternary ammonium compounds and sanguinarine compounds have some merit, but studies of their efficacy in plaque and gingivitis reduction are mixed.[53] Viadent rinse contains sanguinaria extract in combination with zinc chloride. Although sanguinarine has shown effectiveness against plaque-forming bacteria in vitro, results from controlled clinical trials using the rinse alone or in conjunction with Viadent dentifrice have been mixed. Widely divergent findings ranging from significant reduction of plaque and gingivitis to negligible or no effect have been reported in numerous short-term and several long-term clinical studies.[43]

Clinical trials with mouthrinses containing cetylpyridinium chloride alone or in combination with domiphen bromide have reported reductions in plaque accumulation.[55] Based on available data, the potential for oral toxicity with these agents is low, and the potential for a gingival health benefit exists.[7,41,56] However, studies consistent with ADA guidelines have not been evaluated, and further study is needed to substantiate antigingivitis efficacy. At least one study has reported no difference in plaque control and gingival health between a cetylpyridinium rinse and placebo when the former was used as a prebrushing rinse.[56] It was suggested that the order of rinsing and brushing may be relevant: reduced activity may have been influenced by the interaction of the cationic surfactant with anionic detergents in the toothpaste. Rinsing after brushing or at a time separate from brushing may be indicated. Cepacol, Scope, Clear Choice, and Oral-B Anti-Plaque Rinse are examples of products in this category. Because cetylpyridinium is chemically related to chlorhexidine, it too may stain teeth but to a much lesser degree.[56] Staining is usually associated with overuse.

Another approach to plaque control does not rely on antimicrobial activity but is based on principles of surfactant action to loosen plaque. Plax, intended for use as a prebrushing rinse, has been reformulated. The new product, Advanced Formula Plax, contains an enhanced level of detergent (sodium lauryl sulfate) and the addition of detergent builders tetrasodium pyrophosphate and sodium benzoate. Findings reported in clinical trials with the original formula were contradictory. While there were early reports of efficacy for plaque removal in short-term clinical trials,[57,58] a number of studies reported results comparable to those of placebo.[59–61] A more recent clinical study that evaluated the new formula showed it to effect statistically significant reductions in subjects' plaque levels compared with placebo.[62]

Mouthrinses claiming anticalculus or tartar-control activity contain the same active ingredients as anticalculus dentifrices. While the ADA regards inhibition of supragingival calculus as a nontherapeutic use and does not evaluate mouthrinse anticalculus claims, the FDA included these mouthrinses in the aforementioned 1990 call for data on ingredients contained in products bearing antiplaque and antiplaque-related claims and will eventually rule on safety and effectiveness for this indication.[11]

Patients should be cautioned that use of a mouthrinse with plaque or calculus control properties does not substitute for normal oral hygiene. These products are adjunctive to proper toothbrushing and flossing, and in most cases, further research is necessary to determine how efficacious their antiplaque activity is. In the meantime, the benefits of fluoride should not be overlooked in favor of a plaque-control formula without fluoride.

Mouthrinses are intended for use twice daily after brushing, with the exception of Advanced Formula Plax, which should be used prior to brushing. In general, an amount equal to 1–2 tbsp of rinse should be swished vigorously in the mouth and between the teeth for about 30 seconds and then expectorated; the rinses should not be swallowed. Patients should be advised to refrain from smoking, eating, or drinking for 30 minutes following use. These products are generally safe when used as directed, but occasional adverse reactions (eg, burning sensation, irritation) have been reported. Overuse should be discouraged. Consultation with a health professional is indicated if irritation occurs and persists after use of the product is discontinued. Unsupervised use is contraindicated in patients with mouth irritation or ulceration. These products should be kept out of the reach of children.[55]

Tooth Whiteners Tooth whiteners, which claim to bleach teeth, contain oxidizing ingredients such as hydrogen peroxide, carbamide peroxide, or perhydrol urea in gel or liquid form. These products were previously marketed as cosmetics but are now considered drugs by the FDA. The drug classification makes the products subject to rigorous new drug application requirements to document their safety and effectiveness. Safety concerns relate to the long-term exposure of oral tissue to oxidizing agents. These concerns include (1) the possibility of soft tissue damage or delayed wound healing, (2) the potential for damage to tooth pulp, and (3) the potential for mutating or enhancing the carcinogenic effects of other agents (eg, tobacco).[63] The CDT approved safety and efficacy guidelines for peroxide-containing oral hygiene products for dentist-prescribed/home use whitening agents and has accepted two professional products intended for office use.[64,65] The ADA accepts none of the available nonprescription products for unsupervised consumer use as a tooth-whitening agent.[64]

Early reports of dentist-supervised home bleaching of natural teeth began with the use of nonprescription products containing 10% topical carbamide peroxide (Gly-Oxide and Proxigel) that were intended for oral wound cleansing.[66] Patients were instructed to expose extrinsically stained teeth to the peroxide gel by using custom-made mouth trays coated with a thin gel film. Anecdotal reports of successful tooth bleaching emerged. One double-blind study reported effective whitening with minimal and reversible adverse effects (eg, unpleasant taste, burning palate and gingiva, gingival ulceration and tooth sensitivity) during treatment.[63] Products specifically marketed to dentists for home tooth bleaching (Platinum Professional Toothwhitening System, Rembrandt Lighten Gel) also contain 10% carbamide peroxide as the active oxidizing agent. Patients should be strongly discouraged from attempting tooth bleaching without a dentist's direct supervision because serious adverse effects (ie, loss of surface enamel) resulting from misuse or overuse of such products have been reported.[67]

Periodontal Disease

Periodontal disease is associated with oral hygiene status, not age. As life spans increase and people retain more teeth later in life, both the number of teeth at risk and the time for risk of periodontal disease increases.[1]

Etiology and Pathophysiology

The primary etiologic cause of periodontal disease is accumulated bacterial plaque.[68] The basic pathologic process is inflammatory. The more common forms of periodontal disease are gingivitis (an inflammation of the gingiva), which is the mildest form, is reversible, and affects nearly everyone; acute necrotizing ulcerative gingivitis (ANUG); and periodontitis, which, when severe, can cause significant, irreversible alveolar bone loss.

Gingivitis The etiology of gingivitis is thought to be associated with the accumulation of supragingival plaque. The marginal gingiva (the border of the gingiva surrounding the neck of the tooth) is held firmly to the tooth by a network of collagen fibers. Microorganisms present in the plaque in the gingival sulcus (the space between the gingiva and the tooth) are capable of producing harmful products such as acids, toxins, and enzymes that damage cellular and intercellular tissue. Dilatation and proliferation of gingival capillaries, increased flow of gingival fluid, and increased blood flow with resultant erythema of the gingiva are found in early stages. The gingiva may also enlarge, change contour, and appear puffy or swollen as a result of the inflammation. (See color plates, photograph 3.) The inflamed gingiva generally bleeds readily when probed or during toothbrushing; pink-tinted toothbrush bristles should be a sign to patients of possible gingivitis. In the early stage of gingivitis, it is possible to reverse the inflammatory process with effective oral hygiene.

In time and with neglect, the condition becomes chronic as capillaries become engorged, venous return is slowed, and localized anoxemia gives a bluish hue to areas of the reddened gingiva. Chronic gingivitis may be localized to the area around one or several teeth, or it may be generalized, involving the gingiva around all the teeth. The inflammation may involve just the marginal gingiva, or it may be more diffuse and involve all the gingival tissue surrounding the tooth. Changes in gingival color, size, and shape, and ease of gingival bleeding, are common indications of chronic gingivitis that the patient as well as the pharmacist can recognize. The flat knife-edge appearance of healthy gingiva is replaced by a ragged or rounded edge. The presence of red cells in extravascular tissue and the breakdown of hemoglobin also deepen the color of gingival tissue. Progression of these conditions is usually slow and insidious, and often painless.

Left untreated, chronic gingivitis is a common precursor to the more advanced inflammatory condition of chronic destructive periodontal disease, or periodontitis. Bacterial species that predominate in periodontitis but are not present in healthy periodontium have been found in low proportions in gingivitis. Progression of pathophysiology in gingivitis may favor the growth of bacterial species implicated in the genesis of periodontitis.

Acute Necrotizing Ulcerative Gingivitis ANUG, also referred to as Vincent's stomatitis and trench mouth, is an acute bacterial infection characterized by necrosis and ulceration of the gingival surface with underlying inflammation. The disease most commonly starts in the gingiva between teeth and displays "punched-out" papillae (the raised interproximal gingiva). The interdental and marginal gingivae exhibit a necrotic and grayish slough while the adjacent gingiva usually exhibits marked erythema. The disease may involve a single tooth, a group of teeth, or the entire oral cavity. Accompanying symptoms often include severe pain, bleeding gingival tissue, halitosis, foul taste, and increased salivation. Lymphadenopathy, fever, and malaise may accompany the localized symptoms.

ANUG is seen most frequently in the United States in teenagers and young adults. Predisposing factors include anxiety, emotional stress, smoking, malnutrition, and poor oral hygiene. Factors resulting in decreased host resistance that alter the host-bacteria relationship have been implicated.[69] Professional dental treatment is indicated and consists of local debridement and systemic drug therapy coupled with elimination of predisposing factors.

Periodontitis Periodontitis and gingivitis, the two most common periodontal diseases, can be distinguished in the following way. Whereas gingivitis is the inflammation of the gingiva without loss or migration of epithelial attachment to the tooth, periodontitis occurs when the periodontal ligament attachment and alveolar bone support of the tooth have been compromised or lost.[70] This process involves apical migration of the epithelial attachment from the enamel to the root surface. (See color plates, photograph 4.)

The American Academy of Periodontology (AAP) has classified periodontal disease in adults as follows[70]:

- *AAP classification*: Type I, Type II, Type III, and Type IV;
- *Epidemiologic*: moderately and rapidly progressing;
- *Clinical (based on response to treatment)*: refractory and recurrent.

The AAP describes Type I adult periodontitis as gingivitis characterized by changes in color, form, position, and surface appearance, and by the presence of bleeding or exudate. Type II is slight periodontitis characterized by the progression of gingival inflammation into deeper tissues and the alveolar bony crest. The periodontal pocket is 3–4 mm deep, and there is slight loss of connective attachment and alveolar bone. Type III is moderate periodontitis characterized by a noticeable loss of bone support and possible increased tooth mobility. Type IV is advanced periodontitis characterized by a major loss of alveolar bone support usually accompanied by increased tooth mobility.[70]

Adult periodontitis, especially slight or moderate, is very common. Most adults with periodontitis have moderately progressing disease, and perhaps 10% have rapidly progressing disease. As shown in the AAP classification system, diagnosis of adult periodontal disease can be based on the response to therapy.[70] Recurrent periodontitis is the destruction of the attachment apparatus occurring in a patient who has been successfully treated in the past. It often results from inadequate maintenance therapy and is relatively common. It appears to occur in localized areas but may be generalized in immunodeficient patients. Refractory, progressive periodontitis displays a continuous progression that is resistant to therapy.[70]

The AAP has classified periodontal disease in juveniles as either localized or generalized. However, periodontitis in juveniles is relatively rare. Localized juvenile periodontitis (LJP) affects less than 1% of teenagers and young adults; children in the 10- to 15-year age range are at greatest risk.[70] LJP is characterized by pocket formation, attachment loss, and alveolar bone loss primarily affecting the first molars and incisors of the permanent dentition. Occasionally, premolars and second molars are involved. These patients rarely display gingivitis and have little or no plaque or calculus. LJP displays a marked familial tendency and is associated with a particular type of bacteria. Generalized juvenile periodontitis (GJP) affects a slightly older age group and is even less prevalent than LJP. Severe gingival inflammation with extensive plaque and calculus deposits distinguishes GJP from LJP.

A dental periodontal examination includes an assessment of the gingiva and attachment apparatus and an examination of the entire periodontium with a charting of all teeth in the dental record. The gingiva is assessed visually and by gingival bleeding measurements. Pocket depth and attachment levels are measured by periodontal probing. Tooth mobility measurements and a radiographic survey of alveolar bone levels should also be included.[70] Patients have a good prognosis if an initial comprehensive course of therapy is successful. Unfortunately, alveolar bone loss is irreversible. Prospects for disease control are not good if plaque and calculus control is poor or if resolution of inflammation is inadequate despite comprehensive treatment.[70]

Preventive Measures for Periodontal Disease

Adequate removal and control of supragingival plaque is the single most important factor in reversing gingivitis and preventing and controlling periodontal disease. If the accumulation of supragingival plaque is not controlled, it proliferates and invades subgingival spaces. At the same time, as specific types of bacteria are associated with plaque at different stages of accumulation, the composition of the bacterial flora changes to a more complex mix of organisms.[71] The transition from supragingival to subgingival plaque accumulation is significant because the patient cannot remove the subgingival plaque adequately by mechanical means. Thus, the accumulation of supragingival plaque over time can eventually result in gingivitis. Although not all periodontitis is preceded by gingivitis, the progression from supragingival plaque to gingivitis to periodontitis is relatively common, so that controlling gingivitis is a reasonable approach to limiting periodontitis.[44]

Dental Caries

Etiology and Pathophysiology

Dental caries is a destructive microbial disease that affects the calcified tissues of the teeth. Certain plaque bacteria generate acid from dietary carbohydrates; the acid demineralizes tooth enamel, leading to the formation of carious lesions that will eventually destroy the tooth if left untreated. Dental caries formation requires growth and implantation of cariogenic microorganisms (eg, *Streptococcus mutans*, *Lactobacillus casei*, and *Actinomyces viscosus*) on exposed surfaces. If oral hygiene is neglected, dental plaque containing these organisms remains on the tooth surfaces, allowing the carious process to proceed.

The carious process is characterized by alternating periods of destruction and repair. Demineralization is caused by organic acids, such as lactic acid, produced (usually anaerobically) by microorganisms present in dental plaque. Low molecular weight carbohydrates (sugars) readily diffuse into plaque and are quickly metabolized by the bacteria, resulting in a lowered plaque pH. The pH is reduced to a level that can cause demineralization of dental enamel. Repeated and frequent sugar intake will keep plaque pH depressed and thus support the demineralization. This demineralization is chronic in nature. A carious lesion starts slowly on the enamel surface and initially produces no clinical symptoms. Once the demineralization progresses through the enamel to the softer dentin, the destruction is much more rapid and becomes clinically evident as a carious lesion. At this point, the patient can become aware of the process by visualization or by symptoms of sensitivity to stimuli, such as heat, cold, or percussion (chewing). If untreated, the carious lesion can result in damage to the dental pulp itself (with continuous pain as a common symptom) and, eventually, in necrosis of vital pulp tissue. Because an opening exists between the pulp and surrounding supporting tissues via the apical foramen, the infectious process can progress apically and result in bone loss, abscesses, cellulitis, or osteomyelitis. Saliva, rich in calcium and phosphate ions, has a role in remineralizing early carious lesions. Fluoride ion in the mouth also promotes remineralization and thus retards enamel dissolution.

Although sucrose is the most cariogenic sugar, other types of fermentable carbohydrates, such as fructose and lactose, also are cariogenic.[10] Oral hygiene products such as mouthrinses and dentifrices may contain low concentrations of saccharin, a potent noncariogenic sugar substitute, that appear to present no hazard.[7] The FDA limit on saccharin is 1.0 g per day for adults; ingestion from normal use of both mouthrinse and dentifrice would result in a total saccharin exposure of only about 20–40 mg per day.[7] Other sugar substitutes such as sorbitol, xylitol, and aspartame are currently used to sweeten a wide variety of products. Claims for the noncariogenicity of sorbitol need substantiation through further clinical trials.[1] Xylitol has been shown to be noncariogenic, and aspartame appears to be so. Some clinical trials have reported that xylitol-containing chewing gum is cariostatic.[72] Gum chewing is associated with increased salivary flow, which apparently produces a beneficial buffering effect against acids in the oral cavity.[73]

Preventive Measures for Dental Caries

Because a combination of diet (carbohydrate substrate), oral bacteria, and host resistance is involved in the process, intervention to prevent dental caries should be aimed at modifying these factors.[7] Frequency of refined carbohydrate intake should be reduced; plaque, which supports cariogenic bacterial growth, should be removed as discussed previously; and host resistance should be increased through appropriate exposure to fluoride ion. The declining prevalence of dental caries in children may be attributed to a combination of these interventions (eg, increased exposure to fluoride in drinking water, dentifrices, and mouthrinses; changed patterns of diet; and improved oral hygiene).[10]

The Role of Fluoride Fluoride is thought to help prevent dental caries through a combination of effects. Incorporated into developing teeth, fluoride systemically reduces the solubility of dental enamel by enhancing the development of a fluoridated hydroxyapatite (which is more resistant to demineralizing acids) at the enamel surface. The topical effect may aid in remineralizing early carious lesions during repeated cycles of demineralization and remineralization. There is some evidence that fluoride interferes with the bacterial cariogenic process. Fluoride that is chemically bound to organic constituents of plaque may interfere with plaque adherence and may inhibit glycolysis, the process by which sugar is metabolized to produce acid. Another possible mechanism proposes that fluoride may have specific bactericidal action on cariogenic bacteria in the plaque.[2]

Fluoridation of the public water supply is an effective and economically sound public health measure that has played a major role in decreasing the incidence of caries. More than half of the US population resides in communities whose public water supply contains either naturally occurring or added fluoride at optimal levels for decay prevention (eg, 1 ppm or 1 mg/L).[74] Besides the reduction of dental caries in children, benefits of fluoridation extend through adulthood, resulting in fewer decayed, missing, or filled teeth; greater tooth retention; and a lower incidence of root caries. Systemic fluoride supplementation in children is based on the preventive mechanism of fluoride when incorporated into developing enamel. Current concepts of the action of fluoride relative to its presence in saliva and plaque provide a rationale for its topical application to prevent caries in all age groups. It must be noted, however, that any decision to supplement fluoride intake must take into account the concentration of fluoride present in the drinking water.[20,75]

Nonprescription topical fluoride-containing products such as dentifrices, mouthrinses, and self-applied gels provide a means of increasing contact of fluoride with the tooth surfaces, where fluoride exerts its greatest protection (see product table "Topical Fluoride Products").[76] But although brushing with a fluoride dentifrice provides anticaries protection, the fluoride does not reach the surfaces between teeth adequately. Thus, patient groups with high caries activity or risk (eg, orthodontic or medically compromised patients, patients with a nonfluoridated water supply, and patients with exposed root surfaces) may especially benefit from multiple sources of fluoride application. Fluoride-containing dental products are thought to be of greatest benefit when used in areas with a nonfluoridated public water supply; however, they can help reduce the caries incidence even in patients residing in communities with a fluoridated water supply.[20] The FDA has proposed that the following statement be applied to fluoride-containing dental care products: "The combined daily use of a fluoride treatment ('rinse' or 'gel') and a fluoride toothpaste can aid in reducing the incidence of dental cavities."[77]

Fluoride Dentifrices Use of fluoride-containing dentifrices is the one method of caries prevention common to all countries that show a reduction in caries (see product table "Dentifrice Products").[78] Fluoride-containing toothpaste and gel dentifrice formulations with abrasive systems compatible with delivery of the fluoride compound are accepted by the ADA as being safe and effective in caries prevention. Powder dentifrices were in question as vehicles for fluoride delivery because of concern that the amount of fluoride ion delivered to the teeth may vary significantly with patient application. The FDA proposed classifying powdered fluoride-containing dentifrices in Category III but continues to evaluate data.[34,35]

Sodium monofluorophosphate (0.76% or 0.80%) has been the most widely used fluoride compound because of its compatibility with a variety of abrasive systems; most dentifrices contain 0.24% sodium fluoride.[20] The FDA has classified as Category I and equated the efficacy of 0.22% sodium fluoride, 0.76% sodium monofluorophosphate, and 0.4% stannous fluoride dentifrices containing 1,000 ppm fluoride ion in a compatible base.[77] It found inadequate evidence to support differences in clinical effectiveness among these different fluoride agents. Moreover, in a review of approximately 51 studies comparing a fluoride toothpaste (either sodium fluoride or sodium monofluorophosphate) with placebo, no major differences were found and both agents produced an overall average caries reduction rate of 21–22%.[79]

Included among the ADA-accepted dentifrices are the standard 1,000-ppm and 1,100-ppm fluoride ion concentrations as well as a more recent 1,500-ppm fluoride ion product. This extra-strength monofluorophosphate product is clinically and statistically superior to its regular-strength counterpart.[80] However, because of concerns about excessive fluoride ingestion in children, the current ADA limit of 260 mg of fluoride per dentifrice container has been retained, and the ADA has required that the following directions appear on the Extra-Strength Aim carton:

- Not for use by children under 2 years of age;
- To prevent swallowing, children 6 years of age or

younger should be supervised while using the dentifrice;
- Brush teeth thoroughly, at least once daily.[80]

Fluoride Mouthrinses and Gels ADA-accepted nonprescription fluoride mouthrinse products for topical home use include ACT, ACT for Kids, Reach Fluoride Dental Rinse, Fluorigard, Oral-B Rinse Therapy Anti-Cavity Treatment, and Slimer Fluoride Anti-Cavity Rinse.[65] These mouthrinses are therapeutic in that their common ingredient, 0.05% sodium fluoride, is a consistently effective anticaries agent. A number of fluoride gels are accepted by the ADA as well. Active ingredients of the gel formulations intended for home use are neutral or acidulated 1.1% sodium fluoride or 0.4% stannous fluoride.

Fluoride mouthrinsing enables patients to apply fluoride interproximally. Studies of fluoride mouthrinsing have given consistently positive results. Studies in which subjects used 0.05% sodium fluoride rinse once daily have demonstrated a significant reduction in caries incidence (by 17–47%), especially among children living in areas with nonfluoridated water.[81] Orthodontic patients may benefit because they are at risk of developing decalcified areas while under treatment and their ability to clean interdental spaces thoroughly may be inhibited.[81]

Fluoride rinses provide a therapeutic fluoride treatment; they should not be confused with a mouthrinse, and package directions should be followed closely. When recommending a nonprescription sodium fluoride mouthrinse, the pharmacist should stress that:

- The fluoride rinse should be used after brushing the teeth with toothpaste and should be expectorated;
- A measured dose of the rinse (most commonly 10 mL) should be vigorously swished between the teeth for 1 minute;
- Nothing should be taken by mouth for 30 minutes after use;
- The mouthrinse can benefit the patient for as long as the patient has natural dentition;
- The fluoride is preventive in action and will not cure already-carious teeth.[82]

The self-applied fluoride gels are used once daily after the teeth are brushed with a fluoride dentifrice. The gel is a fluoride treatment and should not be confused with a gel form of fluoride dentifrice. The gel is brushed on the teeth, left for 1 minute, and then expectorated, not swallowed. Some concern has been raised about whether unsupervised home use of the fluoride gels is justified.[81]

Orofacial Pain

Toothache

Toothache usually indicates dental pathology involving tooth substance, dental pulp, or the supporting periodontium. Pain may also be referred to the teeth from the sinuses, eyes, or ears. Untreated dental caries will progress to destroy the barrier of enamel and dentin, allowing bacteria to reach the pulp. The inflammatory response to bacteria in the pulp will stimulate free nerve endings, resulting in pulpalgia or common toothache. The nociceptors in dental pulp are capable of only one perception in response to any stimulus strong enough to elicit a response.[83] That perception is pain. Pain may be intermittent, often indicating viable pulp with reversible damage. If pain is continuous and throbbing, this usually indicates irreversible pulp damage.

The FDA has limited the definition of an agent for the relief of toothache to "ingredients placed in a tooth cavity to relieve throbbing, persistent pain resulting from an open cavity in the tooth."[84] Currently, there are no Category I agents for this purpose. Topical oral mucosal anesthetics/analgesics classified as Category I for relief of pain associated with minor irritation or injury to soft tissue are not considered effective for relieving toothache from a cavity and have been classified as Category III for this purpose. Also, the FDA has reclassified eugenol from Category I to Category III, citing the need for controlled clinical investigations that demonstrate its effectiveness in relieving toothache.[84] The ADA accepts eugenol and clove oil for professional use by the dentist; however, although 85% eugenol has historically been used as a nonprescription toothache remedy, the ADA has not accepted eugenol or clove oil as safe and effective nonprescription drugs for toothache. These drugs are generally ineffective in the hands of the patient and can cause damage to viable pulp and soft tissue.

The FDA advisory review panel has recommended that beeswax not be included as an inactive ingredient in products intended for use in an open tooth cavity.[84] Such occlusive inactive ingredients are discouraged because they form a physical barrier and may prevent the escape of fluids and gases from a degenerating pulp. Of equal concern is the potential for patients to use the product as a temporary filling and to delay seeking professional treatment.

The patient with toothache should be advised to seek professional dental assistance. If swelling or fever is present, this usually indicates the need for antibiotic therapy. If the patient wears a removable prosthesis that attaches to the painful tooth, removing the appliance may help temporarily. Nonprescription analgesics such as ibuprofen, aspirin, or acetaminophen may be taken internally for short-term pain relief; however, none of these products, and particularly not aspirin, should ever be placed locally on gingival tissue or in a cavity; doing so can result in chemical burns of sensitive tissue. (See color plates, photograph 5.) Even if aspirin, ibuprofen, or acetaminophen is effective in relieving pain due to toothache, the patient should seek professional dental help as soon as possible.

Hypersensitive Teeth

Tooth hypersensitivity affects approximately 40 million adults at some time, and about one fourth of these adults experience a chronic condition.[36] Hypersensitive teeth result from exposed areas of the root at the cementoenamel junction. Exposed dentin allows stimuli to reach the nerve fibers within the pulp. Causes of dentinal hypersensitivity may relate to braces, a postsurgical condition, gum recession, trauma, or excessive brushing with an abrasive dentifrice or hard bristle brush. Pain may be intense and may condition patients to limit oral hygiene, which in turn will contribute to plaque accumulation and the progression of oral plaque diseases.[85] A patient who has self-diagnosed sensitive teeth should be referred to a dentist for consultation because there may be an underlying cause for pain that requires immediate treatment. However, once the dentist diagnoses the pain as dentinal hypersensitivity, this condition can be treated with a desensitizing dentifrice.

A tooth desensitizer acts on the dentin to block the perception of stimuli that are not usually perceived by subjects with normal teeth. Because the most common cause of tooth sensitivity is exposed dentin, a desensitizing dentifrice must inhibit sensitization while being nonabrasive. Two well-controlled clinical studies and three supportive studies provided sufficient data to the FDA to establish the effectiveness of 5% potassium nitrate for protection against painful sensitivity of the teeth due to cold, heat, acids, sweets, or contact. As a tooth desensitizer, 5% potassium nitrate remains the only Category I agent at this time.[84] Dibasic sodium citrate in pluronic gel and 10% strontium chloride were classified as Category III pending further evidence of effectiveness.

Patients should be advised to apply at least a 1-in. strip of dentifrice to a soft bristle brush and to use the product twice daily for optimum effectiveness. Brushing thoroughly for at least 1 minute will apply the desensitizing agent to all sensitive surfaces. Onset of effect is not immediate and may take several days to 2 weeks. These dentifrices should be used until the sensitivity subsides or as long as a dentist recommends. The patient should then switch to a low-abrasion dentifrice. Patients with hypersensitive teeth should avoid any toothpaste that is highly abrasive or promoted for its whitening effect.

The FDA has proposed a Category I classification for the combination of a Category I fluoride ingredient with 5% potassium nitrate for use in relieving dentinal hypersensitivity and preventing dental caries.[86] Such a product (eg, Sensodyne for Sensitive Teeth and Cavity Prevention, Crest Sensitivity Protection Mild Mint Paste) would be a good recommendation. However, dentifrices containing 5% potassium nitrate are not recommended for children under 12 years of age.

Fractured Dentition and Restorations

Fractures of the natural dentition should be treated by a dentist without delay. Besides being aesthetically unappealing (especially if it involves an anterior tooth), fractured teeth can result in pulp exposure, pain, irritation to adjacent soft tissues, malocclusion, rapid carious breakdown, compromised mastication, and infection. Loose, displaced, or broken dental restorations (fillings) and nonremovable prostheses (crowns and bridges) may result in loss of normal function, tooth breakdown, or malocclusion. Only a dentist can evaluate and treat these conditions adequately. Minor chips in the tooth's crown may be adequately repaired with restorative materials and techniques. However, a large fracture may require endodontic treatment (root canal therapy), extensive restorative procedures, or extraction of the tooth.

Oral Mucosal Lesions

Oral Malignancies

Approximately 30,000 people are diagnosed with oral cancer each year in the United States. This represents approximately 4% of all cancers. Because of the serious consequences, oral cancer must always be considered in the differential diagnosis of persistent oral lesions. Accounting for 90% of oral malignancies is squamous cell carcinoma. Most oropharyngeal squamous cell carcinomas occur in persons over 50 years of age.[1] Clinically, oral carcinomas can appear as red or white lesions, ulcerations, or tumors.

As with other carcinomas, the cause of oral and perioral carcinomas is unknown; however, certain lifestyle behaviors have been identified as risk factors. Smoking, the use of smokeless tobacco products, and the excessive consumption of alcoholic beverages contribute to a higher risk for intraoral cancer. Snuff use in particular, if started at an early age, seems to be associated with a higher incidence of oral cancer.[7] Unprotected sun exposure contributes to the increasing incidence of cancers of the face and lips. It is very important that the pharmacist question patients who seek product recommendations for treatment of persistent oral lesions and refer such individuals to a physician or dentist for evaluation.

Canker Sores and Cold Sores

Two of the most common oral problems for which patients will seek advice and nonprescription treatment are canker sores and cold sores (fever blisters). Both conditions yield to symptomatic self-treatment, and the conditions should be self-limiting unless a secondary infectious process occurs. Patients frequently and actively seek a pharmacist's recommendations for nonprescription products to relieve symptoms of canker sores and cold sores. This provides an excellent opportunity for the pharmacist to intervene on the patient's behalf. However, although many nonprescription products are available for symptomatic treatment of cold sores and canker sores, none has been shown conclusively to decrease the recurrence rate of lesions or to be curative.

Canker Sores Canker sores, also referred to as recurrent aphthous ulcers or recurrent aphthous stomatitis, affect approximately 20% of Americans, with the greater incidence in stressed populations and a slightly higher incidence in women than in men.[87] The cause of aphthous ulcers is unknown; however, evidence suggests that they may result from a hypersensitivity to bacteria found in the mouth. Precipitating or contributing factors may be food allergy, genetic predisposition, stress, hormonal changes, nutritional deficiency (possibly related to iron, B_{12}, or folic acid deficiency), systemic disease, or trauma (eg, chemical irritation, biting the inside of cheeks or lips, or injury caused by toothbrushing or braces).[88] Evidence also suggests that cell-mediated immunity may play a role. Recent studies suggest that aphthous ulcers are caused by a dysfunction of the immune system and may be initiated by a trigger event such as a minor trauma.[88]

Aphthous lesions appear as an epithelial ulceration on nonkeratinized mucosal surfaces of movable mouth parts, such as the tongue, the floor of the mouth, the soft palate, or the inside lining of the lips and cheeks. Rarely, lesions affect keratinized tissue such as gingiva. Some patients may experience a painful sensation before the lesion actually appears. Patients may develop single or multiple lesions. Most aphthous lesions persist for 7–14 days and heal spontaneously without scarring.[88] Canker sores are neither viral in origin nor contagious.

Canker sores usually range from 0.5 to 3.0 cm in diameter; however, larger lesions can develop in clusters. Individual aphthous lesions are usually round or oval in shape and either flat or crater-like in appearance. (See color plates, photograph 6.) The color is usually gray to grayish-yellow with an erythematous halo of inflamed tissue surrounding the ulcer. The lesions can be very painful and may inhibit normal eating, drinking, swallowing, and talking, as well as routine oral hygiene. Although many patients have recurrent episodes of oral lesions with periods of remission, some patients may chronically experience one or more lesions in the mouth for very long periods. There is usually no fever or lymphadenopathy accompanying aphthous lesions; however, these symptoms may arise if a secondary bacterial infection is present.

The main goal in treating canker sores is to control discomfort and protect the sores from irritating stimuli so that the patient can eat, drink, and perform routine oral hygiene. If predisposing factors can be identified, they should be eliminated if possible. Coating the ulcers with topical oral protectants such as Orabase, denture adhesives, or benzoin tincture can be effective in protecting lesions, decreasing friction, and affording temporary symptomatic relief.[20] These products can be applied as needed. The ADA accepts both Orabase Plain and benzoin tincture as topical oral mucosal protectants.

Topical application of local anesthetic/analgesic pastes or gels also affords temporary pain relief. Benzocaine and butacaine are the most commonly used local anesthetics in nonprescription products. However, benzocaine is a known sensitizer (allergen) and should not be used by patients with a history of hypersensitivity to other benzocaine-containing products. The FDA has classified topical oral anesthetic/analgesic products containing 5–20% benzocaine, 0.05–0.1% benzyl alcohol, 0.05–0.1% butacaine sulfate, 0.05–0.1% dyclonine, 0.05–0.1% hexylresorcinol, 0.04–2.0% menthol, 0.5–1.5% phenol, 0.5–1.5% phenolate sodium, and 1–6% salicyl alcohol as safe and effective for temporary relief of pain associated with canker sores.[84]

Pharmacists should discourage the sustained use of potentially inflammatory products containing substantial amounts of menthol, phenol, camphor, and eugenol as anesthetic, counterirritant, or antiseptic treatments for canker sores. These agents may cause tissue irritation and damage or systemic toxicity, especially if overused.[50] None of these ingredients has been accepted as safe and effective by the ADA for treating canker sores.

Products that release nascent oxygen (eg, 10–15% carbamide peroxide, 3% hydrogen peroxide, and perborates) can be used as debriding and cleansing agents to exert temporary relief of canker sore discomfort. Such products can be used up to four times daily (after meals) but should be used for no more than 7 days. Depending on the product form, they are suitable either for direct application or as an oral rinse. It is important that the patient follow specific package directions. The solution should be expectorated and never swallowed. Safety of long-term use is not established, and if no improvement is seen in a week or if the condition worsens, professional consultation is indicated. Reports of tissue irritation, decalcification of enamel, and black hairy tongue are associated with chronic use.[89]

Systemic nonprescription analgesics (eg, aspirin, ibuprofen, and acetaminophen) afford additional relief of discomfort. Aspirin should not be retained in the mouth before swallowing or placed in the area of the oral lesions because of the high risk for chemical burn with necrosis. (See color plates, photograph 5.)

Saline rinses (1–3 tsp of table salt in 4–8 oz of warm tap water) may be soothing and can be used prior to topical application of a medication. If a nutritional deficiency is suspected as a contributing factor, nutritional supplements may be used. Zinc in astringent mouthrinses is of equivocal value in promoting healing. Silver nitrate should not be used to cauterize lesions because it lacks value and may stain teeth and damage healthy tissue.

Cold Sores Cold sores or fever blisters are lesions that are generally caused by the herpes simplex type 1 virus (HSV-1). They are referred to as herpes simplex labialis because they commonly occur on the lip or on areas bordering the lips; the usual site is at the junction of mucous membrane and skin of the lips or nose. The lesions are recurrent, painful, and cosmetically objectionable. About half of all patients who have sustained a primary (initial) HSV-1 infection will experience recurrent local lesions after some unpredictable latent interval, the lesions often arising in the same location repeatedly. After the primary infection, the virus apparently remains in host cells. The primary infection is reported most often in childhood. Patients may relate a history of primary herpetic stomatitis, which usually manifests itself by vesicles (blisters) in the mouth. However, most primary oral infections of herpes seem to be subclinical, and most patients are unaware of their previous primary exposure.

Cold sores are often preceded by a prodrome in which the patient notices burning, itching, tingling, or numbness in the area of the forthcoming lesion. The lesion first becomes visible as small, red papules of fluid-containing vesicles 1–3 mm in diameter. Often, many lesions coalesce to form a larger area of involvement. An erythematous, inflamed border around the fluid-filled vesicles may be present. A mature lesion often has a crust over the top of many coalesced, burst vesicles; its base is erythematous. The presence of pustules or pus under the crust of a cold sore may indicate a secondary bacterial infection and should be evaluated promptly and treated with an appropriate antibiotic.

Cold sores are self-limiting and heal without scarring, usually within 10–14 days. The recurrence rate and extent of lesions vary greatly from patient to patient. Some patients may experience several large lesions every few weeks; other patients may have only a single small lesion at infrequent intervals. Patients will often associate predisposing factors such as sun or wind exposure, fever, systemic infectious diseases (colds and flu), menstruation, extreme physical stress and fatigue, or local trauma with the onset of cold sores. Those who identify sun exposure as a precipitating event should be advised to use a lip sunscreen product routinely.

HSV-1 is contagious and thought to be transmittable by direct contact. Fluid from herpes vesicles contains live virus and may serve to transmit the virus from patient to patient.[20] Herpes simplex type 2 virus (HSV-2), which causes genital lesions, is sexually transmitted. However, it has been demonstrated in herpes lesions of the lip and can be caused by oral-genital contact or hand-to-mouth transfer.

The primary goals in treating cold sores are the same as for canker sores: to control discomfort, allow healing, and prevent complications. The cold sore should be kept moist to prevent drying and fissuring. Cracking of the lesions may render them more susceptible to secondary bacterial infection, may delay healing, and usually increases discomfort. Skin protectant ingredients (eg, allantoin, petrolatum, and cocoa butter) can relieve dryness and keep lesions soft. Topical local anesthetics (eg, benzocaine and dibucaine) in bland, emollient vehicles aid in relieving the discomfort of itching and pain. If there is evidence of secondary bacterial infection, topical application of a thin layer of triple antibiotic ointment (eg, Mycitracin or Neosporin) three to four times daily is recommended, along with systemic antibiotics if indicated. Systemic nonprescription analgesics may provide additional pain relief.

The FDA review of OTC products for fever blisters and cold sores classified external analgesics, alcohols, ketones, and amine and caine-type local anesthetics as Category I.[90] A partial listing of Category I ingredients includes benzocaine 5–20%, dibucaine 0.25–1%, dyclonine hydrochloride 0.5–1%, benzyl alcohol 10–33%, camphor 0.1–3%, menthol 0.1–1%, etc.[90] These ingredients, which suppress cutaneous sensory receptors, offer analgesic, anesthetic, and antipruritic effects in relieving the pain and itching of fever blisters and cold sores. Higher concentrations of certain ingredients (ie, camphor >3% and menthol >1%) that stimulate cutaneous sensory receptors and produce a counterirritant effect are contraindicated.[91] Fever blisters and cold sores are not considered steroid-responsive dermatoses, so the use of topical steroids is also contraindicated.[20] The FDA has proposed the use of topically applied nonprescription skin protectants or externally applied analgesic/anesthetic drug products as the only currently effective nonprescription treatment for relieving the discomfort of fever blisters.[92]

Products that are highly astringent should be avoided. Tannic acid and zinc sulfate are not generally recognized as safe and effective and are misbranded when present in products for the topical management of fever blisters and cold sores.[91] Because frequent applications of tannic acid to the lip and oral cavity could cause a patient to ingest it when eating or drinking, the FDA was concerned about the drug's potential for oral mucosal absorption and toxicity. This concern prompted the FDA to require further clinical data to support the safety and effectiveness of astringents in the symptomatic treatment of cold sores and fever blisters.[90] At the time the final rule was issued in 1993, no data had been submitted to this effect.[91]

Numerous orally administered products (eg, preparations containing *Lactobacillus acidophilus*, *Lactobacillus bulgaricus*, the essential amino acid L-lysine, citrus bioflavinoids, or pyridoxine) have also been proposed for the treatment of cold sores. However, evidence conclusively demonstrating their efficacy is lacking. The FDA determined in a final ruling that "no orally administered active ingredient has been found to be generally recognized as safe and effective for OTC use to treat or relieve the symptoms or discomfort of fever blisters and cold sores."[92]

Lesions should be kept clean by gently washing with mild soap solutions. Hand washing is important in preventing lesion contamination and minimizing autoinoculation of HSV. Factors that delay healing (eg, stress, local trauma, wind, sunlight, and fatigue) should be avoided.

Minor Oral Mucosal Injury or Irritation

Minor wounds or inflammation resulting from dentures, orthodontic appliances, minor dental procedures, accidental injury (eg, biting the cheek or suffering abrasion from sharp, crisp foods), or other irritations of the mouth or gums may be treated with various drugs. Combination preparations to treat minor oral mucosal injury may contain (1) a single anesthetic/analgesic with either a single astringent, an oral mucosal protectant, or a denture adhesive; or (2) benzocaine combined with menthol or phenol preparations. Topical analgesic/anesthetics are applied for pain relief. Astringents cause tissues to contract, or arrest secretions by causing proteins to coagulate on a cell surface.[84] Oral mucosal protectants are pharmacologically inert substances that coat and protect the area. Debriding agents/oral wound cleansers may be used to (1) aid in the removal of debris or phlegm, mucus, or other secretions associated with sore mouth; (2) cleanse minor wounds or minor gum inflammation; and (3) cleanse canker sores.[93] Labeling of these products includes the following warning:

> Do not use this product more than 7 days unless directed by a dentist or doctor. If sore mouth symptoms do not improve in 7 days; if irritation, pain, or redness persists or worsens; or if swelling, rash, or fever develops, see your doctor or dentist promptly.[84]

The FDA has determined that no ingredient is generally recognized as safe and effective for use as a nonprescription oral wound-healing agent.[94] The ingredients reviewed by the OTC panel include allantoin, carbamide peroxide in anhydrous glycerin, water-soluble chlorophyllins, and hydrogen peroxide in aqueous solution. However, the nonmonograph status of these ingredients applies to their use as oral wound-healing agents only. After a thorough review process, the FDA has determined that four active ingredients are generally recognized as safe and effective for use as nonprescription oral health care debriding agents/oral wound cleansers. This proposed ruling applies to carbamide peroxide in anhydrous glycerin, hydrogen peroxide, sodium perborate monohydrate (1.2 g), and sodium bicarbonate.[93] Furthermore, allantoin is recognized as a safe and effective skin protectant. In another segment of the tentative final monograph on Oral Health Care Drug Products, the FDA reviewed oral antiseptic products and, pending submission of further data to support efficacy, classified no ingredients as Category I for oral antiseptic use (ie, to decrease the chance of infection in minor oral irritation).[12]

Dentists may suggest that their patients use oxidizing mouthrinses or drops as an adjunctive treatment of specific conditions or as a postoperative aid to cleaning and to relieving discomfort. Peroxides and perborates release molecular oxygen. Hydrogen peroxide and carbamide peroxide do so immediately upon contact with tissue enzymes (catalase and peroxidase), but tissue and bacterial exposure to the oxygen is very brief.[20] The foaming of the liberated oxygen exerts a mechanical action, which loosens particulate matter and cleanses debris from wounds. The efficacy of oxidizing products in killing anaerobic bacteria in the treatment of infections and periodontitis is equivocal and has not been established.[20]

For direct application, drops of the liquid (carbamide peroxide in anhydrous glycerin or hydrogen peroxide as a 3% aqueous solution) are placed on the affected area and allowed to remain in place for 1 minute. As a rinse, carbamide peroxide drops are placed on the tongue, mixed with saliva, and swished in the mouth for 1 minute. A 3% aqueous solution of hydrogen peroxide should be mixed with an equal amount of water before rinsing the mouth. Some products (eg, Peroxyl Rinse and Perimed) are a 1.5% solution of hydrogen peroxide and should be used full strength. Sodium perborate monohydrate powder (1.2 g) should be dissolved in 1 oz of water and used immediately. In all cases, it is important to follow package directions carefully. The solution should be spit out, not swallowed.

Prolonged rinsing with oxidizing products could lead to soft tissue irritation, decalcified tooth surfaces, and black hairy tongue.[18] Alternatives are a sodium bicarbonate rinse (½ to 1 tsp in 4 oz of water) or a salt water rinse (1–3 tsp of salt in 4–8 oz of warm tap water). Mucolytic action is related to the alkalinity of the sodium bicarbonate solution. As a debriding agent/oral wound cleanser, the solution is swished in the mouth over the affected area for at least 1 minute and then spit out. A saline rinse can be used safely for cleansing and soothing.

Oral Infections

Dentopyogenic Infections

Dentopyogenic infections are pus-producing infections that are associated with a tooth or its supporting structures. Symptoms and severity are determined by factors such as the anatomic features of the infection site, local and systemic host resistance, virulence of the causative organisms, and time between onset of infection and treatment. The symptoms of these infections vary greatly, from minor generalized pain, throbbing, and sensitivity to fever, malaise, swelling, localized pain, erythema, warmth at the infection site, and septic shock. The severity ranges from small, well-localized abscesses with no systemic signs of infection to a diffuse, rapidly spreading cellulitis or osteomyelitis with high morbidity. Patients with severe symptoms associated with dentopyogenic infections usually seek dental attention as soon as possible; however, persons with minimal symptoms may unwisely delay dental treatment and attempt self-treatment. Dentopyogenic abscesses, even if well-localized and seemingly not serious, may progress to more severe acute or chronic infections, requiring surgical intervention with or without systemic antibiotic therapy.

The four common dental abscesses are periapical, periodontal, pericoronal, and subperiosteal.

Periapical Abscess A periapical abscess, located around the apex of a tooth root, originates from a necrotic, infected dental pulp and gains access to the periapical area via the apical foramen. The two most common causes of dental pulp infection and necrosis with subsequent periapical abscess are dental caries that expose the pulp to oral bacteria, and trauma that causes a decrease or stoppage of blood flow to and from the pulp.

Periodontal Abscess A periodontal abscess is usually a result of periodontitis. Periodontitis leads to the destruction of supporting tooth structures and the subsequent formation of deep periodontal pockets. The bacteria associated with periodontitis move toward the apex of the tooth within the deepening pocket. If host resistance decreases or if the bacteria are forced into the surrounding tissue by external trauma or occlusion of the pocket, the accumulated bacteria within this pocket form an abscess in surrounding tissue.

Pericoronal Abscess Pericoronal abscesses are most often associated with mandibular third molars (lower wisdom teeth). Mandibular third molars in the process of erupting or those that do not fully erupt often have gingiva covering a portion of the crown. This gingival tissue can be traumatized by the opposing upper third molar when the patient bites down. An abscess in the tissue surrounding the lower molar may also be caused by food, bacteria, and debris collecting beneath this flap of gingiva. Patients with healthy wisdom teeth may need a child-size toothbrush in addition to a regular toothbrush to reach that area effectively for thorough cleaning.

Subperiosteal Abscess A subperiosteal abscess is a bone abscess located beneath the thin connective tissue (periosteum) covering the bone that surrounds or underlies a tooth socket. These infections are most common after a tooth extraction.

Candidiasis

Candidiasis is often called "the disease of the diseased" because it appears in debilitated patients, immunocompromised patients, and patients taking a variety of drugs. Predisposing factors include physiologic factors (early infancy, pregnancy, and old age); endocrine disorders (diabetes mellitus, hypothyroidism, hypoparathyroidism, and hypoadrenalism); malnutrition and malabsorption syndromes (iron deficiency anemia, pernicious anemia, postgastrectomy, and alcoholism); malignant diseases (leukemias and granulocytopenia); drugs causing depression of defense mechanisms (immunosuppressives, corticosteroids, cytotoxics, and radiation therapy); drugs causing xerostomia (anticholinergics, antidepressants, antipsychotics, antihypertensives, and antihistamines with anticholinergic activity contributing to a dry mouth); and other changes in the host environment (trauma, chemical damage, postoperative states, and chronic use of broad-spectrum antibiotics).

Candida albicans, a fungus commonly found in normal oral flora, is by far the most common opportunistic pathogen associated with oral infections. The acute pseudomembranous form of candidiasis is often referred to as thrush, and it is characterized by white plaques with a milk curd appearance. These plaques, which are attached to the oral mucosa, can usually be detached easily, displaying erythematous, bleeding, sore areas beneath. (See color plates, photograph 7.) Thrush is most common in infants and debilitated patients.

Acute atrophic candidiasis, sometimes referred to as antibiotic tongue or antibiotic sore mouth, is characterized by erythematous, painful, sometimes bleeding areas of the mouth. The entire upper surface of the tongue or the entire oral cavity may be involved. This form is thought to be similar to thrush but lacks the white plaques. Broad-spectrum antibiotic therapy of long duration is the most common predisposing factor.

Chronic atrophic candidiasis, sometimes referred to as denture stomatitis or denture sore mouth, is commonly found in patients with full or partial dentures. Symptomatically, this form is characterized by generalized inflammation of the denture-bearing area. The tissue may be granular in appearance, or erythematous and edematous with soreness or a burning sensation.[95] Inflammation secondary to the trauma of ill-fitting dentures is usually localized to the specific area of the trauma; inflammation secondary to *Candida* is generalized to the entire denture-bearing tissue area. It appears that the candidal organisms adhere to the denture material or reside in pores of the denture material and can reinfect the mouth.[96] If infected, the denture needs to be cleaned with an antifungal denture cleanser. Failure to remove the denture at bedtime and to clean it regularly worsens this condition. Angular cheilitis (inflammation of the corners of the mouth) is commonly associated with chronic atrophic candidiasis and other forms of oral candidiasis.[95]

Candidiasis requires prompt treatment with local or systemic antifungal therapy. Patients with suspected candidiasis should be referred for medical or dental evaluation. Listerine has exhibited anti-*Candida* properties when used as an antifungal rinse for treatment of patients wearing removable dentures. It may also be useful for the prevention of oral candidiasis in immunocompromised patients.[97]

Halitosis

Halitosis, an offensive odor emanating from the oral cavity, may be symptomatic of oral pathology. Odor results from bacterial action of food debris. Because some degree of oral malodor is normal in a healthy individual (eg, morning breath), foul breath can be a useful diagnostic aid, as in the case of trench mouth. The source of halitosis may be either oral or nonoral. Common oral causes include odoriferous decaying food particles, cellular and nutritional debris, plaque-coated tongue, periodontal disease, xerostomia, and stomatitis. Poor oral or denture hygiene, trench mouth, caries, postsurgical states, extraction wounds, purulent infections, chronic periodontitis, side effects of medication, and smoking can contribute to it. Common nonoral causes of halitosis include pulmonary disease such as purulent lung infections, tuberculosis, bronchiectasis, sinusitis, tonsillitis, and rhinitis. Other nonoral causes include the elimination of chemical substances from the blood through the lungs upon exhalation; examples include alcoholic breath or acetone breath in severely hyperglycemic diabetics.

Any patient who complains of severe or lingering halitosis without a readily identifiable cause (eg, smoking) should be advised to see a dentist for a thorough evaluation of possible pathology. Masking foul taste and odor with cosmetic mouthrinses may delay necessary dental or medical assessment and needed treatment.

Therapeutic Considerations in Special Populations

Geriatric Patients

The percentage of the US population aged 65 and older is increasing, and this increase is predicted to continue well into the 21st century. Projections for the year 2030 suggest that 20% of the population will be over age 65 and that 3%, or about 8.8 million people, will be over age 85.[98] Edentulism (toothlessness) is decreasing; more than half of older Americans have retained natural dentition. This has many dental implications. Topical fluoride application in the form of dentifrice, rinse, or gel is indicated for the prevention of coronal and root caries as long as there is natural dentition. Pharmacists should continue to recommend fluoride anticaries products to their older patients.

In counseling geriatric patients on oral health care, it becomes very important to consider medication profiles. Because the elderly are more likely to be taking multiple medications, the likelihood of drug-induced or disease-related changes in oral physiology increases.

Xerostomia

About 20% of the elderly are affected with xerostomia, a condition in which salivary flow is limited or completely arrested. Xerostomia was thought to be an age-related, degenerative process. However, it has been shown that healthy, nonmedicated geriatrics may experience a change in saliva composition but not necessarily a decreased flow.[99] The usual causes of xerostomia are disease (eg, Sjögren's syndrome, diabetes, and depression), drugs (eg, antihypertensives, antidepressants, and diuretics), or functional activity (eg, breathing through the mouth or smoking). Radiation therapy of the head and neck can cause atrophy of the salivary glands. Drugs with anticholinergic activity or drugs that cause depletion of salivary flow volume have been implicated. Older persons are more likely to be taking multiple medications for chronic diseases; however, if xerostomia is drug induced and the medication can be changed, the condition may be reversed. Pharmacists should review medication profiles (prescription and nonprescription) for patients complaining of dry mouth to determine if the condition is drug induced.

Xerostomia can produce difficulty in talking and swallowing, stomatitis and burning tongue, increased caries, periodontal disease, or reduced denture-wearing time, depending on the status of dentition. Treatment should be directed toward the control of dental decay and the relief of soft tissue distress. The commercially available artificial salivas relieve soft tissue discomfort and are more effective and longer lasting than simple rinses and lozenges (see product table "Artificial Saliva Products").

Artificial saliva preparations are designed to mimic natural saliva both chemically and physically. Because they do not stimulate natural salivary gland production, however, they must be considered as replacement therapy, not as a cure for xerostomia. Artificial saliva closely resembles natural saliva and is formulated with the following properties:

- *Viscosity*: Carboxymethylcellulose and glycerin are used to mimic natural saliva viscosity.
- *Mineral content*: All products contain calcium and phosphate ions, and some also contain fluoride. With normal use, no product has demonstrated the ability to remineralize enamel; therefore, the ADA does not recognize any such claims made by the manufacturers.
- *Preservatives*: Salivart does not contain preservatives because it is packaged as a sterile aerosol. Other products do contain preservatives, such as methyl- or propylparaben, which may cause hypersensitivity reactions in certain patients.
- *Palatability*: Flavorings such as mint or lemon and/or sweeteners such as sorbitol and xylitol are commonly used.

Artificial salivas can be used on an as-needed basis. Xerostomic patients with a history of caries susceptibility should use a professionally designed topical fluoride program in addition to artificial saliva products. These patients should also use very soft toothbrushes and avoid mouthrinses with high alcoholic content, given that alcohol contributes to xerostomia.

Among the ADA-accepted artificial salivas are Salivart, Glandosane Synthetic Saliva, Moi-Stir Mouth Moistener and Moi-Stir Oral Swabsticks, Saliva Substitute, and Optimoist Oral Moisturizer.[65]

Denture Problems

Conditions such as denture stomatitis (an inflammation of the oral tissue in contact with a removable denture), inflammatory papillary hyperplasia, and chronic candidiasis can be caused by ill-fitting dentures, trauma, and poor denture hygiene. Denture stomatitis, a distressing and common finding in denture wearers, may also be attributed to infection with *C albicans*, which can be found resident on the denture base.[96] Dentures accumulate plaque, stain, and calculus by a process very similar to that which occurs with natural teeth.[100] The denture plaque mass in contact with oral tissues produces predictable toxic results. Poor denture hygiene contributes to fungal and bacterial growth and so not only affects the patient aesthetically (unpleasant odors and staining), but also seriously affects the patient's oral health (inflammation and mucosal disease) and ability to wear the dentures successfully.[95]

Loose, misfitting, or broken removable dental prostheses (partial or full dentures) can also contribute to accelerated bone loss, ulceration, irritation, tumorous growths, and compromised oral function. Refitting, relining, or repairing dentures to ensure proper functioning requires professional dental treatment.

Denture Cleansers Patients should be instructed to clean dentures thoroughly at least once daily to remove unsightly stain, debris, and potentially harmful plaque. Only products specifically formulated for denture cleansing should be used; household cleansers (used for soaking) are not appropriate and may either be ineffective or damage denture material (see product table "Denture Cleanser Products"). The use of whitening toothpastes meant for natural dentition should be discouraged because their abrasivity is too high for them to be used safely on denture material.

A combination regimen of brushing and soaking is recommended.[101] Brushing with a denture brush, adapted to the denture's contour, and low-abrasion denture paste or powder will mechanically remove plaque and debris. These abrasive products should be used with care, avoiding any excessive force or pressure that could damage acrylic resin. The brushing routine can be followed by soaking the denture in an alkaline peroxide cleansing solution to help remove remaining plaque and bacteria. Plaque removal is then enhanced by brushing the denture after it has soaked; instructions for doing so are included on some products.[102] The denture should be thoroughly rinsed before reinsertion in the mouth.

Denture cleansers are either chemical or abrasive in their cleaning action. The three types of chemical cleansers are alkaline peroxides, alkaline hypochlorites, and dilute acids. The abrasive cleaners are available as pastes, gels, or powders. The ideal denture cleansing product would:

- Remove both organic and inorganic denture deposits effectively;
- Possess bactericidal and fungicidal activity;
- Be nontoxic;
- Do no harm to denture materials.[96]

Because the ideal product does not yet exist, it is necessary to assess product characteristics in conjunction with patient circumstances. More than one product may be required to meet patient needs adequately.

Alkaline peroxide cleaners are the most commonly used chemical denture cleansers. These powders or tablets become alkaline solutions of hydrogen peroxide when dissolved. The ingredients are alkaline detergents and perborates, the latter of which cause oxygen release for a mechanical cleaning effect. Geriatric or handicapped patients may prefer an alkaline peroxide soak solution for daily, overnight cleaning. These products are most effective on new plaque and stains that are soaked for 4–8 hours. The alkaline peroxides have few serious disadvantages and do not damage the surface of acrylic resins.[102]

Alkaline hypochlorites (bleach) remove stains, dissolve mucin, and are both bactericidal and fungicidal. Denture plaque consists of cells embedded in a matrix that serves as a surface on which calculus may develop. Hypochlorite cleansers act directly on the organic plaque matrix to dissolve its structure, but they cannot dissolve calculus once formed.[102] The most serious disadvantage of hypochlorite is that it corrodes metal denture components such as the framework and clasps of removable partial dentures, solder joints, and possibly the pins holding the teeth.[96] The addition of anticorrosive phosphate compounds has greatly reduced this effect, but it is recommended that these products be used for 15-minute soaks to limit exposure[102] and not be used more often than once a week.

Dilute acids, often 3–5% hydrochloric acid, dissolve the inorganic (calcium) phosphate and are effective against calculus and stain on dentures. However, they too corrode metal components and are harmful to fabrics, eyes, and skin if spilled during handling.[102] Therefore, these products are used in the dental office for professional cleaning but are not deemed suitable for routine patient home use.

Although many studies have been conducted on denture-cleansing products, only a few comparative trials have been published, and differences in methodology make direct comparisons of results very difficult. Published findings report that plaque accumulation of less than 24 hours is easier to remove but is not necessarily removed effectively by all products, even within the same class of cleaners. The relative ineffectiveness of all products tested during a short soaking time is often contrary to advertising claims. The following denture cleansers are among those currently accepted by the ADA as safe and effective: Complete, Efferdent, Efferdent paste, Fresh N' Brite, and 2 Layer Efferdent.[13]

All denture-cleansing products should be completely rinsed off the denture before insertion. Contact with oral or other mucous membranes may result in serious tissue irritation or possibly severe chemical burns from the alkaline or acid product.[102] All denture cleansers should be kept out of the reach of children because of the potential for eye or skin irritation or toxicity from accidental ingestion.[102] Patients should not soak or clean dentures in hot water or hot soaking solutions because distortion or warping may occur. Stains that are resistant to proper denture brushing and soaking in available solutions should be evaluated by a dentist.[102]

Denture Adhesives Denture adhesives may be the most overused dental products purchased by patients. Chronic bone resorption of the mandibular and maxillary ridges that support a denture occurs with even the best-fitting denture. Furthermore, pathologic changes in soft tissue under the denture, such as ulcers and fibrous lesions, and accelerated bone resorption have been reported with the inappropriate use of denture adhesives and ill-fitting dentures.[103] Periodic dental examinations are necessary to evaluate bone resorption and ensure proper denture fit. Although denture adhesives may increase denture retention in some persons, the need for adhesives increases as the quality of the denture adaptation to underlying soft tissue deteriorates.[103] Excessive application of adhesives could also cause denture repositioning with resultant malocclusion. The adhesive can actually interfere with correct positioning in relation to supporting bone. Patients who believe that daily use of denture adhesives is necessary to attain denture security and comfort should be referred to their dentist for evaluation.

Denture adhesives are usually composed of materials that swell, gel, and become viscous (eg, karaya, pectin, or methylcellulose); materials that are antibacterial (eg, sodium borate or hexachlorophene); and materials that serve as preservatives, fillers, or wetting or flavoring agents (eg, propylparaben, magnesium oxide, sodium lauryl sulfate, or petroleum derivatives) (see product table "Denture Adhesive Products"). Adhesive powders either have a vegetable gum base or are composed of synthetic polymers. Adhesive pastes usually contain karaya gum, petroleum jelly, colorings, and flavorings.

The ADA has accepted some denture adhesive products provided that the labeling indicates that they are to be used only temporarily or upon the recommendation of a dentist. All accepted denture adhesives contain the following warning label:

> [Product name] is acceptable as a temporary measure to provide increased retention of dentures. However, an ill-fitting denture may impair your health—consult your dentist for periodic examination.

The ADA has accepted the following denture adhesives as safe and effective: Co-Re-Ga, Wernet's Denture Adhesive Cream, Wernet's Powder, Super Wernet's Powder, Extra Strength Effergrip, Firmdent, Orafix Special Denture Adhesive, Perma-Grip, Rigident Cream, and Secure.[13]

Denture Reliners and Cushions Extended use of reliners or cushions for dentures invariably harms the patient and damages the denture. These products change the positioning of the denture, creating high-pressure points that can result in denture distortion, malocclusion, temporomandibular joint problems, decreased mastication function, and altered aesthetics.[103] Denture reliners and cushions have also been associated with bone resorption, traumatic ulcers, and gingival inflammation of the denture-bearing tissues.

The ADA does not accept any of these products as safe and effective, and it discourages their use. The FDA Bureau of Medical Devices requires the following warning label on these products:

> **WARNING** For temporary use only. Long-term use of this product may lead to faster bone loss, continuing irritation, sores, and tumors. For use only until a dentist can be seen.

Patients with dentures need periodic professional dental evaluations. As time passes, it is normal to expect the original fit to need adjustment. Patients who feel their dentures are loose or otherwise uncomfortable should be referred to their dentist for evaluation. Any patients who are considering purchasing a denture reliner or cushion because of actual or perceived denture problems should be encouraged to see their dentist as soon as possible.

Denture Repair Kits

Initial fitting and periodic refitting of dentures require extensive dental knowledge and skill. Patients should not attempt to glue or otherwise repair cracked, broken, or distorted dentures. Broken dentures can be evaluated and repaired only by a dentist. Pharmacists should discourage the use of denture repair kits and advise patients to (1) save all pieces of the denture or appliance to take to the dentist, and (2) seek professional treatment without delay. Prolonged periods without wearing a partial denture can result in position changes among the remaining teeth and a loss of fit.[104]

Denture repair kits may contain methacrylate or other types of glue or acrylic materials. The FDA requires the following label on these products:

WARNING For emergency repairs only. Long-term use of home-repaired dentures may cause faster bone loss, continuing irritation, sores, and tumors. This kit is for emergency use only. See Dentist Without Delay.

Pediatric Patients

The 20 primary teeth that will erupt are present but not visible in a baby's jaws at birth. It is important to start oral hygiene early in life. A wet gauze pad may be used to wipe the baby's gums after each feeding to remove plaque and milk residue. The deciduous teeth will usually start to erupt at about 6 months of age. Decay is a possibility at any time. "Baby bottle caries" results when an infant is allowed to nurse continuously from a bottle of juice, milk, or sugar water when put to bed. The prolonged time that teeth are in contact with the cariogenic liquid promotes caries. When the teeth have erupted, a soft child-size toothbrush can be used for cleaning. Parents must do the brushing and should take care to use only a very small amount of fluoride toothpaste or none at all. Children at this age will swallow the toothpaste, which will contribute to overall systemic fluoride ingestion.

Teething Discomfort

Teething is the eruption of the deciduous teeth through the gingival tissues. Usually this process is uneventful. However, when teething causes sleep disturbances or irritability, symptomatic treatment may be considered. Topical local anesthetics such as benzocaine and frozen teething rings may provide symptomatic relief. Systemic nonprescription analgesics (eg, acetaminophen) may be used at appropriate doses. When teething is accompanied by fever, nasal congestion, or malaise, a dentist or physician should be contacted to rule out an infectious process.

The FDA review of nonprescription drug products for relief of oral discomfort has included benzocaine and phenol preparations as Category I topical anesthetic/analgesics for teething pain (see product table "Oral Discomfort Products"). Labeling reads: "For the temporary relief of sore gums due to teething in infants and children 4 months of age and older."[84] Products containing 5–20% benzocaine in solution or suspension should be applied to the affected area not more than four times daily. Teething preparations containing phenol or phenolate sodium equivalent to 0.5% phenol in aqueous solution or suspension may be applied to the affected area up to six times daily. These preparations are not indicated for children under 4 months of age.[84] Moreover, products for teething must carry a warning that states that fever and nasal congestion are not symptoms of teething and may indicate the presence of an infection. ADA-accepted products include Baby Orajel Teething Pain Medicine and Orabase Baby Analgesic Teething Gel. These alcohol-free products contain 7.5% benzocaine.

Pediatric Toothbrushes

Soft bristles are recommended for children's toothbrushes. A child's toothbrush is smaller than an adult's and is available in a baby (for children up to age 6 or 7) and junior (age 7 to teens) size. Toothbrush size and shape should be individualized according to the size of the child's mouth. Children can usually remove plaque more easily with a brush having short and narrow bristles. No matter what type of toothbrush is used, however, children are usually unable to brush by themselves until they are 4 or 5 years old, and they may require supervision until 8 or 9 years of age to clean effectively.

Dental Fluorosis

Fluoride dentifrices contribute to the total amount of fluoride ingested by children. Other sources are dietary, recommended systemic supplements, and any other topical fluoride preparations. When chronic fluoride ingestion from all sources is considered, children who live in a community with an optimally fluoridated water supply may exceed optimal daily amounts. This places them at risk for mild forms of dental fluorosis, a mottled appearance of surface enamel. Although a mild degree of fluorosis is an aesthetic concern, more severe cases can result in pitting and surface defects.[105] (See color plates, photograph 8.)

In 1994 the ADA revised its recommendations for fluoride supplement dosing in children. The new schedule slightly lowers the dose amounts, recommends beginning treatment not earlier than age 6 months, and extends the age limit from 13 to 16 years. Evaluation of current studies reporting on the intake of fluoride among children prompted the revision.[45]

Studies of dentifrice ingestion by children show great variation in the amount of dentifrice retained and consistently show that younger children are more likely than older ones to swallow some dentifrice.[81] Limiting ingestion of fluoride dentifrice is advised. Parents should apply the toothpaste (only a pea-sized amount) to a child-size toothbrush and should brush the teeth of preschoolers until the children can manage it properly themselves. Children should be taught to rinse thoroughly and expectorate after brushing.[81] Only regular-strength fluoride toothpaste is recommended for use by children under 6 years of age.

A similar problem lies with fluoride rinsing in that children 3–5 years of age may swallow significant amounts of rinse each time they swish. A usual dose of 0.05% rinse contains 2 mg of fluoride ion and may contribute to mild fluorosis in the presence of a fluoridated public water supply. Ethanol content of most nonprescription fluoride rinses ranges from 6 to 8% and may pose a hazard for very young children. Alcohol-free formulations are now available. Fluoride rinses should be used only by children 6 years of age and older who have mastered the swallowing reflex. These products should be kept out of the reach of children, and children under 12 years of age should be supervised when rinsing. High-dose ingestion requires prompt medical assistance. Toxicity is related to fluoride content and ethanol content. Parents should be able to identify the product and estimate the amount ingested.[76]

Finally, fluoride gels are not recommended for children under 6, and children under 12 should use these products only under supervision.

Orthodontia

Fixed orthodontic appliances require very careful attention to oral hygiene to prevent gingivitis and caries. Patients with these appliances need a combination of toothbrush types to clean all surfaces effectively. Use of powered toothbrushes or oral irrigating devices may help to remove plaque and debris around orthodontic bands. It may be advisable for orthodontic patients to use a nonprescription fluoride mouthrinse while undergoing treatment.

Patients with removable orthodontic appliances should consult their orthodontist about using a denture cleanser. Some dental practitioners have recommended a denture cleanser in addition to brushing to remove plaque, tartar, odor-causing bacteria, and stain that accumulates on orthodontic appliances.[106]

Pregnancy Gingivitis

Pregnant patients are more susceptible to both dental caries and gingivitis. Caries generally can be related to changes in eating habits, such as frequent snacking and treats. Careful attention to frequent brushing and flossing is indicated to clear plaque and acid.[104]

Physiologic changes during pregnancy may contribute to changes in the soft oral tissues and result in an increased incidence and severity of gingivitis. An inflammatory condition so common that it is called pregnancy gingivitis is characterized by red, swollen gingival tissue that bleeds easily. This gingivitis is caused by local factors, as it is in any patient. Pregnancy modifies the host's response, however, making gingival tissue more sensitive to bacterial dental plaque. Hormone level or increased production of prostaglandins has been implicated in the heightened inflammatory response.[1] Pregnancy gingivitis can be prevented or resolved with thorough plaque control. The severity of the inflammatory response and resulting gingivitis will decrease postpartum, returning to prepregnancy levels after approximately 1 year.

The pharmacist will quite often be alerted very early in the pregnancy owing to counseling on prescription prenatal vitamins. Besides monitoring the pregnant patient's medications for safety, the pharmacist has an opportunity to advise a dental checkup and careful attention to brushing and flossing to avoid oral health complications.

Value-Added Pharmacy Services

Pharmacists can offer patients good oral health services in several other ways. As an initial step, pharmacists can contact local community dental practitioners and indicate a willingness to work together for optimal patient oral health care. The pharmacist may also want to consider one or more of the activities listed below:

- Contact the local public health agency to determine the level of community water fluoridation. In that way, the pharmacist can assist dental and medical practitioners in prescribing supplements and patients in selecting fluoride-containing dentifrices, mouthrinses, and gels.[105]
- Monitor total fluoride ingestion in children, noting the use of fluoride prescription supplementation and family use of nonprescription fluoride products. Because systemic supplements may be prescribed by both the dentist and the pediatrician, the pharmacist is in a unique position to coordinate children's fluoride supplementation.[105]
- Stock the oral health care section to highlight products accepted or recognized by the ADA, and advise patients of the significance of the ADA acceptance program.
- Make available, as an informational/educational addition to the oral health care section, the many types of brochures and patient information leaflets that the ADA provides on various oral health concerns.
- Take the initiative in counseling patients on the proper selection and use of nonprescription oral health care products. Because of the tremendous amount of advertising in this area, patients need knowledgeable and objective advice and assistance to be able to distinguish among product claims.
- Remember that older patients may be vision impaired and that lighting in the nonprescription product area becomes important for reading label directions and warnings.
- Include records of pertinent dental health information (eg, dentures, orthodontics, and fluorosis) on patient profiles.

Case Studies

Case 25–1

Patient Complaint/History

JR, a 30-year-old male, picks out several nonprescription products and brings them to the pharmacy counter. He asks which product should be used to treat a crusted erythematous sore that is visible on the skin bordering his upper lip. He reveals that several days ago, after sensations of tingling and burning occurred at the lesion site, a cluster of small blisters appeared. The sore has since enlarged and formed a crust; it now hampers speaking and eating. Other symptoms include itching and pain at the site. JR expresses concern for his overall health because he was told this type of lesion indicates an infection with the virus that causes chickenpox.

During conversation with the patient, the pharmacist determines that the lesions are recurrent. JR acknowledges that this outbreak is the third such episode this year: one episode occurred on a 10-day winter vacation in the Caribbean; two other episodes occurred this past summer. He is very interested in preventing future occurrences and asks about preventive medications, specifically pyridoxine (vitamin B_6), which he heard can minimize or prevent these outbreaks.

The nonprescription drugs brought to the counter for the pharmacist's evaluation and recommendation include hydrocortisone 1% topical cream; Blistex Lip Ointment; Orabase Lip Healer cream; Vaseline petroleum jelly; pyridoxine 50-mg tablets. JR mentions that he is allergic to aspirin.

Clinical Consideration/Strategies

The following considerations/strategies are provided to aid the reader in (1) determining whether treatment of the patient's condition with nonprescription medications is warranted, (2) selecting the appropriate nonprescription medication, and (3) developing a patient counseling strategy to ensure optimal therapeutic outcomes:

- Assess the patient's complaint.
- Assess individually the appropriateness of the four topical products (creams/ointments) and the pyroxidine for treating the lesion.
- Determine which ingredients in these products will have little positive impact on the symptom complex or in preventing secondary complications.
- Assess the specific value, or lack of value, that topical steroids have in treating a fever blister.
- Assess the specific value, or lack of value, that orally administered pyroxidine has in treating the symptoms.
- Propose a nonprescription topical medication regimen that is based on patient-specific factors and focuses on products containing emollients and local analgesics/anesthetics.
- Provide the patient with appropriate information regarding product use (eg, dose, frequency of administration, and duration of therapy).
- Define the role of oral nonprescription analgesics (acetaminophen, ibuprofen, naproxen, ketoprofen) in managing pain associated with fever blisters/cold sores.
- Develop a patient education/counseling strategy that will:
  - Explain the etiology of the lesion as well as the tendency for recurrence, predisposing factors, and preventive measures;
  - Define reasonable therapeutic goals in treating the lesion;
  - Emphasize the importance of keeping the lesion and hands clean;
  - Support the logic for changes in the nonprescription medication regimen selected by the patient;
  - Define techniques and procedures for using the nonprescription medication regimen that was recommended by the pharmacist to provide symptomatic relief and prevent complications.

Case 25–2

Patient Complaint/History

DM, a 25-year-old female who is the head of a household with two children and geriatric parents, had previously reported tooth pain in two quadrants. She correlated this pain with drinking coffee in the morning and brushing her teeth. Upon the pharmacist's suggestion, she went to her dentist and was diagnosed as having hypersensitive teeth. Her dentist gave her a sample of a dentifrice for hypersensitive teeth and also advised her to use a nonprescription fluoride rinse. Although the patient did not like the taste of the dentifrice, she used up the sample; however, she is still experiencing pain.

DM, who is at the pharmacy today to pick up her mother's prescription, mentions her disappointment with the dentifrice provided by her dentist. She also has some questions she forgot to ask the dentist: Can the whole family use this new toothpaste? Can she use the same fluoride rinse that her children use? Currently, the children (6 and 10 years old) use a fluoride rinse before breakfast each day.

Clinical Consideration/Strategies

The following considerations/strategies are provided to aid the reader in (1) determining whether treatment of the patient's condition with nonprescription medications is warranted, (2) selecting the appropriate nonprescription medication, and (3) developing a patient counseling strategy to ensure optimal therapeutic outcomes:

- Determine which ingredients are appropriate for treating hypersensitive teeth.
- Recommend alternative products for relief of the symptoms.
- Develop a patient education/counseling strategy that will:
  - Address the patient's concerns about the apparent failure of the desensitizing dentifrice that was recommended by the dentist;
  - Optimize proper use of the nonprescription medication regimen that was recommended to provide symptomatic relief for hypersensitivity and prevention of caries;
  - Include consideration of prevention of caries in other family members.

Summary

Because dental disease is the most frequently encountered health problem in the United States, and because pharmacists see many people with dental problems, today's pharmacist needs a well-developed knowledge of oral health care products and their use. The pharmacist-dentist team can improve oral health in the community. With useful references such as the *Journal of the American Dental Association*, *Clinical Products in Dentistry*, and the special dental issue of *Pharmacy Times* every July; with awareness of ongoing FDA and ADA evaluations of nonprescription dental products; and with open lines of communication to dental practitioners, pharmacists can better serve their patients as oral health consultants and members of the dental health care team.

References

1. Harris NO, Christen AG. *Primary Preventive Dentistry*. 3rd ed. Norwalk, Conn: Appleton & Lange; 1991: 67–8, 91–3, 115–21, 148, 156–7, 338–43, 399, 406, 419, 470–1, 487.
2. Striffler DF, Young WO, Burt BA. *Dentistry, Dental Practice, and the Community*. 3rd ed. Philadelphia: WB Saunders Co; 1983: 123, 140, 204–5, 236.
3. Rosendahl I. Drugstores cling to OTC/HBC lead. *Drug Topics*. 1995 May 8: 52–61.
4. NIH consensus development conference: health implications of smokeless tobacco use. *Am Pharm*. 1986 Apr; NS26(4): 18–20.
5. Glover ED et al. Implications of smokeless tobacco use among athletes. *Physician and Sportsmedicine*. 1986; 14(12): 95–104.
6. McHugh WD. Role of supragingival plaque in oral disease initiation and progression. In: Loe H, Kleinman DV, eds. *Dental*

Plaque Control Measures and Oral Hygiene Practices. Oxford, England: IRL Press; 1986: 1–12.

7. Pader M. *Oral Hygiene Products and Practice.* New York: Marcel Dekker, Inc; 1988: 45–59, 89, 101, 226–8, 333–8, 426–53, 489–504.
8. Greenwell H, Bissada NF, Wittwer JW. Periodontics in general practice: professional plaque control. *J Am Dent Assoc.* 1990: 642–6.
9. Low SB, Ciancio SG. Reviewing nonsurgical periodontal therapy. *J Am Dent Assoc.* 1990; 121: 467–70.
10. Kidd EAM, Joyston-Bechal S. *Essentials of Dental Caries.* Bristol, England: IOP Publishing Ltd; 1987: 3–15, 82.
11. *Federal Register.* 1990 Sep 19; 55: 38560–2.
12. *Federal Register.* 1994 Feb 9; 59: 6084.
13. Council on Dental Materials, Instruments, and Equipment; and Council on Dental Therapeutics. *Clinical Products in Dentistry: A Desktop Reference.* Chicago: American Dental Association; 1993: 1–3, 7–9, 27, 35.
14. Nathan A, Anderson C. Oral health: part 2. oral hygiene. *Pharm J.* 1991 May 25; 246: 657–8.
15. Mandel, ID. The plaque fighters: choosing a weapon. *J Am Dent Assoc.* 1993; 124(4): 71–4.
16. Lazarus G. Colgate's smile still bright in toothbrush sales. *Chicago Tribune.* Mar 27, 1995; 4: 2.
17. Toothbrush may be link to sore throat, infections. *Med World News.* 1986 Mar 10; 27(5): 68.
18. Council on Dental Materials, Instruments, and Equipment; and Council on Dental Therapeutics. *Clinical Products in Dentistry: A Desktop Reference.* Chicago: American Dental Association; 1992: 27–9.
19. Bratel J, Berggren U, Hirsch JM. Electric or manual toothbrush? *Clin Prev Dent.* 1988; 10(3): 23–6.
20. Council on Dental Therapeutics. *Accepted Dental Therapeutics.* 40th ed. Chicago: American Dental Association; 1984: 64–5, 79, 321–4, 386–8, 395–420, 402–11.
21. Mueller LJ et al. Rotary electric toothbrushing: clinical effects on the presence of gingivitis and supragingival dental plaque. *Dent Hyg.* 1987 Dec; 613: 546–50.
22. Glavind L, Zeuner E. The effectiveness of a rotary electric toothbrush on oral cleanliness in adults. *J Clin Periodontol.* 1986; 13: 135–8.
23. Coontz EJ. The effectiveness of a new home plaque-removal instrument on plaque removal. *Compend Cont Educ Dent.* 1985; 6(suppl): 117–22.
24. Frandsen A. Mechanical oral hygiene practices. In: Loe H, Kleinman DV, eds. *Dental Plaque Control Measures and Oral Hygiene Practices.* Oxford, England: IRL Press; 1986: 100.
25. Newman MG et al. Effectiveness of adjunctive irrigation in early periodontitis—multi-center evaluation. *J Periodontol.* 1994 Mar, 65: 224–9.
26. Greenstein G. Effects of subgingival irrigation on periodontal status. *J Periodontol.* 1987 Dec; 58: 827–36.
27. Carranza FA Jr. *Glickman's Clinical Periodontology.* 7th ed. Philadelphia: WB Saunders Co; 1990: 706.
28. Lamberts DM, Wunderlich RC, Caffesse RG. The effect of waxed and unwaxed dental floss on gingival health: part I. plaque removal and gingival response. *J Periodontol.* 1982; 53: 393–9.
29. Hill HC, Levi PA, Glickman I. The effects of waxed and unwaxed dental floss on interdental plaque accumulation and interdental gingival health. *J Periodontol.* 1973; 44: 411–3.
30. Perry DA, Pattison G. An investigation of wax residue on tooth surfaces after the use of waxed dental floss. *Dent Hyg.* 1986; 60: 16–9.
31. Kiger RD, Nylund K, Feller RP. A comparison of proximal plaque removal using floss and interdental brushes. *J Clin Periodontol.* 1991; 18: 681–4.
32. Mauriello S et al. Effectiveness of three interproximal cleaning devices. *Clin Prev Dent.* 1987; 9: 18–22.
33. Controlling plaque limits periodontal disease. *US Pharm.* 1987 Aug; 12: 70–6.
34. *Federal Register.* 1988 Jun 15; 53: 22443–6.
35. *FDC Reports.* 1994 Mar 14; 3: 15.
36. Kanapka JA. Over-the-counter dentifrices in the treatment of tooth hypersensitivity. *Dent Clin North Am.* 1990 Jul; 34: 545–60.
37. Sears C. Baking soda toothpastes. *Am Health.* 1994 Apr; 13: 19.
38. A guide to good dental care. *Consumer Rep.* 1992 Sep; 57: 602–4.
39. *Federal Register.* 1980 Mar 28; 45: 20670.
40. Marsh PD. Dentifrices containing new agents for the control of plaque and gingivitis: microbiological aspects. *J Clin Periodontol.* 1991; 18: 462–7.
41. Hogg SD. Chemical control of plaque. *Dent Update.* 1990 Oct; 17: 330, 332–4.
42. van der Ouderaa F, Cummins D. Anti-plaque dentifrices: current status and prospects. *Int Dent J.* 1991; 41(2): 117–23.
43. Balanyk TE. Sanguinarine: comparisons of antiplaque/antigingivitis reports. *Clin Prev Dent.* 1990; 12(3): 18–25.
44. Council on Dental Therapeutics. Guidelines for acceptance of chemotherapeutic products for the control of supragingival dental plaque and gingivitis. *J Am Dent Assoc.* 1986; 112: 529–32.
45. Jakush J. New fluoride schedule adopted. *ADA News.* 1994 May 16: 12, 14.
46. Lobene RR et al. Reduced formation of supragingival calculus with the use of fluoride–zinc chloride dentifrice. *J Am Dent Assoc.* 1987; 114: 350.
47. Zacherl WA, Pfeiffer HJ, Swancar JR. The effect of soluble pyrophosphates on dental calculus in adults. *J Am Dent Assoc.* 1985; 110: 737–8.
48. Naleway CA, Whall CW Jr. What benefits do tartar control dentifrices provide your patrons? *Pharm Times.* 1987 Jul; 53: 32–7.
49. Beacham BE, Kurgansky D, Gould WM. Circumoral dermatitis and cheilitis caused by tartar control dentifrices. *J Am Acad Dermatol.* 1990 Jun; 22: 1029–32.
50. *Federal Register.* 1982 May 25; 47: 22809, 22842–4.
51. *Federal Register.* 1995 Jan; 60: 4536–41.
52. *NDMA Executive Newsletter.* 1994 Dec 9; 43: 2.
53. Mandel ID. Antimicrobial mouthrinses—overview and update. *J Am Dent Assoc.* 1994 Aug; 125: S2–S10.
54. American Dental Association. Council on Dental Therapeutics accepts Listerine. *J Am Dent Assoc.* 1988; 117: 515–7.
55. Gossel TA. Counseling the consumer on antiplaque mouthrinses. *US Pharm.* 1988 Dec; 13: 46–8, 51.
56. Moran J, Addy M. The effects of a cetylpyridinium chloride prebrushing rinse as an adjunct to oral hygiene and gingival health. *J Periodontol.* 1991; 62: 562–4.
57. Balley L. The effect of a detergent-based pre-brushing dental rinse on plaque accumulation. *J Clin Dent.* 1990; II(1): 6–10.
58. Emling RC, Yankell SL. An analysis of the clinical plaque removal efficacy of a pre-brushing dental rinse in a three center study design. *J Clin Dent.* 1990; II(1): 11–6.
59. Grossman E. Effectiveness of a prebrushing mouthrinse under single-trial and home-use conditions. *Clin Prev Dent.* 1988; 10: 3–6.
60. Beiswanger BB et al. The relative plaque removal effect of a prebrushing mouthrinse. *J Am Dent Assoc.* 1990; 120: 190–2.
61. Freitas BL, Collaert B, Attstrom R. Effect of the pre-brushing rinse, Plax, on dental plaque formation. *J Clin Periodontol.* 1991; 18: 713–5.
62. Schiff TS, Border LC. The effect of a new experimental prebrushing dental rinse on plaque removal. *J Clin Dent.* 1994; 4: 107–10.
63. Howard WR. Patient-applied tooth whiteners: are they safe, effective with supervision? *J Am Dent Assoc.* 1992; 123: 57–60.
64. Council on Dental Therapeutics. Guidelines for the acceptance of peroxide-containing oral hygiene products. *J Am Dent Assoc.* 1994 Aug; 125: 1140–2.

65. Council on Dental Therapeutics. *Accepted Products Categorical Listing*. Chicago: American Dental Association; 1995 Mar: 9–11, 21, 38.
66. Haywood VB, Heymann HO. Nightguard vital bleaching. *Quintessence Int.* 1989; 20: 173–6.
67. Cubbon T, Ore D. Hard tissue and home tooth whiteners. *CDS Rev.* 1991 Jun; 84(5): 32–5.
68. Barrington EP, Nevins M. Diagnosing periodontal diseases. *J Am Dent Assoc.* 1990 Oct; 121: 460–4.
69. Pinkham JR. *Pediatric Dentistry: Infancy through Adolescence.* Philadelphia: WB Saunders Co; 1988: 507–8.
70. Genco RJ, Goldman HM, Cohen DW, eds. *Contemporary Periodontics.* St. Louis: CV Mosby; 1990: 63–81, 348–59.
71. Loe H. The specific etiology of periodontal disease and its application to prevention. In: Carranza FA, Kenney EB, eds. *Prevention of Periodontal Disease.* Chicago: Quintessence Publishing Co; 1981: 15–22.
72. Bar A. Caries prevention with xylitol. *World Rev Nutr Diet.* 1988; 55: 1–27.
73. Consensus: oral health effects of products that increase salivary flow rate. *J Am Dent Assoc.* 1988; 116: 757.
74. Fluoride: still a good public health value. *Pharm Times.* 1990 Jul; 56: 105–7, 111.
75. Pray WS. Fluoridation: the battle continues. *US Pharm.* 1990 Oct; 15: 20–4.
76. Adair SM. Risks and benefits of fluoride mouthrinsing. *Pediatrician.* 1989; 16: 161–9.
77. *Federal Register.* 1985 Sep 30; 50: 39859, 39872.
78. Glass RL. Fluoride dentifrices: the basis for the decline in caries prevalence. *J R Soc Med.* 1986; 79(suppl) 14: 15–7.
79. Mellberg JR. Fluoride dentifrices: current status and prospects. *Int Dent J.* 1991 Feb; 41: 9–16.
80. Council on Dental Therapeutics. Council on Dental Therapeutics accepts Extra-Strength Aim. *J Am Dent Assoc.* 1988; 117: 785.
81. Ripa LW. A critique of topical fluoride methods (dentifrices, mouthrinses, operator-, and self-applied gels) in an era of decreased caries and increased fluorosis prevalence. *J Public Health Dent.* 1991 Winter; 51: 23–41.
82. Gossel TA. The role of fluorides in preventing cavities. *US Pharm.* 1986 Mar; 11: 28–32, 34.
83. Maher WP. Anatomy of a toothache. *Pharm Times.* 1992 Mar; 58: 43–9.
84. *Federal Register.* 1991 Sep 24; 56: 48308–10, 48315–6, 48325, 48335–46.
85. Gossel TA. Hypersensitive teeth: OTCs take the pain away. *US Pharm.* 1991 May; 16: 23–32.
86. *Federal Register.* 1992 May 11; 57: 20115.
87. Pray WS. Oral mucosal lesions. *US Pharm.* 1990 Feb; 15: 21–2, 24–5, 66.
88. Antoon JW, Miller RL. Aphthous ulcers—a review of the literature on etiology, pathogenesis, diagnosis, and treatment. *J Am Dent Assoc.* 1980 Nov; 101: 603–8.
89. Gossel TA. Debriding agents and oral wound cleansers. *US Pharm.* 1990 Feb; 15: 28–36.
90. *Federal Register.* 1990 Jan 31; 55: 3372, 3379.
91. *Federal Register.* 1993 May 10; 58: 27638.
92. *Federal Register.* 1992 Jun 30; 57: 29173.
93. *Federal Register.* 1988 Jan 27; 53: 2453, 2456.
94. *Federal Register.* 1986 Jul 18; 51: 26113.
95. Budtz-Jorgensen E, Bertraum U. Denture stomatitis: I. the etiology in relation to trauma and infection. *Acta Odontol Scand.* 1970; 28: 71–92.
96. Abelson DC. Denture plaque and denture cleansers: review of the literature. *Gerodontics.* 1985; 1: 202–6.
97. Ciancio S. Expanded and future uses of mouthrinses. *J Am Dent Assoc.* 1994 Aug; 125: S29–32.
98. Niessen LC, Williams GC. Aging in America: implications for dentistry. *Pharm Times.* 1988 Jul; 54: 36–40.
99. Baum BJ. Changes in salivary function in older subjects. In: Ferguson DB, ed. *Frontiers of Oral Physiology.* Vol 6. *The Aging Mouth.* Basel, Switzerland: Karger; 1987: 126–34.
100. Gossel TA. Counseling patients on denture cleansing products. *US Pharm.* 1988 Jun; 13: 56–8, 61–2, 76.
101. Zacharczenko N. Dentures and denture care. *Pharm Times.* 1991 Jul; 57: 42.
102. Council on Dental Materials, Instruments, and Equipment. Denture cleansers. *J Am Dent Assoc.* 1983; 106: 77–9.
103. Gossel TA. The proper use of denture adhesives and reliners. *US Pharm.* 1987 Sep; 12: 42, 46, 48, 51.
104. Klatell J, Kaplan A, Williams G Jr. *Family Guide to Dental Health.* New York: Macmillan; 1991: 37, 83.
105. Baker KA, Levy SM. Review of systemic fluoride supplementation and consideration of the pharmacist's role. *Drug Intell Clin Pharm.* 1986; 20: 935–42.
106. Wilson M. Fighting plaque. *Am Drug.* 1988 Sep; 198: 102–4.

CHAPTER 26

Dermatologic Products

Dennis P. West and Phillip A. Nowakowski

Questions to ask in patient assessment and counseling

Dermatitis and Scaly Dermatoses

- *How long have you had this condition?*
- *What skin areas, including mucous membranes, hair, and nails, are involved?*
- *How does the affected area feel (eg, itchy, painful)? Is it dry or oozing?*
- *Do you scratch the affected area? If so, how often? What time of day is it worse?*
- *Has your condition changed in appearance?*
- *Have you ever had this condition before? Does it seem to come and go?*
- *Have you ever had other skin conditions?*
- *Do others in your family have a similar condition?*
- *Do you or any family members have allergies, asthma, or hay fever?*
- *Do you notice a seasonal change in your condition?*
- *What is your occupation?*
- *Is there anything such as engaging in work activities or hobbies; cleaning house; changing soaps, deodorants, or shampoos; wearing jewelry; or taking medications that seems to make the condition worse?*
- *Have you consulted a physician about your condition? If so, what treatment was suggested? Did you, or are you currently, following any suggested treatment? How effective have any previous treatments been for this condition?*
- *Are you currently using any prescription or nonprescription medications? If so, what are they?*
- *What is your (the patient's) age?*

Skin Infections

- *What area of the skin is affected? How extensive is the area involved?*
- *Is the skin broken? Is there pus? Is it painful?*
- *How long have you had this condition? Have you ever had it before?*
- *Has the condition developed as the result of a previous rash or skin condition?*
- *Has the condition worsened?*
- *Are any other members of your family affected?*
- *Do you have a fever or any flulike symptoms?*
- *Do you have diabetes? Do you have any other medical conditions?*
- *Do you have any allergies to topical medications?*
- *What treatments have you tried for this condition? Were they effective?*
- *What oral or topical medications are you currently using? Have they been effective?*

Skin Hyperpigmentation Products

- *Have you been using a skin hyperpigmentation product? If so, for how long?*
- *For what type of "skin spot" do you use it?*
- *How long have you had that mole?*
- *Has the mole changed color or increased in size?*
- *Do you have any medical problems?*
- *Is there any possibility that you are pregnant?*
- *Are you taking any medications, including birth control pills?*

Hair Loss (Alopecia)

- *How long ago did you begin to lose your hair? What areas of the scalp are involved? How extensive are the areas involved?*
- *Do others in your family suffer from hair loss?*
- *What treatments for hair loss have you already tried? Did you see any improvement in the condition?*
- *Have you been diagnosed as having an autoimmune disorder, nutritional deficiency, or endocrine disorder?*
- *Have you undergone chemotherapy or used a hormonal medication?*
- *(If female) Have you recently given birth?*
- *Have you suffered any trauma to the scalp?*

Skin conditions are common, with an estimated 5 in 100 people suffering from a chronic skin, hair, or nail disorder and many others encountering acute or seasonal conditions. The pharmacist is often the first health care professional the patient consults concerning conditions such as dermatitis, dry skin, dandruff, seborrhea, psoriasis, hyperpigmentation, and hair loss. Therefore, when recommending the use of an appropriate nonprescription product or referring the patient to a physician, the pharmacist must consider the cosmetic, psychologic, and work- or recreation-related aspects of a dermatologic disorder in addition to the underlying pathology.

Anatomy and Physiology of Skin

As the largest organ of the body, the skin is involved in numerous physical and biochemical processes.[1] Skin thickness is variable but averages about 1–2 mm; skin is thickest on the palms of the hand and soles of the feet and thinnest on the eyelids and scrotum. Although it is exposed to a wide variety of chemical and environmental insults, skin demonstrates remarkable resiliency and recuperative ability.

Skin Regions

Human skin is composed of three functionally distinct regions: epidermis, dermis, and hypodermis. Figure 1 shows these three regions and their components.

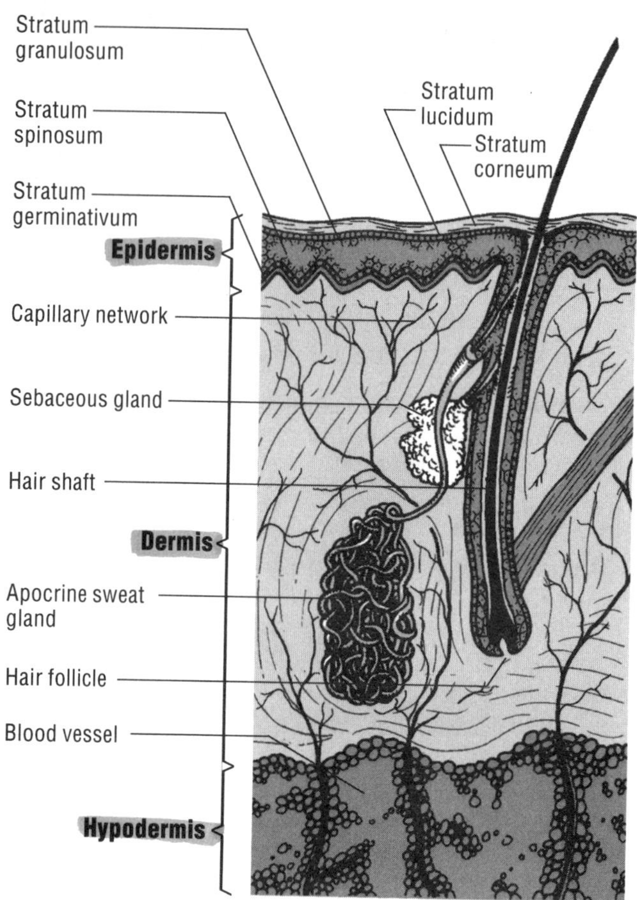

FIGURE 1 Cross section of human skin.

Epidermis

The epidermis (outermost region), which is compact, avascular, and composed of stratified squamous epithelial cells, comprises five distinct layers. Innermost, in close association with the dermis, is the basal cell layer (stratum germinativum). This layer consists of columnar/cuboidal epithelial cells, or keratinocytes, which divide and move upward. The basal cell region is predominately involved in mitotic processes of epidermal regeneration and repair. As keratinocytes migrate to the skin surface, they change from living cells to dead, thick-walled, flat, nonnucleated cells that contain keratin, a fibrous, insoluble protein.

Above the basal cell layer is the prickle cell unit (stratum spinosum), which is thicker in the palms and soles than in other anatomic skin sites. This layer is composed of prickle cells, polygonal epithelial cells that are produced by cellular division and contain keratinocytes, the pigment-forming melanocytes that contain melanin precursors, and melanin granules.

Above the prickle cells is the granular region (stratum granulosum), which is actually several thicknesses of flattened polygonal cells. These cells are rich in granules of keratohyalin.

A translucent, thin area (stratum lucidum), present in the palms and soles, lies between the stratum granulosum and the stratum corneum. The stratum lucidum is a narrow band of flattened, closely packed cells believed to be derived from keratohyalin.

The outermost layer, the stratum corneum, is composed of flat, scaly, dead (keratinized) tissue. Its outermost cells are flat (squamous) plates that are constantly shed (desquamated) and replaced by new cells generated by the mitotic processes of the basal cell layer. Specifically, newer cells push older ones closer to the surface. In the process, the older cells are flattened, lose water, become more compact, and gradually lose their nuclei before taking their place on the skin surface, where they are shed. Because the keratinized, or "horny," layer of the stratum corneum is constantly being shed and regenerated, the epidermis is maintained at a uniform thickness. The complete cycle, from basal cell formation to shedding, is 28–45 days.

Editor's Note: This chapter is based, in part, on the 8th edition chapter "Dermatitis, Dry Skin, Dandruff, Seborrheic Dermatitis, and Psoriasis Products," written by Joseph R. Robinson and Laura J. Gauger, as well as the 10th edition chapter "Dermatologic Products," written by Joye Ann Billow. The present chapter has also been updated and expanded to include discussions of viral and fungal skin infections and skin hyperpigmentation, the core material of which appeared in the 10th edition chapters "Topical Anti-Infective Products," written by Dennis P. West and Susan V. Maddux, and "Personal Care Products," written by Donald R. Miller and Mary Kuzel.

The stratum corneum is the body's primary barrier to insults from the environment. Lipid components of its cells may store fat-soluble materials rather than allow them to pass into the systemic circulation.

Flexibility of the stratum corneum depends on its water content, which is normally between 10% and 20% by weight. A variety of factors, including humidity, temperature, surfactants, and physical and chemical trauma, influence the water content of the stratum corneum.[2] Keratin can absorb many times its weight in water, and so it retains water to maintain the skin's flexibility and integrity. Intracellular spaces of the stratum corneum contain a complex mixture of hygroscopic substances (free amino acids, pyrrolidine carboxylic acid, urea, uric acid, ammonia, creatinine, sodium, calcium, potassium, magnesium, phosphate, chloride, lactate, citrate, formate, sugars, organic acids, and peptides) called the natural moisturizing factor, which holds water and allows the absorption of water-soluble drugs. When water content drops below 10%, chapping occurs and the stratum corneum becomes brittle and cracks easily. This allows irritants and bacteria to penetrate more easily, causing inflammation and possibly infection.

Dermis

About 40 times thicker than the epidermis, the dermis supports the epidermis physically and separates it from the lower fatty layer. The dermis consists mainly of elastic and connective tissue (collagen and elastin) embedded in a mucopolysaccharide substance. Fibroblasts and mast cells are found throughout. A network of nerves and capillaries is found in the dermis; this network comprises the neurovascular supply to dermal appendages (hair follicles, sebaceous glands, and sweat glands). Because this layer of skin contains nerve fibers, it is responsible for cutaneous sensations. The sensation of itching arises in the upper portion; that of stinging, in the middle portion; and that of pain, in the portion closest to the layer of subcutaneous fat. Main regions of the dermis are the papillary and reticular layers. The papillary layer, adjacent to the epidermis, is rich in blood vessels, and the papillae probably assist in bringing nutrients to the avascular epidermis. Below the papillae, the reticular layer contains coarser tissue that connects the dermis with the hypodermis.

Hypodermis

The hypodermis, or subcutaneous tissue, is the innermost area of the skin. It is composed of loose connective tissue and adipose tissue firmly anchored to the dermis. Subcutaneous tissue is of varying thickness and provides necessary pliability for human skin. This layer also includes a fatty component that facilitates thermal control and food reserve and provides cushioning or padding.

Skin Components

Hair Follicles

A follicle is basically an inward tubular insertion of the epidermis into the dermis. Within the follicle is a fiber (hair shaft) of keratinized epithelial cells that grows at the base of the follicle as a result of cell multiplication in the papilla. Capillaries are present and provide nutrients to the hair.

Sebaceous Glands

Most sebaceous (sebum-producing) glands are located in the same anatomic area as the hair because they are usually adjacent to follicles and are fully activated at puberty. Sebaceous glands that are not associated with hair follicles may be found in genital areas, around the nipples, and on the border of the lips. Ducts of these glands are lined with epithelial cells that are continuous with basal cell layers of the epidermis. Sebum, which covers the hair and skin surface, is a mixture of free fatty acids (mainly palmitic and oleic), triglycerides, waxes, cholesterol, squalene, other hydrocarbons, and traces of fat-soluble vitamins. With sweat, sebum forms an emulsion that includes the surface waste products of cutaneous cells.

Sweat Glands

Two types of sweat glands are identified in association with dermal anatomy: the apocrine and eccrine glands. Both are considered exocrine because their secretions (sweat) reach the skin surface.

Apocrine sweat glands are generally attached to hair follicles by ducts that lead down into coiled, secretory glandular tubules. These tubules are covered with myoepithelium, allowing contraction in response to adrenergic stimulation. Such stimulation, as in stress, releases a milky secretion that contains proteins, sugars, and lipids. This secretion is odorless until skin bacteria act on its contents, producing the characteristic body odor ascribed primarily to 3-methyl-2-hexanoic acid, one of the dozens of chemicals isolated from human sweat. Apocrine glands are present around the nipples, in axilla, and in the anogenital region. The glands do not function in body temperature regulation but instead are responsive to hormone secretion. Consequently, their onset of action is associated with puberty.

Eccrine glands are independent of hair follicles and develop from the epithelium of the skin surface, extending in a coil to the dermis. Secretory epithelia are located in the hypodermis, and the ducts ascend through the epidermis. Eccrine glands are present over most of the body surface, except for genital areas and legs, and are especially numerous on palms and soles. Eccrine sweat production is controlled by a heat regulatory center of the hypothalamus. Emotional stress and cholinergic drugs can also trigger eccrine sweating. The volume of eccrine sweat produced is much greater than that of apocrine sweat.

Nails

Nails are modifications of the keratinized region of epidermal tissue. The nail bed, on which the nail plate lies, derives from basal epidermis. At its periphery, the body of the plate is surrounded by the nail matrix. This matrix is derived from the nail groove, which, in turn, is derived from the basal cell layer of the epidermis. At the base of the nail is the white area called the lunula (Figure 2).

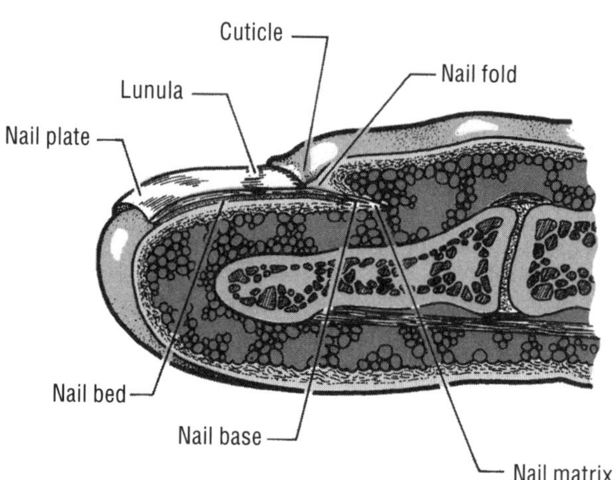

Figure 2 Anatomic features of the nail. Adapted with permission from *Integumentary Systems.* Roanoke, Va: CMRI; 1992: 22.

Skin Surface

Secretions that accumulate on the skin surface are weakly acidic, with a pH of 4.5 to 5.5 (the acid mantle).[1] This pH varies slightly from individual to individual and from one area of the body to another; it is somewhat higher in areas where perspiration evaporates slowly.[3]

Various microorganisms live on the surface of intact skin. Individual species that make up the flora exist in a normal ecologic balance. Skin flora is diverse, including aerobic and anaerobic bacterial species. Some individuals have a consistently high skin microbial population.

Skin Functions

Normal skin and its appendages (hair and nails) have a variety of functions, the most important being to serve as a protective barrier between the body and the environment. The ability of the skin to protect the body from harmful external agents such as pathogenic organisms and chemicals[4] depends on a variety of factors, including the age, immunologic status, and underlying disease states of the individual; the use of certain oral or topical medications; and the preservation of an intact stratum corneum.[5]

The acid mantle has been postulated to be a protective mechanism because many microbes tend to grow better at a pH of 6–7.5. Infected areas of skin typically have higher pH values than areas of normal skin. Several fatty acids (propionic, caproic, and caprylic) found in sweat and sebum help inhibit microbial and fungal growth. Therefore, the importance of the acid mantle concept lies not solely in the inherent pH of the acid mantle but also in the specific compounds responsible for the acidity.

Another protective mechanism is the buffer capacity of skin surface secretion. When pH is altered, the skin tends to readjust to a normal pH. Moreover, normal skin flora acts as a defense mechanism by controlling the growth of potential pathogenic organisms and their possible invasion of the skin and body.

The skin also contributes to sensory experiences and is involved in temperature control, pigment development, and the synthesis of some vitamins. It is also important in hydroregulation because it controls moisture loss from the body and moisture penetration into the body.

Skin hydration is important to the health and normal function of the skin. If the stratum corneum becomes dehydrated, it loses elasticity and its permeation characteristics become altered. The stratum corneum can be hydrated by water transfer from lower regions of the skin and by water accumulation (perspiration) induced by occlusive coverings such as tight, impervious bandages or oleaginous pharmaceutical vehicles (eg, petrolatum). Generally, such moisture accumulation seems to "open" the compactness of the stratum corneum for renewed suppleness and more effective penetration by some drug molecules.

Percutaneous Absorption of Drugs

A drug must be released from its vehicle if it is to exert an effect at the desired site of activity (the skin surface, the epidermis, or the dermis). Release occurs at the interface between the skin surface and the applied layer of product. The physical-chemical relationship between the drug and the vehicle determines the rate and amount of drug released. Considerations such as the drug's solubility in the vehicle, its diffusion coefficient in the vehicle, and its partition coefficient into sebum and stratum corneum are significant to its efficacy.[6] A drug with a strong affinity for the vehicle has a lower rate and extent of percutaneous absorption than does a drug with weaker affinity for its vehicle. Thus, a drug with a proper balance of polar and hydrocarbon moieties (ie, a partition coefficient approaching 1) penetrates the stratum corneum more readily than one that is either highly polar or highly lipoidal because that portion of the skin possesses both hydrated proteins and lipids.

Other factors influencing drug release include degree of hydration of the stratum corneum, pK_a of the drug, pH of the drug vehicle and the skin surface, drug concentration, thickness of the applied layer, and temperature. As temperature increases at the site of application, blood flow in the area also increases, as does the rate of percutaneous absorption. These factors apply to drug release from all topical forms (eg, powders, ointments, pastes, emulsified creams or lotions, gels, suspensions, and solutions).

Oily hydrocarbon bases such as petrolatum are transiently occlusive, promote hydration, and generally increase molecular transport. Hydrous emulsion bases are less occlusive. Water-soluble bases (polyethylene glycols) are minimally occlusive, may attract water from the stratum corneum, and may decrease drug transport. Powders with hydrophilic ingredients presumably decrease hydration because they promote evaporation from the skin by absorbing available water.

Substances are transported from the skin surface to

TABLE 1 Selected dermatologic terms useful in the assessment of skin lesions

Term	Type of lesion[a]	Definition
Crust (scab)	Secondary	Dried exudate containing proteinaceous and cellular debris from erosion or ulceration of primary lesions
Erythema	Primary	Reddened skin
Fissure	Secondary	A split in the epidermis extending into the dermis
Lichenification	Secondary	Thickening and hardening of the skin into an irregular plaque due to excessive rubbing or scratching
Macule	Primary	Flat, nonpalpable, discolored lesion less than 1 cm in diameter. Lesions larger than 1 cm are termed *patches*
Necrosis	Secondary	Dead cells or groups of cells caused by severe trauma or an infectious process
Papule	Primary	A solid, circumscribed, elevated lesion less than 1 cm in diameter
Plaque	Primary	A palpable, papular, relatively flat lesion more than 1 cm in diameter
Pustule	Primary	A circumscribed, elevated lesion less than 1 cm in diameter containing pus. A larger lesion is termed an *abscess* or *furuncle*
Scale	Secondary	Accumulation of loose, desquamated, hyperkeratitic epidermal cells
Ulcer	Secondary	An erosion of the epidermis exposing the dermis. Deep ulcers may result in destruction of the dermis
Vesicle	Primary	A sharply circumscribed, elevated lesion containing fluid. Diameter of a vesicle may be up to 1 cm. A fluid-filled cavity of diameter greater than 1 cm is termed a *blister* or *bulla*

[a]Primary lesions are changes in the skin as a result of the undisturbed disease process. Secondary lesions are the result of external influences on the primary lesion. Primary and secondary lesion frequently coexist.

Adapted from Cahn RL, Longe RL. *The Skin: Assessment*. Palo Alto, Calif: Syntex Laboratories; 1986: 4–5.

the general circulation through percutaneous absorption. The routes of such transport have not been proved, but it is presumed that they involve passage through skin between the keratinized units of the stratum corneum and through skin appendages (hair follicles, sweat glands, and sebaceous glands). The major mechanism of drug absorption is by passive diffusion through the stratum corneum, followed by transport through deeper epidermal regions and then the dermis.

Depending on the physical-chemical properties of a drug, the sebum, and various skin regions, drug movement into and through the skin meets with varying degrees of enhancement or inhibition. The stratum corneum provides the greatest resistance and is often a rate-limiting barrier to percutaneous absorption. Because it is nonliving tissue, the stratum corneum may be viewed as having the general characteristics of an artificial and semipermeable membrane, and molecular passage through it occurs mostly by passive diffusion. Once a molecule has crossed the stratum corneum, there is much less resistance to its transport through the rest of the epidermis and into the dermis.

When the stratum corneum is hydrated, drug diffusion is generally accelerated. Hydration swells the stratum corneum, loosening its normally tight, densely packed arrangement and making diffusion easier. Because occlusion increases hydration of the stratum corneum, it enhances the transfer of most drugs. The increased amount of water present in the skin under such conditions probably further enhances the transfer of polar molecules.

TABLE 2 Characteristics of selected forms of dermatitis and dry skin

Condition	Symptoms	Location	Signs
Atopic dermatitis	Itching, scratching	2 mo: chest, face 2 y: scalp, neck, and extremities 2–4 y: neck, wrist, elbow, knee 12–20 y: flexors, hands	Red, raised vesicles; dry skin; oozing Less acute lesions; edema; erythema Dry, thickened plaques; hyperpigmentation
Contact dermatitis (irritant and allergic)	Acute: itching Chronic: stiffness, dry	Irritant: contact areas Allergic: exposed contact areas (transferable by touch)	Irritant (mild, acute): red, oozing blisters Irritant (mild, chronic): dry, thick, fissured skin Irritant (severe): blisters, ulcers Allergic: unusual pattern of lesions; sharp margins with angles and straight lines
Hand dermatitis	Itching, dry	Sides of fingers, occasionally palms	Red, dry, chapped, fissured skin
Dry skin (chapped)	Often none; moderate to severe itching	Lower legs, backs of hands, forearms, occasionally entire body	Dry, fine scale; patches, diffuse or round; if severe, fissures

Adapted from Ricciatti–Sibbald DJ. In: Clark C, ed. *Self-Medication: A Reference for Health Professionals*. 4th ed. Ottawa: Canadian Pharmaceutical Association; 1992: 65.

Wounds, burns, chafed areas, and dermatitis can alter the integrity of the stratum corneum and result in artificial shunts of the percutaneous absorption process. Scarring and inflammation can also enhance absorption. Because this might result in potentially dangerous systemic drug levels by percutaneous absorption, caution should be used in applying topical medication to damaged skin, especially if large surface areas are involved.

Dermatitis

Dermatitis is a nonspecific term that describes a number of dermatologic conditions that are inflammatory and generally characterized by erythema. The terms *eczema* and *dermatitis* are often used interchangeably to describe a group of inflammatory skin disorders of unknown etiology. When the cause of a particular skin condition is elucidated, the disorder is given a specific name. Known causes of dermatitis include allergens, irritants, and infections. However, there are several distinct forms of dermatitis for which the causes remain unclear.

Dermatitis may be either acute or chronic. Initially, the signs and symptoms are similar for most forms of dermatitis. These signs may include pruritus (itching), erythema (redness), and edema (swelling). Edema may be accompanied by fluid-filled vesicles, which often break and cause weeping or oozing from the skin. Evaporation of water from the exudate results in crusting and scaling. Over time, the weeping may diminish, giving way to a dry, scaly condition. Lesions may be patchy in distribution. When the dermatitis is acute, it is common to observe vesicles on an erythematous base in the lesional area[7]; the dermatitis is further characterized as weeping or oozing (Table 1). If the dermatitis is chronic, weeping present in the acute phase has subsided, the skin is dry and scaly, and fissures may appear. If itching results in excessive scratching, the epidermis may appear thickened and ridged (lichenification). Infections may occur as sequelae to pruritus-induced scratching. Pigment production may be altered, and hyper- or hypopigmentation may become evident.[2]

The most common forms of dermatitis include atopic dermatitis, contact dermatitis (irritant or allergic), and hand dermatitis ("dishpan hands"). Table 2 lists the primary characteristics of these conditions as compared with dry skin.

Specific Conditions

Atopic Dermatitis

Atopic dermatitis, also called eczema, occurs primarily in infants, children, and young adults and is the most common dermatologic condition seen in children. It is often associated with other skin conditions, such as dry skin, hand dermatitis, and contact dermatitis. Depending on the patient's age, areas affected are commonly the face and the skin folds on the inside of the knees and elbows. The primary symptom of atopic dermatitis is intense itching that is often intermittent, leading to vigorous itch-scratch cycles.[8] The skin may show inflammation and produce scales.

Etiology and Characteristics Atopic dermatitis is not contagious but is known to be genetically linked. If one parent has the condition, the child has greater than a 25% chance of developing it also; if both parents have atopic dermatitis, the child has greater than a 50% chance of developing it. Although the etiology of the condition is unknown, patients and their families often have associated asthma, hay fever, or chronic allergic rhinitis.[9] Unfortunately, the avoidance of contact with allergens and the administration of oral antihistamines bring limited relief to the patient with this disease.

Although atopic dermatitis is often first manifested in infancy, it is rarely present at birth. If it does develop early in life, it occurs in the first year of life—often beginning at 2–3 months of age—in approximately 80% of the cases. It initially appears as redness and chapping of the infant's cheeks, which may continue on a chronic basis. Remission usually occurs between the second and fourth year, with recurrences often diminishing in intensity or even disappearing as the child approaches adulthood.[2]

Atopic dermatitis may be exacerbated by various factors, such as irritants, allergens, extremes of temperature and humidity, dry skin, emotional stress, and cutaneous infections. The patient should be encouraged to identify the role of these factors (if any) so that they may be minimized or avoided.

Irritants, which include solvents, industrial chemicals, fragrances, soaps, fumes, tobacco smoke, paints, bleach, wool, and astringents, may cause burning, itching, or redness of the skin.[10] Patients with atopic dermatitis are exquisitely sensitive to low concentrations of irritants that would not generally cause a reaction on normal skin.

Allergens—typically, plant or animal proteins from food, pollens, or pets—may aggravate atopic dermatitis. However, the role of food allergies in exacerbating atopic dermatitis is not clear. It is claimed that up to 20% of children with atopic dermatitis are affected by allergic reactions to foods through either ingestion or skin contact,[10] and specific hypersensitivities to milk products and eggs have been identified. However, the dietary management needed to achieve strict avoidance often poses overwhelming compliance problems. Moreover, while dietary restriction may show some improvement in the condition initially, decreasing long-term benefits are usually the outcome and complete resolution is unlikely to occur. Thus, it is probably best to reserve dietary management for those patients who have severe symptoms and are unresponsive to other treatments.[2,11]

Patients with atopic dermatitis are often intolerant of sudden and extreme changes in temperature and humidity. High humidity may result in increased perspiration, which may lead to increased itching. Low humidity, often found in heated buildings during the winter, dries the skin and increases itching. Use of humidifiers in dry environments will provide some benefit, especially if their use is not accompanied by excessively warm ambient temperatures.

Similar to asthma, emotional stress is an exacerbating factor in some patients. A calm environment and biofeedback techniques may prove beneficial for some of these patients.

Secondary or associated cutaneous infections are common, are often difficult to prevent, and usually aggravate the condition. Patients should be counseled to seek medical attention promptly when signs of bacterial or viral skin infection such as pustules, vesicles (especially exudate or pus-filled), crusting (dried exudate), and herpes simplex (fever blisters or cold sores) are noted.[10]

Assessment and Treatment Because atopic dermatitis is primarily a disease of the young, patient age is important in assessment. The pharmacist should determine whether the patient (or patient's family) has a history of atopic disorders. Inquiries should be made regarding onset and duration of the eruption. Anatomic location and distribution of the lesions should be taken into account. A classic case of infantile or childhood atopic dermatitis involves the cheeks and extensor surfaces of the forearms and legs. (See color plates, photographs 9A, B, and C.) Lesions are typically symmetric in atopic dermatitis patients.

If atopic dermatitis is not extreme and the patient is not a child under 2 years of age, initial treatment may be attempted with nonprescription measures. There is a general understanding that prescription topical products should not be used on children under 2 years of age except under the advice and supervision of a physician. Part of the rationale is that infants have higher body surface area-to-weight ratios than older individuals, as well as immature hepatic enzyme systems, and are therefore at increased risk for systemic effects from topically applied drugs.

Regardless of patient age, the stratum corneum in patients with atopic dermatitis contains less moisture than normal skin. As a result, excessive bathing with soap and water, with its concomitant frequent warming (vasoconstriction from hot water) and cooling (evaporation from skin surface), may actually increase the dryness of the skin and aggravate the dermatitis. Therefore, the first step is to ensure that bathing is not too frequent, preferably no more often than every other day, and to substitute sponge baths with tepid water for full-body bathing several days per week. Because of the significant drying effect of most soaps, mild cleansers (eg, Cetaphil) are recommended and better tolerated.

Treatment of acute weeping or oozing lesions is directed toward drying the lesions. Wet tap-water compresses should be applied for 20 minutes, four to six times daily. Bathing with tepid water containing colloidal oatmeal may be soothing. Hydrocortisone in an oil-in-water base may be used. If the condition does not resolve or if it involves a large area of the body, a physician should be consulted.

Treatment of chronic or dry lesions focuses on measures to maintain skin hydration and decrease itching. Colloidal oatmeal may be used for bathing, or a water-miscible bath oil may be added to the water near the end of the bath. The skin should be gently patted dry because vigorous rubbing produces irritation. An emollient should be applied while the skin is still damp. Ointments with a petrolatum or water-in-oil base maintain hydration best; however, atopic patients may often sweat after the application of heavy ointments, which then adds to the propensity for itching. Oil-in-water preparations are often more cosmetically acceptable, but they may need to be applied more often, and if used, they should have a good emollient effect and not produce dryness. Topical hydrocortisone may be used for inflammation and itching, preferably in an ointment base. If the condition is not relieved, a physician should be consulted.[11]

For itching, simply telling a patient not to scratch is generally not effective. Therefore, adjunctive measures may be used to minimize scratching and the damage it produces. Fingernails should be kept short, smooth, and clean. Scratching may increase at night, even while the patient is sleeping; therefore, wearing cotton gloves or socks on the hands at night helps lessen the resultant mechanical damage related to scratching. For some patients, itching may disrupt sleep. Antihistamines are of limited value in decreasing the itching, but those with a significant sedative effect (eg, diphenhydramine) may be used to promote sleep. A major limitation with the use of classic antihistamines is the undesired drowsiness or residual sedation or "hangover" effect that may be experienced the following morning.[11]

Contact Dermatitis

Contact dermatitis, one of the most common ailments directed to pharmacists for consultation, refers to a rash that results from an allergen or irritant contacting susceptible skin. It is further categorized into either irritant or allergic contact dermatitis,[12] with irritants accounting for 70–80% of all cases. Although the cause of each type is different, the signs, symptoms, and treatment of both are very similar. As with other forms of dermatitis, itching is usually the primary symptom.[13] The acute phase of contact dermatitis is often red, vesicular, and oozing. The chronic phase is likely to be dry, thickened, and fissured.

Although many cases of contact dermatitis involve exposed skin such as the hands and face, lesions may appear at virtually any location. Lesions are often asymmetric in distribution and sharply demarcated, reflecting where contact with the substance occurred.

Etiology and Characteristics Irritant contact dermatitis is a nonallergenic and nonimmunologic irritation. Inflammation may be produced by exposure to many substances if concentration and duration of contact are sufficient. A primary or strong irritant, such as a strong acid or alkali, generally elicits a response on first exposure; the injury it causes to the skin may not be limited to erythema and vesiculation but may result in ulceration and tissue necrosis. Mild irritants, such as soaps, detergents, and cosmetics, generally require repeated or extended contact to cause a significant inflammatory response. A secondary irritant that is not irritating to the skin when applied alone may cause irritation in combination with an agent that enhances absorption, such as a surfactant or keratolytic. Previously damaged skin is more easily irritated than undamaged skin.[7,14]

Environmental conditions play a role in the skin's resistance to irritants. High humidity as well as occlusion produces greater skin hydration and thus greater permeability.[7]

Allergic contact dermatitis is an immunologically mediated and delayed hypersensitivity reaction to contact allergens. It involves contact of the skin with an allergenic material functioning as a hapten, which becomes attached to protein carriers on specific cells in the epidermis. An initial sensitizing exposure is necessary for the reaction to occur. On subsequent contact with the allergen, reactive skin areas typically present an eczematous clinical picture, which usually appears within minutes to hours after exposure. Although it may often diminish substantially with old age, susceptibility to allergic contact dermatitis may last virtually a lifetime.[14]

The most common contact allergen comes from the *Rhus* genus of plants (eg, poison ivy, oak, and sumac). The offending agent is urushiol, a resin found in the leaves, stems, and roots of the plants. It is estimated that 70% of those exposed to urushiol become sensitized to it. In addition, particles in smoke and indirect contact with pets may cause allergic contact dermatitis in very sensitive persons.[2,14] (See Chapter 32, "Poison Ivy, Oak, and Sumac Products.")

A number of metals (eg, cobalt, chromium, and nickel) may cause allergic contact dermatitis. This sensitivity is important to keep in mind because nickel, often with cobalt as a contaminant, is widely used in costume jewelry, watches, and blue jean studs. Chromium is present in cement and may pose an occupational hazard to construction workers and masons.[14] Rubber has often been implicated as an allergenic substance; however, it is not the rubber or latex itself that typically causes the reaction, but rather the chemical accelerators and antioxidants used in processing the rubber.

Assessment and Treatment It is important to identify the offending substance when possible because its removal will usually result in improvement of the condition. Asking questions about the patient's environment and practices (eg, home, work, recreation, laundry products, the wearing of unwashed new clothes, and medication use) may allow a possible irritant or allergen to be identified. Unfortunately, the cause of allergic contact reactions is often elusive. For example, chemicals in the form of airborne pollutants, including substances such as cigarette smoke and vaporized cooking oils, may function as contact sensitizers.

An accurate assessment is made on the basis of the character, configuration, and location of the rash and itching. Skin patch testing may be useful in assessing some allergic contact reactions.[15] Accurate assessment may be difficult, however, if the contact dermatitis is superimposed over another dermatologic condition. Moreover, skin that is in a reactive state may be more easily reactive to other irritating or allergenic substances, making assessment and treatment more complicated.[16] For example, a minor cutaneous bacterial infection may produce a rash and be treated with a topical antibiotic such as neomycin. Because such agents are commonly sensitizing, the neomycin may produce allergic contact dermatitis at the treatment site. Thus, while the infection itself may heal, the allergic contact dermatitis produced by the neomycin persist. Not recognizing that the initial infection has resolved, the patient may continue to use the offending neomycin-containing product, thus setting up a vicious reaction cycle.[7,17]

A few of the other agents that may act as sensitizers include iodine-containing products, sulfonamides, mercury-containing antiseptics, and ethylenediamine. Health care workers may be sensitized to glutaraldehyde as well as to formaldehyde. Many topical skin preparations used for medicinal effect, including some used for itching and skin rashes, may also be a source of allergens. Local anesthetics containing esters such as benzocaine have been used topically for pruritus, local pain, and sunburn and can sensitize individuals. Benzocaine can also cross-react with related chemicals such as hair dyes and with sunscreens containing para-aminobenzoic acid to produce allergic contact dermatitis. Topical products containing pramoxine may sometimes be recommended as an alternative to benzocaine.

Topical antihistamines such as diphenhydramine may also cause sensitization. Once a patient has become sensitized by topical diphenhydramine, oral administration of the agent may also produce dermatitis.[18]

To patients who have experienced topical allergic reactions to cosmetics (particularly those containing unrefined lanolin), fragrances, hair care products, nail polish, hair dyes, deodorants, and soaps, a wide range of hypoallergenic cosmetics and soapless cleansers may be recommended.

The duration of therapy is often relatively short because the condition usually improves upon withdrawal of the allergen or irritant. However, a patient may be sensitive to, or irritated by, more than one drug or chemical. Therefore, before recommending any product for the treatment of contact dermatitis, the pharmacist should first encourage the patient to try to identify possible offending substance(s).

Choice of treatment for contact dermatitis depends on the severity of the condition. Mild to moderate dermatitis is usually amenable to treatment with nonprescription agents. The involved area should usually be washed gently, but well, to remove traces of the offending agent. If the area is oozing, compresses of cool tap water applied for 20 minutes, four to six times daily, may be recommended to aid in drying the lesions. Application of calamine lotion between compress applications and use of colloidal oatmeal baths may be soothing and help relieve itching. Topical hydrocortisone cream may be added to the regimen to reduce inflammation and itching. If the condition does not begin to improve in a couple of days or if it worsens, a physician should be consulted.[2,17] Similarly, a person with a severe reaction or involvement of large areas of the body should also be referred to a physician.

Hand Dermatitis

Etiology and Characteristics Hand dermatitis (hand eczema) is the simplest and most localized form of irritant contact dermatitis.[19] It often occurs in individuals whose occupation requires frequent hand washing or contact with moisture and mild irritants (eg, hairdressers, bartenders, food handlers, and medical personnel). It often begins under a ring that traps residue of an irritant. It may then spread to the adjacent fingers, palm, and the other hand. Because the dermatitis is often related to occupational exposure to irritants, it may be chronic and recurrent.

Hand dermatitis is marked by erythema, dryness, chapping, and, in severe cases, oozing vesicles that form crusts and pruritus of the dorsa of the hands. In severe, untreated cases, fissures may allow infection that can proceed to tissue necrosis.[2,14]

Treatment Acute (ie, red, oozing, and edematous) and subacute (ie, red and scaling but no weeping) hand dermatitis are usually treated in the same manner. Wet dressings may be applied, followed by hydrocortisone ointment. After the acute condition subsides, a nonmedicated emollient or hydrocortisone ointment should continue to be applied at least four times a day until the skin condition has healed or resolved completely.

Treatment of chronic (ie, dry, scaling, and fissured) hand dermatitis initially focuses on maintaining skin hydration by applying emollients often, especially after immersion in water. A water-in-oil emollient should be used, alternating with hydrocortisone ointment, if necessary. Because skin infection may occur in all types of hand dermatitis, medical attention should be sought if the condition does not improve within 1–2 weeks.[2]

A number of adjunctive measures, such as wearing vinyl (not rubber) gloves while doing "wet work," can be recommended in the management of hand dermatitis. Patients should be reminded, however, that wearing a glove with a hole in it will trap irritants next to the skin and is worse than wearing no glove at all. Thin, noncolored, plain cotton liners worn under vinyl gloves may prevent irritation from the vinyl and absorb perspiration. When washing the hands, the patient should use lukewarm water and a minimal amount of soap. The patient should also avoid creams and lotions because they may be too drying and may contain common allergens such as unrefined lanolin or fragrances.

Dry Skin

Almost everyone has experienced dry or chapped skin. In some people, it is a seasonal occurrence; in others, the condition is chronic. Although dry skin is not life-threatening, it is annoying and uncomfortable because of the attendant pruritus and, in some cases, pain and inflammation. In addition, dry skin is more prone to bacterial invasion than is normal skin.

Etiology and Characteristics Dry skin (xerosis) is characterized by one or more of the following symptoms: roughness, scaling, loss of flexibility, fissures, inflammation, and pruritus. The condition tends to appear most often on lower legs, dorsa of the hands, and forearms. Dry skin is especially prevalent during the winter months and is often referred to as "winter itch." It may occur secondary to prolonged detergent use, malnutrition, or physical damage to the stratum corneum. It may also signal a systemic disorder such as hypothyroidism or dehydration.

It is a common misconception that dry skin is caused by a lack of natural skin oils; on the contrary, dry skin is caused by a lack of water in the stratum corneum. The pathophysiology of dry skin, therefore, can be described by examining the factors involved in skin hydration. One is frequent or prolonged bathing or showering with hot water, as well as excessive use of soap, all of which increase dryness of the skin. Soap removes the skin's natural oils, and the short duration of contact with water is usually insufficient to hydrate dry skin. Another factor is environmental conditions. Low humidity allows the outer skin layer to lose moisture, become less flexible, and crack when flexed, thus leading to an increased rate of moisture loss. High wind velocity also causes skin moisture loss. A third factor is physical damage to the stratum corneum, which dramatically increases transepidermal water loss. However, partial recovery occurs within 1 or 2 days with the formation of a temporary barrier consisting of incompletely keratinized cells to provide approximately 50% of normal function and moisture retention, and total function is usually restored in 2–3 weeks.

Dry skin occurs with an increased incidence among elderly people. With advancing age, the epidermis changes because of abnormal maturation or adhesion of the keratinocytes, resulting in a superficial, irregular layer of corneocytes. This may be described as a thinning of the entire epidermis, which produces a roughened skin surface. The skin's hygroscopic substances also decrease in quantity with advancing age. Hormonal changes that accompany aging result in lowered sebum output and therefore lowered skin lubrication.[20]

Two dermatologic conditions that are difficult to differentiate from simple dry skin are asteatotic eczema and ichthyosis vulgaris. Asteatotic eczema is characterized by dry and fissured skin, inflammation, and pruritus. Sebaceous secretions are scanty or absent. The condition is more common during dry winter weather and in elderly individuals as an extension of the dry skin condition.

Ichthyosis vulgaris affects 0.3–1.0% of the population and is usually identified in the first few months of life. It is a genetic disorder (autosomal dominant) that should be suspected when a patient complains of a familial tendency to excessive dryness and chapping. Patients may also have an associated history of atopic disease. Symptoms include dryness and roughness of the skin, accompanied by small, fine, white scales. The condition tends to appear on the extensor aspects of the arms and legs. Dryness of the cheeks, heels, and palms may also be noted. In severe forms of the disease, a classic fish scale appearance of the stratum corneum is noted. Extreme cases have been seen in circuses where individuals are billed as "alligator," "porcupine," or "lizard" people.[7,21] Ichthyosis vulgaris may be placed at the most extreme end on a continuum of dermatitis conditions, with common dry skin at the least severe end.

It should be noted that ichthyosis vulgaris and related ichthyoses do not respond to steroid therapy although the short-term use of topical steroids may reduce inflammation and pruritus.[21]

Treatment The key to treating dry skin is to maintain skin hydration. Full-body bathing may be cut back to every other day or less often/or replaced by sponge baths or quick showers with warm rather than hot water. Bath products such as colloidal oatmeal, oilated oatmeal, or bath oil added near the end of the bath may be used to enhance skin hydration. Oil-based emollients should be applied immediately after bathing while the skin is damp and should be reapplied frequently. More severe cases of dry skin may require a urea- or lactic acid-containing product to enhance hydration. Topical hydrocortisone ointment may be applied on a short-term basis to reduce inflammation and itching. If resolution does not occur within 1 or 2 weeks, a physician should be consulted.[2]

Pharmacologic Agents for Dermatitis and Dry Skin

Nonprescription products for dermatitis and dry skin include bath products, emollients, hydrating agents, keratin-softening agents, astringents, antipruritics, protectants, and hydrocortisone (see the product tables "Dry Skin Products" and "Dermatitis Products"). Keratolytics are usually avoided in dermatitis unless extensive lichenification has occurred; these agents and those that reduce the mitotic activity of the epidermis, such as tars, should be used cautiously, if at all, because of their irritant properties.

Bath Products

Bath Oils Bath oils generally consist of a mineral or vegetable oil plus a surfactant. Mineral oil products are adsorbed better than vegetable oil products. Adsorption onto and absorption into the skin increase as temperature and oil concentration increase. Bath oils are minimally effective in improving a dry skin condition because they are greatly diluted in water. Their major effect is the slip or lubricity they impart to the skin, which may be important to the patient. This effect may be maximized by adding the oil near the end of the bath and patting the skin dry rather than rubbing it. When applied as wet compresses, however, bath oils (1 tsp in 1/4 cup of warm water) help lubricate dry skin and may allow a decrease in the frequency of full-body bathing.[2,22]

Bath oils make the tub and floor slippery, creating a safety hazard especially for elderly patients or children. They also make cleansing the skin with soaps more difficult. There is no clear superiority of one type of bath oil product over another; however, patients with dermatologic disorders should generally avoid products with fragrance.

Oatmeal Products Colloidal oatmeal bath products contain starch, protein, and a small amount of oil. They are less effective than bath oils; however, oilated oatmeal products combine the effect of oatmeal and a bath oil. Colloidal oatmeal is claimed to be soothing and antipruritic, and it does have a lubricating effect.

Cleansers Bath soaps generally contain salts of long-chain fatty acids (commonly oleic, palmitic, or stearic acid) and alkali metals (eg, sodium and potassium). Combined with water, these products act as surfactants and will remove many substances from the skin, including the lipids that normally keep the skin soft and pliable. Some authorities recommend special soaps that contain extra oils to minimize the drying effect of washing; however, these soaps usually lather and clean poorly. Unscented Dove is one example of a cleansing agent with minimal drying effect to skin.[2,20]

Glycerin soaps, which are transparent and more water soluble, have a higher oil content than standard toilet soaps because of the addition of castor oil. They are also closer to a neutral pH and are therefore regarded as less drying than soaps, which are alkaline. Although there is little objective proof of their superiority, the glycerin soaps are advertised for and well accepted by people with skin conditions.

Mild cleansers such as Cetaphil may be recommended if soap should be avoided. Most of these products consist primarily of surfactants and may contain an oil. They foam mildly on application, and on gentle wiping they leave a thin layer of lipid material on the skin, which helps to retain water in the stratum corneum.

Emollients/Moisturizers

Emollients are occlusive agents and moisturizers that are used to prevent or relieve the signs and symptoms of dry skin. These products act primarily by leaving an oily film on the skin surface through which moisture cannot readily escape. Some of the most commonly used emollients include petrolatum, lanolin, mineral oil, and dimethicone.

Some clinicians believe that minimizing transepidermal water loss is not enough to maintain adequate hydration. Therefore, a patient may be advised to hydrate the skin by soaking the affected area in water for 5–10 minutes, patting it dry, and applying an occlusive agent while the skin is still damp. In this way, moisture is retained more adequately in the skin.

Cosmetically, emollients make the skin feel soft and smooth by helping to reestablish the integrity of the stratum corneum. Lipid components make the scales on the skin translucent and flatten them against the underlying skin. This eliminates air between the scales and the skin surface, which is partly responsible for a dry, flaky appearance.[23]

Frequency of application depends on the severity of the dry skin condition as well as on the hydration efficiency of the occlusive agent. For dry hands, the patient may need to apply the occlusive agent after each hand washing as well as at numerous other times during the day. However, care should be exercised to avoid excessive hydration, which may lead to tissue maceration. In addition, although most commercial formulations generally are bland, contact with the eye or with broken or abraded skin should be avoided because formulation ingredients may cause irritation. This is especially true with emulsion systems because the surfactants in them denature protein and may thus produce further irritation.

Petrolatum is an effective occlusive agent and has been given Category I status by the Food and Drug Administration (FDA) as a skin protectant. Mineral oil is not as effective a barrier, and silicones are even less effective. Unfortunately, petrolatum should not be applied over puncture wounds, infections, or lacerations because its high occlusive ability may lead to maceration and further inflammation. Application to intertriginous areas, mucous membranes, and acne-prone areas should also be avoided. Similar precautions should be taken with dimethicone.

Lanolin, a natural product derived from sheep wool, is found in many nonprescription moisturizing products. Some patients develop an allergic reaction to this substance, presumably because its wool wax fraction is recognized as antigenic. Patients with a previous history of allergic reactions to lanolin should generally avoid lanolin-containing products. However, refined lanolin-containing products are generally less likely to be sensitizing and may even be tolerated by those with a history of allergic contact reactions to unrefined lanolin.

Emollient products are available in a wide variety of formulations. Ointments containing petrolatum are very greasy and generally lack consumer appeal because of their texture, difficulty of spreading and removing, and staining properties. Ointments are also inappropriate for an oozing dermatitis. Lotions and creams are either water-in-oil or oil-in-water emulsions. The higher the lipid content, the greater the occlusive effect. In most cases, the less effective but more aesthetic oil-in-water emulsions are preferred for their cosmetic acceptability to patients. These agents help alleviate the pruritus associated with dry skin by virtue of their cooling effect as water evaporates from the skin surface. Moreover, there is enough oil in most oil-in-water emulsions to form a continuous occlusive film on the skin surface.[2,23]

Attempts have been made to formulate products that try to function like sebum. Because sebum and skin surface lipids contain a relatively high concentration of fatty acid glycerides, vegetable and animal oils such as avocado, cucumber, mink, peanut, safflower, sesame, turtle, and shark liver are included in dry skin products, presumably because of their unsaturated fatty acid content. However, although the use of these oils contributes to skin flexibility and lubricity, their occlusive effect is less than that of petrolatum.

The prevention and care of dry skin may become a major focus for the pharmacist as the aged population continues to increase in numbers. There is also a heightened awareness among those caring for elderly people that prophylactic dry skin care can reduce morbidity by minimizing the risk of skin breakdown and thus can ultimately reduce the cost of dermatologic health care.[23,24]

Humectants

Humectants or hydrating agents are hygroscopic materials that may be added to an emollient base. Their function is to draw water into the stratum corneum to hydrate the skin. Water may come from the dermis or from the atmosphere; however, high relative humidity (80% or greater) is necessary for the latter to occur. Humectants are distinct from emollients, which serve to retain water already present. Commonly used hydrating agents are glycerin, propylene glycol, and phospholipids.

Because of glycerin's hygroscopic properties, high concentrations may actually increase water loss by drawing water from the skin rather than from the atmosphere. However, at concentrations of 50% or less, humectants such as glycerin help decrease water loss by keeping water in close contact with skin and accelerating moisture diffusion from the dermis to the epidermis. In addition, glycerin provides lubrication to the skin surface.

Propylene glycol is a viscous, colorless, odorless solvent with hygroscopic properties. It is less viscous than glycerin and is included in many skin care formulations for its humectant action. However, it can cause skin irritation, usually on a concentration-dependent basis.

Phospholipid products contain lecithin, which is a water-binding compound normally present in the skin. Each phospholipid molecule can complex with up to 15 molecules of water. Hydrolysis yields fatty acids, which help retain water.

Keratin-Softening Agents

Chemically altering the keratin layer softens skin and cosmetically improves its appearance. This treatment approach does not need a substantial addition of water, but all the attendant dry skin symptoms may not be alleviated unless water is added to the keratin layer. Agents used as keratin softeners in nonprescription dry skin products are urea, lactic acid, and allantoin.

Urea Urea (carbamide) in concentrations of 10–30% is mildly keratolytic and increases water uptake in the stratum corneum, giving it a high water-binding capacity. Urea has a direct effect on stratum corneum elasticity because of its ability to bind to skin protein. It accelerates fibrin digestion at about 15% and is proteolytic at 40%. It is considered safe and has been recommended for use on crusted necrotic tissue. Concentrations of 10% have been used on simple dry skin; 20–30% formulations have been used for treating more resistant dry skin conditions. Urea-containing creams are claimed to produce good hydration and help remove scales and crusts. They are also less oily than some occlusive preparations. However, urea preparations can cause stinging, burning, and irritation, particularly on broken skin.

Alpha-Hydroxy Acids Lactic acid is an alpha-hydroxy acid that has been useful in concentrations of 2–5% for treating dry skin conditions. Lactic acid increases the hydration of human skin and may act as a modulator of epidermal keratinization rather than as a keratolytic agent. Lactic acid may be added to urea preparations for both its stabilizing and its hydrating effects.

Other alpha-hydroxy acids, found in many fruits, are under investigation for a number of common skin conditions such as dry skin, acne, and fine wrinkles from aging. These acids include malic acid (in apples), citric acid (in oranges and lemons), tartaric acid (in grapes), and glycolic and gluconic acids (in sugar cane).[25]

Allantoin Allantoin and allantoin complexes are claimed to soften keratin by disrupting its structure. Allantoin is a product of purine metabolism and is considered to be a relatively safe compound. However, it is less effective than urea. The FDA has recommended that allantoin be considered safe and effective as a skin protectant for adults, children, and infants when applied in concentrations of 0.5–2.0%.[7]

Astringents

Astringents are substances that retard the oozing, discharge, or bleeding of dermatitis when applied to the unhealthy skin or mucous membranes. They work by coagulating protein. When applied as a wet dressing or compress, they cool and dry the skin through evaporation. They cause vasoconstriction and reduce blood flow in inflammation. They also cleanse the skin of exudates, crust, and debris. Because they generally have a low cell penetrability, their activity is limited to the cell surface and interstitial spaces. The protein precipitate that forms may serve as a protective coat, allowing new tissues to grow underneath.[7]

The FDA has identified two astringent solutions as being safe and effective. These are aluminum acetate (Burow's solution) and witch hazel (hamamelis water). Aluminum acetate solution (USP) contains approximately 5% aluminum acetate. The solution must be diluted 1:10 to 1:40 with water before use. It is commercially available in tablet or powder form. Witch hazel is no longer listed in the official compendia, but it has been used for centuries as an astringent solution. A natural product prepared from the twigs of *Hamamelis virginiana*, it contains tannins, trace amounts of volatile oils (which give it a characteristically pleasant odor), and 14–15% alcohol, all of which contribute to its astringent activity. The product may be applied as often as necessary in the treatment of minor skin irritations. Numerous other ingredients, including alum and zinc oxide, have been promoted as astringents. However, data demonstrating their safety and effectiveness for use as astringents are lacking.[26]

The patient may soak the affected area in the astringent solution two to four times daily for 15–30 minutes. Alternatively, the patient may loosely apply a compress of washcloths or small towels soaked in the solution and then wrung gently so they are wet but not dripping. The dressings should be rewetted and reapplied every few minutes for 20–30 minutes, four to six times daily. Isotonic saline solution, tap water, or diluted white vinegar (¼ cup per pint of water) may also be used in this fashion.[2,7]

Antipruritics

The itching associated with dermatitis may be mediated through several different mechanisms, which may explain how three major classes of pharmacologic agents—local anesthetics, antihistamines, and steroids—are useful as antipruritics. Cooling the area through application of a soothing, bland lotion may also reduce the extent of the pruritus, but this action is only transitory in its effect.

The itching sensation is mediated by the same nerve fibers that carry pain impulses. Local anesthetics block conduction along axonal membranes, thereby relieving itching as well as pain. However, because local anesthetics may also cause systemic side effects, they should not be used in large quantities or over long periods of time, particularly if the skin is raw or blistered. Nonprescription topical anesthetics that appear to be safe and effective are dyclonine and benzocaine; agents such as benzocaine (5–20%) may be applied to the affected area three or four times daily. However, these agents may have a sensitizing effect in a small number of persons.

Itching may also be mediated by various endogenous substances, including histamine. Accordingly, topical antihistamines such as diphenhydramine, tripelennamine, and pyrilamine are effective in alleviating this symptom. Their activity stems from an ability to compete with histamine at H_1-receptor sites and to exert a topical anesthetic effect. Local anesthesia may be the more important mechanism of action because the cause of itching in many conditions (eg, atopic dermatitis) has not been established and may not be related to histamine release at all. Antihistamines are considered safe and effective for use as nonprescription external analgesics. However, because of their significant sensitizing potential, the FDA does not recommend the topical use of these agents for more than 7 consecutive days except under the advice and supervision of a physician.[14,27]

Oral antihistamines have been used to treat the itching of dermatologic disorders with variable results. Some researchers claim that the antipruritic effect is a result of the sedative side effect; others claim the efficacy is owing to antihistaminic activity, although with a delay in onset of several days. If histamine is involved, it has already reached and stimulated the receptor sites to produce itching, and a finite time is required for the antihistamine to displace it. In either case, central nervous system depression may be a problem, as may the anticholinergic side effects in patients with conditions such as prostatic hypertrophy or glaucoma.[14,17]

Protectants

Skin protectants are substances that protect injured or exposed skin surfaces from harmful or annoying stimuli. Zinc oxide (1–25%) is one of the most widely used and clinically accepted skin protectants, and it is claimed to be mildly astringent and antiseptic as well. It may be applied as a paste (Lassar's), ointment, or lotion (calamine). Other protectants in general use include aluminum hydroxide and bismuth subnitrate. Patients should be cautioned that covering the lesions or applying a product with an occlusive barrier may increase the degree of tissue maceration and prevent heat loss, resulting in discomfort. Any powder-based aqueous product that dries weeping through water adsorption or astringency should be used with caution. These agents have a tendency to crust, and removing the crusts may cause bleeding and infections.[7,14]

Topical Hydrocortisone

Hydrocortisone is the only corticosteroid available without a prescription for the topical treatment of dermatitis. Primarily because of its vasocontricting effect, it relieves the redness, heat, pain, swelling, and itch associated with various dermatoses. Official indications for its use include temporary relief of itching associated with minor skin irritations, inflammation, and rashes caused by dermatitis, seborrheic dermatitis, insect bites, poison ivy, poison oak, poison sumac, soaps, detergents, cosmetics, and jewelry.

When hydrocortisone was initially switched from prescription to nonprescription status in 1980, the concentrations available were 0.25 and 0.5%. However, efficacy of hydrocortisone preparations of less than 0.5% concentration has not been established. Concentrations of 0.5–1% are regarded as appropriate for the treatment of localized dermatitis, and in August 1991, the FDA approved the nonprescription marketing of hydrocortisone in strengths up to 1%.[28]

Hydrocortisone should be applied sparingly by massaging it well, but gently, into the affected area three or four times a day. An ointment formulation is best for chronic, non-oozing dermatoses.

Before recommending a hydrocortisone-containing product, the pharmacist should be certain that the area of application is not infected. Signs of bacterial infection include redness, heat, pus, and crusting. Fungal infections may be marked by erythema and scaling. Topical hydrocortisone may mask the symptoms of these dermatologic infections and allow the infection to progress.

Topical hydrocortisone will rarely produce systemic complications because systemic absorption is relatively minimal. Approximately 1% of hydrocortisone solution applied to normal skin on the forearm is absorbed systemically. Absorption increases in the presence of skin inflammation or with the use of occlusive dressings. Certain local adverse effects such as skin atrophy may arise with prolonged use because collagen production is inhibited, which thereby weakens the skin's "infrastructure." In practice, however, clinically detectable atrophy rarely occurs with hydrocortisone in the concentrations available without a prescription; it is more common with the more potent products available by prescription only. Because response to topical steroids decreases with continued use, intermittent courses of therapy are advised.[2]

Product Selection Guidelines

When deciding on which product to recommend for dermatitis or dry skin, the pharmacist must evaluate the active ingredients and the vehicle. Primary active ingredients contained in nonprescription skin products are water and oil. However, a wide variety of secondary ingredients are added to enhance product elegance and stability, and many of them have the potential for producing contact dermatitis through either an irritant or sensitizing effect. These agents may include:

- *Emulsifiers*: cholesterol, magnesium aluminum silicate, polyoxyethylene lauryl ether (Brij), polyoxyethylene monostearate (Myrj), polyoxyethylene sorbitan monolaurate (Tween), propylene glycol monostearate, sodium borate plus fatty acid, sodium lauryl sulfate, sorbitan monopalmitate (Span), or triethanolamine plus fatty acid;
- *Emulsion stabilizers (thickening agents)*: carbomer, cetyl alcohol, glyceryl monostearate, methylcellulose, spermaceti, or stearyl alcohol;
- *Preservatives*: cresol or the parabens.

The type of vehicle (eg, ointment, cream, lotion, gel, solution, or aerosol) may have a significant effect on dermatitis. The following guidelines may be used to choose an appropriate vehicle:

- "If it's wet, dry it." If a drying effect is desired, solutions, gels, and occasionally creams may be recommended. It must be noted, however, that components of these systems may quickly diffuse into the underlying tissue and possibly cause irritation.
- If slight lubrication is needed, creams and lotions are preferred.
- "If it's dry, wet it." If the lesion is very dry and fissured, ointments are the vehicle of choice. However, they

should be avoided in intertriginous areas because of their maceration potential. Also, in an acute process, ointments may cause further irritation because of their occlusive effect.
- Aerosols, gels, or lotions may be recommended when the dermatitis affects a hair-covered area of the body.

A large number of cosmetic dry skin formulations are commercially available. These may contain natural oils, vitamins, or a variety of fragrances that have a psychologic appeal. However, the fragrances and dyes found in many of these formulations may be irritating or allergenic to sensitive dry skin and should be avoided.

Efficacy of any skin care product may need to be sacrificed or compromised somewhat to achieve patient acceptance. The most efficacious product that the patient will accept should be recommended.

Topical nonprescription products come in various package sizes and strengths. Table 3 lists the amount of drug needed to cover a given area of the body three times daily over a 1-week period. By being aware of such details, the pharmacist can serve the patient economically as well as therapeutically.

Scaly Dermatoses

Dandruff, seborrheic dermatitis (seborrhea), and psoriasis are described as chronic, scaly dermatoses. They may be placed on a spectrum ranging from dandruff, a minor problem that is primarily cosmetic, to psoriasis, a clinical condition that can have significant physical, psychologic, and economic consequences. (See Table 4 for the distinguishing features of these three dermatoses.)

TABLE 3 Amount of topical medication needed for three times daily application for 1 week

Part of the body	Cream/ ointment (g)	Lotion/solution/gel (mL)
Face	5–10	100–120
Both hands	25–50	200–240
Scalp	50–100	200–240
Both arms or both legs	100–200	240–360
Trunk	200	360–480
Groin and genitalia	15–25	120–180

Adapted from Bingham EA. Topical dermatologic therapy. In: Rook A, Parish LC, Beare JM, eds. *Practical Management of the Dermatologic Patient.* Philadelphia: JB Lippincott; 1986: 227–8.

Nonprescription products are appropriate for all degrees of dandruff. Many cases of seborrheic dermatitis will respond to the same nonprescription drug regimen used to treat dandruff. Psoriasis that involves mild inflammation may be responsive to nonprescription treatment. However, initial diagnosis and management of acute flare-ups require the attention of a physician.[29]

Specific Conditions

Dandruff

Dandruff is a chronic, noninflammatory scalp condition that results in excessive scaling of scalp epidermis. Dandruff is clinically visible in approximately 20% of the population. Severity declines in the summer and is not proved to be aggravated by emotional states. Authorities disagree over whether inadequate shampooing exacerbates dandruff; however, there is agreement that a consistent washing routine is important in managing the condition.[29,30]

Etiology and Characteristics Dandruff is not a true disease; rather, it is a physiologic event and condition much like the growth of hair and nails, except that the end product is visible on the scalp and has a substantial cosmetic and social stigma associated with its presence. It correlates with the proliferative activity of the epidermis. Dandruff generally appears at puberty, reaches a peak in early adulthood, levels off in middle age, and declines in advancing years (occurring only rarely after age 75).

Dandruff is characterized by accelerated epidermal cell turnover, an irregular keratin breakup pattern, and the shedding of cells in large scales. It is normal for epidermal cells on the scalp to continually slough off just as they do on other parts of the body. It is also normal for the epidermal cell turnover rate to be greater on the scalp than on other parts of the body. In dandruff patients, however, the epidermal cell turnover rate on the scalp is about twice that of normal scalp.[7] This rate also assists in distinguishing dandruff from seborrhea and psoriasis; psoriasis has a higher rate than seborrhea, which has a higher rate than dandruff.

Dandruff is diffuse rather than patchy; it is not inflammatory; and pruritus is common. Scaling, the only visible manifestation of dandruff, is the result of an increased rate of horny substance production on the scalp and the sloughing of large scales. Dandruff scales often appear around a hair shaft because of the epithelial growth at the base of the hair. This phenomenon does not occur on the normal scalp because the horny substance breaks up in a much more uniform fashion. The horny layer of the scalp normally consists of 25–35 fully keratinized, closely coherent cells per square millimeter arranged in an orderly fashion. However, in dandruff, the intact horny layer has fewer than 10 normal cells per square millimeter, and nonkeratinized cells are common. With dandruff, crevices occur deep in the stratum corneum, resulting in cracking, which generates relatively large scales. If the large scales are broken down to smaller units, the dandruff becomes less visible.

As the rate of keratin cell turnover increases, so too

TABLE 4 Distinguishing features of dandruff, seborrhea, and psoriasis

	Dandruff	Seborrhea	Psoriasis
Location	Scalp	Adults and children: head and trunk Children only: back, intertriginous areas	Scalp, elbows, knees, trunk, and lower extremities
Exacerbating factors	Generally a stable condition, exacerbated by inadequate washing, dry climate	Exacerbated by many external factors, notably stress and low relative humidity	Exacerbated by mechanical irritation, stress, climate, drugs, infection, endocrine factors
Appearance	Thin, white, or grayish flakes; even distribution on scalp	Patchy lesions with margins; mild inflammation; oily, yellowish scales	Usually symmetrical, red, patchy plaques with sharp border; silvery-white scale; small bleeding points when removed. Difficult to distinguish from seborrhea in early stages or in intertriginous zones
Inflammation	Absent	Present	Present
Epidermal hyperplasia	Absent	Present	Present
Epidermal kinetics	Turnover rate is two times faster than normal	Turnover rate is about five to six times faster than normal	Turnover rate is about five to six times faster than normal
Percentage of incompletely keratinized cells	Rarely exceeds 5% of total corneocyte count	Commonly makes up 15–25% of corneocyte count	Commonly makes up 40–60% of corneocyte count

Information extracted from:

Wright DE. In: Clark C, ed. *Self-Medication: A Reference for Health Professionals*. 3rd ed. Ottawa: Canadian Pharmaceutical Association; 1988: 87.

McGinley KJ et al. *J Invest Dermatol*. 1969; 53: 107.

Kligman AM et al. *J Soc Cosmet Chem*. 1974; 25: 73.

does the number of incompletely keratinized cells, a situation characterized by the retention of nuclei in keratin layer cells. Incompletely keratinized cells in dandruff appear in clusters, possibly as a result of tiny inflammatory foci that are incited when capillaries discharge a load of inflammatory cells into the epidermis, causing accelerated epidermal growth in a small area. These microfoci are found on all scalps but are increased proportionately in dandruff.[7]

The specific cause of accelerated cell growth seen in dandruff is unknown. There is continuing debate over whether dandruff is a result of elevated microorganism levels—particularly of the yeast *Pityrosporum ovale*.[30]

Treatment Dandruff is more of a cosmetic than a medical problem, and treatment is fairly straightforward. The patient needs to understand that there is no direct cure for dandruff and that the condition can usually be well controlled. Washing the hair and scalp with a nonmedicated shampoo every other day or even daily is often sufficient to control dandruff. If it is not, medicated nonprescription antidandruff products may be recommended. With medicated shampoos, contact time improves effectiveness. The patient should be counseled to allow medicated shampoo to remain on the hair for approximately 1 minute before rinsing and repeating. Thorough rinsing is important in the use of all shampoo products.

A cytostatic agent such as pyrithione zinc, selenium sulfide, or coal tar is recommended. These agents reduce the epidermal turnover rate. However, the coal tar–containing shampoos may tend to discolor light hair as well as clothing and jewelry and thus may not appeal to some patients. Next, a keratolytic shampoo containing salicylic acid or sulfur may be used. If dandruff proves resistant to these agents, the patient should be referred to a physician for treatment.[29,31]

Seborrheic Dermatitis

Seborrheic dermatitis is a general term for a group of eruptions that occur predominantly in the areas of greatest sebaceous gland activity (eg, the scalp, face, and trunk). This condition affects approximately 12 million Americans. Seborrhea occurs mostly in middle-aged and elderly persons, particularly men. It is often found in persons with parkinsonism, endocrine states associated with obesity, zinc deficiency, and human immunodeficiency virus infection. Quadriplegics and persons who have experienced a cerebrovascular accident (stroke) or a myocardial infarct (heart attack) also seem prone to seborrhea. Because nonprescription therapy is effective in a significant percentage of cases, the pharmacist can play a key role in the management of seborrhea.[32]

Etiology and Characteristics Seborrhea is marked by accelerated epidermal proliferation and sebaceous gland activity.[19] The distinctive characteristics of the disorder are its common occurrence in hairy areas (especially the scalp); the appearance of dull, yellowish-red lesions, which are well demarcated; and the associated presence of oily-appearing, yellowish scales. Pruritus is common.[33] The most common form, seborrhea of the scalp, is characterized by greasy scales on the scalp that often extend to the middle third of the face with subsequent eye involvement. (See color plates, photograph 10.) Lesions may also appear in the external auditory canal and around the ear. When seborrhea of the scalp occurs in newborns and infants, it is referred to as cradle cap and is treated primarily by gentle massaging with baby oil followed by a nonmedicated shampoo to remove the scales. Pruritus does not appear to accompany cradle cap, and the condition often clears spontaneously by 8–12 months of age.[11,29,32]

The cause of seborrhea is unknown although predisposition appears to be a genetic trait. Emotional and physical stress serve as aggravating factors. Proposed etiologic factors have included vitamin B complex deficiency, food allergies, autoimmunity, climate changes, and low relative humidity. The characteristic accelerated cell turnover and enhanced sebaceous gland activity give rise to the prominent scale displayed in the condition; however, there is no clear-cut quantitative relationship between the degree of sebaceous gland activity and susceptibility to seborrhea.

It is almost universally accepted that seborrhea is merely an extension of dandruff, and the controversy regarding the involvement of *P ovale* extends to seborrhea. Some researchers, however, dispute the link with dandruff, offering evidence that seborrhea is a separate condition. Incompletely keratinized cells commonly make up 15–25% of the corneocyte count in seborrheic dermatitis but rarely exceed 5% in dandruff.[7,32]

Assessment The differential assessment of seborrheic dermatitis is usually straightforward. However, whereas dandruff is considered a relatively stable condition, seborrhea fluctuates in severity, often as a result of stress. Involvement of eyebrows and eyelashes, with concurrent blepharitis, is associated with seborrhea but not with dandruff. Moreover, dandruff is considered a noninflammatory condition whereas seborrhea is usually accompanied by erythema and sometimes crusting.

Lesion distribution is a key factor in distinguishing seborrhea from psoriasis. Seborrhea commonly involves the face and generally is not found on the extremities, whereas psoriasis is rarely found on the face but is commonly found on bony prominence such as the elbows and knees. However, the scalp is generally involved in both conditions, and if this is the only site of involvement, differential assessment is difficult. Physical appearance of scales may help to differentiate the two disorders. Seborrhea is usually marked by oily, yellow scales whereas psoriatic scales are generally dry and silvery in appearance. Additionally, the presence of the Auspitz sign (small bleeding points) is indicative of psoriasis.

Fungal infections may be mistaken for seborrhea. Thus, proper assessment is important because fungal infections may be worsened by seborrhea therapy using hydrocortisone. If the lesion is located in the groin, tinea cruris (jock itch) must be considered, especially during warm weather. Scalp lesions must be evaluated for the possibility of tinea capitis (ringworm of the scalp).[7]

Treatment The treatment of seborrheic dermatitis is similar to that of dandruff. Seborrhea generally responds to shampoos containing pyrithione zinc, selenium sulfide, salicylic acid, or coal tar. However, frequent use of selenium sulfide may make the scalp oily and may actually exacerbate the seborrheic condition.

A primary difference between the treatment of dandruff and that of seborrhea is the use of topical corticosteroids. These products are not indicated for dandruff but may be used in the management of seborrheic dermatitis whenever erythema is persistent after therapy with medicated shampoos. Hydrocortisone lotions for scalp dermatitis are available without a prescription. The patient should be instructed to apply the hydrocortisone product two to three times a day until symptoms subside and then intermittently to control acute exacerbations. The patient should also be instructed in the proper technique of application. The hair should be parted and the product applied directly to the scalp and massaged in thoroughly. This process should be repeated until desired coverage of the affected area is achieved. The absorption of medication into the scalp is enhanced if the lotion is applied after shampooing; skin hydration promotes drug absorption.

The patient should be encouraged to minimize prolonged and continued use of hydrocortisone in the treatment of seborrheic dermatitis because a rebound flare may occur when prolonged therapy is discontinued. If the condition worsens or if symptoms persist for more than 7 days, a physician should be consulted. At this point, a more potent topical steroid may be indicated.[7]

If the seborrhea spreads to the ear canal, eyelashes, or eyelids, a physician should be consulted for appropriate therapy. This may include the use of prescription otic and ophthalmic agents.

Nonprescription products used to treat seborrhea are to be avoided for children under 2 years of age, except under the advice and supervision of a physician.[34]

Psoriasis

Psoriasis is estimated to afflict 1–3% of the US population. Lesions are often localized but may become gener-

Color Plates

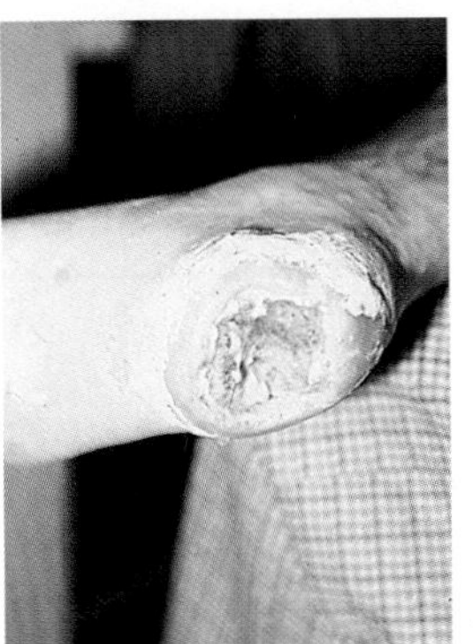

1

1 Gangrene of the foot is a serious and common complication of diabetes caused by trauma that has gone unrecognized because of neuropathy (loss of sensation) or vascular lesions. Eventually, the trauma may lead to gangrene when the necrotic (dead) skin is removed and ulceration results (as shown). (See Chapter 18, "Diabetes Care Products and Monitoring Devices.")

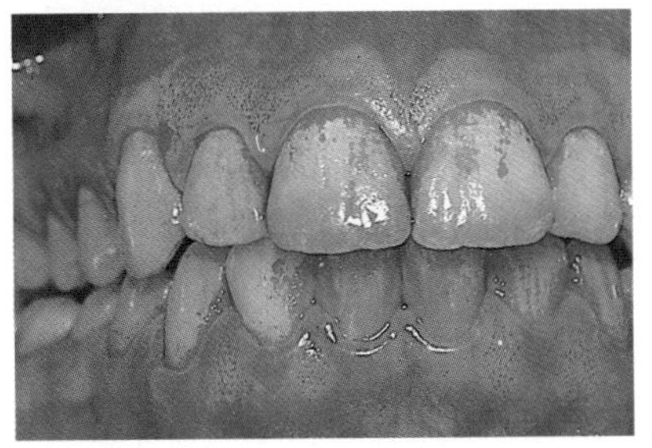

2

2 Disclosing agents, such as erythrosin (FD&C Red No. 3), aid patients in evaluating the effectiveness of their brushing and flossing by staining mucinous film and plaque on teeth. These agents reveal the presence and extent of deposits on teeth that otherwise appear clean. (See Chapter 25, "Oral Health Products.")

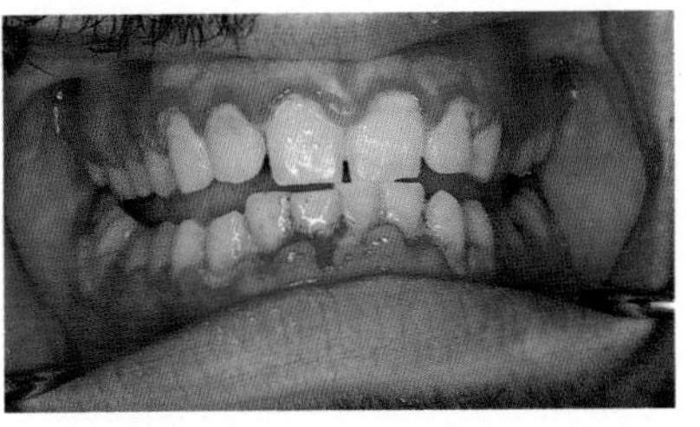

3

3 Chronic gingivitis, an asymptomatic inflammation of the gingivae (gums) at the necks of the teeth, is an early stage of periodontitis and is usually caused by poor oral hygiene. The gingivae are erythematous (red) and may have areas that appear swollen and glossy. In addition, mild hemorrhage may occur during teeth brushing. (See Chapter 25, "Oral Health Products.")

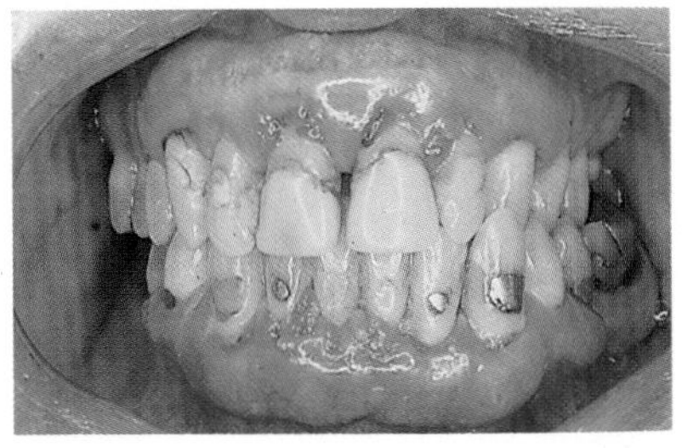

4

4 Chronic periodontitis (pyorrhea), an inflammation of the tissues surrounding the teeth, including the gingivae, periodontal ligaments, alveolar bone, and the cementum (bony material covering the root of a tooth), is caused by plaque accumulation resulting from poor oral hygiene. The gingivae may be erythematous and swollen and may recede from the necks of the teeth. The condition is not painful and usually is accompanied by halitosis, loosening of the teeth, and mild hemorrhage during teeth brushing. (See Chapter 25, "Oral Health Products.")

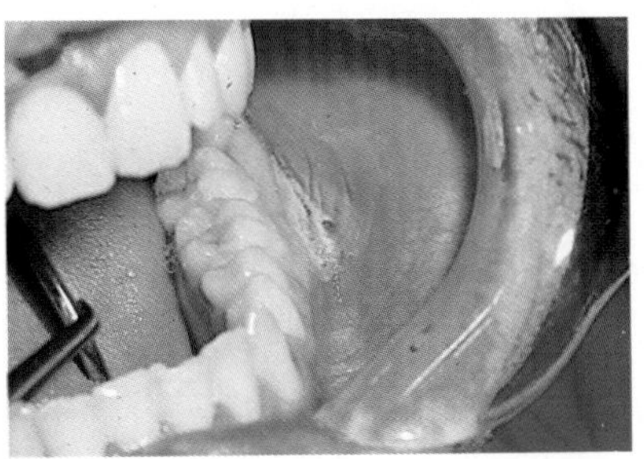

5

5 Aspirin burn results from the topical use of aspirin to relieve toothache. An aspirin tablet is placed against the tooth, where it is held in place by pressure from the buccal (cheek) mucosa. The mucosa becomes necrotic and is characterized by a white slough that rubs away, revealing a painful ulceration. (See Chapter 25, "Oral Health Products.")

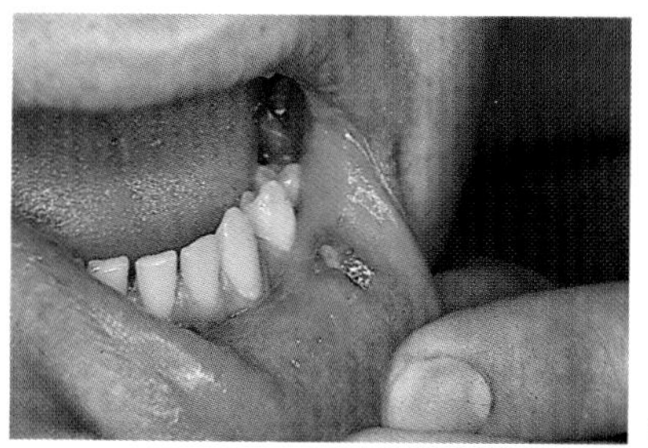

6

6 Aphthous ulcers (canker sores) are recurrent, painful, single or multiple ulcerations of bacterial origin. The central ulceration is sharply demarcated, often has a yellow to white surface of necrotic debris, and is surrounded by an erythematous margin. (See Chapter 25, "Oral Health Products.")

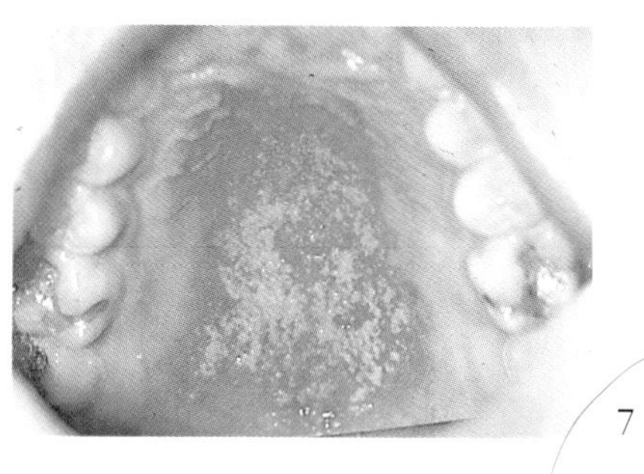

7

7 Candidiasis (candidosis, moniliasis, thrush), an infection caused by overgrowth of *Candida albicans*, tends to occur in people with debilitating or chronic systemic disease or those on long-term antibiotic therapy. Candidiasis commonly presents as a whitish-gray to yellowish, soft, slightly elevated pseudomembrane-like plaque on the oral mucosa; the plaque is often described as having a milk curd appearance. If the membrane is stripped away, a raw bleeding surface remains. A dull, burning pain is often present. (See Chapter 25, "Oral Health Products.")

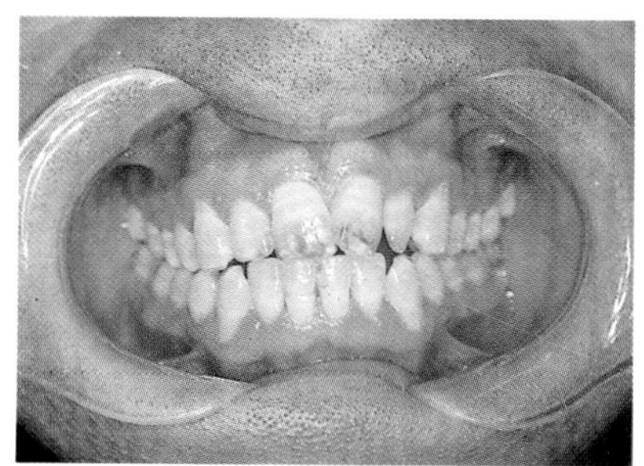

8

8 Dental fluorosis (mottled enamel) occurs during the time of tooth formation and is caused by the long-term ingestion of drinking water containing fluoride at concentrations greater than 1 ppm. Discoloration of the teeth varies, depending on the level of fluoride in the water, and ranges from white flecks or spots to brownish stains, small pits, or deep irregular pits that are dark brown in color. (See Chapter 25, "Oral Health Products.")

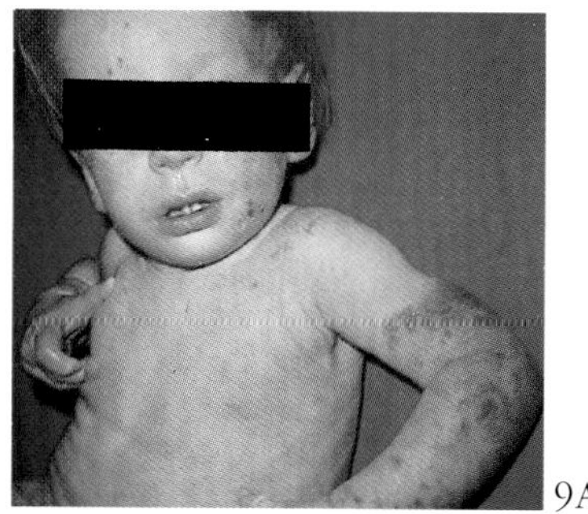

9A

9A, B, and C Atopic dermatitis (eczema) is an inflammatory condition that occurs on the extensor surface of the elbows and knees (**A**) during the first year of life and then involves predominantly the flexors (**B**). The hands, feet, and face are often involved as well (**C**). The dermatitis is characterized by erythema, scale, increased skin surface markings, and crusting; secondary infection is common. (See Chapter 26, "Dermatologic Products.")

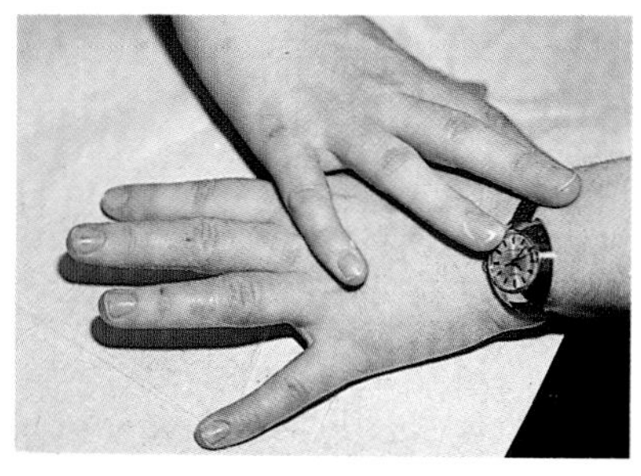

9B

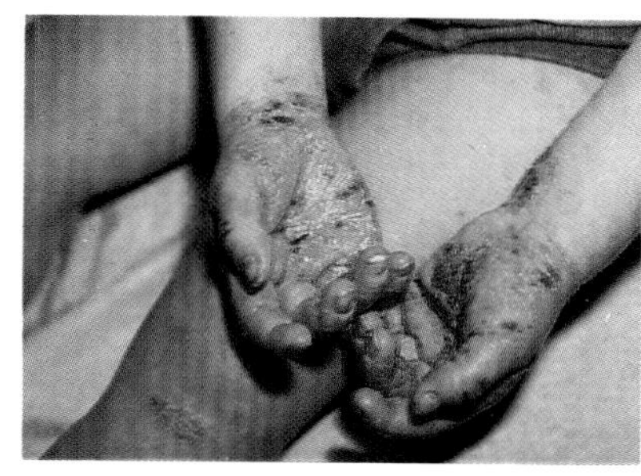

9C

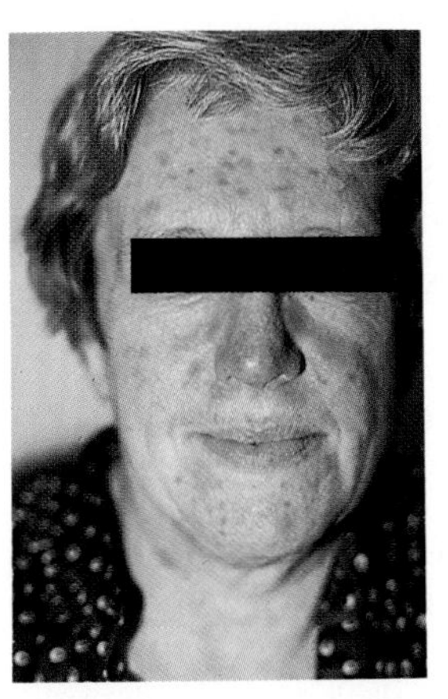
10

10 Seborrhea (seborrheic dermatitis) is a red scaling condition of the scalp, midface, and upper midchest of adults. This dermatitis is marked by characteristic greasy, yellowish scaling and is associated with erythema. (See Chapter 26, "Dermatologic Products.")

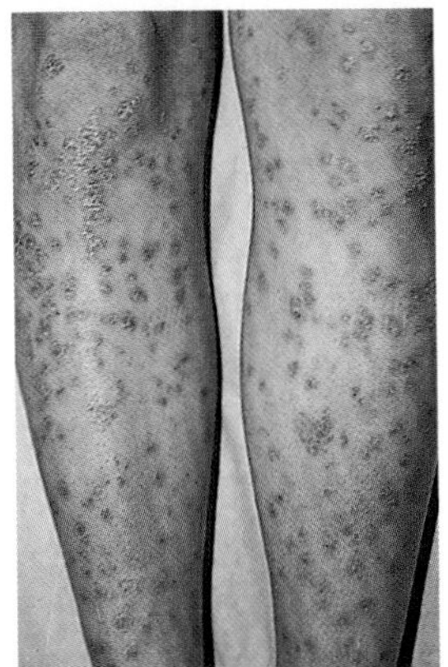
11A

11A, B, and C Psoriasis is a scaling condition in which erythematous plaques (red raised areas) are covered by a thick adherent scale. The borders of the lesions are well developed and vary from guttate (very small drop-shaped plaques) to much larger plaques: (**A**) guttate; (**B**) medium-sized plaques; (**C**) large plaques. (See Chapter 26, "Dermatologic Products.")

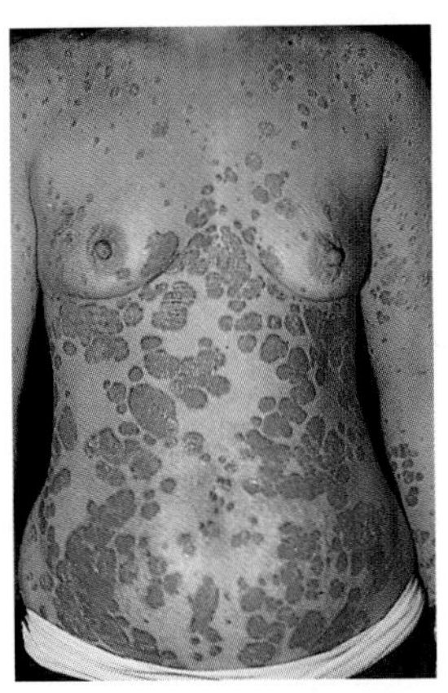
11B

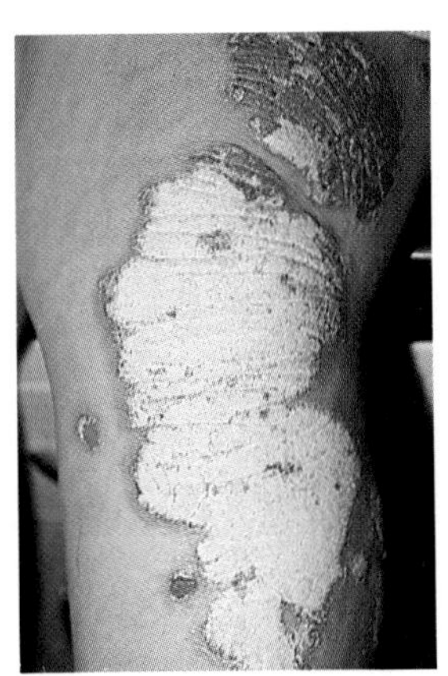
11C

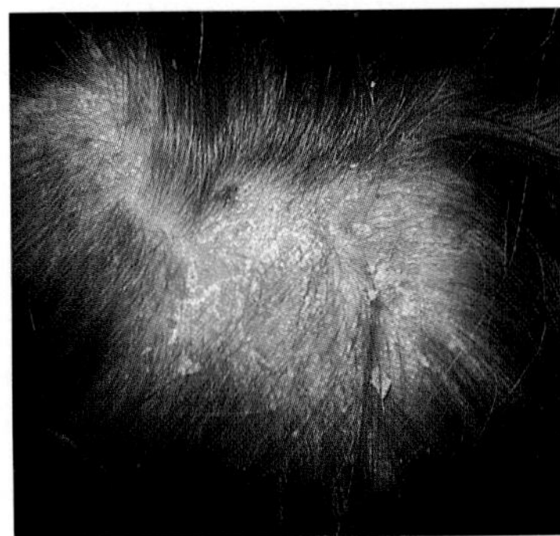
12

12 Tinea capitis, a fungal infection of the scalp, is marked by scale on the scalp with local breaking or loss of hair; erythema (redness) is usually not observed. (See Chapter 26, "Dermatologic Products.")

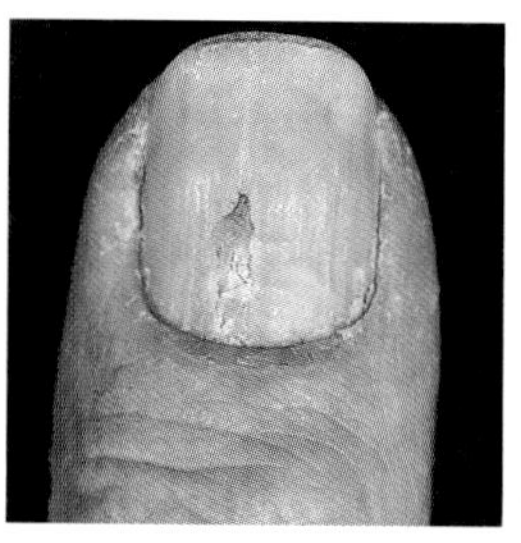

13

13 Paronychia is usually caused by overexposure of the nails to water, causing cuticle loss and inflammation around the nail folds. Approximately 50% of cases involve candidal infection. (See Chapter 26, "Dermatologic Products.")

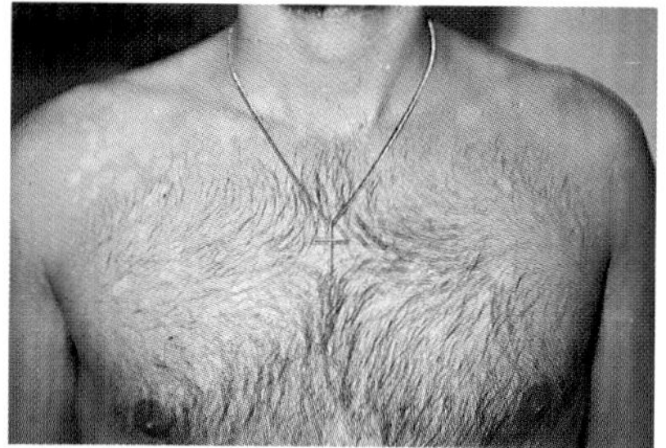

14A

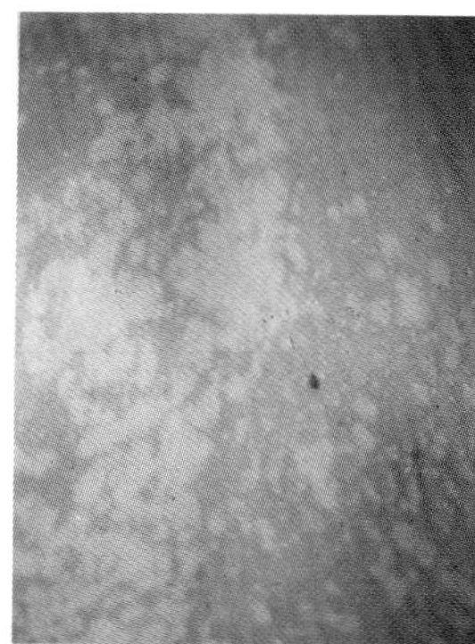

14B

14A and B Tinea versicolor is caused by a yeast organism that overgrows locally, resulting in hyperpigmentation or hypopigmentation (**A**). These mildly scaling eruptions characteristically occur on the chest, upper back, and arms (**B**). (See Chapter 26, "Dermatalogic Products.")

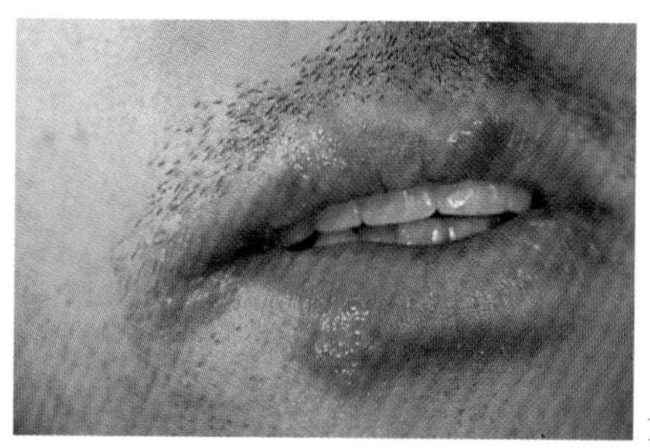

15

15 Herpes simplex lesions of the mouth and the eye usually start as a small cluster of vesicles (tiny blisters) that subsequently heal over with a serosanguinous (blood-tinged) crust. Local stinging, burning, and pain often herald the onset of lesions. Eye involvement should always be referred to an ophthalmologist. (See Chapter 26, "Dermatologic Products.")

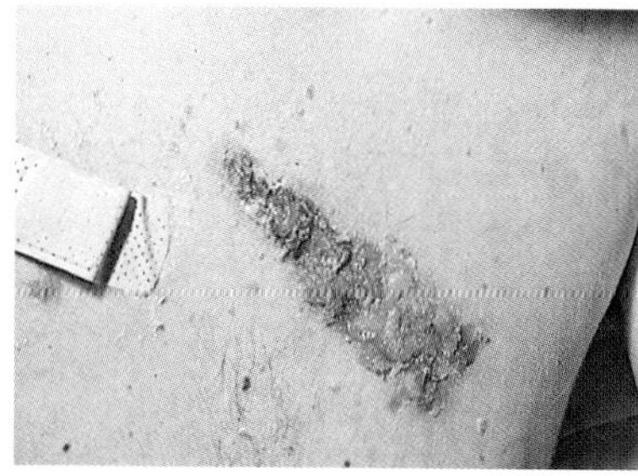

16A

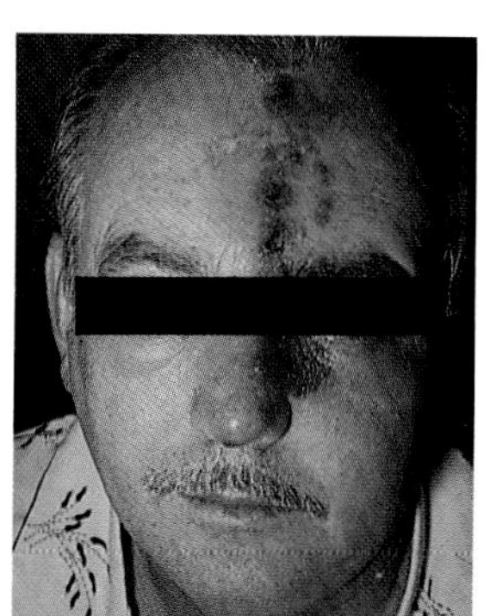

16B

16A and B Herpes zoster is a reactivation of previous chickenpox virus that has remained latent in the nerve roots. Pain precedes small clusters of vesicles (blisters) on an erythematous base that are distributed along the cutaneous (skin) area supplied by the infected nerve (**A**). The inflammation characteristically stops in the midline of the body (**B**). (See Chapter 26, "Dermatologic Products.")

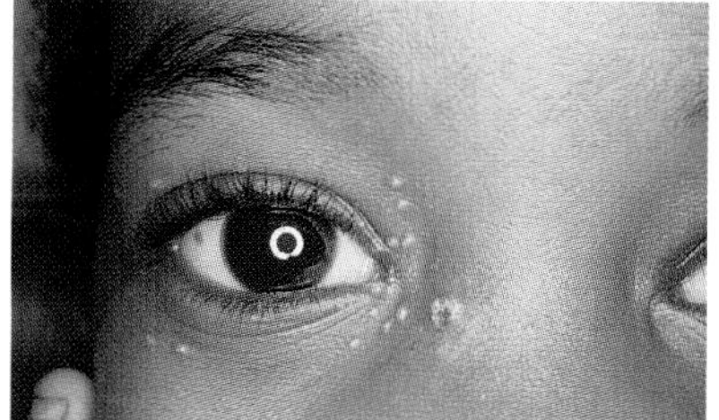

17

17 Molluscum contagiosum is a viral tumor caused by a poxvirus containing DNA. The virus is manifested by one or more small (3–5 mm), pink, slightly raised lesions that are usually found on the abdomen, inner thigh, or perianal area. The mature lesion has a slight depression on the top and a soft core that can be expressed. (See Chapter 26, "Dermatologic Products.")

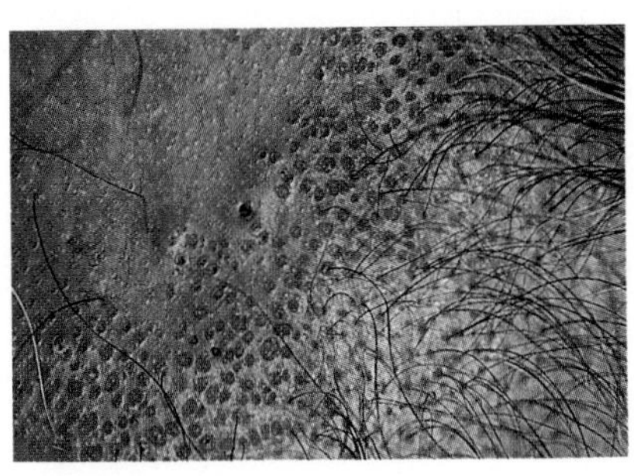

18

18 Comedonic acne (noninflammatory) occurs when follicles become plugged with sebum, forming a comedone on the surface. The black color is caused by oxidation of lipid and melanin, not dirt as is commonly believed. (See Chapter 27, "Acne Products.")

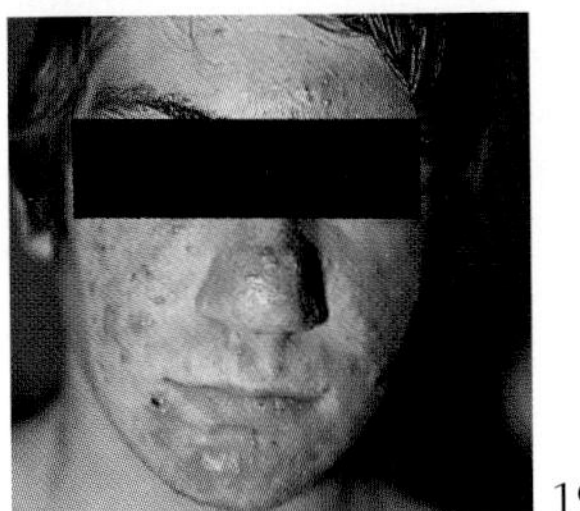

19

19 Pustular acne (inflammatory) presents as inflamed papules that are formed when superficial hair follicles become plugged and rupture at a deeper level. Superficial inflammation results in pustules; deep lesions cause large cysts to form with possible resultant scarring. (See Chapter 27, "Acne Products.")

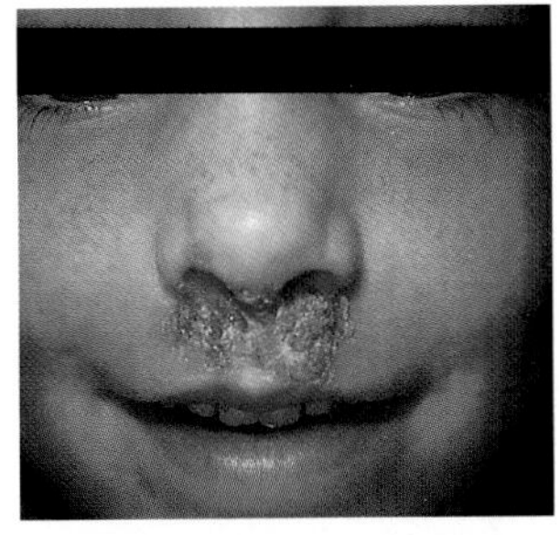

20

20 Impetigo is a bacterial infection characterized by honeycomb crusts on erythematous bases. A bullous (blistering) form can also occur. (See Chapter 28, "First-Aid Products and Minor Wound Care.")

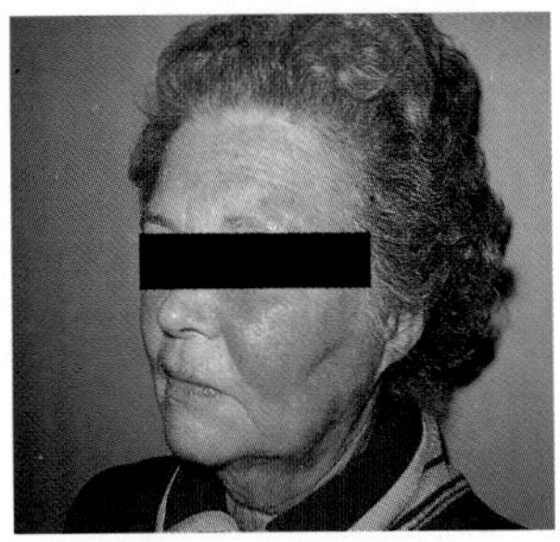

21

21 Erysipeloid is a streptococcal infection that often involves the face or extremities. The infected area is red and raised, with local warmth and edema. The margins of the infected area change rapidly, often forming serpiginous (irregular) patterns. (See Chapter 28, "First-Aid Products and Minor Wound Care.")

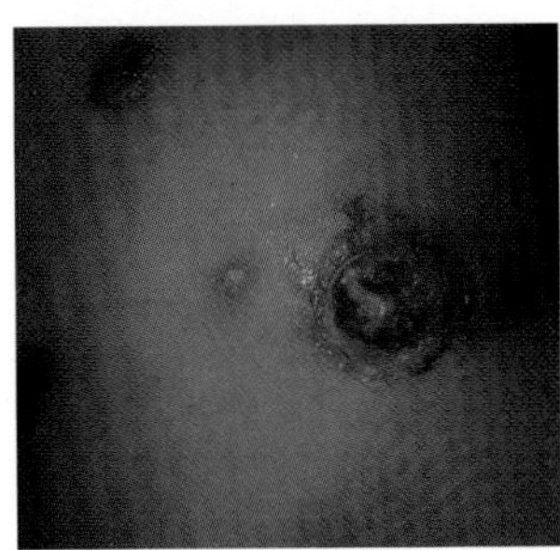

22

22 Infections of the hair follicles are usually caused by staphylococcal or streptococcal organisms. Superficial infections (folliculitis) can occur; deeper infections are called furuncles (small boils). Carbuncles form when adjacent hair follicles are involved. (See Chapter 28, "First-Aid Products and Minor Wound Care.")

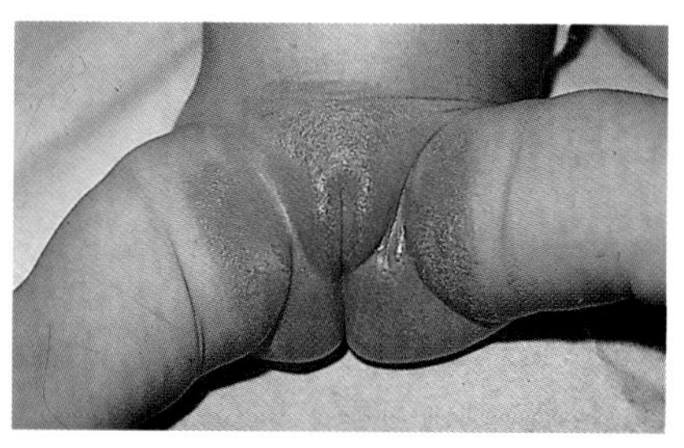
23

23 Diaper dermatitis presents as erythema of the groin (crease area around the genitals) and is common in infants. The case shown here was caused by a contact allergen. Contact irritants, such as urine and feces, and secondary bacterial and yeast infections may also cause problems in this area. (See Chapter 29, "Diaper Rash, Prickly Heat, and Adult Incontinence Products.")

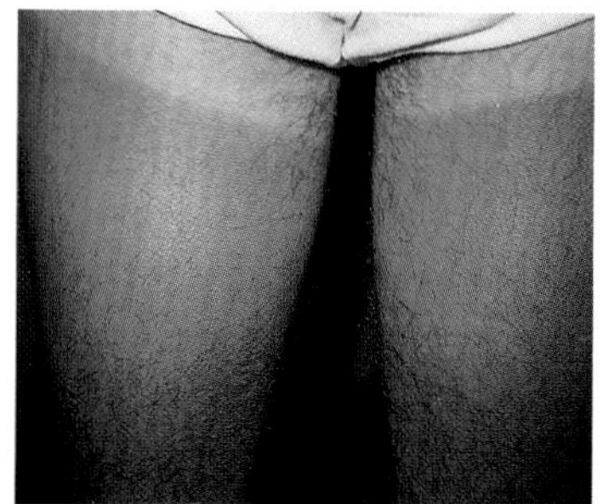
24

24 Miliaria rubra (heat rash) is an obstruction of sweat glands. Superficial involvement results in only tiny vesicles (blisters) appearing on the skin surface (miliaria crystallina). When deeper inflammation is present, the surrounding erythema is characteristic of miliaria rubra. (See Chapter 29, "Diaper Rash, Prickly Heat, and Adult Incontinence Products.")

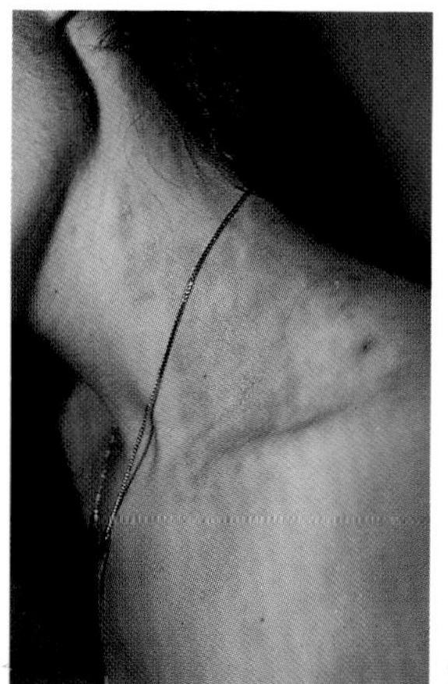
25

25 Sunburn presents as an erythema that occurs after excessive sun exposure; severe burns can result in large blister formation. Proper sunscreen application can provide photoprotection for susceptible patients. (See Chapter 31, "Burn and Sunburn Products.")

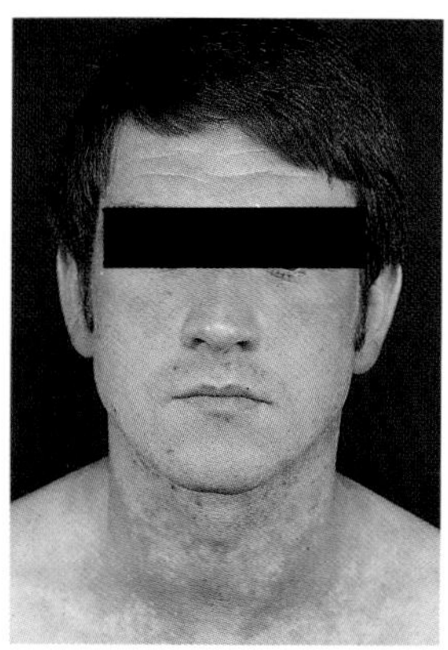
26

26 Cosmetic-induced photosensitivity can be caused by ingredients in certain topical colognes and perfumes. This immunologic reaction produces a local erythema that leaves characteristic postinflammatory pigmentation. (See Chapter 31, "Burn and Sunburn Products.")

27

27 Drug-induced photosensitivity is a reaction that occurs on sun-exposed surfaces of the head, neck, and dorsum (back) of the hands. The erythema does not occur on photoprotected areas (under the nose and chin, behind the ears, and between the fingers). (See Chapter 31, "Burn and Sunburn Products.")

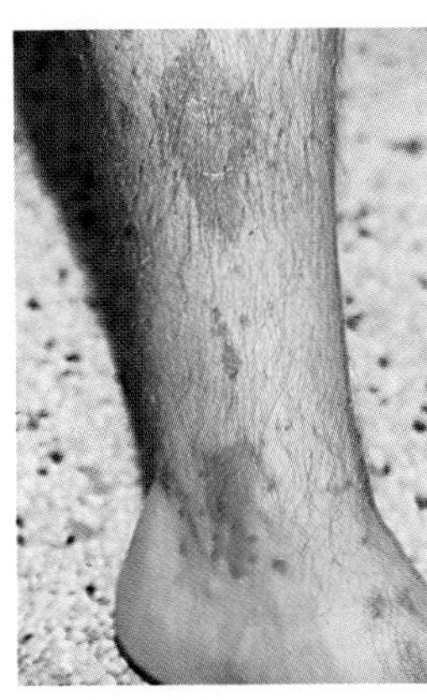

28A

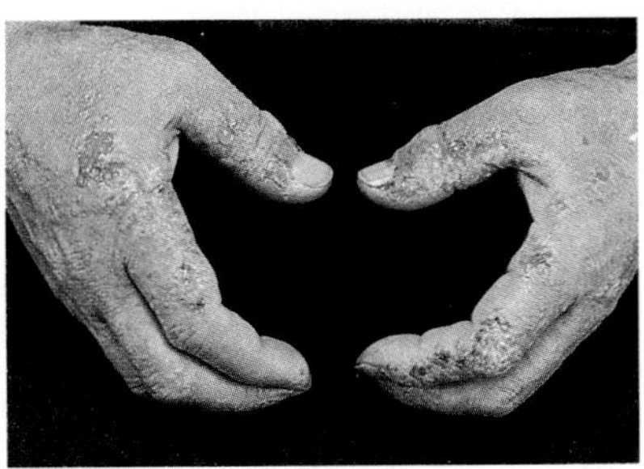

28B

28A and B Poison ivy causes a linear erythema that can develop into large blisters (**A**, **B**). Similar reactions can also be caused by poison oak and poison sumac. (See Chapter 32, "Poison Ivy, Oak, and Sumac Products.")

29

29 Insect bites are often characterized as small clusters of itchy red papules. A small, overlying, superficial vesicle may be present. (Chapter 33, "Insect Sting and Bite Products.")

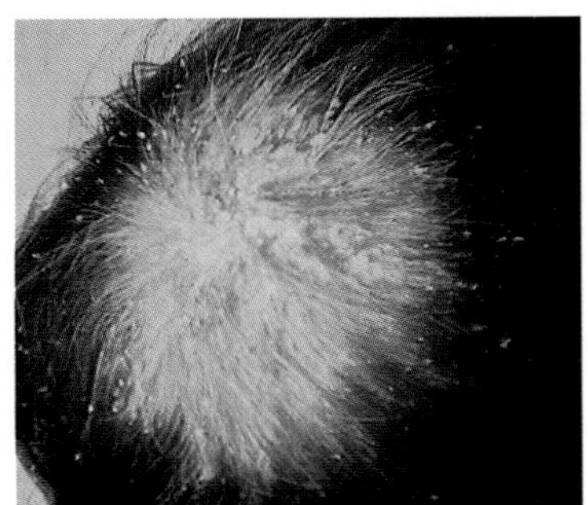

30A

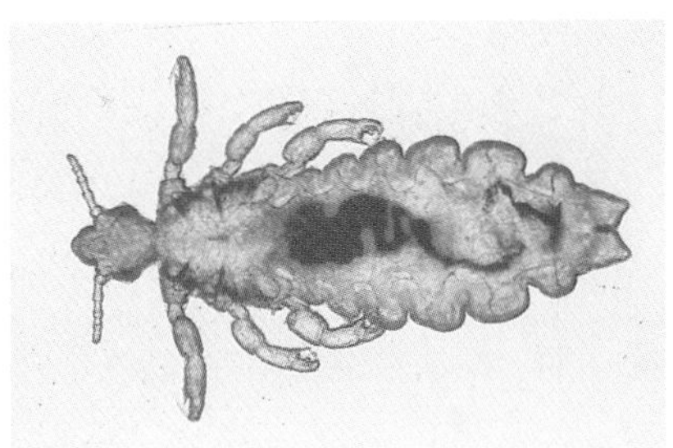

30B

30A and B Pediculosis humanus capitis is a louse infestation of the scalp. Examination of the scalp hair in this infestation shows tiny nits (eggs) attached to the hair shaft (**A**). The organism shown is only occasionally seen (**B**). (See Chapter 33, "Insect Sting and Bite Products.")

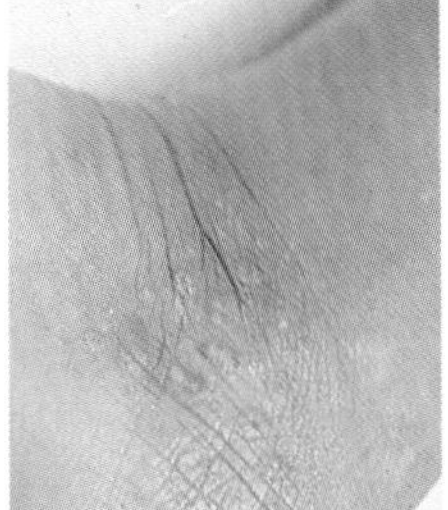

31

31 Scabies is caused by a small mite that burrows under the superficial skin layers. Small linear blisters that cause intense itching can be seen between the finger webs, on the inner wrists, in the axilla, around the areola (nipple) of the breast, and on the genitalia. (See Chapter 33, "Insect Sting and Bite Products.")

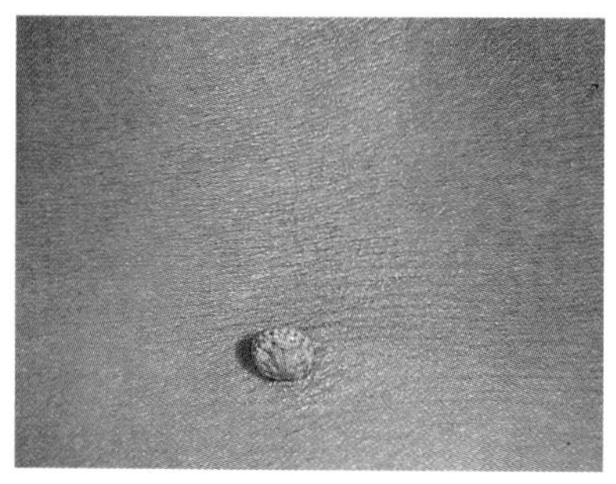

32

32 Ticks can attach to human skin and burrow into superficial skin layers. With careful examination, the back of the organism is usually visible on the skin surface. Ticks are vectors of several systemic diseases. (See Chapter 33, "Insect Sting and Bite Products.")

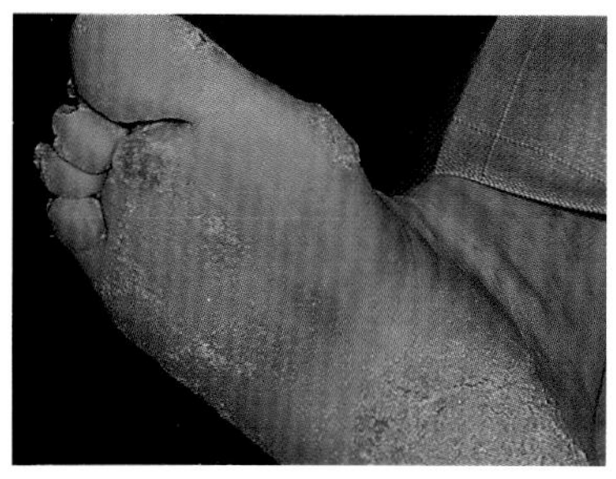

33

33 Calluses are thickened scales that often form on joints and weight-bearing areas. A callus on the plantar surface of the foot is shown here. (See Chapter 34, "Foot Care Products.")

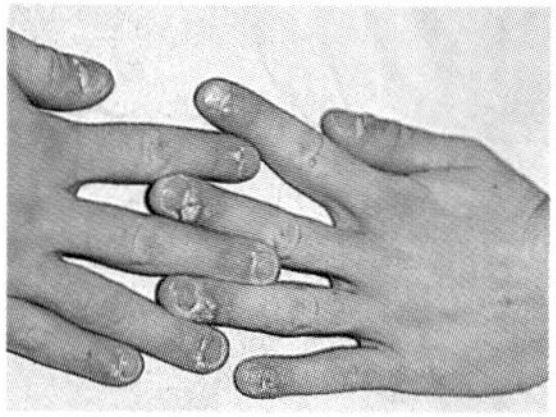

34

34 Common warts are viral-induced lesions that present as localized rough accumulations of keratin (hyperkeratosis) containing many tiny furrows. If the wart's surface is pared, small bleeding points can be seen. (See Chapter 34, "Foot Care Products.")

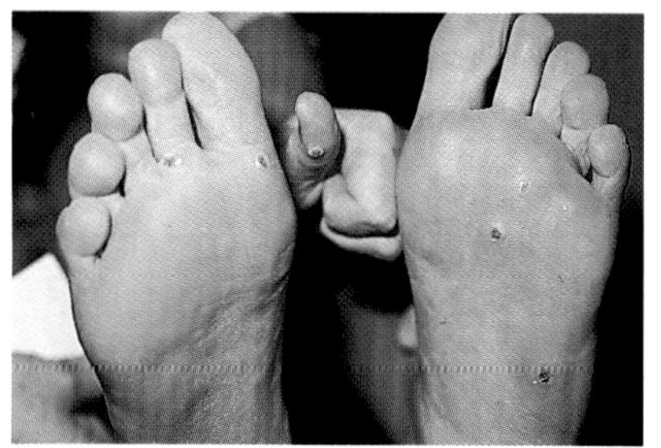

35

35 Plantar warts, caused by a viral infection, are often found on the plantar surface of the foot and present with hard localized accumulations of keratin. The punctate bleeding points seen when the lesions are pared distinguish plantar warts from calluses. (See Chapter 34, "Foot Care Products.")

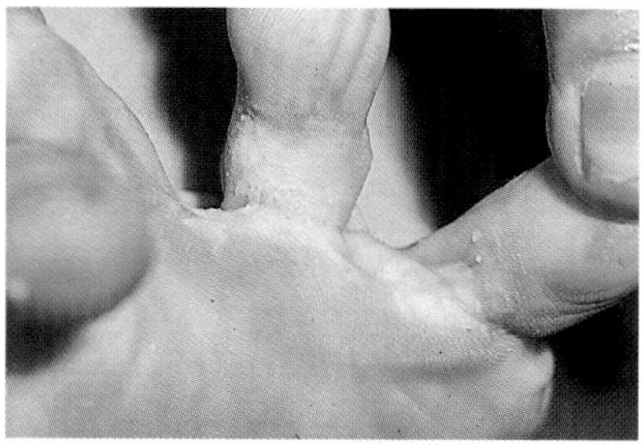

36

36 Tinea pedis infection of the toes characteristically starts between the fourth and fifth web space and spreads proximally. Scaling can progress to maceration with resultant small fissures. (See Chapter 34, "Foot Care Products.")

alized over much of the body surface.[35] Remissions and exacerbations are unpredictable. Approximately 30% of persons with psoriasis find that lesion involvement may clear spontaneously. In fact, psoriasis can be so mild that some people do not even know they have it. However, unrelenting generalized psoriasis may cause enough psychologic distress to affect lifestyle and career choice adversely. With an associated psoriatic arthritis, it may even result in disability and deformity.[36] Treatment of severe psoriasis can also produce a significant physical and economic burden.[29,37]

Etiology and Characteristics Psoriasis is a papulosquamous erythematous skin disease marked by the presence of silvery scales. These scales cover lesions that are flat topped and pink or dull red in color. Edges of the lesions are sharply delineated, and individual diameters may vary from a few millimeters to 20 cm or more. When psoriatic scales are removed mechanically, small bleeding points (the Auspitz sign) appear. Psoriatic skin is more permeable to many substances than is normal skin; for example, it may lose water 8–10 times faster. In fact, when large areas of the body surface are involved, skin water loss may be as much as 2–3 L daily in addition to normal perspiration loss. Evaporation of this volume of water requires more than 1,000 calories. For this reason, psoriatic patients may show increased metabolic rates at the expense of tissue catabolism, and muscle wasting may occur.[7]

Psoriatic lesions tend to appear on the scalp, elbows, knees, fingernails, lower back, and the genitoanal region. Lesions may develop at sites of trauma (Koebner's phenomenon) such as vaccination or skin tests, scratch marks, or surgical incisions, and they have even been reportedly produced by shock and noise. In fact, the response to skin trauma is so predictable that it can be used in the assessment of up to 40% of persons afflicted. For example, assessment is difficult when scaling is not evident, but scales can usually be induced by light scratching if the patient demonstrates evidence of Koebner's phenomenon. It has been shown that both the epidermis and dermis must be damaged before this reaction occurs and that the reaction generally occurs within 6–18 days following the injury.[7]

Many patients and clinicians do not mention pruritus as a symptom of psoriasis. However, several surveys indicate that itching is a significant manifestation of the disease in 30–70% of cases, and the name *psoriasis* originates from the Greek word for *itch*.[37]

Psoriasis assumes several different pathologic forms, the most common being psoriasis vulgaris. This is the chronic, plaquetype psoriasis of the general description. The plaques may be any size and may be quite extensive.[29]

Guttate psoriasis accounts for about 17% of psoriatic cases. It is characterized by many small, teardrop-shaped lesions distributed more or less evenly over the body. These lesions may later coalesce to form large characteristic plaques. (See color plates, photographs 11A, B, and C.) Psoriasis in children is usually of the guttate variety and may be precipitated by various systemic diseases such as streptococcal tonsillitis. Acute attacks of guttate psoriasis have also been noted to occur at puberty and following childbirth. When the psoriatic condition is initiated by a guttate attack, the disease carries a slightly better prognosis than that of a slower and more diffuse onset.[7]

Another type of psoriasis is known as pustular psoriasis. It is marked by localized, sterile pustules on the palms and soles. In severe or generalized cases (von Zumbusch's type), the entire skin may be involved and the condition may become life-threatening.[37]

Flexural psoriasis involves the intertriginous folds. Often no other lesions are present, which makes it difficult to distinguish the condition from seborrheic dermatitis. Again, the Auspitz sign is usually detectable in psoriasis but is not demonstrated in seborrheic dermatitis. Because of moisture and friction associated with the affected areas, treatment is often difficult as well.[29]

Erythrodermic psoriasis is a severe complication that can be life-threatening. The entire skin surface can become red with little evidence of scales. Massive shunting of blood to the skin surface can cause heat and water loss extensive enough to cause cardiac failure.[29,37]

Psoriasis is primarily manifested in the epidermis; mucous membranes are rarely involved. Besides skin, tissues known to be clinically involved are the synovium and nails. In many patients with coexisting joint disease and psoriasis, the arthritic component is not easily distinguishable from rheumatoid arthritis. About 7% of psoriatic patients, however, have a unique form of arthritis, psoriatic arthritis, which is recognized as a distinct clinical entity. Psoriatic arthritis is distinguished from rheumatoid arthritis in several respects. Its onset is often in the distal rather than proximal joints of the fingers or toes, and this involvement is associated with psoriasis of the nails in 80% of persons affected. Nail involvement includes onycholysis (separation of the nail from the nail bed), pitting, and yellow discoloration. Unlike rheumatoid arthritis, psoriatic arthritis is often asymmetric in its joint involvement. Usually, the rheumatoid factor is absent and prognosis is better than it is with rheumatoid arthritis.

The duration of psoriasis is variable. Lesions may last a lifetime or may disappear quickly. When they disappear, they may leave the skin either hypopigmented or hyperpigmented. The disease course is marked by spontaneous exacerbations and remissions, and it tends to be chronic and relapsing.

Although it is not contagious from one patient to another, there seems to be an inherited predisposition to psoriasis, given that about 30% of psoriatic patients show an associated family history. Evidence supports an autosomal dominant mode of inheritance, and genetic markers as determined by the major histocompatibility locus antigen system have been identified. Persons with psoriasis also have a higher than usual incidence of occlusive vascular episodes, which seems to correlate with the extensiveness of the lesions. Environmental factors are not to be underestimated. Controlled exposure to sunlight usually improves the condition. Many investigators agree that emotional stress often affects psoriasis adversely. It is well documented that antimalarial agents, beta-blockers, and lithium can exacerbate or precipitate a psoriasis-like eruption. Abrupt withdrawal of corticosteroids in psoriatic patients may precipitate a severe rebound flare.[29,37]

No age group is exempt from psoriasis; incidence

of initial onset peaks in the late 20s and then declines with advancing age. It is also distributed almost equally between men and women. Psoriasis is common to all races and geographic regions; however, its incidence is lower in people living in countries close to the equator and in Japanese and Native Americans.[37]

Major Pathophysiologic Events The pathophysiology of the psoriatic lesion is very complex, involving not only the epidermis but also the dermis and the body's immune system. Three major pathophysiologic events are involved in the disease process: accelerated epidermal proliferation and metabolic activity, proliferation of capillaries in the dermal region, and invasion of the dermis and epidermis by inflammatory cells.

Accelerated epidermal proliferation leading to excessive scaling is one hallmark of psoriasis. Normal epidermal cell turnover is 25–30 days; in a psoriatic plaque, it is 3–4 days. According to one theory, accelerated epidermal proliferation is due to a shortening of cell division cycle time. Data have been collected showing that the germinative cell cycle of the psoriatic epidermal cell is 12 times faster than the normal cycle (37.5 versus 457 hours). These data, however, have been disputed. A second theory is that the germinative layer in human epidermis is composed of three distinct populations of epidermal cells. In normal skin, only one of these populations may be actively cycling, but in psoriasis, all three epidermal cell populations may be involved in active proliferation.[7]

When one considers the extent of epidermal proliferation in psoriasis, it logically follows that an expanded vascular system is needed to satisfy increasing metabolic requirements. In psoriasis, capillaries in the dermal region proliferate. Resultant capillary loops are arranged vertically at the center of the plaque and are responsible for the minor bleeding when adherent scales are lifted from the skin (the Auspitz sign). It has been postulated that psoriatic plaque may generate a substance responsible for this capillary proliferation, enabling the lesion to expand.[7]

The third major pathophysiologic event in psoriasis is invasion of the dermis and epidermis by inflammatory cells. Mononuclear cells and polymorphonuclear (PMN) leukocytes can be found in the dermis; PMN leukocytes also tend to infiltrate the epidermis. Extracts of psoriatic scale have been shown to contain factors that can induce directed migration (chemotaxis) of these inflammatory cells. Moreover, mononuclear cells and PMN leukocytes from psoriatic patients have been shown to exhibit enhanced responsiveness to chemoattractants. Lithium carbonate increases the total mass of circulating PMN leukocytes and is therefore associated with an induction or exacerbation of psoriatic symptoms. The presence of inflammatory cells in psoriatic skin may induce epidermal proliferation and has led to many theories about the possible role of the immune system in the pathogenesis of psoriasis.[7]

Assessment Assessment of simple psoriasis usually is straightforward. Sites of involvement, the dry silvery appearance of scales, and a small area of bleeding after gentle scale removal are characteristic. Pruritus and joint involvement may also be present. Information regarding precipitating factors such as disease, pregnancy, a recent vaccination, emotional stress, or physical trauma is useful in a preliminary assessment.

It is important to differentiate psoriasis from other diseases that may have similar symptoms but call for different treatment. When the scalp or the flexural and intertriginous areas are involved, psoriasis must be differentiated from a fungal infection or seborrhea. A fungal organism may be identified from lesion scrapings; when nails are involved, differentiation requires laboratory analysis. Psoriasis of the scalp may be distinguished from seborrhea by the Auspitz sign and by the difference in scale appearance and color. Also, the psoriatic plaque has a full, rich, red color with a depth of hue and opacity not typically seen in seborrhea or dermatitis. In dark skin, this distinction may be lost. If lesions are present in the groin, axilla, and inframammary region, assessment based on visual inspection may be difficult, and histopathology may be required.

Treatment Careful questioning of the patient and examination of lesions, when feasible, are essential in determining whether the complaint is psoriasis and amenable to nonprescription therapy. Pruritic dry skin is very common in psoriasis, and emollients and lubricating bath products often provide relief for these symptoms. Gentle rubbing with a soft cloth following the bath helps remove scales. If this is insufficient, self-treatment may progress to the use of keratolytics, coal tar, and topical hydrocortisone.[29] Vigorous rubbing, which can aggravate the lesions, should be avoided.

Acute localized flares, characterized by strongly erythematous lesions, call for soothing local therapy with emollients and hydrocortisone. Tars, salicylic acid, and aggressive UV radiation therapy must be avoided at this stage because of potential exacerbating effects. After the flare has subsided and the usual thick-scaled plaques appear, therapy with agents such as keratolytics may be used. Many patients respond well to simple measures while others are refractory even to aggressive treatments.[7]

In the case of psoriatic arthritis, the psoriatic lesions are treated topically; the joint involvement is usually treated with nonsteroidal anti-inflammatory agents.[29,37] Unfortunately, there is no effective treatment for nail psoriasis.

The FDA recommends that only mild cases of psoriasis be self-treated. If a nonprescription product is used, the pharmacist should counsel the patient to consult a physician if the condition does not improve in 1–2 weeks or if it worsens. Individuals with severe cases involving large areas of the body should be under a physician's care.[7] Severe or generalized psoriasis sometimes necessitates day care or hospitalization of the patient.

Psoriasis cannot be cured, but signs and symptoms can usually be controlled adequately with appropriate patient education and treatment. The patient should be reassured that, in most cases, control is possible. Such reassurance increases compliance with treatment regimens that are often burdensome and prolonged. Also, if the pharmacist can help the patient gain some understanding and acceptance of the condition, it may reduce the patient's emotional stress and therefore decrease psychogenic exacerbations. Prevention of flares, achieved by minimizing identified precipitating factors such as

TABLE 5 Concentrations of approved nonprescription ingredients for products for the treatment of dandruff, seborrheic dermatitis, and psoriasis

Ingredient	Dandruff (%)	Seborrheic dermatitis (%)	Psoriasis (%)
Coal tar	0.5–5	0.5–5	0.5–5
Pyrithione zinc (brief exposure)	0.3–2	0.95–2	—
Pyrithione zinc (residual)	0.1–0.25	0.1–0.25	—
Salicylic acid	1.8–3	1.8–3	1.8–3
Selenium sulfide	1	1	—
Sulfur	2–5	—	—

[a]For control of dandruff, salicylic acid may be combined with sulfur, provided each ingredient is present within the approved concentrations.

Reprinted from *Federal Register*. 1982; 47: 54646–84.

emotional stress, skin irritation, and physical trauma, should be emphasized.

Pharmacologic Agents for Scaly Dermatoses

The final monograph on nonprescription dandruff, seborrheic dermatitis, and psoriasis products was released by the FDA on December 4, 1991, and became effective on December 4, 1992.[38] Active ingredients cited as Category I include the following:

- *Dandruff*: coal tar preparations, pyrithione zinc, salicylic acid, selenium sulfide, sulfur, and sulfur in combination with salicylic acid;
- *Seborrheic dermatitis*: coal tar preparations, pyrithione zinc, salicylic acid, and selenium sulfide;
- *Psoriasis*: coal tar preparations and salicylic acid (Table 5). Topical hydrocortisone is also found useful in the self-treatment of seborrhea and psoriasis.

Not found to be effective for these uses and designated as nonmonograph were 28 additional nonprescription ingredients commonly found in dandruff, seborrhea, and psoriasis products. These ingredients should soon be of historic interest as products are reformulated (see product table "Dandruff, Seborrhea, and Psoriasis Products").

High-potency topical corticosteroids may be used to treat seborrhea and psoriasis under physician supervision. Prescription drug treatment for psoriasis also includes topical anthralin, antimetabolites (such as methotrexate), psoralens combined with long-wave UV phototherapy, retinoids (such as etretinate), topical calcipotriene (vitamin D_3 analog), and systemic corticosteroids.

Cytostatic Agents

Cytostatic agents work by decreasing the rate of epidermal cell replication, which, in turn, increases the time required for epidermal cell turnover. Increasing the time for cell turnover makes it possible to normalize epidermal differentiation and to bring about a dramatic decline in visible scales. Thus, cytostatic agents represent a direct approach to controlling dandruff and seborrhea.

Pyrithione Zinc Pyrithione zinc's action is likely due to a nonspecific toxicity for epidermal cells. The pyrithione moiety is apparently the active part of the molecule. Product effectiveness is influenced by several factors. For one thing, pyrithione zinc is strongly bound to both hair and the external skin layers; the extent of binding correlates with clinical performance. For another, the drug does not penetrate into the dermal region. Third, its absorption increases with contact time, temperature, concentration, and frequency of application. Some consider pyrithione zinc to be slower acting than selenium sulfide.[7]

For pyrithione zinc products intended to be applied and washed off after a brief exposure, the FDA allows concentrations of 0.3–2% for treating dandruff and 0.95–2% for treating seborrhea. Concentrations for products intended to be applied and then left on the skin or scalp are 0.1–0.25% for treating both dandruff and seborrhea.[38] Shampoos and soaps are currently available in 1 and 2% concentrations.

Before using one of these products, the patient should

be advised to shampoo with a nonmedicated, nonresidue shampoo to remove scalp and hair dirt, oil, and scale. Most shampoos leave a residue on the hair shaft and scalp that may aggravate scalp disorders such as dandruff, seborrhea, and psoriasis. Nonresidue shampoos (eg, Prell, Breck, and Johnson and Johnson Baby Shampoo) do not interfere with these scalp conditions; rather, they leave the scalp clean and receptive to optimal effects from medicated shampoos. A nonresidue shampoo application and rinse may be followed by a pyrithione zinc shampoo worked into the scalp vigorously for at least 5 minutes and then rinsed out thoroughly. This treatment should be repeated twice weekly for 2 weeks and then once weekly as needed.[29]

Long-term use of 1–2% pyrithione zinc products has not been associated with toxicity. This may be because pyrithione zinc is relatively insoluble in water and is not easily absorbed through the skin or mucous membranes. Nevertheless, patients should be cautioned against using this agent on broken or abraded skin since rare cases of contact dermatitis have been reported.

Selenium Sulfide Selenium sulfide is thought to have a direct antimitotic effect on epidermal cells. Like pyrithione zinc, it is more effective with longer contact time and thus should be applied in a similar manner. The product must be rinsed from the hair thoroughly or discoloration may result, especially in blond, gray, or dyed hair. Frequent use of selenium sulfide tends to leave a residual odor and an oily scalp.

Selenium sulfide has been approved in a 1% concentration as an active ingredient in nonprescription products to treat dandruff and seborrhea.[38] A higher concentration is available by prescription for use in resistant cases.

Cytostatic toxicity from selenium sulfide is minimal, but the product can cause irritation of scalp and adjacent skin areas and should be avoided if such irritation occurs. Contact with the eyes should be avoided because of the potential for irritation. If such contact does occur, the patient should flush the eyes with copious amounts of water. Selenium sulfide is toxic if ingested. Because of the risk of systemic toxicity, it should only be applied to intact skin.[39]

Coal Tar

Coal tar products have long been popular for the treatment of dandruff, seborrhea, and psoriasis. Many nonprescription products are available. Crude coal tar, which consists of a heterogeneous mixture of more than 10,000 different compounds, is produced by the destructive distillation of bituminous coal. Its composition varies depending on the source of the coal and the process used. Crude coal tar is the most active; the refined tars, less so; and liquor carbonis detergens, the least active.[29]

Its mechanism of action is not known, but coal tar has been attributed with antiseptic, antipruritic, keratoplastic, antiparasitic, antifungal, antibacterial, antimitotic, vasoconstrictive, and photosensitizing capabilities. Its beneficial activity in the conditions under consideration seems to depend on the dispersion of scales and its ability to reduce the number and size of epidermal cells produced.

Crude coal tar (1–5%) and UV radiation therapy have been used in the treatment of psoriasis since 1925 in a method known as the Goeckerman treatment. A therapeutic benefit of both the tar alone and the irradiation alone has been demonstrated, but the combination is more effective than either agent by itself. Remissions lasting up to 12 months have been reported after 2–4 weeks of therapy. The coal tar is removed from the skin before irradiation takes place; otherwise, the UV radiation will not reach the skin. For many years, the therapeutic response to this form of therapy was believed to be caused by phototoxicity, but this theory has been challenged. Now it is thought that the beneficial effect of coal tar may lie in its ability to cross-link with DNA. Coal tar in combination with UV radiation may also increase prostaglandin synthesis in the skin, which may contribute to its beneficial effect. Combinations of 1% crude coal tar with long-wave UV (UV-B) radiation and of 6% crude coal tar with UV-B radiation have been shown to be equally effective. Hence, only modest levels of coal tar are needed.[7]

Coal tar is available in creams, ointments, pastes, lotions, bath oils, shampoos, soaps, and gels. This wide variety of products has partly resulted from an attempt to develop a cosmetically acceptable product, one that masks the odor, color, and staining properties of crude coal tar that most patients find aesthetically unappealing. Liquor carbonis detergens is a 20% tincture of coal tar that has been useful in the development of acceptable tar products. It is used in concentrations of 3–15%.

Tar gels represent a unique product form that appears to deliver the beneficial elements of crude coal tar in a form both convenient to apply and cosmetically acceptable. These gels are nongreasy, nonstaining, and nearly colorless. The pharmacist should caution the patient, however, that these gels may have a drying effect on the skin, necessitating the use of an emollient.

Certain side effects are associated with the use of coal tar. These include folliculitis, particularly of the axilla and groin; staining of the skin and hair, particularly blond, gray, and dyed hair; photosensitization; and dermatitis due to irritation.[40] Certain patients may even show a worsening of the condition being treated when they are exposed to coal tar products. This is of particular concern in the acute phase of psoriasis, when topical steroids are recommended to reduce inflammation before coal tar preparations are used.[29]

Some known active photosensitizers of coal tar include acridine, anthracene, and pyridine. If the patient is currently using other photosensitizing drugs such as tetracyclines, phenothiazines, thiazides, or sulfonamides, the pharmacist should give appropriate warnings. Moreover, the patient should not use extensive exposure to sunlight or sunlamps to simulate the Goeckerman treatment since this procedure requires careful monitoring of UV radiation exposure. Generally, patients should be cautioned that the use of coal tar may increase their tendency to sunburn for up to 24 hours after application. However, before advising the patient to avoid sun exposure, the pharmacist should ask what directions were given by the physician because patients are commonly told to apply the coal tar in the evening and then spend time in the sunlight on the following day.

Crude coal tar and UV radiation are both thought to have carcinogenic potential, particularly in the anogenital area. However, there have been no reports of an increased frequency of skin cancer in psoriatic patients treated for many years with coal tar and UV radiation. Because of the short contact time, the FDA considers the benefits of coal tar to outweigh the risks for use in shampoo formulations and has granted approval for coal tar in concentrations of 0.5–5% in the self-treatment of dandruff, seborrhea, and psoriasis.[38]

Keratolytic Agents

Keratolytic agents are used in dandruff and seborrhea products to loosen and lyse keratin aggregates, thereby facilitating their removal from the scalp in smaller particles. These agents act by dissolving the "cement" that holds epidermal cells together. Vehicle composition, contact time, and concentration are important factors in the success of a keratolytic agent. The keratolytic concentrations in nonprescription scalp products are not sufficient to impair the normal skin barrier but do affect the abnormal, incompletely keratinized stratum corneum.

Keratolytic agents may produce several adverse effects, and the patient should be counseled accordingly. These agents have a primary, concentration-dependent irritant effect, particularly on mucous membranes and the conjunctiva of the eye. They also have the potential of acting on hair keratin as well as on skin keratin. Thus, hair appearance may be altered as a result of extended use. The directions and precautions for the use of keratolytic shampoos are similar to those for shampoos containing cytostatic agents.

Salicylic Acid Salicylic acid decreases skin pH, causing increased hydration of keratin and thus facilitating its loosening and removal. Since contact time is minimal for a shampoo, extensive absorption/adsorption of the agent by the skin should not occur.

Topical salicylic acid is useful for psoriasis when thick scales are present. A patient should soak the psoriatic lesion(s) in warm water for 10–20 minutes before applying the preparation, which may then be covered by an occlusive dressing. However, application over extensive areas should be avoided because of the potential for percutaneous absorption and systemic toxicity. Initially, lower concentrations should be used to minimize the possibility of causing irritation and worsening the condition.[7]

Salicylic acid has been approved in concentrations of 1.8–3% for the self-treatment of dandruff, seborrhea, and psoriasis.[38] At these concentrations, the keratolytic effect typically takes 7–10 days. In higher concentrations for other uses, the keratolytic effect may be evident in 2–3 days.

Sulfur Sulfur is believed to function by an inflammatory process, causing increased sloughing of cells and reduced corneocyte counts.[41]

Sulfur has been approved in concentrations of 2–5% for the self-treatment of dandruff only. Although it is approved as a single-entity active ingredient, sulfur is often combined with salicylic acid. For the control of dandruff, the sulfur–salicylic acid combination is useful if both ingredients are present within the approved concentrations.[38] While not an official indication, this combination has also been commonly used for the self-treatment of seborrhea.[32]

Topical Hydrocortisone

Topical hydrocortisone (0.25–1%) is available without a prescription and has been promoted for the temporary relief of itching due to body and scalp dermatoses. Hydrocortisone is generally efficacious as an antipruritic agent when used in concentrations of at least 1%. It is not indicated, nor is there evidence that it is effective, in the treatment of dandruff. However, it may be useful for seborrhea accompanied by inflammation and should be reserved for scalp seborrhea unresponsive to medicated shampoos.[32]

Nonprescription hydrocortisone products play an important role in the management of psoriasis. A major problem with hydrocortisone and all topical steroids is that there is usually a prompt rebound when topical steroid therapy is discontinued, and the psoriasis may reappear as the more severe pustular form. Relapse occurs more quickly after use of topical corticosteroids than after use of tar or anthralin therapy. Nevertheless, these agents are more appealing to the patient on cosmetic grounds, which are a consideration in long-term therapy.[37]

Topical corticosteroids have several effects (eg, anti-inflammatory, antimitotic/antisynthetic, antipruritic, vasoconstrictive, and immunosuppressive) on cellular activity. Efficacy may be enhanced by an occlusive dressing. However, continued use of topical steroids beyond 2 or 3 weeks may render the drug less effective. If the patient does not respond adequately to hydrocortisone, physician referral is appropriate because the use of more potent steroids may be in order. Selection of the proper prescription steroid may be complex owing to the common assumption that potency and adverse effects are linked directly to halogenation.[42,43]

Adverse effects associated with the use of topical steroids include local atrophy of the skin after prolonged use and the aggravation of certain cutaneous infections. The possibility of systemic sequelae exists and is enhanced by the use of the more potent compounds, by occlusive dressings, or by application to large areas of the body. Because children have a greater surface area-to-body mass ratio, they are at greater risk for developing systemic complications. In general, however, the concentrations of hydrocortisone available in nonprescription preparations are unlikely to cause systemic sequelae.[42,43]

Pharmacists play a vital role in patient care by prudently advising patients about the safe and appropriate use of nonprescription topical hydrocortisone preparations. The patient should be instructed to apply the hydrocortisone as a thin film two to four times a day at the onset of therapy and intermittently thereafter to control exacerbations. The medication should be thoroughly but gently massaged into the skin. Continued and frequent use of hydrocortisone is to be discouraged because topical steroids may become less effective with prolonged use, may promote local rebound, may cause adverse local effects, and, most importantly, may not induce remissions of psoriasis. The patient should be instructed to rely primarily on other treatments and to use topical hydrocortisone only when necessary.

The systemic use of corticosteroids is contraindicated in all but the most severe forms of psoriasis. This restriction is owing to the undesirable side effects that accompany systemic use of steroids as well as to the fact that, after therapy is stopped, the disease is almost certain to be worse than it was initially.[37] Intralesional injections of steroids have a limited use in treating isolated lesions and nail psoriasis.[29]

Other Agents

Detergents are not generally considered to be active ingredients in antidandruff products. However, for mild forms of dandruff, frequent and vigorous washing with a nonmedicated shampoo may help control excess scaling. Massaging the scalp produces a dispersion of scales into smaller, less visible subunits. Detergents may contribute to this effect by virtue of their surfactant activity. Detergents found in shampoos include sodium lauryl sulfate, polyoxyethylene ethers, triethanolamine, and quaternary ammonium compounds such as benzalkonium chloride, benzethonium chloride, and isoquinolinium bromides.[7]

Although ordinary vitamin D is of no known value in treating psoriasis, topical calcipotriene (a synthetic vitamin D_3 analog) is now available by prescription. This product is useful for treating localized lesions and can be combined with other forms of treatment.[44–46]

Product Selection Guidelines

Dandruff and Seborrheic Dermatitis

Guidelines for nonprescription therapy are as follows:

- If possible, the patient should shampoo daily at first and then at least every other day.
- If shampooing every other day does not control the condition, a medicated shampoo should be used.
- The patient should be instructed to wet the hair first and then lather a generous amount of medicated shampoo into the entire scalp, paying special attention to the hairline and other areas of activity, such as around the ears, nose, and eyebrows. The shampoo should be left on the scalp and skin for about 1 minute and then rinsed off. The process should then be repeated. It is important that the patient ensure adequate contact time.
- The patient should be reassured that dandruff and seborrhea are extensions of normal physiologic events and cautioned that total control using therapeutic agents may not always be achievable. If the patient has tried one medicated shampoo without success, the next alternative should be a product with a different mechanism of action.
- If the erythema or itching persists after a trial period with a medicated shampoo, a hydrocortisone lotion or gel may be added to the regimen. It should be applied sparingly once a day and worked into the scalp thoroughly. Improvement should be seen within the first week.
- Recalcitrant cases, cases involving large areas of the body, and cases in children under 2 years of age should be referred to a physician for evaluation.

Psoriasis

Psoriasis is not a trivial medical problem, and psoriatic patients should be under a physician's care. The pharmacist's role in the management of psoriasis is that of a knowledgeable consultant. When deciding which product to recommend for a psoriatic condition, the pharmacist must consider the area to which the agent is going to be applied. Response to topical medications shows striking anatomic regional variation.

Psoriasis of the Scalp Previous guidelines for nonprescription therapy with a medicated shampoo for dandruff and seborrhea are applicable to the treatment of scalp psoriasis with regard to tar- as well as salicylic acid–based products. Again, sufficient contact time is the key to successful therapy, the goal of which is the removal of scales. In addition, although 1% hydrocortisone products for scalp itching and erythema may be used, significant lesions or widespread involvement dictates that the patient be treated by a physician.

Psoriasis of the Body, Arms, and Legs Because dry skin often accompanies psoriasis, emollients are widely used in mild as well as severe psoriasis.

Salicylic acid products may be more cosmetically acceptable than coal tar products to some patients and may encourage compliance. Such products are most useful if thick scales are present. Soaking the affected area in warm water for 10–20 minutes before applying a salicylic acid product enhances drug activity.

Coal tar products may be applied to the body, arms, and legs at bedtime. Because coal tar stains most materials, the patient should be advised to use appropriate bed linen and clothing during applications. The overnight application is followed by a bath in the morning to remove residual coal tar and also to loosen psoriatic scales.

Topical hydrocortisone ointment may be applied sparingly to lesions and massaged into the skin thoroughly but gently.

Intertriginous Psoriasis Because intertriginous areas such as the armpits and genitoanal region are sensitive to irritants such as coal tar and salicylic acid, these agents should be used carefully, if at all, to treat psoriasis in these areas. Instead, hydrocortisone cream may be applied sparingly two or three times a day and should be used less often as improvement occurs.

Skin Infections

Cutaneous infections may be caused by bacteria, fungi, viruses, or parasites. Many bacterial and fungal infections are amenable to topical therapy. The condition should be carefully assessed before a treatment is selected or the patient counseled.

Specific Conditions

Bacterial Skin Infections

See Chapter 28, "First-Aid Products and Minor Wound Care," for a discussion of bacterial skin infections.

Fungal Skin Infections

Fungal skin infections, often called dermatomycoses, are among the most common cutaneous disorders.[47] Characteristically, they exhibit single or multiple lesions that may produce mild scaling or deep granulomas (inflamed, nodular-sized lesions). Infections are superficial, affecting the hair, nails, and skin, and are generally caused by three genera of fungi: *Trichophyton*, *Microsporum*, and *Epidermophyton*. Species of *Candida* may also be involved.[48]

Tinea Pedis Tinea pedis, also known as athlete's foot or ringworm of the feet, is caused by several species of fungi. (See Chapter 34, "Foot Care Products.")

Tinea Capitis Transmitted by direct contact with infected persons or animals, ringworm of the scalp is caused by species of *Microsporum* or *Trichophyton*. Most cases occur in children. Depending on the causative organism, the clinical presentation varies from noninflamed areas of hair loss to deep, crusted lesions that may lead to scarring and permanent hair loss. (See color plates, photograph 12.) These large lesions, similar to carbuncles in appearance, are called kerions.

Tinea Cruris Tinea cruris (also called jock itch) is caused by *Epidermophyton floccosum*, *Trichophyton rubrum*, or *Trichophyton mentagrophytes*. It occurs on the medial and upper parts of the thighs and the pubic area and is more common in males. The lesions have specific margins that are elevated slightly and are more inflamed than the central parts; small vesicles are found at the margins. Acute lesions are bright red, and chronic cases tend to be hyperpigmented; there is usually fine scaling present. This condition is generally bilateral with significant pruritus.

Tinea Corporis Species of *Trichophyton* or *Microsporum* cause ringworm of the skin. There is a higher incidence of tinea corporis among persons living in humid climates. The lesions, which involve glabrous (smooth and bare) skin, begin as small, circular, erythematous, scaly, pruritic areas. They spread peripherally, and the borders may contain vesicles or pustules. Tinea corporis should be differentiated from noninfectious dermatitis; the lesions may be similar in appearance.

Moniliasis (Candidiasis) Moniliasis or candidiasis, caused mainly by *Candida albicans*, usually occurs in intertriginous areas such as the groin, axilla, interdigital spaces, under the breasts, and at the corners of the mouth. Involvement of the mucous membranes may be known as thrush, vaginal candidiasis, balanitis, or pruritus ani, depending on the area affected. Lesions are either moist, red, and oozing or dry and scaly; they have sharp borders and are surrounded by satellite vesicles and/or pustules. Candidal paronychia is most common in people whose activities involve routine immersion of the hands in water. (See color plate, photograph 13.) Infection, malignancy, and systemic diseases such as diabetes may lower general resistance and allow candidal infections to flourish. Certain drugs, including oral antibiotics and steroids, may also contribute to candidal infection when used over prolonged periods of time.

Tinea Versicolor Tinea versicolor is a common superficial fungal infection of the stratum corneum caused by *Pityrosporum orbiculare*. This organism is part of the normal flora in most individuals but is capable of becoming pathogenic under certain conditions. The most distinctive clinical feature of this infection is the change in pigmentation at the affected sites, ranging from white to medium brown. The shade of the macular lesions depends on the pigmentation of the individual; lesions usually occur on seborrheic areas of the body in a confetti-like configuration. (See color plates, photographs 14A and B.) Because mild scaling and pruritus are the only other sequelae, tinea versicolor is generally considered a disease of cosmetic concern.

Viral Skin Infections

Viral infections may occur directly in or on the skin and commonly present as warts, molluscum contagiosum, herpes simplex,[49,50] or varicella-zoster infections (usually shingles [herpes zoster] in adults and varicella [chickenpox] in children).

Herpes Simplex Herpes simplex virus infection usually involves the skin and mucous membranes. The causative agent is a large virus, *Herpesvirus hominis*. (See color plates, photograph 15.) Two types of herpesvirus are involved: type 1 (HSV-1), which causes fever blisters (cold sores) and is most commonly found in the perioral area, and type 2 (HSV-2), which is most commonly seen as genital lesions. The virus is latent after the primary infection and may subsequently be triggered and reactivated by multiple factors, such as sunlight, menses, stress, fever, mechanical irritation, and systemic bacterial infection. Lesions are characterized by grouped vesicles that are clear, may become pustular, and then crust and heal within 7–10 days. There is often a painful, burning sensation associated with the lesions. Prior to the eruption, it is common to experience prodromal itching and tingling sensations at the site of the impending eruption.

Varicella-Zoster Infections *Herpes varicella* (chickenpox) is acute, highly contagious, and generalized, and it develops in the nonimmune host; shingles (caused by the same virus) is localized and painful, and it develops in the partially immune host. Not surprisingly, immunosuppressed patients are quite vulnerable to the varicella-zoster virus. It is spread by respiratory droplets and direct lesion contact, and it is most common during winter and spring seasons in children who are less than 10 years old.

Chickenpox acutely erupts on the trunk and face as red macules and rapidly progresses to papules, vesicles, pustules, and crust formation. In addition to skin, vesicles may also develop on mucous membranes, especially in the mouth. Severe pruritus may be present; fever and malaise are common.

Shingles probably results after reactivation of the latent virus, which resides in the dorsal root or cranial nerve ganglion cells. Patients with shingles usually have a past history of chickenpox. Unlike herpes simplex, neither shingles nor chickenpox is normally a recurrent disease. Lesions usually occur along a single dermatome; they appear acutely as grouped vesicles on an erythematous base following the course of the nerve(s) involved. The involved area may coalesce to form larger plaquelike lesions that may be very painful. (See color plates, photographs 16A and B.) Appearance of lesions may be preceded by itching, tenderness, and pain in the involved region. Symptoms may include malaise and burning or stinging sensations. Peripheral neuropathy (nerve pain), which may develop and persist over weeks or months, is treatable with the external analgesic agent capsaicin. (See Chapter 5, "External Analgesic Products.")

Molluscum Contagiosum Molluscum contagiosum is a viral tumor caused by a poxvirus containing DNA. The disease is contracted by direct contact with an infected person, by contact with a fomite, or by autoinoculation.

The virus is manifested by one or more small (3–5 mm), pink, slightly raised lesions that are usually found on the abdomen, inner thigh, or perianal area. The mature lesion has a slight depression on the top and a soft core that can be expressed. (See color plates, photograph 17.)

Assessment of Skin Infections

Before recommending a topical product for self-medication of cutaneous infections, the pharmacist should assess the nature of the patient's complaint. Noninfectious processes, including drug-induced eruptions, should be taken into account.[51] In cases of infectious etiology or of a possible secondary infection, antimicrobial agents should generally be considered.

Referral to a physician should be considered, especially if:

- There is doubt as to the causative factor or organism.
- Initial treatment has not been successful, or the condition is getting worse.
- Applications of topical drug products have been used for prolonged periods over large areas, especially on denuded skin (creating a potential for systemic toxicity).
- Exudate is excessive and continuous.
- Widespread infection has occurred.
- There is a predisposing illness, such as diabetes, systemic infection, or an immune deficiency.
- Fever, malaise, or both occur.
- A primary dermatitis (allergic dermatitis, psoriasis, or seborrhea) exists and becomes secondarily infected.
- Lesions are deep and extensive.
- Lancing is needed to aid drainage of exudate or provide pain relief.

Treatment of Skin Infections

Viral Cutaneous Infections

There are currently no nonprescription products specifically used as antiviral agents for cutaneous viral infections. Most of the products that are used are antiseptic products for relieving symptoms and preventing secondary bacterial infection. (See Chapter 28, "First-Aid Products and Minor Wound Care.")

Topical preparations that enhance vesicular drying may reduce discomfort. For chickenpox, tepid oatmeal or starch baths, topical calamine lotion, and oral antihistamines may relieve pruritus. Oral acetaminophen may be given for fever.

For shingles, treatment objectives are to relieve pain and minimize the risk of complications such as infection, scarring, nerve pain and damage, and eye involvement. Nonadherent dressings can be used to protect the lesional area from irritation. Soothing compresses may be used during the vesicular stages. Oral analgesics and occlusive dressings may help relieve pain; opioids may be necessary. Oral antihistamines may help relieve itching, and oral and topical antibiotics may be used for secondary infections. After resolution of the skin lesions, topical capsaicin, a neuropeptide-active compound capable of relieving peripheral neuropathic pain, may be used. Topical antibacterial and antifungal products are often used to treat as well as to prevent secondary infection. Topical antiseptic drug products are used to help prevent cutaneous infections.

Cutaneous Antifungal Agents

Topical anti-infectives are used to treat and prevent fungal infection of various tissues (skin, hair, nails, and mucous membranes). The active ingredients in most of these products are antifungal agents that either inhibit sterol synthesis or bind to sterols in the organism's cell membrane, causing cell leakage and eventually cell death. Because this product classification is so broad, the present focus is on products for use in the prevention and self-treatment of fungal skin infections (see product table "Topical Antifungal Products").

Clioquinol (3%), clotrimazole (1%), haloprogin (1%), miconazole nitrate (2%), povidone–iodine (10%), tolnaftate (1%), and various undecylenates (10–25%) are considered safe and effective by the FDA for nonprescription use.[52] However, in a proposed notice of rulemaking, effective February 26, 1993, the FDA determined that certain topical antifungals should not be generally recognized as safe and effective for nonprescription use (Table 6).[53] Similarly, in a final rule published December 18, 1992, the FDA established that "any over-the-counter (OTC) topical antifungal drug product for use in the treatment and/or prevention of diaper rash is not generally recognized as safe and effective and is misbranded."[54] This final rule became effective June 18, 1993.

Agents used for cutaneous fungal infections are found in ointments, creams, powders, and aerosols. Creams or solutions are the most efficient and effective antifungal product forms for delivery of the active agent into the epidermis. Sprays and powders are less effective because they are often not rubbed into the skin. They are probably more useful as adjuncts to a cream or solution or as prophylactic agents in preventing new or recurrent infections.

When a cream or solution is used to treat an active fungal infection, it is important that the patient clean the affected area first and then massage the product thoroughly into the entire affected area. In treating tinea pedis, for example, the patient must apply the product between all toes, to the skin around every toenail, and

TABLE 6 Nonprescription topical antifungal ingredients

Topical nonprescription antifungal drug products generally recognized as safe and effective	
Clioquinol	Providone iodine
Clotrimazole	Tolnaftate
Haloprogin	Undecylenates
Miconazole nitrate	

Topical nonprescription antifungal drug products not generally recognized as safe and effective[a]	
Alcloxa	Phenol
Alum, potassium	Phenolate sodium
Aluminum sulfate	Phenyl salicylate
Amyltricresols, secondary	Propionic acid
Basic fuchsin	Propylparaben
Benzethonium chloride	Resorcinol
Benzoic acid	Salicylic acid
Benzoxiquine	Sodium borate
Boric acid	Sodium caprylate
Camphor	Sodium propionate
Candicidin	Sulfur
Chlorothymol	Tannic acid
Coal tar	Thymol
Dichlorophen	Tolindate
Menthol	Triacetin
Methylparaben	Zinc caprylate
Oxyquinoline	Zinc propionate
Oxyquinoline sulfate	

[a]Effective February 26, 1993.

to the entire sole of the foot. Because the infection almost always includes both feet, the patient should treat both feet with identical thoroughness, even if erythema and scaling are predominant on one foot.

Chloroxylenol In 0.5–3.75% concentrations, chloroxylenol (parachlorometaxylenol) is classified as safe for use for up to 13 weeks for the treatment of athlete's foot, jock itch, or ringworm. However, additional safety data (for long-term, repeated use) and clinical efficacy data are needed before the FDA can place chloroxylenol in Category I.[52]

Undecylenic Acid Undecylenic acid has the greatest antifungal activity of the fatty acids. It is a fungistatic agent, requiring prolonged exposure at relatively high concentrations to be effective. It is used as a zinc, calcium, or copper salt in ointment, cream, powder, and aerosol forms (2–5% acid, 20% salt) for an additive antifungal effect.

Haloprogin Haloprogin products include haloprogin 1% cream and solution. Haloprogin is an effective alternative for the treatment of athlete's foot, jock itch, and ringworm. The compound has significant activity against several species of *Trichophyton* and *Microsporum* as well as *Candida albicans, Epidermophyton floccosum, Streptococcus pyogenes*, and *Staphylococcus aureus*.[55]

Haloprogin has been shown to be superior to placebo[56] and equal in effectiveness to tolnaftate.[56,57] One investigator found higher cure rates and fewer relapses with haloprogin than with tolnaftate when laboratory criteria (potassium hydroxide slide preparations and cultures) were used; however, clinical cure rates were equal.[58] Side effects of the topically applied drug, which are relatively rare and minor, include burning, itching, and scaling of the skin. Should these side effects occur, use of the preparation should be discontinued.

Miconazole and Clotrimazole Miconazole nitrate and clotrimazole are imidazole-structured topical antifungals originally approved for prescription use but now reclassified as nonprescription agents. They are active against fungi and some gram-positive bacteria but not against gram-negative bacteria.[59] Their broad spectrum includes a common dermatophyte, the organism causing tinea versicolor, and *C albicans*.

Treatment with miconazole and clotrimazole results in a low rate of recurrent infection when therapy is continued for 2 weeks or more, depending on the clinical disorder.[60,61] However, the onset of recurrence may simply be delayed in several cases. Allergic contact sensitization is rare, and other side effects are usually self-limiting on discontinuation of the preparation.

Selenium Sulfide Selenium sulfide is usually effective in the treatment of tinea versicolor. It is a potential irritant, and contact with the eyes and sensitive skin areas should be avoided. Although selenium sulfide is not absorbed in significant amounts when applied to the skin, it is hazardous if swallowed, producing central nervous system effects and respiratory and vasomotor depression. Areas affected by tinea versicolor should be lathered with the agent for 5 minutes only and washed off thoroughly. This treatment should be repeated daily for 2 weeks or until a response is noted; it should then be tapered to twice weekly and then once weekly according to response. Patients with recurrent tinea versicolor may use the product on a weekly basis indefinitely.

Tolnaftate Tolnaftate is a topical antifungal agent that is effective against most superficial dermatophytes but ineffective in the treatment of tinea versicolor and *C albicans*. Complete clearing of cutaneous lesions may take more than a month of therapy. The mechanism of action appears to be inhibition of fungal cell wall synthesis.[62] Topically, applied tolnaftate has a low incidence of toxicity; however, if local irritation occurs, treatment should be discontinued. (See Chapter 34, "Foot Care Products.")

Clioquinol Clioquinol, formerly called iodochlorhydroxyquin, has both antifungal and antibacterial properties. Its antibacterial properties have been used to treat cutaneous infections such as pyoderma, folliculitis, and impetigo; its antifungal properties have been used to treat mucocutaneous mycotic conditions such as athlete's foot, jock itch, ringworm, and moniliasis.[63] As an irritant and a known allergen, clioquinol may cause transient stinging or pruritus as well as allergic contact dermatitis. If these symptoms persist, discontinuation of the product is recommended. Several prescription product forms (lotion, cream, and ointment) contain a combination of clioquinol and hydrocortisone. The FDA requires the following special warning statements: "Do not use on children under 2 years of age" and "Do not use for diaper rash."[52]

Patient Counseling

For viral and fungal infections, regularly scheduled applications of medications throughout a complete course of therapy are important. Proper application technique should be described to the patient to prevent over- or undermedication. If irritation occurs, the patient should be instructed to contact a physician. In addition to information about nonprescription drug usage, the pharmacist may also provide information that will help control or eradicate the infection and minimize the likelihood of recurrent infections. Such information should address proper care of the infected skin site, appropriate laundry techniques and products, minimal use of occlusive clothing, and avoidance of habits or behavior that leads to recurring infections.

Moreover, the patient should be told the expected duration of therapy and the conditions that would indicate a need for physician-directed care (eg, the development of a secondary bacterial infection). In general, the patient should see substantial improvement in 1 week; if this does not occur, the patient should be referred to a physician. Recurring skin infections may be a sign of undiagnosed diabetes, immunodeficiency, or other organic problems and should be referred to a physician.

Skin Hyperpigmentation

Hyperpigmentation is usually a benign phenomenon but may occasionally represent a sign of systemic disease. As a facial disorder, it can be viewed by the patient as disfigurement and may lead to psychologic disorder. Thus, agents that can reduce pigment when applied topically are used widely around the world, especially where hyperpigmented skin is in noticeable contrast to surrounding normal skin color. Although these products serve a cosmetic function, it is important to emphasize that they are drugs and have potential toxicity and side effects.

Physiology of Skin Hyperpigmentation

Normal skin color is contributed by melanocytes in the basal layer of epidermis. Melanocytes produce melanosomes, which are pigment granules that contain a complex protein called melanin, a brown-black pigment. Melanocytes can be viewed as tiny one-celled glands with long projections to pass pigment particles into keratinocytes, which, in turn, synthesize keratin. As keratinocytes migrate upward, they carry pigment and deposit it on the skin surface. Melanocytes are also present in hair bulb cells, and they pass pigment granules on to the hair.

Melanin functions as an efficient sunscreen. It prevents damaging UV rays from entering deeper regions of the skin and minimizes the risk of sunburn and DNA damage. Solar radiation stimulates melanocytes to provide more melanin protection to minimize DNA damage, and this results in gradual skin darkening or a "tan." There is little variation in the number of melanocytes regardless of skin color, but people with heavily pigmented skin have more active cells.[64]

Etiology of Hyperpigmentation

Systemic as well as localized skin diseases may cause pigment cells to become overactive, resulting in a darkening of the skin, or to become underactive, with a resultant lightening of the skin. Endocrine imbalances caused by Addison's disease, Cushing's disease, hyperthyroidism, pregnancy, and estrogen therapy (including oral contraceptives) are capable of altering skin pigmentation. Metabolic alterations affecting the liver and certain nutritional deficiencies can be associated with diffuse melanosis.[65] Inflammatory dermatoses or physical trauma to the skin, such as from a thermal burn, may cause a postinflammatory hyperpigmentation that may last for a prolonged period of time. Also, certain drugs such as chlorpromazine and hydroxychloroquine have an affinity for melanin and may cause hyperpigmentation.

Freckles are spots of uneven skin pigmentation that first appear in childhood and are exacerbated by the sun. Melasma (also called chloasma) is a condition in which macular hyperpigmentation appears, usually on the face or neck. Melasma is often associated with pregnancy ("the mask of pregnancy") or the ingestion of oral contraceptives, and sun exposure also enhances its development. Lentigines, hyperpigmented spots that may appear at any age anywhere on the skin or mucous membranes, are caused by an increased deposition of melanin and an increased number of melanocytes. They are darker than freckles and not induced by UV radiation. However, solar or "senile" lentigines, also called age spots and commonly but incorrectly known as liver spots, appear on the exposed surfaces, especially in fair-skinned people, and are induced by UV radiation.

Assessment of Hyperpigmentation

Several types of hyperpigmentation, including freckles, melasma, and lentigines, are amenable to self-treatment.[66] However, the pharmacist must inquire about concurrent drug therapy and systemic illnesses before recommending a nonprescription product. Diffuse pigmentation disorders and those caused by systemic factors should not be self-treated without prior evaluation by a physician. Similarly, lesions that are changing in size, shape, or color should not be self-treated but should be referred promptly to a physician.

Treatment of Hyperpigmentation

Freckles, melasma, and lentigines may be diminished by topical nonprescription skin-bleaching agents. Such products are directed at inhibiting melanin production within the skin.[67] To avoid negating the effects of treatment, the pharmacist must emphasize to patients the importance of avoiding even minimal exposure to sunlight and of using sunscreen agents as well as protective clothing on an indefinite, ongoing basis, even after discontinuing the bleaching agent.

Systemic therapy is required for widespread pigmentation disorders. Physician-directed management of hyperpigmentation may include topical prescription agents composed of ingredients known to cause lightening of the skin, such as tretinoin (retinoic acid), hydroquinone, and a corticosteroid such as dexamethasone. This combination of ingredients may sometimes be effective for the treatment-resistant problem of postinflammatory hyperpigmentation. Monobenzone should not be used for hyperpigmentation because it produces irreversible loss of pigment in normal as well as hyperpigmented skin.

Pharmacologic Agents for Hyperpigmentation

Historically, a number of topical agents have been used in skin-bleaching preparations.[68] These agents have included hydroquinone, the monobenzyl and monomethyl ethers of hydroquinone, ammoniated mercury, ascorbic acid, and peroxides (see product table "Hyperpigmentation Products"). However, only preparations containing hydroquinone were submitted to the FDA Advisory Review Panel on Over-the-Counter Miscellaneous External Drug Products.[65]

Hydroquinone The FDA has recommended that only hydroquinone (*p*-dihydroxybenzene) in concentrations of 1.5–2.0% be available for nonprescription use.[66] Hydroquinone produces reversible hypopigmentation of the skin and hair of mice, guinea pigs, and humans by a complex mechanism of action. Hydroquinone and its derivatives are oxidized by tyrosinase to form highly toxic free radicals that cause selective damage to the lipoprotein membranes of the melanocyte, thereby reducing conversion of tyrosine to dopa and subsequently to melanin.[69]

Several studies demonstrate that topical preparations of 2–5% hydroquinone are effective in producing cutaneous hypopigmentation.[65] The 2% concentration is safer and has produced results equivalent to those of higher concentrations. Side effects are mild when topical hydroquinone is used in low concentrations. Tingling or burning on application and subsequent erythema and inflammation were observed in 8% of patients using a 2% concentration and in 32% of patients using a 5% concentration.[70] Higher concentrations frequently irritate the skin and, if used for prolonged periods, may cause side effects including epidermal thickening, pitch-black pigmentation, and colloid milium (yellowish papules associated with colloid degeneration).[65,71]

The effectiveness of hydroquinone varies among patients, and treatment must usually be maintained faithfully on a prolonged basis to maintain the desired level of lightening once it has been achieved. Results are best on lighter skin and lighter lesions. In African Americans, the response to hydroquinone depends on the amount of pigment present. Additionally, the earlier that hydroquinone is used to treat hyperpigmentation, the more likely that results will be satisfactory. When hypopigmentation does occur after treatment with hydroquinone, melanin production is generally reduced by about 50%.[65] Hyperpigmented areas fade more rapidly and completely than surrounding normal skin. Although treatment may not lead to complete disappearance of hypermelanosis, the results are often satisfactory enough to reduce self-consciousness. A disadvantage of treatment with hydroquinone is that it tends to overshoot the intended degree of hypopigmentation and may produce treated areas that are lighter than the surrounding normal skin color. Therefore, the patient must carefully observe the degree of lightening as the treatment progresses and must subsequently decrease applications when sufficient lightening has occurred.

When treatment is begun, melanin production may actually increase briefly. A decrease in skin color usually becomes noticeable in about 4 weeks; however, the time of onset varies from 3 weeks to 3 months. Hypopigmentation lasts for 2–6 months but is reversible. Darker lesions repigment faster than lighter lesions. Although sunscreens may help, even visible light may cause some darkening, and sun protection should preferably be opaque.[72] Some hydroquinone products are available in an opaque base (Eldopaque) or together with a sunscreen (Selaquin).

In some cases, lesions become slightly darker before fading. A transient inflammatory reaction may develop after the first few weeks of treatment. Occurrence of inflammation makes subsequent lightening more likely although inflammation can occur without the development of hypopigmentation. The appearance of mild inflammation need not be considered an indication to stop therapy except in the patient whose reaction increases in intensity. In such situations, sensitization should be considered. Topical hydrocortisone may be used temporarily to alleviate the inflammatory reaction. Contact with the eyes should be avoided. A patch test can be done to test for allergy to hydroquinone; however, a majority of reactions are irritant rather than allergic in nature.

If hydroquinone is accidentally ingested, it seldom produces serious systemic toxicity. However, oral ingestion of 5–15 g has produced tremor, convulsions, and hemolytic anemia.[73]

Reversible brown discoloration of nails has been reported occasionally following the application of 2% hydroquinone to the back of the hand.[74] Discoloration is probably caused by formation of oxidation products of hydroquinone. Hydroquinone is readily oxidized in the presence of light and air. Discoloration or darkening of the cream is an indication of product deterioration and a possible decline in the strength of available hydroquinone.[65] Thus, the preferable method of packaging is in small squeeze tubes.

Hydroquinone is dosed as a thin topical application of a 2% concentration rubbed gently but well into affected areas twice daily. If no improvement is seen within 3 months, its use should be discontinued and the advice of a physician sought.[66] Once the desired benefit is achieved, hydroquinone can be applied as often as needed in a once- or twice-daily regimen to maintain lightening of the skin. Because of the lack of safety data, hydroquinone is not recommended for children under age 12 except under the supervision of a physician.

Hydroquinone Adjuvants and Combinations

Because hydroquinone is oxidized by contact with air, antioxidants such as sodium bisulfite may be added to the formulation. Hydroquinone is incompatible with alkali or ferric salts.[72] Iodochlorhydroxyquin or oxyquinolone sulfate may be added as antimicrobial preservatives.[65] The inclusion of a sunscreen agent is rational and appropriate, provided that combination products are advertised not primarily as sunscreens but as skin-bleaching agents with added sunscreen.

Monobenzone

Monobenzone, the monobenzyl ether of hydroquinone, is restricted to prescription-only use. Its action and onset time are similar to that of hydroquinone except that a complete and permanent depigmentation may occur. Its use is restricted to depigmenting remaining areas of normally pigmented skin in patients with extensive vitiligo (a condition resulting in patches of depigmentation, often with hyperpigmented borders).

Ammoniated Mercury

Ammoniated mercury was in common use as a skin-bleaching agent decades ago. However, chronic application of ammoniated mercury can cause systemic mercury poisoning, sensitization is relatively common, and efficacy data are lacking. Therefore, ammoniated mercury is not approved by the FDA for nonprescription use as a skin-bleaching agent.[75]

Product Selection Guidelines

Before selecting a nonprescription skin-bleaching product, the pharmacist should be sure that a physician has confirmed the patient's need for it. These products are intended to lighten only limited areas of hyperpigmented skin and should be used only in areas of brownish discoloration; nevi (moles) and reddish or bluish areas, such as port wine discolorations, are not amenable to skin-bleaching treatment. In addition, these products should not be used on areas that are independently changing in size, shape, or color. If the product is effective, results should be noticeable within 2 weeks to 3 months. Hydroquinone may be applied to a small area of unbroken skin and should be assessed at 24 hours to observe for irritation or allergic reactions. It should not be applied near the eyes or to damaged or sunburned skin.

Hair Loss (Alopecia)

Hereditary hair loss (androgenetic alopecia) is the most common form of hair loss, affecting about one third of the US male population and about one sixth of the female population. US consumers spend hundreds of millions of dollars each year on proven and unproven methods of treating hair loss.

Physiology of Hair Growth

A strand of hair is a cylinder of tightly keratinized cells that grows at the base of the follicle[76] (Figure 1). The hair follicle, which anchors the hair strand to the skin, contains cells that produce new hairs. These germinative cells, located at the base of the follicle next to the dermal papilla, make up the follicular matrix; the matrix cells eventually keratinize to form hair.

Hair follicle activity is cyclic. In the growing phase (anagen), the follicle lengthens, the dermal papilla grows in size, and a new hair is formed. During the catagen phase—a transition phase between the growing and resting phases—cell proliferation ceases, the hair follicle shortens, and a bulbous enlargement forms at the base of the hair. The resting phase (telogen) is demonstrated as this shortened follicle, which contains a mature hair with an unpigmented, club-shaped root. Telogen, or terminal, hairs are very loosely held in place. Duration of the anagen phase in any individual normal scalp follicle is genetically determined and ranges from 2 to 5 years with an average duration of 1,000 days.[77] The average duration of the telogen phase, however, is 100 days, resulting in a ratio of anagen to telogen hairs of 9:1. Typically, up to 100 hairs are lost from the scalp each day as telogen hairs are shed.

The average rate of human scalp hair growth is estimated to be 0.37 mm per day. The type of hair growth depends on follicle location and the person's age and gender. Vellus hair is soft, fine, usually unpigmented, and less than 2 cm long (eg, abdominal hair), whereas terminal hair is coarse, of greater length, and pigmented (eg, scalp hair). The human scalp contains approximately 100,000 hair follicles.[78] Blonds apparently have greater than the usual number of follicles, and redheads, fewer. By the third decade, density of hair follicles usually decreases to half of that found in a newborn.[78]

Etiology and Characteristics of Hair Loss

In hereditary hair loss, the follicle becomes gradually smaller, the anagen phase becomes shorter, and increased shedding of telogen hairs occurs. As telogen hairs are shed, they are gradually replaced by vellus-like hairs.[79] The rate of progression and the pattern of hair loss appear to be genetically determined. In women, hereditary hair thinning is usually located on the top center of the scalp. Male-pattern hair loss and/or gradual hair thinning usually occurs at the top rear of the head (vertex).

Nonhereditary hair loss can occur following a pregnancy or be induced by certain drugs or severe nutritional deficiencies. Iatrogenic causes of hair loss include chemotherapy and discontinuation of hormonal agents. Other pathophysiologic causes include autoimmune disorders, endocrine disorders such as hypothyroidism, and certain diseases that cause scarring of the scalp. Hair care products and hair grooming methods that cause scarring or burns on the scalp have also been known to induce hair loss.

Treatment of Hair Loss

Topical minoxidil 2%, as a hydroalcoholic solution, is the only nonprescription agent currently approved by the FDA for use in regrowth of hair. The agency is also currently reviewing data on a higher concentration of this agent; if approved, the higher potency product would be available only by prescription. Only hereditary hair loss in men and women is amenable to topical minoxidil treatment; this agent is not indicated for use in children.

The nonprescription formulation marketed by Pharmacia & Upjohn, Inc, is packaged separately for use in men (blue package with short applicator) and women (salmon package with long applicator). Barre-National, Inc, Bausch & Lomb Pharmaceutical Division, and Lemmon Company each market a generic nonprescription minoxidil product. These products are labled for the treatment of male pattern baldness (see product table "Hair Regrowth Products").

Possible mechanisms of action for topical minoxidil have been investigated. In studies of male pattern baldness, hypertrophy of preexisting hair follicles at treatment sites was noted after 12 weeks of treatment with a higher concentration of topical minoxidil than is currently marketed.[80] Additionally, in vitro studies have shown that this agent has direct stimulatory effects on epidermal cells: an increased synthesis of epidermal cells was reported.[81] It appears that minoxidil directly stimulates folliclular hypertrophy and prolongs the anagen phase. In another study using a higher than marketed concentration, an increase in mean hair shaft diameter could be attributed to minoxidil.[82] After up to 12 months of therapy, a reduction in the percentage of telogen hairs was also noted in a subset of these same patients.

The therapeutic effect of minoxidil was also studied in one type of macaque monkey that exhibits baldness similar to that seen in humans with hereditary hair loss.[83] In early anagen phases, topical minoxidil induced accelerated cyclic turnover of vellus follicles and simultaneous enlargement of regrowing follicles. "Transformed vellus follicles" in the bald scalp were able to recover their ability to produce thick hair. The macques with more recent onset of hair loss experienced more dramatic results than did those with long-standing hair loss.

Earlier studies of hypertrichosis reported an association between localized hair growth and local increases in cutaneous blood flow.[84–86] In a study of minoxidil's effect on blood circulation, cutaneous blood flow to the scalp was measured by laser doppler velocimetry and photopulse plethysmography before and after application of the agent in concentrations of 0%, 1%, 3%, and 5%.[87] Both measurement techniques indicated that the 5% solution stimulated microcirculation of the scalp. In addition, laser doppler velocimetry suggested that the 1% and 3% solutions increased blood flow in a dose-related fashion.

In men, minoxidil is more likely to be effective when less than one fourth of the scalp surface has already experienced hair loss or thinning. Even with continued treatment, all of the hair usually does not grow back; however, progressive loss of hair is usually slowed.

Study data for males 18–49 years of age indicate that about one fourth of the patients experienced moderate or better hair regrowth after using topical minoxidil. One third of the patients, however, attained only minimal hair regrowth. Minimal regrowth means some new hairs are visible but not enough to cover thinning areas; further, the hair density (ie, how closely the hairs grow) in treated areas will be less than that in the untreated part of the head where significant hair loss has not occurred. With moderate regrowth, hairs may cover some or all of the thinning area and may grow more closely together; however, the hair density in the treated area will again be less than that on the rest of the head. A minority of the patients had dense regrowth, which, by definition, covers or almost completely covers thinning areas. In this case, hair density is equal to that of the untreated part of the head. The placebo vehicle also showed a modest response: about one tenth of the patients had moderate or better regrowth, and about one third had minimal regrowth.

In women, topical minoxidil is more effective if less than about one third of the scalp is thinning. Study data for women 18–45 years of age indicate that about one fifth of the women experienced moderate regrowth after using topical minoxidil, whereas more than one third experienced only minimal regrowth. In comparison, the placebo vehicle showed a 7% response rate for moderate regrowth and a 33% rate for minimal regrowth.

The most common side effect associated with this agent, local itching at the site of application (about 7% of patients), may be related to the hydroalcoholic vehicle. Although a measurable amount of minoxidil is absorbed through the skin, systemic side effects are rare. Scalp psoriasis, severe sunburn, or scalp abrasions, however, may increase absorption of minoxidil. Further, additional precaution should be taken if corticosteroids or any agents known to increase cutaneous absorption of a drug are used concurrently with this product.

A potential effect of minoxidil on systemic endocrine function has been sought but not found. Measurement of plasma testosterone and excretion of urinary hydroxysteroids and ketosteroids in hypertensive patients treated with oral minoxidil did not reveal any effects of the therapy.[77] Further, serum cortisol, testosterone, and thyroid indices are apparently unchanged by topical minoxidil.[88] However, unstable cardiac patients should not use the product unless supervised by a physician.

Patient Counseling

Patients should be advised that most treatment regimens for hair loss do not alter its progression, especially if the hair loss has gone on for some time. Some patients might instead be interested in transplantation of hair. This process, which involves surgical transplantation of multiple, small, full-thickness grafts from normal areas of hair growth to bald areas, has been successful in selected cases.[89] Quality-made hair pieces are also an option for some patients.

The pharmacist should inform patients who wish to use nonprescription minoxidil that the longer the hair thinning or loss has gone on, the less likely it is that treatment will elicit a regrowth response. Beginning treatment early after the onset of thinning optimizes the therapeutic response and thus stops the progression of hair loss. Early treatment, therefore, is virtually as important as the therapeutic endpoint of hair regrowth. The pharmacist should also emphasize that treatment must be continuous and indefinite to maintain regrowth. If treatment is interrupted, regrowth will typically be lost within 4 months or less, and progression of hair loss will begin again.

Patients should be advised to apply 1 mL of the solution to the scalp twice daily, being careful not to allow the solution to come in contact with the eyes or mucous membranes.[90] Such contact might result in burning or itching of these areas. Local itching at the site of application is also the most common side effect associated with minoxidil. After application of the solution, the scalp should be kept dry for 4 hours. If the scalp becomes wet within this 4-hour period, (ie, from swimming, exercise, or rain), the patient should reapply the medication to a dry scalp. Hair grooming and styling products (eg, sprays, mousses, and gels) or permanents, coloring agents, or relaxing agents usually do not affect the efficacy of topical minoxidil.[90] These products can be applied after the medication has dried.

The pharmacist should advise patients that it usually takes up to 12 months to assess whether an optimal response is being achieved. Patients should be cautioned that overuse (more than twice daily applications) will not achieve better regrowth or a more rapid response. They should also be cautioned to keep product containers out of the reach of children because acute ingestion of minoxidil is hazardous.

Case Studies

Case 26–1

Patient Complaint/History

PL, a 28-year-old female, presents to the pharmacist with a complaint of dry, scaly elbows; she requests recommendations for treatment of the condition. She reveals that she has used various nonprescription topical hydrocortisone ointments with some success; however, soon after she stops using the medication, the condition reappears. The patient says that the condition, which started about 2–3 years ago, improves in hot weather and worsens during cold weather or stressful periods in her life.

PL's current lesions are raised, circular, well-circumscribed, silver-scaled plaques, which are approximately 5 cm in diameter. If the scales are rubbed off, the exposed area appears red and sometimes bleeds very slightly; itching is also present. Years ago, the patient's mother was diagnosed as having psoriasis that supposedly cleared spontaneously.

Clinical Considerations/Strategies

The following considerations/strategies are provided to aid the reader in (1) determining whether treatment of the patient's condition with nonprescription medications is warranted, (2) selecting the appropriate nonprescription medication, and (3) developing a patient counseling strategy to ensure optimal therapeutic outcomes:

- Assess the patient's condition.
- Based on your assessment and the patient's complaints, decide if referral to a physician or dermatologist is warranted.
- Given that the patient prefers to self-medicate, decide what information, other than that obtained from the patient's history and physical observations, is needed before recommending therapy.
- Determine what type of therapy to recommend.
- Based on the therapy recommendations, determine the following:
  - What inconveniences, if any, the patient might encounter and what advice the patient should receive to deal with the inconveniences;
  - The therapeutic goals and the appropriate counseling to provide the patient about these goals;
  - What potential adverse effects, if any, might occur.
- Identify resources available to the patient that provide additional information about her condition.

Case 26–2

Patient Complaint/History

SP, a 20-year-old healthy male who presents to the pharmacist with a complaint of irritated hands, requests assistance in choosing a product to treat the condition. The patient, a college student, is working this summer as a construction laborer; his main tasks are mixing and transporting brick mortar. He does not wear gloves while working. After performing these tasks for the past 3–4 weeks, he noticed his hands had become progressively irritated.

Physical observation reveals that the patient's hands appear dry with minimal fissuring at the flexures; no vesicles, weeping, or infection is apparent; the forearms are uninvolved. SP says that his hands itch periodically and feel tight, as though the skin would crack with any movement.

Clinical Considerations/Strategies

The following considerations/strategies are provided to aid the reader in (1) determining whether treatment of the patient's condition with nonprescription medications is warranted, (2) selecting the appropriate nonprescription medication, and (3) developing a patient counseling strategy to ensure optimal therapeutic outcomes:

- Determine what additional information is needed from the patient before therapy can be recommended.
- Determine what nondrug measures may be helpful.
- Recommend a nonprescription product to relieve the dryness and itching.
- Develop a patient education/counseling plan that will:
  - Explain the therapeutic goals for the recommended product;
  - Explain the adverse effects, if any, of the recommended therapy.

Summary

Many patients are afflicted with dermatitis, dry skin, dandruff, seborrhea, and psoriasis. It is important that these patients be assessed before self-treatment is undertaken. Therapy effective for one disorder may exacerbate another. The pharmacist performs a valuable service by educating patients about the clinical disorder and choosing the most effective nonprescription therapy, or by providing an appropriate physician referral.

Superficial fungal infections of the skin are very common and are responsive to nonprescription therapy. Pharmacist-provided patient education and advice is of great value to this patient population. Unfortunately, direct-acting pharmacologic agents are unavailable for nonprescription therapy of cutaneous viral infections; however, symptomatic treatment is available for nonprescription therapy and requires pharmacist advice and consultation.

Although hyperpigmentation disorders are not as common as some other dermatologic disorders, patients may be significantly affected psychologically by what is perceived as a cosmetic disfigurement. Fortunately, most of these hyperpigmented disorders are amenable to nonprescription therapy, and pharmacist-provided education is essential to treatment success.

References

1. Odland GF. Structure of the skin in physiology. In: Goldsmith LA, ed. *Physiology, Biochemistry, and Molecular Biology of the Skin*. New York: Oxford University Press; 1991: 3–62.
2. Ricciatti-Sibbald DJ. Dermatitis. In: Clark C, ed. *Self-Medication: A Reference for Health Professionals*. 3rd ed. Ottawa: Canadian Pharmaceutical Association; 1988: 67–85.
3. Jellinek JS. *Formulation and Function of Cosmetics*. 2nd ed. New York: John Wiley; 1970: 4–14.
4. Guy RH, Hadgraft J. In: Bronaugh RL, Maibach HI, eds. *Percutaneous Absorption*. 2nd ed. New York: Marcel Dekker; 1989: 13–26.
5. Roth RR, James WD. *J Am Acad Dermatol*. 1989; 20: 367–90.
6. Cascella PJ, Powers JE. *US Pharm*. 1988; 13(12): 26.
7. Robinson JR. Dermatitis, dry skin, dandruff, seborrheic dermatitis, and psoriasis products. In: *Handbook of Nonprescription Drugs*. 9th ed. Washington, DC: American Pharmaceutical Association; 1990: 811–40.
8. Lung DYM et al. In: Fitzpatrick TB et al, eds. *Dermatology in General Medicine*. 4th ed. New York: McGraw-Hill; 1993: 1543–64.
9. Campion RH, Parish WE. In: Campion RH, Burton JL, Ebling FJG, eds. *Textbook of Dermatology*. 5th ed. Oxford, England: Blackwell Scientific Publications; 1992: 589–610.
10. Pearce M. Atopic dermatitis. *Pharm Times*. 1990 May: 88–92.
11. David TJ, Devlin J, Ewing CI. Atopic and seborrheic dermatitis: practical management. *Pediatrician*. 1991; 18: 211–7.
12. Wilkinson JD, Rycroft RJG. In: Campion RH, Burton JL, Ebling FJG, eds. *Textbook of Dermatology*. 5th ed. Oxford, England: Blackwell Scientific Publications; 1992: 611–42.
13. Belsito D. In: Fitzpatrick TB et al, eds. *Dermatology in General Medicine*. 4th ed. New York: McGraw-Hill; 1993: 1531–42.
14. Keefner KR, DeSimone EM. Contact dermatitis: skin reactions to irritants. *US Pharm*. 1991 Jun; 16 (skin care suppl): 36–9.
15. Wahlberg JE. Patch testing. In: Rycroft RJG, Menne T, Frosch PJ, eds. *Textbook of Contact Dermatitis*. 2nd ed. Berlin: Springer-Verlag; 1995: 241–68.
16. Angelini G. Topical drugs. In: Rycroft RJG, Menne T, Frosch PJ, eds. *Textbook of Contact Dermatitis*. 2nd ed. Berlin: Springer-Verlag; 1995: 477–503.
17. Gossel TA. Therapeutic relief of contact dermatitis. *US Pharm*. 1990 May; 15: 12–6.
18. Fisher AA. Allergic contact dermatitis associated with OTC topical anesthetics and antihistamines. *Pharm Times*. 1991 May; 57: 65–8.
19. Burton JL. In: Campion RH, Burton JL, Ebling FJG, eds. *Textbook of Dermatology*. 5th ed. Oxford, England: Blackwell Scientific Publications; 1992: 537–88.
20. Fitzpatrick JE. Common inflammatory skin diseases of the elderly. *Geriatrics*. 1989 Jul; 44: 40–6.
21. Shwayder T, Ott F. All about ichthyosis. *Pediatr Clin North Am*. 1991 Aug; 38: 835–57.
22. Gossel TA. Dry skin. *US Pharm*. 1990 Jan; 15: 20–4.
23. Lazar AP, Lazar P. Dry skin, water, and lubrication. *Dermatol Clin*. 1991 Jan; 9: 45–51.
24. DP Hamacher. Facial moisturizers. *NARD*. 1991 Aug; 113: 63.
25. Jackson EM. AHA-type products proliferate in 1993. *Cosmet Dermatol*. 1993; 6: 22–4.
26. *Federal Register*. 1982; 47: 39444–8.
27. *Federal Register*. 1979; 44: 69768–866.
28. *Federal Register*. 1991; 56: 43025–6.
29. Wright DE. Psoriasis, seborrheic dermatitis and dandruff. In: Clark C, ed. *Self-Medication: A Reference for Health Professionals*. 3rd ed. Ottawa: Canadian Pharmaceutical Association; 1988: 87–98.
30. Dolnick E. A flaky concern. *Hippocrates*. 1989 Jan–Feb; 3: 28–30.
31. Cauwenbergh G et al. Treatment of dandruff with a 2% ketoconazole scalp gel: a double-blind placebo-controlled study. *Int J Dermatol*. 1986 Oct; 25: 541.
32. Gossel TA, Slattery CD. Self-treatment of seborrhea. *US Pharm*. 1991 Mar; 16: 24–34.
33. Plewig G. In: Fitzpatrick TB et al, eds. *Dermatology in General Medicine*. 4th ed. New York: McGraw-Hill; 1993: 1569–74.
34. *Federal Register*. 1982; 47: 54646–84.
35. Christophers E, Sterry W. In: Fitzpatrick TB et al, eds. *Dermatology in General Medicine*. 4th ed. New York: McGraw-Hill; 1993: 489–514.
36. Winchester R. In: Fitzpatrick TB et al, eds. *Dermatology in General Medicine*. 4th ed. New York: McGraw-Hill; 1993: 515–27.
37. Pray WS. Psoriasis: it can be dangerous. *US Pharm*. 1991 Jun; 16 (skin care suppl): 28–34.
38. *Federal Register*. 1991; 56: 63554–69.
39. *AHFS 95 Drug Information*. Bethesda, Md: American Society of Health System Pharmacists; 1995: 2436–7.
40. *AHFS 95 Drug Information*. Bethesda, Md: American Society of Health System Pharmacists; 1995: 2469–72.
41. *AHFS 95 Drug Information*. Bethesda, Md: American Society of Health System Pharmacists; 1995: 2466–8.
42. Vonderweidt J. Sorting out topical corticosteroids. *US Pharm*. 1988 Jul; 13: 54–65.
43. Trozak DJ. Topical corticosteroid therapy in psoriasis vulgaris. *Cutis*. 1990 Oct; 46: 341–50.
44. Araujo OE, Flowers FP, Brown K. Vitamin D therapy in psoriasis. *DICP Ann Pharmacother*. 1991 Jul–Aug; 25: 835–9.
45. McQueen KD. Is vitamin D effective in treating psoriasis? *DICP Ann Pharmacother*. 1991 Jul–Aug; 25: 753–4.
46. *AHFS 95 Drug Information*. Bethesda, Md: American Society of Health System Pharmacists; 1995: 2473.
47. Hay RJ, Roberts SOB, MacKenzie DWR. In: Campion RH, Burton JL, Ebling FJG, eds. *Textbook of Dermatology*. 5th ed. Oxford, England: Blackwell Scientific Publications; 1992: 1127–216.
48. Martin AG, Kobayashi GS. In: Fitzpatrick TB et al, eds. *Dermatology in General Medicine*. 4th ed. New York: McGraw-Hill; 1993: 2437–9.
49. Stone MS, Lynch PJ. In: Sams WM Jr, Lynch PJ, eds. *Principles and Practice of Dermatology*. New York: Churchill Livingstone; 1990: 119–27.
50. Elliott GW, Sams WM Jr. In: Sams WM Jr, Lynch PJ, eds. *Principles and Practice of Dermatology*. New York: Churchill Livingstone; 1990: 99–112.
51. Bruinsma W, ed. *A Guide to Drug Eruptions*. 6th ed. Amsterdam: Free University Press; 1995.
52. *Federal Register*. 1989; 54: 51136.
53. *Federal Register*. 1992; 57: 38568.

54. *Federal Register.* 1992; 57: 60429–31.
55. McEvoy GK, ed. *1995 AHFS Drug Information.* Bethesda, Md: American Society of Health-System Pharmacists; 1995: 2403.
56. Hermann HW. *Arch Dermatol.* 1972; 106: 839.
57. Katz R, Cahn B. *Arch Dermatol.* 1972; 106: 837.
58. Carter VH. *Curr Ther Res.* 1972; 14: 307.
59. Hildrick-Smith G. *Adv Biol Skin.* 1972; 12: 303.
60. Mandy SJ, Garrott TC. *JAMA.* 1974; 230: 72.
61. Fulton JE Jr. *Arch Dermatol.* 1975; 111: 596.
62. Barrett-Bee KJ et al. *J Med Vet Mycol.* 1986; 24:155–60.
63. Harvey SC. In: Gennaro AR, ed. *Remington's Pharmaceutical Sciences.* 18th ed. Easton, Pa: Mack Publishing; 1990: 1236.
64. Grimes PE, Davis LT. Cosmetics in Blacks. *Dermatol Clin.* 1991; 9: 53–68.
65. *Federal Register.* 1978; 43: 51546–55.
66. *Federal Register.* 1982; 47: 39108–17.
67. Engasser PG, Maibach HI. Cosmetics and dermatology: bleaching creams. *J Am Acad Dermatol.* 1981; 5: 143–7.
68. Bleehan SS, Ebling FJG, Campion RH. In: Campion RH, Burton JL, Ebling FJG, eds. *Textbook of Dermatology.* 5th ed. Oxford, England: Blackwell Scientific Publications; 1992: 1561–622.
69. Jimbow K et al. Mechanism of depigmentation by hydroquinone. *J Invest Dermatol.* 1974; 62: 436–49.
70. Arndt KA, Fitzpatrick TB. Topical use of hydroquinone as a depigmenting agent. *JAMA.* 1965; 194: 965–7.
71. Hoshaw RA, Zimmerman KG, Menter A. Ochronosis-like pigmentation from hydroquinone bleaching creams in American Blacks. *Arch Dermatol.* 1985; 121: 105–8.
72. Arndt KA. In: *Manual of Dermatologic Therapeutics.* 5th ed. Boston: Little, Brown; 1995: 105–11.
73. *AHFS 95 Drug Information.* Bethesda, Md: American Society of Health System Pharmacists; 1995: 2489–90.
74. Mann RJ, Harman RM. Nail staining due to hydroquinone skin lightening creams. *Br J Dermatol.* 1983; 108: 363–5.
75. *Federal Register.* 1990; 55: 46914–21.
76. Ebling FJ. Biology of hair follicles. In: Fitzpatrick TB, Eisen AZ, Wolff K et al. *Dermatology in General Medicine.* New York: McGraw-Hill Book Company; 1987: 213–9.
77. Earhart RN, Ball 1, Nuss DD et al. Minoxidil-induced hypertrichosis: treatment with calcium thioglycolate depilatory. *South Med J.* 1977; 70: 442–3.
78. Rook A, Dawber R. Diseases of the hair and scalp. Oxford: Blackwell Scientific Publications; 1982: 9–17.
79. Rook A, Dawber R. Diseases of the hair and scalp. Oxford: Blackwell Scientific Publications; 1982: 90–112.
80. Headington JT, Novak E. Clinical and histological studies of male pattern baldness treated with topical minoxidil. *Curr Ther Res.* 1984; 36: 1098–106.
81. Cohen RL, Alves MEAF, Weiss VC et al. Direct effects of minoxidil on epidermal cells in culture. *J Invest Dermatol.* 1984; 82: 90–3.
82. Abell E, Cary MM. The pathogenic effect of minoxidil in male pattern alopecia. *J Invest Dermatol.* 1986; 86: 459.
83. Uno H, Cappas A, Schlagel C. Cyclic dynamics of hair follicles and the effect of minoxidil on the bald scalps of stumptailed macaques. *Am J Dermatopathol.* 1985; 7: 283–97.
84. Burton JL, Schutt WH, Caldwell IW. Hypertrichosis due to diazoxide. *Br J Dermatol.* 1975; 93: 707–11.
85. Ressmann AC, Butterworth T. Localized acquired hypertrichosis. *AMA Arch Dermatol.* 1952; 65: 458–63.
86. Ebling FJ, Rook A. Hair. In: Rook A, Wilkinson DS. Textbook of dermatology. Oxford: Blackwell Scientific Publications; 1979: 1733–824.
87. Wester RC, Maibach Hl, Guv RH et al. Minoxidil stimulates cutaneous blood flow in human balding scalps: pharmacodynamics measured by laser doppler velocimetry and photopulse plethysmography. *J Invest Dermatol.* 1984; 82: 515–7.
88. Weiss VC, West D, Fu TS et al. Alopecia areata treated with topical minoxidil. *Arch Dermatol.* 1984; 120: 457–63.
89. Roenigk HH. Combined surgical treatment of male pattern alopecia. *Cutis.* 1985; 35: 570–7.
90. Rogaine product information. Kalamazoo, Mich: Pharmacia & Upjohn, Inc; 1996.

CHAPTER 27

Acne Products

Joye Ann Billow

Questions to ask in patient assessment and counseling

- *How old are you?*
- *How long have you had acne?*
- *Is the acne a problem on areas other than your face (eg, neck, shoulders, chest, or back)?*
- *Have you consulted a physician about your acne? If so, what treatment was suggested? Are you currently following it?*
- *Are you currently using any medications, either prescription or nonprescription? If so, what are they?*
- *Have you already tried acne treatments? If so, which ones? How did you use them? For how long did you use them? How effective were they?*
- *Do you prefer one type of acne treatment product (eg, lotion, cream, gel, or soap) over another?*
- *What type of cosmetics, including makeup, aftershave, or hair preparations, do you use? Do they seem to aggravate the acne?*
- *How often do you wash your face? How (eg, with pads or washcloths) do you wash? What type of soap do you use?*
- *How often do you shampoo your hair? What type of shampoo do you use?*
- *Do you notice a seasonal change in the number or severity of acne lesions?*
- *Are you routinely exposed to environmental conditions such as heat or humidity or cooking oils in the air?*

Acne vulgaris, the most common adolescent skin disorder, is often linked to the onset of puberty. Involving the oil glands and hair follicles of the skin, primarily on the face and trunk, the disease is characterized by whiteheads, blackheads, acne pimples, and acne blemishes (Table 1).[1] Whiteheads and blackheads are noninflammatory lesions also known as closed and open comedones. The inflammatory lesions are composed of papules, pustules, and nodules. Nodules with necrotic, purulent contents, which were previously misnamed cysts, may lead to pitting and scarring if left untreated.

The incidence of acne is nearly universal; approximately 85% of all people between the ages of 12 and 25 years will develop it to some degree.[2] Acne typically develops in males aged 16–18 and in females aged 15–17. Acne lesions may precede other signs of puberty and may be diagnosed as early as age 7. Papular lesions generally appear during the mid-teen years and nodular lesions appear in the late teens. In males, acne generally clears by the mid-20s. However, in females it may persist through the third and fourth decades (in each case, among approximately 30% of women) and may worsen during menopause.[3] It may be exacerbated by cosmetics (acne cosmetica) at any age.[4] Acne may also disappear spontaneously in adults for reasons that are not readily apparent.

Although acne is not a physical threat, it may have a significant negative psychosocial impact on an adolescent during a time when physiologic changes necessitate emotional and social adjustments. Acne may precipitate problems of low self-esteem, social phobias, and depression and may even trigger obsessive–compulsive disorders or psychosis. However, medical treatment may manage acne symptoms and thus alleviate these psychosocial conditions.[5] It is estimated that more than 60% of US teenagers use nonprescription products to treat acne and that more than 65% of reported sales of acne remedies occur in pharmacies.[6] Thus, the pharmacist can be instrumental in assisting teenagers to make informed choices about a treatment that may greatly affect their cosmetic and psychosocial well-being. This contact also represents a tremendous opportunity for pharmacists to introduce a new group of consumers to the value of pharmaceutical care.

Etiology and Pathophysiology

Acne vulgaris has its origin in the pilosebaceous units in the dermis (Figure 1A). These units, consisting of a hair follicle and the associated sebaceous glands, are connected to the skin surface by a duct (the infundibulum) through which the hair shaft passes. The sebaceous glands produce sebum, a complex mixture of triglycerides, squalene, and wax esters. The sebum passes to the skin surface through the infundibulum, and then spreads over the skin to retard water loss and maintain hydration of the skin and hair. Because the sebaceous glands are more common on the face, back, and chest, acne tends to occur most often in these areas.

At puberty, the production of androgenic hormones increases in both sexes. The increase of circulating testosterone is taken up, in part, by the sebaceous glands and converted to dihydrotestosterone, which is considered to be the tissue androgen responsible for acne.

TABLE 1 Definition and classification of selected acne terms

Term	Definition	Comment
Whitehead	A condition of the skin that occurs in acne, characterized by a small, firm, whitish, closed elevation of the skin	Also known as a closed comedo; is a noninflammatory lesion
Blackhead	A condition of the skin that occurs in acne, characterized by a black coloration at the skin surface	Also known as an open comedo; is a noninflammatory lesion
Acne pimple	A small, prominent, inflamed elevation of the skin resulting from acne	May occur as a papule or pustule; is an inflammatory lesion; may progress to a necrotic, purulent nodular lesion

The sebaceous glands, under the influence of increased androgen levels, increase in size and activity, producing larger amounts of sebum. At the same time, keratinization of the follicular walls increases and causes mechanical blockage of sebum flow, resulting in the dilation of the follicle and the entrapment of sebum and cellular debris. This results in a microcomedo, the initial pathologic lesion of acne (Figure 1B).

Although androgens are the major stimulus to sebaceous gland development and sebum secretion, patients with acne do not necessarily have abnormal androgen levels. It is theorized that acne-prone patients have increased end-organ sensitivity to normal levels of androgens, facilitating the hypertrophic changes.[7]

The epithelial tissue, an extension of the surface epidermis, forms the lining of the infundibulum and becomes thinner as it extends into the deeper portions of the duct. Normally, the epithelial tissue continually sheds cells, which are carried to the skin surface by the flow of sebum. However, in acne, the shed epithelial cells are more distinct and durable, and they stick together to form a coherent horny layer that blocks the follicular channel.[8] This impaction may plug and distend the follicle to form a microcomedo.

As more cells and sebum accumulate, the microcomedo enlarges and becomes visible; it is called a closed comedo (whitehead) because its contents do not reach the surface of the skin (Figure 1C). Two processes may then follow, one leading to noninflammatory acne and the other leading to inflammatory acne. Most individuals experience a combination of the two types.

If the plug enlarges and protrudes from the orifice of the follicular canal, it is called an open comedo (blackhead) because its contents open to the surface (Figure 1D). The tip of the plug of the open comedo may darken because of melanin (not dirt or oxidized fat) produced by the epithelial cells lining the infundibulum. Open comedones may be carefully expressed with a clean comedo extractor. To prevent infection, care should be taken to avoid using dirty extractors or squeezing with dirty fingers. Acne characterized by the presence of closed or open comedones is called noninflammatory acne. (See color plates, photograph 18.)

Inflammatory acne is characterized by inflammation around the comedo, which may rupture to form a papule (Figure 1E). Papules are inflammatory lesions appearing as raised, reddened areas on the skin. These lesions may enlarge to form pustules, which also appear as raised, reddened areas but are filled with pus (Figure 1F). The pustules can rupture spontaneously. More extensive penetration into surrounding and underlying tissue produces necrotic, purulent nodular lesions.

Inflammatory acne typically begins with closed comedones. As the microcomedo develops, it distends the follicle so that the cellular lining of the walls is spread and thinned. Primary inflammation of the follicle wall may develop with the disruption of the epithelial lining and lymphocyte infiltration into and around the follicular wall.[9] If the follicle wall ruptures spontaneously or is ruptured by picking or squeezing, and if the contents are discharged into the surrounding tissue, a more severe inflammatory reaction results. The epithelial cells, sebum, and any microorganisms present represent foreign substances capable of eliciting an inflammatory reaction. The results may be abscesses, which, in the process of healing, may cause scars or pits.

Theories explaining the development of inflammatory acne suggest that the initial inflammation of the follicle wall results from the presence of free fatty acids derived from the sebum.[9] In the presence of bacterial lipolytic enzymes in the sebaceous glands, triglycerides in the sebum are split, releasing the free fatty acids.

The main microorganism found in the sebaceous duct is an anaerobic rod, *Propionibacterium acnes*. While *P acnes* is a normal part of the flora, colony counts are higher in those patients with acne than in those without acne. *P acnes* is not considered a pathogen; however, it is a major contributor to the production of inflammatory acne lesions. This is because it produces a polymorphonuclear PMN leukocyte chemoattractant, which allows PMN leukocytes to enter the sebaceous follicle to ingest the bacteria, releasing hydrolytic enzymes and inflammatory free fatty acids.[3] The effectiveness of oral antibiotics (eg, erythromycin, clindamycin, minocycline, meclocycline, tetracycline, or doxycycline) and topical antibiotics (eg, tetracycline, erythromycin, or clindamycin) in treating inflammatory acne is possibly owing to their ability to suppress the bacterial population of the sebaceous duct, thus reducing free fatty acid formation and concentration.[10]

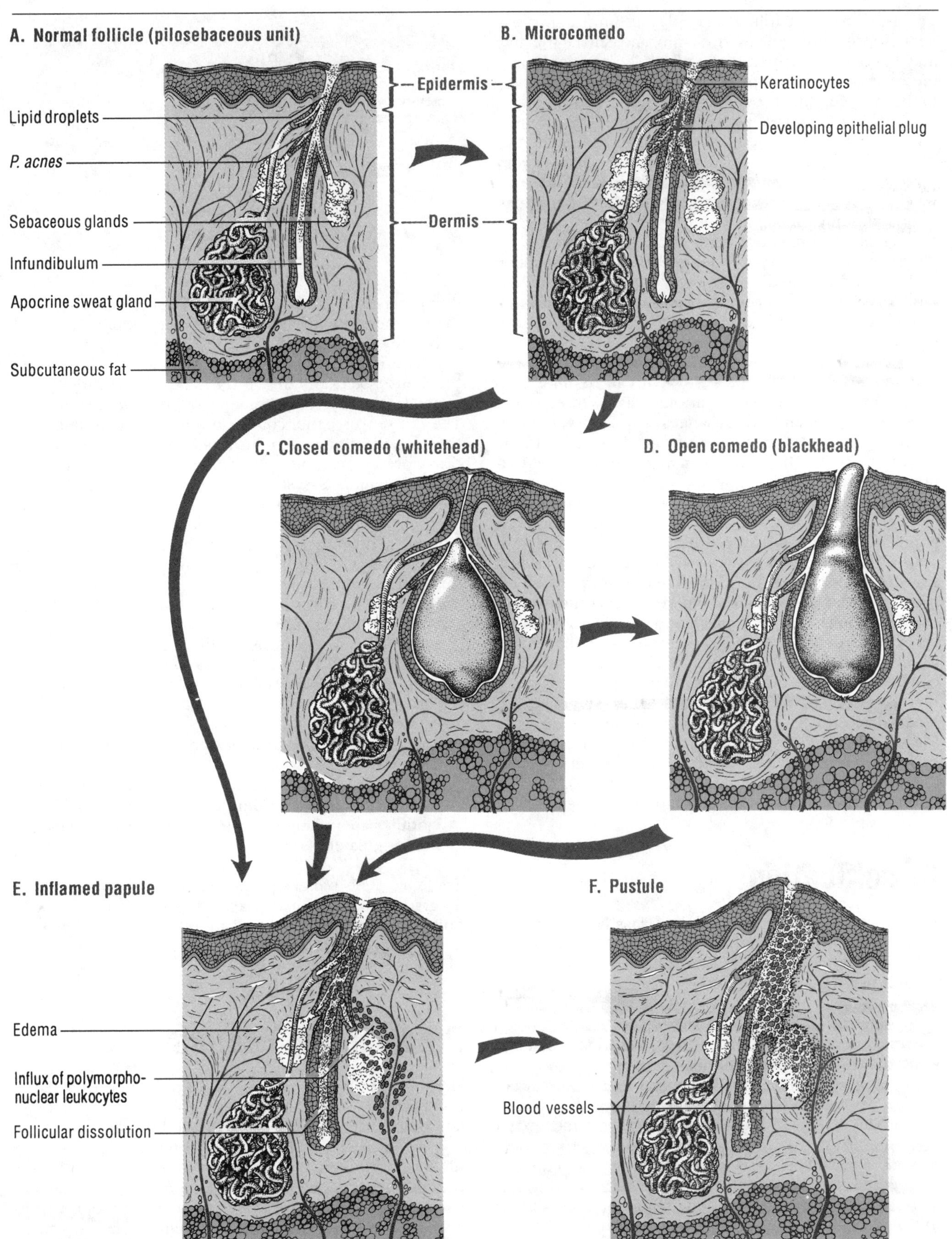

Figure 1 Pathogenesis of acne. Adapted with permission from Fulton JE, Bradley S. *Cutis*. 1976; 17: 560.

The hair in the follicle may play a significant role in comedo development. If it is thin and small, the hair may become entrapped in the plug. The heavier hair of the scalp and beard typically push the developing plug to the surface, thus preventing comedo formation.

Picking or squeezing inflamed follicles or attempting to express closed comedones may rupture the follicle walls and thus produce inflammatory lesions. The pustules or purulent nodules of inflammatory acne are much more likely to cause permanent scarring than those of noninflammatory acne. (See color plates, photograph 19.) Thus, inflammatory acne should be treated by a physician. Treatment typically requires both nonprescription and prescription medication. Prescription drugs such as antibiotics (oral and topical), tretinoin, or isotretinoin, as well as the possible excision and drainage of inflammatory lesions, may be required.

Rosacea (acne rosacea, or "adult acne") is a generalized disorder of the blood vessels. It can be differentiated from acne vulgaris in various ways. Onset is not typically linked to endocrine changes associated with surges in androgen levels, which occur from adolescence to the early to mid-20s. The condition may occur in early adulthood or at any time later. Symptoms may be progressive and may consist of sensitivity to touch, reddening of the face, enlarged blood vessels, and formation of solid red papules or pustules. Factors that may aggravate symptoms include alcohol ingestion, overexposure to sunlight, spicy foods, smoking, hot drinks, temperature extremes, friction, irritating cosmetics, and systemic corticosteroid use. Symptoms tend to diminish and flare in a somewhat cyclic pattern. Lesions tend to be localized to the central portion of the face (eg, center of forehead, nose, and chin). Comedones are not typically present.

As with acne vulgaris, there is no cure for rosacea. Medical referral is required, and treatment is directed toward relieving symptoms. If untreated, symptoms may progressively worsen. Oral antibiotics (eg, erythromycin, tetracycline), topical metronidazole gel (0.75%), or oral isotretinoin may be required to treat the lesions.[11]

Classification

Various systems have been used to classify the severity of acne vulgaris, but none is universally accepted. In the Pillsbury grading scale, Roman numerals from I to IV indicate the level of severity. Grade I, the mildest form of acne, consists of primarily comedones with a small number of inflamed pustules and is often localized on one portion of the face. Grade II acne is confined mainly to the face but displays a marked increase in the number of inflammatory lesions. In grade III acne, the lesions can be found on the upper torso (eg, chest, upper back, and shoulders) as well as on the face; papules and pustules predominate and some scar formation is likely. Grade IV acne, the most severe form, consists of necrotic, purulent nodules and is often called cystic acne, nodulocystic acne, or acne conglobata. Moderate to severe scarring is likely.[12,13]

One problem with the Pillsbury classification system is that the number of acne lesions is not considered. This may result in a person with several pustules being classified as having a more severe case of acne than someone with a large number of comedones and only a few or no pustules.

TABLE 2 Severity grading of inflammatory acne lesions

Severity	Papules/Pustules	Nodules
Mild	Few to several	None
Moderate	Several to many	Few to several
Severe	Numerous and/or extensive	Many

The issue of acne classification was addressed by the Consensus Conference on Acne Classification convened by the American Academy of Dermatology in 1990. The consensus panel concluded that a strictly quantitative classification of acne cannot be established and that "acne grading can best be accomplished by the use of a pattern–diagnosis system, which would include a global (total) evaluation of lesions and their complications such as drainage, hemorrhage, and pain."[14] The division of acne into inflammatory and noninflammatory types has not been changed. However, the opinion is that noninflammatory acne, presenting as comedones only, can rarely be classified as severe even if the comedones are present in large numbers.

Inflammatory acne is defined as the presence of one or more of the following lesions: papules, pustules, and nodules. The parameters for defining the lesions are as follows:

- Papules are inflammatory lesions smaller than 5 mm in diameter.
- Pustules are similar in size to papules but have a visible central core of purulent material.
- Nodules are inflammatory lesions with a diameter of 5 mm or greater.[14]

The consensus panel's proposed classification of severity grades for inflammatory acne, based on a lesion count approximation, is presented in Table 2. A designation of "very severe" is reserved for the most destructive forms of acne.

Predisposing Factors

Many women with acne experience a premenstrual flare-up of symptoms. Hormonal changes associated with ovulation and pregnancy are also related to flare-ups. Oral contraceptives containing androgenic progestins with higher androgenic activity have been implicated in the production of acne, as have certain cyclic progestins used in menopausal hormone replacement therapy. It is also possible that severe or prolonged stress or other emotional extremes may exacerbate the condition.

Hydration decreases the size of the pilosebaceous duct orifice, which explains why acne is exacerbated in conditions of high humidity or in situations that induce frequent and prolonged sweating.

Local irritation or friction may increase the incidence and severity of acne symptoms. Rough or occlusive clothing, headgear straps, athletic equipment, and other friction-producing devices can aggravate acne (acne mechanica). Even resting the chin or cheek on the hand often or for long periods creates localized conditions conducive to lesion formation in acne-prone individuals.[8]

Acne cosmetica is a low-grade, mild form of acne on the face, cheek, and chin. The lesions of acne cosmetica typically are closed, noninflammatory comedones and cannot be easily distinguished from similar lesions of acne vulgaris. This form of acne is more common in women than in men because women are more likely to use cosmetics. Some products may contain oils that are comedogenic (eg, lanolin, mineral oil, or cocoa butter). Oil-based cosmetics may be occlusive and plug the follicles, thus exacerbating or even initiating acne.

Pomade acne, most often seen in African Americans and manifested by comedones along the hairline on the forehead and temples, is reported to be caused directly by the long-term use of hair dressings that contain occlusive petrolatum or liquid petrolatum.

Drug-induced acne (acne medicamentosa) is not a true acne. Drugs can exacerbate preexisting acne vulgaris. Corticosteroids, both systemic and topical, may also induce hypertrophic changes by sensitizing the follicle and producing "steroid acne." Other systemic drugs known to precipitate acne eruptions include androgens, oral contraceptives containing norgestrel or norethindrone, iodides, bromides, ethionamide, azathioprine, dantrolene, haloperidol, halothane, isoniazid, lithium, phenytoin, thyroid preparations, and trimethadione.[2,15]

Occupational exposure to dirt or certain industrial chemicals such as coal tar and petroleum derivatives may cause occupational acne. The term "McDonald's" or "french fryer's" acne refers to acne initiated or exacerbated by vaporized oils present as air contaminants.[16]

There is little evidence to support a direct relationship between diet and acne. Several studies have demonstrated that chocolate does not affect acne even though some clinicians and patients remain unconvinced. Other clinicians think that dietary restrictions are unwarranted because no convincing evidence has been presented to implicate nuts, fats, colas, or carbohydrates. However, an indirect relationship has been proposed between acne and a diet that is high in fat and refined carbohydrates and low in fiber, suggesting that dietary habits may be a risk factor in acne as well as in more serious illnesses.[17] The practical approach is for people to avoid any particular food that seems to exacerbate their acne.

As with many other medical conditions, heredity may predispose a person to the development of acne. Not unexpectedly, the chances are higher that offspring will develop acne if both parents suffered from it rather than only one parent.[18]

Treatment

Acne is rarely cured, but its symptoms can be controlled to varying degrees. In most cases, available therapeutic regimens and patient compliance will reduce symptoms and minimize permanent scarring. Because acne persists for long periods, often from adolescence to the early 20s or beyond, treatment must be long-term, continuous, and consistent.

Goals

The objectives of any acne treatment should include the following:

- Ensuring patient compliance;
- Relieving physical and social discomfort;
- Removing excess sebum from the skin with proper cleansing;
- Preventing closure of the pilosebaceous orifice;
- Using irritants to unblock ducts;
- Reducing lipase activity;
- Minimizing conditions conducive to the development of acne, such as the presence of physical irritants and the use of oil-based cleansers and cosmetics;
- Educating the individual in the proper use of and need for patience with both the nondrug and drug portions of the treatment regimen.

Self-Treatment versus Referral

Self-treatment should be limited to patients who experience noninflammatory acne of mild to moderate severity that is limited to observed whiteheads and blackheads. It is most appropriate if lesions are not extensive (fewer than 10 on one side of the face). Self-treatment should include attention to exacerbating factors such as cosmetic use, high humidity, and overexposure to irritating chemicals. Self-treatment of acne is most effective in patients who are mature enough to understand that treatment will be long-term and that symptoms can be controlled to varying degrees but not cured.

Depending on the answers provided in response to the patient assessment and counseling questions that introduce this chapter, the pharmacist may find the following pointers useful when advising the patient about self-treatment:

- If acne lesions are present where clothes, headbands, helmets, or other devices cause friction, preventing friction-induced irritation should be discussed with the patient. Irritation may also occur as a result of routinely resting the face or chin on the hand; this habit should be avoided or minimized if it is problematic.
- If oil-based cosmetic products are used, water-based products should be considered. If the hair is oily, frequent shampooing with a water-based shampoo is encouraged.
- If face washing is frequent or if a drying soap is used, gentle washing two to three times daily with a mild facial soap and soft washcloth is generally recommended. Medicated soaps are of equivocal value. Mild abrasive soaps may be helpful in treating noninflammatory acne.

- If exposure to environmental factors (eg, dirt, dust, oil, or chemical irritants) seems to exacerbate the acne, the patient should be counseled on how to minimize or avoid these exposures.
- Regardless of the degree of acne severity, the patient should be advised against squeezing, pinching, or picking at acne lesions, especially inflammatory ones. Such behavior aggravates the condition and may result in scarring.

There are situations in which self-treatment is inadequate and physician referral is required. For example, inflammatory acne consisting of observed papules, pustules, and nodules that are extensive (more than 10 lesions on one side of the face) should be referred to a physician, preferably a dermatologist. If the acne is thought to be associated with the use of a drug with comedogenic (eg, androgenic) activity, a pharmacist or physician should be contacted. If acne lesions persist beyond the mid-20s or develop in the mid-20s or later, the symptoms may signal rosacea rather than acne vulgaris. These conditions need to be medically differentiated because the approach for treating rosacea, although similar to that for treating acne vulgaris in some ways, also has unique elements.

Suppressing or altering hormonal activity, correcting disfiguring effects, and using prescription drugs to treat acne must be directed by a physician.

Nondrug Measures

The starting point in treating acne is proper skin hygiene. The preferred method of removing excess sebum from the skin is a conscientious program of daily washing, the purpose of which is to produce a mild drying of the skin and, perhaps, mild erythema. The affected areas should be thoroughly but gently washed at least twice daily with warm water, medicated or unmedicated soap, and a soft washcloth; they should then be patted dry. More frequent washing is appropriate if the skin is oily. Washing should not be excessively vigorous because it may worsen the condition and cause acne mechanica. Washing should cause barely noticeable peeling that can loosen comedones. If it produces a feeling of tautness in the skin, the intensity and frequency of washings should be reduced and use of a less drying soap should be considered.

Ordinary facial soaps that do not contain moisturizing oils are usually satisfactory. Soaps containing antibacterial agents have been suggested for controlling acne, but no conclusive evidence of their clinical value has been presented. Although salicylic acid, sulfur, and sulfur in combination with resorcinol or resorcinol monoacetate are safe and effective for self-treating acne, their benefit as ingredients in soaps is questionable because little, if any, residue is left on the skin after thorough washing.[19]

Soap substitutes containing surfactants (ionic or nonionic) have been suggested for acne because they are less drying to the skin. However, because a mild degree of drying is desirable, an ordinary facial soap should be tried first. Some cleansing preparations contain pumice, polyethylene, or aluminum oxide particles to add abrasive action. For example, there are cleansing sponges that assist in removing the outer layer of dead skin cells by gentle abrasion. Used gently, these abrasive agents may be helpful in treating noninflammatory acne. Abrasives should be avoided in inflammatory acne, however, because of increased irritation. If it is inconvenient to wash during the day, cleansing pads that contain alcohol, acetone, and a surfactant are often convenient to use at school or work.

Because acne treatment begins with removing excess sebum from the skin, topically applied products such as cosmetics and hair dressings should be water based rather than oil based. Hair should be shampooed often because acne is usually accompanied by an oily scalp.

Pharmacologic Agents

The Category I (generally recognized as safe and effective by the Food and Drug Administration [FDA]) active topical antiacne ingredients include 0.5–2% salicylic acid, 3–8% sulfur, and a combination of 3–8% sulfur with either 2% resorcinol or 3% resorcinol monoacetate.[1] Benzoyl peroxide, although proposed and initially classified as a Category I ingredient, was temporarily reclassified to Category III (more data needed) because of concern over its tumorigenic potential. Safety studies are ongoing to determine whether benzoyl peroxide enhances the ability of UV radiation to produce skin cancer. In the meantime, the product remains on the market as an effective product, but a rule proposed by the FDA will require additional warning statements and directions on the label.[20] (See product table "Acne Products" for a list of medications that contain these antiacne ingredients.)

Salicylic Acid

Salicylic acid is a mild comedolytic agent that is available in various nonprescription acne products in concentrations of 0.5–2%. Pharmacologically, it acts as a surface keratolytic.[2] The keratolytic effect and possible enhanced absorption of other agents provide the rationale for the topical use of salicylic acid; however, its safety is questionable when used over large areas for prolonged periods of time.[20]

The use of salicylic acid in cleansing preparations is considered adjunctive acne treatment in reducing comedonal lesions and improving the overall condition.[21] A recent review indicates that salicylic acid pads are safe, effective, and superior to benzoyl peroxide in preventing and clearing both the comedones and inflammatory lesions of acne.[22]

Sulfur

Sulfur has met the criteria of the FDA Advisory Review Panel for Over-the-Counter Topical Acne Products although the claim for its antibacterial effects was disallowed.[1] Alternate forms of sulfur, such as sodium thiosulfate, zinc sulfate, and zinc sulfide, are not recognized in the monograph as safe and effective.

Sulfur, in a precipitated or colloidal form, is included in acne products as a keratolytic in concentrations of 3–10%.

Sulfur is generally accepted as an effective agent for promoting the resolution of existing comedones, but on continued use it may have a comedogenic effect.

Sulfur-containing products are applied in a thin film to the affected area once or twice daily. They have a noticeable color and odor, characteristics that must be considered when their selection and use are being recommended. Compliance may be enhanced by recommending fleshtone products or suggesting usage after school and at bedtime.

Resorcinol and Resorcinol Monoacetate

Although resorcinol and resorcinol monoacetate are not considered to be efficacious as single agents in the treatment of acne, they have been offered in concentrations of 1–2%. There is some question as to whether percutaneous resorcinol absorption may precipitate systemic toxicity when these agents are applied to extensive areas of the body. The FDA advisory review panel concluded that, when used alone, these agents in lower concentrations are safe but not effective in the topical treatment of acne. Therefore, the FDA placed such products in Category II (not generally recognized as safe and effective, or unacceptable indications).[13]

Sulfur Combined with Resorcinol or Resorcinol Monoacetate

The FDA includes the combination of 3–8% sulfur with 2% resorcinol or 3% resorcinol monoacetate in the Category I list of active ingredients for nonprescription acne products.[1] The precise mechanism by which this combination helps to resolve acne lesions has not been determined. The agents function primarily as keratolytics fostering cell turnover and desquamation.

The sulfur–resorcinol products have the characteristic color and odor noted for the sulfur-only products. Additionally, resorcinol may produce a dark brown scale on some darker skinned individuals, who should be forewarned and reassured that the reaction is reversible when the medication is discontinued.

Benzoyl Peroxide

Having determined that additional studies are needed to address concerns about benzoyl peroxide's possible tumor-initiating and promotion potential, the FDA has delayed final action on this medication pending such further study.[1,23,24] Part of the reason for this uncertainty is attributed to reports that benzoyl peroxide is a tumor promoter and progressor, but is neither an initiator nor a complete carcinogen.[25,26] Thus, while studies are being conducted and analyzed, the FDA is unable to state that this ingredient is unsafe for use. The FDA acknowledges that this research, as well as a final determination on benzoyl peroxide's safety, may take several years.[27] In the meantime, benzoyl peroxide has been placed in Category III because currently available data are insufficient to classify it as safe as well as effective.

Benzoyl peroxide, one of the most effective and widely used topical nonprescription medications available for treating acne, may act in several ways. It causes irritation and desquamation, which prevents closure of the pilosebaceous orifice. Its irritant effect causes an increased turnover rate of the epithelial cells lining the follicular duct, which increases sloughing and promotes resolution of the comedones. Its oxidizing potential may contribute to bacteriostatic and bactericidal activity, suppressing the local population of *P acnes* and reducing the formation of irritating free fatty acids. It also exhibits irritant, drying, and sensitizing effects and may bleach hair and fabrics.

Benzoyl peroxide is available most commonly in concentrations of 2.5%, 5%, and 10% in such diverse dosage forms as lotions, gels, creams, cleansers, masks, and soaps. Benzoyl peroxide products in concentrations of 4%, 5.5%, and 20% are also available. Clinical response to all concentrations is similar in terms of reducing the number of inflammatory lesions. However, the different formulations are not equivalent. The drying effect of the alcohol gel base enhances benzoyl peroxide's effectiveness; therefore, this form is superior to a lotion of the same concentration. Some products, mainly the gels, are available by prescription only. Although the washes and cleansers containing benzoyl peroxide are widely used as acne treatment adjuncts, they have been found to have little or no comedolytic effect.[21]

Instructions for the proper use of topical nonprescription benzoyl peroxide products include the following:

- The affected area or area likely to be affected should be gently cleansed with a nonmedicated soap and patted dry, and a small quantity of the preparation should be smoothed over the area once or twice daily.
- Because some individuals are sensitive to benzoyl peroxide, the initial applications may be limited to one or two small areas at the 2.5% or 5% concentration to determine whether discomfort will occur.
- The initial application should be left on the skin for only 15 minutes and washed off. The time benzoyl peroxide is left on the skin should then be increased in 15-minute increments as tolerance allows. Once it is tolerated for 2 hours, it can be left on the skin overnight. The once-a-day application may be all that is needed. A morning dose may be applied if tolerated.
- Fair-skinned individuals should initiate therapy with the 2.5%, 4%, or 5% strength and apply it only once daily during the first few weeks of therapy.
- Benzoyl peroxide should be used with great care near the eyes, mouth, lips, and nose, as well as near cuts, scrapes, and other abrasions, because it is highly irritating.
- The drug should not be used concurrently with other topical products unless recommended by a physician or pharmacist.
- The drug should be used externally only.
- Excessive dryness, marked peeling, some skin sloughing, erythema, or edema suggests that lower concentrations should be used for shorter periods of time. Cool compresses may relieve the discomfort of inflamed skin.
- Use of the drug may bleach hair and clothing.
- Use of the drug may cause transient stinging and burning, but this is not generally a cause for alarm unless it persists or becomes worse.

- If excessive stinging and burning occur after application, the preparation should be removed with soap and water and not reapplied until the next day.
- Other sources of irritation, such as sunlamps and excessive exposure to the sun, should be avoided.
- The full therapeutic effect may not be experienced for 4–6 weeks, so users should be encouraged to be patient and compliant.

Other Combination Products

Assorted nonprescription combinations of benzoyl peroxide, sulfur, salicylic acid, and resorcinol have been used to treat acne. The efficacy of these combination products over the single-ingredient products has not been clearly demonstrated. However, these combination products, as well as an extensive list of other acne product ingredients, may soon be of only historical interest if the FDA does not recognize them as safe and effective for acne self-therapy.

Other Treatments

Although sunlight and artificial UV radiation were once thought to be beneficial in acne treatment by virtue of their drying and peeling effect, they are largely ineffective and not currently recommended. Sunlight can, in fact, aggravate acne. Additionally, excessive exposure to UV radiation hastens skin aging and wrinkling and contributes to an increased risk of skin cancer.

Formulation Considerations

The formulation that carries topical acne medication to the skin can influence the drug's effectiveness. Therefore, particular attention should be paid to this aspect of product selection when advising a patient.

Cleansing bars, liquids, suspensions, lotions, creams, and gels are the vehicles generally used for antiacne preparations. Cleansing products alone are of little value since they leave little residue of active ingredient on the skin. Lotions and creams should have a low fat content so that they do not counteract drying (astringent effect) and peeling (keratolytic effect). They are an acceptable alternative to the more effective gels, and are recommended for dry or sensitive skin and for use during dry winter weather. In general, gels are the most effective formulations because they are astringents and remain on the skin the longest. Nonfatty gels dry slowly if formulated in a completely aqueous base. Ethyl or isopropyl alcohol added to liquid preparations and gels hastens their drying to a film. The drying effect of the volatile solvents may enhance the effectiveness of the various preparations, but the solvents' greater irritant effect may be unacceptable to the patient.[28]

Thickening agents in preparations should not dry to a sticky film. The solids in most preparations leave a film that is not noticeably visible and does not need coloring to blend in with the skin. However, some products are intended to hide blemishes by depositing an opaque film of insoluble masking agents such as zinc oxide on the skin. These products are tinted to improve their cosmetic effect; however, they rarely produce a satisfactory color match.

In general, cream formulations should be recommended for individuals with fair complexions and gels for those with dark complexions.

Patient Counseling

Various therapeutic approaches may be used to treat acne. Familiarity with these approaches will help in advising individuals.

The questions at the beginning of this chapter provide an overview of baseline information to aid the pharmacist in advising and counseling an acne patient. Before counseling the patient on treatment, the pharmacist should try to determine whether the patient is suffering from acne vulgaris or another dermatological condition. The pharmacist should then decide whether the condition merits self-treatment or warrants physician referral.

Before recommending self-treatment, the pharmacist should evaluate the patient's attitude toward treatment and willingness to comply with a skin care program that involves a continued daily regimen of washing affected areas and applying or ingesting medication. The pharmacist should clearly explain the basis for the recommendation. Comedonal and mild papular acne can usually be successfully self-treated, whereas moderately severe papular, pustular, and nodular acne require the attention of a physician, preferably a dermatologist.

Once the decision has been made as to which approach to recommend, the pharmacist should explain acne as a medical condition, describe the treatment program, and correct any misconceptions the patient might have. The patient should be advised about scalp and hair care; the use of cosmetics; and, above all, the need for long-term, conscientious care. (See the appendix at the end of the chapter for sources of patient brochures on skin care, acne vulgaris, and acne rosacea.) The patient should also be advised of the following points when appropriate:

- A proper diet is important in maintaining health, but many of the myths about diet and acne are unfounded.
- Stressful situations may play a role in acne flare-ups but do not cause acne.
- Sexual activity plays no role in the occurrence or worsening of acne.

Because acne cannot be cured but only controlled, reassurance and emotional support are often necessary to reduce patient concern.

Case Studies

Case 27–1

Patient Complaint/History

JW, a 19-year-old male, presents to the pharmacist with typical symptoms of moderate acne. His facial lesions consist of numerous noninflammatory comedones on the cheeks, nose, and forehead as well as several inflammatory pustules on the chin. The patient, who will accompany his family on a Caribbean cruise the following week, asks for help in selecting a nonprescription acne product to clear the flare-up on his chin.

JW reveals that he is taking an oral antibiotic to treat the acne and that the prescribing dermatologist suggested supplementation with nonprescription products. The choice of product was left up to the patient, who indicates he has never used nonprescription acne products. Pharmacy records show that JW has been compliant in taking tetracycline 250 mg one capsule daily; he is not currently taking other medications.

Clinical Considerations/Strategies

The following considerations/strategies are provided to aid the reader in (1) determining whether treatment of the patient's condition with nonprescription medications is warranted, (2) selecting the appropriate nonprescription medication, and (3) developing a patient counseling strategy to ensure optimal therapeutic outcomes:

- Assess the presence of external exacerbating factors that can be controlled by the patient.
- Assess the potential value of a supplemental nonprescription acne product.
- Determine the ingredient(s) in nonprescription acne products that would be most likely to produce a positive outcome and that would be well tolerated if used properly.
- Determine the most appropriate dosage form and strength for this patient.
- Assess nonpharmacologic measures that should be added to the treatment regimen.
- Assess the use of adjunctive nonprescription acne preparations that may be appropriate for the upcoming vacation environment.
- Develop a patient education/counseling strategy that will:
  - Foster thorough understanding of the pathogenesis as well as etiologic and confounding factors of acne;
  - Explain the importance of proper hygiene of affected areas;
  - Explain the importance of nonpharmacologic measures and identify exacerbating situations to avoid or minimize;
  - Explain the value and proper use of nonprescription drug therapy;
  - Support/justify the use of recommended supplementary nonprescription product(s);
  - Optimize the proper use of the recommended product(s);
  - Encourage the patient to comply with the suggested pharmacologic and nonpharmacologic measures.

Case 27–2

Patient Complaint/History

CL, a 34-year-old female, presents to the pharmacist with what appears to be noninflammatory acne. The skin of her cheeks is red and rough with lesions that are typical of closed comedones. The patient reveals that the condition has worsened over the past year. She requests a recommendation for a nonprescription acne product.

CL goes on to reveal that she rarely had acne blemishes as a teenager and does not regard herself as having had acne. She mentions that the condition, which seems to worsen before her menstrual period, also seems to be associated with eye irritation. Physical observation reveals a few small telangiectasias (spider veins) on the patient's cheeks.

CL's current medications include the following: Lo/Ovral-28 one tablet qAM for 21 days, one inert tablet for 7 days; Tavist-D one tablet q12h prn.

Clinical Considerations/Strategies

The following considerations/strategies are provided to aid the reader in (1) determining whether treatment of the patient's condition with nonprescription medications is warranted, (2) selecting the appropriate nonprescription medication, and (3) developing a patient counseling strategy to ensure optimal therapeutic outcomes:

- Determine whether the lesions are actually acne vulgaris.
- Assess whether the condition may be a side effect induced by current medications.
- Attempt to determine the presence of exacerbating factors.
- Evaluate the patient to determine whether a relationship may exist between the facial lesions, ocular irritation, and telangiectasias.
- Assess the feasibility and appropriateness of a medical referral.
- Assess the potential of any nonprescription acne product to produce positive results.
- Determine the ingredient(s) in nonprescription acne products that would most likely produce a positive outcome.
- Determine the most appropriate dosage form for this patient.
- Develop a patient education/counseling strategy that will:
  - Foster a thorough understanding of the etiology and pathogenesis of the condition;
  - Support/justify the use of the recommended nonprescription product(s);
  - Optimize the proper use of the recommended product(s);
  - Encourage the patient to seek the advice of a dermatologist to confirm your assessment.

Summary

Acne vulgaris occurs almost universally in young adults from their early teens to their mid-20s, and it occasionally appears in prepubertal and older people. Generally, acne cannot be cured; however, it may be controlled enough to improve cosmetic appearance and prevent the development of severe acne with its resultant scarring. With empathy and reassurance, acne patients may understand that the condition will not exist forever but that care must be given to the affected areas for a long time for improvement to occur.

References

1. *Federal Register.* 1991 Aug 16; 56: 41018–20.
2. Leyden JJ, Shalita AR. Rational therapy for acne vulgaris: an update on topical treatment. *J Am Acad Dermatol.* 1986 Oct; 15(pt 2): 907–15.
3. Rothman KF, Lucky AW. Acne vulgaris. *Adv Dermatol.* 1993; 8: 347–75.
4. Bennett RW, Popovich NG. Treatment of acne vulgaris. *US Pharm.* 1989 Jan; 14: 40–51.
5. Koo JYM, Smith LL. Psychologic aspects of acne. *Pediatr Dermatol.* 1991; 8(3): 185–8.
6. Gossel TA. OTC anti-acne medications. *US Pharm.* 1990 Oct; 15: 24–34.
7. Arndt KA, ed. *Manual of Dermatologic Therapeutics with Essentials of Diagnosis.* 2nd ed. Boston: Little, Brown and Co; 1978: 3–15.
8. Kligman AM. An overview of acne. *J Invest Dermatol.* 1974; 62: 268–87.
9. Frienkel RK. Pathogenesis of acne vulgaris. *N Engl J Med.* 1969 May 22; 280: 1161–2.
10. Frienkel RK et al. Effect of tetracycline on the composition of sebum in acne vulgaris. *N Engl J Med.* 1965 Oct 14; 273: 850–4.
11. Patient counseling. Facial skin problems may be rosacea. *Am Pharm.* 1992 Jan; NS32(1): 9–10.
12. Pillsbury DM. *A Manual of Dermatology.* Philadelphia: WB Saunders; 1971: 173–4.
13. *Federal Register.* 1982 Mar 23; 47: 12430–77.
14. Pochi PE et al. Report of the Consensus Conference on Acne Classification. *J Am Acad Dermatol.* 1991 Mar; 24(3): 495–500.
15. Pochi PE. The pathogenesis and treatment of acne. *Annu Rev Med.* 1990; 41: 187–98.
16. Popovich NG. Acne: control is a slow process. *US Pharm* (skin care supplement). 1991 Jun; 16: 20–7.
17. Rosenberg EW, Kirk BS. Acne diet reconsidered. *Arch Dermatol.* 1981 Apr; 117: 193–5.
18. Pochi PE. Treatment of teenage acne. *Drug Ther.* 1991 Jan; 21: 56–62.
19. *Federal Register.* 1985 Jan 15; 50: 2172–82.
20. *NDWA Executive Newsletter.* 1995 Feb 17; 4–95: 7.
21. Shalita AR. Comparison of a salicylic acid cleanser and a benzoyl peroxide wash in the treatment of acne vulgaris. *Clin Ther.* 1989; 11(2): 264–7.
22. Zander E, Weisman S. Treatment of acne vulgaris with salicylic acid pads. *Clin Ther.* 1992; 14(2): 247–52.
23. Slaga TJ et al. Skin-tumor promoting activity of benzoyl peroxide, a widely used free radical-generating compound. *Science.* 1981; 213: 1023–5.
24. Kurokawa Y et al. Studies on the promoting and complete carcinogenic activities of some oxidizing chemicals in skin carcinogenesis. *Can Lett.* 1984; 24: 299–304.
25. Schweizer J et al. Benzoyl peroxide promotes the formation of melanotic tumors in the skin of 7,12-dimethyl benz[a]antracene-initiated syrian golden hamsters. *Carcinogenesis.* 1987; 8(3): 479–82.
26. Swauger JE et al. Role of the benzoyloxyl radical in DNA damage mediated by benzoyl peroxide. *Chem Res Toxicol.* 1991 Mar–Apr; 4: 223–8.
27. *Federal Register.* 1991 Aug 7; 56: 37622–35.
28. Ives TJ. Benzoyl peroxide. *Am Pharm.* 1992; NS32(8): 33–8.

Appendix: Acne Information Sources

- National Rosacea Society
  220 South Cook Street, Suite 201
  Barrington, IL 60010
  708–382–8971
  Patient brochures on acne rosacea.
- Dermatological Division
  Ortho McNeil Pharmaceutical Corporation
  US Route 202
  PO Box 300
  Raritan, NJ 08869–0602
  908–218–6000
  Patient brochures on tretinoin therapy.
- Roche Laboratories
  340 Kingsland Street
  Nutley, NJ 07110
  201–235–5000
  Patient brochures on isotretinoin therapy.
- The Upjohn Company
  7000 Portage Road
  Kalamazoo, MI 49001
  616–323–4000
  Patient brochures on acne vulgaris.
- Westwood Pharmaceuticals Inc
  100 Forest Avenue
  Buffalo, NY 14213
  716–887–3400
  Patient brochures on acne vulgaris.

CHAPTER 28

First-Aid Products and Minor Wound Care

Edwina Chan and Raymond Benza

Questions to ask in patient assessment and counseling

- *What type of wound is present? Is the wound acute (an abrasion, puncture, or laceration) or chronic (a pressure ulcer, arterial ulcer, or venous ulcer)?*
- *Where is the wound located? How extensive is the area involved?*
- *Are there foreign objects or dead tissue present at the wound site?*
- *What is the color of the wound bed? What is the condition of the wound margins and the surrounding skin?*
- *Is there redness, warmth, swelling, and/or pain in the affected area?*
- *Is pus present in the area? If so, what color is it and does it have an odor?*
- *Do you have a fever or any flulike symptoms?*
- *Do you have diabetes or any other medical conditions?*
- *What medications are you currently taking?*
- *What measures or medications have you used to self-treat the wound? Were they effective?*
- *Do you have any allergies to topical medications? Do you have any other allergies?*

The skin is a versatile, multifunctional organ whose intricate workings depend on a delicate balance between structure and function. When a wound alters or disturbs this balance, prompt restoration is required to ensure body homeostasis. This is accomplished through the process of wound healing, a complex cascade of localized biochemical and cellular events regulated by the immune system and orchestrated by the skin. Although the skin is well adapted to heal minor wounds over time, proper cleansing and the use of antibiotics, antiseptics, and dressing facilitate healing and prevent scar formation.

The approach to wound care has dramatically changed over the last decade. In the past, problems related to wound healing were approached empirically, and solutions were usually based on anecdotal experience. Popular opinion dictated that wounds be left exposed to air to encourage drying and scab formation. Occlusive dressings were expressly avoided because it was thought that the moist, warm environment they created promoted bacterial colonization. Today, despite clear evidence to support the benefits of a moist wound-healing environment,[1,2] clinical practice has lagged behind in instituting moist wound-healing therapy. Traditional gauze dressings, which promote dehydration of the wound, continue to predominate over the newer, synthetic products that provide a moist environment. Thus, the goal of this chapter is to educate pharmacists and health care providers as to the principles of the moist wound-healing method and its proper implementation through the use of selected first-aid products.

This goal will be accomplished through a review of skin anatomy and function, the physiology of wound healing, classifications and type of wounds and superficial skin infections, management of wounds and dermal-related infections through the use of drugs and/or dressings, and, finally, a schematic approach to triaging wounds. This chapter should enable pharmacists to communicate effectively with physicians on wound-related issues as well as to provide a firm foundation for effective outpatient counseling on basic wound processes and treatments.

Skin Anatomy

The skin is composed of two anatomic layers, the epidermis and the dermis, supported by a variably thick subcutaneous layer called the hypodermis (Table 1). (See Figure 1 in Chapter 26, "Dermatologic Products.") The epidermis, the most superficial layer of the skin, is normally in direct contact with the outside environment. Approximately 0.04 mm thick and avascular, it consists of five layers of stratified squamous epithelium (keratinocytes).[3] This stratified organization results from the upward migration of dividing cells from the stratum germinativum (basilar layer lying adjacent to the dermis) toward the stratum corneum (uppermost layer); as the cells migrate, they lose their nucleus, die, and become tightly packed and keratinized. This keratinized layer provides a tough, resistant, waterproof covering for the skin. Aside from its protective function, the epidermis serves several other functions as well, as it contains the cell types necessary for immune regulation (Langerhans' cells), skin color (melanocytes), and proprioception (Merkel's cells). Skin appendages, including the sweat glands and hair follicles, are also derived from the epidermis.

Editor's Note: This chapter is based, in part, on portions of two 10th edition chapters: "Topical Anti-Infective Products," written by Dennis P. West and Susan V. Maddux, and "Ostomy and Wound Care Products," written by Michael L. Kleinberg and Moya J. Vazquez.

The dermis is the layer directly below the epidermis. It is approximately 0.5 mm thick[3] and contains a rich vascular supply, multiple nerve endings, lymphatics, collagen proteins, and connective tissue. It also contains two main cell types, fibroblasts and macrophages.[4] The main function of fibroblasts is to produce collagen, a structural support protein necessary for scar formation. Macrophages, on the other hand, are multifunctional cells that are vital for wound repair. They serve as both immune and growth regulators, functions that are necessary for the sterilization, debridement, and eventual healing of the wound. The dermis also contains the basilar projections of epidermally derived sweat glands and hair follicles.

The subcutaneous tissue contains mostly adipocytes and is also the origination site for dermal blood vessels. Its major function is to provide insulation, padding, and protection against mechanical injury. It also stores calories in the form of fat, and it provides the skin with a moderate degree of mobility, protecting it against friction and shear-related injury.[3]

TABLE 1 Structure and function of the skin

Epidermis
Thickness of 0.04 mm
No blood supply
Composed of epithelium
Resident florae
Appendages: hair follicles, sebaceous glands, sweat glands
Five layers (two are stratum corneum and stratum germinativum or basement layer)

Dermis
Thickness of 0.5 mm
Main support structure
Contains nerve endings, lymphatics, vasculature
Normally moist
Extension of epidermal appendages

Subcutaneous tissue (hypodermis)
Variable thickness
Reservoir for fat storage
Temperature insulator
Shock absorber
Stores calories
Contains all structures and appendages found in dermis

Reprinted from Bryant R. Wound repair: a review. *J Enterostomal Ther.* 1987; 14(6): 262–3.

Skin Function

The skin has five basic functions: protection, sensation, thermoregulation, immunomodulation, and vitamin D production.[5] Its protective features are twofold: It provides the body with a barrier against physical injury from chemicals, sunlight, dehydration, and bacterial invasion, and it also acts as a "shock absorber" against mechanical trauma. The skin modulates sensation through its vast network of pressure and touch receptors localized primarily in the dermis and subcutaneous layers. Its thermal regulation lies in its ability to modify fluid and electrolyte balances. Specialized cells within the epidermis act as antigen-processing sites, thus forming the basis of the skin's immunomodulation activity. In addition, vitamin D_3, which is important for calcium homeostasis, is synthesized in the epidermis by a process in which an endogenous cholesterol 7-dehydrocholesterol is photolyzed by ultraviolet radiation.

The skin also has several other specialized features. Its surface is inhabited by bacteria (skin flora), including *Staphylococcus epidermidis* and *Staphylococcus aureus* as well as *Candida albicans*.[5] These skin flora serve to protect against invasion by other pathogenic bacteria. The pH of the skin is acidic (range between 4.2 and 5.6),[5] which allows it to regulate the number and activity of the skin flora. This feature is important as these normal flora can become pathogenic under certain conditions.

Wound-Healing Process

Physiology of Wound Healing

Wound healing begins immediately after injury and consists of three overlapping stages (Figure 1): the inflammatory, proliferative, and maturation (remodeling) stages.[6]

Inflammatory Phase

The inflammatory phase is the body's immediate response to injury. This phase, which lasts approximately 3–4 days, is responsible for preparing the wound for subsequent tissue development and consists of two primary parts, hemostasis and inflammation.

In the initial portion of the inflammatory phase, the wound becomes hypoxic and acidotic. Hemostasis is then initiated by the release of thromboplastin from injured cells. Thromboplastin, in turn, activates the body's intrinsic clotting system. The activated clotting factors, along with recruited platelets, form a clot within the first several hours. The newly formed clot stops the bleeding and allows healing to progress. The recruited platelets are crucial to the initial phases of healing because they release cytokines such as platelet-derived growth factor (PDGF) and transforming growth factor beta (TGF-beta). These cytokines stimulate chemotaxis of polymorphonuclear neutrophil (PMN) leukocytes, monocytes, and fibroblasts. Cytokines will also subsequently promote mitogenesis and collagen synthesis.[7]

After hemostasis is achieved, an active inflammatory phase begins, the primary function of which is to cleanse the wound. Inflammation begins with the recruitment of PMN leukocytes within the first 24–48 hours. PMN leukocytes, which require oxygen to function, phagocytize debris and bacteria in the wound. Yet the wound can heal in the absence of these cells. This is because platelets release bradykinin, histamine, and prostaglandins into the wound during this time, initiating an intense vasodilatation of the vessels surrounding the wound and thereby flooding the wound in a type of rinsing action with water, plasma proteins, electrolytes, antibodies, and complement.[7] As a result, the wound becomes erythematous and edematous. After the first 24 hours, blood monocytes are recruited into the wound by released chemotactic factors and become tissue macrophages. Without these macrophages, the wound would not heal. Macrophages function as phagocytes, releasing more chemotactic factors and, most importantly, releasing growth factors. These growth factors stimulate epithelial mitogenesis and endothelial angiogenesis. They also induce fibroblasts to synthesize collagen,[8,9] which provides a healthy bed of granulation tissue for future epithelial cells.

The final portion of the inflammatory phase involves epithelial migration into the wound. Epithelial cells from the stratum germinativum migrate from the intact wound edges and epithelial appendages to cover the denuded area of the wound. As mentioned earlier, the successful migration and adherence of epithelial cells to the wound require a clean, healthy bed of granulation tissue. Once these epithelial cells become established on their granulation bed, they provide the initial (one-cell-thick) layer of new skin for the wound.[10] Epithelial cells can migrate under the clot and eschar (scab) in the wound, but, in doing so, they delay healing time and promote scar formation.

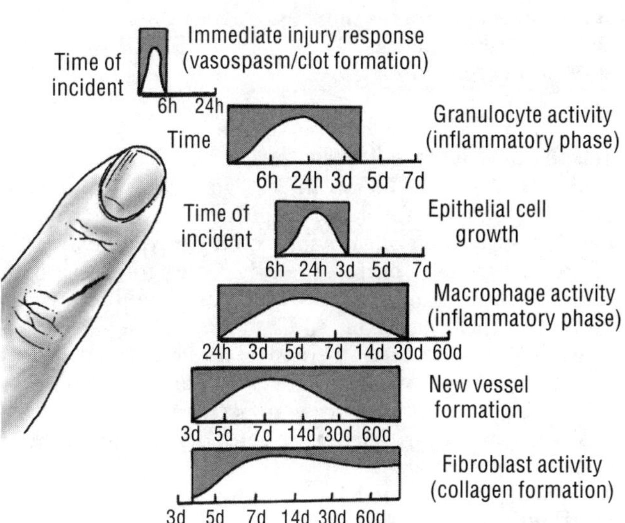

FIGURE 1 The chronology of early wound healing: activity of wound healing components. Adapted with permission from Trott A. Surface injury and wound healing. In: *Wounds and Lacerations: Emergency Care and Closure*. St Louis: Mosby-Year Book; 1991: 15.

Proliferative Phase

The next phase of healing is the proliferative phase, in which the wound is filled with new connective tissue and covered with new epithelium. This phase starts on about day 3 and continues for about 3 weeks. It involves the formation of granulation tissue, which is a collection of new connective tissue (fibroblasts and newly synthesized collagen), new capillaries, and inflammatory cells. The formation of this matrix involves several key coexisting and ongoing processes, including neoangiogenesis (capillary formation) and collagen synthesis.[1] The process of neoangiogenesis is stimulated by the acidic environment of the wound and directed by a variety of cytokines produced by stimulated macrophages, platelets, and endothelial cells, including TGF-alpha, TGF-beta, and angiogenesis growth factor. Collagen synthesis by fibroblasts is also directed by cytokines produced by stimulated macrophages, including PDGF, TGF-alpha and TGF-beta, fibroblast growth factor, monocyte/macrophage-derived growth factor, and interleukin-2.[11] Collagen synthesis also requires oxygen, zinc, iron, and vitamin C. As granulation tissue is being laid down, epithelial cells, which began to migrate during the inflammatory phase, resurface the wound defect. It is important to remember that epithelial cells do not migrate across a dry or necrotic surface. The final portion of this phase involves the action of cytokine-recruited smooth muscle cells, which begin the process of wound contraction. This involves the mobilization and pulling together of the wound edges.

Maturation Phase

The final phase of healing is known as the maturation or "remodeling" phase. The longest phase, it begins at about week 3, when the wound is completely closed by connective tissue and resurfaced by epithelial cells, and can continue for approximately 2 years after the injury. It involves a continual process of collagen synthesis and breakdown, replacing earlier, weak collagen with high tensile strength collagen.[10] The end result is a scar with approximately 70–80% of the original strength of the skin it replaced.

As stated previously, all the healing phases involve and make use of cell-derived growth factors or cytokines. The cytokines are polypeptides that promote cellular growth, chemotaxis, proliferation, and differentiation as well as collagen synthesis, contraction, and eventual healing of the wound.[11] These features make cytokines an attractive new source of first-aid products to facilitate wound healing. One such product is topical silver nitrate impregnated with epidermal growth factor, which has been shown in animal models to shorten healing time when applied to burns.[12,13] Topical TGF-beta has also been used to reverse the deleterious effects of glucocorticoids on wound tensile strength and hypocellularity.[14] The description, source, and cellular targets of these cytokines are beyond the scope of this chapter.

Factors Affecting Wound Healing

Several local and systemic factors can affect how efficiently and to what extent a wound will heal. Some of the important systemic factors that can affect the healing process include[5]:

- Inadequate tissue perfusion and oxygenation at the site of the wound;

- The patient's overall nutritional status, age, and weight;
- The presence or absence of local infection;
- Coexisting diabetes mellitus;
- Certain medications;
- Wound characteristics.

Tissue Perfusion and Oxygenation

Adequate tissue perfusion and oxygenation promote and enhance phagocytosis and angiogenesis, which stabilize cell structure and stimulate collagen synthesis. Lack of adequate tissue perfusion and oxygenation results in impaired collagen synthesis, decreased epithelial proliferation and migration, and reduced tissue resistance to infection. Decreased perfusion and oxygenation can result from hypovolemia, severe anemia (hematocrit ≤ 20 g/dL), peripheral vascular occlusive disease, congestive heart failure, or severe lung disease resulting in resting hypoxemia.[15]

Nutrition

Maintenance of adequate nutrition is extremely important in providing the building blocks for wound repair. Protein, carbohydrates, vitamins, and trace elements are needed for collagen production and cellular energy. Vitamins A and C are important for producing and maintaining wound integrity. Vitamin A stimulates collagen synthesis and epithelialization, and can help reverse the harmful effects of steroids on wound repair (with the exception of steroid-induced failure of wound contraction).[16] Vitamin C is necessary to maintain proper cellular membrane integrity.[16] Zinc also promotes cell proliferation.[17]

Age and Weight

A patient's age and body composition are also important systemic factors affecting proper wound repair. Aging can cause a delayed inflammatory response and is associated with increased capillary fragility, reduced collagen synthesis, and neovascularization.[18] Aging is also associated with slow epithelialization. Patients who are obese (>20% of ideal body weight) experience the same difficulties as those who are elderly.[5] They also have more problems with poor perfusion (adipose tissue lacks extensive vascular tissue) and delayed development of tensile strength.[15]

Infection

All traumatic wounds are contaminated with bacteria to some degree; such contamination is usually restrained by phagocytic action. However, an infection will develop if the following four factors are present: (1) a high level of bacterial contamination (eg, greater than 10^5 bacteria per gram of wound tissue), (2) a compromised tissue microenvironment (eg, eschar, necrosis), (3) systemic conditions (eg, age, steroid therapy, malnutrition), and (4) immunoincompetence.[10,19]

The presence of localized infection in the wound delays collagen synthesis and epithelialization and prolongs the inflammatory phase, causing additional tissue destruction. Bacteria in the wound compete with fibroblasts and macrophages for the available oxygen supplies, thus impeding the roles of these cells in wound restructuring. The most common bacteria implicated in community-acquired wound infections include gram-positive *S aureus*, *Streptococcus faecalis*, and pyogenes. Gram-negative *Escherichia coli*, *Pseudomonas aeruginosa*, and *Klebsiella* species are often associated with hospital-acquired or chronic wounds. Anaerobic organisms such as *Bacteroides* species are particularly infective in wounds with necrotic or poorly perfused tissue.[10]

The classic signs and symptoms of a local wound infection include erythema, edema, induration, pain, crepitance, and the presence of purulent or odorous exudate in the affected area.[15] Fever, flulike symptoms, and leukocytosis are frequently associated with systemic infections. Wound cultures should be taken to identify the infecting organisms when the classic clinical signs of infection are present. Usually, if these signs are severe, there will be fever and systemic leukocytosis.[15]

Coexisting Diabetes Mellitus

Patients who have coexisting diabetes mellitus may have particular difficulties with proper wound healing. Poorly controlled diabetes is usually associated with reduced collagen synthesis, impaired wound contraction, delayed epidermal migration, and reduced PMN leukocytes chemotaxis and phagocytosis. Strict professional attention should be given to wounds in diabetes patients because of these inherent difficulties.[15]

Medications

Pharmacists can play a key role in identifying potential detriments to proper wound closure. Certain medications, for example, can act directly to impede healing through their interaction at various stages of the healing process. Corticosteroids (topical or systemic) reduce phagocytosis, angiogenesis, and collagen synthesis.[20] Antineoplastic drugs and radiation therapy interfere with the cellular division necessary for fibroblast function and reepithelialization.[21] Immunosuppressive agents and anticoagulants can also interfere, especially in the early inflammatory phase. Patients who are taking these medications should be carefully followed by a wound care specialist to ensure that proper healing occurs.

Wound Characteristics

Local characteristics of the wound site are also factors in the regulation of wound healing. Local features that may impair wound closure include the presence of necrotic tissue (eschar) or foreign bodies (eg, glass, dirt), the lack of moisture, and the presence of infection.[15] Pharmacists who are aware of and can recognize problems with these local factors can, through careful counseling, do their part to ensure proper wound healing.

Wound Classification and Type

Classification of wound type is necessary for implementing proper and specific wound therapy; hence, it is imperative that pharmacists who are recommending outpatient first-aid products be aware of these classifications. Wounds can be classified according to their acuity and/or depth.

Using the acuity classification, wounds can be either acute or chronic.

Acute Wounds

Acute wounds are usually abrasions, punctures, lacerations, or burns. Burns are discussed in Chapter 31, "Burn and Sunburn Products."

Abrasions

Abrasions usually result from a rubbing or friction injury to the epidermal portion of the skin and extend to the uppermost portion of the dermis. These wounds should be cleansed with soap and water and then covered with a sterile, semipermeable dressing that is nonadhering to the wound bed.[22]

Punctures

Punctures usually result from a sharp object that has pierced the epidermis and lodged in the dermis or deeper tissues. It is important for a physician to inspect these wounds to ensure that no foreign bodies are retained and to update tetanus prophylaxis, if necessary. If no debris are present, the wounds should then be cleansed with either water or sterile saline. These wounds should be left open, elevated, and soaked with soapy water daily to allow for proper healing.[22]

Lacerations

The last acute form of injury is laceration, which results from sharp objects cutting through the various layers of the skin. Lacerations should also be inspected by a physician, debrided, and flushed; again, tetanus prophylaxis is important. If they are clean, these wounds can be sutured to facilitate their contracture. If they are grossly contaminated by foreign particles or inorganic matter or if they show evidence of early infection, these wounds should instead be left open and covered with a sterile, nonadhering, semipermeable dressing to facilitate healing by secondary closure,[22] as detailed in the section Wound Dressings.

Chronic Wounds

Those wounds classified as chronic include pressure ulcers or decubiti, and arterial and venous ulcers. Among these, pressure ulcers deserve special attention as they often require intense supervision and professional aid to heal properly.

Pressure Ulcers

Pressure ulcers, which are commonly encountered in bedbound or neurologically impaired, immobile patients,[23] are initiated by three forces that are usually present in these patients. These forces include pressure, shear, and friction (Figure 2). Pressure is the perpendicular force exerted on a unit of body tissue; shear refers to those forces that move fascia and skin in opposition to each other; and frictional forces are produced when two surfaces move across one another (eg, skin and sheets).[10] Acting together, these three forces result in the avulsion of local arteries supplying blood to an area of skin (Figure 3). Once perfusion decreases, tissue hypoxia ensues, resulting in skin necrosis and decubiti formation.

Demographic risk factors for the development of these forces include obesity, malnutrition, incontinence, and generalized debilitation. Common areas of involvement include the bony prominences of the body, especially the sacrum, trochanters, heels, and elbows.[24]

Pressure ulcers can be further subdivided according to their depth (Table 2) or color. Because color classifications are often used by the lay public to describe these wounds, it is particularly important for the pharmacist to recognize these descriptions in order to counsel patients properly and facilitate appropriate management. Red wounds usually involve a partial-thickness loss of the skin layers (see the section on Classification of Wound Depth). The wound base is moist, red, painful, and free of necrotic tissue[24]; the base is red and granular. Yellow wounds involve tissue loss that extends through the dermis. The wound exhibits devitalized tissue that appears yellow or grayish in the base.[25] Moisture is usually present and the wound is painless. Black wounds are usually covered by eschar, a thick, black, leatherlike crust of dead tissue,[25] which blocks visualization of the wound base.

Pharmacists should counsel patients that the management of decubiti should be closely supervised by individuals trained to treat these particular wounds. The selection of products to assist in this treatment is based on the extent and depth of the wound, as detailed in the section Classification of Wound Depth. Close attention should be given to alleviating the cause of these wounds, keeping in mind the forces that initiated them and the risk factors that promote those forces.

Arterial and Venous Ulcers

Arterial and venous ulcers are the second form of chronic wounds (Table 3). Arterial ulcers are usually secondary to severe peripheral vascular occlusive disease. They are commonly encountered in the lower extremities and are painful. Venous ulcers are secondary to incompetent venous valves. Incompetent valves allow fibrin to leak from the blood vessels and form obstructive rings around capillaries; this causes tissue ischemia and breakdown.[26]

Classification of Wound Depth

Wound depth classification is used primarily by health care personnel and is based on the extent or number of skin layers damaged during the wound-initiating process. This classification has been divided, for simplicity sake, into four descriptive stages. Stage I does not involve loss of any skin layers and consists primarily of reddened, unbroken skin. Stage II includes the development of a blister or partial-thickness skin loss involving all the epidermis and part of the dermis. Stage III, full-thickness skin loss, includes damage to the entire epidermis, dermis, and dermal appendages. Stage IV is an extension of stage III but further involves the subcutaneous tissue and underlying muscle, tendon, and bone.

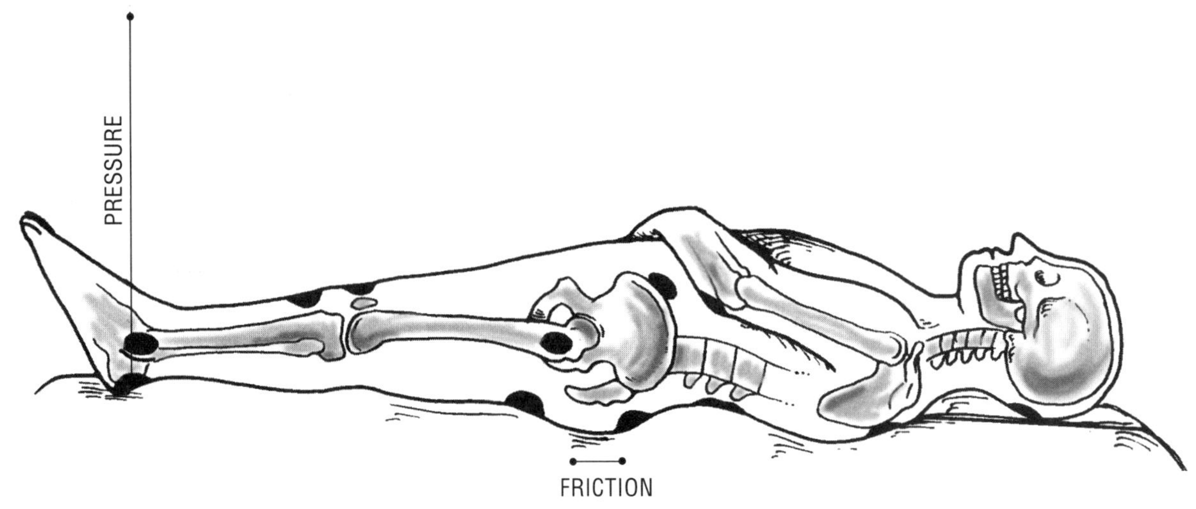

KEY:
Major points of pressure over bony prominences
Forces acting on skin

FIGURE 2 Stresses on skin.

Understanding these stages helps in the selection of appropriate dressings for proper wound closure (Table 4 and Figure 4).

Wound Management

As stated earlier, the proper management of all wounds depends on the type, depth, location, degree of contamination, presence of comorbid conditions, and preexisting medical therapy. Once these factors have been noted and discussed, specific management decisions can be made. The goals of wound management should include a stepwise approach that involves cleansing of the wound, selective use of antiseptics and antibiotics, and closure with an appropriate dressing (see product table "First-Aid Antibiotic and Antiseptic Products").

Uncontaminated wounds require only basic supportive measures, including the use of mild soap and water for proper cleansing. To help prevent superficial skin infection in minor cuts, scrapes, and burns, topical nonprescription antibiotic and antiseptic preparations can be useful but should be viewed as extensions of supportive treatment. More serious or deeper tissue infection (eg, puncture wounds, severe burns) requires physician consultation to assess the need for systemic or topical prescription antibiotics.

Pharmacologic Agents

First-Aid Antiseptics

Antiseptics are chemical substances designed for application to intact skin up to the edges of a wound for disinfection purposes.[27] When effective antisepsis is combined with proper wound care technique, including gentle handling of tissue, the infection rate is low—about 1.6%.[27] Ideally, antiseptics should exert a sustained effect against all microorganisms without causing tissue damage. However, even when used in therapeutic concentrations, these agents have been shown to be leukocytotoxic. Increased intensity and duration of inflammation, tissue necrosis, endothelial damage, and thrombosis have been observed in wound models treated with various antiseptics.[28] Thus, the current recommendation in the literature is to avoid using antiseptics on open wounds but to use them instead for what they were originally intended: disinfection of intact skin.

Antiseptics, which are subject to the Food and Drug Administration's (FDA's) ongoing review of over-the-counter (OTC) topical antimicrobial products, encompass four groups of products that may contain the same active ingredients but are labeled and marketed for different intended uses. The first group covers products that are generally intended for use by health care professionals as patient preoperative skin preparations, personnel hand washes, and surgical hand scrubs. The second group encompasses antiseptic hand washes purchased by consumers for personal use in the home. The third group includes first-aid antiseptics to help prevent infection in minor scrapes, cuts, and burns (Table 5). The fourth group covers hand cleansers used by food handlers to prevent disease caused by contaminated food.

The FDA's proposed classification of first-aid antiseptic ingredients for safety and effectiveness was published in July 1991.[29] With the myriad of antiseptic active ingredients available for use, only five ingredients—alcohol (60–95%), isopropyl alcohol (50–91.3%), iodine topical solution (USP), iodine tincture (USP), and povidone-iodine complex (5–10%)—are recognized as

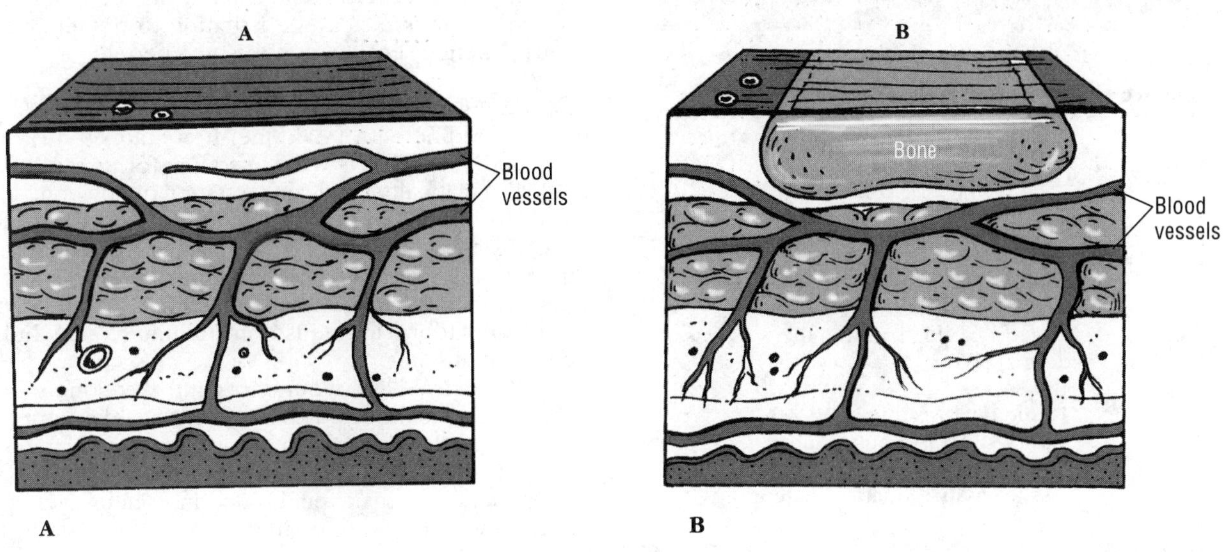

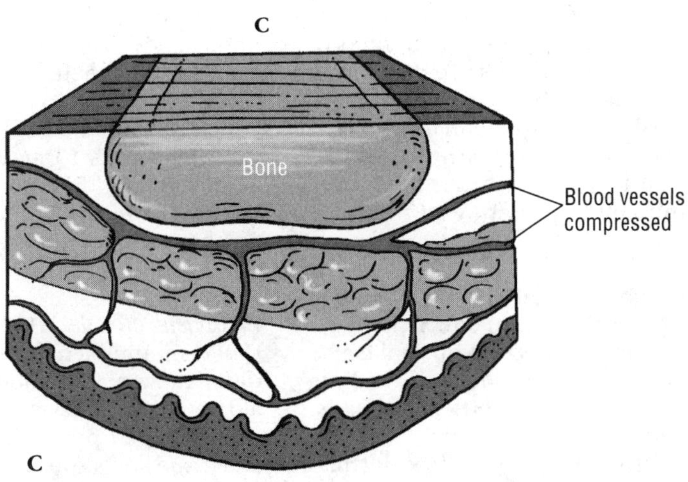

FIGURE 3 Diagrammatic representation of the decubitus ulcer developmental process. A: Normal skin is kept healthy by capillary blood supply. B: In some places of the body, large bony prominences lie close to the skin, especially at the hips, sacrum, heels, elbows, etc. C: When a patient is lying down, the skin is compressed between the bones and the bed, which impedes the blood supply to that area of the body. At this point, there is great risk of developing decubitus ulcers. Adapted with permission from Szycher M, Lee SJ. Modern wound dressings: a systemic approach to wounds. *J Biomater Appl.* 1992; 7(2): 142–213.

safe and effective (Category I) for use both as preoperative skin preparations by health care professionals and as first-aid products. Only two of these ingredients, alcohol and povidone-iodine, are considered Category I for all antiseptic uses (Table 5). Other common agents such as hydrogen peroxide, phenolic compounds, hexylresorcinol, and quaternary ammonium compounds are considered Category I for use as first-aid products only. The following discussion of antiseptic agents is confined to their use as first-aid antiseptics.

Alcohol Alcohol has good bactericidal activity in a 20–70% concentration. For first-aid uses, it decreases the risk of infection in minor cuts, scrapes, and burns. Caution must be used, however, when applying it to the intact skin surrounding the wound since direct application of alcohol to the wound bed can cause tissue irritation. Alcohol usually contains denaturants that will dehydrate the skin when applied topically at high concentration. It is also highly flammable and must be kept away from fire or flame. Alcohol wash may be used one to three times daily and may be covered with a sterile bandage after the washed area has dried.[30]

Isopropyl Alcohol Isopropyl alcohol, which has somewhat stronger bactericidal activity and lower surface tension

TABLE 2 Decubitus ulcer assessment scale

Grade of score	Comments
0	Erythema/induration noted (potential sore)
1	Blister skin formation; erythema that does not disappear within 30 minutes after pressure is relieved
2	Superficial skin break in the dermal layers
3	Tissue necrosis involving loss of subcutaneous tissue
4	Tissue cavity formation, extending to bones

than ethanol, is generally used for its cleansing and antiseptic effects on the skin. It can be used undiluted or as a 70% aqueous solution. Denaturants are not added because isopropyl alcohol itself is not potable. However, isopropyl alcohol has a greater potential for drying the skin (astringent action) because its lipid solvent effects are stronger than those of alcohol. Like alcohol, it is flammable and must be kept away from fire or flame.

Iodine Iodine's broad antimicrobial spectrum against bacteria, fungi, virus, spores, protozoa, and yeast is attributed to its ability to oxidize microbial protoplasm.[30] An iodine solution (USP) of 2% iodine and 2.5% sodium iodide is used as an antiseptic for superficial wounds. An iodine tincture (USP) of 2% iodine, 2.5% sodium iodide, and about 50% alcohol is less preferable than the aqueous solution because it is irritating to the tissue. Strong iodine solution (Lugol's) must not be used as an antiseptic.

In general, bandaging should be discouraged after iodine application to avoid tissue irritation.[30] Iodine solutions stain skin, may be irritating to tissue, and may cause allergic sensitization in some people.

Povidone-Iodine Povidone-iodine is a water-soluble complex of iodine with povidone. It contains 9–12% available iodine, which is what accounts for its rapid bactericidal activity. Reduced concentration of povidone-iodine at 0.001% (eg, vaginal douches) has been shown to be less toxic to leukocytes than to bacteria, so this antiseptic not only reduces bacterial counts but also allows for normal immune responses that promote wound maturation.[31] Povidone-iodine is nonirritating to skin and mucous membranes.

When used as a wound irrigant, povidone-iodine is absorbed systemically, with the extent of iodine absorption being related to the concentration used and the frequency of application. Final serum level is also dependent upon the patient's intrinsic renal function. When severe burns and large wounds are treated with povidone-iodine, iodine absorption through the skin and mucous membranes can result in excess systemic iodine concentrations and can cause transient thyroid dysfunction, clinical hyperthyroidism, and thyroid hyperplasia. If renal function is normal, however, the absorbed iodine is rapidly excreted, and signs of hyperthyroidism do not develop. Thus, povidone-iodine should be used with discretion when treating large wounds.[32]

Detergents formed by the combination of surfactants with povidone-iodine have been found to damage wound tissue and potentiate infection. Therefore, these combination products are not recommended for scrubbing wounds.[32]

Hydrogen Peroxide Hydrogen peroxide (topical solution, USP), an antimicrobial oxidizing agent (along with sodium and zinc peroxides), is the most widely used first-aid antiseptic. Enzymatic release of oxygen occurs when the hydrogen peroxide comes into contact with blood and tissue fluids. Mechanical release (fizzing) of the oxygen has a cleansing effect on a wound, but organic matter reduces its effectiveness. The duration of action is only as long as the period of active oxygen release. Using

TABLE 3 Ischemic ulcers

	Arterial	Venous
Cause of ulcer	Arterial occlusion curtails blood flow	Incompetent perforator valves
Initiating factor	Arteriosclerosis; atherosclerosis	Deep vein thrombosis
Location	Toes, heels	Above medial malleolus
Pain	Extreme; increases with leg elevation	Medium; decreases with leg elevation
Pedal pulses	Usually absent	Usually present
Appearance	Punched-out lesion with pale or white bed	Irregular lesion with brown and blue color

Adapted with permission from Szycher M, Lee SJ. Modern wound dressings: a systemic approach to wounds. *J Biomater Appl.* 1992; 7(2): 142–213.

TABLE 4 Options in wound management

Description (brand name)[a]	Use indications	Advantages	Disadvantages
Transparent adhesive films			
Semiocclusive translucent dressings with partial or continuous adhesive composed of polyurethane or copolyester thin film (eg, ACU-derm, Op-Site, Uniflex) (See Figure 6C)	Stages I, II, shallow stage III Clean, granular wounds Minimally exuding wounds Autolysis Can use with absorption products and alginates Can be used in conjunction with some enzymatic debriders	Semiocclusive Gas permeable Easy inspection Autolysis Protection Impermeable to fluids/bacteria Conformable Self-adherent Reduce pain Moist environment Resist shear	For uninfected wounds only Not absorptive May cause periwound trauma on removal With continuous adhesive, may reinjure wound on removal With large amounts of exudate, maceration may occur
Nonadherent dressings			
Nonadherent, porous dressings. Lightly coated dressings allow easy flow-through of exudate (eg, Adaptic, Telfa)	Skin donor sites Stage II, shallow stage III Staple/suture lines Abrasions Lacerations	Readily available Less adherent than plain gauze	Need secondary dressing May have traumatic/painful dressing removal Some impregnated dressings may delay healing May require frequent dressing changes Some may cause exudate pooling
Alginates			
Hydrophilic, nonwoven dressings of calcium-sodium (percentages vary between products) alginate fibers. Alginates are processed from brown seaweed into pad or twisted fiber form. Exudate transforms fibers to gel at wound interface (eg, Kaltostat, Sorbsan)	Light to heavy exuding wounds Stages II, III, IV Moist wound environment Autolysis Skin donor sites	Absorptive Reduce pain Nonocclusive Moist wound environment Conformable Easy, trauma-free removal Can use on infected wounds Accelerate healing time Less frequent dressing changes Potential to aid in control of minor bleeding	Require secondary dressing Characteristic odor May need wound irrigation May desiccate May promote hypergranulation
Exudate absorbers			
Hydrophilic dressings that absorb exudate dead cells and bacteria (eg, Debrisan Beads, Hydragran)	Stages II, III Exuding wounds Nontunneling deep wounds Infected wounds	Absorb exudate Moist environment Nonocclusive Reduce odor Conformable Inert Clean debris Many distributed in unit dose packs	Contraindicated with tunneling May be difficult to remove May increase wound pH May sting on application Need secondary dressing Application techniques vary

continued

TABLE 4 Options in wound management

Description (brand name)	Use indications	Advantages	Disadvantages
Debriding agents			
Debriders digest necrotic tissue by differing methods (eg, Elase, Santyl)	Stages II, III, some stage IV Dermal ulcers Second- and third-degree burns	Nonsurgical method of debridement Some will not damage healthy tissue	May require frequent dressing changes Require secondary dressing May require cross-hatching of eschar Some may damage healthy tissue Application techniques vary significantly Need moist wound environment Some require refrigeration
Gauze dressings			
Nonocclusive fiber dressing with loose, open weave	Stages II–IV Minimal to heavy exuding wounds/topicals Infected wounds Debridement Wound rehydration	Readily available Deep wound packing May use with infected wounds/topicals Mechanical debridement Nonocclusive Conformable	Wound bed may desiccate if dressing dry Nonselective debridement May cause bleeding/pain on removal Need secondary dressing Frequent dressing changes Some dressings may "shed"
Hydrogels/Gels			
Nonadherent, nonocclusive dressings with high moisture content that come in the form of sheets and gels (eg, Elasto-Gel, Vigilon) (See Figure 6D)	Stages II, III, some approved for stage IV Granular or necrotic wound beds Autolysis Some used on partial- and full-thickness burns	Nonadherent Most are nonocclusive Trauma-free removal Varying absorption capabilities Conformable Some can be used in conjunction with topicals Thermal insulation Reduce pain Moist environment	Most require secondary dressings May macerate periwound skin Some products may dehydrate Slow to minimal absorption rate in most Most require frequent/daily dressing change
Composite/Island dressings			
Nonadherent absorptive center barrier with adhesive at perimeter (eg, Airstrip, Viasorb)	Stages II, III Moderate to heavy exuding wounds Autolysis Suture/staple lines	Nonadherent over wound Semiocclusive No secondary dressing required Impermeable to fluids/bacteria Protective Reduce pain	May cause periwound trauma on removal

TABLE 4 *continued*

Description (brand name)	Use indications	Advantages	Disadvantages
Foams			
Semipermeable, absorptive, nonwoven, inert polyurethane foam dressings (eg, EPIGARD, LYOfoam) (See Figure 6E)	Stage II, shallow stage III Minimal to moderate drainage Autolysis Donor sites First- and second-degree burns Contraindicated for third-degree burns	Most are nonadhesive Some can be used with infected wounds/topicals Thermal insulation Reduce pain Nonocclusive Moist environment Conformable Less frequent dressing changes Trauma-free removal Absorbent	Most require secondary dressing May require cutting May cause wound desiccation May be difficult to determine wound contact surface
Hydrocolloids			
Wafer dressings composed of hydrophilic particles in an adhesive form covered by a water-resistant film or foam (eg, Comfeel, ULTEC) (See Figure 6F)	Stages I, II, and shallow stage III Clean, granular wounds Autolysis Minimal to moderate exuding wounds Can use with absorption products and alginates	Occlusive Manage exudate by particle swelling Autolysis Long wear time Self-adherent Impermeable to fluids/bacteria Conformable Protective Thermal insulation Reduce pain Moist environment	For uninfected wounds only May cause periwound trauma on removal Difficult wound assessment Characteristic odor Impermeable to gases Some may leave residue on skin or in wound
Carbon-impregnated (odor control) dressings			
Dressings with an outer layer of carbon for odor control (eg, LYOfoam "C" Odor Absorbent Dressing)	Malodorous wounds	Control odor	Require appropriate seal or odor may escape Carbon is inactivated when it becomes wet
Biosynthetics			
Semipermeable dressings that are designed to adhere to a clean or debrided wound and remain in place without removal throughout the course of reepithelialization (eg, BioBrane II)	Partial-thickness burns Donor sites Meshed autografts	Gas permeable Adherent to wound May be used in conjunction with topical antibacterial agents Reduce pain Wound visible	Permeable to fluids/bacteria May require secondary dressing or skin staples May adhere to skin at removal Not for use on necrotic tissue

[a]The brand names listed for each type of wound dressing are given as examples of available products; however, these brand names do not constitute an all-inclusive list of available wound-dressing products.

Adapted with permission from an unpublished document prepared by McIntosh A, Raher E. Silver Cross Hospital, Joliet, Ill, 1991.

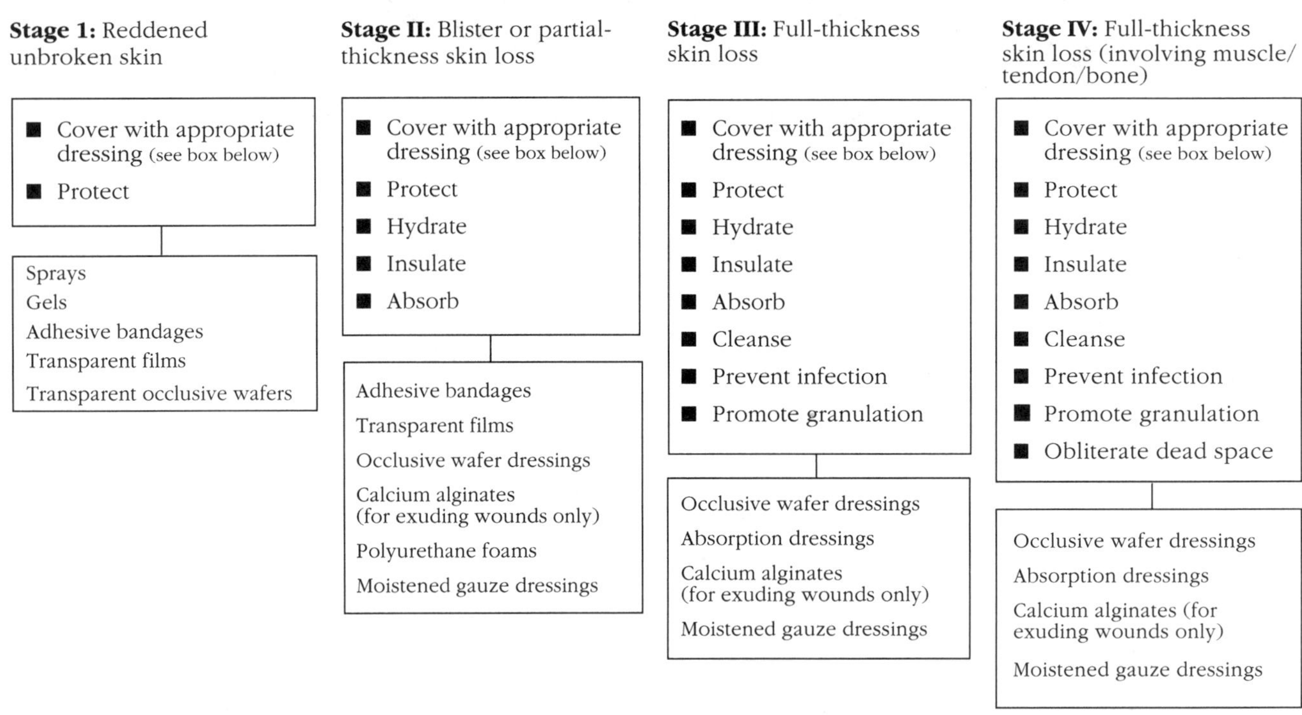

FIGURE 4 Guidelines for product selection based on wound severity. Adapted with permission from Jeter KF, Tintle TE. Wound dressings of the nineties: indications and contraindications. *Clin Podiatr Med Surg*. 1991; 8(4): 805.

hydrogen peroxide on intact skin is of minimal value because the release of nascent oxygen is too slow.

Hydrogen peroxide should be used where released gas can escape; therefore, it should not be used in abscesses, nor should bandages be applied before the compound dries.

Phenolic Compounds In very dilute solutions, phenol is an antiseptic and a disinfectant. It has local anesthetic activity and is claimed to be an antipruritic in concentrations of 1:100–1:200 (eg, phenolated calamine lotion). In aqueous solutions of more than 1%, however, it is a primary irritant and should not be used on the skin except as a keratolytic or peeling agent.

Camphorated Phenol Oily solutions of phenol and camphor are often used as nonprescription first-aid antiseptics. Such products contain relatively high concentrations of phenol (4%) and must be used with caution. If oleaginous phenolic solutions are applied to moist areas, the phenol is partitioned out of the vehicle into water, resulting in caustic concentrations of phenol on the skin. To avoid such damaging effects, these products should be applied only to dry skin.

Hexylresorcinol Hexylresorcinol (0.1%) is more effective than phenol as an antibacterial agent and is less toxic. It has been used in mouthwashes. The FDA has judged it safe and effective (Category I) as a first-aid antiseptic.[29] But even though it is used in low concentrations, it may be irritating.

Quaternary Ammonium Compounds The FDA's monograph for proposed first-aid antiseptics includes the quaternary ammonium compounds benzalkonium chloride, benzethonium chloride, and methylbenzethonium chloride (Table 5). These compounds are considered Category I for use as first-aid products. Quaternary ammonium compounds are cationic surfactants that have antimicrobial effects on gram-positive and gram-negative bacteria but not on spores.[30] Gram-negative bacteria are more resistant than gram-positive ones; thus, they need a longer period of exposure. The antimicrobial activity of these compounds consists of disrupting cell membranes and denaturing the lipoproteins of microbes. Quaternary ammonium compounds are sometimes included in topical anti-infective products. In addition to their antiseptic properties, these agents are used for their cleansing properties: they emulsify sebum and have a detergent effect that assists in removing dirt, bacteria, and desquamated epithelial cells. The "quats" can be inactivated by various anionic adjuvant ingredients (eg, soaps and viscosity-building agents).

These compounds are formulated as creams, dusting powders, and aqueous or alcoholic solutions. Stock solutions are available for dilution to proper concentration for topical use. If used undiluted, these preparations may cause serious skin irritation. Quaternary compounds are irritating to the eyes, so caution must be used when applying them to skin near the eyes. For use on broken or diseased skin, concentrations of 1:5,000–1:20,000 may be used. For use on intact skin and minor abrasions, a concentration of 1:750 is recommended.

TABLE 5 Classification of antiseptic uses

Category I Antiseptic Agents	First-aid use	Consumer use (antiseptic and wash)	Health care use: Preoperative skin preparation	Health care use: Personnel hand wash	Health care use: Surgical hand scrub
Alcohol (60–95%)	✔	✔	✔	✔	✔
Benzalkonium chloride (0.1–0.13%)	✔				
Benzethonium chloride (0.1–0.2%)	✔				
Camphorated metacresol complex	✔				
Camphorated phenol complex	✔				
Combination of eucalyptol (0.091%), menthol (0.042%), methylsalicylate (.955%) and thymol (0.063%)	✔				
Hexylresorcinol (0.1%)	✔				
Hydrogen peroxide topical solution (USP)	✔				
Iodine tincture (USP)	✔		✔		
Iodine topical solution (USP)	✔		✔		
Isopropyl alcohol (50–91.3%)	✔		✔		
Methylbenzethonium chloride (0.13–0.5%)	✔				
Phenol (0.5–1.5%)	✔				
Povidone-iodine complex (5–10%)	✔	✔	✔	✔	✔

First-Aid Antibiotics

Topical nonprescription antibiotic agents such as tetracyclines or the combination of bacitracin, neomycin, and polymyxin B sulfate help prevent infection in minor cuts, wounds, scrapes, and burns.[30] When applied to dirty, contaminated wounds up to 4 hours after insult, topical antibiotic combinations have been demonstrated to reduce the likelihood of wound infection by (1) removing the cause of tissue breakdown (infection and inflammation); (2) reducing pain; (3) removing necrotic tissue, the presence of which delays healing; (4) assisting in wound closure; and (5) fostering the healing process.[33]

Topical antibiotic preparations should be applied to the infected wound bed after cleansing and before application of a sterile dressing. Special caution should be taken when applying these preparations to large areas of denuded skin, however, because the potential for systemic toxicity can increase. Prolonged use of these

TABLE 6 Nonprescription topical antibiotic product guide

Ingredient	Product	Dosage form
Bacitracin + neomycin + polymyxin (B+N+P)	Maximum Strength Neosporin Neosporin Ointment Bactine First-Aid Mycitracin Triple Antibiotic N.B.P. Septa Neomixin Medi-Quick Triple Antibiotic	Ointment
Bacitracin + neomycin	Neosporin Cream	Cream
Bacitracin + polymyxin	Polysporin	Ointment, powder, spray
Bacitracin	Baciguent Various generic products	Ointment
Neomycin	Myciguent Various generic products	Cream
Tetracycline	Achromycin	Ointment
Chlortetracycline	Aueromycin	Ointment

agents may result in secondary fungal infection.[30] If healing does not occur within 5 days, the patient should consult a physician.

Currently recognized in the FDA's most recent monograph for first-aid antibiotics,[34] which was last amended in June 1990, are six ingredients considered to be generally safe and effective for use (Category I): bacitracin, neomycin, polymyxin B sulfate, tetracycline hydrochloride, chlortetracycline hydrochloride, and combination products containing oxytetracycline hydrochloride (Table 6).

Bacitracin Bacitracin is a polypeptide bactericidal antibiotic that inhibits cell wall synthesis in several gram-positive organisms.[35] The development of resistance in previously sensitive organisms is rare. Minimal absorption occurs with topical administration. The frequency of allergic contact dermatitis (erythema, infiltration, papules, edematous or vesicular reaction) is approximately 2%.[36] Topical nonprescription preparations usually contain 400–500 U per gram of ointment and are applied one to three times a day.[30]

Neomycin Neomycin is an aminoglycoside antibiotic; it exerts its bactericidal activity by irreversibly binding to the 30S ribosomal subunit to inhibit protein synthesis in gram-negative organisms and some species of *Staphylococcus.* Neomycin has been demonstrated to decrease the severity of clinical infection 48 hours after treatment in tape-stripped wounds.[33] Resistant organisms may develop. Neomycin applied topically produces a relatively high rate of hypersensitivity; reactions occur in 3.5–6% of patients.[37] Some patients with positive results to neomycin on skin tests also react to bacitracin. Because these two agents are not chemically related, these responses apparently represent independent sensitization rather than cross-reactions.[37] Although neomycin is not absorbed when applied to intact skin, application to large areas of denuded skin has been known to cause systemic toxicity (ototoxicity and nephrotoxicity).[30]

Neomycin is available in cream and ointment forms, alone or in combination. It is most frequently used in combination with polymyxin and bacitracin to prevent the development of neomycin-resistant organisms. Because neomycin is a relatively common cause of allergic contact dermatitis and is not essential to topical antibacterial coverage of skin infections, it is rarely recommended by the dermatologic community. The combination of bacitracin and polymyxin B sulfate is more widely accepted for clinical use in dermatology than the triple antibiotic combination of bacitracin, polymyxin B sulfate, and neomycin.[33]

The concentration of neomycin commonly used in nonprescription products is 3.5 mg/g. Applications are made one to three times a day.

Polymyxin B Sulfate Polymyxin B sulfate is a polypeptide antibiotic effective against several gram-negative organisms because it alters the bacterial cell wall permeability.[35] However, its effect on healing is unknown. Polymyxin B is a rare sensitizer.[36] Concentrations of 5,000 U/g and 10,000 U/g are available in nonprescription combination preparations. Applications are usually made one to three times a day.

Tetracyclines Tetracycline, chlortetracycline, and oxytetracycline are broad-spectrum antibiotics that, like neomycin, exert their bacteriostatic effects by binding to the 30S ribosomal subunit to inhibit bacterial protein synthesis. Tetracycline derivatives have activity against gram-positive and most gram-negative bacteria except *Proteus* and *Pseudomonas* species. Because of the high incidence of bacterial resistance, topical tetracycline and chlortetracycline are often ineffective for the treatment of primary bacterial infection. Toxicity is rare when applied topically; however, hypersensitivity reaction may be triggered in allergic patients even by topical application. If redness, irritation, swelling, or pain persists or increases in the applied area, it is recommended that use of tetracycline be discontinued.[30] Because tetracycline products oxidize in the presence of light on human skin, they may turn the skin a reversible yellow-brown color and may stain clothing.

Currently, 3% ointments of tetracycline and chlortetracycline are available as nonprescription agents. In its first-aid monograph for nonprescription first-aid antibiotics, the FDA included oxytetracycline only in combination with polymyxin B sulfate in ointment or powder form. These products are usually applied one to three times per day and may be covered with a sterile bandage afterwards.

Antimicrobial Selection Guidelines

Before recommending a topical product for self-medication of cutaneous infections, the pharmacist should assess the nature of the patient's complaint. Noninfectious processes, including drug-induced eruptions, should be considered. Antimicrobial agents should generally be recommended in cases of infectious etiology and where secondary infection may occur.

Referral to a physician should be considered in the following situations:

- There is doubt as to the causative factor or organism.
- Initial treatment has not been successful or the condition is getting worse.
- Topical drug products have been applied for prolonged periods over large areas, especially on denuded skin (creating the potential for systemic toxicity).
- Exudate is excessive and continuous.
- Widespread infection has occurred.
- There is predisposing illness, such as diabetes, systemic infection, or an immune deficiency.
- Fever, malaise, or both occur.
- A primary dermatitis (allergic dermatitis, psoriasis, or seborrhea) exists and becomes secondarily infected.
- Lesions are deep and extensive.
- Lancing is needed to aid drainage of exudate or provide pain relief.

Wound Dressings

Traditional wound management involves leaving the wound open to air or covering it with an occlusive textile dressing (gauze). However, this type of management leads to several important problems. It promotes eschar formation, which impedes reepithelialization of wounds and creates unwanted scars (Figure 5A). It also offers excessive exudate control, which dehydrates wounds and delays healing. Removal of these dressings tears away not only the eschar, but also the new tissue under the eschar. Finally, this treatment promotes bacterial entry into the wound, increasing the incidence of infection and delaying healing. These cumulative problems have led physicians and nurses to develop new treatment strategies based on the creation of a moist wound environment (Figure 5B). Such an environment prevents eschar development, removes excess exudate without dehydration, and prevents bacterial invasion of the wound. Accordingly, it makes use of semipermeable dressings that promote optimal moisture, exudate removal, and gas exchange. This technique has been shown to accelerate healing and prevent scarring.[1,2,10] Additionally, it reduces pain and promotes epithelialization and the healing of chronic wounds.

Prior to the discussion of wound dressing, a brief mention should be made as to the techniques of wound closure. These techniques should be used for the more extensive wounds that fall under a physician's supervision. Closure of the wound depends on the degree of contamination and extent of the wound. Primary closure with sutures or adhesives is used only for clean, uncontaminated wounds. Secondary closure is used mainly for contaminated wounds; wounds are left open so they can be filled in by the normal healing process under the close supervision of a physician. Tertiary closure (delayed primary closure) is for contaminated and extensive wounds. With this approach, wounds are left open for several days to initiate the healing process and are then later sealed by primary closure techniques.[10]

The primary goal in wound healing is to minimize scarring, and scarring is closely related to the type of dressing used; occlusive dressings result in less scarring than gauze dressings.[26] The timing of the dressing placement is also important; immediate occlusion leads to resurfacing of epithelium faster than delayed occlusion.[26] Turner has developed a set of criteria for the optimal dressing[22]: the ideal dressing (1) removes excess exudate, (2) maintains a moist environment, (3) is permeable to oxygen, (4) thermally insulates the wound, (5) protects the wound from infection, (6) is free of particulate or toxic contaminants, and (7) can be removed without disrupting delicate new tissue.[22] A plethora of solutions and coverings for wounds are available today, and the range of choices may be overwhelming to an individual trying to choose an appropriate dressing. Jeter and Tintle have developed a schema to assist clinicians in choosing the most appropriate dressing for their patients' wounds (Figure 4).[38]

Most superficial wounds (minor abrasions and lacerations) that pharmacists encounter may simply require the application of adhesive bandages such as Band-Aids. Pharmacists should consider the various features of these

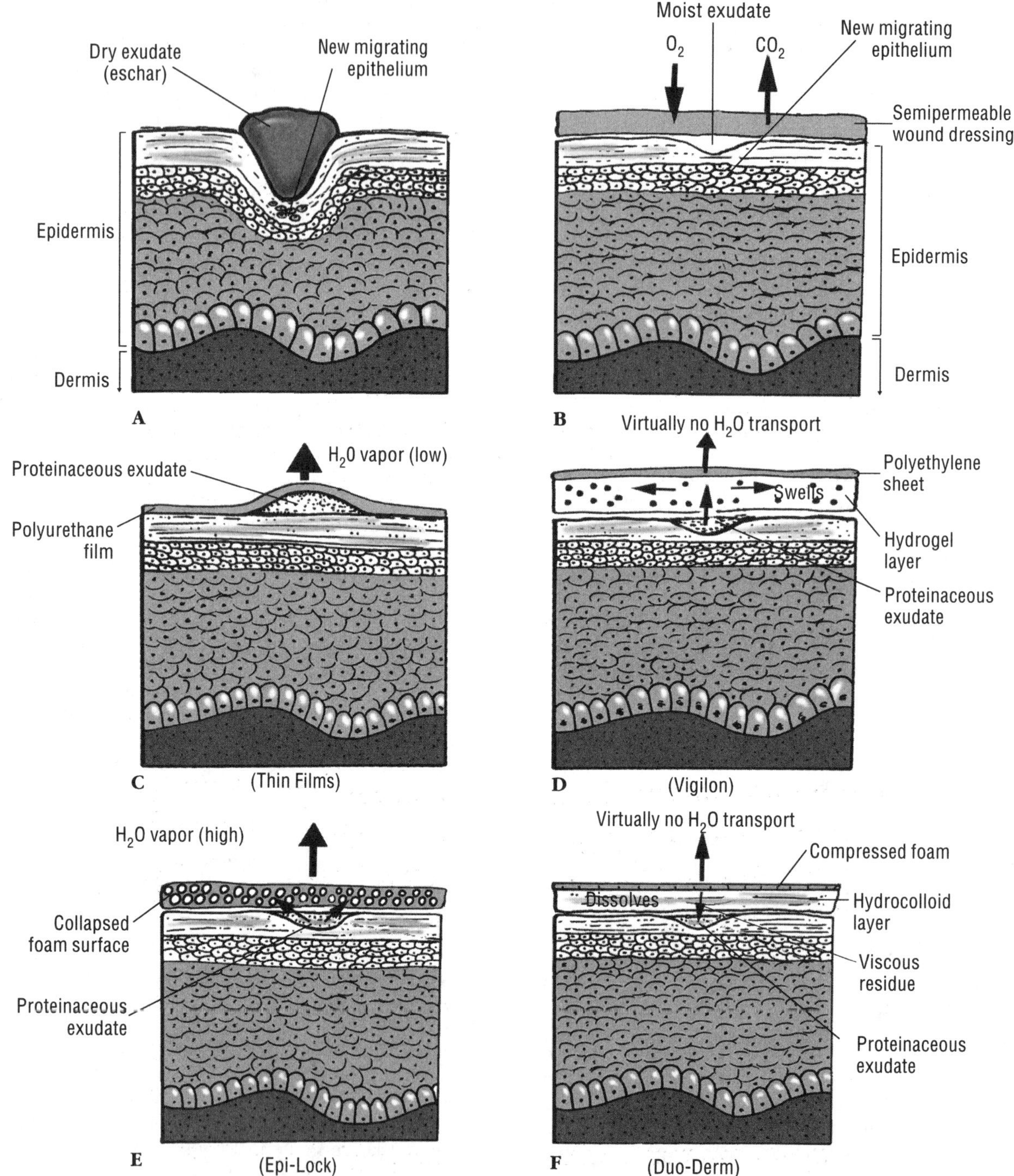

FIGURE 5 Mechanisms by which semipermeable wound dressings create a moist environment for wound healing. A: Regenerating epidermal cells are forced to "tunnel" below the dry wound eschar to attain wound closure. This tunneling delays wound closure. B: Semipermeable wound dressings prevent formation of eschar by maintaining an optimal moisture level at the wound bed. Unhindered by the presence of a dry eschar, migrating epithelial cells are able to migrate and close the wound. C: Mechanism of water vapor transmission in thin films. D: Mechanism of action of a hydrogel wound dressing (Vigilon). E: Mechanism of action of a hydrophilic polyurethane foam dressing (Epi-Lock). F: Mechanisms of action of a hydrocolloid wound dressing (DuoDerm).

Adapted with permission from Szycher M, Lee SJ. Modern wound dressings: a systemic approach to wounds. *J Biomater Appl.* 1992; 7(2): 142–213.

bandages (eg, contour, size, padding, allergenicity, impregnation with medication) in their recommendations for patients. As discussed previously, the more extensive wounds require the pharmacist to triage the patient to a physician or a wound care specialist for further evaluation. Table 4 and Figure 5C–F describe and illustrate the major categories of wound care products available today and provide an overview of their indications, advantages, and disadvantages. Although none of these products meets all of Turner's criteria, many do approach his description of the optimal dressing.

Treatment of Acute Wounds

After performing an initial assessment of an acute wound (Figure 6), the pharmacist should counsel the patient to do the following:

- Position the wound above the level of the heart to slow bleeding and relieve throbbing pain.
- If it is dirty, clean the wound with mild soap and water or a mild wound cleanser that is not toxic to cells, avoiding antiseptic solutions unless they are extremely dilute.
- Occlude the wound with a dressing that will keep the wound site moist and is an appropriate size and contour for the affected body part.
- Avoid disrupting the dressing unnecessarily; change it only if it is dirty or not intact. (Frequent changes may remove resurfacing layers of epithelium and slow the healing process.)
- Use a mild analgesic to control pain.
- Observe the wound for signs of infection. (Redness, swelling, and exudate are a normal part of healing; foul odor is not.)
- Consult a physician if infection is suspected.
- Consult a physician if the wound occurred in dirty conditions and the patient's tetanus immunization status is uncertain.

Treatment of Chronic Wounds

The basic instructions for treating acute wounds may not apply to chronic wounds. For that reason, patients who have chronic wounds should be advised to seek medical advice concerning wound care. These patients should also:

- Consult a physician about any slow-healing wound because the underlying defect in healing probably requires systemic treatment as well as local wound care;
- Prevent pressure ulcers by repositioning the body regularly and often and using pressure-relieving devices;
- Watch for early signs of skin redness over bony prominences as prompt intervention can prevent skin breakdown.

Superficial Skin Infections

Bacterial skin infection may occur secondary to a contaminated wound or may present as a primary pyodermic infection. Pyoderma is a broad term that refers to cutaneous bacterial infection characterized by crusted, oozing lesions with variable amounts of purulence and tenderness.[39] If the infection is deep or extensive, systemic toxicity may occur as manifested by an elevation in temperature and leukocytosis. Pyodermic infection may be either primary (no previous dermatoses exist) or secondary (a predisposing problem preceded the infection). Cultures of primary cutaneous lesions most often reveal *S aureus* and Group A *Streptococcus*. Gram-negative *P aeruginosa* may be present in secondary pyodermas, which are especially prevalent on warm, moist skin such as axillae, ear canals, and interdigital spaces.

Normally, the stratum corneum has only about 10% water content, which is enough to ensure elasticity but is generally below that needed to support luxuriant microbial growth.[4] However, an increase in moisture content may allow microbial growth, leading to infection. A break in the intact skin surface has a deleterious effect on the skin's defensive properties, allowing large numbers of pathogenic organisms to be introduced into the inner layers. In addition, the risk of infection may be increased by excessive scrubbing and irritation of the skin (especially with strong detergents), excessive exposure to water, prolonged occlusion, excessively elevated skin temperature, or local injury. Therefore, the presence and severity of microbial skin infection generally depend on the number of pathogenic organisms present, the condition of the skin's defense mechanisms, and the supportive nutrient environment for those organisms.

Types of Infection

The main pyodermic infections are impetigo, ecthyma (ulcerative impetigo), erysipeloid, folliculitis, furuncles and carbuncles, and erythrasma.[40]

Impetigo (Primary)

Impetigo is a very superficial infection of the skin due to either *S aureus*, Group A beta-hemolytic *Streptococci*, or a mixed infection. Impetigo is most common in preschool children and young adults. Direct contact with the infected exudate may result in transmission of the organisms. Predisposing factors include crowded living conditions, poor hygiene, and neglected minor trauma. Lesions first appear as small red spots that may evolve into characteristic vesicles filled with amber fluid. Exudate accumulates and forms yellow or brown crusts (scabs) on the skin surface, often surrounded by erythematous skin. Eruptions may be annular (circular) with clear central areas, or they may be clustered or grouped. Lesions typically last for days, accompanied by variable pruritus. Satellite lesions occur by autoinoculation. Face, arms, legs, and buttocks are common affected areas. Glomerulonephritis with certain streptococcal strains may be a complication.[40] (See color plates, photograph 20.)

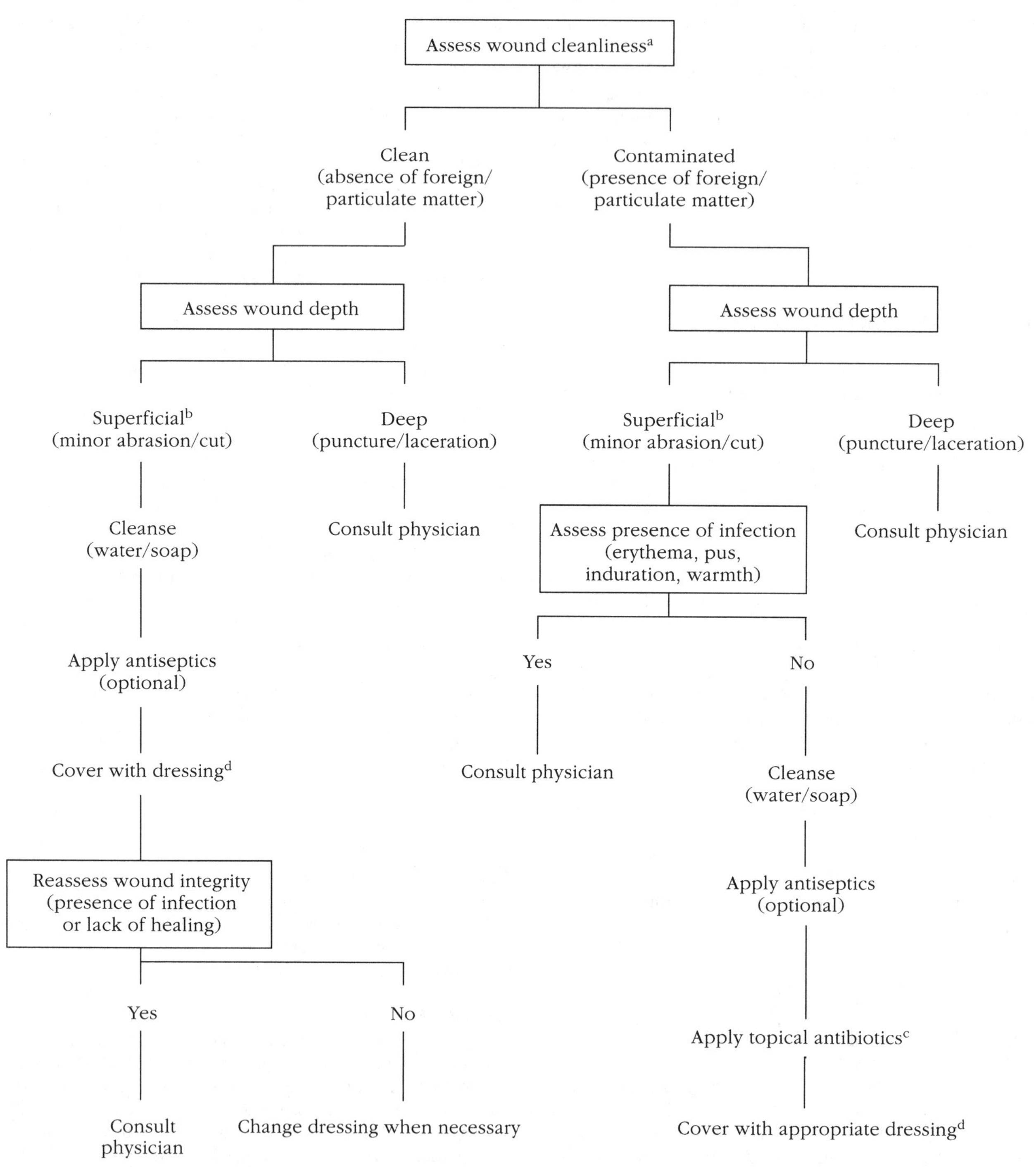

[a]Ensure that patient's tetanus immunization is up-to-date.
[b]Consider physician referral if affected area involves the face, mucous membrane, or genitalia or if patient has comorbid conditions.
[c]If healing does not occur within 5 days, consult physician.
[d]Refer to Table 4 and Figure 4.

FIGURE 6 Initial assessment of acute wounds.

Ecythma (Ulcerative Impetigo)

Ecythma refers to an ulcerative bacterial infection caused most frequently by Group A *Streptococci* or *Staphylococci* or both. Children, adolescents, and elderly persons are commonly affected. Ecythma is a lesion of neglect, which develops in excoriations, insect bites, minor trauma in elderly patients, soldiers, sewage workers, alcoholics, and homeless people. The lesion usually begins as an erythematous pustule that rapidly erodes and becomes crusted. These lesions extend much deeper into the dermis than those in impetigo. They have a scattered, discrete arrangement and are commonly distributed on ankles, dorsa of feet, thighs, and buttocks. Lesions are pruritic and tender; they last for weeks and often heal with a scar.[40]

Erysipeloid

Erysipeloid ("crab dermatitis") is an acute but slowly evolving cellulitis occurring at sites of inoculation, most commonly the hands. Often occupational, it is associated with handling fish, shellfish, meat, poultry, hides, and bones. Infection follows an abrasion, scratch, or puncture wound that occurs while organic material containing *Erysipelothrix rhusiopathiae*, a gram-positive rod, is being handled. The incubation period is 1–4 days. The highest incidence occurs in adult men during summer and early fall. Erysipeloid has a characteristic, violaceous, sharply marginated lesion composed of macules and plaques. The lesion is slightly tender and warm but not hot. Skin symptoms include itching, burning, throbbing, and pain. Occasional lymphangitis or lymphadenitis may occur. Erysipeloid is usually self-limited, subsiding in about 3 weeks. Relapse may occur. Endocarditis or septic arthritis may rarely complicate bacteremia.[40] (See color plates, photograph 21.)

Folliculitis

Folliculitis is a superficial, often bacterial inflammation of hair follicles that heals without scarring. Skin areas regularly exposed to tar, grease, mineral oil, adhesive plaster, and plastic occlusive dressings are most susceptible to folliculitis. *S aureus* folliculitis is aggravated by shaving (eg, beard area, axillae, legs). Skin lesions commonly last for days. They appear dirty yellow or gray with erythema. Affected areas are usually nontender or slightly tender and pruritic.[40] (See color plates, photograph 22.)

Furuncles and Carbuncles

A furuncle is an acute, deep-seated, tender, erythematous, inflammatory nodule that evolves from a staphylococcal folliculitis. A carbuncle is a conglomerate of multiple coalescing furuncles. Children, adolescents, and young adults are frequently affected, and there is an increased incidence in boys. A chronic staphylococcal carrier state in nostrils or perineum, friction from collars or belts, obesity, and bactericidal defects (eg, defects in cellular chemotaxis) are all predisposing factors. Chronic cases of these pyodermas should be referred to a physician for evaluation of a possible underlying disease.[40]

In these pyodermas, the lesion may start as superficial folliculitis but may develop into deep nodules. The initial erythema and swelling stage is followed by a thinning of the skin around the primary follicle, centralized pustulation, destruction of the pilosebaceous structure, discharge of the central necrotic plug, and eventual ulcer formation. The fully established furuncle is bright red, indurated, and erythematous. These lesions commonly last for days, with associated skin symptoms of throbbing pain and, invariably, exquisite tenderness. Constitutional symptoms include low-grade fever and malaise. At times, furunculosis is complicated by bacteremia and possible hematogenous seeding of heart valves, joints, spine, long bones, and kidneys. Some patients are subject to recurrent furunculosis.[40] (See color plates, photograph 22.)

Erythrasma

Erythrasma is a chronic bacterial infection that is caused by *Corynebacterium minutissimum* and affects the intertriginous areas of the toes, groin, and axillae. Adults are generally affected, with a higher incidence in obese middle-aged blacks. Predisposing factors include diabetes and a warm, humid climate. The skin lesions are sharply marginated, brownish-red, scaly eruptions that may last for months to years. Irritation may be the only skin symptom.[28]

Treatment of Skin Infections

For the treatment of primary impetigo, a systemic or topical prescription antibiotic such as mupirocin is highly effective and preferred.[33,41] Topical nonprescription antibiotic preparations with neomycin, bacitracin, and polymyxin B sulfate seem to be most effective when lesions are superficial and are not extensive.[35] Cleaning the area with mild soap and water and gently removing loose crusts should improve response to topical therapy. Because streptococcal infection can occur in other tissues (eg, renal, heart valve) concurrent with impetigo, most physicians treat impetigo infections with systemic as well as topical products.

For the treatment of ecthyma, folliculitis, and erysipeloid, a systemic antibiotic is usually indicated.[40] The role of topical nonprescription antibiotics in these infections is very limited; their usage is confined to very superficial infections, and their efficacy may be questionable. Furuncles and carbuncles may be resolved with incision, drainage, and the prescription of systemic antibiotics by a physician. Minor cases of erythrasma may respond to showers with povidone-iodine soap.[40] However, in most cases, systemic or topical prescription antibiotics are preferred.

Case Studies

Case 28–1

Patient Complaint/History

A mother presents to the pharmacist with her 5-year-old son NN, who injured his upper left arm 24 hours earlier by scraping it on a tree branch. The wound, which is about 1 in. long, contains no foreign matter or necrotic tissue; however, the pinkish skin surrounding the wound indicates that the slight abrasion is inflamed. NN says that the wound feels warm but does not hurt.

The mother asks whether a triple antibiotic ointment is appropriate to use on the wound. She previously scrubbed the wound with Dial soap and water, applied hydrogen peroxide with a cotton ball, and covered the wound with an adhesive bandage. She has also taken the child's temperature several times and reports that the temperature measurements were normal.

NN's patient profile shows no current medical problems or known drug allergies. The mother confirms that the child is not taking any medications.

Clinical Considerations/Strategies

The following considerations/strategies are provided to aid the reader in (1) determining whether treatment of the patient's condition with nonprescription medications is warranted, (2) selecting the appropriate nonprescription medication, and (3) developing a patient counseling strategy to ensure optimal therapeutic outcomes:

- Assess the appropriateness of the mother's cleaning of the wound. If warranted, propose an alternative cleaning procedure.
- Explain to the mother why the wound is warm and the skin surrounding it is pink.
- Respond to the mother's question about using the triple antibiotic ointment on the wound.
- Identify symptoms that would warrant contacting the child's physician.
- Develop a patient education/counseling strategy that will:
  - Explain the appropriate technique and procedure for cleaning the wound and maintaining wound hygiene;
  - Explain how to monitor the wound and what changes in the wound's appearance warrant contacting the child's physician;
  - Explain when and how to apply topical medications to the wound;
  - Explain the appropriate type of dressing to use in covering the wound, how often to change the dressing, and when to stop using a dressing.

Case 28–2

Patient Complaint/History

JJ, a 25-year-old male college student, presents to the pharmacist with a 2-day-old wound. The puncture wound, located on his left leg above the knee, was treated by a physician; the wound did not require stitches. The wound, however, is now oozing a yellowish liquid that has a slight odor. JJ says that he is taking acetaminophen 1,000 mg q6h for minor pain associated with the wound; he does not have a fever.

When questioned about his care of the wound, the patient responds that he is following the physician's instructions: cleaning the wound with antiseptic soap and water and applying Polysporin daily. Because his mother told him that covering the wound would speed up the healing, JJ is also covering the wound with gauze dressing and adhesive tape.

JJ's patient profile shows that he has been taking Florinef Acetate (fludrocortisone acetate) 0.1 mg daily for the past 5 years. The patient appears to be thin and underweight.

Clinical Considerations/Strategies

The following considerations/strategies are provided to aid the reader in (1) determining whether treatment of the patient's condition with nonprescription medications is warranted, (2) selecting the appropriate nonprescription medication, and (3) developing a patient counseling strategy to ensure optimal therapeutic outcomes:

- Determine the cause of the exudate and odor.
- Determine why the wound is not healing as expected.
- Identify the most common microorganisms that infect this type of wound.
- Determine whether the patient should see his physician again.
- Develop a patient education/counseling strategy that will:
  - Explain the appropriate procedure for cleaning and dressing the wound;
  - Explain how to monitor the wound and what changes in the wound's appearance warrant contacting a physician;
  - Explain that, even when treated superficially with topical antibiotics, some wounds become infected by nonsusceptible bacteria.

References

1. Winter GD. Formation of scab and rate of epithelialization on superficial wounds in the skin of the domestic pig. *Nature.* 1962; 193: 293–4.
2. Hinman CC, Maibach HI, Winter GD. Effect of air exposure and occlusion on experimental skin wound. *Nature.* 1963; 200: 377.
3. Bryant R. Wound repair: a review. *J Enterostomal Ther.* 1987; 14(6): 262–3.
4. Bauer EA, Tabas M, Goslen JB. Skin: cells, matrix and function. In: Kelly WN, ed. *Textbook of Internal Medicine.* 1st ed. Philadelphia: JB Lippincott; 1989: 971–4.
5. Norris SO. Physiology of wound healing and risk factors that impede. *AACN Clin Issues Crit Care Nurs.* 1990; 1(3): 545–52.
6. Cooper DM. Optimizing wound healing: a practice within nursing's domain. *Nurs Clin North Am.* 1990; 25(1): 165–80.
7. Skover GR. Cellular and biochemical dynamics of wound repair: wound environment in collagen regeneration. *Clin Podiatr Med Surg.* 1991; 8(4): 723–56.
8. Servold SA. Growth factor impact on wound healing. *Clin Podiatr Med Surg.* 1991; 8(4): 937–96.
9. Howell SM. Current and future trends in wound healing. *Emerg Med Clin North Am.* 1992; 10(4): 655–63.
10. Szycher M, Lee SJ. Modern wound dressings: a systemic approach to wounds. *J Biomater Appl.* 1992; 7(2): 142–213.
11. McGrath MH. Peptide growth factors and wound healing. *Clin Plast Surg.* 1990; 17(3): 421–32.
12. Brown GL et al. Enhancement of wound healing by topical treatment with epidermal growth factor. *N Engl J Med.* 1989; 321: 76–9.
13. Hunt TK, LaVan FB. Enhancement of wound healing by growth factors. *N Engl J Med.* 1989; 321: 111–42.
14. Pierce GF et al. Transforming growth factor beta reverses glucocorticoid-induced wound healing deficits in rats: possible

regulation in macrophages by platelet-derived growth factor. *Proc Natl Acad Sci.* 1989; 86: 2229–33.

15. Albritton JS. Complications of wound repair. *Clin Podiatr Med Surg.* 1991; 8(4): 773–85.
16. Reed BR, Clark R. Cutaneous tissue repair: practical implications of current knowledge. *J Am Acad Dermatol.* 1985; 13: 919–36.
17. Chvapil M. Zinc and other factors of the pharmacology of wound healing. In: Hunt TK,ed. *Wound Healing and Wound Infection: Theory and Surgical Practice.* New York: Appleton-Century-Crofts; 1980: 143–5.
18. Tepelidis NT. Wound healing in the elderly. *Clin Podiatr Med Surg.* 1991; 8(4): 817–26.
19. Rodgers KG. The rational use of antimicrobial agents in simple wounds. *Emerg Med Clin North Am.* 1992; 10(4): 55–66.
20. Ahonen J, Jiborn H, Zederfedlt B. Hormonal influence on wound healing. In: Hunt TK, ed. *Wound Healing and Wound Infection: Theory and Surgical Practice.* New York: Appleton-Century-Crofts; 1980: 100–2.
21. Mulder GD, Daly T. In: Cloth LC, McCullough JM, Feeder J, eds. *Wound Healing Alternatives in Management.* Philadelphia: FA Davis; 1990: 43–51.
22. Turner TD. Recent advances in wound management products. In: Turner TD, ed. *Advances in Wound Management.* London: John Wiley & Sons; 1986.
23. Guggisberg E et al. New perspectives in the treatment of decubitus ulcers. *J Palliat Care.* 1992; 8(2): 5–12.
24. Romanko KP. Pressure ulcers. *Clin Podiatr Med Surg.* 1991; 8(4): 857–68.
25. Jordon R. *Wound Management: A Treatment Plan.* Paper presented at the Kirklin Clinic: Nursing Continuing Education Seminar; July 1994.
26. Bolton L, van Rijswijk L. Wound dressings: meeting clinical and biological needs. *Dermatology.* 1991; 3(3): 146–61.
27. McKenna PJ et al. Antiseptic effectiveness with fibroblast preservation. *Ann Plast Surg.* 1991; 27: 265–8.
28. Leaper DJ. Prophylactic and therapeutic role of antibiotics in wound care. *Am J Surg.* 1994; 167(1A suppl): 155–205.
29. *Federal Register.* 1991 Jul; 56: 33677.
30. Brown CD, Zitelli JA. A review of topical agents for wounds and methods of wounding: guidelines for wound management. *J Dermatol Surg Oncol.* 1993; 19: 732–7.
31. Goldenheim PD. An appraisal of povidone–iodine and wound healing. *Postgrad Med J.* 1993; 69(suppl 3): S97–105.
32. Swaim SF. Bandages and topical agents. *Vet Clin North Am.* 1990; 20(1): 47–65.
33. Bolton L, Fattu AJ. Topical agents and wound healing. *Clin Dermatol.* 1994; 22(1): 95–120.
34. *Federal Register.* 1987; 52: 47312–4.
35. Sanford JP. *Guide to Antimicrobial Therapy.* Dallas: Antimicrobial Therapy; 1994.
36. Gette MT, Marks JG, Maloney ME. Frequency of post-operative allergic contact dermatitis to topical antibiotics. *Arch Dermatol.* 1992; 128: 365–7.
37. Hirschmann JV. Topical antibiotics in dermatology. *Arch Dermatol.* 1988; 124: 1697.
38. Jeter KF, Tintle TE. Wound dressings of the nineties: indications and contraindications. *Clin Podiatr Med Surg.* 1991; 8(4): 799–816.
39. Tabas M, Goslen JB, Bauer EA. Infections of skin. In: Kelly WN, ed. *Textbook of Internal Medicine.* 1st ed. Philadelphia: JB Lippincott; 1989: 1046.
40. Fitzpatrick TB et al. In: *Color Atlas and Synopsis of Clinical Dermatology: Common and Serious Diseases.* 2nd ed. New York: McGraw Hill; 1992: 82–96.
41. Strock LL et al. Topical bactroban (mupirocin): efficacy in treating burn wounds infected with methicillin-resistant staphylococci. *J Burn Care Rehab.* 1990; 11: 454–9.

CHAPTER 29

Diaper Rash, Prickly Heat, and Adult Incontinence Products

Gary H. Smith, Victor A. Elsberry, and Martin D. Higbee

Questions to ask in patient assessment and counseling

Diaper Rash

- *Do you use disposable diapers or a diaper service?*
- *Do you use cloth diapers? How do you launder them?*
- *Do you use double diapers or plastic pants?*
- *How often do you change the baby's diapers?*
- *How do you clean the baby's skin during a diaper change?*
- *What products have you tried for the rash?*
- *Does the baby have a fever?*
- *Has the baby had diarrhea recently?*
- *Has the baby ever had a yeast infection in the diaper area?*
- *Has any new type of food recently been added to the baby's diet?*
- *Is there a family history of allergic disorders?*
- *Is the baby being given any medication? If so, what and by what route?*

Prickly Heat

- *Where is the rash located and what does it look like?*
- *How long has the rash been present?*
- *Does the patient sleep in a warm and humid room?*
- *How much clothing does the patient wear during the day and night?*
- *What products have you already tried for the rash?*

Adult Urinary Incontinence

- *Has the incontinence been evaluated by a physician?*
- *What type of urinary incontinence does the patient have?*
- *What time of the day is protection needed most? Least?*
- *Does the patient need assistance in changing or using absorbent materials?*
- *What products have been used to treat or prevent rash? Odor?*

Editor's Note: This chapter is based, in part, on a chapter with a similar title that appeared in the 10th edition but was written by Gary H. Smith.

Diaper rash and prickly heat (miliaria rubra) are acute, transient, inflammatory skin conditions that occur in many infants, young children, and adults, especially those who are urine incontinent. Both conditions cause burning and itching that can result in restlessness, irritability, and sleep interruptions. Prevention is the best cure.

For skin to function efficiently, it should remain dry, smooth, and slightly acidic. The skin of most adults is 1.5–4 mm thick, including the dermis and epidermis. Infants' skin, however, is only about 1 mm thick[1] and thus is more delicate and susceptible to injury. Because the epidermis (the outermost skin layer), which accounts for 5% of the total skin thickness, is only 0.05–0.1 mm thick in infants, the external barrier that protects the infant from the environment is very thin and vulnerable.[1] The infant's thin skin, which is exposed to a greater degree of hydration, is also more susceptible to absorption of topically applied agents that are potentially toxic.[1,2]

Diaper Rash

Diaper rash, or diaper dermatitis, is one of the most common dermatitides in infants. A 1986 survey of 1,089 infants aged 1–20 months showed a frequency of diaper rash approaching 65%, with most cases being mild or of minor severity. Only about 5% of the infants had severe dermatitis; the remainder of the cases were classified as moderate. The incidence of diaper rash peaked between 9 and 12 months of age.[3] A 1992 study of 200 infants between 3 and 24 months of age found the frequency of episodes of diaper dermatitis to be 15.2%, with the peak incidence occurring between 3 and 6 months of age (19.4%).[4] Diaper rash can also develop in incontinent adults.

In 1990, the Food and Drug Administration (FDA) modified the advisory review panel's definition of diaper rash, defining it as an inflammatory skin condition in the diaper area (perineum, buttocks, lower abdomen, and inner thighs) caused by one or more of the following factors: moisture, occlusion, chafing, continued contact with urine or feces or both, or mechanical or chemical irritation. Mild conditions appear as simple erythema. More severe conditions include papules, vesicles, oozing, and ulceration.[5–8]

Etiology

Urine and feces have long been implicated as contributors to the development of diaper rash. Normal newborns begin urinating within 24 hours after birth. Urination occurs up to 20 times daily until approximately 2 months of age and as often as eight times daily from 2 months to 8 years of age. Defecation also occurs several times daily in infants. Breast-fed infants tend to urinate less often and have a lower incidence of diaper-area dermatitis than bottle-fed infants.[9] Furthermore, the urine and feces of nursing infants tend to be less alkaline and therefore less irritating than those of bottle-fed infants.[3,10] A 1993 study has shown that early introduction of solid food has no effect on the incidence of diaper rash in infants who are breast-fed or bottle-fed.[10] However, high-protein foods may make the urine and stools more acidic and produce an "acid scald."[11] Such foods in the baby's diet may also be contributing factors in diaper rash. Complications may occur, including secondary infections caused by various microorganisms.

The distribution of diaper rash may be positional. If the baby lies on its stomach, the rash may be ventral; if the baby lies on its back, the rash may be dorsally located. It may spread to the entire diaper area, depending on the cause of the rash and the promptness of therapy. The diaper area is vulnerable to inflammation because the skin is thin, warm, and moist and is exposed to irritants and bacteria.

The pathologic changes vary with the causative factors and the severity of the dermatitis. Diaper rash may range from mild erythema with or without maceration and chafing to vesicles, pustules, or bullae. Deeper nodular and infiltrated lesions may develop, depending on the primary cause of the dermatitis. Seborrhea, psoriasis, and atopic dermatitis may predispose the skin to irritation and infection.

Ammonia

According to the ammonia theory of diaper rash, ammonia formed from the action of bacteria on urine increases the environmental pH and activates fecal enzymes that facilitate entry of irritants into the skin.[4] However, the FDA believes that this theory, although perhaps not yet totally disproved, has been discredited by recent studies. None of the data submitted to the FDA is sufficiently compelling to support claims based on the activity of antimicrobials against specific urea-splitting bacteria.

Infant urine does not cause significant skin irritation for up to 48 hours, but skin damage can occur after 10 days of continuous exposure.[12] Feces, in the absence of urine or ammonia, have been shown to cause skin irritation. The presence of feces in the diaper area is substantially more likely to promote diaper rash than is the presence of urine. This explains the increased occurrence of diaper rash in infants with diarrhea or frequent stools.[3,4,12,13]

Moisture Retention

Skin wetness, measured as transepidermal water loss, has been shown to be a factor in the development of diaper dermatitis.[14] If a soiled diaper is not changed promptly, the stratum corneum in the diaper area becomes waterlogged. This saturation causes keratotic plugging of the sweat glands, which results in sweat retention and may produce vesicles and irritation (ie, prickly heat or miliaria). Thus, the role of urine in the genesis of diaper rash may simply be a function of overhydration of the skin in the diaper area. Wet skin is more permeable than dry skin to low-molecular weight compounds and therefore is more susceptible to irritation.[4,14,15]

Mechanical and Chemical Irritants

Tightly fitting diapers covered with plastic pants or disposable diapers with a plastic bottom increase moisture and temperature in the diaper area and prevent air from circulating around the skin. This environment not only causes prickly heat and more maceration than occurs with the use of cloth diapers alone, but also is conducive to irritation and secondary infection. Irritation results from chafing, as when rough cloth or tight or stiff plastic diapers constantly rub against the skin, and eroded skin is more susceptible to infection. Frequent changing of diapers may prevent or minimize irritation.

Chemical irritants from various sources may precipitate a rash in the diaper area. (See color plates, photograph 23.) Feces remaining in contact with the skin cause irritation, especially if the infant's diet promotes the elimination of irritating substances and unabsorbed foodstuffs or causes diarrhea. Preparations applied to the diaper area, such as proprietary antiseptic agents and harsh soaps containing phenol, tars, salicylic acid, or sulfur, also may cause diaper rash. Diapers rinsed inadequately after washing may retain residues from detergents or bleach that can irritate the diaper area or cause allergic reactions. Precautions should be taken to avoid exposing the sensitive skin of infants and young children to these irritating substances.

Complications of Diaper Rash

Fungal and bacterial infections are the most common complications of diaper rash. These cutaneous infections are often secondary to untreated or improperly treated diaper dermatitis. The moist, warm, alkaline environment created by unchanged diapers is conducive to the development and multiplication of pathogenic bacteria and fungi.[12] If the skin is eroded or macerated or if the normal balance of the skin's bacterial flora is disturbed, these organisms may become pathogenic and cause infection in the diaper area.[9]

Fungal Infection

Fungal infections of the diaper area have long been considered a secondary complication of diaper dermatitis, but recent evidence suggests that they may be a primary cause. Therefore, they should be considered in all cases of severe diaper dermatitis.[3,16] Fungal infections caused by *Candida albicans* are the most common complications of diaper rash. *C albicans*, which may be part of the normal colonic flora, has been cultured from the feces of up to 20% of normal infants[9,16,17]; a strong correlation exists between the presence of *C albicans* in the stool and the severity of the diaper dermatitis.[9] *C albicans* proliferates to produce a characteristic, bright red, sharply marginated rash with satellite pustules and erosions. The only precise method of diagnosis, however, is culturing the organism from scrapings or swabs of the skin lesions. A potassium hydroxide preparation from skin scrapings may be highly suggestive of *C albicans* infection.[13]

In newborns younger than 2 weeks, candidal diaper dermatitis is usually accompanied by oral thrush. Both conditions probably result from a maternal candidal vaginal infection before and during delivery. The lesions are usually erythematous and are surrounded by characteristic satellite pustules. They may become eroded and begin weeping. A physician should be consulted for appropriate treatment of this condition.

The systemic use of some broad-spectrum antibiotics may predispose the infant to diaper candidiases caused by an overgrowth of *C albicans* in the stool. Infants with severe diaper dermatitis who are concurrently receiving a broad-spectrum antibiotic should be evaluated for candidiasis by a physician.[18] Infectious complications of diaper rash caused by other dermatophytes, including *Epidermophyton floccosum*,[19–21] *Trichophyton rubrum*,[22] and *Trichophyton verrucosum*,[23] have also been reported.

Bacterial Infection

Bacterial infection of the diaper area is caused most commonly by *Staphylococcus aureus* and is often seen as a form of folliculitis. Classic lesions are follicular micropustules that coalesce with adjacent lesions to form lakes or pustules. Occasionally, bullous or encrusted impetigo, characterized by large, blister-like lesions or honeycomb crusting, may occur. In some cases, group A *Streptococcus pyogenes* may be the pathogen. An infant with a suspected bacterial infection in the diaper area should be referred to a physician for appropriate diagnosis and treatment.[3]

Viral Infection

Herpetiform diaper dermatitis has recently been reported and should be considered when a parent of an infant has an active herpes simplex infection.[24] Jacquet's diaper dermatitis is a primary irritant diaper dermatitis characterized by well-demarcated ulcers or erosions with elevated borders. Its frequency has decreased with the increased use of disposable diapers.[25] Cytomegalovirus diaper rash has now been reported in infants born with congenital human immunodeficiency virus (HIV) and therefore should be considered in such patients.[26]

Other Diaper Dermatitides

Other conditions that may present as diaper dermatitis include granuloma gluteale infantum,[27] Kawasaki syndrome,[28] atopic dermatitis, infantile seborrheic dermatitis, acute histiocytosis X, psoriasis vulgaris, congenital syphilis, acrodermatitis enteropathica, and biotin deficiency.[29] Kawasaki syndrome should be suspected if an erythematous, desquamating perineal rash appears in diapered infants or young children who also have symptoms such as fever, lymphadenopathy, a "strawberry geographic" tongue, or a rash elsewhere, especially on the ears and fingertips. Perianal pseudoverrucous papules and nodules are usually described in association with urostomies but have also been described in children as the result of fecal or urinary incontinence.[30]

Ulceration of the penile meatus may be a painful complication of diaper rash in babies who are circumcised. The pain associated with this condition may lead to reflex inhibition of micturition and secondary distention of the bladder.

Assessment of Diaper Rash

The pharmacist may be able to determine the cause of many conditions by questioning the parents. For example, the pharmacist should determine whether nondisposable cloth diapers are being used and whether diapers are being laundered with detergents containing irritants. In general, if diaper dermatitis is confined to the diaper area and does not present symptoms of fungal or bacterial infection, the pharmacist may recommend a nonprescription protectant product. If the infant has had diaper rash for only a few days, treatment by the parent may be recommended. If diaper rash persists 1 week or more after the infant has been treated with protectants and diapers have been changed frequently, or if the rash recurs often or is resistant to nonprescription treatment, the rash may be caused by a problem other than the diaper and a physician should be consulted. If the infant has had persistent diarrhea, appears irritable, or has a fever, a physician should be consulted because the problem may be more serious than simple diaper rash.

If the rash occurs on areas outside the diaper area (groin, intergluteal fold, and lower abdomen), infants should be diagnosed and treated by a physician. A condition such as atopic dermatitis, psoriasis, seborrheic dermatitis, allergic contact dermatitis, or scabies may be present. If the lesions are follicular micropustules or bullae or if they look like impetigo, a bacterial infection may be the cause.

In addition to explaining the steps that must be taken to prevent diaper rash as well as prickly heat, the pharmacist may recommend several nonprescription products suited to the child's condition. However, if the rash has persisted and appears to be complicated by infection or another process, the pharmacist should suggest that the child be taken to a physician.

Treatment of Diaper Rash

Primary Treatment

The active treatment of diaper rash involves (1) removing the source of irritation, (2) reducing the immediate skin reaction, (3) relieving discomfort, and (4) preventing secondary infection and other complications. The FDA has stated that ordinary mild diaper rash, characterized by erythema of the buttocks, perineum, and lower abdomen, responds to very frequent diaper changes, cleansing with water, and removal of plastic occlusion.[6–9] Thus, the area should be kept as dry and clean as possible; the diaper should be loose and well ventilated, and should be changed as quickly as possible after becoming soiled; and the diaper area should be dried completely before a new diaper is used. Plain water should be used to cleanse the diaper area to avoid sensitizing chemicals in soaps and commercial wipes. Cornstarch is a safe and effective dusting powder; it does not promote the growth of bacteria or fungi, as was once thought.[31] Careful use of a hair blow-dryer on a low setting to dry the area is effective and safer than a heat lamp. The use of a good protective agent, such as zinc oxide paste (Lassar's paste), Desitin, or white petrolatum, provides a barrier to protect the skin from moisture. Plastic pants should be avoided.

The pharmacist should be able to advise parents about which products to use for a particular kind of dermatitis and what specific care is required. As with most forms of therapy, the simplest regimen is the one most likely to be followed consistently. A baby's skin is sensitive, and many babies may be irritated by or allergic to some available products.

Pharmacologic Agents

In 1990,the FDA issued notices of proposed rulemakings for the four types of product ingredients used in the treatment of diaper rash and prickly heat (see product table "Diaper Rash and Prickly Heat Products"). These products include antimicrobials, external analgesics, skin protectants, and antifungals.[5–8] The FDA provided guidelines for study protocols to demonstrate safety and efficacy in clinical trials.

In a final rule dated December 18, 1992, the FDA declared that diaper rash claims should be removed from all nonprescription antifungals and external analgesics because adequate evidence of their safety and efficacy was lacking. As of June 18, 1993, any claim that such products are safe or efficacious in treating or preventing diaper rash has been considered misbranding. The FDA has encouraged the voluntary removal of such products from the market as soon as possible. Approved new drug applications are required for such products to be marketed as prescription drugs.

External Analgesics The FDA considered deficient any clinical data demonstrating that nonprescription external analgesics are safe and effective in treating or preventing diaper rash. It further noted that since infants and young children, the potential users of these products, cannot adequately communicate symptoms to a parent or caregiver, no objective assessment of need can be appropriately determined.

Antifungals The FDA also determined that antifungal active ingredients should not be included in nonprescription diaper rash products. This is because fungal infections associated with diaper rash are not suitable for diagnosis and treatment by parents or caregivers and therefore should be brought to the attention of a physician for diagnosis and treatment.

Antimicrobials The FDA currently classifies no nonprescription antimicrobial ingredients in diaper rash products as Category I (safe and effective). It further encourages manufacturers to remove all ingredients in diaper rash products that are not classified as Category I. Category II products include boric acid, hexachlorophene, *p*-chloromercuriphenol, phenol, and resorcinol. One or more Category III products may eventually receive Category I classification, but this remains to be determined. Category III products include benzalkonium chloride, benzethonium chloride, calcium undecylenate, chloroxylenol, methylbenzethonium chloride, oxyquinoline sodium propionate, and triclosan.

Protectants Protectants help prevent or treat diaper rash by acting as a physical barrier to irritants and by sealing out or absorbing moisture. Several protectants are classified as Category I. These include allantoin, calamine, and cod liver oil (in combination); dimethicone, kaolin, and lanolin (in combination); mineral oil; petrolatum; talc; topical cornstarch; white petrolatum; and zinc oxide. Category II products include bismuth subnitrate, boric acid, sulfur, and tannic acid. Category III products include aldioxa, aluminum acetate, aluminum hydroxide, microporous cellulose, cholecalciferol, cocoa butter, colloidal oatmeal, cysteine hydrochloride, dexpanthenol, glycerin, live yeast cell derivative, peruvian balsam oil, protein hydrolysate, racemethionine, shark liver oil, sodium bicarbonate, vitamin A, zinc acetate, and zinc bicarbonate.

Zinc oxide, an excellent protectant found in many products used to treat diaper rash, is a mild astringent with weak antiseptic properties. Many preparations contain various concentrations of zinc oxide and petrolatum. Zinc oxide paste USP, the simplest of these formulations, contains 25% zinc oxide, 25% cornstarch, and 50% white petrolatum. This combination serves as a highly protective and water-absorptive base; parents should be informed that this paste is most easily removed with mineral oil. Many preparations contain zinc oxide in a higher concentration than that contained in Lassar's paste. (Desitin contains 40% zinc oxide.) Most of the preparations also contain one or more of various other protectant medications, such as cod liver oil, vitamins A and D, lanolin, peruvian balsam, and silicone.

In general, these products are popular and are promoted primarily for the treatment of diaper rash. Only recently have there been controlled studies with these products.[32] Reports from Leeming/Pacquin[32] show Desitin Ointment to be superior to bland soap and unmedicated talcum powder in the treatment of diaper rash. Only two reports have compared one product with the other.[33,34] Lantiseptic Ointment (*p*-chloromercuriphenol [1:1,500] in a lanolin and petrolatum base) was shown in a controlled study to be equal or superior to vitamin A and D ointment in the treatment of diaper rash. Although several anecdotal reports indicate that vitamin A and D ointment or ointments containing cod liver oil may be beneficial in preventing and treating diaper rash, no evidence exists that any of these products is superior to zinc oxide paste or white petrolatum, either of which can be used alone as a protectant and as an initial treatment for diaper rash. Use of these products avoids subjecting the infant to compounds that may cause skin sensitization, such as peruvian balsam. However, whereas zinc oxide paste is absorptive because of the powders in its base, which enable it to take up moisture and thus keep the skin dry, white petrolatum is oleaginous and hydrophobic and cannot absorb any moisture. Therefore, petrolatum may trap moisture beneath it and keep the diaper area hydrated, a condition that is not desirable in cases of prickly heat. White petrolatum is also more irritating to the skin than zinc oxide paste. Of the two products, the one that will keep the diaper area driest and cause the least irritation is zinc oxide paste.

The powdered protectant agents that have been used most often in treating diaper rash and prickly heat are talc, magnesium stearate, calcium carbonate, cornstarch, kaolin, zinc stearate, and microporous cellulose. Talc is a natural hydrous magnesium silicate that allays irritation, prevents chafing, and absorbs sweat. Talc, a finely milled powder that will not cake in the folds and cause maceration by friction, is similar to ointments and creams in that it adheres well to the skin. Magnesium stearate has been included in some dusting powders promoted for use in infants because of its ability to adhere to the skin and to serve as a mechanical barrier to irritants. Calcium carbonate, cornstarch, kaolin, zinc stearate, and microporous cellulose are also included in diaper rash products for their moisture-absorbing properties. When applied after each diaper change, these products serve primarily to keep the diaper area dry. They should be applied with a cotton fluff to spread evenly. However, powders should never be applied to an acute oozing dermatitis because they may promote secondary crusting and infection.

Although it recognized that diaper rash products in a powdered form have been used extensively for many years, the FDA proposed an additional warning for them because of the numerous reported incidents of accidental baby powder inhalation that have appeared in the literature.[7] Inhalation of the dust by the infant may be harmful and could lead to chemical pneumonia. Therefore, parents should be instructed to use powders cautiously and apply them carefully. The FDA has proposed the following warnings for products containing talc: "Do not use on broken skin," and "Keep powder away from child's face to avoid inhalation, which can cause breathing problems." In addition, the FDA has proposed directions for applying powder products: "Apply powder close to the body away from child's face. Carefully shake the powder into the diaper or into the hand and apply to diaper area." A recent report substantiates the potential hazards of powders.[35]

Hydrocortisone The medical community's recognition of the value of topical hydrocortisone for diaper dermatitis does not warrant its use for infants on a nonprescription basis. Because occlusive dressings facilitate the absorption of topically applied steroids, these medications should not be used in the diaper area. When steroids are applied topically to inflamed or abraded skin, increased absorption may cause systemic levels to be higher than when the steroids are applied to normal skin. Also, chronic use of steroids (eg, 0.1% triamcinolone cream) can cause thinning of the skin, with resultant striae and easy bruising.[5–8] Because 0.25%, 0.5%, and 1.0% hydrocortisone ointments and creams are available for nonprescription use, pharmacists should caution parents concerning their use for diaper rash. It has been suggested that hydrocortisone should be reserved for cases in which zinc oxide ointment or similar products and standard preventive measures have not been sufficient. Hydrocortisone is not recommended for use on children under 2 years of age except under the advice and supervision of a physician. The topical use of hydrocortisone for the infant patient without a physician's intervention does not appear to be warranted.

Treatment of Secondary Complications

A rash in the diaper area that does not clear up in a reasonable amount of time may indicate the presence of a secondary bacterial or fungal skin infection. Although, various topical antiseptic agents have been used to treat staphylococcal and streptococcal infections, the FDA believes that antimicrobial (antiseptic) drug products have significant limitations in treating the secondary infections that may accompany irritation caused by diaper rash.[5] Such infections should not be treated with nonprescription drugs. The infant with a suspected bacterial or fungal infection in the diaper area or with diaper rash that has persisted for a week or more should be taken to a physician for appropriate diagnosis and treatment. Some physicians recommend treating these infections in the diaper area with systemic antibiotics or topical antifungals.

Nonprescription topical antibiotics have an adjunctive role, at best, in the treatment of these bacterial infections. Systemic antibiotics are the treatment of choice for impetigo. Quaternary ammonium compounds, such as benzalkonium chloride, are included as antibacterial agents in commercial products; however, their effectiveness has been questioned because these cationic surfactants are inactivated by organic matter included in urine and feces. In addition, these antibacterial compounds may act as irritants in some cases, exacerbating the inflammation and causing discomfort when applied. Antibiotic ointments should be used only when clearly indicated because they may cause hypersensitivity reactions and foster the evolution of resistant organisms. Topical neomycin, a dermal sensitizer, for diaper rash should not be used owing to the high incidence of adverse reactions to neomycin, the increased probability of its absorption through inflamed and occluded skin, and the availability of more appropriate topical antibiotics. Secondary infections that may be caused by bacteria or species of *Candida* or other fungi should be diagnosed and treated by a physician.

Topical 2% miconazole cream and 1% haloprogin cream have been shown to be effective in treating candidal diaper rash.[36,37] Hydroxyquinoline can be applied topically for its antibacterial and antifungal activity. Calcium undecylenate is used for its antifungal activity. Nystatin, amphotericin B, haloprogin cream, and hydroxyquinoline are prescription-only products; aluminum acetate solution, miconazole, clotrimazole, chlorhexidine, and calcium undecylenate are available without prescription. The FDA has concluded that the complications of common diaper rash should be diagnosed and treated by a physician and that antifungals are therefore not suitable for the nonprescription treatment or prevention of diaper rash.

Product Selection Guidelines

Pharmacists should advise patients about the correct use of any product they recommend. Some general precautions should be mentioned, such as use of products prior to their expiration dates and care in applying topical preparations that might sting already irritated skin. If powders are recommended, parents, caregivers, or patients themselves should be instructed to apply them carefully to prevent their accidental inhalation, which could lead to chemical pneumonia. When soaks and solutions (such as aluminum acetate solution) are used, the unused portion should be discarded after each use; that is, only a fresh preparation should be used each time.

Above all, pharmacists should caution parents about the general use of any medication for a baby's skin. The best therapy for diaper dermatitis is to keep the skin clean and dry. This is true for both infants and adults.

Few infants escape diaper rash. The pharmacist may help by teaching parents the proper procedures for preventing diaper rash and prickly heat. Parents should understand that using medications indiscriminately is not the proper way to treat either condition and is ill-advised. Drugs alone cannot stop or prevent diaper rash or prickly heat. Many newborns, infants, and young children may be hypersensitive to various medications, and more harm than good can result from their use.

Prevention of Diaper Rash

Proper Hygiene in Diaper Area

Good prophylactic practices depend on parental cooperation and responsibility. A diaper should be changed as soon as it is soiled; leaving a wet diaper on for several hours increases the chances of diaper rash. The apparently unsoiled part of the diaper should never be used to wipe the baby. This practice spreads microorganisms over the skin, and they may proliferate when the child next urinates or defecates. If frequent changes are impossible, the infant should be kept belly down to reduce the tendency for feces and urine to become compressed under the gluteal area. Nondisposable cloth diapers should be made of soft material and should be fastened loosely to prevent rubbing. Plastic pants should be used as seldom as possible because they are occlusive and impede airflow through the diaper. The use of plastic pants at night and for extended periods should be discouraged, and daily baths should be encouraged.

Infants often urinate soon after they are put to bed for the night. Parents can reduce the time a child is exposed to a wet diaper and the amount of urine accumulated at night by changing the diaper within several hours after putting the child to bed.

The diaper area should be cleaned at each diaper change. Mild soap should be used for cleaning the diaper area and for bathing. It is important that skin folds that entrap perspiration and feces be cleaned thoroughly and rinsed well with clean water. The various diaper wipe products now available may contain antiseptics, soap, and lanolin that may contribute to the rash. Convenience may dictate their use, but caution should be exercised because irritants may be present and because a hypersensitivity reaction may occur. Therefore, if such products must be used, unscented, hypoallergenic wipes are recommended. The diaper area should be completely dry before a clean diaper is put on. Exposing the diaper area to warm, dry air for a few minutes between changes helps to keep the skin dry. A bland ointment or dusting powder (such as zinc oxide ointment, cornstarch, or talcum powder) may be recommended after washing.

Just because an infant wears diapers, however, does not mean that powders and ointments should be applied. If a problem occurs, it should be treated; if it recurs, prophylaxis is warranted. In clinical practice, a significant number of infants with a history of diaper rash fall into this category. This is especially true in those cases of diaper rash induced by antibiotics or specific food groups and in infants with atopic dermatitis. However, most babies who develop diaper rash do respond to treatment and do not need prophylaxis. Babies who require continued prophylaxis should have it stopped periodically to determine whether it is still necessary.[7]

Proper Washing of Cloth Diapers

Diapers should be washed with mild soap. The use of harsh detergents and water softeners should be avoided. After they are washed, diapers should be rinsed thoroughly. If an automatic washing machine is used, repeating the rinse cycle is recommended. Air drying diapers in the sun helps kill bacteria. Ironing dry, washed diapers will reduce any surviving bacteria or fungi.

Adding a disinfectant during the washing process effectively reduces the bacterial count. Adding ordinary laundry bleach to the wash may substantially reduce the number of organisms. The use of clorophene (*o*-benzyl-*p*-chlorophenol) in the first rinse water in a concentration of 1 part clorophene to 2,500 parts water is also effective in treating and preventing diaper dermatitis. Acidification of diapers may also be helpful; this can be accomplished by rinsing the diapers a final time in a solution made by adding one cup of vinegar to a half-filled washing machine tub. The diapers are then added and soaked for 30 minutes.

Use of Disposable versus Cloth Diapers

Over the past 10–15 years, there has been a trend away from the use of cloth diapers. Market research and surveys of parents have shown that 53–71% use only disposable diapers, 22–43% use both, and less than 7% use cloth diapers exclusively.[3,38,39] About 16 billion disposable diapers are bought each year in the United States. The majority of these are Pampers or Luvs from Procter & Gamble or Huggies from Kimberly–Clark.[39]

Several studies have been conducted to compare the incidence of diaper rash in infants diapered with cloth versus infants diapered with the different types of disposable diapers.[3,40–47] Cloth diapers cleaned by a diaper service were associated with the lowest incidence of diaper rash; disposable diapers showed a similar low incidence; and home-laundered diapers, which were not rinsed with a bacteriostatic agent, were associated with the highest incidence. These reports show the necessity of using a bacteriostatic agent either in the rinse water or in the diaper pail. Diapers containing fecal material should be rinsed well in the toilet before being placed in the diaper pail. Commercial diaper services provide essentially sterile diapers.

Over the last 10 years there has been considerable effort on the part of disposable diaper manufacturers to improve their products. Since it has been shown that the major causes of diaper rash are skin wetness, skin damage from fecal protease and lipase enzymes, and pH increase when urine and feces are together in the same area, the focus has been on the development of diapers that control skin wetness and pH.[12,13] The disposable diaper Ultra Pampers contains absorbent gelling material (AGM) consisting of cross-linked sodium polyacrylate. Diapers containing AGM are designed to absorb moisture and bind it tightly to a gel matrix, to provide a buffering system with the AGM's partially neutralized carboxylic acid structure, and to reduce the potential for urine and feces to mix, thereby providing better pH control. Infants who wear the AGM diapers have been found to be substantially drier and to have significantly less diaper rash and less severe diaper rash than infants wearing either conventional disposable or home-laundered diapers. Cloth diapers do not appear to be superior to the improved disposable diapers.[38,41–47]

In a 1988 study in day care centers, 180 children wearing conventional disposable or AGM disposable diapers were evaluated for frequency of diarrhea, antibiotic use, and diaper dermatitis. The children who had diarrhea and were diapered with AGM diapers had a statistically significantly lower grade of diaper rash than infants who had diarrhea and were diapered with conventional diapers. Among children who were taking antibiotics and children who had diarrhea and were also taking antibiotics, diaper dermatitis was less severe in the children wearing AGM diapers than in those wearing conventional diapers. However, the difference was not statistically significant in either case.[43]

Atopic dermatitis occurs in about 10% of children as an inherited skin disease. Because the skin of such children is erythematous and pruritic, it is very sensitive to substances that irritate or dry it. Infants with atopic dermatitis need to maintain epidermal hydration to prevent the skin from becoming brittle and more sensitive to toxins and infections. A 1987 randomized study of 1,800 infants was conducted to evaluate the effects of AGM diapers compared with conventional cellulose disposable diapers and cloth diapers on infants with atopic dermatitis. While there were no differences between AGM diapers and conventional cellulose disposable diapers, infants in the cloth diaper group had consistently worse diaper rash than did the other two groups. Diaper rash in the control group (infants without atopic dermatitis) did not differ with the type of diaper used. However, a comparison of all infants in the atopic dermatitis group with all infants in the control group showed that the control group had less rash at all times during the 30 weeks of the study, indicating that any type of diaper increases the risk of rash or makes it more severe in infants with atopic dermatitis.[47]

Overall, studies appear to favor AGM diapers but fail to reveal any statistical difference between conventional disposable diapers and home-laundered cloth diapers. No comparison was made with commercial diaper services, nor were mothers of the infants in the cloth diaper groups given any specific washing instructions. The cost of the more expensive AGM diapers must be weighed against the slightly increased benefit in the prevention of diaper dermatitis. In 1991 the cost for home-laundered cloth diapers was approximately $526; the cost for a diaper service, $1,268; and the cost for disposable diapers, $1,352.[39]

In 1991 the Consumers Union evaluated the various disposable and cloth diapers. Ratings were consistently higher for disposable diapers than for cloth diapers in the areas of leakage, dryness, and fastening quality. Improved design and placement of elastic barriers make disposable diapers more resistant to leakage. Absorbent gel in the padding improves the diaper's ability to keep the infant dry.[39] However, it was noted that all disposables are subject to padding shifts; that is, the padding sags or clumps when it is wet, leaving some area of the diaper without padding. This is not the case with the cloth diapers.

An additional concern is that disposable diapers, for the most part, are not biodegradable and may present an ecologic hazard. Even those that are promoted as biodegradable (eg, green-label Nappies and Tender Care) are really not because they depend on air, water, and sunlight to degrade. Most landfills do not provide these ingredients. Composting may be an alternative method for disposal of these diapers, but further research is needed.[39]

The prompt changing of soiled or wet diapers is still the best method of preventing diaper rash, irrespective of the type of diaper used.

Prickly Heat (Miliaria)

The lesions associated with prickly heat result from obstruction of the sweat gland pores. Retained sweat causes the dilation and rupture of the epidermal sweat pores, producing swelling and inflammation of the dermis. (See color plates, photograph 24.) The term *prickly heat* was coined because the lesions usually produce some itching but mostly stinging. Prickly heat occurs primarily during hot, humid weather or during a febrile illness with profuse sweating. It may also occur as a result of excessive clothing, polyester clothing, and overcovering, especially at night in warm, humid rooms. Prickly heat may occur during infancy, childhood, or adulthood.

In infants, the lesions most often appear in intertriginous areas and under plastic pants, diapers, and adhesive tape. In children and adults, the dermatitis is seen on areas of skin that have been heavily occluded with clothing. The lesions, which are erythematous papules, may become pustular and are usually localized to the sites of occlusion.

In the treatment of prickly heat, the primary goal is to cool the patient to reduce sweating and, in patients with fever, to administer antipyretics. Clothing should be made of light material and should not rub the skin. Light clothing and coverings are recommended to allow air to reach the skin. Air-conditioning the environment helps to lower humidity and temperature. Maceration and irritants may be reduced with baths or sponge baths at least two times a day and the use of a bland talc dusting powder. Frequent diaper changes and the elimination of excessive soap or chemical irritants help to reduce the discomfort associated with prickly heat.

Adult Urinary Incontinence

Urinary incontinence is defined as the involuntary loss of urine sufficient in amount or frequency to be a social or health problem.[48] The consequences of this problem are considerable. First, many elderly persons are embarrassed by such a condition and refrain from discussing their urinary problems with their primary health care providers. Second, elderly people often accept the myth that urinary incontinence is a normal consequence of aging rather than a symptom of underlying disease or anatomic change. This acceptance leads to depression and low self-esteem. Social isolation occurs since the incontinent elderly patient refuses social interaction because of the embarrassment and rejection that often accompanies urinary incontinence, and intimate contact and sexual activity with their partners can also decrease.

Thus, the patient's social and psychologic well-being are compromised. Third, attempts to limit episodes of involuntary urine loss by restricting fluid intake cause dehydration and hypotension, while skin irritation and ulceration due to long exposure to urine results in "diaper rash" and, perhaps worst of all, pressure ulcers.[48] Also, the caregivers of incontinent elderly patients are stressed because of the tedious and time-consuming care needed to deal with the problem at home. Often the loss of urine control leads to premature institutionalization or elder abuse.[48,49] It is therefore important that health care professionals, patients, and caregivers recognize that urinary incontinence is a symptom and not a single disease process. Urinary incontinence *must* always be medically evaluated inasmuch as it can often be treated and resolved.[48,49]

Physiologic Changes in the Urinary Tract

Age-related changes in the bladder and urinary tract may contribute to an elderly person's vulnerability to urinary incontinence. This is especially true for women. With age, the kidney's ability to concentrate urine diminishes, resulting in larger urine volumes. In addition, age-related hypotrophic changes in bladder tissue lead to frequent urination and nocturia, while decreases in the muscle tone of the bladder, as well as of the bladder sphincters and pelvic muscles, contribute to the potential for decreased urine control. This, in combination with diminished mobility and reaction time, sets the stage for many elderly persons to develop urinary incontinence.[49,50]

Certain chronic and acute illnesses encountered in the aged may enhance the potential for urinary incontinence. Parkinson's disease, stroke, and conditions of cerebrovascular degeneration can disrupt parasympathetic control of the bladder, leading to bladder instability and a decline in bladder capacity.[50] Conditions that cause peripheral neuropathy, such as vascular disease, diabetes mellitus, and nutritional deficiencies, may also decrease bladder capacity, leading to an increased need to urinate.[50]

In women, the decline of estrogen with age brings about a decrease in bladder outlet and urethral resistance, as well as a decline in pelvic musculature, all of which increase the likelihood of urinary incontinence. Additionally, estrogen loss results in atrophic changes in the vaginal and urethral mucosa, disrupting the vaginal flora and leading to atrophic vaginitis and chronic urethritis. These conditions may cause urinary frequency and urgency, dysuria, urinary tract infections, and urinary incontinence.[49,50] The woman's short urethra exerts less resistance to intravesicular pressure than does the longer male urethra. Also, childbirth, gynecologic procedures, and obesity weaken the pelvic floor muscles, thereby decreasing support for the bladder; as a consequence, the anatomy of the bladder becomes distorted, resulting in cystocele, rectocele, or uterine prolapse. These conditions result in chronic obstruction to the bladder, again leading to incontinence.[50] For their part, men often have prostatic enlargement, which also results in urethral obstruction leading to decreased urinary flow rates, increased residual volumes, detrusor instability, and overflow incontinence.[49] Urologic surgical procedures, such as prostatectomy, may also contribute to urine leakage in men.

As would be expected from the above discussion of predisposing factors, the incidence of urinary incontinence is high among the elderly population, afflicting 30% of those in the community, 35% of those in hospitals, and approximately 60% of those in nursing homes.[48] The annual costs associated with this problem are also staggering: $7 billion for care in the community and $3.3 billion for nursing home residents, based on 1987 costs.[51]

Types of Urinary Incontinence

Part of the difficulty in understanding and communicating about urinary incontinence is the number of synonyms used to describe the same condition. The basic types of incontinence and their associated synonyms are as follows[48]:

- *Detrusor instability*: detrusor hyperactivity, detrusor overactivity, detrusor hyperreflexia, unstable bladder, spastic bladder, uninhibited bladder, urge incontinence.
- *Stress incontinence*: sphincter insufficiency, outlet impotence.
- *Overflow incontinence*: detrusor areflexia, atonic bladder, impaired contractility, urge incontinence.
- *Functional incontinence*: reflex incontinence.
- *Iatrogenic incontinence*.
- *Mixed incontinence*.

Other terms occasionally used to describe the type of urinary incontinence manifested are *transient* and *established*.[52,53] Transient incontinence usually occurs suddenly and is secondary to acute illness, such as urinary tract infections, or to any disease that causes acute confusion (respiratory disease, myocardial infarction, septicemia, etc) or immobility such that the person cannot reach a toilet independently or in time.[52,53] Established incontinence is persistent and related to neurologic or other chronic conditions, such as prostatic hypertrophy, cystocele, or uterine prolapse.[50,52,53] Another term often used by the public is *urge incontinence*, which is a sudden desire to void, resulting often in uncontrolled urine loss. This term is medically im precise since both detrusor instability and overflow incontinence have associated urgency as a symptom.[48]

Pathophysiology

Detrusor instability is a common form of incontinence due to uninhibited contractions of the detrusor muscle, bundles of smooth muscle fibers that form the body of the bladder and cause urine expulsion when they contract.[48] The primary symptoms of detrusor instability are an urgent sensation to void urine and an inability to delay voiding when the sensation occurs. The etiology of this incontinence is most often related to local irritants or central nervous system diseases, such as dementias, stroke, Parkinson's disease, and demyelinating diseases (eg, multiple sclerosis).[52,54]

Stress incontinence is the most frequently encountered type of urinary incontinence in women. It is characterized by involuntary leakage of small amounts of urine during sudden increases in intra-abdominal pressure, as occurs with sneezing, laughing, coughing, exercise, and lifting.[48,52,54] This is thought to be caused by hypermobility of the bladder neck or weakness of the bladder sphincter and pelvic floor muscles.[48] Hypermobility refers to displacement of the bladder neck and urethra during exertion, and it occurs when supporting pelvic muscles have been weakened as a result of childbearing and aging. The weakening of the sphincter can be secondary to surgery or trauma, or may be neurogenic in etiology.[48]

Overflow incontinence results in dribbling, urgency, and sometimes stress incontinence. It occurs when the bladder cannot be emptied properly because of obstruction (prostate hypertrophy, cystocele, fecal impaction) or a contractile state (diabetes mellitus, drugs) and is thus overdistended.[48,52]

Functional incontinence is associated with the inability to reach toileting facilities in time or to perform toileting tasks. Causes of this type of incontinence are many and include impaired cognitive function or perception, stroke, diminished mobility, environmental barriers, and psychologic unwillingness to toilet in the proper place.[48,52,54]

Iatrogenic causes of incontinence should be considered since many medications are capable of causing transient incontinence. Incontinence may result from the medical use of physical restraints that make toileting without assistance impossible. Drugs with anticholinergic action (phenothiazines, antihistamines, antidepressants) may inhibit bladder function (emptying). Decongestants may cause retention of urine by stimulating alpha and beta receptors, which enhances bladder filling and increases bladder sphincter tone. Alpha-receptor agonists used for hypertension treatment may also enhance the action of adrenergic receptors in the bladder. Diuretics, particularly if given late in the evening, may overwhelm the elderly person's ability to toilet; and sedating medications (hypnotics) may decrease the older patient's awareness of bladder filling.[48,54]

It is important for health care professionals to understand that urinary incontinence is rarely one isolated type of incontinence but rather is often a mixture of types. Elderly women frequently have stress incontinence with an element of detrusor instability (urge incontinence). Fifty percent of men with outlet obstruction (prostate enlargement) have detrusor instability.[48,52,54]

Treatment of Incontinence

After medical evaluation has occurred and diagnosis has been established, treatment with appropriate agents and nonpharmacologic measures can be implemented for each type of urinary incontinence. Most medications used to treat these disorders are prescription products, but in some cases, nonprescription medications may be appropriate. Most nonprescription items sold for urinary incontinence involve medications to control or treat skin breakdown (diaper rash), agents to control odor, and absorbent products. However, owing to the public's general lack of sufficient medical knowledge about the different types of urinary incontinence, some patients (or their caregivers) may attempt self-diagnosis and treatment without consulting their primary care provider. This could obviously lead to inappropriate assessment and treatment. Thus, it is imperative that pharmacists inquire about a proper medical evaluation before recommending nonprescription products, including absorbent products.

Type-Specific Approaches

Detrusor Instability Detrusor instability may be treated with anticholinergic medications, which facilitate urine storage by decreasing uninhibited detrusor contractions. Most often a prescription medication such as oxybutynin chloride, flavoxate hydrochloride, or hyoscyamine will be initiated for this type of incontinence.[48,52] However, diphenhydramine is occasionally used as initial drug therapy. (See Chapter 8, "Cold, Cough, and Allergy Products.") Pharmacists should counsel patients about the potential side effects that occur more frequently with diphenhydramine than with the aforementioned prescription products; sedation, dry mouth (a problem for denture use), constipation, and confusion can be significant problems in elderly patients. In addition, the patient should be instructed to do pelvic floor muscle exercises and encouraged to adhere to a "timed voiding" schedule to increase the efficacy of treatment.[48] Contraindications to the use of diphenhydramine (and other anticholinergic medications) include many conditions that occur more often in elderly individuals (eg, narrow-angle glaucoma, peptic ulcer, urinary tract obstruction, and hyperthyroidism) than in other patients.

Stress Incontinence Stress incontinence is often treated with agents that increase outflow resistance through alpha-receptor stimulation that enhances contraction of the bladder neck muscles. Commonly recommended drugs are often nonprescription agents such as ephedrine, pseudoephedrine, phenylephrine, and phenylpropanolamine. (See Chapter 8, "Cold, Cough, and Allergy Products.") Caution should be used, however, when initiating such therapy in patients with hypertension and/or cardiac arrhythmias, and the patient should be advised to monitor blood pressure and pulse, and to report any new occurrences of heart palpitations or fainting. As in detrusor instability, the use of pelvic floor muscle exercises and a timed voiding schedule will assist in controlling this type of incontinence.[48]

In women, estrogen therapy may also be used; benefits are seen in 4–6 weeks. Estrogen can be used in combination with alpha-adrenergic agonists. Pharmacists should counsel about the common side effects of estrogen therapy, such as weight gain, fluid retention, increased blood pressure, and vaginal spotting. Should medical treatment fail, surgical correction may be possible.[48]

Overflow Incontinence The treatment of overflow incontinence is directed by the underlying cause. In these cases, surgery is often necessary. Prescription agents such as bethanechol chloride with or without metoclopramide may be initiated where the bladder has insufficient contractile strength.[48] Catheterization, a last resort, is used when medical and surgical corrections have failed.[48]

Functional and Iatrogenic Incontinence Functional and iatrogenic incontinence require evaluation of the patient's entire medical status and medication history. Side effects from medications can often be eliminated by initiating alternative treatments. Underlying dysfunctions such as rheumatoid arthritis and decreased mobility can be remedied by medical as well as environmental changes that make toileting accessible and possible within the limitations of the patient's functional status. Often an assessment by physical or occupational therapists can remedy many problems dealing with the physical limitations of the patient.

Absorbent Products

The use of protective undergarments and pads is aimed at protecting clothing, bedding, and furniture while allowing independence and mobility of the patient. But while absorbent products are very beneficial, they should be used only after a thorough and complete examination.[52] If patients or caregivers prematurely initiate the use of absorbent protective products, they treat the symptom and obscure the cause. Since correction may be possible, the premature acceptance of urinary incontinence may have significant financial, social, and psychologic consequences.

Selection Factors The type of absorbent product used depends on several factors[54]:

- Type and severity of incontinence;
- Functional status;
- Sex;
- Availability of caregivers;
- Patient preference;
- Convenience.

The pharmacist needs to discuss such factors with patients and their caregivers when helping to select absorbent products.

Absorbent garments and pads are available as reusable or disposable products (see product table "Adult Incontinence Garments"). The disposable product market has become a multimillion dollar industry over the last decade.[55] These products work in the same manner as children's disposable diapers. They are designed to absorb urine; provide a moisture barrier to protect clothes, bedding, and furniture; and minimize skin contact with urine. Urine is jelled in the matrix, which minimizes urine contact with skin.

The capacity of each disposable product corresponds to the needs of the patient:

- *Guards/shields*: 2–12 oz (60–360 mL), light to heavy capacity;
- *Briefs*: 28–36 oz (840–1,100 mL), moderate to heavy capacity;
- *Undergarments*: 12–18 oz (360–540 mL), moderate to heavy capacity.

Patients with small amounts of leakage, as occurs in stress or overflow incontinence and following urologic surgical procedures (eg, dribbling), may require only a shield. If larger amounts of urine are lost with incontinence, such as often occurs with detrusor instability, products with large capacity would be more appropriate. Also, many products are designed for overnight (heavy) use, and these tend to have the largest capacities.[55,56]

Another important issue is the functional capacity of the patient. Does the patient use the toilet and change undergarments independently? Is the patient limited in mobility so that the heaviest protection is needed during the night? Will the patient need assistance in changing the products? If so, briefs or diapers with roll-on bed application and adhesive closures may be useful for a caregiver.

Securing the product may also be an important issue. Some garments or shields have adhesive strips or belts to hold them in place. Belts may require assistance from a caregiver. Of course, comfort and leg security from leakage are important. Many product lines offer elastic legs or contoured shapes. The anatomic differences between men and women are another consideration; products designed with these differences in mind should be considered when large-capacity products are used.[55,56]

Protective underpads are often used in conjunction with briefs and undergarments for extended duration activities, such as sleeping and sitting. Both bed and chair pads are available, and the pharmacist should inquire about the need for additional protection. The underpad should have a known capacity, a waterproof duration of several hours, and the ability to remain intact when wet. Bed pads are available in sizes from 16 × 24 in. to 24 × 24 in. It is suggested that for chairs, a pad that is 16 × 18 in. be used.[56]

Complications from Absorbent Products Because the use of absorbent products increases the risk of skin irritation and maceration, such products should be checked every 2 hours. With continual urine loss, it is recommended that the absorbent material be changed every 2–4 hours. The use of skin protectants (barrier creams and ointments) as in diaper rash is appropriate. Should a rash occur, the same treatment as was described previously for infants is indicated.

Odor is an embarrassing problem. Nonprescription products containing chlorophyll (eg, Derifil, Pals, and Nullo) can be recommended to help decrease odor. However, frequent checks and changes are better than efforts to disguise odor.

Pressure ulcers may occur if the patient is immobile. Any skin breakdown with development of a lesion needs to be reported to the primary care provider. This serious complication should not be treated with nonprescription products without medical supervision.

Since most pharmacies do not carry a full line of products for the urine incontinent patient, the pharmacist can direct patients to: Help for Incontinent People (HIP) Inc, PO Box 544, Union, SC 29379; 803–579–7900, 800–BLADDER, or fax 803–579–7902.

Product Selection Guidelines

Although there are not many nonprescription products available for this medical problem, pharmacists nonetheless need to be familiar with this disease process to advise patients and caregivers appropriately. Oral nonprescription medications may be useful in some cases of detrusor instability and stress incontinence. Diphenhydramine and pseudoephedrine can be used, for example, to help control urine loss. However, these should be used only after a thorough evaluation has determined the cause and/or type of incontinence. Inappropriate use of systemic nonprescription products and incorrect use of absorbent undergarments and pads before a proper evaluation has been made results in unnecessary expense, inappropriate treatment, and possibly unnecessary changes in lifestyle and psychologic well-being. It is therefore imperative that pharmacists obtain enough patient history to ensure that requests for nonprescription products are being made under proper medical supervision. Armed with the history and proper diagnosis, the pharmacist can answer questions appropriately and help in the selection and proper use of devices and medications for treatment of this disorder.

Case Studies

Case 29–1

Patient Complaint/History

SB, a 22-year-old female carrying a small infant, enters the pharmacy and is browsing in the ointment section. She explains that her infant daughter has a mild diaper rash and displays an area of the rash. The rash is red and looks slightly inflamed; the redness is confined to the diaper area. Indicating the tube of Neosporin Ointment in her hand, SB asks whether the product will clear up the rash.

Clinical Considerations/Strategies

The following considerations/strategies are provided to aid the reader in (1) determining whether treatment of the patient's condition with nonprescription medications is warranted, (2) selecting the appropriate nonprescription medication, and (3) developing a patient counseling strategy to ensure optimal therapeutic outcomes:

- Assess the appropriateness of the selected ointment.
- Propose an alternative and more appropriate nonprescription medication regimen for the diaper rash.
- Develop a patient education/counseling strategy that will:
  - Define steps that the mother can use to prevent or minimize the recurrence of diaper rash (eg, proper hygiene of the diaper area, use of absorbable diapers, frequent changing of diapers, and use of barrier products);
  - Advise the mother of the differences in appearance of candidal versus staphylococcal diaper rash;
  - Advise the mother of symptoms of candidal or staphylococcal diaper rashes that would warrant referral to a pediatrician.

Case 29–2

Patient Complaint/History

MS, a 72-year-old female, presents to the pharmacy with a complaint of "urine release"; she reveals that the first incident occurred 2 weeks earlier during lunch with friends. The patient goes on to explain that the "leakage" occurs when she laughs, coughs, or sneezes. As a result, she has become depressed and declines social invitations.

MS recalls that a friend who also experienced urine leakage was treated by a physician with a "cold medicine." MS pleads for help, exclaiming "I can't go on like this! I'm missing so much because of this problem, and I'm so depressed and embarrassed."

The patient's known medical problems include hypertension and congestive heart failure for which she has taken hydrochlorothiazide 25 mg once daily for 6 years; digoxin 0.25 mg once daily for 3 years; potassium chloride 20 mEq once daily for 6 years; and ofloxacin 200 mg bid for 7 days. Other medications include an unidentified cough medicine prn; aspirin taken occasionally for headache; and chlorpheniramine sustained-release capsules 8 mg prn for allergies.

Clinical Considerations/Strategies

The following considerations/strategies are provided to aid the reader in (1) determining whether treatment of the patient's condition with nonprescription medications is warranted, (2) selecting the appropriate nonprescription medication, and (3) developing a patient counseling strategy to ensure optimal therapeutic outcomes:

- Determine what additional information is needed and formulate the appropriate questions.
- Based on information provided, assess the most likely explanation for this patient's symptoms/condition.
- Develop a patient education/counseling strategy that will:
  - Provide the patient with information to help her understand the condition;
  - Define a care plan for the patient;
  - If applicable, identify the type of absorbent garment that could be used;
  - Define nonpharmacologic treatments that could resolve the problem;
  - Identify appropriate pharmacologic therapy;
  - Advise the patient of adverse effects that may occur with pharmacologic therapy.

Summary

Pharmacists should be prepared to offer sound advice on a good prophylactic program and to recommend therapy for uncomplicated, uninfected cases of diaper rash, prickly heat, and adult incontinence. They should also be prepared to assess the severity of the rash and be able to recommend appropriate action, whether it be referral to a physician or a treatment plan.

Diaper dermatitis and prickly heat are the two most common dermal afflictions of newborns, infants, and young children, but their incidence and severity may be reduced by following proper procedures. If the dermatitis does not respond within 1 week to frequent diaper changes, frequent exposure to air, and application of a protectant such as zinc oxide paste, a physician should be consulted.

Urinary incontinence is common in the elderly community. Since various processes can cause this complex urinary disorder, the patient should receive a full medical evaluation before treating it. At that point, a variety of treatments, both pharmacologic and nonpharmacologic, can be prescribed depending on the etiology and type of the disorder. The pharmacist can assist the patient or caregiver by providing medication counseling, advice on the complications, and assistance in selecting appropriate absorbent devices for persons with urinary incontinence.

References

1. Weston WL. *Practical Pediatric Dermatology*. 2nd ed. Boston: Little, Brown and Co; 1985: 1–2.
2. Gowdy JM, Ulsamer AG. Hexachlorophene lesions in newborn infants. *Am J Dis Child*. 1976 Mar; 20: 247–50.
3. Jordan WE et al. Diaper dermatitis: frequency and severity among a general infant population. *Pediatr Dermatol*. 1986 Jun; 3: 198–207.
4. Longhi F et al. Diaper dermatitis: a study of contributing factors. *Contact Dermatitis*. 1992; 26: 248–52.
5. *Federal Register*. 1990; 55: 25246.
6. *Federal Register*. 1990; 55: 25234.
7. *Federal Register*. 1990; 55: 25204.
8. *Federal Register*. 1990; 55: 25240.
9. Berg RW. Etiologic factors in diaper dermatitis: a model for development of improved diapers. *Pediatrics*. 1987; 14(suppl 1): 27.
10. Forsyth JS et al. Relation between early introduction of solid food to infants and their weight and illnesses during the first two years of life. *Br Med J*. 1993; 306: 1572–6.
11. Brown CP, Wilson FH. Diaper region irritations: pertinent facts and methods of prevention. *Clin Pediatr*. 1964 July; 3(7): 409–13.
12. Berg RW. Etiologic factors in diaper dermatitis: the role of urine. *Pediatr Dermatol*. 1986 Feb; 3: 102–6.
13. Benjamin L. Clinical correlates with diaper dermatitis. *Pediatrician*. 1987; 14(suppl 1): 21–6.
14. Berg RW et al. Association of skin wetness and pH with diaper dermatitis. *Pediatr Dermatol*. 1994 Mar; 11: 18–20.
15. Zimmerer RE et al. The effects of wearing diapers on skin. *Pediatr Dermatol*. 1986 Jan; 3: 95–101.
16. Rebora A, Leyden JJ. Napkin (diaper) dermatitis and gastrointestinal carriage of *Candida albicans*. *Br J Dermatol*. 1981 Mar; 105: 551–5.
17. Sevim A et al. Relation between the intestinal flora and diaper dermatitis in infancy. *Trop Geogr Med*. 1990 Jun; 42: 238–40.
18. Honig PJ et al. Amoxicillin and diaper dermatitis. *J Am Acad Dermatol*. 1988 Aug; 19: 275–9.
19. Hayden GF. Dermatophyte infection in the diaper area: report of two cases. *Pediatr Infect Dis J*. 1985 May; 4: 289–91.
20. Congly H. Infection of the diaper area caused by *Epidermophyton floccosum*. *Can Med Assoc J*. 1983 Sep; 129: 410–1.
21. Kahana M et al. Dermatophytosis of the diaper area. *Clin Pediatr*. 1987 Mar; 26: 149–51.
22. Cavanaugh RM, Greeson JD. Infection of the diaper area. *Arch Dermatol*. 1982 Jun; 118: 446.
23. Baudraz-Rosselet F et al. Diaper dermatitis due to *Tricophyton verrucosum*. *Pediatr Dermatol*. 1993 Dec; 10: 368–9.
24. Jenson HB, Shapiro ED. Primary herpes simplex virus infection of a diaper rash. *Pediatr Infect Dis J*. 1987 Dec; 6: 1136–8.
25. Hara M et al. Jacquet erosive diaper dermatitis in a young girl with urinary incontinence. *Pediatr Dermatol*. 1991 Jun; 8: 160–1.
26. Thiboutot DM et al. Cytomegalovirus diaper dermatitis. *Arch Dermatol*. 1991 Mar; 127: 396–8.
27. Bluestein J et al. Granuloma gluteale infantum: case report and review of the literature. *Pediatr Dermatol*. 1990 Sep; 7: 196–8.
28. Friter BS, Lucky AW. The perineal eruption of Kawasaki syndrome. *Arch Dermatol*. 1988 Dec; 124: 1805–10.
29. Janniger CK, Thomas I. Diaper dermatitis: an approach to prevention employing effective diaper care. *Cutis*. 1993 Sep; 52: 153–5.
30. Cano LR et al. Perianal pseudoverrucous papules and nodules after surgery for Hirschsprung disease. *J Pediatrics*. 1994 Dec; 125: 914–6.
31. Leyden JJ. Corn starch, *Candida albicans*, and diaper rash. *Pediatr Dermatol*. 1984 Apr; 1: 322–5.
32. Research report. New York: Leeming/Pacquin Pharmaceutical Co; 1974.
33. James WS. A new use for an old ointment: Lantiseptic ointment as a treatment for diaper dermatitis. *J Med Assoc Ga*. 1975 May; 64: 133–4.
34. Bosch-Banyeras JM et al. Diaper dermatitis: value of vitamin A topically applied. *Clin Pediatr*. 1988 Sep; 27: 448–50.
35. Mofenson HC et al. Baby powder—a hazard! *Pediatrics*. 1981 Aug; 68: 265–6.
36. Mackie RM, Scott E. Topical miconazole cream in infantile napkin dermatitis. *Practitioner*. 1979 Jan; 222: 124–6.
37. Montes LF, Hermann HW. Clinical and antimicrobial effects of haloprogin cream in diaper dermatitis. *Cutis*. 1978 Mar; 21: 410–2.
38. Lane At et al. Evaluations of diapers containing absorbent gelling material with conventional disposable diapers in newborn infants. *Am J Dis Child*. 1990 Mar; 144: 315–8.
39. Diaper decisions: which are best for the baby? *Consumer Rep*. 1991 Aug; 551–6.
40. Stein H. Incidence of diaper rash when using cloth and disposable diapers. *J Pediatr*. 1982 Nov; 101: 721–3.
41. Seymour JL et al. Clinical effects of diaper types on the skin of normal infants and infants with atopic dermatitis. *J Am Acad Dermatol*. 1987 May; 17: 988–97.
42. Campbell RL et al. Clinical studies with disposable diapers containing absorbent gelling materials: evaluation of effects on infant skin condition. *J Am Acad Dermatol*. 1987 Dec; 17: 978–87.
43. Campbell RL et al. Effects of diaper types on diaper dermatitis associated with diarrhea and antibiotic use in children in day-care centers. *Pediatr Dermatol*. 1988; 5(2): 83–7.
44. Austin AP et al. A survey of factors associated with diaper dermatitis in thirty-six pediatric practices. *J Pediatr Health Care*. 1988 Nov–Dec; 2: 295–9.
45. Campbell RL. Clinical tests with improved disposable diapers. *Pediatrician*. 1987; 14(suppl 1): 34–8.
46. Davis JA et al. Comparison of disposable diapers with fluff absorbent and fluff plus absorbent polymers: effects on skin hydration, skin pH, and diaper dermatitis. *Pediatr Dermatol*. 1989 Jun; 6: 102–8.
47. Seymour JL. Clinical and microbial effects of cloth, cellulose core, and cellulose core/absorbent gel diapers in atopic dermatitis. *Pediatrician*. 1987; 14(suppl 1): 39–43.
48. Rosenthal AJ, McMurtry CT. Urinary incontinence in the elderly: often simple to treat when properly evaluated. *Postgrad Med*. 1995; 97(5): 109–21.
49. Pickell GC et al. Genitourinary and sexual problems of the elderly. In: Ham RJ et al, eds. *Primary Care Geriatrics: A Case-Based Learning Program*. Littleton, Mass: PSG Inc; 1983: 203–13.
50. Houston KA. Incontinence and the older woman. *Clin Geriatr Med*. 1993; 9(1): 157–71.
51. Hu T. Impact of urinary incontinence on health-care costs. *J Am Geriatr Soc*. 1990; 38: 292–5.
52. Brocklehurst JC. The bladder. In: *Textbook of Geriatric Medicine and Gerontology*, 4th ed. New York: Churchill Livingstone; 1992: 629–46.

53. Plymot KR, Turner SL. In-home management of urinary incontinence. *Home Healthcare Nurse.* 1988; 6(4): 30–4.

54. US Department of Health and Human Services. *Urinary Incontinence in Adults: Clinical Practice Guideline.* Washington, DC: Public Health Service, Agency for Health Care Policy and Research; March 1992.

55. Smith DA. Devices for continence. *Nurs Pract Forum.* 1994; 5(3): 186–9.

56. Brink CA, Wells TJ. Environmental support for geriatric incontinence. *Clin Geriatr Med.* 1986; 2(4): 829–41.

CHAPTER 30

Sunscreen and Suntan Products

Edward M. DeSimone II

Questions to ask in patient assessment and counseling

- *Do you sunburn easily?*
- *How long can you stay in full sun without your skin turning red?*
- *How well do you tan?*
- *Do you normally spend much time outdoors because of your job, sports, or other activities?*
- *Are you currently using a sun protection product?*
- *What products have you used in the past?*
- *Have you ever had a growth on your skin or lip caused by sun exposure?*
- *Have you ever had a reaction to a prescription or nonprescription drug?*
- *Have you ever had a reaction to any sunscreen products?*
- *Are you taking any medications such as a tetracycline, diuretic, or sulfa drug?*
- *Will you be using the product while swimming, skiing, participating in strenuous activities, or working?*

One of the most popular activities since the turn of the century has been to spend leisure time "soaking up the rays of the sun." The popular association in the 1950s of tanned skin with good health spawned a major industry that revolved around suntanning, including suntan lotions, sunless tanning products, and tanning beds and booths. Within the last 20 years, however, research has generated an understanding of the effects of UV radiation and the discovery that this type of radiation is, in fact, harmful.

Whether sun exposure is recreational or occupational, sunburn often occurs, the severity of which depends on an individual's natural skin type as well as on the measures used (eg, protective clothing, sunscreens) to protect the skin. Most people consider sunburn with its accompanying swelling and tenderness, to be a minor, albeit painful, inconvenience. However, repeated exposure to UV radiation is cumulative and can produce serious, long-term problems such as premature aging of the skin. In addition, cumulative exposure from childhood to adulthood, even without a serious sunburn ever developing, may cause both precancerous and cancerous skin conditions. More than 800,000 new cases of skin cancer are diagnosed each year. Although the mortality rate for each type of cancer varies, more than 20% of persons with malignant melanoma die each year. This fact is now clear: avoiding excessive exposure to UV radiation will reduce the incidence of premature aging of the skin, skin cancer, and other long-term dermatologic effects.

With this new understanding of the dangers of UV radiation has come a large variety of sunscreen (rather than suntan) products intended not only to help darken but also to protect the skin from the harmful effects of exposure to the sun. Applied properly, these products block some or most of the sun's harmful UV rays. Unfortunately, the average consumer shows a considerable lack of understanding of both the process of tanning and the necessity of using sunscreens properly. Thus, pharmacists need to educate the public on the safe and effective use of sunscreen and suntan products. To perform this function, pharmacists must be aware of the hazards of UV radiation as well as the criteria for selection and proper use of sunscreen products. They must also become involved in an aggressive education program to help minimize the morbidity and mortality associated with UV radiation.

Ultraviolet Radiation

UV radiation is commonly referred to as UV light. However, *light* technically refers to only the visible spectrum; thus, the correct terminology in this context is *radiation*.[1] The UV spectrum is divided into three major bands: UVC, UVB, and UVA.

UVC Radiation

The wavelength of UVC, also known as germicidal radiation, is within the 200- to 290-nm band. Little UVC radiation from the sun reaches the surface of the Earth because it is screened out by the ozone layer of the upper atmosphere. However, UVC is emitted by some artificial sources of UV radiation, and most of the UVC that strikes the skin is absorbed by the dead cell layer of the stratum corneum.[2] Although UVC does not stimulate tanning, it can cause some erythema (redness) of the skin.[2]

UVB Radiation

The wavelength of the UVB band is between 290 and 320 nm. This is the most active UV radiation wavelength for producing erythema, which is why it is called sunburn radiation. The irradiance (ie, intensity of the radiation reaching the surface) of UVB is most intense from late morning to early afternoon (10 AM–4 PM). To minimize the damaging effects of UVB, exposure to UVR during this time should be avoided.

Cutaneous UVB exposure is responsible for vitamin D_3 synthesis in the skin. Current consensus suggests that this is the only true therapeutic effect of UVB.[3] While vitamin D deficiency does not seem to be a problem for infants in the United States who receive vitamin D–fortified milk, it may be a problem for chronic shut-ins or for elderly individuals who spend little time outdoors if they do not receive adequate vitamin D in their diet or as a vitamin supplement. Its therapeutic benefit notwithstanding, however, UVB is considered to be primarily responsible for inducing skin cancer, and its carcinogenic effects are believed to be augmented by UVA.[4] In addition, UVB is primarily responsible for wrinkling of the skin, epidermal hyperplasia, elastosis (loss of skin elasticity), and collagen damage.[5] The recent discovery of the effects of UVR on the immune system has led to the development of the new field of photoimmunology.[6]

UVA Radiation

The wavelength of UVA radiation ranges from 320 to 400 nm. Although most of the concerns regarding the hazards of sun exposure to date have focused specifically on UVB, concern about the adverse effects of UVA has been slowly developing since the early 1980s.[7] It is now known that UVA radiation penetrates deeper into the skin than UVB, thereby having a greater effect on the dermis than on the epidermis. This deeper penetration can cause both histologic and vascular damage.[8,9] Evidence suggests that subsequent UVA exposure may cause further and more serious acute and chronic damage to the underlying tissue than UVB exposure. UVA is also believed to be involved in suppression of the immune system as well as in damage to DNA.[5,10]

Based on current research into the effects of UVA on the skin and underlying structures, the UVA band has been divided into two subsets: UVA II (320–340 nm) and UVA I (340–400 nm).[11] It has been suggested that the degree of damage caused by UV radiation parallels the degree of erythema across the UV spectrum.[12] That is, the damage at 290 nm is 100 times greater than that at 320 nm and the damage at 320 nm is 100 times greater than that at 400 nm, whereas the damage caused at 320 nm is believed to be 10 times higher than that at 340 nm. Based on these data, after UVB, UVA II radiation is the most damaging to the skin.[13] This has significant implications for sunscreen products and the type of protection they offer.

The results of this research have caused some controversy about the relative importance of UVA effects on skin as compared with those of UVB. Although approximately 20 times more UVA than UVB reaches the earth's surface at noon (30 times more in winter), erythemogenic activity is relatively weak in the UVA band, requiring up to 200 times more UVA energy than UVB energy.[14] In addition, the irradiance of UVA varies by a factor of 4 to 1 throughout the day and 3 to 1 from summer to winter; however, the significance of this variation is being debated.[14] UVA also represents the wavelength in which most photosensitizing chemicals such as 8-methoxypsoralen (8-MOP) are active. This is true throughout the UVA band but especially above 360 nm.

The Process of Burning and Tanning

The degree to which an individual will develop a sunburn or a tan depends on a number of factors, including (1) the type and amount of radiation received, (2) the thickness of the epidermis and stratum corneum, (3) the pigmentation of the skin, (4) the hydration of the skin, and (5) the distribution and concentration of peripheral blood vessels.[15] Most UV radiation that strikes the skin is absorbed by the epidermis.

A sunburn is the result of an inflammatory reaction involving a number of mediators, including histamine, lysosomal enzymes, kinins, and at least one prostaglandin. These mediators produce peripheral vasodilatation as the UV radiation penetrates the epidermis; an inflammatory reaction involving a lymphocytic infiltrate develops. Swelling of the endothelium and leakage of red blood cells from capillaries also occur. Although the exact mechanism is not fully understood, it is believed that UVB radiation produces erythema by first causing damage to cellular DNA. The intensity of the UVB-induced erythema peaks at 12–24 hours after exposure.[15]

Sunburn is, in fact, a burn. It is most often seen as a first-degree (superficial) burn, with a reaction ranging from mild erythema to tenderness, pain, and edema. Severe reactions to excessive UV exposure can sometimes produce a second-degree burn, with the development of vesicles (blisters) or bullae (many large blisters) as well as the constitutional symptoms of fever, chills, weakness, and shock. Shock caused by heat prostration or hyperpyrexia can lead to death. (See Chapter 31, "Burn and Sunburn Products.")

A tan is produced when UV radiation stimulates the melanocytes in the germinating skin layer to generate more melanin and oxidizes the melanin already in the epidermis. Both processes serve as protective mechanisms by diffusing and absorbing additional UV radiation. Although UVB and UVA contribute to the tanning process, they induce pigmentation by different mechanisms. UVB acts by stimulating epidermal hyperplasia as well as a shift of melanin up through the skin. UVA acts by increasing the total amount of melanin in the basal layer. Because of the location of melanin in each case, there is greater photoprotection from UVB-induced pigmentation than from UVA-induced pigmentation.[16] UVA produces a tan through two processes. The first is known as immediate pigment darkening (IPD), which involves photooxidation of existing melanin.[17] It begins to be visible from 5 to 10 minutes after exposure and reaches its maximum effect in 60–90 minutes. The effects of IPD begin to fade very quickly and may be gone within 24 hours. The second process is delayed tanning, or melanogenesis, which involves an increase in the number and size of melanocytes as well as in the number of melanosomes or pigment granules produced by melanocytes. This delayed tanning contributes to the development of a slow natural tan.

UV-Induced Skin Disorders

Consumers use sunscreens primarily to prevent sunburn and to aid in the development of a tan. Sunscreens are also effective in protecting against drug-related UV-induced photosensitivity and other types of photodermatoses. They can also be used to protect exposed areas of the body from premature photoaging and the long-term hazards of skin cancer.

Drug Photosensitivity

Photosensitivity encompasses two types of conditions: photoallergy and phototoxicity. Drug photoallergy, a relatively uncommon immunologic response, involves an increased, chemically induced reactivity of the skin to UV radiation and/or visible light. UV radiation (primarily UVA) triggers an antigenic reaction in the skin, which is characterized by urticaria, bullae, and/or sunburn. This reaction, which is not dose related, is usually seen after at least one prior exposure to the involved chemical agent or drug.

Phototoxicity is also an increased, chemically induced reactivity of the skin to UV radiation and/or visible light. However, this reaction is not immunologic in nature. It is often seen upon first exposure to a chemical agent or drug, it is dose related, and it usually exhibits no drug cross-sensitivity. It is most likely to appear as an exaggerated sunburn.[18] Some of the drugs associated with phototoxicity are tetracyclines (especially demeclocycline), sulfonamides, antineoplastics (eg, 5-fluorouracil), hypoglycemics, thiazides, phenothiazines (especially chlorpromazine), and the psoralens. This type of reaction is not limited to drugs but is also associated with plants, cosmetics, and soaps. (For an additional reference to photosensitivity, see Chapter 31, "Burn and Sunburn Products.")

The efficacy of sunscreen agents in preventing photosensitization has been questioned by some investigators and is apparently under discussion between manufacturers and the Food and Drug Administration (FDA). Although the issue has yet to be resolved, it seems reasonable to assume that, because UVA radiation is primarily responsible for triggering a photosensitivity reaction, a sunscreen effective throughout the entire UVA range, especially above 360 nm, would help to prevent a large number of cases of photosensitivity. Since UVB can also produce photosensitivity, although the incidence is low, it would be best to use a broad-spectrum sunscreen, which protects throughout the entire UVB range as well.

Photodermatoses

Photodermatoses are skin eruptions that are idiopathic (self-originated) or exacerbated (photoaggravated) by radiation of varying wavelengths, including UVA and some visible light. UVB, however, is most often responsible for the reactions. There are more than 20 known disorders classified as photodermatoses; Table 1 lists the most common photodermatoses. Almost all cases of nondrug photodermatosis are manifested as one of four diseases: polymorphic light eruption (PMLE), systemic lupus erythematosus (SLE), solar urticaria, and the porphyrias.[16]

TABLE 1 Most common photodermatoses

Idiopathic disorders

- Actinic prurigo
- Chronic actinic dermatitis
- Polymorphic light eruption Most common ♀
- Solar urticaria

Photoaggravated disorders

- Acne vulgaris
- Atopic dermatitis
- Atopic eczema
- Bullous pemphigoid
- Chloasma
- Dermatomyositis
- Drug photosensitivity
- Erythema multiforme
- Herpes simplex labialis
- Lichen planus
- Psoriasis
- Rosacea
- Seborrheic dermatitis
- Systemic lupus erythematosus

Source:

Pathak MA, Fitzpatrick TB, Parrish JA. In: Fitzpatrick TB et al, eds. *Dermatology in General Medicine*. 3rd ed. New York: McGraw-Hill; 1987: 254–62.

Guercio-Hauer C, Macfarlane DF, Deleo VA. Photodamage, photoaging and photoprotection of the skin. *Am Fam Phys*. 1994 Aug; 50: 327–32.

Kligman LH, Kligman AM. In: Fitzpatrick TB et al, eds. *Dermatology in General Medicine*. 3rd ed. New York: McGraw-Hill; 1987: 1470–5.

The most common of the idiopathic photodermatoses is PMLE. This condition usually manifests itself in a single morphologic form that includes erythema, vesicles, or plaques on skin exposed to UV radiation. It appears to affect approximately 10% of the population, with a first occurrence usually before the age of 30.[18,19] It affects women more often than men and is usually seen in persons who are capable of experiencing a burn, including those persons who tan well.

Another disorder that has shown an increase in recent years is a phytophotodermatitis, also known as "weed wacker dermatitis."[20] This usually occurs when the sap of plants bruised by high-speed weed-cutting machines (used by many homeowners) gets on the skin and the skin is struck by UV radiation. The only protection is to cover the skin with clothing.

In addition to the idiopathic photodermatoses, UV radiation can precipitate or exacerbate more than 20 photoaggravated dermatologic conditions, including herpes simplex labialis (cold sores), SLE and associated skin lesions, and chloasma, which may affect pregnant women and women taking oral contraceptives.

Avoidance of UV radiation is the best way to prevent the occurrence or exacerbation of all photodermatoses.

It is generally believed that sunscreens with the widest range of UV absorbance may afford the next best protection.

Premature Aging

One of the long-term hazards of radiation is premature photoaging of the skin. This type of aging is genetically determined; for example, Caucasians are more susceptible than African Americans. The condition, which is most easily characterized by wrinkling and yellowing of the skin, is called premature photoaging because the obvious physical findings are similar to those seen in natural aging. However, histologic and biochemical differences distinguish these degenerative changes from those associated with normal aging. Conclusive evidence reveals that prolonged exposure to UV radiation in susceptible individuals results in elastosis (degeneration of the skin due to breakdown of the skin's elastic fibers). Pronounced drying, thickening, and wrinkling of the skin may also result.[21] Other physical changes include cracking, telangiectasia (spider vessels), solar keratoses (growths), and ecchymoses (subcutaneous hemorrhagic lesions).[22]

As with normal aging of the skin, solar damage has been generally believed to be irreversible. However, there is some evidence that, in certain cases, sun protection allows for true repair of existing damage.[23] In addition, one of the most promising areas in the treatment of photoaged skin is the use of topical retinoids, especially tretinoin (Retin-A). Investigators have reported significant reversal of minor photodamage to the skin with the use of tretinoin.[24] Current recommendations are to start with 0.025% cream applied twice weekly. If there is no excessive dryness, the dose can then be increased gradually until it is applied twice a day. If the drug is still well tolerated, the dose can continue to be increased over a period of months to years since it requires long-term therapy. Sunscreens appear to help by keeping additional UV radiation from reaching the skin structures. Not only does this help prevent a worsening of the condition, but it also appears to aid in the reversal of some of the skin damage.[13] Patients should be counseled to use a sunscreen product of no less than sun protection factor (SPF) 15 during treatment.[21] Additional studies are being conducted to measure the long-term effects of such treatment. However, it is now believed that up to 80% of all photoaging damage occurs by the age of 20.[25]

Skin Cancer

Numerous epidemiologic studies have been conducted since the 1950s that demonstrate a strong relationship between chronic, excessive, and unprotected sun exposure and human skin cancer. Skin cancer is the most common type of cancer by far, accounting for approximately 33% of all malignancies. Chronic, unprotected sun exposure accounts for up to 90% of skin cancer. About 80% of all skin cancers occur on the most exposed areas of the body, such as the face, head, neck, and back of hands.

The two most common types of nonmelanoma skin cancer (NMSC) are basal cell carcinoma and squamous cell carcinoma. Other UV-induced disorders include premalignant actinic keratosis (which usually develops into squamous cell carcinoma if left untreated), keratoacanthoma, and malignant melanoma. It is estimated that approximately 800,000 individuals will have been diagnosed with basal cell (640,000) and squamous cell carcinomas (160,000) in the United States in 1995.[26] The rate at which these carcinomas grow and invade tissue is relatively low, and more than 99% are curable with early detection and treatment. By contrast, there will have been an estimated 34,000 new cases of malignant melanoma in 1995, representing 5% of all skin cancers. The mortality rate from malignant melanoma is estimated to be as high as 20–25% among all those who develop the condition.[26]

During the 1980s, a large number of studies linking skin cancer with UV exposure were reported. This relationship has become accepted by most health professionals. Since 1990, however, additional studies have produced some evidence that while the relationship does exist, the type of cancer varies significantly according to the causes and contributing factors.

For example, studies have shown conclusively that skin cancer occurs more often in Caucasians than in other ethnic groups.[2] This is believed to be because individuals with darker pigmentation have more melanin in the skin; melanin functions to absorb UV radiation, thereby preventing the radiation from penetrating into the tissue. Accordingly, Gallagher et al reported the corroboration of other researchers in the finding that individuals with blonde or red hair, a history of freckling, and light skin with a tendency to burn rather than tan are at greater risk of developing squamous cell carcinoma.[27]

Another risk factor was found to be a history of severe sunburn. Gallagher et al reported that occupational sun exposure increased the risk of squamous cell carcinoma, but only during the 10 years before the cancer developed.[27] Another finding of this study—that lifetime or recreational UV exposure showed no effect—is contrary to current opinion. In a parallel study on basal cell carcinoma, however, Gallagher et al reported an elevated risk from childhood (5–15 years of age) sun exposure but not from recreational exposure at other ages and no effect from occupational sun exposure.[28] As in the study on squamous cell carcinoma, freckling was also shown as a risk factor for basal cell carcinoma. One of the implications from the data on sun exposure is that avoidance of the sun as an adult may not alter the chances of developing basal cell carcinoma later in life. Kricker et al also reported no association between basal cell carcinoma and occupational sun exposure but did find an association with recreational exposure.[29]

Of all the skin cancers, melanoma has stimulated the most interest in recent years. Melanoma exhibits a pathophysiology different from the NMSCs. Risk factors include light skin, large numbers of melanocytic nevi (moles), and excessive sun exposure.[30] One finding, also noted by Kricker et al for basal cell carcinoma,[29] is the development of melanoma on any area of the body subjected to intense, intermittent sun exposure, such as the legs and trunk. It seems clear that there is an increased (but modest) risk of developing melanoma if frequent sunburn episodes occur.[31]

These recent studies have raised many new questions and identified new confounding factors. Most researchers agree that follow-up corroborating studies need to be done before a definitive relationship between the type of sun exposure and the type of skin cancer can be made. However, there is no question that skin cancer is linked to sun exposure.

One factor affecting skin cancer has been generally accepted: its relationship to latitude. It has been shown that the incidence of skin cancer increases steadily in populations closer to the equator. The quantity of harmful UV radiation that reaches the Earth's surface increases as the angle of the sun to a reference point on Earth approaches 90° and the distance of the sun to the Earth decreases.[32] In the United States as elsewhere, a constant rate of increase in the incidence of skin cancer is found as one approaches the equator from north to south; the incidence approximately doubles for every 3°48' reduction in latitude.[33]

Until all the other major factors affecting skin cancer are conclusively identified, it is recommended that avoidance of UV radiation exposure, the use of hats and other coverings, and the use of sunscreens continue to be the norm to minimize future skin damage.

Sunscreen Products

FDA Review of Sunscreen Agents

The Advisory Review Panel on Topical Analgesic, Antirheumatic, Otic, Burn, and Sunburn Prevention and Treatment Drug Products issued the advance notice of proposal rulemaking (ANPR) on over-the-counter (OTC) sunscreen agents in 1978.[34] At that time, sunscreen manufacturers reformulated their products and changed their labeling to conform to the ANPR proposals. Since then, the FDA has received hundreds of comments addressing 108 issues concerning these agents. Because of the number of comments received in response to the ANPR and significant new developments in the area of photobiology, the FDA delayed issuing guidelines. In May of 1993, the FDA published the long-awaited tentative final monograph (TFM).[35] The FDA will accept comments on the TFM until early 1996; the final monograph will probably be issued several years after that deadline.[36] In the interim, manufacturers are not bound by the proposals in the TFM; they may follow those specific proposals that they like and ignore those that they do not like. Based on the initial responses to the TFM, manufacturers are unhappy with many of the new proposals.

One of the problems for pharmacists and consumers is that confusion may arise concerning the best product to use, given that product formulation and labeling may now follow the ANPR or the TFM. The TFM allows for the following labeling claims on sunscreen product packaging[35]:

- Helps prevent sunburn;
- Helps prevent lip damage;
- Helps prevent skin damage;
- Helps prevent freckling;
- Helps prevent uneven coloration;
- Permits tanning.

Each claim and the specific language used depends on the SPF of the product.

Each indication also appears to be general enough to be understood by the average consumer. The FDA did receive several comments in this regard, suggesting that professional labeling be created that would not be available to consumers. Such information, intended for health professionals only, would deal with the use of sunscreens specifically as therapeutic agents—that is, for patients at risk of developing photosensitivity, photodermatoses, skin cancer, and other conditions. While the TFM makes no recommendation on professional labeling, it does invite comment on this issue.

Throughout the remainder of this chapter, the new proposals will be contrasted to the old where they apply. It should be noted that many of the proposals in the TFM relate to manufacturing issues and are beyond the scope of this chapter.

Classification as Drug Products

Prior to the OTC review, sunscreens were considered to be cosmetics. The TFM addresses a troublesome gray area that has allowed the proliferation of cosmetics claiming to offer sun protection.[35] It stipulates that sunscreen products will be classified as drugs rather than cosmetics because they are intended to be used therapeutically to prevent damage to the skin or lips and can alter physiologic functions such as the production of melanin. However, cosmetics that contain sunscreen agents will be classified as cosmetics so long as the terms *sunscreen* or *SPF* or an SPF value do not appear on the label and no therapeutic claims are made.

Official Names of Sunscreen Agents

Considerable confusion has existed in the literature concerning whether to call each sunscreen by its chemical name, proprietary name, or official compendial name. The TFM clarifies this by stating that the FDA revoked its designated list of official names in 1984 and that the agency "will not routinely designate official names."[35] The FDA's official policy is that drug names "will ordinarily be either the compendial name of the active ingredient or, if there is no compendial name, the common and usual name of the active ingredient." If no official name exists, the name published in the *USP Dictionary of USAN and International Drug Names* will be considered the established name. The names used for the sunscreens in Table 2 are recognized by the FDA.

Sunscreen Efficacy

Minimal Erythema Dose

It is difficult to ascertain the efficacy of sunscreens on humans because individual responsiveness to UV radiation varies greatly. The standardized measure that is used is the minimal erythema dose (MED), defined as the "minimum UV radiation dose that produces clearly marginated erythema in the irradiated site, given as a single exposure."[15] It is a dose of radiation and not a grade of

TABLE 2 Sunscreens considered to be safe and effective

Sunscreen agent	Absorbance range (nm)	Maximum range (nm)	Approved concentration (%)
ABA and derivatives			
Aminobenzoic acid (ABA) (formerly known as PABA)	260–313	288.5	5–15
Glyceryl aminobenzoate[a] (formerly known as glyceryl *p*-aminobenzoate)	264–315	295	2–3
Padimate O	290–315	310	1.4–8
Ethyl 4-[bis(hydroxypropyl)] aminobenzoate[a]	280–330	308–311	1–5
Anthranilates			
Menthyl anthranilate[a]	260–380[b]	340[b]	3.5–5
Benzophenones			
Dioxybenzone	260–380[c]	282[d]	3
Oxybenzone	270–350	290[e]	2–6
Sulisobenzone	260–375	285[f]	5–10
Cinnamates			
Cinoxate	270–328	310	1–3
Diethanolamine methoxycinnamate[a] (formerly known as diethanolamine *p*-methoxycinnamate)	280–310	290	8–10
Octyl methoxycinnamate[a] (formerly known as ethylhexyl *p*-methoxycinnamate)	290–320	308–310	2–7.5
Octocrylene (formerly known as 2-ethylhexyl 2-cyano-3,3-diphenylacrylate)	250–360	303	7–10
Dibenzoylmethane derivatives			
Avobenzone[g,h]	320–400	360	3
Salicylates			
Octyl salicylate[a] (formerly known as 2-ethylhexyl salicylate)	280–320	305	3–5
Homosalate	295–315	306	4–15
Trolamine salicylate	260–320	298	5–12
Miscellaneous			
Digalloyl trioleate	270–320	300	2–5
Lawsone with dihydroxyacetone (DHA)[a]	290–400	—	0.25 (lawsone); 3 (DHA)
Phenylbenzimidazole sulfonic acid[a] (formerly known as 2-phenylbenzimidazole-5-sulfonic acid)	290–320	302	1–4
Red petrolatum[a,i]	290–365	—	30–100
Titanium dioxide[j]	290–770	—	2–25

[a]United States Adopted Names Council has not issued an official name for this agent.
[b]Values are for concentrations higher than those normally found in nonprescription drugs.
[c]Values are achieved when used in combination with other sunscreen agents.
[d]Second peak occurs at 327 nm.
[e]Second peak occurs at 329 nm.
[f]Second peak occurs at 324 nm.
[g]Agent is currently marketed through a new drug application.
[h]Agent is commercially available in a 3% concentration in combination with 3% oxybenzone and 7.5% octyl methoxycinnamate.
[i]A 0.03-mm film absorbs UV radiation below 320 nm. At 334 nm, 16% of radiation is transmitted to the skin; at 365 nm, 58% is transmitted.
[j]Agent scatters, rather than absorbs, radiation in the 290- to 770-nm range.

Source: *Federal Register*. 1978 Aug; 43: 38206–69; *Federal Register*. 1993 May; 58: 28194–302; Shaath NA. Encyclopedia of UV absorbers for sunscreen products. *Cosmetic Toiletries*. 1987 Mar; 102: 21–36.

erythema. The MED is indicative not only of the amount of energy reaching the skin but also of the responsiveness of the skin to the radiation. For instance, 2 MEDs will produce a bright erythema; 4 MEDs, a painful sunburn; and 8 MEDs, a blistering burn. There may also be different MEDs on different parts of the body because of variations in the thickness of the stratum corneum. In addition, the MED for African Americans with heavy pigmentation has been estimated to be up to 33 times higher than that for Caucasians with light pigmentation.

Sun Protection Factor

Another important measure is the SPF, derived by dividing the MED of protected skin by the MED of unprotected skin. For example, if an individual requires 25 mJ/cm^2 of UVB radiation to experience 1 MED on unprotected skin but requires 250 units of radiation to produce 1 MED after applying a given sunscreen, the product would be given an SPF rating of 10. The higher the SPF, the more effective the agent in preventing sunburn. If it normally takes 60 minutes for someone to experience 2 MEDs (a bright erythematous sunburn), a sunscreen with an SPF of 6 will allow that individual to stay in the sun six times longer (or 6 hours) before receiving this same sunburn (assuming the sunscreen is reapplied at the recommended intervals). The SPF is product specific since it is calculated based on the final formulation of the product and cannot be determined on the basis of the active ingredient alone.

Table 3 presents the newly revised skin type classifications and relationships of sunburn and tanning history to SPF and product category designations. These are part of the labeling requirements based on a product's SPF and an individual's natural response to UV radiation. There are several major changes from the ANPR, the most significant involving an upward shift in the recommended SPF for each skin type. Previously, the recommended minimum SPF for a person who "burns moderately and tans gradually" was 4–5.[34] The TFM changes this to 8–12.[35] In the most sun-sensitive category, the recommended SPF goes from 8 or more to 20–30. These changes reflect a new understanding of the important role of higher SPF products.

Perhaps the most controversial proposal in the TFM, and one that will affect the greatest number of sunscreen consumers, sets a maximum SPF of 30 for all commercial sunscreen products. Since 1978, SPFs have climbed all the way to a high of 50, triggering debate about whether products with an SPF greater than 30 offer any advantage to users. For example, a product with an SPF of 15 blocks out 93% of UVB. Raising the SPF to 30 increases UVB protection to only 96.7%, and an SPF-40 blocks out 97.5%. There is a belief that to achieve this small gain in protection (from 30 to 40) might require up to 25% more sunscreen ingredients. This could add to the problems of possible systemic effects and local adverse effects, as well as to a significant increase in cost. A comment to the FDA stated that a hypothetical SPF of 70 would increase UVB protection to only 98.6%.

On the other side of the issue are those who argue in favor of no SPF limits for medical reasons. It has been pointed out that patients with SLE and other lupus-related disorders require a minimum SPF of 40 to prevent triggering the disease.[35] Another comment to the FDA stated that patients taking photosensitizing drugs require an SPF of 45 to provide adequate protection.

In response, the FDA has decided that an SPF of 30 provides adequate all-day protection for all skin types, including patients with UV-induced disorders. In determining protection from photosensitivity, the wavelength at which the product absorbs or reflects the UV radiation is more important than the SPF. For example, there is no evidence that an SPF of 40 will protect against photosensitivity if the reaction is triggered at 370 nm and the product absorbs only up to 340 nm.

The question remains as to whether an SPF of 30 provides adequate protection for all individuals and whether the risks of higher SPF products outweigh the benefits. It is interesting to note here that in a study of actinic keratoses, the use of a waterproof, ultra high (SPF 29) sunscreen product reduced the incidence of new growth development compared with placebo.[37] Since actinic keratoses develop into squamous cell carcinomas, the implication is that regular sunscreen use will reduce the incidence of these cancers. The study results show a

TABLE 3 Sunburn and tanning history

Skin type[a]	Sunburn/tanning history	Recommended SPF	Recommended PCD[a,b]
I	Always burns easily; never tans	20–30	Ultra high
II	Always burns easily; tans minimally	12–<20	Very high
III	Burns moderately; tans gradually	8–<12	High
IV	Burns minimally; always tans well	4–<8	Moderate
V	Rarely burns; tans profusely	2–<4	Minimal
VI[c]	Never burns; deeply pigmented (insensitive)	—	—

[a]Optional labeling information according to the TFM.

[b]Product category designation (PCD).

[c]Skin type VI, which is not part of the proposed *Recommended Sunscreen Product Guide*, is included in this table because the TFM addresses it with the other skin types; however, this skin type is used only under the general testing procedures for the selection of test subjects.

Adapted from *Federal Register*. 1993 May; 58: 28194–302.

greater reduction in both patients with lighter skin and patients with a greater number of preexisting actinic keratoses at the time of the study. There was even a protective effect for individuals with naturally darker skin.

Measures of UVA Protection

With concern about the long-term adverse effects of UVA growing, the utility of the SPF value has been questioned. The SPF provides a measure of a person's erythemogenic response to UVB when using a sunscreen. However, UVA is at least 200 times less potent than UVB in producing erythema, and its effects on the skin are somewhat different from those produced by UVB.[14] Recent investigations have shown that sunscreens with similar SPFs show significant differences in their abilities to protect against UV-induced immunologic injury to the skin.[38] Current data suggest that high SPF products block significant amounts of UVA. However, among products of equal SPF, UVA blockage may vary considerably. At present, the SPF is not considered to be a reliable measure of UVA protection. As a temporary measure, the TFM allows a product to make a claim of UVA protection so long as the ingredients have an absorption spectrum that extends to at least 360 nm.[35]

One area of considerable discussion and debate is how best to measure UVA protection. The FDA received many comments as well as several proposals in this regard. The key is to create an index of protection analogous to the SPF. The FDA stated in the TFM that the various UVA protection factors being proposed by sunscreen manufacturers are not yet "meaningful."[35] It is believed that a useful and understandable UVA protection factor will be part of the final monograph.

Substantivity

The efficacy of a sunscreen is related to its substantivity—that is, its ability to remain effective during prolonged exercise, sweating, and swimming. This property can be a function of the active sunscreen, the vehicle, or both. Generally speaking, products with cream-based (water in oil) vehicles appear more resistant to removal by water than those with alcohol bases and will reduce desquamation of the skin. It should be remembered, however, that part of a sunscreen's effectiveness may relate to the ability of the active agent to bind with constituents of the skin. This binding characteristic may be independent of the vehicle. Oil-based products have traditionally been the most popular and are the easiest to apply. However, they tend to have lower SPF values.

The ANPR contained three categories of substantivity: sweat resistant, water resistant, and waterproof.[34] The TFM eliminates "sweat resistant" as a category. The FDA is concerned about the health risks to subjects who must be exposed to a temperature of 35°–38°C (95°–100°F) and to 70–80% humidity with little air movement. Under the TFM, any product that falls into one of the two other categories of substantivity can still be labeled as either "resists removal by perspiring" or "perspiration resistant."[35] The TFM guidelines for sunscreen product substantivity are[35]:

- *Water resistant*: retains its sun protection for at least 40 minutes in water;
- *Very water resistant*: retains its sun protection for at least 80 minutes in water.

The category of *very water resistant* is intended to replace *waterproof*, which is currently in use. This is one of the areas in which manufacturers do not agree with the FDA and have chosen to continue to label products as waterproof until either the agency changes its mind or the final monograph is published.

In addition, the TFM proposes that products making claims of substantivity be labeled with both the static SPF (measured under dry conditions) and the SPF under water-testing guidelines. For example, a product that has a static SPF of 30 and meets *water resistant* test standards with an SPF of 20 will be labeled as follows:

> SPF = 30 before perspiring or going into the water.
> SPF = 20 after 40 minutes of perspiring or activity in the water.

Although some comments claimed that requiring dual SPFs would confuse consumers, the FDA believes that allowing dual SPFs to be optional would be even more confusing. There are products on the market that claim longer periods of protection than the FDA definitions allow, such as "8 hour" or "all day" protection. This type of extended substantivity is not covered by the TFM and will need to be addressed in the final monograph.

Formulation Factors

Although pharmacists cannot control the formulation of the various commercially available sunscreen products, a knowledge of the specific active and inactive ingredients and their concentrations may help them differentiate a good product from a mediocre one. Several factors affecting the efficacy of nonprescription sunscreen products are related to the vehicle/solvent system. For example:

- The partition coefficient relative to the skin should favor passage of the sunscreen to the skin.
- The pH of the solvent can vary the fraction of ionized and nonionized sunscreen agent, thereby rendering it less effective or even ineffective.
- The solvent system should provide a high degree of substantivity.
- The sunscreen must remain stable for the desired period of protection.

While acknowledging that an ideal vehicle does not exist, the ANPR described such a vehicle as follows:

> An ideal sunscreen vehicle would be stable, neutral, nongreasy, nondegreasing, nonirritating, nondehydrating, nondrying, odorless, and efficient on all types of human skin. It would also hold at least 50% water, be easily compounded of known chemicals, and have infinite stability during storage.[34]

It also recommended that all inactive ingredients be included on product labels. This labeling would allow evaluation by the consumer, pharmacist, and physician for several factors, including sensitivity to any product ingredients.

Types of Sunscreen Agents

Two definitions for therapeutic sunscreen types have been proposed[35]:

- *Sunscreen active ingredient*: an active ingredient that absorbs at least 85% of the radiation in the UV range at wavelengths from 290 to 320 nm, but that may or may not allow transmission of radiation to the skin at wavelengths longer than 320 nm.
- *Sunscreen opaque sunblock*: an opaque sunscreen active ingredient that reflects or scatters all light in the UV and visible range at wavelengths from 290 to 777 nm and thereby prevents or minimizes suntan and sunburn.

Based on these definitions, topical sunscreens can also be divided into two major subgroups: chemical and physical. Chemical sunscreens work by absorbing and thus blocking the transmission of UV radiation to the epidermis. Physical sunscreens are generally opaque and act by reflecting and scattering UV radiation rather than absorbing it.

Many sunscreen products contain a combination of sunscreen agents. A single product containing an agent that absorbs primarily UVA radiation is also available (see product table "Sunscreen and Suntan Products").

The TFM lists 20 chemical compounds (compared with 21 in the ANPR[18]) as safe and efficacious for nonprescription use as topical sunscreens.[35] All of these sunscreens are included in Table 2.

Chemical Sunscreens

Aminobenzoic Acid and Derivatives For many years, aminobenzoic acid (ABA; formerly known as para-aminobenzoic acid, or PABA) has been used in many sunscreen products. ABA is an effective UVB sunscreen, especially when formulated in a hydroalcoholic base (maximum of 50–60% alcohol). The SPF of such formulations increases proportionally as the concentration of ABA increases from 2 to 5%. There is evidence that some UVA is also blocked at the 5% or higher level.[39]

One advantage of ABA is its ability to penetrate into the horny layer of the skin and provide lasting protection. It has significant substantivity on sweating skin although not so much on skin that is immersed in water. The primary advantage of ABA derivatives over ABA is that they do not stain clothing.

The disadvantages of alcoholic solutions of ABA include (1) contact dermatitis, (2) photosensitivity, (3) stinging and drying of the skin, and (4) yellow staining of clothes upon exposure to the sun.[40] It is perhaps ironic that certain sunscreen agents such as ABA, which are intended to prevent photosensitivity reactions, can themselves induce photosensitivity and contact dermatitis. Some of the drugs that may induce cross-sensitivity to ABA and its derivatives include thiazide diuretics, sulfonamides, and "caine" anesthetics such as lidocaine and benzocaine. Patients who have experienced a photosensitivity reaction to any of these drugs should not use a sunscreen containing ABA or any of its derivatives.

Of all the available sunscreens, glyceryl para-aminobenzoate is associated with the highest risk of inducing allergic contact dermatitis. Because of this risk and because it is a very irritating substance, it is not currently found in any commercially available nonprescription sunscreen product.

There have been recent reports of significant phototoxic reactions to another ABA ester, padimate A. Because of these adverse reaction reports, all manufacturers in the United States have removed padimate A from their products; the European Union has banned its use. Accordingly, the TFM places padimate A in concentrations of 5% and higher in Category II (not generally recognized as safe and effective) and in concentrations lower than 5% in Category III (available data are insufficient to classify it as safe and effective; further testing is required).

Anthranilates The anthranilates are ortho-ABA derivatives. Menthyl anthranilate, the menthyl ester of anthranilic acid, is a weak UV sunscreen with maximal absorbance in the UVA range. It is usually found in combination with other sunscreen agents to provide broader UV coverage.

Benzophenones There are three agents in the benzophenone group: dioxybenzone, oxybenzone (benzophenone-3), and sulisobenzone (benzophenone-4). As a group, these agents are primarily UVB absorbers with maximum absorbance between 282 and 290 nm. However, their absorbance extends well into the UVA range, with oxybenzone up to 350 nm and dioxybenzone up to 380 nm. Because of their extended spectrum of action, benzophenones are often found in combination with other sunscreens to provide a very broad spectrum of coverage.

Owing to the possibility of allergic reactions to ABA and its derivatives and to the wider spectrum of action of the benzophenones, more sunscreen products contain benzophenones in their formulations. Because of this and the fact that oxybenzone, found in some cosmetic formulations, is a sensitizing agent, there has been a rise in reports of sensitivity to the benzophenones.[41]

Cinnamates There are four sunscreens in this group. Three of the four agents—cinoxate, diethanolamine methoxycinnamate, and octyl methoxycinnamate—have similar absorbance ranges as well as maximum absorbances. The exception is octocrylene, which has an absorbance range of 250–360 nm, well into the UVA range. Octocrylene is currently found in many more commercial sunscreen preparations than it was in the past, possibly reflecting its broader spectrum of absorbance. Unfortunately, cinnamates do not adhere well to the skin and must rely on the vehicle in a given formulation for their substantivity.

Salicylates Salicylic acid derivatives are weak sunscreens and must be used in high concentrations. They do not adhere well to the skin and are easily removed by perspiration or swimming.

Physical Sunscreens

Physical sunscreens scatter rather than absorb UV and visible radiation (290–777 nm). They are most often used on small and prominently exposed areas by people who cannot limit or control their exposure to the sun (eg, lifeguards). The nose and tops of the ears are often coated with a white or colored substance containing zinc oxide or titanium dioxide. Manufacturers have not yet developed a way to make physical sunscreens transparent while maintaining similar efficacy. (Such a product would also not be consistent with the FDA definition of a physical sunscreen.) The effectiveness of physical sunscreens is related to the thickness with which they are applied. Their disadvantages are that they can discolor clothing and may occlude the skin to produce miliaria (prickly heat) and folliculitis. Because titanium dioxide increases the effective SPF of a product and extends the spectrum of protection well into the UVA range, the number of commercial products containing this agent has increased.

Zinc oxide was inadvertently skipped when the advisory review panel initially evaluated the various sunscreen agents. It was subsequently categorized as a Category I skin protectant and an inactive sunscreen agent. Based on the FDA's later decision that data on zinc oxide's effectiveness as a sunscreen agent are insufficient, the TFM has placed this agent in Category III.[35]

UVA Sunscreens

Dibenzoylmethane derivatives are the first of a new class of sunscreen agents effective throughout the entire UVA range (full spectrum). The first of these new agents is avobenzone (butyl methoxydibenzoylmethane, originally known as Parsol 1789), which has maximum absorbance at approximately 360 nm.[42] This agent entered the market through a new drug application (NDA). Although avobenzone absorbs UV radiation through all of the UVA spectrum, its absorbance falls off sharply at 370 nm. There is still the possibility of a photosensitivity reaction from those chemicals that are highly reactive in the 370- to 400-nm range. There is currently only one product on the market containing avobenzone: Shade UVAGuard, which contains avobenzone 3% (320–400 nm), oxybenzone 3% (270–350 nm), and octyl methoxycinnamate 7.5% (290–320 nm), and has an SPF of 15.

Combination Products

The FDA has not recommended any limits on the number of sunscreen agents that may be used together in a nonprescription product. Since the SPF is product specific and not dependent on the sunscreen active agent alone, the TFM has eliminated a required minimum strength for single active ingredient sunscreen products. There is, however, a concern by the FDA that additional sunscreen agents must contribute to the efficacy of a product and not be included merely for marketing promotion purposes. Therefore, the TFM does include a minimum concentration for each sunscreen agent when used in combination.[35]

Suntan Products and Devices

Two types of products fall under the general heading of suntan products: those that contain a sunscreen and those that do not. Products without a sunscreen are easily identified by the absence of an SPF value on the label. These products are considered cosmetics and are used for coloring the skin rather than for any therapeutic indications. Thus, they are formulated with oily vehicles that tend to concentrate UV radiation onto the skin. Although they are also formulated with emollients, this type of suntan product provides no protection whatsoever against all the short- and long-term hazards of UV radiation exposure. However, all suntan products that contain sunscreen active ingredients can still be considered suntan products, even those with the highest SPFs. Thus, the TFM allows the claim of "permits tanning" on products with an SPF of 2 to <12, while a product with an SPF of 12 to <20 "limits tanning."

Pigmenting Agents

Oral Agents

During the past several years, a number of products have claimed to be effective oral tanning compounds. Their active ingredients are the dyes canthaxanthin and beta-carotene, which are chemically similar to one another. Beta-carotene and canthaxanthin are both approved by the FDA as color additives in foods and drugs, and beta-carotene is also approved for use in cosmetics. Canthaxanthin is a synthetic dye that is similar to those dyes found naturally in fruits, vegetables, and flowers. Both agents are used to enhance the appearance of foods such as pizza, barbecue and spaghetti sauces, soups, salad dressings, fruit drinks, baked goods, pudding, cheese, ketchup, and margarine. However, they are present in food in lower concentrations than they are in oral products that claim to produce tanning. For example, the daily dietary intakes of beta-carotene and canthaxanthin as food colorants are about 0.3 mg and 5.6 mg, respectively[43]; in one brand of tanning tablet, however, the daily intakes are 12 mg and 100 mg, respectively.

The dyes alter skin tone by coloring the fat cells under the epidermal layer. Because of variations in fat cells and epidermal thickness, the extent of the tan varies from person to person. Canthaxanthin is dosed by body weight, with a 20-day schedule necessary to achieve a significant change in skin tone. This process is followed by doses of one to two capsules per day to maintain the color. The promotional literature cautions the user that if the palms turn orange, too much of the product is being consumed.

According to the 1960 Color Additive Amendment, any new use of a color additive must be submitted to the FDA for approval.[44] The FDA has not yet approved either beta-carotene or canthaxanthin for artificial tanning. One major concern is the discoloration of the feces to brick red, which could mask gastrointestinal bleeding. A second concern is the long-term adverse effects that may be associated with the large doses recommended. Although beta-carotene is used on a prescription basis to help prevent photosensitivity in patients with erythropoietic protoporphyria, there is no evidence documenting the safety of canthaxanthin at the high doses found in oral tanning products. In fact, a recent case has been reported of fatal aplastic anemia associated with canthaxanthin ingestion from an oral tanning product. Reported cases of retinopathy, hepatitis, and urticaria associated with the use of oral tanning agents has prompted the FDA to issue further warnings on such products.[45]

In addition, Canada, which previously allowed the nonprescription sale of canthaxanthin for tanning purposes, has decided that there is insufficient evidence of its safety and no longer allows such sales.

Topical Dyes

Another type of pigmenting agent is dihydroxyacetone (DHA). For years, DHA has been the major ingredient in products that claim to tan without sun. DHA produces a reddish brown color by binding with specific amino acids in the stratum corneum. The intensity of the tan is related to the thickness of the skin. If the product is not washed off the hands immediately after application, however, the palms may also develop this tan (turn orange). In addition, dry areas such as elbows and kneecaps will absorb the DHA more readily, resulting in uneven coloration. The color fades after 5–7 days with desquamation of the stratum corneum.

The FDA has determined that DHA alone is ineffective as a sunscreen and that it should be classified as a cosmetic. However, in combination with lawsone, a major dye component of henna, the combination is classified as a weak sunscreen. This combination will not directly affect melanin production, and in one study, the SPF of such products was calculated to be less than 2[40]; the TFM requires that a sunscreen product have a minimum SPF of not less than 2.[35] There are currently no products on the market containing this combination. Several sun-less tanning products combine DHA with various sunscreen agents, which at least helps prevent photodamage for those persons who intend to spend some time in the sun.

Tan Accelerators

Tan accelerators are cosmetic products that claim to stimulate a faster and deeper tan. There are several of these products currently on the market. Their major ingredient is tyrosine, an amino acid necessary for the production of melanin. Product literature recommends application of these products once daily for at least 3 days before sun exposure. However, one study that tested two commercial products using indoor UV radiation found no evidence of benefit.[46] The TFM recognizes this fact and states that "any product containing tyrosine or its derivatives and claiming to accelerate the tanning process is an unapproved new drug."[35]

Melanotropins

A hormone known as alpha-melanotropin or alpha-melanocyte-stimulating hormone (ALPHA-MSH) has been located within the human central nervous system. The role of ALPHA-MSH in humans, if any, has not yet been identified. However, this hormone is produced by the pituitary gland of numerous vertebrates and has been shown to affect skin color through its action on melanocytes. Alpha-melanotropin is currently under investigation to determine whether it can affect skin tanning.[47]

Tanning Booths and Sunbeds

The availability of tanning booths and sunbeds may prompt questions from patients concerning their safety. Since 1980, manufacturers have shifted the composition of UV radiation emitted by these devices from UVB to UVA. The newer types of tanning devices use UV radiation sources composed of more than 96% UVA and less than 4% UVB, a considerably different mix of UV radiation than that obtained from natural sunlight.[11] Some tanning devices in commercial use are almost exclusively UVA although all of them contain a minimal amount of UVB necessary to stimulate tanning. The emission spectrum of tanning devices varies significantly, and the user has no way of knowing the effects to be expected.[48]

It would appear that UVA, if used properly, could generate a tan without producing an erythematous sunburn. However, there is a concern about UVB contamination of UVA lamps. It is believed that even 1% UVB emission can cause a significant increase in the incidence of skin cancer. In addition, some UVA lamps produce more than five times as much UVA per unit of time than does sunlight.[13] There is a small but growing body of evidence that the use of sunlamps and sunbeds is related to the rising incidence of malignant melanoma worldwide.[49,50] It has been speculated that the lack of sufficient corroborating data is partly owing to a latent period between exposure and the development of melanoma. The effects of the transition to predominantly UVA sunlamps and sunbeds since 1980 may only just now be beginning to surface.

UVA also presents other hazards, such as deeper tissue penetration than UVB, as described earlier. UVA radiation may trigger the eruption of cold sores. In addition, it can produce a photosensitivity reaction in patients who have ingested or applied photosensitizing agents. There has even been a recent report of a phototoxic reaction with the use of a home tanning bed.[51] Moreover, because UVA is less likely to produce the overt burning (erythema) of UVB, patients may become complacent and forgo the use of eye goggles; this practice will produce eye burns and may increase the risk of subsequently developing cataracts. In one study on eye injuries from UV tanning devices, ophthalmologists treated 152 patients over a 12-month period for a variety of ocular injuries, primarily of the cornea and retina.[52] Only 24% of patients wore safety goggles while using the devices.

The FDA sets standards for sunlamp products and UV lamps.[53] These regulations deal with such issues as timers, exposure time, and device labeling, as well as the use of goggles with specified transmittance limits. Despite all these precautions and warnings, however, these FDA regulations do not include any specified limits on the amount or ratio of UVA and UVB emitted from tanning devices. Patients should be advised that the possibility of long-term hazards related to UVA has not yet been fully assessed and that there are currently no accepted health benefits from tanning devices.

Sunglasses

Concern has been expressed regarding the relationship between UV radiation and eye damage such as cataracts or long-term retinal damage.[54] UV radiation may also cause temporary injuries such as photokeratitis (a painful type of snow blindness associated with highly reflective surfaces). One of the most recent problems to surface involves an increase in the incidence of uveal (iris plus ciliary body) melanoma.[55] These concerns are all the more serious because of the erroneous belief that all sunglasses screen out UV radiation. In response, the Sunglass Association of America, working with the FDA, has developed a voluntary labeling program. Abbreviated information concerning the UV radiation screening properties is directly attached to each pair of sunglasses, while brochures describing the appropriate use of each type of lens are available at outlets selling the sunglasses. Based on its UV radiation filtration properties, each pair of sunglasses is placed in one of three categories[56]:

- *Cosmetic* sunglasses block at least 70% of UVB, 20% of UVA, and less than 60% of visible light. They are recommended for activities in nonharsh sunlight, such as shopping.
- *General purpose* sunglasses block at least 95% of UVB, at least 60% of UVA, and 60–92% of visible light. With shades that range from medium to dark, they are recommended for most activities in sunny environments, such as boating, driving, flying, or hiking.
- *Special purpose* sunglasses block at least 99% of UVB, 60% of UVA, and 20–97% of visible light. They are recommended for activities in very bright environments, such as ski slopes and tropical beaches.

Product Selection Guidelines

The most important thing a pharmacist needs to know before recommending a sunscreen product is the patient's natural skin type and tanning history. The pharmacist should also find out from the patient how much time is normally spent out of doors in occupational and recreational pursuits. Other questions the pharmacist might ask are presented at the beginning of this chapter. Using this information, as well as knowing both the active and inactive ingredients in the various products and the products' SPFs, the pharmacist can feel comfortable in recommending a sunscreen product.

Efficacy Considerations

Sun Protection Factor

Patients with less natural skin protection should use products with higher SPFs. A product with an SPF-15 will prevent sunburn while also allowing for a gradually developing tan. A product of SPF-30 should be recommended for patients who burn easily, cannot tan, or cannot afford any degree of sunburn or overexposure to UV radiation of any type. Patients who have a personal or family history of certain dermatologic problems, such as atopic dermatitis or sunburn with short exposure, or who have any type of skin cancer or precancerous dermatologic lesion should use a total blocking agent or a sunscreen with an SPF of 30 or higher when prolonged exposure to sunlight is expected. Studies have shown that even low protective sunscreens (SPF-2) can reduce the incidence of nonmelanoma skin cancers from 36% to 54% if properly used beginning in childhood.[57] However, some investigators and clinicians have suggested that products with an SPF of less than 6 not be recommended routinely to patients[40]; because of the hazards associated with UV radiation, they recommend instead the selection of a product with an SPF of 15 or higher. Any product in the 15–50 SPF range will significantly reduce the total amount of UVB and UVA radiation received.

The current public health emphasis is on reducing total lifetime exposure to UV radiation. While pharmacists need to assess the patient's particular situation in selecting the best sunscreen product, in the vast majority of cases an SPF of 30 is the best choice. However, for patients with UV-induced disorders or taking photosensitizing drugs, a sunscreen that absorbs throughout the UVA range is probably a better choice than the highest SPF product. A broad-spectrum sunscreen, while effective throughout the UVB range, is required to have absorption activity only through 360 nm and not through 400 nm. Therefore, it may not provide complete protection, especially against photosensitivity.

Broad-Spectrum Sunscreens

The question of what constitutes a true broad-spectrum sunscreen remains. A number of commercial products claim to be broad spectrum; the TFM allows such claims if the product contains ingredients that absorb or reflect UVB (290–320 nm) *and* absorb up to 360 nm.[19] Products with equal SPFs may still differ significantly in total UV protection, depending on the absorbances of the various sunscreens they contain. Most currently available broad-spectrum products have a minimum of two sunscreen ingredients while many others incorporate three or even four sunscreens.

Although UVA II is more damaging to the skin than UVA I, the lack of a standardized UVA protection factor does not allow such considerations to be taken into account in product selection. Thus, there is no one generally accepted measure to evaluate the actual efficacy of a product that claims to provide UVA protection. The best recommendation would be to select a product that contains a combination of sunscreen agents that protect throughout the entire UVB range and across the widest possible UVA range. A product that contains avobenzone, claims to be broad spectrum, and has an SPF of at least 15 is an excellent choice for patients with UV-induced disorders or taking photosensitizing drugs. Currently, Shade UVAGuard is the only such product on the market. A very broad spectrum of coverage can also be obtained by using an ABA derivative combined with one of the benzophenones, octocrylene, or menthyl anthranilate. There are a number of broad-spectrum combinations on the market.

Substantivity

A very important factor in product selection is the product's substantivity. Given three products of equal SPF but varying substantivity, the best and most cost-effective selection is the product that is most substantive. A *very water resistant/waterproof* product needs to be reapplied only after 80 minutes of swimming or continuous water exposure, whereas a water-resistant product must be reapplied after 40 minutes of swimming or continuous water exposure. A product that makes no claims of substantivity probably requires reapplication after every 30 minutes of perspiration. The less substantive a product, the more likely it is to be rubbed off by any type of contact.

Lip Protection

One of the most common locations for oral cancer is the lips. Because there are few melanocytes in the lips, they burn rather than tan and are prone to the development of cancer that has been associated with exposure to UV radiation. The lips also can become dry and chapped.

More than a dozen sunscreen products are on the market to prevent burning of the lips (or nose). Although they differ in ingredients and UVA and UVB spectrum, these products carry the same labeling, including the SPF, as do the sunscreen lotions (with the exception that they do not require "for external use only"). The SPF of these products is usually at least 15. Studies have shown that lip protection not only helps prevent drying and burning of the lips but also helps prevent the development of cold sores (fever blisters) triggered by the herpes simplex virus in patients who are susceptible to recurrent cold sores. Because these products are available in stick or lipstick form, they are convenient to carry and use, and they can be reapplied as often as necessary. Lipsticks are perhaps the most often neglected sunscreen product.

Sunscreens for Children

Special consideration is needed when recommending a sunscreen product for young children. The consensus is that the absorptive characteristics of human skin in children under 6 months of age are different from those of adult skin. Related to this is the belief that the metabolic and excretory systems of children under 6 months of age are not fully developed to handle any sunscreen agent absorbed through the skin. Therefore, only persons over 6 months of age are considered to have adult human skin. The TFM has made two specific, age-related recommendations regarding the labeling of nonprescription sunscreens[35]:

- Children under 6 months of age should be seen by a doctor.
- Children under 2 years of age should use sunscreen products with a minimum SPF of 4.

Caregivers should be extremely wary regarding sun exposure in children, especially those under 6 months old. Regular use of an SPF-15 product starting after 6 months of age and continuing through 18 years can reduce the incidence of skin cancer over a lifetime by as much as 78%.[57] Even better would be a product with an SPF of 30. Such usage would also result in a reduction in sunburn and a reduced risk of premature skin aging and other skin problems.

Precautions

Staining

There has been some concern about sunscreen products staining clothing or the vinyl and fiberglass found in boats. This is no longer a major concern because staining is primarily associated with ABA, which currently exists in only a few commercial products and whose esters (eg, padimate O) do not cause staining. However, to be used safely, sunscreen products containing ABA should be allowed to dry before the skin comes into contact with clothing, vinyl, or fiberglass. This is probably a good rule to follow regardless of the sunscreen used. The only other sunscreen that has potential for staining is DHA, which is found in some tanning and sunscreen products. Again, product labels warn that, to prevent staining, the skin should be allowed to dry thoroughly before coming into contact with clothing.

Contact Dermatitis and Other Skin Considerations

Photosensitivity and contact dermatitis are more likely to occur with ABA and its esters. Other sunscreens have also been reported to produce both conditions, although to a lesser degree. These sunscreens include the benzophenones, the cinnamates, homosalate, avobenzone, and menthyl anthranilate. In addition, patients who are allergy prone and have allergies to various drugs, such as benzocaine, thiazides, or sulfonamides, may also develop an allergic reaction to either ABA or its esters.

Other general cosmetic considerations also need to be taken into account because anything that will motivate an individual to use a sunscreen is a welcome advantage. For example, at least one third of the commercial products currently available are labeled noncomedogenic, fragrance free, and hypoallergenic. Products that are noncomedogenic are those that do not plug the pores and therefore do not exacerbate acne. This is especially important for teenagers, who generally spend more time out of doors than other age groups and would generally prefer not to use comedogenic sunscreens. Regarding fragrance-free and hypoallergenic properties, many individuals are sensitive to various ingredients, including fragrances, emulsifiers, and preservatives. In a recent randomized, placebo-controlled study of adverse reactions to sunscreens, 16% of subjects developed a local reaction to the topically applied product.[58] Of those subjects, 53% agreed to be patch tested and photopatch tested. None of these individuals showed a sensitivity to the sunscreen agents. Instead, all the reactions were found to be caused by formulation ingredients such as fragrances and preservatives. This seems to reinforce the belief that while some individuals are sensitive to certain sunscreen products, most of that sensitivity may be due to nonsunscreen ingredients. While it may not be possible to figure out what specific ingredient an individual is sensitive to, patients who have a history of sensitivity to these types of ingredients would do well to use a fragrance-free, hypoallergenic product.

Some individuals have normally dry skin. Sunbathing can further exacerbate this problem. Ethyl and isopropyl alcohols, which are included in a number of commercial sunscreen products, can also dry the skin and should be avoided in these patients.

A product that promises sunless tanning and has an SPF rating contains DHA with a sunscreen, whereas a product that promises sunless tanning and has no SPF most likely contains DHA alone. Such products may create a false sense of security. The individual might look tan, but these products provide no sunscreen protection, and overexposure to UV radiation may thus result in a serious burn.

Patient Counseling

Pharmacists can provide a great service by counseling consumers about the suntanning process and the proper selection and use of sunscreens. In one study involving almost 500 persons, a considerable amount of misinformation was found to exist concerning sunscreen use.[59] For example, 51% of those surveyed did not know the definition of SPF or its significance; 26% were not even aware of the existence of sunscreens before the study; and of the 41% who used sunscreens, one third thought those products would promote tanning.

The rays of the sun are the most direct and damaging between 10 AM and 3 PM. It is best to avoid sunning during this period, especially at the beginning of the season before any protective tan has developed. Closely related to this is the misconception that one cannot burn on an overcast or cloudy day. Although varying amounts of visible sunlight may not pass through cloud cover and the clouds tend to filter out the infrared radiation that contributes to the sensation of heat, this reduction in heat sensation provides a false sense of security against a burn.[60] In fact, very little UV radiation is filtered and most (70–80%) will penetrate clouds. In addition, the intensity of exposure increases as one moves closer to the equator. People in the southern part of the United States are at greater risk from the harmful effects of UV radiation than those in northern areas. Also, the irradiance of UVB increases by 4% for every 1,000 feet of altitude. This may be of particular concern to skiers and individuals living and working in higher elevations.

Another potential problem is that UV radiation reflects off of various surfaces. Fresh snow will reflect 85–100% of the light and radiation that strikes it, creating the need for sunglasses when one is skiing on a sunny day. This reflected radiation is also why a skier can receive a significant sunburn, even on a cloudy day, and thus should use a sunscreen. Similarly, sand and white-painted surfaces, while not as reflective as snow, nevertheless reflect a significant amount of the radiation striking them. Therefore, a person sitting in the shade of a beach umbrella may still be bombarded by UV radiation reflecting off the sand. This contributes to the overall radiation received, and a severe sunburn may result. Water reflects no more than 5% of UV radiation and allows the remaining 95% to penetrate and burn the swimmer. Therefore, time in the water, even if the swimmer is completely submerged, should be considered as part of the total time spent in the sun. In addition, although dry clothes reflect almost all UV radiation, wet clothes allow transmission of approximately 50% of UV radiation. However, if light passes through dry clothing when held up to the light, UV radiation will also penetrate that clothing. Tightly woven material offers the greatest protection.

If properly applied, products with an SPF of 15–30 allow an individual to stay out in the sun for long periods and slowly develop a tan over several days to weeks. It is important to remember, however, that as an individual tans, a natural protection against burning also develops. Therefore, an individual who insists on tanning should begin the summer using a product with an SPF of at least 15 and switch to a product with a lower SPF (eg, 12, then 10, then 8, etc) as the natural tan progresses. This change will allow a more rapid deepening of the tan while helping to build up natural protection in the skin. The person can, however, continue to use the product with the SPF of 15; it will simply take longer to achieve the desired tan.

Patients should be advised that, although tanning and thickening of the skin serve as protective mechanisms against future injury, peeling of the skin removes part of this protection. The amount of exposure to the sun as well as the SPF of the product being used must be reevaluated as tanning and peeling occur.

The two major causes of poor sun protection with sunscreen use are application of inadequate amounts and infrequent reapplication. In a recent report on sunscreen application to eight areas of the face, the degree of complete coverage ranged from 8% periorbital and 18% ears to 80% forehead and 94% cheeks.[61] Sunscreens must be liberally applied to all exposed areas of the body and reapplied as often as the label recommends for maximum effectiveness. Although these two factors drive up the cost of sunscreen use, the long-term benefits of proper sunscreen use far outweigh the costs.

The FDA standard for application of sunscreens is 2 mcL/cm^2 of body surface area. This means that, for sufficient protection, the average adult in a bathing suit should apply nine portions of sunscreen of approximately ½ teaspoon each, or approximately 4½ teaspoons total. The sunscreen should be distributed as follows[62]:

- Face and neck: ½ teaspoon;
- Arms and shoulders: ½ teaspoon to each side;
- Torso: ½ teaspoon each to front and back;
- Legs and top of feet: 1 teaspoon to each side.

Because of the cost of sunscreen products and the need to apply them often and in sufficient amounts, people may use far less sunscreen than is necessary to provide adequate protection. One study demonstrated that the effective SPF of commercial products was only 50% of the labeled value when subjects were allowed to apply sunscreen according to their own assessment of need.[63] One simple way to find out if patients are using sunscreen properly is to ask how long the current bottle they are using has lasted. When applied properly, according to the above-suggested dosing guidelines and in accordance with the appropriate substantivity of the product, a sunbather could easily use about 1 oz every 80–90 minutes. This would amount to several ounces a day and several bottles per week. Incredibly, many frequent sunbathers use only one bottle in an entire season. This demonstrates the importance of individuals receiving adequate counseling from pharmacists to get the protection they desire.

The TFM proposes that the directions for use of products that make no substantivity claims read as follows[35]:

- Apply liberally/generously/smoothly/evenly [*manufacturer may select one or more of these terms*] before sun exposure.
- Reapply after swimming, excessive sweating/perspiring [*manufacturer may select one term*], or any time after toweling dry.

Reapplying a sunscreen does not extend the amount of time a person can spend in the sun. Outdoor exposure to UV radiation should be within the limits of the SPF value of the sunscreen. Moreover, although some sunscreen products now have an SPF of 50, the use of an SPF-30 offers adequate protection to the average person. The best all-purpose, general recommendation for providing optimal protection from immediate as well as long-term injury from sun exposure is a product with an SPF of 30. This will allow the development of a slow tan with safety. Children should use SPF-30 sunscreens daily whenever they play outdoors, not just when swimming. Pharmacists should emphasize these recommendations during consultation.

Recently, questions have arisen as to whether the substantivity of a sunscreen may affect the temperature-regulating ability of the body. One study reported that exercising in hot weather after applying a sunscreen product may increase the risk of overheating.[64] Under hot, humid conditions, there is increased sweating but poor evaporation. When the humidity is low, overheating during exercise may still occur, possibly because the oily vehicle of the sunscreen may block the pores. Therefore, sunbathers should be cautious when exercising in hot weather after applying a sunscreen product.

There has been one report of individuals ingesting ABA in doses of up to 1 g daily to prevent phototoxic reactions.[65] However, there is no evidence demonstrating the safety or efficacy of ABA when used in this manner. Moreover, oral ingestion of ABA has been associated with a lowered white blood cell count, drug fever, and organ damage, and thus should be vigorously discouraged.

The TFM also proposed that labeling of all sunscreens contain the following warnings[35]:

- For external use only, not to be swallowed.
- Avoid contact with eyes. If contact occurs, rinse eyes thoroughly with water.
- Discontinue use if signs of irritation or rash appear. If irritation or rash persists, consult a doctor.

Consumers should be advised that if itching, redness, or a rash develops while using a particular product, they should discontinue using the product and contact a pharmacist.

Case Studies

Case 30–1

Patient Complaint/History

KL, a 23-year-old female student who has blonde hair and numerous freckles on her face, presents to the pharmacist and asks about the SPF of sunscreen products. She is holding a suntan product with an SPF of 2 as well as a sunscreen product with an SPF of 15. During questioning by the pharmacist, KL explains that she plans to go to the beach in 2 days. She admits that she does not tan easily and has experienced several severe sunburns in the past. However, she usually wears a tee shirt over her swimsuit when she body surfs or swims.

KL is presently on day 4 of a 10-day course of Bactrim therapy for a urinary tract infection. No one in her family has had skin cancer.

Clinical Considerations/Strategies

The following considerations/strategies are provided to aid the reader in (1) determining whether treatment of the patient's condition with nonprescription medications is warranted, (2) selecting the appropriate nonprescription medication, and (3) developing a patient counseling strategy to ensure optimal therapeutic outcomes:

- List factors that may predispose the patient to sunburn.
- Determine the best sunscreen or suntan product for this patient.
- Determine other protective measures that the patient can take at the beach to prevent or minimize the risk of sunburn.
- Explain the meaning of SPF to the patient.
- Identify key points about the recommended sunscreen product(s) to discuss with the patient.
- Assess the long-term consequences for this patient if she does not follow the recommendations for protecting her skin on an ongoing basis.
- Develop a patient education/counseling strategy that will:
  - Ensure that the patient understands how to apply and use (ie, amount and frequency of application) the recommended sunscreen or suntan products;
  - Ensure that the patient understands the importance of using such products as well as the long-term adverse effects of not using them.

Case 30–2

Patient Complaint/History

EF, a 31-year-old male grocery broker, plays golf two to three times a week. He is in the pharmacy today looking at sunscreen products. He explains that he usually protects his head and neck from sun exposure by wearing a hat; however, he would like to keep a sunscreen product in his golf bag in case he forgets his hat.

Physical observation of the patient reveals that he is balding and has numerous nevi; further, his neck is red and appears to be sunburned. EF admits that he tans gradually and that his father had several lesions removed from his head and neck 4 years earlier. The patient cannot remember if his father's lesions were basal cell or squamous cell "skin cancers."

EF is presently taking Dyazide every other day for mild hypertension.

Clinical Considerations/Strategies

The following considerations/strategies are provided to aid the reader in (1) determining whether treatment of the patient's condition with nonprescription medications is warranted, (2) selecting the appropriate nonprescription medication, and (3) developing a patient counseling strategy to ensure optimal therapeutic outcomes:

- List factors that may predispose this patient to sunburn.
- Determine the best sunscreen or suntan products for this patient.
- Determine other protective measures that the patient can take to prevent sunburn during golf outings.
- Identify key points to discuss with the patient about the recommended sunscreen or suntan product(s).
- Assess the long-term consequences for this patient if he does not follow the recommendations for protecting his skin on an ongoing basis.
- Develop a patient education/counseling strategy that will:
  - Ensure that the patient understands how to apply and use (ie, amount and frequency of application) the recommended products;
  - Ensure that the patient understands the importance of using such products as well as the long-term adverse effects of not using them.

Summary

Tanning or burning of the skin can result from recreational sunbathing or outdoor activities such as yard work or sports; it can also be an occupational hazard. Whatever the circumstances, the hazards of long-term exposure to UV radiation are well documented, and sustained efforts to educate the public are needed to minimize these hazards.

The key to proper protection is the identification of skin type and tolerability to UV radiation exposure. With this information, a product with the appropriate SPF can be selected. Because products with the same SPF provide equivalent efficacy against sunburn, other factors that may help determine product selection may be taken into account. These factors are skin sensitivity, product substantivity, price, ability of product to damage fabrics, and the therapeutic use of the product.

Current evidence strongly suggests that a broad-spectrum product with the highest SPF is best for most people. However, avoidance of unnecessary exposure to UV radiation is the primary preventive measure.

Once a product is selected, it should be applied at least 30 minutes before exposure to the sun (up to 2 hours before with ABA and its esters) to allow binding to the skin. The product should be applied often, especially after heavy sweating and swimming.

If the individual's ultimate goal is to develop a deep tan, the best approach is slow and cautious. Increasing exposure to the sun gradually while avoiding peak sun times provides natural protection to the skin through melanin formation and skin thickening and thus allows for gradual tanning with minimal burning. With proper use of sunscreen products and judicious tanning, both the short- and long-term hazards of exposure to the sun can be minimized.

References

1. Kochevar IE, Pathak MA, Parrish JA. In: Fitzpatrick TB et al, eds. *Dermatology in General Medicine.* 3rd ed. New York: McGraw-Hill; 1987: 1441–51.
2. Pathak MA, Fitzpatrick TB, Parrish JA. In: Fitzpatrick TB et al, eds. *Dermatology in General Medicine.* 3rd ed. New York: McGraw-Hill; 1987: 254–62.
3. Forbes PD et al. In: Jackson EM, ed. *Photobiology of the Skin and Eye.* New York: Marcel Dekker; 1986: 67–84.
4. Willis I, Menter JM, Whyte HJ. The rapid induction of cancer in the hairless mouse utilizing the principle of photoaugmentation. *J Invest Dermatol.* 1981 May; 76: 404–8.
5. Cole CA, Van Fossen R. In: Urbach F, ed. *Biological Responses to Ultraviolet A Radiation.* Overland Park, Kan: Valdenmar; 1992: 335–45.
6. Kripke ML. Ultraviolet radiation and immunology: something new under the sun—Presidential Address. *Cancer Res.* 1994 Dec; 54: 6102–5.
7. Kligman LH. In: Urbach F, Gange RW, eds. *The Biological Effects of UV-A Radiation.* New York: Praeger; 1986: 98–110.
8. Gilchrest BA et al. Histologic changes associated with ultraviolet A-induced erythema in normal human skin. *J Am Acad Dermatol.* 1983 Aug; 9: 213–9.
9. Staberg B et al. Direct and indirect effects of UVA on skin vessel leakiness. *J Invest Dermatol.* 1982 Dec; 79: 358–60.
10. Ruenger TM, Epe B, Moeller K. Repair of ultraviolet B and singlet oxygen-induced DNA damage in xeroderma pigmentosum cells. *J Invest Dermatol.* 1995; 104: 68–73.
11. Mutzhas MF, Cesarini JP. In: Passchier WF, Bosnjakovic BFM, eds. *Human Exposure to Ultraviolet Radiation: Risk and Regulations.* Amsterdam, the Netherlands: Elsevier Science Publishers; 1987: 345–52.
12. McKinlay AF, Diffey BL. A reference action spectrum for ultraviolet induced erythema in human skin. *CIE-J.* 1987; 6(1): 17–22.
13. *Consensus Development Conference Statement on Sunlight, Ultraviolet Radiation, and the Skin.* Bethesda, Md: National Institutes of Health; May 8–10, 1989.
14. Urbach F. Ultraviolet A transmission by modern sunscreens: is there a real risk? *Photodermatol Photoimmunol Photomed.* 1993; 9: 237–41.
15. Gange RW. In: Fitzpatrick TB et al, eds. *Dermatology in General Medicine.* 3rd ed. New York: McGraw-Hill; 1987: 1451–7.
16. Morison WL et al, Photobiology. *J Am Acad Dermatol.* 1991 Aug; 25: 327–9.
17. Pathak MA. In: Urbach F, Gange RW, eds. *The Biological Effects of UV-A Radiation.* New York: Praeger; 1986: 156–67.
18. Bernhard JD et al. In: Fitzpatrick TB et al, eds. *Dermatology in General Medicine.* 3rd ed. New York: McGraw-Hill; 1987: 1480–507.
19. Taylor CR, Hawk JL. Recognizing photosensitivity. *Ann Rheum Dis.* 1994 Nov; 53: 705–7.
20. Reynolds NJ et al. Weed wacker dermatitis. *Arch Dermatol.* 1991 Sep; 127: 1419–20. Letter.

21. Guercio-Hauer C, Macfarlane DF, Deleo VA. Photodamage, photoaging and photoprotection of the skin. *Am Fam Phys.* 1994 Aug; 50: 327–32.
22. Kligman LH, Kligman AM. In: Fitzpatrick TB et al, eds. *Dermatology in General Medicine.* 3rd ed. New York: McGraw-Hill; 1987: 1470–5.
23. *Consensus Conference Statement on Photoaging/Photodamage.* St Louis: American Academy of Dermatology; 1988 Mar: 1–12.
24. Kligman AM. The treatment of photoaged human skin by topical tretinoin. *Drugs.* 1989 Jul; 38: 1–8.
25. Leyden JJ. Clinical features of aging skin. *Br J Dermatol.* 1990; 122(suppl 35): 1–3.
26. *Skin Cancer Facts and Figures—1995.* New York: Skin Cancer Foundation; 1995: 1–2.
27. Gallagher RP et al. Sunlight exposure, pigmentation factors, and risk of nonmelanocytic skin cancer: II. squamous cell carcinoma. *Arch Dermatol.* 1995 Feb; 131: 164–9.
28. Gallagher RP et al. Sunlight exposure, pigmentary factors, and risk of nonmelanocytic skin cancer: I. basal cell carcinoma. *Arch Dermatol.* 1995 Feb; 131: 157–63.
29. Kricker A et al. A dose-response curve for sun exposure and basal cell carcinoma. *Int J Cancer.* 1995; 60: 482–8.
30. Williams ML, Pennella R. Melanoma, melanocytic nevi, and other melanoma risk factors in children. *J Pediatr.* 1994 Jun; 124: 833–45.
31. Marks R, Whiteman D. Sunburn and melanoma: how strong is the evidence? *Br Med J.* 1994 Jan; 308: 75–6.
32. Urbach F et al. *Tenth International Cancer Congress* (Abstracts). Philadelphia: JB Lippincott; 1970: 109–10.
33. Averbach H. Geographic variation in incidence of skin cancer in the United States. *Public Health Rep.* 1961 Apr; 76: 345–8.
34. *Federal Register.* 1978 Aug; 43: 38206–69.
35. *Federal Register.* 1993 May; 58: 28194–302.
36. Rippere J. Personal communication on the status of the final monograph. Bethesda, Md: FDA, Office of OTC Drug Evaluation; May 31, 1995.
37. Naylor MF et al. High sun protection factor sunscreens in the suppression of actinic neoplasia. *Arch Dermatol.* 1995 Feb; 131: 170–5.
38. Mommaas AM et al. Analysis of the protective effect of topical sunscreens on the UVB-radiation-induced suppression of the mixed-lymphocyte reaction. *J Invest Dermatol.* 1990 Sep; 95: 313–6.
39. Roelandts R et al. A survey of ultraviolet absorbers in commercially available sun products. *Int J Dermatol.* 1983 May; 22: 247–55.
40. Pathak MA. Sunscreens: topical and systemic approaches for protection of human skin against harmful effects of solar radiation. *J Am Acad Dermatol.* 1982 Sep; 7: 285–312.
41. Ferguson J, Collins P. Photoallergic contact dermatitis to oxybenzone. *Br J Dermatol.* 1994; 131: 124–9.
42. Kaidbey K, Gange RW. Comparison of methods for assessing photoprotection against ultraviolet A in vivo. *J Am Acad Dermatol.* 1987 Feb; 16: 346–53.
43. Fenner L. The tanning pill, a questionable dye job. *FDA Consumer.* 1982 Feb; 16: 23–4.
44. Tanning pills. Talk paper. Rockville, Md: US Department of Health and Human Services, FDA; Jul 1981.
45. Bluhm R et al. Aplastic anemia associated with canthaxanthin ingested for "tanning" purposes. *JAMA.* 1990 Sep; 264: 1141–2.
46. Jaworsky C, Ratz JL, Dijkstra JWE. Efficacy of tan accelerators. *J Am Acad Dermatol.* 1987 Apr; 16: 769–71.
47. Levine N et al. Induction of skin tanning by subcutaneous administration of a potent synthetic melanotropin. *JAMA.* 1991 Nov; 266: 2730–6.
48. Daxecker F, Blumthaler M, Ambach W. Ultraviolet exposure of cornea from sunbeds. *Lancet.* 1994 Sep; 344: 886. Letter.
49. Autier O et al. Cutaneous malignant melanoma and exposure to sunlamps or sunbeds: an EORTC multicenter case-control study in Belgium, France and Germany. *Int J Cancer.* 1994; 58: 809–13.
50. Westerdahl J et al. Use of sunbeds or sunlamps and malignant melanoma in southern Sweden. *Am J Epidemiol.* 1994; 140(8): 691–8.
51. Cohen JB, Bergstresser PR. Inadvertent phototoxicity from home tanning equipment. *Arch Dermatol.* 1994 Jun; 130: 804–6. Letter.
52. Injuries associated with ultraviolet tanning devices—Wisconsin. *MMWR.* 1989 May; 38: 333–5.
53. Sunlamp products and ultraviolet lamps intended for use in sunlamp products. 21 CFR 1040.20 (1992): 519–22.
54. Taylor HR et al. Effect of ultraviolet radiation on cataract formation. *N Engl J Med.* 1988 Dec; 319: 1429–33.
55. Horn EP et al. Sunlight and risk of uveal melanoma. *J Natl Cancer Inst.* 1994 Oct; 86: 1476–8.
56. *SAA UV Labeling Policy.* Norwalk, Conn: Sunglass Association of America; 1989.
57. Stern RS, Weinstein MC, Baker SG. Risk reduction for nonmelanoma skin cancer with childhood sunscreen use. *Arch Dermatol.* 1986 May; 122: 537–45.
58. Foley P et al. Frequency of reactions to sunscreens: results of a longitudinal population-based study on the regular use of sunscreens in Australia. *Br J Dermatol.* 1993; 128: 512–8.
59. Johnson EY, Lookingbill DP. Sunscreen use and sun exposure: trends in a white population. *Arch Dermatol.* 1984 Jun; 120: 727–31.
60. Pathak MA et al. In: Fitzpatrick TB et al, eds. *Dermatology in General Medicine.* 3rd ed. New York: McGraw-Hill; 1987: 1507–77.
61. Loesch H, Kaplan DL. Pitfalls in sunscreen application. *Arch Dermatol.* 1994 May; 130: 665–6.
62. Sunscreens. *Consumer Rep.* 1980 Jun; 45: 353–6.
63. Stenberg C, Larko O. Sunscreen application and its importance for the sun protection factor. *Arch Dermatol.* 1985 Nov; 121: 1400–2.
64. Wells TD, Jessup GT, Langlotz KS. Effects of sunscreen use during exercise in the heat. *Physician Sportsmed.* 1984 Jun; 12: 132–42.
65. Letter to the editor. *JAMA.* 1984 May; 251: 2348.

CHAPTER 31

Burn and Sunburn Products

Robert H. Moore III and John D. Bowman

Questions to ask in patient assessment and counseling

- *What caused the burn—chemicals, sun exposure, electricity, or heat?*
- *How severe is the burn? Is the skin broken and/or blistered?*
- *When did the burn occur?*
- *Where is the burn? Does it affect the eyes, genitalia, face, hands, or feet?*
- *Is the burn oozing?*
- *Is the burn painful?*
- *How large is the burned area?*
- *Do you have any other injuries or symptoms?*
- *What treatments have you used on the burn?*
- *How long have you been using this treatment?*
- *What effect has this treatment had?*
- *Do you have any other medical problems?*
- *Are you currently taking any oral prescription or nonprescription medication?*
- *Are you currently or have you recently been using any topical medication for a condition other than the burn?*

Burns of all types and degrees of severity account for approximately 2.3% of all injuries in the United States each year and affect about 1.75 million people. In 1982, more than 100,000 victims were hospitalized for burns, and more than 10,000 burn-related deaths occurred. However, because of the effectiveness of fire control measures, flame-retardant clothing, and improved safety standards for housing, these numbers are decreasing each year. Additionally, improved therapy, better understanding of burn pathophysiology, and the availability of burn centers have reduced morbidity and mortality associated with severe burns. More than 92% of people with burn injuries receive medical attention. Of these, 46.2% have injuries that restrict their activity and 22.8% have injuries that confine them to bed. Burn injuries occur more often in persons under 17 years of age, persons with low income, and persons with less than 12 years of formal education.[1,2] During 1991, residential fires were the second leading cause of injury deaths (after motor vehicle injuries) among children aged 1–9 years, and the sixth leading cause of injury deaths among those 65 years of age and older.[3]

The pharmacist will encounter a large number of patients with minor burns and sunburns amenable to self-treatment and should have the knowledge and skills necessary to advise those patients about treatment. The pharmacist should also know when the burn injury is severe enough to require referral to a physician.

Etiology

There were 3,683 deaths in 1991 owing to residential fires. This represents a 37% decline in deaths from this type of fire since 1970. The highest death rates occurred in children younger than 5 years of age and in persons 70 years of age or older. The three leading causes of fire in the pediatric deaths were the children playing with fire-ignition sources such as matches (37%), faulty or misused heating devices (19%), and faulty or misused electrical sources (11%). Among the elderly, the causes were careless smoking (33%), faulty or misused heating devices (19%), and faulty or misused electrical sources (12%). Of those 3,683 deaths in 1991, 48% occurred in the months March through December. The increased occurrence of deaths during the winter months reflects the use of space heaters, portable heaters, fireplaces, and Christmas trees.[3]

More than 80% of minor burns occur in the home. Sixty-three percent of household burns are on the hands and arms, and 34% are on the face and legs. Of the minor burns that occur outside the home, sunburn is the most common. The incidence and significance of sunburn has been underrated, and the injury goes unreported in most burn surveys because the public often does not consider sunburn in the same context as thermal, electrical, and chemical burns. Most minor burns do not require medical intervention, and symptoms may be managed by the patient with appropriate care and nonprescription drug therapy.

Anatomy and Physiology of the Skin

The skin is the largest organ of the human body, accounting for approximately 17% of the body weight of an average person. The skin performs a number of vital physiologic functions. It protects the body from injury, serving as a barrier against many foreign bodies, including microorganisms. By synthesizing melanin, the skin also protects the underlying tissues from certain forms of irradiation. Additionally, the skin is a sense organ, receiving sensory input—especially touch and temperature—from the proximal environment. Oil, which lubricates and prevents excessive drying of the skin, is

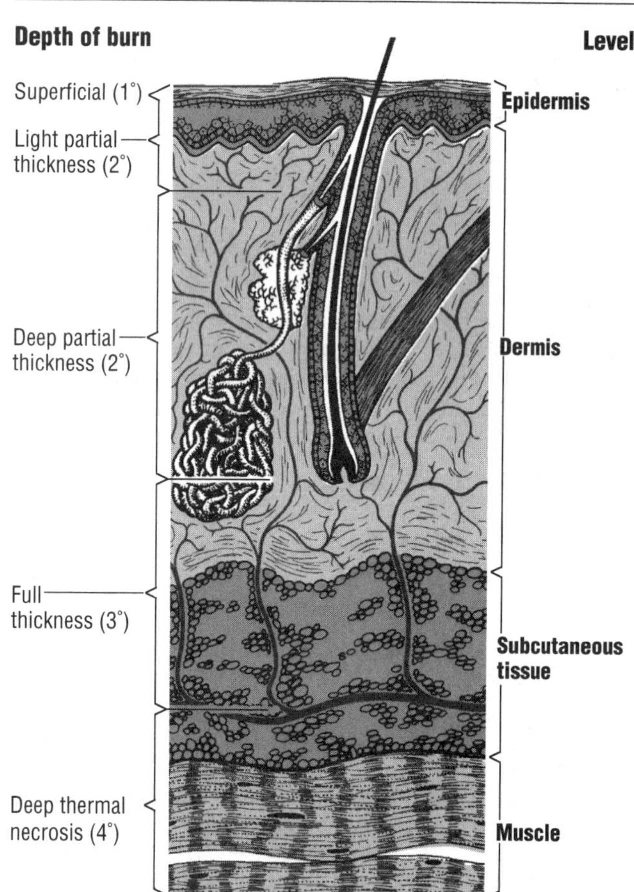

FIGURE 1 Cross section of skin showing depth of burns.

produced in the sebaceous glands. Fat deposits in the subcutaneous tissue play a role in lipid biotransformation. Cholecalciferol (vitamin D_3), which is involved in calcium regulation, is produced in the skin through exposure to UV radiation. The skin plays a major role in thermoregulation because cutaneous blood flow and perspiration are important in maintaining the core temperature of the body at a normal level. These two factors are also involved with maintaining water balance in the body.

Figure 1 shows a cross section of the anatomy of the skin. Also illustrated are the depths of injury caused by thermal burns.

Categorization of Burns

Burns are tissue injuries caused by thermal (flame and scalding), electrical (flash and contact), chemical, and irradiation contacts. Burn injury of the skin results in cell death, denaturation of proteins and subsequent cellular dysfunction, vascular permeability with localized edema, and cutaneous vasodilation.

Determining the area and degree of a burn is not simple, even for burn specialists. The American Burn Association currently identifies three major categories of burn injuries:

- *Major* burn injuries are second-degree burns over a body surface area (BSA) greater than 25% in adults or 20% in children; all third-degree burns over a BSA of 10% or greater; all burns involving hands, face, eyes, ears, feet, and perineum; all inhalation injuries; electrical burns; complicated burn injuries involving fractures or other major trauma; and burns on all high-risk patients (ie, those who are elderly or who have debilitating diseases).
- *Moderate*, uncomplicated burn injuries are second-degree burns over a BSA of 15–25% in adults or 10–20% in children; third-degree burns over a BSA of 2–10%; and burns not involving eyes, ears, face, hands, feet, or perineum.
- *Minor* burn injuries are second-degree burns over a BSA of 15% or less in adults or 10% or less in children; third-degree burns over a BSA of less than 2%; and burns not involving eyes, ears, face, hands, feet, or perineum. Minor burns exclude electrical injuries, inhalation injuries, and burns on all high-risk patients.

The severity of a burn is determined quantitatively by the percentage of BSA affected and by the depth of the burn (Figure 1).

The percentage of the adult body that has been burned can be estimated by the rule of nines (Figure 2). The total BSA is divided into 11 areas, each accounting for 9% or a multiple of 9. The head accounts for 9% of the BSA (the front and the back of the head are each considered 4.5%); the arms are 9% each; the legs are 18% each; and the trunk is 36% (18% front, 18% back). The perineum is considered 1%. The rule of nines is

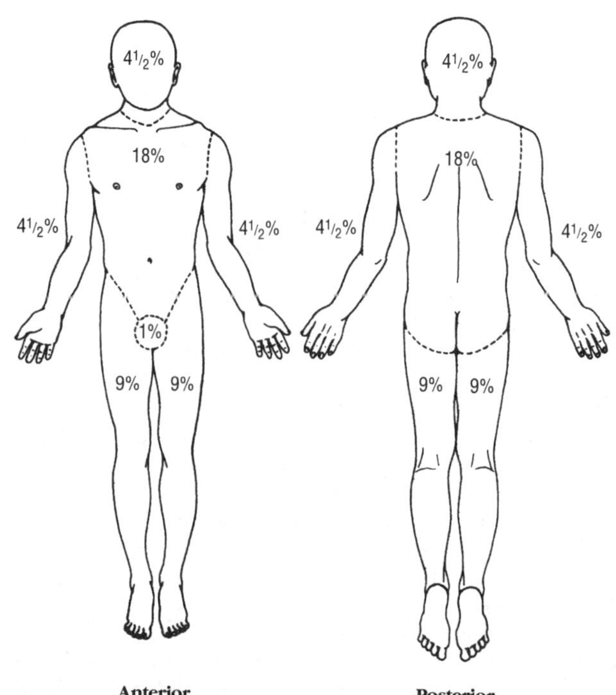

FIGURE 2 Rule-of-nine method for quickly establishing the percentage of adult body surface burned. Adapted with permission from *The Guide to Fluid Therapy*. Deerfield, Ill: Baxter Laboratories; 1969: 111.

TABLE 1 Changes in body surface area with age (%)

	Age					
Surface	**Birth**	**1 y**	**5 y**	**10 y**	**15 y**	**Adult**
Head	19	17	13	11	9	7
Neck	2	2	2	2	2	2
Trunk (anterior)	13	13	13	13	13	13
Trunk (posterior)	13	13	13	13	13	13
Buttocks	5	5	5	5	5	5
Perineum	1	1	1	1	1	1
Arms	8	8	8	8	8	8
Forearms	6	6	6	6	6	6
Hands	5	5	5	5	5	5
Thighs	11	13	16	17	18	19
Legs	10	10	11	12	13	14
Feet	7	7	7	7	7	7

reliable for adults but is inaccurate for children and persons with small body surfaces. Table 1 illustrates how the distribution of BSA changes with age. This table allows for the quick estimation of the BSA of a burn on a child. If the burn is second degree or greater and covers more than 1% of the BSA, a physician should be consulted.

The depth of a burn has traditionally been described as first, second, or third degree (Table 2). A classification of fourth degree is currently being used to describe burns affecting all layers of the skin as well as underlying muscle. The terms *superficial, partial thickness,* and *full thickness* are used with greater frequency. The inflammatory response to a burn injury evolves over the first 24–48 hours, so the initial appearance of the injury can lead to an underestimation of its actual severity.

First-degree burns are superficial, involving only the epidermis (partial thickness). In most circumstances, there is no blistering. Redness, warmth, and slight edema are present. The burn may be painful because the sensory nerve endings are intact. First-degree burns tend to heal spontaneously within 3–10 days with no scarring. Symptomatic relief of pain and fever and avoidance of additional injury are usually the only treatment required. Sunburn is classified most often in this category.

Second-degree burns involve the entire depth of the epidermis and may extend into the dermis (deep partial thickness). Second-degree burns are characterized by erythema, blistering, and oozing. Pain is usually more intense than in first-degree burns because of the irritation to the nerve endings. With superficial second-degree burns, healing is generally spontaneous, occurring within about 3 weeks, and there is minimal or no scarring. Deep second-degree burns involve more of the dermis, so these burns take longer to heal (up to 6 weeks) and may cause thick scar formation (hypertrophic scarring or cheloid).

Third-degree (full-thickness) burns destroy both the dermis and epidermis and may extend into underlying tissues. Usually the burn is not edematous because the vascular supply to the area has been de-

TABLE 2 Classification of burn by depth

Type	Tissue affected	Characteristics
First degree	Epidermis	Superficial, erythematous, local pain, no blistering, no scarring, little epidermal alteration. Heals within 3–10 days
Second degree	Epidermis and the most superficial portion of dermis	Erythematous, local pain, elevated vesicle (blister) formation, little or no irreversible damage to dermis, depigmentation in some cases. Usually heals fully in 3–4 weeks with no scarring. Considered a partial-thickness burn.
Third degree	Entire depth of dermis and epidermis; may penetrate into subcutaneous tissue	Extensive and partially irreversible damage to entire depth of dermis and epidermis (and possibly subcutaneous tissue), leathery/white mottled appearance, too severe to blister. Less painful than some first- or second-degree burns because of destruction of nerve endings. Infection a significant risk. Heals over several months. Scarring probable; skin grafting may be necessary to minimize scarring. Considered a full-thickness burn.
Fourth degree	All layers of skin (full thickness) and underlying tissue, including muscle	Charred, dry. Great risk of severe gram-positive or gram-negative infection. Takes months to heal. Skin grafting necessary.

stroyed. The affected area will have a leathery, white, or charred appearance. Because nerve terminals are destroyed, pain will be absent or diminished in comparison with the other degrees of burns. Healing occurs slowly over months, and grafting is often required to achieve wound closure. Scarring usually results.

The term *fourth-degree burn* is used to describe burn wounds that are full skin thickness with damage to underlying tissue, including muscle. The damaged tissue is dry and charred, and there is a high risk of infection. Healing takes months and usually requires skin grafting. Scarring is prominent.

Flame burns may be partial thickness, full thickness, or a mixture of the two. Scald burns are usually partial thickness but can be full-thickness, especially in children. Superheated steam can cause full-thickness burns. Many steam cleaners contain chemicals that can produce a chemical injury as well. Thermal damage to the respiratory tract can also result from exposure to steam. Inhalation of hot gases can lead to immediate upper airway obstruction as well as to obstruction of the lower bronchioles owing to slowly developing edema. Smoke inhalation may produce extensive lung damage because of toxic particles. Injury to small airway alveolar capillaries can cause progressive respiratory failure. Flash burns are most often partial-thickness injuries to exposed areas. Chemical burns can be partial or full thickness. If not properly treated, chemical burns will occasionally extend slowly for several hours after exposure; thus, all efforts should be made to remove the chemical to prevent further injury. Electrical burns result from exposure to heat of up to 9,000°F (5,000°C). Most of the resistance to an electrical burn is at the skin, but electrical burns can cause extensive damage to underlying tissues and may be of any size and depth. Progressive necrosis and sloughing are usually greater than the initial lesion indicates.

Most burn injuries involve less than 20% of the BSA and are not life-threatening. Although deep partial-thickness burns will generally heal in 4–6 weeks, healing accompanied by excessive fibrosis and unsightly scarring may develop. Thus, it is important to assess the depth of the burn correctly and to reassess it at 24–48 hours when the true depth may become apparent. For patients whose injuries range from superficial to moderately deep partial-thickness burns, outpatient care and self-care are often appropriate. Such patients are unlikely to develop complications.

The pharmacist should feel confident in recommending treatment for minor first-degree burns that do not cover an extensive area and do not involve the eyes, ears, face, feet, or perineum, as well as for minor second-degree burns that cover less than 1% of the BSA. Generally, however, all burns greater than first degree should be evaluated by a physician to prevent complications, particularly infections. Any second-degree burn covering a more extensive area should always be referred to a physician. Extreme care should be taken when the burn is electrical, occurs by inhalation, or occurs in a high-risk patient. If the degree or severity of the burn is difficult to determine, the patient should be referred to a physician immediately.

Complications of Burn Injuries

Infection secondary to burns is dangerous and difficult to treat because the burned dead skin, or eschar, may serve as a growth medium for microorganisms. In moderate or major injuries, a burn wound infection may increase the depth of the original injury, delay healing, and invade the host, thereby causing systemic infection. Diffusion of systemic antimicrobial agents from the perfused wound margins into the avascular eschar is variable and unreliable. Prophylaxis with topical antimicrobial therapy has been universally adopted by burn treatment facilities for patients with moderate to severe burns, while systemic antibiotics are generally not used unless symptoms warrant.

Scar contracture is the result of a contractile process occurring in a healed scar. It often produces a cosmetically unacceptable rigid scar that can be deforming or limit functioning. Scar contracture can be minimized by prolonged splinting, range-of-motion exercises, application of pressure such as the wearing of pressure garments, skin grafting of wounds with full-thickness skin, proper surgical incision across joints, and surgical release of formed contractures. A related phenomenon is wound contraction, which is a naturally occurring process by which the edges of an open wound are drawn toward the center, facilitating healing.

Hypertrophic scars, or keloids, are large fibrous growths caused by an abnormal connective tissue response to injury. These can be thought of as unchecked healing. Incidence of hypertrophic scarring is greater in individuals with darker pigmentation.

Sunburn

Excessive exposure to sunlight (especially those rays between 290 and 320 nm) can lead to an acute dermatologic reaction known as sunburn.[4] (See Chapter 30, "Sunscreen and Suntan Products.") Several endogenous vasoactive agents have been suggested as mediators of the erythema seen in sunburn, but none has been definitively shown to cause the reaction. However, there is evidence that the prostaglandins and leukocytes are involved.[4–6]

Sunburn-producing UV radiation is filtered out somewhat by window glass, smoke, and smog but readily passes through light clouds, fog, and clear water. Exposure to UV rays may be enhanced by reflection off snow and sand.

As a normal protective response, the epidermis thickens and melanin production increases when the skin is exposed to sunlight. People vary tremendously in their individual responses to such exposure. For example, many fair-haired individuals will freckle because of uneven melanin deposition. Blonds and redheads are particularly susceptible to sunburn because of a low population of melanocytes. Blacks and other darker-skinned persons can also burn with prolonged exposure to the sun.

Signs and symptoms of sunburn are seen in 1–24 hours following excessive exposure (see color plates, photograph 25). With mild exposure, erythema with subsequent scaling and exfoliation of the skin occurs. Pain and low-grade fever may accompany the erythema. More

TABLE 3 Selected groups of medications associated with photosensitivity reactions

Antidepressants
Amitriptyline
Amoxapine
Clomipramine
Desipramine
Doxepin
Imipramine
Isocarboxazid
Maprotiline
Nortriptyline
Phenelzine
Protriptyline
Trazodone
Trimipramine

Antihistamines
Astemizole
Azatadine
Brompheniramine
Buclizine
Carbinoxamine
Chlorpheniramine
Clemastine
Cyclizine
Cyproheptadine
Dexchlorpheniramine
Dimenhydrinate
Diphenhydramine
Doxylamine
Hydroxyzine
Meclizine
Methapyrilene
Methdilazine
Pheniramine
Promethazine
Pyrilamine
Terfenadine
Trimeprazine
Tripelennamine
Triprolidine

Antihypertensives
Captopril
Diltiazem
Enalapril
Labetalol
Lisinopril
Methyldopa
Minoxidil
Nifedipine

Antipsychotics
Acetophenazine
Chlorpromazine
Fluphenazine
Haloperidol
Mesoridazine
Perphenazine
Prochlorperazine
Promazine
Thioridazine
Thiothixene
Trifluoperazine
Triflupromazine

Coal tar and derivatives (selected brand name products)
Denorex Medicated Shampoo
DHS Tar Gel Shampoo
Doak Tar Shampoo
Estar Gel
Ionil T Plus Shampoo
Neutrogena T/Derm Body Oil
Neutrogena T/Gel Extra Strength Therapeutic Shampoo
Tegrin Shampoo
Zetar Shampoo

Diuretics (thiazides)
Bendroflumethiazide
Benzthiazide
Chlorothiazide
Chlorthalidone
Cyclothiazide
Hydrochlorothiazide
Hydroflumethiazide
Methyclothiazide
Polythiazide
Trichlormethiazide

Estrogens/progestins (includes ingredients in oral contraceptives)

Estrogens
Chlorotrianisene
Diethylstilbestrol
Estradiol
Estrogens, conjugated
Estrogens, esterified
Estropipate
Ethinyl estradiol
Megestrol

Progestins
Medroxyprogesterone
Norethindrone
Norgestrel

Hypoglycemics
Acetohexamide
Chlorpropamide
Glipizide
Glyburide
Tolazamide
Tolbutamide

Nonsteroidal anti-inflammatory drugs
Diclofenac
Diflunisal
Fenoprofen
Flurbiprofen
Ibuprofen
Indomethacin
Ketoprofen
Meclofenamate
Nabumetone
Naproxen
Piroxicam
Sulindac
Tolmetin

Psoralens
Methoxsalen
Trioxsalen

Sulfonamides
Sulfadiazine
Sulfamethizole
Sulfamethoxazole
Sulfapyridine
Sulfasalazine
Sulfinpyrazone
Sulfisoxazole

continued

prolonged exposure causes pain, edema, skin tenderness, and possibly blistering. Systemic symptoms similar to those of thermal burn, such as fever, chills, weakness, and shock, may be seen in persons in whom a large portion of the BSA has been affected. Following exfoliation and for several weeks thereafter, the skin will be more susceptible than normal to burning.

Photosensitization

Some drugs can produce photosensitivity reactions. The drugs alone pose no hazard, but when the patient comes into contact with UV radiation, photosensitivity reactions may occur (see color plates, photographs 26 and 27). These can be manifested as photoallergy or phototoxicity.

Photoallergic reactions, which are immunologic, are most commonly caused by exposure to UV radiation in the UV-A range (320–400 nm).[7] (Chapter 30, "Sunscreen and Suntan Products," provides detailed information on the various bands of UV radiation associated with sunburn and photosensitivity.) With photoallergy, a drug or other chemical absorbs UV radiation. This combination is then acted upon by the immune system as an antigen, eliciting antibody formation. With future use of the drug and exposure to UV radiation, a hypersensitive immunologic response can occur. Usual reactions include erythema, edema, and warmth. Ec-

TABLE 3 Selected groups of medications associated with photosensitivity reactions, *continued*

Tetracyclines Chlortetracycline Demeclocycline Doxycycline Methacycline Minocycline Oxytetracycline Tetracycline **Other agents** ***Anticancer drugs*** Dacarbazine Fluorouracil Flutamide Methotrexate Procarbazine Vinblastine	***Anti-infectives (other)*** Ciprofloxacin Dapsone Enoxacin Ethionamide Flucytosine Gentamicin Griseofulvin Lomefloxacin Nalidixic acid Norfloxacin Ofloxacin Pyrazinamide Sulfonamides Trimethoprim ***Antiparasitic drugs*** Bithionol Chloroquine Quinine Thiabendazole	***Diuretics (other)*** Acetazolamide Amiloride Furosemide Metolazone Triamterene ***Sunscreens*** Benzophenones Cinnamates Homosalate Menthyl anthranilate Oxybenzone PABA esters Para-aminobenzoic acid ***Miscellaneous*** Amiodarone (antiarrhythmic) Benzocaine (local anesthetic) Benzyl peroxide	Carbamazepine (anticonvulsant) Disopyramide (antiarrhythmic) Etretinate (antipsoriatic) Gold salts (antiarthritic) Isotretinoin (antiacne) Lamotrigine (anticonvulsant) Lovastatin (antihyperlipidemic) Nabilone (antiemetic) Phenytoin (anticonvulsant) Quinidine sulfate (antiarrhythmic) Selegiline (antiparkinsonism) Tretinoin (antiacne)

Sources: *Med Lett.* 1993; 37: 946.

Medications That Increase Sensitivity to Light: A 1990 Listing. FDA Pub No 91-8280. Washington, DC: US Department of Health and Human Services, Public Health Service; 1995.

Drug Facts and Comparisons. St. Louis: JB Lippincott Co; 1993.

zema may occur. Topical preparations cause more photoallergic responses than do systemic agents. Table 3 lists 12 groups of medications, including selected, specific drugs that are positively associated with photosensitivity reactions. It is important to remember, however, that not every individual taking these medications will experience an adverse reaction to UV radiation, and those who do will not exhibit the same degree of symptomatic response.

Phototoxicity is more common than photoallergy. Phototoxicity does not produce an immune response, so it may occur the first time an offending or precipitating drug is used. Such a reaction occurs rapidly (within minutes to hours) following exposure to UV radiation, especially UV-A radiation. An exaggerated erythema, relative to the time of exposure, is seen. The effects are maximal within a few hours to a few days. Areas exposed to UV radiation are the only areas of involvement.[7]

Patient Assessment

The pharmacist must accurately assess the status of the patient before intervening with therapy. Of utmost importance is determining whether the burn is amenable to self-medication or calls for referral to a physician. The cause, depth, and location of the burn; the BSA involved; and when the burn occurred should all be taken into consideration. The degree of pain should be assessed, as well as the presence of elevated body temperature and dehydration. If the cause of the burn is unclear, a careful drug history is important since drug photosensitivity or contact dermatitis may be implicated.

Age should also be taken into account. Newborns, young children, and elderly people do not tolerate the effects of burns as well as young adults. Individuals with chronic illnesses, such as diabetes, cardiovascular disease, alcoholism, renal disease, or immunosuppression (acquired immunodeficiency syndrome [AIDS], cancer chemotherapy, corticosteroids, transplant rejection medications, leukemia, etc) are more likely to develop complications than normal persons.

Patients who have received burns to the genitalia, the perineum, and the eye are prone to more serious symptoms and complications. Facial burns may be associated with respiratory injuries due to inhalation, and those that are greater than first degree may also result in permanent scarring. Burns of the hands and feet also deserve special attention, not only because they are often quite painful but also because healing may be delayed in these areas, particularly in patients with a circulatory disorder. In all these cases, patients should be referred to a physician.

TABLE 4 Nonprescription oral analgesics for minor burn pain (adult)

Drug	Dose (mg)	Frequency of administration
Aspirin (eg, Bayer)	325–650	Every 3–4 h, as needed
Acetaminophen[a] (eg, Tylenol)	325–650 1,000	Every 4–6 h, as needed Three to four times a day, as needed
Ibuprofen[b] (eg, Advil, Motrin IB, Nuprin)	200–400	Every 4–6 h, as needed
Naproxen[c] (eg, Aleve)	200[d]	Every 12 h, as needed
Ketoprofen (eg, Orudis KT, Actron)	12.5	Every 4–6 h, as needed

[a]Daily dose should not exceed 4 g. The recommended dose should not be exceeded. Consult physician if use extends beyond 10 consecutive days for adults or beyond 3 days in the presence of fever.

[b]Daily dose of ibuprofen should not exceed 1,200 mg. It should not be taken for pain that persists beyond 10 days or for fever that persists beyond 3 days unless directed by a physician.

[c]Daily dose of naproxen should not exceed 600 mg.

[d]Initial dose of 400 mg may provide better relief.

Self-Treatment of Minor Burns

The goals in treating first- and second-degree burns are to (1) relieve pain associated with the burn, (2) avoid maceration of the tissue, (3) prevent dryness, and (4) provide a favorable environment for healing that minimizes the chances of infection and scarring.

Thermal Burns

Thermal burns include flame, heat, sun, and scald burns. The initial treatment of minor thermal burns is to cool the affected area in cool tap water (no ice) for 10–30 minutes. This phase of treatment does not apply when the depth and extent of the burn is serious because such action would delay emergency treatment. However, perhaps because it decreases vasodilation, immersion has been shown to decrease the area of redness, and thus edema, associated with the burn in the surrounding tissue. This treatment may help to prevent blister formation. If blisters form, medical referral should be made. Aspirin, ibuprofen, naproxen, or acetaminophen can be given to reduce pain (Table 4).

Electrical Burns

The only visible signs of electrical burns may be the points of entrance and exit. The superficial extent of these points may mask extensive underlying tissue damage. Only when an electrical burn is very minor should self-medication be attempted. Otherwise, electrical burns should be referred to a physician. Some electrical burns are actually flash burns, in which no electricity has passed through the victim's body. A flash burn is treated in the same way as a thermal burn.

Chemical Burns

In the case of chemical burns, any clothing on or near the affected area should be immediately removed. The affected area should then be washed with tap water for anywhere from 15 minutes to 2 hours until the offending agent has been removed. If the eye is involved, the eyelid should be pulled back and the eye irrigated with tap water for at least 15–30 minutes. The irrigation fluid should flow from the nasal side of the eye to the outside corner to prevent washing the contaminant into the other eye. When the offending agent is identified, the area poison information center should be contacted immediately for treatment guidelines. In most cases of chemical burns and chemical contact with the eye, further medical attention is encouraged and should be sought as soon as possible. (See Chapter 22, "Ophthalmic Products.")

No attempt should be made to antagonize or neutralize a chemical burn. Such an action may produce an exothermic (heat-generating) chemical reaction, which can damage the injured area more than the original offending agent. It would be inappropriate, for example, to treat a burn caused by an acid by applying a base such as sodium bicarbonate. It should be noted that for certain chemicals, even a small area of contact can produce serious or lethal injury. For example, hydrofluoric acid, an industrial chemical, has caused death within 2 or 3 hours following exposure involving areas as small as 2.5% BSA.[8]

Sunburn

Initial treatment for minor sunburn is to get out of the sunlight and avoid further exposure. Minor sunburn can be relieved to some extent with cool compresses or a cool bath. Administration of nonprescription analgesics (eg, aspirin, ibuprofen, naproxen, or acetaminophen) for treatment of pain is recommended (Table 4).

Heat stroke may occur with excessive exposure to sunlight in a hot and/or humid environment. Because of the complications of heat stroke, patients exhibiting hyperpyrexia, confusion, weakness, or convulsions should be referred to a physician or to an appropriate medical facility immediately.

Cleansing of Burns

After cool moisture is applied to the burned area to help stop the progression of the burn injury, reduce local edema, and relieve pain, the area should be gently cleansed with water and a bland soap, such as a baby wash or a surfactant (eg, Shur-Clens). Alcohol-containing preparations should not be used because they cause pain to denuded skin and are drying. After the burn is cleansed, a nonadherent, hypoallergenic dressing may be applied if the area is small. A skin protectant/lubricant may be applied if the burn is extensive or in an area that cannot be dressed easily (Table 5). If the burn is weeping, soaking it in warm tap water three to six times a day for 15–30 minutes will provide a soothing effect and diminish the weeping. Minor burns usually heal without additional treatment. For second-degree burns, once or twice daily cleansing to remove dead skin is recommended. Patients should be advised to avoid pulling at loose skin or peeling off the burned skin since viable skin may be removed in the process and healing delayed.

TABLE 5 Topical protectant agents used in the treatment of minor burns

Ingredient	Approved concentrations (%)
Allantoin	0.5–2
Cocoa butter	50–100
Petrolatum	30–100
Shark liver oil	3
White petrolatum	30–100

Adapted from *Federal Register*. 1983; 48: 6832.

Dressings for Burns

Sterile, nonadherent gauze dressings are the most convenient way to cover a small burn on an area of the body that is easily bandaged, such as the arm or leg. The following is the recommended sequence for dressing a small burn (normally necessary only with second-degree burns)[9]:

- First, a nonadherent primary layer of sterile, fine-mesh gauze lightly impregnated with sterile petrolatum should be applied over the burn. Petrolatum gauze does not stick to the wound and allows burn exudate to flow freely through the dressing, thus avoiding tissue maceration. Commercially prepared nonadhering petrolatum dressings (eg, Xeroflo or Adaptic) incorporate hydrophilic petrolatum into the gauze to aid permeability.
- Second, an absorbent intermediate layer of piled-up gauze should be applied over the petrolatum gauze. This layer draws and stores exudate away from the wound, protecting the wound against maceration. Cotton or other nonlubricated products should not be applied directly to the burn because they often stick to the burn and are painful and difficult to remove. This layer should be applied loosely to accommodate edema, should it occur.
- Finally, a supportive layer of rolled gauze bandage should be applied over the primary and intermediate gauze layers to hold these layers in place and mildly restrict movement. Elastic or other expandable bandages that tighten after being applied should not be used because they could restrict circulation if edema develops.

The dressing should be changed every 24–48 hours. If the dressing sticks to the wound, soaking in warm water will loosen the gauze from the burn with minimal pain and trauma. Also, removing the sticking gauze slowly will protect the regenerating epithelium and minimize pain. The wound should be examined for signs of infection at each dressing change. The earliest signs of infection may be inflamed wound edges, new blistering, or intensified pain. If the affected skin begins to become macerated (ie, if it feels or looks wet, wrinkled, or fissured), dressing the wound should be temporarily discontinued, and the wound should be exposed to air. Once the pain subsides and healing begins (usually in 4–10 days), wound dressings may be discontinued.

Newer dressings have been designed to incorporate the desirable characteristics of exudate absorption with the occlusiveness provided by the combination of dressings discussed above. Representative products include DuoDerm, Vigilon, and Viasorb. It should be noted that most burn wounds treated on an outpatient basis have little if any exudative drainage. Such wounds usually can be dressed with an occlusive or semiocclusive, nonabsorbent dressing such as Op-Site or Tegaderm.

Pharmacologic Agents

As previously mentioned, most first- and minor second-degree burns heal readily without complications. The purpose of pharmacotherapy in managing minor burns is to make the patient more comfortable and symptom free, and to allow the skin to heal normally (see product table "Burn and Sunburn Products"). Pharmacists should generally limit their treatment recommendations to patients with such burns. The pharmacist should not recommend a product for extensive or deep second-, third-, or fourth-degree burns because this may cause the patient to delay appropriate medical evaluation and treatment. Additionally, inappropriate applications of topical preparations to severe burns must be removed (usually with considerable discomfort) when the patient seeks medical treatment. The pharmacist should also be aware that damaged skin secondary to burns loses some of its barrier function, thus enhancing percutaneous absorption of drugs and other chemicals. This factor increases the possibility of systemic, drug-induced adverse effects.

Protectants

Based on recommendations of its Advisory Review Panel on Over-the-Counter (OTC) Skin-Protectant Drug Products, the Food and Drug Administration (FDA) has recognized the agents in Table 5 as safe and effective (Category I) for the temporary protection of minor burns and sunburn. Skin protectants benefit patients with minor burns by making the wound area less painful. They do this by protecting the burn from mechanical irritation caused by friction and rubbing, and by preventing drying of the stratum corneum. Rehydrating the stratum corneum assists in relieving the symptoms of irritation and permits normal healing to continue. Skin protectants provide only symptomatic relief. The FDA has revised labeling for the indications of skin protectants as follows: "For the temporary protection of minor cuts, scrapes, burns, and sunburn."[10]

In selecting a skin protectant for burns, the pharmacist should choose products that prevent dryness and provide lubrication. Accordingly, the FDA has proposed that bismuth subnitrate, boric acid, sulfur, and tannic acid not be generally recognized as safe and effective when used as skin protectants. Based on advisory panel recommendations, it has also proposed that products with labeling claims of "cures any irritation" or "prevents formation of blisters" not be generally recognized as safe and effective (Category II) either, nor has it recognized claims that certain substances (eg, allantoin, live yeast cell derivatives, or zinc acetate) contained in many skin protectants are effective in accelerating wound healing. Controlled studies conclusively demonstrating that minor wounds treated with any nonprescription treatment healed faster because of these products are lacking.

The provisional FDA-approved skin protectants (Table 5) are considered safe. Liver oils have been used for many years as folk remedies for wound healing. Shark liver oil contains a high concentration of vitamin A and is approved as a skin protectant. Vitamin A and D ointment has been used to treat minor skin burns and abrasions. The FDA recommends that the restriction preventing the use of these products on children under 2 years of age be waived except for those products containing live yeast cell derivatives, shark liver oil, and zinc acetate. Generally, the patient with minor burns may apply a skin protectant as often as needed. If the burn has not improved in 7 days or if it worsens during or after treatment, the patient should consult a physician immediately.

Analgesics

Aspirin, naproxen, and ibuprofen may be used to help alleviate the pain associated with minor burns. As prostaglandin inhibitors and nonsteroidal anti-inflammatory drugs (NSAIDs), these drugs may decrease the erythema and edema in the burned area. For patients who cannot tolerate aspirin, naproxen, or ibuprofen, acetaminophen can provide pain relief. The dose of acetaminophen should not exceed 4 g per day, and prolonged use should be discussed with a pharmacist or physician (Table 4). Although acetaminophen is a weak prostaglandin inhibitor and is not an anti-inflammatory agent, it may still produce beneficial analgesia. Further guidelines for the proper use of internal analgesic agents are included in Chapter 4.

The use of various systemic NSAIDs has been shown to decrease inflammation caused by exposure to UV radiation. However, this effect has been found to last only about 24 hours,[11] possibly because the initial inflammation of sunburn is mediated by prostaglandins whereas the later ensuing inflammation is primarily associated with leukocytes. The combined use of a topical corticosteroid and oral ibuprofen or another NSAID has been found to produce more effective sunburn relief than either agent used alone.[12] Ibuprofen may decrease early inflammation by inhibiting prostaglandin formation, and the corticosteroid provides later relief by decreasing leukocyte infiltration into the area.

Local Anesthetics

The pain of minor burns and sunburn can be attenuated by the judicious use of local anesthetics. The agents that have been approved as safe and effective in providing temporary relief of pain associated with minor burns are found in Table 6.

Benzocaine (5–20%) and lidocaine (0.5–4%) are the two amine local anesthetics that are most often used in nonprescription drug preparations. Dibucaine (0.25–1%), tetracaine (1–2%), butamben (1%), and pramoxine (0.5–1%) are also found in topical anesthetic preparations. The higher concentrations of the local anesthetics are appropriate for burns in which the skin is intact; the lower concentrations are better for skin that has been broken.

Benzocaine produces a hypersensitivity reaction in about 1% of patients. This is a higher incidence than that seen with lidocaine. In contrast, benzocaine is essentially devoid of systemic toxicity whereas systemic absorption of lidocaine can lead to a number of side effects if serum concentrations are high enough. Systemic toxicities due to lidocaine are rare, however, if the product is used on intact skin, on localized areas, and for short periods.

Local anesthetics should be applied no more than three or four times daily. Since their duration of action is short, ranging from about 15 to 45 minutes, continuous pain relief cannot be obtained with these agents. Increasing the number of applications increases the risk of a hypersensitivity reaction or, more important, the chance for systemic toxicity. Local anesthetics should not be used to treat serious burns because their use may delay the seeking of appropriate medical treatment.

TABLE 6 Topical ingredients approved by the FDA in the treatment of minor burns

Types	Approved concentrations (%)
Amine and "caine"-type local anesthetics	
Benzocaine	5–20
Butamben picrate	1
Dibucaine	0.25–1
Dibucaine hydrochloride	0.25–1
Dimethisoquin hydrochloride	0.3–0.5
Dyclonine hydrochloride	0.5–1
Lidocaine	0.5–4
Lidocaine hydrochloride	0.5–4
Pramoxine hydrochloride	0.5–1
Tetracaine	1–2
Tetracaine hydrochloride	1–2
Alcohol and ketone counterirritants	
Benzyl alcohol	10–33
Camphor	0.1–3
Camphor	3–10.8[a]
Camphorated metacresol	
Camphor	3–10.8
Metacresol	1–5
Juniper tar	1–5
Menthol	0.1–1
Phenol	4.7[a]
Phenolate sodium	0.5–1.5
Resorcinol	0.5–3
Antihistamines	
Diphenhydramine hydrochloride	1–2
Tripelennamine hydrochloride	0.5–2

[a]When combined in a light mineral oil, USP vehicle.
Adapted from *Federal Register*. 1983; 48: 5867–8.

Topical Hydrocortisone

Although not FDA-approved for use in treating minor burns, 1% topical hydrocortisone is often used in the first-aid treatment of minor burns covering a small area. An anti-inflammatory agent, hydrocortisone should be used with caution if the skin is broken because its use may allow infections to develop. While low-potency 1% hydrocortisone ointment does not interfere with resurfacing of the skin, topical corticosteroid treatment with high-potency agents has been shown to decrease collagen synthesis and delay reepithelialization in dermal wounds.[13]

Antimicrobials

Antimicrobial therapy is crucial in major burns; however, nonprescription first-aid antibiotic or antiseptic drugs are of limited value, especially on burns in which the skin is intact. These drugs may be used on minor burns in which the skin has been broken. Based on data and information submitted to the rule-making panel for OTC topical antimicrobial drug products, the FDA issued an amended proposed rule for first-aid antiseptics.[14] Those preparations that may be used to help prevent infection in minor burns or sunburn are presented in Chapter 28, "First-Aid Products and Minor Wound Care."

Moderate to severe burn wounds are particularly susceptible to infection. Because the effects of infection can be serious and devastating, any patient in whom infection is evident or whose burn is so severe that the risk of a bacterial infection is likely should be referred to a physician immediately. Prophylactic application of a double or triple antibiotic ointment to minor burns should be done with caution because such use can actually aggravate burns should the patient develop a topical fungal infection or allergic contact dermatitis to one of the antibiotics. Prescription topical antimicrobials are used for major burns.

Vitamins

Vitamin supplementation is commonly used by burn centers for severe burn injuries. The benefits of vitamin supplementation for minor burns are not known. It is known that a frank deficiency of vitamin C (ascorbic acid) or vitamin A will result in impaired wound healing, but there is no evidence that vitamin C dosages beyond normal daily requirements will accelerate wound healing. However, Vitamin C does play a key role in wound healing because it is required for collagen synthesis. Since vitamin C is not stored in the body, it is reasonable to recommend up to 2 g of vitamin C daily from the time of injury until healing is complete.

A number of animal studies indicate that vitamin A enhances healing in a variety of wounds. Following serious injury, there may be an increased requirement for vitamin A. Deficiency states are associated with increased infections. Because vitamin A is stored in large amounts in the liver, supplemental vitamin A should not be continued for long periods. It is unlikely that minor burn injuries will be improved with supplemental vitamin A.

Deficiency of B vitamins may retard wound healing, so this vitamin should be supplemented if nutritional status is poor. Excess vitamin E may delay wound healing and does not play a role in burn injury. Vitamin D is not significantly involved in wound healing.

Zinc administration is not beneficial in those persons who are not zinc deficient. Iron deficiency anemia can decrease the oxygen supply to the healing area and should be corrected if present. Copper deficiency may impair healing and can be corrected through normal dietary intake.

In summary, it would appear that individuals with good nutritional status may not benefit from vitamin or mineral supplementation. However, those persons whose dietary intake may be suboptimal will not be harmed by, and could benefit from, temporary supplementation with standard multivitamin/mineral preparations. Assurance of adequate vitamin C intake is recommended during healing from burn injury.

Counterirritants

Although counterirritants, such as camphor, menthol, and ichthammol, are currently approved for use in minor burn treatment, the FDA is still evaluating these agents and they should not generally be used for such purposes. Although they do reduce pain by stimulating sensory nerve fibers, they also increase blood flow to the area, causing further development of edema in the area. They also further irritate the already sensitized and damaged skin.

Miscellaneous Agents

The ability of topical agents such as aloe vera, vitamin E, and shark liver oil to aid in the healing of minor burns and sunburn has not been substantiated, so these agents are not approved as healing aids. Small studies suggest that so-called inert topical preparations may alter wound healing in either a positive or a negative manner. Topical nitrofurantoin, a liquid detergent, and some petrolatum-containing products have been shown to retard epithelial healing, while an oil-in-water cream, Neosporin Ointment, Silvadene Cream, and benzoyl peroxide lotion 10% and 20% have increased the rate of healing.[13]

Product Formulation

Rarely will a product that is intended to treat minor burns contain only one ingredient. The FDA Advisory Review Panel on Over-the-Counter Skin-Protectant Drug Products concluded that two or more skin-protectant ingredients may be combined, provided that:

- Each is present in sufficient quantity to act additively or synergistically to produce the claimed therapeutic effect when the ingredients are within the effective concentration range specified for each in the monograph;
- The ingredients do not interact with or reduce the effectiveness of each other by precipitation, change in acidity or alkalinity, or some other manner that hinders the claimed therapeutic effect;
- The partition of the active ingredients between the skin and the vehicle in which they are incorporated is not impeded, and the therapeutic effectiveness of each ingredient remains as claimed or is not decreased.[12]

Additionally, this panel recognized that skin protectants are suitable vehicles for delivering active ingredients classified in other categories, such as external analgesics (Chapter 5) and sunscreens (Chapter 30). Under these circumstances, the skin protectant may serve a different purpose and is expected to meet the criteria established for this other purpose (analgesic or sunscreen).

Product Selection Guidelines

An initial step in treating the patient with a minor burn is to recommend the short-term administration of an oral analgesic, preferably one with anti-inflammatory activity, such as aspirin, naproxen, or ibuprofen. If the patient cannot tolerate these agents, acetaminophen would be a short-term alternative. Aspirin, naproxen, or ibuprofen may be especially beneficial in the patient with mild sunburn, especially in the first 24 hours after overexposure to UV radiation.

If a local anesthetic or topical hydrocortisone is appropriate therapy, the pharmacist should recommend the most appropriate products. Such products are available as ointments, creams, solutions (lotions), and sprays (aerosols).

Ointments are oleaginous-based preparations that provide a protective film that impedes the evaporation of water from the wound area. This helps keep the skin from drying. However, if the skin is broken, an ointment may not be appropriate because of its impermeability. The presence of excessive moisture trapped beneath the application may promote bacterial growth. Thus, ointments are more appropriate for minor burns, in which the skin is intact. Creams are emulsions that allow some fluid to pass through the film, so they provide less of a medium for bacterial growth and are best applied to broken skin. Generally, creams are also a little less messy and less difficult to apply than ointments. To prevent contamination of the preparation, ointments and creams should not be applied directly onto the burns from the container.

Lotions can be easily spread and may be more easily applied when the area of the burn is large. However, lotions that produce a powdery cover should not be used on a burn. These tend to dry the area, are difficult (and possibly painful) to remove, and provide a medium for bacterial growth under the caked particles.

Generally, aerosol and pump sprays are more costly than other topical dosage forms. But sprays offer the advantage of precluding the need to touch the injured area physically, so there is less pain associated with applying the medication. Application requires holding the container approximately 6 in. from the burn and spraying for 1–3 seconds. This method decreases the chances of chilling the area. However, sprays are not usually protective in that the aerosol is typically water- or alcohol-based and will evaporate.

Case Studies

Case 31–1

Patient Complaint/History

SH, a 16-year-old female who has a fair complexion, blue eyes, and reddish-blond hair, presents to the pharmacist with an apparent sunburn. She requests advice on products to relieve the burning and stinging sensations. Physical observation reveals erythema on the face, arms, neck, and legs in a pattern consistent with overexposure to UV. Because she wanted to develop a tan and eliminate facial acne prior to an upcoming social event, the patient used the services of a local tanning salon the day before for less than an hour.

SH's current medications include benzoyl peroxide 5% lotion hs and tetracycline 250 mg one capsule daily for acne prophylaxis.

Clinical Considerations/Strategies

The following considerations/strategies are provided to aid the reader in (1) determining whether treatment of the patient's condition with nonprescription medications is warranted, (2) selecting the appropriate nonprescription medication, and (3) developing a patient counseling strategy to ensure optimal therapeutic outcomes:

- Assess possible causes of the erythema, including excessive UVA sunlamp exposure, drug-induced photosensitization, and contact dermatitis.
- Attempt to determine any change in soaps, cosmetics, or other topical interventions that might account for contact dermatitis.
- Assess the appropriateness of the nonprescription medication currently used to manage acne symptoms.
- Support/justify any change in the current nonprescription medication regimen.
- Consider referring the patient to her prescriber for reevaluation of the tetracycline therapy.
- Develop a patient education and counseling strategy that will:
  - Optimize the patient's understanding of the etiology and pathogenesis of acne;
  - Optimize the patient's understanding of nondrug measures for acne management;
  - Optimize the patient's understanding of the optimal use of nonprescription acne products, the warnings/precautions pertinent to these products, and the adverse effects associated with them;
  - Foster understanding of the risk related to overexposure to UVA and UVB radiation, especially in the presence of photosensitizing chemicals.

Case 31–2

Patient Complaint/History

WD, a 43-year-old female, comes to the pharmacy counter and requests help in selecting a topical product for a recent thermal burn. She burned her hand and forearm earlier that morning when hot oil from a frying pan splashed onto her right hand and forearm. Because the patient does not have medical insurance, she hopes to find an aloe-containing product to relieve the pain associated with the burn.

Physical observation of the patient reveals thermal injury to the entire back of the right hand, scattered areas on the fingers of the right hand, and areas of the forearm comprising about one fourth of its dorsal surface. The burn areas are erythematous with some small elevated blisters present in some of the areas; the hand and forearm appear edematous.

WD is not currently taking any medications; she is allergic to codeine and penicillin.

Clinical Considerations/Strategies

The following considerations/strategies are provided to aid the reader in (1) determining whether treatment of the patient's condition with nonprescription medications is warranted, (2) selecting the appropriate nonprescription medication, and (3) developing a patient counseling strategy to ensure optimal therapeutic outcomes:

- Assess the degree of severity and extent of the burn injuries.
- Based on the previous assessment, make appropriate recommendations.
- Taking into consideration the patient's reluctance to seek medical attention, determine whether recommending a nonprescription topical product is appropriate.
- If deemed appropriate, recommend nonprescription products to treat the burn.
- Discuss with the patient the potential consequences of failing to obtain appropriate medical care for an acute injury of this type.
- Determine the pharmacist's duty in this situation.

Summary

To assess the patient's burn accurately and recommend appropriate treatment, the pharmacist should be able to do the following:

- Understand the etiology and pathophysiology of burns and sunburns;
- Recognize the complications associated with burns and sunburns;
- Deliver initial care to the patient with a minor burn;
- Recommend appropriate nondrug therapy for the burn patient;
- Recommend appropriate pharmacotherapy for the burn patient;
- Recommend referral to a physician, if necessary.

In addition to providing accurate information and product recommendations, the pharmacist should be able to instruct the burn patient on how to care for the burn to optimize healing, manage symptoms, and minimize complications.

References

1. Types of injuries by selected characteristics: United States 1985–87. *Vital and Health Statistics*. Pub No 10–175 NCHS. Washington, DC: US Department of Health and Human Services; December 1990: 9–35.
2. US Department of Health, Education, and Welfare. Reports of the epidemiology and surveillance of injuries. DHEW Pub No (HSM) 73-10001. Atlanta: Centers for Disease Control; 1982.
3. Deaths resulting from residential fires—United States, 1991. *MMWR Morb Mortal Wkly Rep*. 1994 Dec; 43: 901–4.
4. Fitzpatrick TB, Freedberg IM. *Dermatology in General Medicine*. 3rd ed. New York: McGraw-Hill; 1987: 1425.
5. Greaves MW, Sondergaard J. Pharmacologic agents released in ultraviolet inflammation studied by continuous skin perfusion. *J Invest Dermatol*. 1970 May; 54: 365–7.
6. Mathur GP, Gandhi VM. Prostaglandins in human and albino rat skin. *J Invest Dermatol*. 1972 May; 58: 291–5.
7. Pathak MA, Fitzpatrick TB, Parrish JA. Photosensitivity and other reactions to light. In: Braunwald E et al, eds. *Principles of Internal Medicine*. 11th ed. New York: McGraw-Hill; 1987: 254–62.
8. Greco RJ et al. Hydrofluoric acid–induced hypocalcemia. *J Trauma*. 1988; 28: 1593–6.

9. Epstein MF, Crawford JD. Cooling in the emergency treatment of burns. *Pediatrics.* 1973 Sep; 52: 430–2.
10. Skin protectant drug products for over-the-counter human use: tentative final monograph. *Federal Register.* 1983 Feb; 48: 6820–33.
11. Greenberg RA et al. Orally given indomethacin and blood flow responses to UVL. *Arch Dermatol.* 1975 Mar; 111: 328–30.
12. Eaglestein WH, Ginsberg LD, Mertz PM. Ultraviolet irradiation-induced inflammation: effects of steroids and nonsteroidal anti-inflammatory agents. *Arch Dermatol.* 1979 Dec; 115: 1421–3.
13. Eaglestein WH, Mertz BA, Alvarez OM. Effect of topically applied agents on healing wounds. *Clin Dermatol.* 1984 Jul/Sep; 2: 112–5.
14. Topical antimicrobial drug products for over-the-counter human use: tentative final monograph for First Aid Antiseptic Drug Products. *Federal Register.* 1991 Jul; 56(140): 33644–80.

CHAPTER 32

Poison Ivy, Oak, and Sumac Products

Henry Wormser

Questions to ask in patient assessment and counseling

- *How long have you had the rash?*
- *Have you recently been camping, walking in the woods, or working in the garden?*
- *Have you ever had a rash from poison ivy, poison oak, or poison sumac?*
- *When did you notice the rash?*
- *Where is the rash located? How extensive is it?*
- *Would you describe the rash or affected skin?*
- *Do the skin lesions contain fluid? Are they oozing?*
- *What treatments have you tried? Were they effective?*
- *Are you allergic to any medication or product ingredient?*

Poison ivy, poison oak, and poison sumac dermatitis are allergic contact dermatitides that are often assessed by pharmacists and treated with nonprescription drugs. These conditions may be acute or chronic, depending on the extent of the patient's exposure and the degree of the patient's sensitivity to the allergens.

Etiology

Causative Plants

There are more than 60 plants and parts of plants that may cause allergic reactions in hypersensitive individuals.[1]

The Anacardiaceae family of trees and shrubs, which contains both noxious and useful plants, grows in many parts of the world. This botanical family includes the Japanese lacquer tree (*Rhus verniciflua*), which grows in Japan, China, and Indochina and from which a rich furniture lacquer is obtained; the cashew nut tree (*Anacardium occidentale*), which grows in India, Pakistan, the East Indies, Africa, and Central and South America; and the mango tree (*Mangifera indica*), which grows in tropical areas. Cross-sensitivity may occur on skin contact with parts of or products from these plants, such as cashew nut shells or oil, mango rinds, and furniture painted with natural lacquer.

Four species of the Anacardiaceae family are most commonly encountered in the United States and cause the more severe cases of allergic contact dermatitis: poison ivy (*Toxicodendron radicans*), western poison oak (*Toxicodendron diversilobum*), eastern poison oak (*Toxicodendron quercifolium*), and poison sumac (*Toxicodendron vernix*).[2] Poison ivy, which grows as either a shrub or a trailing vine, is identified by its characteristic clusters of three lobe-shaped leaflets, each 3–15 cm long, arranged on stalks; its white, ball-shaped berries that appear in the fall; and its usual climbing nature and hair roots when it appears as a vine (Figure 1). Abundant in North America, the plant grows everywhere in the United States except at altitudes above 4,000 feet and in Alaska, Hawaii, and the desert areas of California and Nevada.

Poison oak has blunt-tipped leaflets that are hairy on both sides and cluster in threes. These leaflets are somewhat shorter (3–7 cm) than those of poison ivy. The plant commonly appears as either an unsupported, erect bush or a vine, and the center leaf of the cluster resembles an oak leaf. Western poison oak grows along the Pacific Coast from New Mexico to Canada. Eastern poison oak is indigenous to regions from New Jersey to Florida and from central Texas to Kansas, growing primarily in sandy soil (Figure 2).

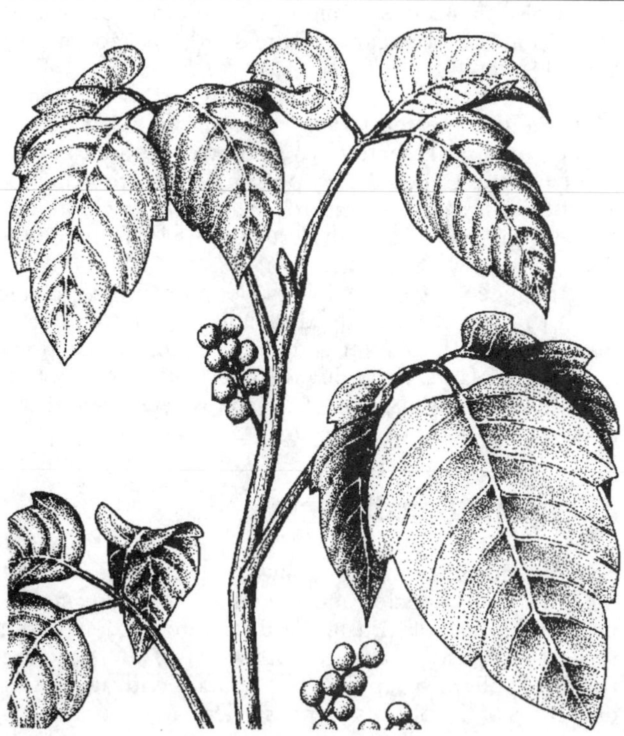

FIGURE 1 Poison ivy.

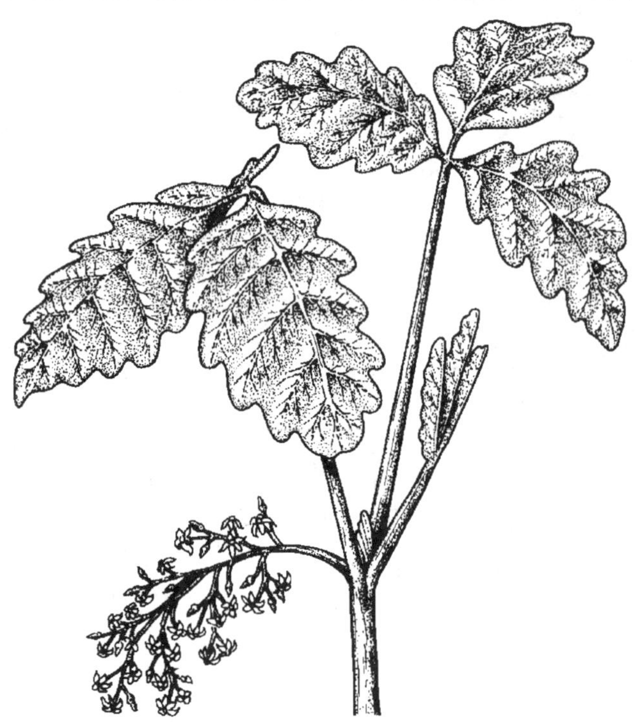

FIGURE 2 Poison oak.

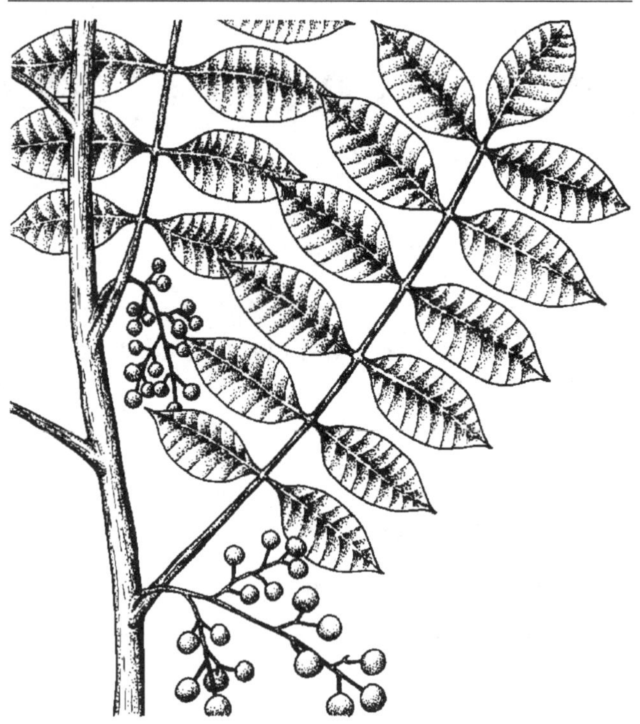

FIGURE 3 Poison sumac.

Poison sumac, also known as poison dogwood or poison elder, has pointed, pale green leaves in 7- to 13-leaf clusters arranged on each side of a red-ribbed leaf stalk[3] (Figure 3). The leaves are smooth edged, oval, and about 10 cm long. A coarse, woody shrub or small tree, poison sumac is commonly found in swamps and along ponds and streams of the southern and eastern United States.[4,5]

Formerly, the species were assigned to the genus *Rhus*; hence, the term *rhus dermatitis* is used to describe the topical reactions caused by exposure to these plants. In the United States, poison ivy and poison oak are the main causes of rhus dermatitis. In England and western Europe, primrose dermatitis is more common than poison ivy dermatitis.[6]

Irrespective of the etiology (ie, poison ivy, poison oak, or poison sumac), the dermatitides and treatments discussed in this chapter generally pertain to reactions to all three plants. Accordingly, unless otherwise noted, the following discussions of poison ivy also pertain to poison oak and poison sumac.

Allergenic Constituents

Toxicodendrol, a phenolic oily resin, is present in all the poisonous species and contains a complex active principle, urushiol. Urushiol is distributed widely in the roots, stems, leaves, and fruit of the plant, but not in the flowers, pollen, or epidermis.[7] Contact with the intact epidermis of the plant is harmless; dermatitis occurs only after contact with a damaged plant or its sap. However, the epidermis of these plants is very fragile, and relatively minor friction or force such as high winds will injure the plant. The oleoresin may then collect on the surface as a black sticky sap. Dead and dried plants may be dangerous as well because their leaves and vines are also easily damaged.

Because neither toxicodendrol nor urushiol is volatile, the dermatitis cannot be contracted through the air unless the plants are burned. Smoke from burning plants carries a substantial amount of the irritating oleoresin and may cause serious external and systemic reactions in susceptible individuals. Inhalation may produce severe trauma to the oral and nasal mucosa and lung tissue.

Researchers have identified four allergens in poison ivy, the chemical structures of which have been identified and elucidated.[8–10] Although all four allergens possess a 1,2-dihydroxybenzene or pyrocatechol nucleus with either a 15- or a 17-carbon atom side chain at position 3, their chemical structures differ primarily by the degree of unsaturation of the alkyl side chains. The allergens include a saturated component (3-pentadecylcatechol, or 3-PDC), a mono-olefin, a diolefin, a triolefin, and a tetraolefin. The concentrations and ratios of these compounds vary considerably among species of toxicodendrol-containing plants and within different growing environments. The most reactive compounds are those containing one or more double bonds.[11] Certain individuals who are hypersensitive to 3-PDC show cross-reactivity with other compounds such as resorcinol, hexylresorcinol, and the hydroquinones, but not with phenol itself.[12]

As little as 1 mcg of crude urushiol may cause dermatitis in hypersensitive individuals.[13] Direct contact with the plant is not necessary; contact may be made with the allergens via an article that injured the plant or via soot particles that contain allergenic material from the plant. The urushiol may be active for months on tools, sports equipment, shoes, and clothing, especially in a dry atmosphere. Stroking a pet whose fur is contaminated is also a common cause of allergic reaction. It has been estimated that 50–85% of the adult population of the United States is sensitive to urushiol. Thus, as many as 50 million people per year may be affected. The contact dermatitis also represents a major cause of occupational disability among outdoor workers such as firefighters, forestry personnel, and horticulturists.

Although the highest incidence of rhus dermatitis occurs in spring and summer, when the plant leaves are young, soft, and more easily injured, the dermatitis also occurs in autumn and winter.[3] In autumn, yellow leaves on the plant still have allergenic properties. Once they wither and fall, the leaves are much less allergenic. Winter episodes of the dermatitis often occur around Christmas in tree nursery employees and in people who cut their own trees; such episodes are caused by contact with the roots or vines of toxicodendron plants growing on the trees.

Mechanism of Contact Dermatitis

Development of contact dermatitis requires that an individual be sensitized to the toxic agent by a previous exposure; therefore, an allergic reaction does not occur on first contact with the plant. Accordingly, contact dermatitis has two phases: a *sensitization* phase, during which a specific hypersensitivity to the allergen is acquired, and an *elicitation* phase, during which subsequent contact with the allergen elicits a visible dermatologic response.[14]

In the sensitization phase, components of the allergen urushiol are presumably oxidized to the o-quinone derivatives, which react readily with human epidermal proteins by nucleophilic addition to form complete antigens. It has been suggested that the urushiol components go through a process of redox cycling and depletion of reducing equivalents to form reactive radical species, which serve as the ultimate haptenes.[15] Each allergen then leaves the skin through the lymphatic system and is carried to the reticuloendothelial system. There, in response to the antigenic stimulus, special globulins and antibodies are synthesized and T lymphocytes are sensitized.

In the elicitation phase, repeated contact with the allergen again produces the antigenic conjugate, this time causing a noticeable reaction with the activated T lymphocytes. The reaction appears to be triggered by the association of specific immunologic elements (effector cells and lymphokines) carried by the blood to the skin.

The degree of hypersensitivity to the toxic agent varies. Dark-skinned people seem less susceptible to the dermatitis. Young people are more susceptible than the elderly, and newborns are readily sensitized if they come in contact with sap from the plants.[1] The interval between contact with the allergen and appearance of the rash and associated symptoms varies with the individual's degree of sensitivity, as well as with the amount of allergen contacted and the thickness of the skin at the site of contact. Reaction time—the time between contact with the allergen and the first sign of reaction—is usually 2–3 days but not less than 12 hours. This interval is characteristic of delayed hypersensitivity reactions involving cell-mediated immunity.

Dermatologic lesions vary from simple maculae to vesicles and bullae. Contrary to popular belief, fluid in the vesicles and bullae is not antigenic. Histologically, nonspecific inflammatory changes occur in the dermis; and edema, followed by intraepidermal vesicles, develops in the epidermis in the acute stage of the disease. Premature bursting of the vesicles may lead to secondary bacterial infection.

Patient Assessment

Signs and Symptoms

Although the limbs, face, and neck are common sites of the dermatitis, all skin areas that come in contact with the allergen may be affected. Distribution of lesions may be erratic, especially if the allergen is in the clothes or is transferred to various parts of the body by the fingers. The dermatitis may appear early in one area of the body and later in another. Males have been known to transfer the offending oleoresin from their hands to their genitalia and even to the genitals of their sex partner during intercourse. Often, parts of the body that are in contact with a heavy concentration of the antigen show more severe reactions and remain hypersensitive for several years. Similarly, areas where the skin is thicker (eg, the palms of the hands or the soles of the feet) may take longer to erupt.

Poison ivy produces an allergic eczematous contact dermatitis. The initial reaction after exposure to the antigen is erythema or rash. The development of raised lesions (erythematous maculae and papules) follows, and finally, fluid accumulates in the raised lesions of the epidermis, forming vesicles and bullae. (See color plates, photographs 28A and B.) The lesions are more severe than those of dermatitides caused by other plants. The initial lesions are usually marked by mild to intensive itching and burning because of the fine nerve endings in the epidermis. The affected area, often hot and swollen, oozes and eventually dries and crusts.[16] Secondary bacterial infections may occur. Unlike certain other plant-induced allergic contact dermatitides, poison ivy rash is not photoactivated.

Most cases of the dermatitis are self-limiting and disappear in 14–20 days. Again, the duration and severity depend on the degree of sensitization and on the frequency and degree of reexposure to the allergen.

Chewing poison ivy leaves may result in edematous swelling and pain of the tongue, cheeks, palate, and pharynx. If the leaves are then swallowed, swelling and pain may occur in the anal region.[17] Very rare complications include eosinophilia, kidney damage, toxic shock syndrome, urticaria, erythema multiforme, dyshidrosis, marked pigmentation, and leukoderma (loss of melanin pigmentation occurring in patches).

Rhus dermatitis may be assessed not only from the morphologic appearance of its lesions but also from their distribution. Linear streaking is common and occurs naturally as the skin brushes against the poisonous plant. Because toxicodendron plants are not photosensitizers, the dermatitis can occur on covered as well as uncovered parts of the body.

Diagnostic Testing

Diagnostic patch testing is a valuable tool in investigating allergic contact dermatitis[18–20]; however, substances used in patch testing may sensitize the patient during testing. The currently accepted device for patch testing is a small aluminum disk, 8 mm in diameter, known as the Finn chamber. The Finn chamber is charged with a small ribbon of a petrolatum-based allergen or, if the allergen is a liquid, a small disk of filter paper containing one to several drops of the test allergen. (In the case of rhus oleoresin, a 1:50 solution in absolute alcohol is used.) The Finn chamber is then applied to the patient's back for 2 days with an adhesive, nonallergenic tape.[21]

Patch testing should be performed only by allergists or other individuals thoroughly familiar with accepted techniques. This procedure should never be done during the acute phase of any dermatitis as it will exacerbate the symptoms. Furthermore, because approximately 75% of the US population has been sensitized to urushiol, patch testing should not be a routine procedure.

Patch testing results alone are not diagnostic. To interpret test results properly, practitioners must also consider the patient's history of exposure to the causative plants and any physical findings, as well as their own clinical experience.

Treatment

Preventive Measures

The best way to prevent any allergic contact dermatitis is to avoid the allergen completely. People should learn to recognize and avoid poison ivy and related plants. They should observe and search surrounding terrain carefully when hiking and before choosing a picnic area or campsite. Susceptible individuals should wear protective clothing (eg, long sleeves, long pants, socks, and shoes) when exposure to the offending agents is probable. After an outing, they should carefully launder their clothing with a detergent and hot water. They should also wash with alcohol or another suitable organic solvent any object that may have come in contact with the plants to remove the oleoresin. As previously noted, any unremoved oleoresin will remain potent on the object's surface for a considerable time.

When a poisonous plant is in a garden or yard, it should be destroyed chemically or removed physically. Herbicide sprays may be used any time poison ivy is in full leaf, but June and July are the preferred months. Ordinarily, spraying should begin no later than mid-August because poison ivy begins to go dormant then and the herbicides are ineffective. At least three to four sprayings at intervals of 2–8 weeks are necessary to kill all the plants.[22] The herbicides that are most effective against poison ivy include amitrole (aminotriazole); ammonium sulfamate; 2,4-dichlorophenoxyacetic acid (2,4-D); 2,4,5-trichlorophenoxyacetic acid (2,4,5-T); ammonium thiocyanate; borax; carbon disulfide; coal tar; creosote oils; fuel oil and similar petroleum distillates (eg, kerosene and diesel fuel); sodium chlorate; and sodium arsenite.

Applying herbicides is the easier and less dangerous method of plant removal, but once root growth is well established, it is much more difficult to eradicate the plants with chemicals. Moreover, there are areas where herbicides cannot be used (eg, around some grasses, hedges, and shrubbery). In such situations, digging and pulling up the plants by the roots is the only satisfactory method of removal. Whichever method is chosen, however, individuals should always wear appropriate protective gear. Roots, stems, and leaves should be buried rather than incinerated.

Once contact with poison ivy is made, the antigen enters the skin rapidly. Thorough washing with an alkaline soap or organic solvents such as alcohol or acetone within 5–10 minutes of exposure is necessary to prevent absorption of the antigen. A product that was originally designed to remove radioactive dust from the skin in the event of a nuclear catastrophe has been marketed as a skin cleanser (Technu Poison Oak-n-Ivy Cleansing Treatment).

Another topical preventive measure includes the application of barrier creams prior to contact.[12] However, many investigators and clinicians question the effectiveness of barrier creams.[23–25]

Thirty-four barrier preparations were tested over a 2-year period on a group of people highly susceptible to rhus dermatitis.[12] The preparations contained substances such as potassium permanganate, hydrogen peroxide, sodium perborate, iodine, and iron and silver salts. The investigator concluded that none of the preparations could prevent the dermatitis. This suggests that the antigen reacts rapidly and quite selectively with the skin and that the antigen–antibody reaction occurs and progresses before effective preventive action can be taken.

Although enthusiastic anecdotal claims have been made for zirconium oxide, tests have found it to be completely ineffective for preventing the dermatitis.[12] In addition, several researchers found that extensive, sarcoidlike granulomas of glabrous skin developed because of allergic hypersensitivity to insoluble zirconium oxide.[26–28] More recently, some success has been obtained with some formulations of organoclay (a quaternary ammonium salt of bentonite),[29] polyamine salts of linoleic acid dimer[30] (Stokoguard), and a product marketed under the name Ivy Shield.[31]

Hyposensitization Therapy

Specific hyposensitization may be tried by administering repeated and gradually increasing doses of toxicodendron antigens before and during the poison ivy season. Various forms of these antigens, administered either by mouth or by intramuscular injection, have been investigated. For equivalent effects, larger amounts are required of the oral antigen than of the parenteral formulation because the antigen may undergo partial inactivation and imperfect absorption when taken orally. Sustained release is probably the major factor in the greater efficacy of intramuscular antigen injection. Nevertheless, such prophylaxis is neither complete nor permanent, given that the original sensitivity returns approximately 6 months after the therapy ends.[32,33] Nor is this approach approved by the Food and Drug Administration (FDA). Most products used for hyposensitization therapy became commercially available before the FDA tightened regulations; thus, these products are exempt from FDA safety and efficacy testing.

Hyposensitizing by administering parenterally crude extracts or oleoresins from the plants has also been generally ineffective. This is because potency of the extracts varies, and recommended doses of the antigens are usually far below those required. Three or four injections cannot provide the clinical protection needed for moderately or extremely hypersensitive persons.

Because hyposensitization is temporary, maintenance doses of the antigen should be administered at predetermined intervals. If successful, hyposensitization results in milder and shorter reactions that are less likely to spread to other parts of the body. In fact, the only objective proof of successful hyposensitization is a negative or weak positive reaction to the antigens at a site that previously gave a strong positive reaction.

Administering an antigenic substance to a hypersensitive individual involves great risk. The exact course of treatment must be individualized to the person's sensitivity level and capacity to tolerate the antigen without serious allergic reactions. Further, the dermatitis must be diagnosed by a dermatologist before hyposensitization can begin. Prophylactic administration of toxicodendrol antigens has no effect on contact dermatitis caused by other substances. Finally, if the dermatitis appears during prophylactic treatment, the treatment should be stopped for the duration of the eruption.

Topical Treatment

The initial symptoms of the dermatologic reaction may be discomforting and alarming. While the urge to treat them aggressively is strong, moderation is recommended as simplicity and safety are key elements of treatment. Many claims for products used for self-medication take credit for the body's own natural reparative and homeostatic processes; in most cases, the contact dermatitis is self-resolving. Thus, the major treatment objectives of therapy are to:

- Protect the damaged tissue until the acute reaction has subsided;
- Prevent both excessive accumulation of debris and complications resulting from oozing, scaling, and crusting, without disturbing normal tissue;
- Relieve itching and thus prevent scratching, excoriation, and secondary bacterial infection.

Mild Dermatitis

Linear streaks of papules and vesicles often characterize mild poison ivy dermatitis. These lesions and their accompanying pain and itching can be treated by an antipruritic lotion such as calamine or zinc oxide. A combination of 1% menthol and equal parts of calamine, zinc oxide, and rubbing alcohol can be soothing.[34]

Soaks, baths, or wet dressings can also be effective in soothing pain and itching. A diluted (1:40) aluminum acetate solution (Burow's solution, or Domeboro), a saline solution, or a sodium bicarbonate solution can be used in this manner for 30 minutes, three or four times a day. Burow's solution for topical use (USP) is usually a 1:10 or 1:40 dilution of aluminum acetate solution in water.[35] In addition, the application of either warm or very cold water may provide relief. A simple suggestion is to encourage parents of children with poison ivy dermatitis to clip the child's fingernails. Short, clipped fingernails and good hygiene will go a long way to prevent secondary infections.

Topical preparations containing local anesthetics or antihistamines are available; however, their routine use is somewhat controversial because of their sensitizing capabilities. Nonprescription topical steroids such as hydrocortisone are also available and have proven safe and effective for use in mild dermatitis.[36] Greasy ointments should not be used when vesicles are present and oozing. Also, creams are more aesthetic.

Moderately Severe Dermatitis

Moderately severe poison ivy dermatitis is characterized by the presence of bullae and edematous swelling of affected body parts, in addition to the papules and vesicles present in milder cases. To reduce discomfort, large bullae may be drained by puncturing their edges with a sterilized needle; this should preferably be done by a trained medical professional. The tops of the lesions should be kept intact because they protect the underlying, denuded epidermis of the lesions as they dry. The patient should be reassured that fluid from the lesions will *not* spread the dermatitis and that the dermatitis is *not* contagious. Application of cool compresses of Burow's solution (1:10) to edematous areas may be helpful.

Lesions on the face can be treated by applying wet dressings. If the eyelids are affected, cold compresses of a dilute boric acid solution can be used.[1] Lotions should be avoided because they tend to cake, causing discomfort. Men may find that shaving, although uncomfortable, is more comfortable and aesthetic than the accumulation of crust and debris in the beard.

During the healing phase, application of a soothing cream (eg, Curél Therapeutic Moisturizing Cream or Aveeno Moisturizing Cream) helps prevent crusting, scaling, and thickening of the lesions. However, any cream that is recommended should be of neutral pH to avoid discomfort. Following exposure to a plant sensitizer, some patients may have a heightened sensitivity to various ingredients (eg, dye, perfume, or preservatives) of a certain formulation; this may be particularly true of emulsions. In such a case, the patient has a reaction to the medication, assumes the cause is the poison ivy, and responds by applying still more medication, which perpetuates the cycle.

Taking two to six tepid tub baths using oatmeal or a commercially available colloidal preparation (eg, Aveeno Bath Treatment) may be soothing. Because these preparations make the bathtub very slick, patients who use them should be warned to place a nonskid mat in the tub. They also should be reminded to read the package instructions carefully before using the products.

Severe Dermatitis

A patient experiencing a widespread reaction over the body that is associated with major swelling or eye involvement should be referred to a physician for prescription therapy with either potent topical or systemic anti-inflammatory steroids.

Topical treatment of severe poison ivy dermatitis is similar to that recommended for moderately severe dermatitis.[1] Physicians will often prescribe topical corticosteroids such as 0.5% or 1.0% hydrocortisone, 0.1% betamethasone valerate (Valisone), 0.05% betamethasone dipropionate (Diprosone), 0.01% fluocinolone acetonide (Synalar), or 0.1% or 0.5% triamcinolone acetonide (Aristocort or Kenalog).

Systemic treatment usually involves prescription drugs such as anti-inflammatory steroids. Corticosteroids such as prednisone and methylprednisolone are commonly administered orally over 7 days to 3 weeks in a gradually descending dosage schedule. The starting dose should be based on the patient's age and ideal body weight. The tapering regimen is relatively safe because it is short term and does not lead to significant hypothalamic-pituitary-adrenal suppression. However, pharmacists must counsel patients to adhere to the directions and complete the entire course of dose-tapering steroid therapy. Certain patients may develop nervousness, irritability, insomnia, gastrointestinal intolerance, or weight gain. Unfortunately, it is difficult to predict who will have these reactions.

Oral antihistamines such as diphenhydramine, chlorpheniramine, or tripelennamine may be useful for their systemic antipruritic effects.[1,37] However, the anticholinergic side effects of antihistamines could exacerbate preexisting conditions of patients who have prostatic hypertrophy, narrow-angle glaucoma, stenosing peptic ulcer, bladder neck obstruction, and a tendency toward constipation. It should be noted that histamine plays only a minor role in contact dermatitis allergic reactions, so the benefits of these agents may be less than the risks.

Respiratory emergencies resulting from inhalation of dust or smoke from burning plants are extremely rare except among forest firefighters, but such occurrences require immediate attention. Patients may experience shortness of breath, dyspnea, or stridor as a result of pharyngeal or laryngeal edema. Treatment should be directed toward maintaining a patent airway and administering intravenous corticosteroids.

Pharmacologic Agents

Four major types of pharmacologic agents—local anesthetics, antipruritics, antiseptics, and astringents—are used as topical nonprescription products for poison ivy dermatitis (see product table "Poison Ivy, Oak, and Sumac Products").

Local Anesthetics

Local anesthetics affect sensation by interfering with the transmission of impulses along sensory nerve fibers. Many free nerve endings, nerve fibers, and specialized endings (receptors) are present in the epidermis. The topically applied anesthetics act only at the application site.

Benzocaine and pramoxine hydrochloride are the most common local anesthetics found in nonprescription products for poison ivy and poison oak. Poorly soluble local anesthetics (eg, benzocaine) are less likely to be absorbed and to produce systemic toxicity than are more soluble local anesthetics (eg, tetracaine hydrochloride). However, regardless of which agent is selected, the high serum concentrations necessary to produce systemic toxicity are difficult to achieve with nonprescription topical anesthetics. If a contact dermatitis worsens after the topical application of a local anesthetic, the affected area should be washed thoroughly with mild soap and water, and use of the anesthetic should be discontinued. Side effects of topically applied local anesthetics can include dermatitis (characterized by cutaneous lesions), urticaria and edema, and anaphylactic reactions. (See Chapter 31, "Burn and Sunburn Products.")

Antipruritics

Topically applied antipruritics, including antihistamines, counterirritants, and hydrocortisone, are agents that help to alleviate itching.

Antihistamines

Antihistamines such as diphenhydramine (Benadryl) relieve the discomfort of itching by competing with histamine at the H_1 receptor (one of two broad classes of histamine receptors). They also produce a mild local anesthetic effect if applied topically. For instance, application of a 1–2% concentration of topical diphenhydramine to the affected area three times a day should effectively relieve itching. The topical use of antihistamines does not produce anticholinergic adverse effects or systemic toxicity. However, like the "caine" anesthetics, antihistamines may occasionally act as sensitizers and aggravate a contact dermatitis.

Antihistamines are more effective as antipruritics when taken orally, particularly when itching is generalized. However, an individual who is sensitized to a topical agent should not take it orally.

Counterirritants

Counterirritants, which contain products such as menthol, phenol, and camphor, produce a sensation of coolness and reduce irritation. The sensation is difficult to explain because these chemicals produce local hyperemia and, when applied to severely damaged skin, may actually cause irritation. However, low concentrations of these drugs (ie, 0.1%), particularly menthol, relieve irritation by the depression of cutaneous receptors. (See Chapter 5, "External Analgesic Products.")

Hydrocortisone

Hydrocortisone is a naturally occurring glucocorticoid synthesized endogenously in the adrenal cortex. Although topical corticosteroids are useful for a variety of dermatitides, their effectiveness on poison ivy dermatitis is acknowledged. The FDA's Advisory Review Panel on Over-the-Counter External Analgesic Drug Products reported that short-term topical use of 0.5–1% hydrocortisone is unlikely to exacerbate cutaneous bacterial, fungal, or viral infections. The panel also reported that allergic reactions to hydrocortisone at these concentrations are rare. Additionally, the panel found evidence that prolonged administration of 0.5–1% hydrocortisone does not appear to cause toxic effects by systemic absorption, even when applied to large areas of damaged or abraded skin.[38]

Nonprescription hydrocortisone products approved by the FDA for use on rashes and minor skin irritations carry the following label:

> "For the temporary relief of minor skin irritations, itching, and rashes due to eczema, dermatitis, insect bites, poison ivy, poison oak, poison sumac, soaps, detergents, cosmetics, and jewelry and for itchy genital and anal areas but not for ophthalmic use."

Recommended dosage for adults and children 2 years of age and above is 1% hydrocortisone applied to the affected area three or four times a day. Children under 2 years of age should be treated only under the advice and supervision of a physician.

Antiseptics

Antiseptics contained in poison ivy and poison oak products are intended for prophylaxis against secondary bacterial infections, but their effectiveness is questionable. Of the available antiseptics (eg, phenols, alcohols, and oxidizing agents) and quaternary ammonium compounds (eg, benzalkonium chloride), the latter seem to be more effective. Unfortunately, their activity is decreased by anionic compounds such as soaps.[39]

Astringents

Astringents (eg, witch hazel, aluminum acetate, tannic acid, zinc and iron oxides) are mild protein precipitants that are used to stop oozing, reduce inflammation, and promote healing of the dermatitis. These agents produce these effects either by forming a thick coagulum on the surface of lesions or by coagulating and removing overlying debris. The astringent action may be accompanied by contraction, wrinkling, and blanching of tissue. The cement substance of the capillary endothelium is hardened so that pathologic transcapillary movement of plasma proteins is inhibited, thus reducing local edema, inflammation, and exudation.

As noted previously, Burow's solution is generally diluted with water to produce a 1:10 or 1:40 solution and used as a wet dressing three or four times a day. Therapy may be continued for approximately 5–7 days. However, continuous or prolonged use for extended periods may be inflammatory. Because application of the concentrate can cause skin damage and pain, the pharmacist should make sure that the patient understands how to dilute Burow's solution.

Zinc oxide lotion (15–25%) has mild astringent, protective, and antiseptic actions. Calamine plus zinc oxide is often preferred over zinc oxide alone because of its pink, skinlike coloration. However, continuous use may build a thick layer of material on the skin unless the previous application is gently removed.

Product Selection Guidelines

Selection of products depends on the severity of the dermatitis. Although patients with severe cases of poison ivy dermatitis should be referred to a physician, mild to moderately severe cases can usually be treated with one or more topical products. Systemic use of antihistamines may be combined with application of topical agents to relieve itching. Preparations that contain benzocaine or other local anesthetics should be used with caution.

Lotions, which may contain phenol or menthol, provide prompt relief from itching. However, the pharmacist should caution against their frequent or excessive use. Lotions pile layers of plasterlike material on the skin, which may produce discomfort and can be difficult and painful to remove.

Finally, the pharmacist should inform individuals who are sensitive to toxicodendron plants that certain cosmetics, hair dyes, bleaches, and other topical commercial products contain compounds related to 3-PDC and could cause cross-sensitivity. Such patients should be advised to reduce their use of these products.

Case Studies

Case 32–1

Patient Complaint/History

JJ, a healthy 14-year-old female, has just returned from a 2-week camping trip along the shore of Lake Superior in northern Michigan. She presents to the pharmacist with extensive vesicular and bullous eruptions on approximately 40% of her body; the highest concentration of eruptions is on her arms and legs. She also has weeping lesions on her face as well as on her back and abdomen. JJ reports that the campgrounds were rather primitive and offered few opportunities for freshwater showers. She thinks that she has acquired a serious case of poison ivy, poison oak, or poison sumac.

Clinical Considerations/Strategies

The following considerations/strategies are provided to aid the reader in (1) determining whether treatment of the patient's condition with nonprescription medications is warranted, (2) selecting the appropriate nonprescription medication, and (3) developing a patient counseling strategy to ensure optimal therapeutic outcomes:

- Develop a series of questions to ask the patient that would confirm her assessment of the condition.
- Assess the severity of the condition and determine whether to triage to a physician or treat the condition with nonprescription medications.
- Determine which nonprescription medications are most likely to produce a significant degree of symptomatic relief for this patient.

- Develop a patient education/counseling strategy that will:
  - Ensure that the patient understands how the condition will most likely progress, what symptoms to expect, and when resolution of the symptoms is most likely to occur;
  - Explain what complications may develop and what to do if they occur;
  - Ensure that the patient understands the medical condition, the importance of drug therapy, and when and how to use the recommended nonprescription drug therapy.

Case 32–2

Patient Complaint/History

MS, a 55-year-old single female paraplegic, has been confined to a wheelchair for the past 40 years as a result of poliomyelitis. In addition to asthma for which she uses a medi-inhaler (Ventolin), MS also has diabetes. The diabetes is managed with an oral sulfonylurea (DiaBeta) and a strict diet.

Except for a weekly shopping trip on which her brother accompanies her, the patient stays indoors most of the time. She and her two German shepherd dogs, who are her daily companions and protectors, live in a heavily wooded area near Atlantic City, New Jersey. The dogs are let out twice a day into a sideyard that borders the woods.

Yesterday MS noticed a dry eruption on her hands, arms, and knees; the eruption causes intense itching and interrupts her sleep at night. She is calling the pharmacy today to request advice on treating the dermatologic condition.

Clinical Considerations/Strategies

The following considerations/strategies are provided to aid the reader in (1) determining whether treatment of the patient's condition with nonprescription medications is warranted, (2) selecting the appropriate nonprescription medication, and (3) developing a patient counseling strategy to ensure optimal therapeutic outcomes:

- Speculate on the possible etiology of the patient's dermatitis.
- Discuss with the patient your hypothesis on the etiology of her dermatologic symptoms.
- Assess the severity of the patient's symptoms.
- Determine which nonprescription medications are most likely to produce a significant degree of symptomatic relief.
- Develop a patient education/counseling strategy that will:
  - Help the patient understand her dermatologic condition, how the condition will most likely progress, and when resolution of the symptoms is most likely to occur;
  - Explain what complications may develop and what to do if they occur;
  - Ensure that the patient understands the importance of nonprescription drug therapy and when and how to use the recommended therapy.

Summary

Every year poison ivy, poison oak, and poison sumac produce contact dermatitides in thousands of people. The best approach to treatment is prevention: avoiding contact with the offending plant. Once the dermatitis develops, symptomatic relief is the only therapy. A better understanding of the mechanism of the allergic reaction, cross-sensitivity, and hyposensitization will help in formulating products that are more effective in treating and managing this annoying and often serious disorder.

References

1. Fisher AA, Adams RM. *Contact Dermatitis*. 3rd ed. Philadelphia: Lea and Febiger; 1986: 405–17.
2. Lesser MA. Poison ivy. *Drug Cosmet Ind*. 1952 May; 70: 610–1.
3. Dawson CR. The chemistry of poison ivy. *Trans N Y Acad Sci*. 1956; 18: 427–43.
4. Marderosian AHD. Poison ivy and related dermatitis. *Drug Ther*. 1977 Aug; 112: 57–74.
5. Vietmeyer N. Science has got its hands on poison ivy, oak and sumac. *Smithsonian*. 1985; 16: 89–95.
6. Rook A, Wilson HTH. Primula dermatitis. *Br Med J*. 1965 Jan; 5429: 220–2.
7. Doyle JH. Poison ivy dermatitis. *Pediatr Clin N Am*. 1961; 8: 259–63.
8. Sunthankar SV, Dawson CR. The structural identification of the olefinic components of Japanese lac urushiol. *J Am Chem Soc*. 1954; 76: 5070–4.
9. Symes WF, Dawson CR. Poison ivy "urushiol." *J Am Chem Soc*. 1954; 76: 2959–63.
10. Loev B, Dawson CR. The geometrical configuration of the olefinic components of poison ivy urushiol. The synthesis of a model compound. *J Am Chem Soc*. 1956; 78: 1180–3.
11. Gross M et al. Urushiols of poisonous Anacardiaceae. *Phytochemistry*. 1975; 4: 2263.
12. Kligman AM. Poison ivy (rhus) dermatitis. *Arch Dermatol*. 1958; 77: 149–80.
13. Stevens FA. Status of poison ivy extracts. *JAMA*. 1945 Apr; 127: 912–21.
14. Epstein WL. In: Fitzpatrick TB et al, eds. *Dermatology in General Medicine*. New York: McGraw-Hill, 1979: 1373–83.
15. Schmidt RJ, Khan L, Chung LY. Are free radicals and not quinones the haptenic species derived from urushiols and the other contact allergenic mono- and dihydric alkylbenzenes? The significance of NADH, glutathione, and redox cycling in the skin. *Arch Dermatol Res*. 1990; 282(1): 56–64.
16. Selfon PM. The treatment of acute poison ivy dermatitis among our military field personnel. *Milit Med*. 1963 Sep; 128: 895–900.
17. Silvers SH. Stomatitis venenata and dermatitis of anal orifice from chewing poison ivy leaves (Rhus toxicodendron). *JAMA*. 1941 May; 116: 2257.
18. Kligman AM. The identification of contact allergens by human assay: I. a critique of standard methods. *J Invest Dermatol*. 1966 Nov; 47: 369–74.
19. Kligman AM. The identification of contact allergens by human assay. II. factors influencing the induction and measurement of allergic contact dermatitis. *J Invest Dermatol*. 1966 Nov; 47: 375–92.
20. Kligman AM. The identification of contact allergens by human assay: III. the maximization test: a procedure for screening and rating contact sensitizers. *J Invest Dermatol*. 1966 Nov; 47: 393–409.

21. Rietschel RL. Contact dermatitis and diagnostic techniques. *Allergy Proc.* 1989 Nov–Dec; 10(6): 403–11.

22. Crooks DM, Kephart LW. *Farmers' Bulletin.* Pub No 1972. Washington, DC: US Department of Agriculture; 1951: 30.

23. Shelmire B. Contact dermatitis from weeds; patch testing with their oleoresins. *JAMA.* 1939 Sep; 113: 1085–90.

24. Gisvold O. Effect of some absorbents, precipitants and oxidants upon resin of Rhus toxicodendron. *J Am Pharm Assoc, Sci Ed.* 1941 Jan; 30: 17–8.

25. Howell JB. Evaluation of measures for prevention of ivy dermatitis. *Arch Dermatol & Syphiology.* 1943 Oct; 48: 373–8.

26. LoPresti PJ, Hambrick GW Jr. Zirconium granuloma following treatment of rhus dermatitis. *Arch Dermatol* (Chicago). 1965 Aug; 92: 188–91.

27. Epstein WL, Allen JR. Granulomatous hypersensitivity after use of zirconium-containing poison oak lotion. *JAMA.* 1964 Dec; 190(10): 940–2.

28. Hall NA. O-T-C products for rhus dermatitis—zirconium-containing topical application. *J Am Pharm Assoc.* 1972 Nov; 12: 576–7.

29. Epstein WL. Topical prevention of poison ivy/oak dermatitis. *Arch Dermatol.* 1989 Apr; 125(4): 499–501.

30. Orchard SM, Fellman JH, Storrs FJ. Poison ivy/oak dermatitis: use of polyamine salts of a linoleic acid dimer for topical prophylaxis. *Arch Dermatol.* 1986; 122: 783–9.

31. Basiliere D. Personal communication of unpublished research on Ivy Shield. Haverhill, Mass: Interpro, Inc; 1989.

32. Kligman AM. Hyposensitization against rhus dermatitis. *Arch Dermatol.* 1958; 78: 47–72.

33. Kligman AM. Cashew nut shell oil for hyposensitization against rhus dermatitis. *Arch Dermatol.* 1958; 78: 359–63.

34. Fowler JF. In: Rakel RE, ed. *Conn's Current Therapy.* Philadelphia: WB Saunders; 1992: 786–7.

35. Skin protectant drug products for over-the-counter human use; astringent drug products. *Federal Register.* 1989 Apr; 54: 13480–99.

36. du Vivier AWP. Over-the-counter hydrocortisone. *Practitioner.* 1986; 230: 897–900.

37. Bond CA. In: Young LY, Koda-Kimble MA, eds. *Applied Therapeutics: The Clinical Use of Drugs.* 4th ed. Vancouver, Wash: Applied Therapeutics Inc; 1988: 1413–4.

38. Hydrocortisone: marketing status as external analgesic drug product for over-the-counter human use; notice of enforcement policy. *Federal Register.* 1991 Aug; 156: 43025.

39. Apted JH. Poison ivy dermatitis in Victoria. *Australas J Dermatol.* 1978 Apr; 19(1): 35–6. Letter.

CHAPTER 33

Insect Sting and Bite Products

Farid Sadik

Questions to ask in patient assessment and counseling

- *How extensive are the bites or stings on your body?*
- *Is the reaction limited to the site of the bite or sting?*
- *Have you developed hives, excessive swelling, dizziness, vomiting, or difficulty in breathing since being bitten or stung?*
- *Have you ever been previously stung by a honeybee, wasp, or hornet?*
- *Have you previously had severe reactions to insect bites or stings?*
- *Have you ever consulted a physician?*
- *What have you tried so far, if anything, to treat the reaction?*
- *Have you ever had adverse reactions to topically applied products?*
- *Do you have a personal or family history of allergic reactions such as hay fever?*
- *If a child, what is the patient's age and approximate weight?*

Human contact with various species of insects is inevitable. Summertime outdoor activists such as gardeners, beachgoers, hunters, fishermen, and hikers, as well as individuals whose occupation requires them to remain outdoors and even those who spend time in their backyards, are at risk of insect bites and stings. For about 90% of Americans, many of whom are otherwise healthy, the reactions to these injuries are mild and local in nature. Some reactions are prolonged and annoying, compelling those who have been injured to seek their pharmacist's advice in selecting a nonprescription product that provides symptomatic relief from the resultant local reactions. However, about 1% of the population are allergic to the insect venom, and for them the reaction can be severe and possibly life-threatening. Each year in the United States at least 50 persons die as a result of allergic hypersensitivity to insect stings.[1]

Biting Insects and Arachnids

Insects such as mosquitoes, fleas, bedbugs, lice, and arachnids such as ticks and chiggers (red bugs) bite their prey. They insert their biting organs into the skin to feed by sucking blood from their hosts. In sensitive individuals, the salivary secretions, which contain antigenic substances, produce local erythematous, itching papules with central puncta. (See color plates, photograph 29.)

Mosquitoes

Mosquitoes are found in abundance worldwide, particularly in humid, warm climates. They usually attack exposed parts of the body (face, neck, forearms, and legs). They can, however, bite through thin clothing. When a mosquito alights on the skin, it cuts through the skin with its mandibles and maxillae. A fine, hollow, needle-like, flexible structure (proboscis) is introduced into the cut and probes the tissue for a blood vessel. Blood is sucked directly from a capillary lumen or from previously lacerated capillaries with extravasated blood. During feeding, the mosquito injects into the wound a salivary secretion containing an anticoagulant and antigenic components, which cause the itching.

Fleas

Fleas are tiny (1.5–4 mm long), bloodsucking, wingless, laterally compressed parasites with strongly developed posterior legs used for leaping. Fleas parasitize various avian and mammalian hosts. Body warmth and exhaled carbon dioxide are believed to attract fleas to the host. Most people are bitten about the legs and ankles; bites usually are multiple and grouped. Each lesion is characterized by an erythematous region around the puncture and causes intense itching. Fleas are not only annoying but also responsible for transmitting diseases such as bubonic plague and endemic typhus.

Fleas are found throughout the world (including arctic regions) but breed best in warm areas with relatively high humidity. They may survive and multiply without food for several weeks. However, females need a blood meal to deposit eggs. Places that have been vacant for weeks may be heavily infested, partly because of the hatching of eggs, which are usually deposited in floor crevices or on rugs, particularly those on which pets have been sleeping.

Bedbugs

Bedbugs have a short head and a broad, flat body (4–5 mm long and 3 mm wide). Their mouth parts consist of two pairs of stylets used to pierce the skin. The outer part has barbs that saw the skin, and the inner part is used to suck blood and allow salivary secretions to flow into the wound. Depending on the sensitivity of the bitten individual, the reaction may range from irritation at the site of the bite to a small dermal hemorrhage.

Bedbugs usually hide and deposit their eggs in crevices of walls, floors, picture frames, bedding, and other furniture. They normally hide during the day, become active at night, and bite their sleeping victims. Persons may also be bitten in subdued light by day while sitting in theaters or other public places. A bedbug can engorge itself with blood within 3–5 minutes, and then it typically seeks its hiding place.

Lice

Lice are wingless parasites with well-developed legs. They do not jump like fleas and do not fly. Each leg has a claw that helps the louse cling firmly to hair or clothing fibers while sucking blood. An adult louse inserts its mouth into the skin and injects anticoagulant saliva to allow the flow of blood into its mouth. It feeds for 30–45 minutes every 3–4 hours. Thus, depending on the extent of the infestation, the host may receive hundreds of bites each day. The bites produce papular dermatitis and cause the host to scratch constantly. In addition to being irritating pests, lice may act as vectors of epidemic diseases such as typhus.

Lice infestations (pediculosis) in the United States are common.[2] There are three types of lice that infest humans: head lice (*Pediculus humanus capitis*), body lice (*Pediculus humanus corporis*) and pubic lice (*Phthirus pubis*).

Head Lice

Head lice is the most common lice infestation,[3] affecting more than 10 million Americans annually. The vast majority of cases involve children 1–12 years of age. Outbreaks of lice infestation are common in crowded places such as schools, day care centers, and nursing homes and usually peak after the opening of schools each year between the months of August and November.[4] The National Pediculosis Association recommends schoolwide screenings after school opens, before Christmas, and before school is out for the summer.

Head lice usually infest the head and live on the scalp.[5] (See color plates, photographs 30A and B.) The female deposits 10–150 nits (eggs), which become glued to the hair and hatch in 5–10 days. The nit is about 5 mm in diameter and has yellowish or grayish white color. Once hatched, the louse must begin the feeding process within 24 hours or it dies. The nymph (newly hatched immature louse) resembles an adult and matures within 8–9 days. The lifespan of an adult is about 1 month. The nymph is active and tends to move about the head, whereas the adults are less active.

Transmission of head lice occurs directly through physical contact with an infested individual or indirectly through the sharing of articles such as combs, brushes, towels, caps, and hats.[6] Awareness and action by health officials, school authorities, and parents are essential in stopping the spread of lice. Pharmacists can be effective in this regard and can obtain information on safe treatments and preventive measures for head lice from the National Pediculosis Association, PO Box 610189, Newton, MA 02161; 617–449–NITS.

Assessment of Head Lice Head lice may be assessed by examining the hair for nits, nymphs, or crawling adults. Examination is best done under strong light,[7] and a magnifying glass may be used. Parting the hair with a comb or with fingers protected by gloves may help reveal the nits that have been laid on the hair shaft close to the scalp. The nits are attached with a cementlike substance so they will not brush or comb off with a regular comb. Because hair grows at a relatively constant rate of approximately one-half inch per month, the duration of infestation may be estimated by measuring the distance of the nit from the scalp surface.

As previously noted, head lice infestation often causes itching, a reaction to the bites or fecal deposits of the lice. Scratching the irritation may result in excoriation of the scalp tissue and, possibly, a secondary bacterial or fungal infection. In some instances, pyoderma results, characterized by erythema, crusting, and oozing on the scalp and hair margins. In severe cases, the patient may suffer from swollen glands and mild fever. Prolonged and frequent exposure to bites may lead to immunity to the extent that the infected person may experience little or no reaction to bites.

Treatment of Head Lice Treatment is initiated following assessment. Currently, there are pediculicides available in both prescription and nonprescription products (see product table "Pediculicide Products").

In 1986 the Food and Drug Administration (FDA) approved 1% permethrin cream rinse as a prescription drug[8]; it later approved this product as a nonprescription drug. The 1% permethrin cream rinse is the drug of choice for treating head lice in adults and in children 2 years of age and older, and it may also be used to treat pubic lice.[9,10] Permethrin is a synthetic pyrethroid that acts on the nerve cell membrane of the lice, causing delayed repolarization and paralysis.[11] Its pediculicidal and ovicidal activities as well as its residual persistence on the hair eradicate the head lice and prevent reinfestation. There is a cure rate of up to 99% in patients following a single application. Some patients may require a second application 7 days after the initial treatment. A study has shown that the cure rate following its application is higher than that following the application of 1% gamma benzene hexachloride (lindane), a prescription product.

Before permethrin cream rinse is applied, the hair should be shampooed with regular shampoo, rinsed, and dried. Enough of the undiluted liquid (25–30 mL) is then applied to saturate the hair and scalp and allowed to remain there for 10 minutes. Next, the medication is rinsed out with water, and the hair is towel dried. A specially designed comb, which is included in the package, may be used to remove the nits and nits' shells. The main adverse reaction to permethrin is transient pruritus, burning, stinging, and irritation to the scalp. Permethrin should not be used on infants under 2 years of age or on individuals who are sensitive to pyrethroid, pyrethrin, or chrysanthemums.

Pyrethrins are insecticides extracted from *Chrysanthemum cinerariafolium*. They exert their paralyzing effect by disrupting the nervous transmission in the insect. Their most important distinguishing features are low mammalian toxicity, rapid action, and short residual effect. Pyrethrins are effective in concentrations ranging from 0.17–0.33%, but they lose their potency within 12–24 hours owing to their instability in light. Pyrethrins are usually combined with 2–4% piperonyl butoxide, a chemical that has no insecticidal activity but that potentiates the lethal action of the pyrethrins by blocking detoxification of the drug by the insect. A combination of pyrethrins (0.17–0.33%) with piperonyl butoxide (2–4%) in a nonaerosol product formulation has been generally recognized as safe and effective by the FDA in its tentative final monograph for pediculicide drug products for nonprescription human use. These pediculicides are available in gel, liquid, and shampoo formulations. The medication is applied to the infested area and allowed to remain in place for no less than 10 minutes; it is then thoroughly washed out with warm water. Pyrethrins rarely produce any adverse reactions. However, contact with eyes and mucous membranes should be avoided. Because of their safety and effectiveness, they are a popular ingredient in most household insecticide sprays and aerosols. They are also used in dusting powder for the control of fleas, lice, and ticks on pets.

Gamma benzene hexachloride is a chlorinated hydrocarbon. The drug possesses pediculicidal and ovicidal activities and is available on prescription as a 1% shampoo for treating head and pubic lice. However, extreme caution should be exercised in its use because accidental oral ingestion or overdosing may cause central nervous system stimulation and seizures. The shampoo should not be applied to the face, eyelashes, or eyebrows. Because of its neurotoxicity, the shampoo should not be used on a daily basis. When used according to directions, however, a single shampooing poses no health hazard because the level of gamma benzene hexachloride in the blood is very low.

The proper use of the shampoo requires that any oil-based hair dressing be removed before applying the shampoo because oil may enhance absorption of the drug. Enough shampoo (30–60 mL) is applied to the hair along with enough water to form good lather. The lather is allowed to remain for 4 minutes, after which the hair is rinsed thoroughly and towel dried. When the shampoo is used to treat pubic lice, simultaneous treatment of sexual partners is recommended.

Malathion is an organophosphorus compound that acts as a cholinesterase inhibitor. In addition to being an effective pediculicide and ovicide, it slowly bonds to the hair to provide enough residual effect to prevent reinfestation. It is available on prescription in a 0.5% lotion containing 78% isopropyl alcohol. Consequently, caution must be exercised not to apply the medication near open flames or hair dryers. Malathion is recommended for adults and children 2 years of age and older. However, pregnant women and nursing mothers should avoid using the medication. The lotion is applied to the hair until the hair is moistened, and it is allowed to remain in place for 8–12 hours, after which the hair is shampooed, rinsed, and towel dried. A fine-toothed comb may be used to remove dead lice and nits. The main disadvantage of malathion is its unpleasant odor and the long contact time required with the scalp to exert its activity. However, it has a relatively low toxicity to warm-blooded animals and a short systemic residual effect.

Body Lice

Body lice live, hide, and lay their eggs in clothing, particularly in the seams and folds of underclothing, which they periodically leave to invade the host's body to feed. Infestations occur in individuals who do not change clothing frequently, such as homeless people and soldiers in extended military campaigns. These insects are larger than head lice and twice as long; consequently, the female body louse lays more eggs (as many as 300). Diagnosis of body lice can be made by identifying the adult lice and nits in the seams of clothing. Intense body itching and the scratching it triggers should also provide a clue to the presence of the infestation. Treatment of body lice is similar to that of head lice. However, body lice may be eradicated by measures other than medications. Washing clothing with hot water (125°F [52°C]) or disinfecting them with dry cleaning is effective. Changing clothing and underclothing daily as well as bathing daily should then rid the body of these lice. To relieve itching, an antipruritic lotion may be applied.

Pubic Lice

Pubic lice, commonly called crab lice because of their crablike appearance, may be encountered in all persons, even those with high standards of hygiene. An infestation of pubic lice is identified by the presence of the parasite and its nits. The lice are usually found in the pubic area but may infest armpits and occasionally eyelashes, mustaches, beards, and eyebrows. They may be transmitted through sexual contact, toilet seats, or shared undergarments and sheets. A female adult pubic louse deposits 50 eggs during her lifetime. Treatment of pubic lice is similar to that of head lice.

Sarcoptes scabiei

Scabies, commonly called "the itch," is a contagious parasitic skin infestation caused by *Sarcoptes scabiei*, a very small and rarely seen arachnid mite. It burrows beneath the stratum corneum but neither bites nor stings. Characterized by secondary inflammation and intense itching, this infestation is often associated with poor hygiene, crowded conditions, and venereal disease. Scabies is transmitted through bodily contact with an infested host, clothing, or bed linen. An infected person may easily spread the disease to other family members. It is also possible to acquire scabies from a toilet seat. The female mite, which is responsible for causing scabies, is transmitted readily by close personal contact with an infected person. Once on the skin, the impregnated female burrows into the stratum corneum with her jaws and the first two pairs of legs, forming tunnels up to 1 cm long in which she lays eggs and excretes fecal matter. In a few days, the hatched larvae form their own burrows and develop into adults. The adult mites copulate, and the impregnated females burrow into the stratum corneum to start a new life cycle. The most common infestation sites are the interdigital spaces of the fingers, the flexor surface of the wrists, the external male genitalia, the buttocks, and the anterior axillary folds. (See color plates, photograph 31.) The head and neck are not affected, except in infants. When the mite first burrows in the skin, there is no local reaction; within a month, however, sensitization begins. Intense itching occurs, especially at night, at the infestation site. Unrestrained scratching may cause secondary bacterial infections, such as excoriation and impetigo, furuncles, or cellulitis. Scabies diagnosis may be made by identifying the mite under a microscope and the burrow in the skin. The burrow is visible to the naked eye and appears as a narrow, dark line on a raised bump or blister.

Scabies may be controlled by using any of the following prescription drugs: 25% benzyl benzoate lotion, 1% gamma benzene hexachloride cream or lotion, or 10% crotamiton lotion or cream. The nonprescription drug 5% permethrin cream is also effective against scabies. Before applying the medication, the patient should bathe, vigorously scrubbing the infested area. The preparation should then be applied to the entire body except the face and should remain in place for a specified period of time, after which the patient should bathe again. A second application is usually unnecessary but may sometimes be required. Clothing and bedding used by infested individuals should be washed in hot water. Since the incubation period of scabies is delayed, it is recommended that other members of the household undergo treatment.

Ticks and Lyme Disease

Ticks are arachnid parasites that feed on the blood of humans and of both wild and domesticated animals. During feeding, the tick's mouth parts are introduced into the skin, enabling it to hold firmly. If the tick is removed, the mouth parts are torn from the tick and remain embedded, causing intense itching and nodules, which may be surgically excised. (See color plates, photograph 32.) If the tick is left attached to the skin, it becomes fully engorged with blood and remains for as long as 10 days before it drops off. The local reaction to tick bites consists of itching papules, which disappear within 1 week. Ticks should be removed from the skin intact by using fine tweezers. If fingers are used, they should be protected by using gloves and washed afterwards. Fingernail polish or mineral oil may be applied on the tick to facilitate its removal.

Certain species of ticks can transmit systemic disease such as Lyme disease. This disease was first recognized in 1975 when a number of juvenile rheumatoid arthritis cases occurred in Lyme, Conn; it was described and named by Dr Allen Steere in 1977.[12] Five years later, Dr Willy Burgdorf recognized that Lyme disease is a systemic infection that is caused by a spirochete found in the deer tick (*Ixodes dammini*) and is transmitted into the victim following tick bites. The spirochetes, which were named *Borrelia burgdorferi*, appear as irregular coils that range from 10 to 30 microns in length and from 0.18 to 0.25 microns in diameter.

The deer tick lives in wooded areas and parasitizes white-tailed deer (the primary carrier), mice, dogs, squirrels, and other mammals including humans. It is very small compared with the dog tick; it is about one eighth of an inch in diameter and thus is difficult to find when it parasitizes animals. (See Figure 1 for the life cycle of the deer tick.) The tick inserts its mouth piece into its prey to suck blood. During the feeding process, *B burgdorferi* are released at the bite site and spread throughout the body hematogenously to initiate the infection.[13]

Most of the acute stages of the infection are heralded by a skin rash and flulike symptoms. The rash appears first as a papule at the bite site and may become an enlarged circle with a clear center referred to as a "bull's eye" or erythema migrans. The infection then gradually spreads to various parts of the body. The lesions are usually urticarial in nature and tender. They appear 3–30 days after the bite and disappear spontaneously within 3–4 weeks, but when they are treated with antibiotics, remission occurs within several days. The flulike symptoms include fever, headache, fatigue, muscle and joint pain, and, in severe cases, conjunctivitis. If left untreated, neurologic (aseptic meningitis, headache, stiff neck, paresis, paresthesia), cardiac (tachycardia), and musculoskeletal symptoms may develop and may last up to several months. The last and most durable symptoms are arthritis and a red discoloration of the hands, wrists, feet, or ankles.

Lyme disease can be diagnosed by studying the medical history of the patient and conducting laboratory examinations such as enzyme-linked immunosorbent assays, immunoblotting technique, and indirect fluorescent antibody test. Early diagnosis and prompt treatment of Lyme disease can prevent the development of neurologic, cardiac, and rheumatologic manifestations. The disease is treated with antibiotics such as tetracycline, doxycycline, amoxicillin, and cephalosporins.

Lyme disease can be prevented by (1) avoiding areas that may be infested with deer ticks, especially during the spring and summer months; (2) applying insect repellent containing *N,N*-diethyl-*m*-toluamide (DEET) on the skin as well as on shoe tops and socks; (3) applying the pesticide permethrin on clothes; and (4) treating pets regularly with insecticides.

Chiggers

Chiggers or red bugs are very annoying pests. Only the chigger larvae, which are nearly microscopic, attack the host by attaching to the skin and sucking blood. Once in contact with the skin, the larvae insert their mouth parts into the skin and secrete a digestive fluid that causes cellular disintegration of the affected area, a red papule, and intense itching. Chiggers do not burrow in the skin; however, the injected fluid causes the skin to harden and a tiny tube to be formed. The chigger lies in this tube and continues to feed until engorged, after which it drops off and changes into an adult.

Chiggers are prevalent in southern parts of the United States mainly during summer and fall. They usually live in wooded areas, grass, and brush. Chigger infestation may be prevented by avoiding areas infested with the mite, using insect repellent, and wearing protective clothing. Bathing immediately after exposure is helpful. Removing brush, mowing grass, and spraying the area with lawn pest insecticide are also useful. Treatment is symptomatic and consists of the use of antipruritic topical medications.

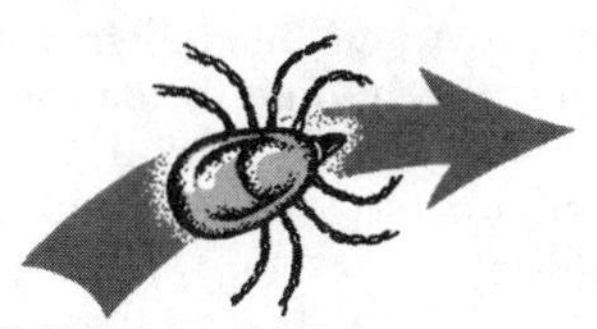
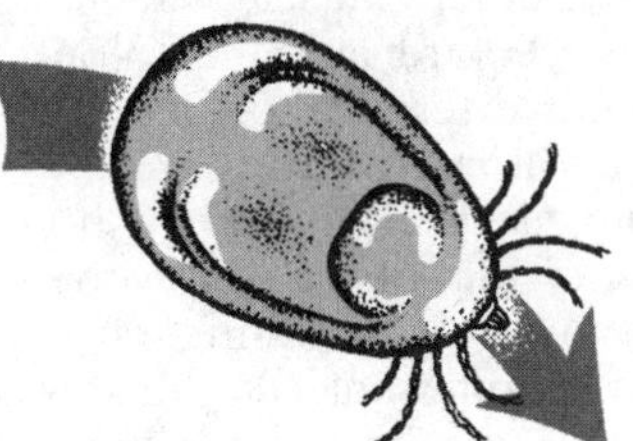

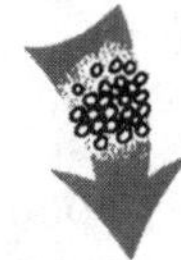
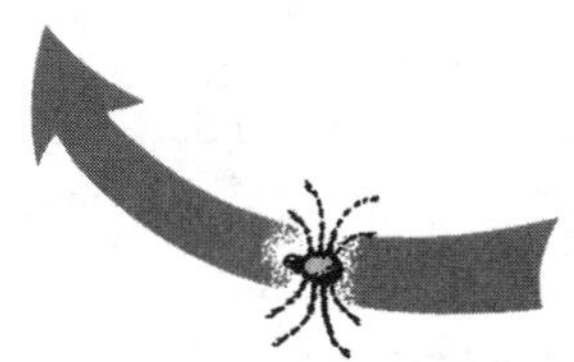
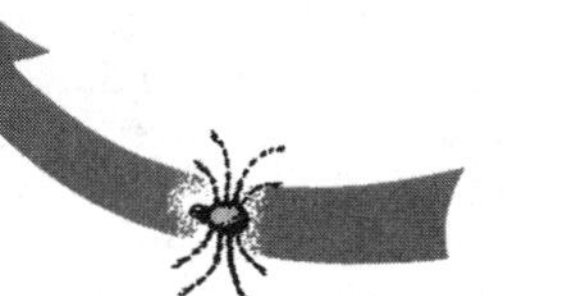

FIGURE 1 Life cycle of the deer tick (*Ixodes dammini*). Reprinted from *Lyme Disease in Wisconsin: An Update*. Madison, Wis: Wisconsin Department of Natural Resources and Department of Health and Social Services; 1989.

Stinging Insects

Stinging insects belonging to the order Hymenoptera (membranous wings) are most often responsible for insect sting hypersensitivity. Among the three families commonly involved are the Apidae, including honeybees (*Apis*) and bumblebees (*Bumbus*); the Vespidae, including paper wasps (*Polistes*), yellow jackets (*Vespula*), and hornets (*Vespa*); and the Formicidae, including imported fire ants (*Solenopsis*) and harvester ants (*Pogonomyrmes*). Although they are small, these insects have a venom as potent as that of snakes. However, whereas death from a snakebite is usually due to toxicity of the venom and occurs within 3 hours to several days, death from an insect sting is usually due not to toxicity of the venom but to allergic hypersensitivity, which could lead to an anaphylactic reaction within 5–30 minutes after the sting. Simultaneous multiple stings of 500 or more may cause death due to toxicity. In the United States, more people die from insect stings than from the bites of other poisonous animals combined.

The stinging insects are nonparasitic and attack only to defend themselves or to kill other insects. They inject the venom into their victims through a piercing organ (stinger), a modified ovipositor delicately attached to the rear of the female's abdomen. (Males do not have an ovipositor and consequently are stingless.) The stinger consists of two lancets made of highly chitinous material and separated by the poison canal. The venom flows through the canal from the venom sac attached to the stinger's dorsal section. The tip of the stinger, which is directed posteriorly, has sharp barbs, and the base enlarges into a bulblike structure. Most species of bees and wasps have two types of venom glands under the last abdominal segment. The larger gland secretes an acidic toxin directly into the venom sac; the smaller one, at the base of the sac, secretes a less potent alkaline toxin. The injected venom is usually a mixture of the two toxins.

When the honeybee stings, it attaches firmly to the skin with tiny, sharp claws at the tip of each foot, arches its abdomen, and immediately jabs the barbed stinger into the skin. The barbs firmly embed the stinger, and when the honeybee pulls away or is brushed off, the entire stinging apparatus (stinger, appendages, venom sac, and glands) is detached from the bee's abdomen. The disemboweled bee later dies. The abandoned stinger, driven deeper into the skin by rhythmic contractions of the venom sac's smooth muscle wall, continues to inject venom. Honeybees are most commonly found in the western and midwestern United States. Wild honeybees usually nest in hollow tree trunks.

The stinging mechanism of wasps, hornets, and yellow jackets resembles that of the honeybee except that the stingers are not barbed. The stingers can be withdrawn easily after the venom is injected, enabling these insects to survive and sting repeatedly. Paper wasps, hornets, and yellow jackets are more commonly found in the southcentral and southwestern United States. Paper wasps tend to nest in high places, under eaves of houses, or on the branches of high trees, whereas hornets prefer to nest in hollow spaces, especially hollow trees. Yellow jackets, considered to be the most common stinging culprits, usually nest in low places such as burrows in the ground, cracks in walls, or small shrubs.

Some ants only bite; others bite and sting simultaneously. Stinging ants (fire ants) (*Solenopsis invicta*) use their mandibles to cling to the skin of their prey; then they bend their abdomen, sting the flesh, and empty the contents of their poison vesicle into the wound. Because they use their mandibles, it is often believed that the bite causes the reaction. Fire ants, which were imported from South America, are now found in the southern and western United States. They live in underground colonies, forming large raised mounds. Fire ants are considered a health hazard. Their sting causes intense itching, burning (hence the name), vesiculation, necrosis, and anaphylactic reaction in hypersensitive persons. It appears that there is very limited or no cross-sensitivity between the venom of fire ants and that of bees, wasps, hornets, and yellow jackets.

Reactions to Insect Bites and Stings

An insect bite or sting is an injury to the skin caused by penetration of the biting or stinging organ of an insect. The reactions are produced mainly by substances contained in the saliva of biting insects or in the venom of stinging insects. Although the pain associated with the skin penetration is brief, the aftereffects vary according to the degree of exposure and hypersensitivity.

Insect Bites

Reactions to biting insects are usually local although the pathogenesis of these reactions has not been well characterized. Some species of mosquitoes have agglutinin and anticoagulant agents in their salivary secretions; others have neither. Many attempts have been made to identify the antigenic factors in mosquito bites by studying whole mosquito extracts. Extracts from *Aedes aegypti* were shown by paper chromatography to contain at least four fractions that can produce skin reactions. Eluates of each constituent caused positive reactions in sensitized individuals.

Reactions to mosquito bites vary in intensity. Wheal formation, erythema, papular reaction, and itching are characteristic. The lesions may have a rapid or slow onset and can be a persistent nuisance for weeks. Hypersensitivity to mosquito bites aggravated by scratching causes papule and nodule formations that may persist and lead to secondary infections such as impetigo, furunculosis, or infectious eczematoid dermatitis. The bite site may influence reaction intensity; bites on the ankles and legs are more severe than bites elsewhere on the body because of the relative circulatory stasis in the legs. Consequently, the tendency toward vesiculation, hemorrhage, eczematization, and ulceration is greater in these areas. Systemic reactions such as fever and malaise also may occur.

Insect Stings

In the past decade, significant progress has been made in understanding the pathogenesis of allergic reactions to the Hymenoptera order of insects. Venoms from these insects have been purified and analyzed. The venoms' mechanisms for causing severe reactions have been investigated, and they are now being used to diagnose and treat allergic reactions to insect stings.

Venom Components

Hymenoptera venom contains a number of allergenic proteins as well as several pharmacologically active molecules. These contents vary among different families within the Hymenoptera order. Therefore, venoms are discussed here in general terms.

The major antigenic proteins are the enzymes hyaluronidase and phospholipase A. Hyaluronidase breaks down hyaluronic acid, which is the binding agent in connective tissue. By altering tissue structure, hyaluronidase acts as a spreading factor, allowing for enhanced penetration of venom substances. Phospholipase A attacks phospholipids in cell membranes. It also contracts smooth muscle, causes hypotension, increases vascular permeability, and destroys mast cells.

Studies have shown that 50–100% of individuals with a history of local or systemic reactions to insect stings will have demonstrable immunoglobulin E (IgE) antibody to venom constituents. The variability among studies in detecting IgE may be owing to differences in laboratory techniques and the lack of positive identification of the insect eliciting the reaction. Studies further show that the presence of venom-specific IgE in the sera of patients with local reactions correlates with the duration of the reaction.

Other venom components include histamine, meletin, apamin, and mast cell degranulating peptide. Of these, only meletin is antigenic, and not all individuals make antibodies against it. Although these mediators do not directly contribute to insect sting anaphylaxis, they do affect the rate at which venom antigens become available to the systemic circulation following a sting. These molecules have direct and indirect effects on mast cell mediator release, vascular permeability, and smooth muscle contractions. Table 1 summarizes the pharmacologic actions of the venom constituents.

Types of Reactions

Reactions to insect stings range from small local reactions limited to the sting site to systemic reactions lead-

TABLE 1 Properties of Hymenoptera venom components

	Histamine	Meletin	Apamin	MCD peptide[a]	Hyaluronidase	Phospholipase A
Pain production	+	+	?	?	0	?
Increased capillary permeability	+	+	+	+	I	+
Smooth muscle contraction	+	+	0	0	0	+
Histamine release	0	+	0	+	0	+
Cellular damage	0	+	?	+	0	+
Antigenic effect	0	+	?	?	+	+

[a] Mast cell degranulating (MCD) peptide.

Key:
+ means indicated reaction occurs.
0 means indicated reaction does not occur.
? means indicated reaction is not demonstrated.
I means indicated reaction occurs indirectly.

ing to death. Several theoretic factors may explain why a local reaction occurs in one instance and a systemic reaction occurs in another. The dose of venom injected at each sting may vary, thereby varying the amount of antigen entering the body. The location of the sting may also be a factor: head and neck stings may cause more laryngeal edema whereas stings on extremities may produce only local reactions. A sting that limits the venom to the intradermal space may present as a local reaction; a sting on a capillary or venule would allow for systemic injection of the venom and may present as a systemic reaction. Reactions may be divided into three categories: local, unusual, and anaphylactic.

Local Reactions Most allergic reactions to insect stings are cutaneous and occur at the sting site. The manifestations are erythema and varying amounts of pain or itching, with symptoms lasting from several hours to several days. Swelling may extend from the sting site and cover an extensive area. Immune mechanisms have been implicated as the cause of the reaction in some patients. However, not all patients studied have shown evidence of immunologically mediated reactions.[14]

Unusual Reactions Occasionally, unusual reactions follow insect stings. Neurologic reactions, renal involvement, serum sickness reactions, encephalopathy, and delayed hypersensitivity skin reactions have been reported. The mechanisms for these reactions have not been clearly elucidated, but immunologic causes have been implicated in some cases.

Anaphylactic Reactions Most allergic reactions from insect stings are cutaneous. Symptoms include erythema, pruritus, urticaria (hives), or angioedema. The most serious sequelae from stings are systemic anaphylactic reactions. These reactions are immunologically mediated, usually occurring within 15 minutes after the sting. In severe cases, hypotension, laryngeal edema, bronchospasm, and respiratory distress may occur, leading to a shocklike state. If these reactions are not treated promptly, death may ensue. Less common anaphylactic reactions may produce nausea, vomiting, or diarrhea.

Anaphylactic reactions are mediated by immunoglobulin E (IgE) antibodies that bind to the specific antigens (allergens) causing the reaction. The insect sting antigens are proteins and glycoproteins contained in insect venom. After an initial exposure to certain antigens, the body responds by making IgE antibodies against the antigens. These antibodies bind to tissue mast cells and blood basophils. Mast cells are primarily located in lung tissue, bronchial smooth muscle, and vascular endothelium. Once these IgE antibodies are bound to the cells, the person is considered sensitized.

When sensitized persons are exposed to antigens to which they are sensitive, under the appropriate circumstances, the IgE on mast cells or basophils will bind the antigens. When this occurs, IgE receptors on the cells are bridged together and the cells release active substances from their granules.[15] Active substances released or immediately generated by degranulation include histamine, serotonin, eosinophil chemotactic factor of anaphylaxis (ECF-A), leukotrienes, and bradykinin.

Histamine is a bioactive amine that increases capillary permeability, contracts bronchial and vascular smooth muscle, and increases nasal and bronchial mucous gland secretion. Serotonin increases vascular permeability in mice, but its role in human anaphylaxis is unknown. Leukotrienes contract smooth muscle. Unlike histamine, which is preformed in the cell granules, leukotrienes are formed after the IgE–antigen interaction occurs and are then released. Antihistamines are ineffective at reversing the effects of leukotrienes, but epinephrine will terminate the muscle contractions they induce. ECF-A is also released by mast cells and causes eosinophils to accumulate in the area of the allergic reaction. Eosinophils can release an enzyme, arylsulfatase B, which inactivates leukotrienes. Bradykinin contracts vascular and bronchial smooth muscle, increases vascular permeability, increases mucus secretion, and stimulates pain fibers.

The severity and type of anaphylactic reaction depends on the location and number of cells degranulating their mediators. Degranulation in specific target organs produces local anaphylaxis. If the reaction is limited to the gastrointestinal tract, diarrhea may occur; if mast cell mediators are released in the nasal mucosa, rhinorrhea may occur; if the mediators are limited to the skin, hives may be the only prominent sign.

Systemic degranulation of mast cells and basophils leads to severe systemic symptoms and is responsible for shock and death occurring after an insect sting. Release of large amounts of mediators can cause a marked increase in capillary permeability, leading to leakage of intravascular fluids and hypotension. This shocklike state can be further compounded by mediator-induced laryngeal edema and bronchoconstriction, resulting in respiratory distress or failure.

Treatment of Systemic Reactions

Because of the wide range of reactions to insect stings and bites, treatment usually depends on the symptoms. For local reactions, a nonprescription product that minimizes scratching by relieving discomfort, itching, and pain may be recommended. Prophylactic products, such as insect repellents, also are available. However, nonprescription drugs are of no value in systemic reactions; such cases need prompt medical attention. Because hypersensitive reactions to insect stings and bites occur rapidly and may be severe, the sooner medical attention is given, the better the chances for recovery.

Systemic reactions caused by insect stings and bites are considered medical emergencies for which aqueous epinephrine (1:1,000; 0.3–0.5 mL) should be injected immediately, either subcutaneously or intramuscularly; it may also be injected directly into the sting site to delay absorption of the venom. Sublingual isoproterenol should not be administered simultaneously because it may induce serious arrhythmia. Parenteral antihistamines may be used for persistent urticaria, angioedema, or laryngeal edema in patients who do not respond to epinephrine. Pressor agents may be used if shock persists. Parenteral corticosteroids administered through the systemic route may be used for patients with protracted anaphylaxis and delayed reactions. Respiratory support should be available if needed; in severe cases, a tracheotomy may be necessary.

The pharmacist should advise hypersensitive individuals of the following:

- If symptomatic, the victim must seek medical attention immediately after an insect sting or bite.
- Basic first aid, such as applying ice to the sting and removing the stinger, is generally helpful.
- Emergency kits for insect stings are available by prescription. Kits containing epinephrine are preferable to those containing antihistamines for treating allergic reactions to stings.
- Receiving injections of venom extract for protection against systemic reactions (desensitization) is useful.
- Insect repellents are not effective against stinging insects.

First Aid

Basic first aid is helpful until medical help is available. Prompt application of ice packs to the sting site helps to slow absorption and reduce itching, swelling, and pain. Removal of the honeybee's stinger and venom sac, which usually are left in the skin, is another measure that should be explained, particularly to allergic individuals. The stinger should be removed before all venom is injected; it takes approximately 2–3 minutes to empty all the contents from the honeybee's venom sac. The sac should not be squeezed; rubbing, scratching, or grasping it releases more venom. Scraping the stinger with tweezers or a fingernail minimizes the venom flow. After the stinger is removed, an antiseptic should be applied.

Emergency Kits

Emergency kits for individuals hypersensitive to insect stings are available by prescription. In addition to tweezers for removing the honeybee stinger, the typical kit includes epinephrine hydrochloride and antihistamines. Kits containing autoinjectable epinephrine syringes are also available.

The pharmacist should carefully explain the directions for and the benefits of using an emergency kit for insect stings, emphasizing that epinephrine is the drug of choice for anaphylactic reactions. The pharmacist should further instruct the patient that such kits no longer require refrigeration but must be stored in the dark at room temperature. A kit should not be left in the glove compartment of a car where heat becomes excessive in cars parked in the sun.

Epinephrine Hydrochloride

Because of its potent and rapid action, epinephrine hydrochloride (1:1,000) injection is preferred to counteract the bronchoconstriction associated with anaphylaxis. It should be administered subcutaneously immediately after stinging. Some insect sting emergency kits have a preloaded (0.3-mL) sterile syringe. Generally, a 0.25-mL dose is injected subcutaneously and, after 15 minutes, another dose is injected if necessary. For individuals with cardiovascular disease, diabetes, hypertension, or hyperthyroidism, the injection should be administered with caution.

Antihistamines

Although they are slow in onset of action and may be ineffective in severe reactions, antihistamines often are used in conjunction with epinephrine hydrochloride. They are administered orally or parenterally.

Preventive Measures

Avoidance of Exposure

Individuals who are hypersensitive to insect stings should take precautions to avoid exposure to these insects. Foods and odors tend to attract insects; therefore, outdoor activities such as picnicking should be engaged in cautiously. Keeping garbage contained and food covered will help keep insects away. Shoes should always be worn in grass and fields. In addition, perfumes and brightly colored clothes attract stinging insects and should not be worn outdoors. Destroying hives of stinging insects located in the vicinity of homes is recommended; aerosol insecticides are designed for this purpose. A common sense approach will lower the risk of stings and subsequent adverse reactions.

Venom Immunotherapy

Hymenoptera venom is used prophylactically to treat patients who have had reactions to stings. Venom immunotherapy, also known as desensitization, is done by subcutaneous injection of small amounts of venom at regularly scheduled intervals. The dose of the venom is gradually increased over many weeks until a predetermined maintenance dose is reached. The optimal doses, frequency of injections, and duration of maintenance therapy are still being investigated. Hymenoptera venom preparations should be used only by physicians experienced in administering allergens to the maximum tolerated dose and/or after allergy consultation.[16] Patients should be advised that if they stop the immunotherapy, they may again be at high risk for anaphylaxis following a sting.

Nonprescription Pharmacologic Agents

Most nonprescription products used for symptomatic relief of insect stings and bites contain one or more pharmacologic agents, which fall into one of three main categories: external analgesics/antipruritics, skin protectants, and antibacterials (see product table "Insect Sting and Bite Products"). Another category of nonprescription products, insect repellents, work in a preventive capacity.

External Analgesics/Antipruritics

This category is subdivided further into three groups: agents with analgesic activity derived from (1) the stimulation of cutaneous sensory receptors (counterirritants), (2) the depression of cutaneous sensory receptors (anesthetics and antihistamines), and (3) the reduction of inflammation (hydrocortisone). These agents are considered safe and effective when used as recommended for adults and children over 2 years of age. They are not recommended for children under 2 years of age except under the advice or supervision of a physician. (See Chapter 5, "External Analgesic Products.")

Counterirritants

Counterirritants reduce pain and itching by stimulating cutaneous sensory receptors to provide a feeling of warmth, coolness, or milder pain, which obscures the more severe pain of the injury. The activity of these agents depends on the concentration. In low concentrations, they may depress the cutaneous receptors and result in an anesthetic effect.

Camphor At concentrations of 0.1–3%, camphor depresses cutaneous receptors, thereby relieving itching and irritation. At higher concentrations of 3–11%, camphor stimulates cutaneous receptors and therefore acts as a counterirritant. Camphor is safe and effective for use as an external analgesic at these concentrations when applied to the affected area no more than three or four times a day. However, camphor-containing products can be very dangerous if ingested. Patients should be warned to keep these (and all drugs) out of the reach of children and to contact a physician or poison control center immediately if ingestion is suspected.

Cresol Camphor complex (camphorated metacresol) is used to reduce pain. However, the drug is not classified by the FDA as effective in treating insect bites and stings.

Ichthammol Ichthammol has bacteriostatic and counterirritant properties. However, its effectiveness for insect stings is difficult to assess in concentrations used in nonprescription products.

Menthol In concentrations of more than 1.25%, menthol acts as a counterirritant and excites cutaneous sensory receptors. However, in concentrations of less than 1%, it depresses cutaneous receptors and exerts an analgesic effect. Menthol is considered a safe and effective antipruritic when applied to the affected area in concentrations of 0.1–1%.

Methyl Salicylate Methyl salicylate stimulates cutaneous receptors when used in concentrations of 10–60%.

Peppermint and Clove Oils When applied externally, peppermint and clove oils act as mild counterirritants, causing a sensation of warmth.

Local Anesthetics

The FDA Advisory Review Panel on Over-the-Counter External Analgesic Drug Products concluded that benzocaine and dibucaine, the local anesthetics used in insect sting and bite products, are safe and effective when used according to label directions. Dermatitis has reportedly resulted from topically applied local anesthetics, including benzocaine. Although adverse reactions from topical applications are often blamed on allergy to the local anesthetics, allergy is an infrequent cause of reaction. Any dermatitis that may occur is caused by frequent contact, and patients should be warned against continued applications for prolonged periods.

Benzocaine Benzocaine was found to be safe and effective for use by adults and children over 2 years of age when applied to the affected area no more than three or four times a day. The concentrations of benzocaine available in nonprescription products range from 5 to 20%.

Cyclomethycaine Sulfate The FDA panel on external analgesic products concluded that cyclomethycaine sulfate is safe but that available data are insufficient to permit final classification of its effectiveness for use as a nonprescription external analgesic.

Dibucaine Dibucaine is another local anesthetic found in insect sting and bite products. Although in the same class as benzocaine, dibucaine products carry specific additional labeling: "**WARNING** Do not use in large quantities, particularly over raw surfaces or blistered areas." This is because convulsions, myocardial depression, and death have been reported from systemic absorption. The recommended dosage for adults and children over 2 years of age is a 0.25–1% solution applied to the affected area no more than three or four times a day.

Phenol Phenol exerts topical anesthetic action by depressing cutaneous sensory receptors. It is caustic when applied in undiluted form to the skin. Phenol aqueous solutions of greater than 2% are irritating and may cause sloughing and necrosis. Phenol is considered safe and effective as a nonprescription external analgesic when applied to the affected area no more than three or four times a day in concentrations of 0.5–1.5% for adults and children 2 years of age and older. Nonprescription products that contain phenol should include the following specific warning: "Do not apply this product to extensive areas of the body or under compresses or bandages."

Ammonium Hydroxide and Trimethanolamine Ammonium hydroxide and trimethanolamine have been claimed to have a neutralizing effect on insect bites and stings. The FDA now regards ammonium hydroxide as Category I.

Antihistamines

Topical antihistamines, which are considered safe and effective external analgesics, relieve pain and itching by depressing cutaneous sensory receptors. Although some absorption occurs through the skin, these ingredients are not absorbed in sufficient quantities to cause systemic side effects even when applied to damaged skin. However, antihistamines are capable of acting as haptenes, producing hypersensitivity reactions.

Continued use of any of these agents over 3–4 weeks increases the possibility of allergic contact dermatitis. In addition, their continued antipruritic action over a period of time is questionable. With this in mind, the FDA panel on external analgesic products recommended that these agents be used for no longer than 7 days except under the advice of a physician. These agents are not recommended for children under 2 years of age.

Both local anesthetics and antihistamines carry the following labeling as recommended by the FDA panel: For temporary relief of pain and itching due to minor burns, sunburn, minor cuts, abrasions, insect bites, and minor skin irritations.

Diphenhydramine Products containing diphenhydramine are Category I in concentrations of 1–2% and may be applied three or four times a day.

Tripelennamine Tripelennamine in concentrations of 0.5–2% may be applied three or four times a day.

Hydrocortisone

Hydrocortisone is an anti-inflammatory agent that is capable of preventing or suppressing the development of edema, capillary dilation, swelling, and tenderness accompanying inflammation. It relieves pain and itching by reducing inflammation. Preparations containing hydrocortisone in concentrations of up to 1% have been approved by the FDA and are considered relatively safe and effective for use as nonprescription products. These preparations should be applied three or four times a day for adults and children 2 years of age and older. Patients should be warned against using topically applied hydrocortisone if they have conditions such as scabies, tinea, bacterial infections, and moniliasis. Not only may the underlying conditions be worsened, but hydrocortisone may also mask these disorders, making accurate diagnosis difficult. Products containing hydrocortisone or its acetate salts carry specific labeling as follows:

> For the temporary relief of minor skin irritations, itching, and rashes due to eczema, dermatitis, insect bites, poison ivy, poison oak, poison sumac, soaps, detergent, cosmetics, and jewelry, and for itchy genital and anal areas.

Aspirin

The topical use of aspirin for insect stings has been reported to be effective in reducing the wheal reaction and its subsequent itching and irritation. The FDA panel on external analgesic products concluded that aspirin is safe, but available data are insufficient to permit final classification of its effectiveness for use as a nonprescription external analgesic. Aspirin possesses no direct topical anesthetic activity; therefore, it exerts no anesthetic and analgesic effect on the sting site.

Skin Protectants

Aluminum Acetate

Aluminum acetate solutions in concentrations of 2.5–5% are condsidered safe and effective for use as external astringents.

Glycerin

The FDA Advisory Review Panel on Over-the-Counter Skin Protectant Drug Products concluded that glycerin is safe and effective for nonprescription use as a skin protectant because of its absorbent, demulcent, and emollient properties. In addition, glycerin is widely used for its solvent properties.

Hamamelis Water

Hamamelis water (witch hazel) possesses astringent properties and may act as a hemostatic for small superficial wounds.

Titanium Dioxide

Titanium dioxide has an action similar to that of zinc oxide (see the following section). However, the FDA has not addressed the safety and effectiveness of this ingredient in insect bite and sting products.

Zinc Oxide and Calamine

Zinc oxide and calamine are used in lotions, ointments, creams, and sprays for their cooling, slightly astringent, antiseptic, antibacterial, and protective actions. Calamine is a mixture of zinc and ferrous oxide. The ferrous oxide acts only as a coloring agent and is not an active ingredient. Zinc oxide and calamine tend to absorb fluids from weeping rashes. The FDA panel on skin protectant products concluded that zinc oxide and calamine are safe and effective in the nonprescription concentration range of 1–25% for use as skin protectants. The preparation, which is recommended for adults, children, and infants, should be applied topically to the affected areas as needed.

Antibacterials

The most commonly used antibacterial agents in nonprescription products for insect stings and bites are benzalkonium chloride, benzethonium chloride, and methylbenzethonium chloride. These quaternary ammonium compounds, which are included to prevent and treat secondary infection that may result from scratching, are classified as safe and effective for first-aid use.

Chlorothymol

Chlorothymol acts as an antibacterial and antifungal agent. However, it is irritating to mucous membranes.

Chloroxylenol

Chloroxylenol is a bacteriostatic agent that primarily acts against gram-positive bacteria. The FDA Advisory Review Panel on Over-the-Counter Antimicrobial Drug Products could not evaluate the safety and effectiveness of chloroxylenol in topical preparations because of insufficient data.

Cresol

Cresol, which has antibacterial action similar to that of phenol, is often used as a preservative.

8-Hydroxyquinoline Sulfate

The 8-hydroxyquinoline sulfate chemical is included in topical preparations for its antibacterial effect.

Salicylic Acid

At concentrations ranging from 2 to 20%, salicylic acid acts as a keratolytic. In addition, it exerts a slight antiseptic action.

Insect Repellents

Insect repellents do not kill insects. Most repellents are volatile, however, and when they are applied to skin or clothing, their vapor tends to discourage the approach of insects and prevent them from alighting. Thus, repellents protect the skin against insect bites (see product table "Insect Repellent Products").

An insect repellent should have an inoffensive odor, protect for several hours, be effective against as wide a variety of insects as possible, be relatively safe, withstand all weather conditions, and have an aesthetic feel and appearance. Oils of citronella, turpentine, pennyroyal, cedarwood, eucalyptus, and wintergreen were previously used in insect repellent formulations. However, after World War II, investigations showed that these agents were relatively ineffective. Although more than 15,000 compounds have been tested, only a few have been found to be effective and safe enough to use on the skin.

The best all-purpose repellent is *N,N*-diethyl-*m*-toluamide, commonly called DEET. Use of products containing DEET is discouraged in children under 2 years of age because of possible toxicity to the central nervous system. Ethohexadiol dimethyl phthalate, dimethyl ethyl hexanediol carbate, and butopyronoxyl are effective repellents, but they are not as effective against as many kinds of insects as DEET. However, a mixture of two or more of these repellents is more effective against a greater variety of insects than is a single repellent. Local reactions to the application of insect repellents have been reported.[17–19]

Repellents may be toxic if taken internally. People who are sensitive to these chemicals may develop skin reactions such as itching, burning, and swelling. Repellents cause smarting when they are applied to broken skin or mucous membranes. They should be applied carefully around the eyes because they may cause a burning sensation. Even though permethrin is a pesticide, it may be used as a clothing spray for protection against mosquitoes and ticks.[20]

The FDA's final rule on insect repellents for nonprescription oral use in humans indicates that these products are not generally recognized as safe and effective and are misbranded.[21] Thiamine hydrochloride (vitamin B_1) has been marketed as an ingredient in nonprescription drug products for oral use as an insect repellent. Oral sulfur tablets have also been suggested. However, there are no data to establish the effectiveness of these or any other ingredients for nonprescription oral use as systemic insect repellents. Labeling claims for such products—for example, "oral mosquito repellent," "mosquitoes avoid you," "bugs stay away," "keep mosquitoes away for 12–24 hours," and "the newest way to fight mosquitoes"—are either false, misleading, or unsupported by scientific data.

Product Selection Guidelines

Medication is often requested after symptoms appear; thus, it is important to determine what symptoms appeared following the sting or bite, how soon the symptoms appeared, how severe the symptoms are, and what other drugs are being used concurrently.

Nonprescription products are of minimal value to hypersensitive individuals. The pharmacist should record all information on such individuals and recommend that the person wear a tag or carry a card showing the nature of the allergy. If the symptoms, such as localized irritation, itching, or swelling, are minor, an appropriate nonprescription product may be recommended. Topical lotions, creams, ointments, and sprays are the main nonprescription product forms used for symptomatic relief of local reactions to insect stings and bites. The main considerations in product selection are reducing the possibility of additional stings or bites, providing proper protection to the affected skin, preventing secondary infection in the affected area, and relieving itching and irritation. The pharmacist may also advise patients of several nonpharmacologic measures to relieve itching and irritation:

- Avoid wearing rough and irritating clothing, especially wool, over the affected area;
- Avoid using strong soaps, highly perfumed soaps, or harsh detergents;
- Apply an occlusive skin protectant to the affected area after bathing;
- Bathe in cool (never warm) water for 10–20 minutes;
- Avoid scratching the affected area; also, keep fingernails trimmed short and filed smooth to minimize possible damage to the affected skin if scratching occurs, especially in the case of children.

Although they are capable of producing topical or systemic adverse reactions, external analgesics and antipruritics are considered to be relatively safe and effective. These nonprescription products are for adults and children 2 years of age and older and should be applied no more than three or four times a day. For children under 2 years of age, there is no recommended usage except under the advice and supervision of a physician.

The labels on external analgesic nonprescription products should indicate the ingredients and their concentrations, the manner of usage and frequency of applications, and the indications for use. The FDA panel on external analgesic products recommended that the labels should also include the following warnings:

- For external use only.
- Avoid contact with eyes.
- If condition worsens or if symptoms persist for more than 7 days, discontinue use of this product and consult a physician.
- Do not use for children under 2 years of age except under the advice and supervision of a physician.

Case Studies

Case 33–1

Patient Complaint/History

RH, a 32-year-old male, was stung by hornets on the arms and back of the neck while trimming shrubs in his front yard. He rushed into the house, where suddenly feeling faint, he quickly sat down in a nearby chair. His wife applied an ice compress to the sting sites, each of which presented as a white ring about one-half inch in diameter with a red spot in the center. Within minutes of the incident he experienced more severe symptoms, including his eyes swelling shut, profuse sweating, difficulty in breathing, and nausea but no vomiting. His ears also turned blue and his arms hung limply by his sides; however, he never lost consciousness.

After being rushed to the hospital emergency room, he was given repeated intramuscular injections of 0.2 mg of adrenaline hydrochloride (1:1,000) and 50 mg of diphenhydramine hydrochloride; he also received 15 mg of prednisone by mouth. Although his symptoms subsided within a few hours, he was hospitalized and released the following morning.

During a conversation with the pharmacist a few days later, RH revealed that he had been stung by hornets and bees on several prior occasions and had suffered only local reactions. His last bee sting had resulted in some shortness of breath, abdominal cramps, and dizziness; these symptoms, however, subsided within 1 hour.

Clinical Considerations/Strategies

The following considerations/strategies are provided to aid the reader in (1) determining whether treatment of the patient's condition with nonprescription medications is warranted, (2) selecting the appropriate nonprescription medication, and (3) developing a patient counseling strategy to ensure optimal therapeutic outcomes:

- Assess the patient's understanding of his progressively severe hypersensitivity reactions to hornet stings as well as the potential consequences of subsequent stings.
- Advise the patient of how a particular foreign protein present in hornet's venom affects the body when it enters the circulatory system.
- Explain the limitations of nonprescription products in treating his degree of hypersensitivity and the need to minimize the risk of hornet stings.
- Explain the importance of always having immediate access to an epinephrine-containing injection (eg, EpiPen Auto-Injector, which contains a 0.3-mg IM dose of 1:1,000 epinephrine in a 2.0-mL disposable prefilled injector).
- Explain the importance of informing family, friends, and coworkers of the severity of the hypersensitivity and the need for immediate medical intervention if the patient suffers a hornet sting.

Case 33–2

Patient Complaint/History

JB, a 17-year-old female, was stung on the feet repeatedly by several fire ants a few hours earlier. She comes to the pharmacy counter and requests advice on relieving the symptoms of a local reaction to the stings. The symptoms, which are limited to the sting sites, include intense itching, inflammation, and mild swelling. JB reveals that her parents recommended applying a cosmetic lotion to the sting sites; however, the lotion offered little symptomatic relief.

Clinical Considerations/Strategies

The following considerations/strategies are provided to aid the reader in (1) determining whether treatment of the patient's condition with nonprescription medications is warranted, (2) selecting the appropriate nonprescription medication, and (3) developing a patient counseling strategy to ensure optimal therapeutic outcomes:

- Advise the patient of proper hygiene of the wound site.
- Consider topical versus systemic therapy to manage the symptoms.
- Evaluate the clinical appropriateness of using the following topical ingredients to treat this reaction: astringents, antibiotics, local anesthetics, steroids, and antihistamines.
- Evaluate the clinical appropriateness of the following oral agents: ibuprofen, antihistamines, prednisone, and amoxicillin.
- Recommend one or more topical products to manage the immediate symptoms.
- Recommend techniques and procedures for proper application of the topical products.

Summary

Stings of honeybees, bumblebees, yellow jackets, hornets, wasps, and ants cause pain, discomfort, illness, and severe local and systemic reactions. In normal individuals, insect stings and bites cause local irritation, inflammation, swelling, and itching that provoke rubbing and scratching. In hypersensitive individuals, anaphylactic reactions may pose serious emergency problems.

People sensitized to insect venom may react violently when stung. They need immediate, active treatment such as the administration of epinephrine hydrochloride. Partial desensitization may be accomplished by insect venom immunotherapy. The pharmacist can play a significant role by advising hypersensitive individuals on emergency procedures for insect stings. The pharmacist should also advise and educate patients in the treatment and prevention of lice infestation, tick-induced diseases, and other insect bites.

A wide variety of nonprescription products is available to treat stings and bites. These products include external analgesics and antipruritics (eg, antihistamines, local anesthetics, counterirritants, hydrocortisone, and aspirin), skin protectants, and antibacterials.

References

1. Wyngaarden JB, Smith LH, eds. *Cecil Textbook of Medicine.* 16th ed. Philadelphia: WB Saunders; 1982: 1805.
2. Fusia AF et al. *Curr Ther Res.* 1987; 41: 881.
3. Sause RB, Galizia VJ. *Pharm Times.* 1989 Sep; 132.
4. Robinson DH, Shephard DA. *Curr Ther Res.* 1980; 27: 1.
5. Zack R. *RN.* 1987 Sep; 30.
6. Rasmussen J. *NARD J.* 1987 Sep; 32.
7. Covington TR. *Facts and Comparisons Drug Newsletter.* 1990; 9: 65.
8. Hussar DA. *Am Pharm.* 1987; 27: 26.
9. Abramowicz M, ed. *Med Lett Drugs Ther.* 1990; 32: 23.
10. Abramowicz M, ed. *Med Lett Drugs Ther.* 1990; 32: 21.
11. Phipps MV. *Am Pharm.* 1991; 31: 53.
12. Steere AC. *N Engl J Med.* 1989; 321: 9, 586.
13. Carlstedt BC, Johnson RC, Kreter B. *US Pharm.* 1990 Apr; 33.
14. Green AW et al. *J Allergy Clin Immunol.* 1980; 66: 186.
15. Ishizaka T. *J Allergy Clin Immunol.* 1981; 67: 90.
16. *FDA Drug Bull.* 1979; 9: 3, 15.
17. Roland EH, Jan JE, Rigg JM. *Can Med Assoc J.* 1985; 132: 155.
18. Reuvini H, Yagupsky P. *Arch Dermatol.* 1982; 118: 582.
19. Edwards DL, Johnson CE. *Clin Pharm.* 1987; 6: 496.
20. Abramowicz M, ed. *Med Lett Drug Ther.* 1989; 31: 45.
21. *Federal Register.* 1985; 50: 25170.

CHAPTER 34

Foot Care Products

Nicholas G. Popovich and Gail D. Newton

Questions to ask in patient assessment and counseling

General Foot Conditions

- *Where is the sore located (on or between the toes or on the sole of the foot)? Is the toenail involved?*
- *Is there any redness, itching, blistering, oozing, scaling, or bleeding from the lesion?*
- *Is the condition painful? Is it too uncomfortable to walk? Do your feet hurt or ache at the end of the day?*
- *During which activities is the pain noticed?*
- *How long have you had the problem? Did it occur gradually?*
- *Did the problem begin with the use of new shoes (sandals or enclosed shoes, jogging or tennis shoes, flat or high heels), socks, or soaps? Do your new shoes seem tighter than they have been in the past or tight at the end of the day?*
- *Can you associate the symptom with a particular type/pair of shoe(s)?*
- *Have attempts at self-treatment with nonprescription inserts failed?*
- *Do your feet sweat a lot? Do you notice an odor when you take off your shoes? Do your feet sweat more when you wear socks or hosiery made of nylon or other synthetic material?*
- *Do you have allergies, asthma, or skin problems?*
- *What is your occupation?*
- *Have you significantly increased repetitive weight-bearing activity? Do you plan to continue this activity?*
- *Do you have a history of a fracture, dislocation, or surgery in the legs or feet?*
- *Did you wear corrective shoes or braces on the legs or feet as a child?*
- *Did you ever injure your foot? If yes, do the current symptoms seem to be related to the prior injury?*
- *How often and in what manner do you trim your toenails?*
- *Have you tried to treat this problem yourself? If so, how?*
- *Did you see your physician about this problem? If so, what did he or she tell you to do? What have you done? Did it help?*
- *Is a physician treating you for any other medical condition, such as diabetes, heart trouble, or circulatory problems?*
- *Do you take insulin? What (other) prescription or nonprescription medications do you take on a routine basis?*
- *Have you ever had vascular surgery or been treated for circulatory problems?*
- *Do you have a family member or other caregiver to assist you with the recommended treatment(s)?*
- *Do you participate in a daily or regular exercise program such as jogging or aerobics?*

Foot Conditions Related to Running/Jogging

- *Is the discomfort getting progressively worse?*
- *Has the discomfort plateaued at a level that continues to affect your running/jogging performance?*
- *Is the discomfort more frequent and severe while running? Is it present while not running?*
- *Is the discomfort causing you to compensate and develop additional injuries?*
- *Have attempts at self-treatment (eg, new shoes, a change of running surface, or a change in training intensity) failed to relieve the symptoms?*

Annual foot care product sales now exceed $300 million. Historically, however, Americans have seemed to use more than just these products to relieve foot problems. For example, in 1988, a Gallup survey of family/general practitioners, dermatologists, and podiatrists identified the foot problems most often encountered and the ways in which patients dealt with them.[1] The four most common foot complaints were corns, calluses, and plantar warts; athlete's foot; sore, aching feet; and ingrown toenails. The survey identified harmful foot practices, such as scraping or cutting corns and calluses, opening blisters or removing the skin cover, improperly trim-

Editor's Note: This chapter is based, in part, on the chapter with the same title that appeared in the 10th edition but was written by Nicholas G. Popovich.

TABLE 1 Mycotic infections

Type	Site(s) of invasion	Example
Superficial	Outermost layer of skin and appendages	Tinea versicolor (caused by *Malassezia furfur*)
Cutaneous	Skin lesion and/or nail	Tinea pedis (caused by *Trichophyton rubrum*)
Subcutaneous	Cutaneous and subcutaneous tissue	Sporotrichosis (caused by *Sporotrichum schenckii*)
Intermediate	Skin, mucous membranes, internal viscera	Vaginal candidiasis (caused by *Candida albicans*)
Deep systemic	Viscera, bone, nerve, skin	Blastomycosis (caused by *Blastomyces dermatitidis*)

Reprinted with permission from Raskin J. In: Conn HF, ed. *Current Therapy*. Philadelphia: WB Saunders; 1976; 611–4.

ming toenails, and (among diabetes patients) inappropriately using hot water to clean and bathe the feet. The survey also identified potentially harmful home remedies for foot problems, including the application of caulk plaster, WD 40 lubricant, Crisco or butter, Clorox or other bleach products, and gasoline or kerosene. Obviously, there is a significant need to educate patients about proper foot care, including self-treatment measures. The pharmacist can serve as a valuable resource in this regard.

Instruction in proper foot care should begin at an early age when good health habits can be nurtured. At birth, an infant's foot has 35 joints, 19 muscles, more than 100 ligaments, and cartilage that will develop into 26 bones. These small components continue to develop and mature until the age of 14–16 for females and 15–21 for males. Women will generally begin to notice changes in their feet in their 30s; men, in their 40s. After years of bearing the body's weight, the feet tend to broaden and flatten, thus stretching ligaments and causing bones to shift positions. These changes subject the feet to stress, which is compounded by prolonged standing: an estimated 40% of the US population spend about 75% of their workday on their feet. Such stresses increase the potential for painful foot conditions. Thus, the simplest rule of foot care is daily inspection of the feet to note any overt signs of early problems.

There are three distinct groups of patients who often encounter foot problems. First are pediatric patients whose difficulty is a congenital malformation or deformity, or a specific disease that affects the foot (eg, juvenile arthritis). These patients need special shoes and foot care provided with the oversight of an orthopedic surgeon or podiatrist. The second group comprises adolescents who experience rapid growth. Growth plates in their feet may become stressed and irritated. Athletic activity at this age can also contribute to problems, especially if there are associated injuries to the feet that are not properly treated. Osteoarthritis, for example, can occur secondary to a foot injury. Third are geriatric patients, who encounter foot problems due to aging (as the foot assumes its final shape) and disease. In particular, diabetes mellitus and arthritis can cause secondary foot problems.

Prevention of foot problems begins with the purchase of comfortable, well-fitted shoes of proper width and length (ie, the toes should not bump into the front of the shoe or be cramped in the toe box). The heel support in the shoe should fit snugly and help hold the foot straight. Depending on the person's activity level, the midsole should provide adequate cushioning and support. Because shoes are mass-produced, a person should try both shoes on at the time of purchase, preferably wearing a pair of socks or stockings of the type that will be worn normally with the new pair of shoes. If people are prone to edema, shoe selection should occur at the end of the day.

Geriatric persons should be advised to wear shoes that are comfortable and provide support, even around the home. A real danger for such patients around the home occurs with slippers. Although slippers are comfortable and easy to get on and off, they tend to get caught on carpeting, throw rugs, or stairs. Consequently, the elderly person may slip or fall, risking serious injury (eg, broken hip or other bone fracture).

In the past two decades, society's attitude toward physical fitness and body awareness has changed dramatically. Millions of people exercise every day; jogging, running, and aerobic exercising are methods used most often to remain or get "in shape." If people do not take adequate precautions, however, problems can arise, particularly involving the feet. Appropriate footwear is one of several factors that should be addressed by joggers and runners to prevent foot problems.

Although foot conditions are generally not life-threatening, except perhaps to persons with diabetes, severely arthritic patients, and those with impaired circulation, such problems may cause a substantial measure of discomfort and impaired mobility and may even indicate a serious disease condition. Corns, calluses, and ingrown toenails are common problems that may contribute to impairment. Hardening of the skin may signal a biomechanical problem and cause abnormal weight distribution in a particular area of the foot; in this case, a podiatric examination is warranted to determine whether an imbalance is present. Human mycotic (fungal) infections may be subdivided into five categories based on the site of invasion (Table 1).[2] The superficial and cutaneous types, such as athlete's foot, usually warrant the pharmacist's advice.

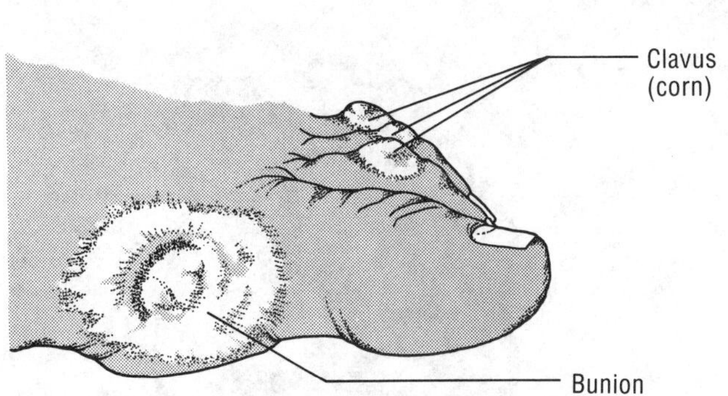

FIGURE 1 Conditions affecting the top of the foot.

Corns, Calluses, and Warts

Corns and Calluses

Corns and calluses are similar in one respect: each produces a marked hyperkeratosis of the stratum corneum. Besides this feature, however, there are marked differences.

A corn (clavus) is a small, raised, sharply demarcated, hyperkeratotic lesion having a central core (Figure 1). It has a yellowish-gray color and ranges from a few millimeters to 1 cm or more in diameter. The base of the corn is on the skin surface; the apex of the corn points inward and presses on the nerve endings in the dermis, causing pain.

Corns may be either hard or soft. Hard corns occur on the surface of the toes and appear shiny and polished. Soft corns are whitish thickenings of the skin, usually found on the webs between the fourth and fifth toes. Accumulated perspiration macerates the epidermis and gives the corn a soft appearance. Soft corns occur because the fifth metatarsal is much shorter than the fourth, and the web between these toes is deeper and extends more proximally than the webs between the other toes.

Hard corns (usually) and soft corns (less frequently) are caused by underlying bony prominences. A bony spur, or exostosis (a bony tumor in the form of an ossified muscular attachment to the bone surface), nearly always exists between long-lasting hard and soft corns. A lesion located over non–weight-bearing bony prominences or joints—such as metatarsal heads, the bulb of the great toe, the dorsum of the fifth toe, or the tips of the middle toes—is usually a corn.[3]

A callus may be broad based or have a central core with sharply circumscribed margins and diffuse thickening of the skin (Figure 1). It has indefinite borders and ranges from a few millimeters to several centimeters in diameter. It is usually raised and yellow, and it has a normal pattern of skin ridges on its surface. Calluses form on joints and weight-bearing areas, such as the palms of the hands and the sides and soles of the feet. (See color plates, photograph 33.)

Pathophysiology

Under normal conditions, the cells in the basal cell layer undergo mitotic division at a rate that is equal to that of the continual surface cellular desquamation. Normal mitotic activity and subsequent desquamation lead to the complete replacement of the epidermis in about 1 month. During corn or callus development, however, friction and pressure increase mitotic activity of the basal cell layer,[4] leading to the migration of maturing cells through the prickle cell (stratum spinosum) and granular (stratum granulosum) skin layers. This produces a thicker stratum corneum as more cells reach the outer skin surface. When the friction or pressure is relieved, mitotic activity returns to normal, causing remission and disappearance of the lesion.

Symptoms

Pressure from tight-fitting shoes is the most frequent cause of pain from corns. As narrow-toed or high-heeled shoes crowd toes into the narrow toe box, the most lateral toe, the fifth, sustains the most pressure and friction and is the usual site of a corn. The resultant pain may be severe and sharp (when downward pressure is applied) or dull and discomforting. Consumer research approximates that about 82% of women aged 35–54 suffer moderate to intense pain from corns and that 35% are consequently limited or restricted in their activities.

Friction (caused by loose-fitting shoes or tight-fitting hosiery), walking barefoot, and structural biomechanical problems contribute to the development of calluses. Structural problems include improper weight distribution, pressure, and the development of bunions with age. Calluses are usually asymptomatic, causing pain only when pressure is applied. Individuals who suffer from calluses on the sole of the foot often liken their discomfort to that of walking with a pebble in the shoe.

Warts (Verrucae)

Warts, or verrucae, are common viral infections of the skin and mucous membranes. Approximately 9 million US citizens contract them each year. They are caused by human papillomaviruses (HPVs), which contain DNA.[5]

Papillomavirus particles assemble in the nuclei of upper-layer keratinocytes and are subsequently released

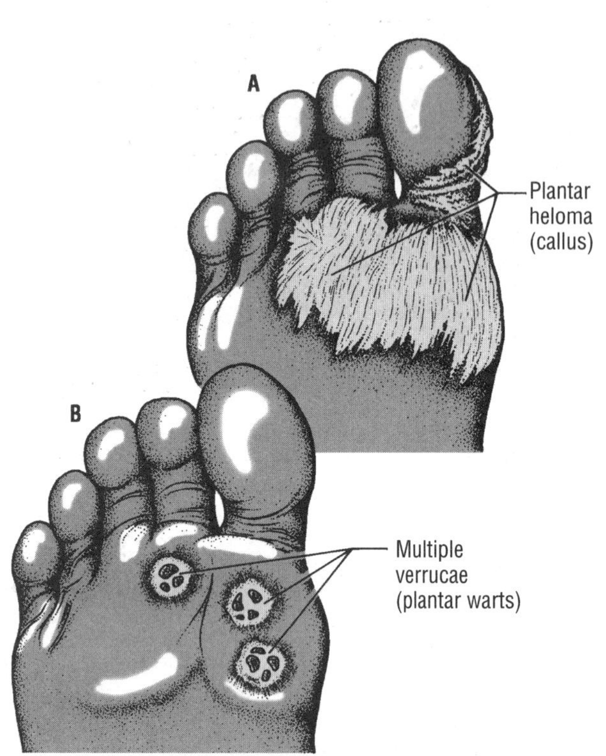

FIGURE 2A and B Conditions affecting the sole of the foot: A, plantar heloma (callus); B, multiple verrucae (plantar warts)

into the milieu within the stratum corneum. It has been demonstrated that HPVs do not bud from the cell membrane and thus lack a thermosensitive lipid envelope like that found in the herpes viruses and the human retroviruses. It is thought that the presence of a stable protein coat allows the HPV to remain infectious outside the host cells for substantial periods of time.

Types

Because warts were induced when extracts from common warts and anogenital warts were injected into different sites, it was hypothesized that all warts were caused by a single agent. In the past decade, however, immunologic techniques in conjunction with DNA purification and restrictive endonuclease digestion have identified at least 50 HPV types,[6] each with its own characteristic histopathology and cytopathology.

Past studies showed that HPV-6 and HPV-11 were responsible for anogenital warts, and that these strains were different from other HPVs in serologic molecular hybridization.[5,7] This prompted the belief that HPV type dictated the kind of wart and that these viruses were confined to specific body locations. Evidence now suggests that HPV types are not restricted to a specific site, but that, for unknown reasons (perhaps epithelial cell receptor specificity), viral particles function in keratinocytes only in specific locations and will induce warts only in these locations.

Common virogenic warts are recognized by their rough, cauliflower-like appearance. They are slightly scaly, rough papules or nodules that appear alone or grouped. They can be found on any skin surface although they most often appear on the hands. (See color plates, photograph 34.) Warts are defined according to their location. Common warts (verruca vulgaris) are usually found on the hands and fingers but may also occur on the face. Periungual and subungual warts occur around and underneath the nail beds, especially in nail biters and cuticle pickers.[5] Juvenile, or flat, warts (verruca plana) usually occur on the face, neck, and dorsa of the hands, wrists, and knees of children. Venereal warts (condyloma lata and condyloma acuminata) typically occur near the genitalia and anus; however, the penile shaft is the most common site of lesions in men. Plantar warts (verruca plantaris) are common on the soles of the feet.[5] (See color plates, photograph 35.)

Plantar warts, hyperkeratotic lesions generally associated with pressure, are more common in older children and adolescents but also occur in adults. They may be confined to the weight-bearing areas of the foot (the sole of the heel, the great toe, the areas below the heads of the metatarsal bones, and the ball), or they may occur in non–weight-bearing areas of the sole of the foot (Figure 2). Calluses are also commonly found on weight-bearing areas of the foot, and because of their smooth keratotic surfaces, they may resemble isolated plantar warts. Therefore, the distinction between a wart and a callus is sometimes unclear. However, unlike a callus, a plantar wart is tender with pressure and interrupts the footprint pattern. Optimally, a podiatrist or dermatologist will have the opportunity to assess the condition and make a differential diagnosis. To do this, the physician may shave away the outer keratinous surface to expose thrombosed capillaries in the papilloma, which appear as black dots or seeds.

Plantar warts, if located on weight-bearing portions of the foot, are under constant pressure and are usually not raised above the skin surface. The wart itself is in the center of the lesion and is roughly circular, with a diameter of 0.5–3.0 cm. The surface is grayish and friable, and the surrounding skin is thick and heaped. Several warts may coalesce and fuse, giving the appearance of one large wart (mosaic wart).

Susceptibility

Three criteria must be met for an individual to develop a wart:

- The papillomavirus must be present.
- There must be an open avenue such as an abrasion through which the virus can enter the skin.
- The individual's immune system must be susceptible to the virus (probably the key reason that certain individuals develop warts and others do not).

Indeed, immunodeficient patients (eg, those maintained on systemic or topical glucocorticoids), once infected, develop widespread and highly resistant warts.[8]

Warts are most common in children and young adults. The peak incidence of warts occurs between 12 and 16 years of age; as many as 10% of schoolchildren under age 16 have one or more warts.[9]

Warts may spread by direct person-to-person contact, by autoinoculation to another body area, or indirectly through public shower floors or swimming pools. It is thought that swimming, especially in warm water with a pH greater than 5, swells and softens the horny skin layer cells on the sole of the foot. The abrasive surface of the pool and diving board also contributes to tissue debridement. Scrapings of the horny layer of plantar warts contain virus particles; therefore, it is conceivable that the heavy traffic area of a pool can be easily contaminated by one person with a plantar wart, making inoculation in that area around the pool likely. The incubation period after inoculation is 1–20 months, with an average of 3–4 months.

Mechanism

Warts begin as minute, smooth-surfaced, skin-colored lesions that enlarge over time. Repeated irritation causes them to continue enlarging. Plantar warts are usually asymptomatic when small and may not be noticed. However, if they are large or occur on the heel or ball of the foot, there may be severe discomfort and limitation of function.

Warts are not usually permanent; approximately 30% clear spontaneously in 6 months, 65% clear in 2 years, and most warts clear in 5 years.[10] The mechanism of spontaneous resolution is not fully understood.

Evaluation

Many foot conditions require a physician's attention, especially those conditions accompanying chronic, debilitating diseases such as diabetes mellitus or arteriosclerosis. Because circulation is impaired in such cases, treatment with nonprescription products, if not properly supervised, may induce more inflammation, ulceration, or even gangrene, particularly in cases of vascular insufficiency in the foot. Persons with diabetes and patients prone to ischemic changes are particularly susceptible to gangrene. (See Chapter 18, "Diabetes Care Products and Monitoring Devices.") In addition, simple lesions may mask more serious abscesses or ulcerations; if left medically unattended, these lesions may lead to such conditions as osteomyelitis, which may require hospitalization and aggressive parenteral antibiotic therapy. If exostoses associated with corns are not excised by a physician, the corns will persist. Sites with many corns, many calluses, or lesions that ooze purulent material (a sign of a secondary bacterial infection) should also be examined by a physician or podiatrist.

Most patients with rheumatoid arthritis eventually have foot involvement, the major forefoot deformities in these patients being painful metatarsal heads, hallux valgus (the deviation of the great toe toward the lateral, or outer side of the foot), and clawfoot. Corrective surgical procedures are often indicated to reduce pain and improve function and mobility. There is little evidence that conventional nonsurgical therapy (eg, orthopedic shoes, metatarsal inserts, conventional arch supports, and metatarsal bars) is effective in these cases.

The pharmacist must be aware that warts may occasionally be confused with more serious conditions, such as squamous cell carcinoma and deep fungal infections. A squamous cell carcinoma may develop rapidly, attaining a diameter of 1 cm within 2 weeks. The lesion generally appears as a small, red, conical, hard nodule that quickly ulcerates. Subungual verrucae, which occur under the nail plate, may exist in conjunction with periungual verrucae. A long-standing subungual verruca may be difficult to differentiate from a squamous cell carcinoma, especially in elderly patients.

In addition to responses to some of the questions suggested in the patient assessment and counseling section at the beginning of this chapter, the patient's medical history and medication profile should include the following information:

- Characteristics (particularly oozing and bleeding of warts) and duration of the condition;
- Similar problems that may have occurred in other family members;
- Any medical treatment being given for the problem or for other conditions (eg, immunosuppressive disorders, diabetes mellitus, or rheumatoid arthritis);
- Any drug allergies.

Medical referral is indicated if:

- Diabetes mellitus, a peripheral circulatory disease, or a medical condition already under a physician's care exists;
- Hemorrhaging or oozing of purulent material occurs;
- Corns and calluses indicate an anatomical defect or fault in body weight distribution;
- Corns and calluses on the foot are extensive or are painful and debilitating;
- Extensive warts at one site exist;
- Proper self-medication for warts has been tried for an adequate period without success;
- Patient has a history of rheumatoid arthritis and complains of painful metatarsal heads or deviation of the great toe.

Self-treatment is appropriate if:

- Chronic, debilitating diseases do not contraindicate the use of foot care products;
- The patient is not diabetic;
- The directions for use of the products can be followed with no difficulty;
- No concurrent medication (eg, immunosuppressives) is being taken that contraindicates the use of these products;
- Corns and calluses are minor;
- Predisposing factors (eg, ill-fitting footwear and hosiery) of corns and calluses are removed;
- Neither an anatomical defect nor faulty weight distribution is indicated by corns or calluses;
- Plantar warts have not spread extensively over the sole of the foot.

Treatment

Pharmacologic Approaches

Corns and Calluses Successful treatment of corns and calluses with nonprescription products depends on eliminating the causes: pressure and friction. This entails using well-fitting, nonbinding footwear that evenly distributes body weight. For anatomical foot deformities, orthopedic corrections must be made. These measures relieve pressure and friction to allow normal mitosis of the basal cell layer to resume, the stratum corneum to normalize after total desquamation of the hyperkeratotic tissue, and topical products to take effect. Before beginning self-treatment, however, a patient should consult a doctor or a pharmacist; if circulatory problems are present or if the patient has diabetes, a medical opinion should definitely be secured.

In the final monograph for over-the-counter (OTC) drug products that remove corns and calluses, the Food and Drug Administration (FDA) adopted the advisory review panel's recommendations that only salicylic acid be categorized as safe and effective for this purpose.[11] The final monograph dictates that products containing salicylic acid in a plaster, pad, disk, or collodion vehicle must be classified as Category I.[11] The FDA recognized that use of the term *plaster* includes disc and pad because these dosage forms are similar in nature. It also indicated that these products are to be advertised to consumers "for the removal of corns and calluses."

In an earlier study, corns were treated with a subdermal injection of fluid silicone.[12] The injected silicone, at times, seems to augment digital and plantar tissues by using a cushioning effect, reducing pain, and decreasing the need for regular palliative treatment.

Warts Many practitioners believe that early and vigorous treatment of warts is best. The urgency for treatment is based on such considerations as the cosmetic effect (facial warts), the number of warts present in an area, the site of the wart (weight-bearing area of the foot), and the age of the patient. Moreover, prolonged treatment with nonprescription products may increase the chance of autoinoculation.

Choice of treatment type depends on the location, size, and type of wart, and on the extent and number of lesions present. It should also take into account the patient's age, immunologic status, and expected compliance with treatment. Other important considerations prior to initiation of treatment are the pain, the inconvenience, and the risk of scarring, as well as the experience of the physician or dermatologist.

No specific effective medication for curing warts is available although topical agents and procedures can sometimes help in their removal and relieve the pain. Topical salicylic acid in three different vehicles has been recognized as the only drug that is safe and effective for self-treatment of common or plantar warts.[13] However, the FDA Advisory Review Panel on Over-the-Counter Miscellaneous External Drug Products recommended that these products be labeled for treating *only* common and plantar warts.[13] It excluded the other wart types from self-therapy because of the difficulty in recognizing and treating them without the supervision of a physician.[13] Indeed, painful plantar warts, as well as multiple flat warts, facial warts, periungual warts, and venereal warts, should all be treated by a physician.[10] Because of the latency factor, warts may reappear several months after they have been "cured."

Pharmacologic Agents

As previously stated, salicylic acid is the only nonprescription drug found by the FDA to be both safe and effective as a keratolytic agent for the treatment of corns, calluses, and plantar warts (see product table "Callus, Corn, and Wart Products"). [11] Although several prescription products (eg, cantharidin, podophyllum, and podofilox) and/or cryotherapy may also be used to treat warts, discussion of these treatments is outside the scope of this chapter.

TABLE 2 FDA final monographs on foot care products for corns, calluses, and warts

Corn and callus remover drug products[a]
Salicylic acid, 12–40% in a plaster vehicle
Salicylic acid, 12–17.6% in a collodion-like vehicle

Wart remover drug products[b]
Salicylic acid, 12–40% in a plaster vehicle
Salicylic acid, 5–17% in a collodion-like vehicle
Salicylic acid, 15% in a karaya gum, glycol plaster vehicle

[a] *Federal Register*. 1990 Aug 14; 55 (157): 33258–62.
[b] *Federal Register*. 1990 Aug 14; 55 (157): 33246–56.

Salicylic Acid Salicylic acid, the oldest of the keratolytic agents, is formulated in many strengths (0.5–40%), depending on its intended use. For the self-treatment of corns, calluses, and warts, its approved concentration ranges in the various topical product forms are listed in Table 2.

Salicylic acid is thought to act on hyperplastic keratin in two ways: (1) it decreases keratinocyte adhesion, and (2) it increases water binding, which leads to a hydration of keratin. Because of the latter effect, the presence of moisture had been thought to be an important component of salicylic acid's therapeutic efficacy, and soaking the area in a warm water bath for 5 minutes before applying salicylic acid was recommended. However, evidence submitted to the FDA indicated that presoaking produced no significant positive effects for any efficacy parameter assessed.[13] In its final rule, the FDA proposed to allow the manufacturers of these products to state as an optional direction to the consumer: "May soak corn/callus (or wart) in warm water for 5 minutes to assist in removal."

In years past, packaging and labeling for corn, callus, or wart removal products warned patients with diabetes or peripheral vascular disease not to use the products except under direct physician supervision. This was because any acute inflammation or ulcer formation caused by the topical salicylic acid could be dangerous. In its final monograph, the FDA determined that the warning should be stronger and should directly caution against using the product under certain conditions rather than including an "except under" condition for use. Consequently, the revised warning is as follows:

> **WARNING** Do not use this product on irritated skin, on any area that is infected or reddened, if you are diabetic, or if you have poor blood circulation.[13]

It is not necessary to encircle surrounding healthy skin with a film of white petrolatum to protect it from irritation caused by the inadvertent application of salicylic acid during treatment. Thus, the FDA has deleted this instruction on salicylic acid product packaging.

Significant percutaneous absorption may occur when salicylic acid is applied over large body areas—for example, during therapy for extensive psoriasis on the face, trunk, or extremities. Absorbed salicylic acid is largely metabolized in the liver and excreted in the urine; patients with impaired liver or kidney function are therefore predisposed to accumulation and salicylate toxicity. However, although occlusive vehicles can enhance the percutaneous absorption of salicylic acid, it is highly unlikely that salicylism will result during corn, callus, or wart therapy with recommended dosages.

Salicylic acid is usually applied to a corn, callus, or common wart in a collodion or collodion-like vehicle. The patient should thoroughly wash and dry the affected area before applying the product. For corns and calluses, the solution is applied once or twice daily as needed for up to 14 days or until the corn or callus is removed. For warts, it is applied once or twice daily as needed for up to 12 weeks or until the wart is removed. For all three conditions, the product is applied one drop at a time until the affected area is well covered. The patient should be advised not to overuse the product.

The liquid form is often the easiest for the patient to apply. However, this treatment mode requires patience and persistence because of the length of time it requires to resolve the problem. It is suggested that the patient keep the adjacent healthy skin dry and clean, and that the collodion film be peeled away every 2 or 3 days to remove keratotic debris.[9]

Salicylic acid may also be delivered to the skin through the use of a plaster disc or pad. This delivery system provides direct and prolonged contact of the drug with the affected area. Salicylic acid plaster is a uniform solid or semisolid adhesive mixture of salicylic acid in a suitable base, spread on appropriate backing material (eg, felt, moleskin, cotton, or plastic), which may be applied directly to the affected area. The usual concentration of salicylic acid in the base is 40%. A small piece of the 40% plaster may be cut to the size of the wart and held in place by waterproof tape. More convenient, however, are corn or callus pads that have small salicylic acid discs for direct application to the skin. The patient selects the appropriately sized disk, places it directly on the affected area, and then covers it with the pad.

For corns and calluses, salicylic acid plasters or discs are generally applied and removed within 48 hours, with a maximum of five treatments over a 2-week period. For warts, these products are applied and removed every 48 hours, with a maximum treatment period not to exceed 12 weeks. The karaya gum, glycol plaster with 15% salicylic acid for wart removal is specifically designed to be applied at bedtime and left on for at least 8 hours; in the morning, it is removed and discarded. This procedure is repeated every 24 hours as needed for up to 12 weeks. If the wart remains, a physician should be consulted.

Collodion Vehicles Topical keratolytics used in treating corns, calluses, and warts are generally formulated in flexible collodion-like delivery systems containing pyroxylin; various combinations of volatile solvents such as ether, acetone, or alcohol; or a plasticizer, usually castor oil. Pyroxylin is a nitrocellulose derivative that remains on the skin as a water-repellent film after the volatile solvents have evaporated. The advantages of collodions are that they form an adherent flexible or rigid film and prevent moisture evaporation; these qualities aid penetration of the active ingredient into the affected tissue and result in sustained local action of the drug. The systems are largely water insoluble, as are most of their active ingredients such as salicylic acid. They are also less apt to run onto surrounding skin than are aqueous solutions. The disadvantages of collodions are that they are extremely flammable and volatile and that, by occluding normal water transport through the skin, they may be mechanically irritating. Also, the collodion's occlusive nature allows systemic absorption of some drugs. Some patients may abuse these vehicles by sniffing their volatile aromatic solvents.

Historically Used Unapproved Agents In its final monograph, the FDA classified drugs used historically for corn, callus, or wart removal as nonmonograph ingredients.[11,13] These drugs include acetic acid, glacial acetic acid, allantoin, ascorbic acid, belladonna extract, benzocaine, calcium pantothenate, camphor, castor oil, chlorobutanol, diperodon hydrochloride, ichthammol, iodine, lactic acid, menthol, methylbenzethonium chloride, methyl salicylate, panthenol, phenoxyacetic acid, phenyl salicylate, vitamin A, and zinc chloride. These ineffective drugs are no longer approved for self-treatment of corns, calluses, or warts and cannot be marketed for use in this regard unless they are the subject of a specifically approved application.

Folk Remedies

Some folk remedies are occasionally attempted for wart treatment, with beneficial effects claimed.[14] There is a long list of such remedies, but a few are worth sharing:

- Rub a dusty, dry toad on warts, and they will disappear.
- Rub the gizzard of a chicken on warts during the decrease of the moon; bury the gizzard in the center of a dirt road.
- Cut a potato and rub it on the warts; then throw the potato over the fence.
- Steal a used washcloth, rub it over the warts, bury it, and the warts will disappear as the cloth rots.
- Rub the wart with castor oil every day.

The perceived beneficial effects of these remedies is most likely owing to the coincidental and spontaneous resolution of the wart in response to natural immune functions. Nonetheless, the pharmacist may be asked about their usefulness.

Adjunctive Therapy

In addition to nonprescription drugs, self-therapy measures include daily soaking of the affected area throughout treatment for at least 5 minutes in warm (not hot) water to remove dead tissue. Dead tissue should be removed gently rather than forcibly after normal washing to avoid further damage. A rough towel, callus file, or pumice stone effectively accomplishes this purpose. Sharp knives or razor blades should not be used because they may cause bacterial contamination and infection. Petroleum jelly need not be applied to healthy skin surrounding the affected area before corrosive products are applied; however, this precaution should be suggested to persons with poor eyesight or other conditions that increase the likelihood of misapplication or accidental spillage.

To relieve painful pressure emanating from inflamed underlying tissue and irritated or hypertrophied bones directly underneath a corn or callus, patients may use a pad such as a Dr. Scholl's with an aperture for the corn or callus. If the skin can tolerate the pads, they may be used for up to 1 week or longer. To prevent the pads from adhering to hosiery, patients may wax them with paraffin or a candle, and then powder them daily with a hygienic foot powder or cover them with an adhesive bandage. If, despite these measures, friction causes the pads to peel up at the edge and stick to hosiery, the pharmacist may recommend that patients cover their toes with the forefoot of an old stocking or pantyhose before putting on hosiery.

Many of the disadvantages associated with older pads have been overcome with the introduction of a new cushioning material. Cushlin, a soft polymer, has been clinically proven to provide immediate, all-day relief from corns and calluses. When applied to the skin, it molds to the shape of the foot and adheres to the skin without leaving a sticky residue. Additionally, its smooth outer surface prevents snags and runs in socks and hosiery.

Pharmacists should advise patients that if at any time the pad begins to cause itching, burning, or pain, it should be removed and a physician or podiatrist be consulted. Patients should also be advised that these pads will provide only temporary relief and will rarely cure a corn or callus.

To avoid the spread of warts, which are contagious, patients should wash their hands before and after treating or touching wart tissue. A specific towel should be used only for drying the affected area after cleaning. Patients should not probe, poke, or cut the wart tissue. If warts are present on the sole of the foot, patients should not walk in bare feet unless the wart is securely covered.

Patient Education and Consultation

Remission of corns, calluses, and warts does not happen quickly; it can take several days to several months. For warts, for example, patients will notice visible improvement within the first or second week of treatment; removal should be complete within 4–12 weeks of product use. Thus, selection of a convenient time to apply the product and adherence to the dosage regimen are important. Topical products should be applied no more than twice daily; the most convenient times are generally in the morning and evening. If the wart remains after a full course of treatment, a physician should be consulted.

The pharmacist should counsel the patient or caregiver on how to use the medication. Because many products contain corrosive materials, they must be applied only to the corn, callus, or wart. If a plaster or pad is used, the pharmacist should first explain how to trim the pad to follow the contours of the corn or callus. The pharmacist should then instruct the patient how to apply the plaster to the skin and cover it with adhesive occlusive tape; how to remove the dressing the next day and soak the foot in warm water; how to remove the macerated, soft white skin of the corn or callus by scrubbing gently with a rough towel, pumice stone, or callus file and not debriding the healthy skin; and how to reapply the plaster.

If a solution is used, the pharmacist should instruct the patient to apply one drop at a time directly to the corn, callus, or wart; to allow the drops to dry and harden so the solution does not run; and to continue the procedure until the entire affected area is covered. Adjacent areas of normal healthy skin should not come in contact with the drug. If they do, the solution should be washed off immediately with soap and water. If the solution is being used on a soft corn between the toes, the toes should be held apart until the solution has dried. The solution should solidify before a dressing is applied. This treatment is to be followed for 3–6 days.

Pharmacists should remind patients that these products are keratolytic and cause skin tissue to slough off, leaving an unsightly pinkish tinge to the skin. Nevertheless, these products should continue to be used and should be discontinued only when a severe inflammatory response (swelling or reddening) or irritation occurs, or when pain occurs immediately upon application.

Because liquid nonprescription preparations contain volatile and irritating ingredients, the patient should be cautious in using them. After use, the container should be tightly capped to prevent evaporation and to prevent the active ingredients from assuming a greater concentration. The volatile delivery systems are quite flammable, and the product should be stored in amber or light-resistant containers away from direct sunlight or heat.

Pharmacists should alert patients that the products that contain collodions are poisonous when taken orally and that these products, as well as all other corn, callus, and wart removal products, should be stored out of children's reach. Collodion-containing products are volatile, have an odor similar to that of airplane glue, and may be subject to abuse by inhalation.

Nonprescription corn, callus, and wart removal products are not recommended for patients with diabetes or circulatory problems. Pharmacists should reinforce contraindications, warnings, and precautions with all patients to avoid the inadvertent use of these products by other individuals who have such conditions.

Bunions

The hallux, or great toe, along with the inner side of the foot, provides the elasticity and mobility needed to walk or run. Thus, the hallux is a dynamic body part. However, this mobility causes several anatomical disorders associated with the foot, such as hallux valgus. Prolonged pressure due to hallux valgus may result in pressure over the angulation of the metatarsophalangeal joint of the big toe, causing inflammatory swelling of the bursa over that joint (Figure 3). This may result in bunion formation (Figure 1).

Bunions, which are swellings of the bursae and/or exostoses, can be caused by various conditions. Pressure may result from the manner in which a person sits, walks, or stands, but pressure from a tight-fitting shoe over a period of time generally aggravates the condition. Friction on the toes from bone malformations (wide heads or lateral bending) is also a major factor in bunion production. Some individuals have a hereditary predisposition to the development of bunions.

Corrective steps to alleviate bunions often depend on the degree of discomfort. Bunions are usually asymptomatic but may become quite painful, swollen, and tender. The bunion itself usually is covered by an extensive keratinous overgrowth.

Bunions are not amenable to topical drug therapy. Nor is the routine, chronic use of oral nonprescription analgesics, particularly ibuprofen, suggested. The patient should correct the etiologic condition by wearing properly fitting shoes or should seek the advice of a podiatrist or orthopedist.

Topical nonprescription padding (eg, moleskin) can be helpful and may be all that is necessary to decrease the irritation of footwear. Eventually, padding can help decrease inflammation around the bunion area. If the pharmacist recommends the use of topical adhesive cushioning to alleviate the pressure on a bunion, instructions should be given on proper use. Before the protective pad is applied, the foot should be bathed and thoroughly dried. The pad should then be cut into a shape that conforms to the bunion. If the intent is to relieve the pressure from the center of the bunion area, the pad should be cut to surround the bunion. Precut pads are available for immediate patient use. Constant skin contact with adhesive-backed pads should generally be avoided, however, unless recommended by a podiatrist or physician.

Alternatively, a nonmedicated, self-adhesive bunion cushion (ie, Bunion Guard) is commercially available. One advantage of this product is that it protects the bunion and can be easily removed prior to showering. The cushion, made of a soft polymer gel, can then be reapplied onto the bunion after showering for up to 3 months. Another advantage of Bunion Guard is that it does not contain an adhesive backing that can be irritating to the patient's skin. The outer surface is smooth and not prone to snag socks and hosiery.

Larger footwear may be necessary to compensate for the space taken up by the pad; not increasing shoe size appropriately may cause pressure in other areas. Also, protective pads should not be used on bunions when the skin is broken or blistered. Abraded skin should receive palliative treatment before pads are applied. If symptoms persist, particularly in diabetic patients, the pharmacist should recommend that these patients consult a podiatrist or orthopedist. Ultimately, surgical treatment may be necessary.

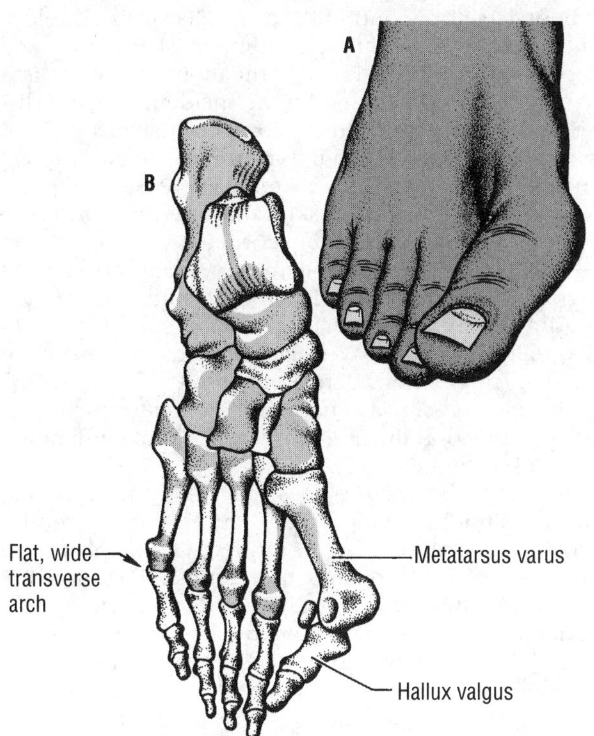

FIGURE 3A and B Two views of hallux valgus: A, gross representation of hallux valgus; B, bone structure of hallux valgus.

Athlete's Foot

The most prevalent cutaneous fungal infection in humans is athlete's foot (dermatophytosis of the foot, or tinea pedis). Athlete's foot afflicts approximately 26.5 million people in the United States every year, and of every 10 sufferers, 7 are male. It is estimated that 70% of the population will be afflicted with athlete's foot in their lifetime and that approximately 45% will suffer with it episodically for more than 10 years. When exposure to infectious environments is equal, the incidence of tinea infections in women approaches that in men.

The clinical spectrum of athlete's foot ranges from mild itching and scaling to a severe, exudative inflammatory process characterized by fissuring and denudation. The prevalent type of athlete's foot, midway between these two extremes, is characterized by maceration, hyperkeratosis, pruritus, malodor, itching, and a stinging sensation of the feet. (See color plates, photograph 36.)

Etiology

Tinea pedis is an infection type of relatively recent onset. It was not common until humans began wearing occlusive footwear, and it was not reported in the medical literature until 1888. Because ringworm fungi (dermatophytes) are generally the causative or initiating organisms, athlete's foot is often synonymous with a ringworm infection.[15] Tinea pedis is most commonly caused by *Trichophyton rubrum*, *Trichophyton mentagrophytes*, or *Epidermophyton floccosum*. *T rubrum* often causes a dry, hyperkeratotic involvement of the feet; *T mentagrophytes* often produces a blister-like or vesicular pattern; and *E floccosum* is capable of producing both of these patterns.

In addition to specific microorganisms, other environmental factors contribute to the disease's development, such as the climatic conditions of the area and the customs of the resident population. Footwear is a key variable, as illustrated by the incidence of the disease in any population that wears occlusive footwear, especially in the summer and in tropical or subtropical climates. Nonporous shoe material increases temperature and hydration of the skin and interferes with the barrier function of the stratum corneum.

The type of dermatophytosis present varies with geographic location.[16] In Vietnam, US soldiers often acquired a disabling, inflammatory *T mentagrophytes* infection although South Vietnamese soldiers did not. In a resident population, dermatophytosis infection is often observed as chronic and noninflammatory whereas the same infection in virgin hosts is markedly inflammatory and self-limited.[16]

Species of dermatophytes that infect humans (eg, *T rubrum* and *T mentagrophytes*) are transmitted either directly by human contact or indirectly by exposure to inanimate objects. It is thought that this infection is acquired most often by walking barefoot on infected floors (eg, hotel bathrooms, swimming pools, or locker rooms) and may be spread within families by exposure to bathroom floors, mats, or rugs. Therefore, tinea pedis is considered to be an exogenously transmitted infection in which cross-infection among susceptible individuals readily occurs.[16]

Pathophysiology

After being inoculated into the skin under suitable conditions, the infection progresses through several stages. These stages include periods of incubation and then enlargement, followed by a refractory period and a stage of involution.

During the incubation period, the dermatophyte grows in the stratum corneum, sometimes with minimal signs of infection. After the incubation period and once the infection is established, two factors appear to play a role in determining the size and duration of the lesions. These factors are the growth rate of the organism and the epidermal turnover rate.[16] The fungal growth rate must equal or exceed the epidermal turnover rate, or the organism will quickly shed.

Dermatophytid infestations remain within the stratum corneum. This resistance to the spread of infection seems to involve both immunologic and nonimmunologic mechanisms. For example, the substance serum inhibitory factor (SIF) appears to limit the growth of dermatophytes beyond the stratum corneum. SIF is not an antibody but a dialyzable, heat-labile component of fresh sera. It appears that SIF binds to the iron that dermatophytes need for continued growth.[16]

Once into the stratum corneum, dermatophytes produce keratinases and other proteolytic enzymes. US combat personnel in Vietnam demonstrated a particularly inflammatory type of *T mentagrophytes* infection associated with elastase production. This indicated that enzymes or toxins produced by these microorganisms account for some of the severe clinical reactions.

Types

Clinically, there are four accepted variants of tinea pedis; two or more of these types may overlap. The most common is the chronic, intertriginous type,[16] characterized by fissuring, scaling, or maceration in the interdigital spaces. Typically, the infection involves the lateral toe webs, usually between the fourth and fifth or third and fourth toes. From these sites, the infection spreads to the sole or instep of the foot but rarely to the dorsum. Warmth and humidity aggravate this condition; consequently, hyperhidrosis (excessive sweating) becomes an underlying problem and must be treated along with the dermatophyte infestation.

Normal resident aerobic diphtheroids may become involved in the athlete's foot process. After initial invasion of the stratum corneum by dermatophytes, enough moisture may accumulate to trigger a bacterial overgrowth. Increased moisture and temperature then lead to the release of metabolic products, which diffuse easily through the underlying horny layer already damaged by fungal invasion. In the more severe cases, gram-negative organisms intrude and may exacerbate the condition, causing skin maceration, white hyperkeratosis, or erosions with increased patient symptomatology.

The second variant of athlete's foot is known as the chronic, papulosquamous pattern.[16] It is usually found on both feet and is characterized by mild inflammation and diffuse scaling on the soles of the feet. Tinea unguium (ie, ringworm of the nails, or onychomycosis) of one or more toenails may also be present and may continue to fuel the infection. The toenails must first be cured with oral drug therapy, such as griseofulvin, itraconazole, or ketoconazole, or removed surgically to rid the area of the offending fungus. Surgery is preferred because oral antifungal therapy is not always effective.

The third variant of tinea pedis is the vesicular type, usually caused by *T mentagrophytes* var *interdigitale*.[16] Small vesicles or vesicopustules are observed near the instep and on the midanterior plantar surface. Skin scaling is seen on these areas as well as on the toe webs. This variant is symptomatic in the summer and clinically quiescent during the cooler months.

The acute ulcerative type is the fourth variant of tinea pedis. It is often associated with macerated, denuded, weeping ulcerations of the sole of the foot. Typically, white hyperkeratosis and a pungent odor are present. This type of infection, which is complicated by an overgrowth of opportunistic, gram-negative bacteria such as *Proteus* and *Pseudomonas*, has been called dermatophytosis complex or gram-negative athlete's foot, and it may produce an extremely painful, erosive, purulent interspace that can be disabling.

Susceptibility

Although there are many pathogenic fungi in the environment, the overall incidence of actual superficial fungal infections is remarkably low. Many degrees of susceptibility, from instantaneous "takes" by a single spore to severe trauma with massive exposure, produce a clinical infection. It appears, however, that trauma to the skin, especially that which produces blisters (from wearing ill-fitting footwear), may be significantly more important to the occurrence of human fungal infections than is simple exposure to the offending pathogens.

Although tinea pedis may occur at all ages, it is more common in adults, presumably because of their increased opportunities for exposure to pathogens. However, it can also occur in children. Individual susceptibility is also affected by other disease processes the patient may have. For example, dermatophytosis infections may be more severe and difficult to ameliorate in patients with diabetes mellitus, lymphoid malignancies, immunologic compromise, and Cushing's syndrome.[16]

Evaluation

The most common complaint of patients suffering from tinea pedis is pruritus. However, if fissures are present, particularly between the toes, painful burning and stinging may also occur. If the foot area is abraded, denuded, or inflamed, there may be weeping or oozing in addition to pain. Some patients may merely remark on the bothersome scaling of dry skin, particularly if it has progressed to the soles of the feet. Small vesicular lesions may combine to form a larger bullous eruption marked by pain and irritation. The only symptoms may be brittleness and discoloration of a hypertrophied toenail.

The only true determinant of a fungal foot infection is the clinical laboratory evaluation of tissue scrapings from the foot. This process involves a potassium hydroxide mount preparation of the scrapings and cuttings on a special growth medium to show the actual presence and specific identity of fungi. The procedure can be ordered and performed only at the direction of a physician, and microscopic confirmation is probably possible only in the dry, scaly type of tinea pedis. The recovery of fungi for diagnosis decreases as athlete's foot becomes progressively more severe. In typical cases of dermatophytosis complex, fungus recovery rates are only about 25–50%.

The pharmacist should question the patient thoroughly regarding the condition and its characteristics to determine symptoms, the extent of disease, previous patient compliance with medications, and any mitigating circumstances, such as diabetes or obesity, that might render the patient susceptible. Persons with diabetes, for example, may present with a mixed dermatophytid and monilial infection. In general, it is not inappropriate to inspect the foot if privacy and sanitary conditions allow, and it is especially appropriate with diabetes patients.

The pharmacist should seek to distinguish tinea pedis from diseases with similar symptoms, such as dermatitis, allergic contact dermatitis, and atopic dermatitis. In children, peridigital dermatitis or atopic dermatitis is more common than tinea pedis. Shoe dermatitis is perhaps the most common form of allergic contact dermatitis from clothing. Since 1950, the increased use of rubber and adhesives in footwear has paralleled the increase in reports of shoe dermatitis in the dermatologic and podiatric literature. Contact allergy to accelerators—the chemical compounds used to speed up the processing of rubber used in sponge-rubber insoles for tennis shoes—has also been reported.[17] In addition to accelerators, antioxidants have been implicated as major chemical allergens, and various phenolic resins used in adhesives are also troublesome. The patient is usually unaware that his or her footwear may be causing the problem.

Hyperhidrosis of interdigital spaces and the sole of the foot is common, as is infection of the toe webs by gram-negative bacteria. In hyperhidrosis, tender vesicles cover the sole of the foot and toes and may be quite painful. The skin generally turns white, erodes, and becomes macerated. This condition is accompanied by a foul foot odor. Infection by gram-negative bacteria is characterized by a soggy wetness of the toe webs and immediately adjacent skin; the affected tissue is damp and softened. The last toe web (adjacent to the little toe) is the most common area of primary or initial involvement because it is deeper and extends more proximally than the web between the other toes. Furthermore, abundant exocrine sweat glands, a semiocclusive anatomical setting, and the added occlusion provided by footwear enhance development of the disease at this site. The pharmacist must be careful not to confuse this condition with soft corns, which also appear between the fourth and fifth toes.

Severe forms of tinea pedis may progress to disintegration and denudation of the affected skin and to profuse, serous, purulent discharge. Denudation may involve all the toe webs, the dorsal and plantar surfaces of the toes, and an area about 1 cm wide beyond the base of the toes on the plantar surface of the foot. When the disease is out of control, its progression is observed on the dorsum of the foot and the calf in the form of tiny red follicular crusts. Paradoxically, this condition may be caused by the use of reputed germicidal soaps such as pHisoHex, Dial, and Safeguard. It was hypothesized that these soaps reduce the presence of harmless saprophytes and thus promote an overgrowth of resistant pathogens (eg, *Pseudomonas aeruginosa* and *Proteus mirabilis*) by removing their competitors.

If the patient has used a nonprescription antifungal product appropriately for 4 weeks without satisfactory results, a disease other than tinea pedis may be involved. Therapeutic failure may be owing to gram-negative athlete's foot, which no nonprescription antifungal product will ameliorate. Persons suffering from such an infection, as well as from hyperhidrosis, allergic contact dermatitis, or atopic dermatitis, should consult a podiatrist or physician for treatment.

The pharmacist should be aware of the implications of the following conditions and be able to recommend to the patient the appropriate course of action:

- If the toenail is involved, topical treatment is ineffective and will not allay the condition until the disease's primary focus is treated with oral griseofulvin, itraconazole, or ketoconazole or until other preventive measures are instituted (eg, surgical avulsion of the nail).
- If vesicular eruptions are oozing purulent material that could indicate a secondary bacterial infection, topical astringent therapy and/or antibiotic therapy may be appropriate.
- If the interspace between the toes is foul smelling; whitish; painful; soggy; or characterized by erosions, oozing, or serious inflammation, and especially if the condition is disabling, the patient should be referred to a physician.

- If the foot is seriously inflamed or swollen and a major portion of it is involved, supportive therapy must be instituted before an antifungal agent may be applied.
- If the patient is a child who presents with an eczematous eruption of the feet, including that complicated by blisters and/or pyoderma, self-treatment should not be recommended.
- If the patient is under a physician's supervision for a disease such as diabetes or asthma, in which normal host defense mechanisms may be deficient, nonprescription products should not be recommended before medical consultation.

Pharmacologic Treatment

Before self-medication can be effective, the type of tinea pedis and the appropriate treatment must be determined. Self-treatment of an acute, superficial tinea foot infection may be effective if certain conditions are met. In acute, inflammatory tinea pedis, characterized by reddened, oozing, and vesicular eruptions, the inflammation must be counteracted before antifungal therapy can be instituted. This step is especially important if the eruptions are caused by a secondary bacterial infection.

Hydrocortisone, in conjunction with clioquinol (formerly iodochlorhydroxyquin), has demonstrated favorable results toward resolving uncomplicated cutaneous fungal infections (tinea cruris, tinea pedis, and moniliasis). Erythema and itching were relieved more with the combination of these two drugs than with either drug alone or the placebo cream. However, with the availability of nonprescription topical hydrocortisone products, it is conceivable that their indiscriminate use to relieve the itching and redness of athlete's foot could complicate and delay appropriate medical care. Topical hydrocortisone by itself is contraindicated in the presence of fungal infections because it may complicate and delay healing. Nor should the pharmacist recommend the use of a nonprescription topical hydrocortisone cream in conjunction with a nonprescription antifungal product to relieve the itching associated with athlete's foot.

Self treatment is effective only if the patient understands the importance of compliance with all facets of the treatment plan. Specific antifungal products must be used appropriately in conjunction with other treatment measures, including general hygienic measures and local drying. Local hygienic measures should not be minimized as a useful adjunct to specific antifungal therapy.

In its final rule for topical antifungal drug products for OTC human use,[18] the FDA agreed with its Advisory Review Panel on Over-the-Counter Antimicrobial Drug Products[19] that, to best serve all consumers, a nonprescription product must provide more than temporary symptomatic relief of athlete's foot and related infections. Such products must contain a Category I antifungal ingredient capable of killing the fungus (Table 3) (see also product table "Athlete's Foot Products"). The panel required each antifungal ingredient to have at least one well-designed clinical trial demonstrating its effectiveness in the treatment of athlete's foot to be classified as Category I.[19]

Clioquinol

Clioquinol has demonstrated efficacy in treating athlete's foot. The FDA classified it as Category I—safe and effective for topical nonprescription use in the treatment of this condition. Evaluations of clioquinol used alone and in combination with hydrocortisone indicate the following effectiveness: clioquinol-hydrocortisone combination > clioquinol alone > hydrocortisone alone > placebo.

Clioquinol has a low incidence of side effects; however, it may cause itching, redness, and irritation. Even though the possibility of its percutaneous absorption is low, clioquinol may interfere with thyroid function tests. Thus, patients undergoing these tests must be questioned carefully to assess their prior use of iodine-containing clioquinol.

Clotrimazole and Miconazole Nitrate

Clotrimazole and miconazole nitrate are imidazole derivatives that demonstrate fungistatic/fungicidal activity (depending upon concentration) against *T mentagrophytes, T rubrum, E floccosum,* and *Candida albicans.* These agents act by inhibiting the biosynthesis of ergosterol and other steroids, and by damaging the fungal cell wall membrane and altering its permeability so that essential intracellular elements may be lost. These drugs have also been shown to inhibit oxidative and peroxidative enzyme activity, which results in intracellular buildup of toxic concentrations of hydrogen peroxide; this may then contribute to the degradation of subcellular organelles and to cellular necrosis. In *C albicans*, these drugs have been shown to inhibit the transformation of blastospores into invasive mycelial form.

Both of these former prescription drugs have been reclassified as nonprescription. Both are suggested for application twice daily, once in the morning and once in the evening. Controlled studies have demonstrated their efficacy for athlete's foot as well as for other kinds of fungal skin infections. (See Chapter 6, "Vaginal and Menstrual Products," and Chapter 26, "Dermatologic Products.") Both would be expected to demonstrate efficacy comparable to that of tolnaftate (see next section) for tinea pedis, and in the event of treatment failure in which patient factors (eg, noncompliance or improper foot hygiene) have been ruled out as a cause, both can be suggested as alternative treatment modalities. Rare cases of mild skin irritation, burning, and stinging have occurred with their use.

Tolnaftate

Tolnaftate has demonstrated clinical efficacy since its commercial introduction into the United States in 1965, and it has become the standard topical antifungal medication. Tolnaftate is the only nonprescription drug approved for both the prevention and treatment of athlete's foot.[18] It acts on typical fungi responsible for tinea pedis, including *T mentagrophytes* and *T rubrum.* It is also effective against *E floccosum* and species of *Microsporum.* Although its exact mechanism of action has not been reported, it is believed that tolnaftate distorts the hyphae and stunts the mycelial growth of the fungi species. Tolnaftate is effective in tinea pedis but not in onychomycosis. For treatment of tinea pedis, concomitant administration of oral griseofulvin, itraconazole, or ketoconazole is often necessary.

Tolnaftate is valuable primarily in the dry, scaly

TABLE 3 FDA-approved topical antifungal drugs for over-the-counter use[a]

Drug	Concentration (%)
Haloprogin	1
Clioquinol	3
Miconazole nitrate	2
Tolnaftate	1
Undecylenic acid and its salts	10–25
Povidone-Iodine	10

[a]*Federal Register.* 1993 Sep 23; 58 (183): 49890–9.

type of athlete's foot. Superficial fungal infection relapse has occurred after tolnaftate therapy has been discontinued. Relapse may be caused by inadequate duration of treatment, patient noncompliance with the medication, or use of tolnaftate when oral griseofulvin or ketoconazole should have been used. Because tolnaftate does not possess antibacterial properties, its value must be viewed with skepticism for use in the soggy, macerated type of athlete's foot in which bacteria are probably involved.

Tolnaftate is well tolerated when applied to intact or broken skin in either exposed or intertriginous areas, although it usually stings slightly when applied. Delayed hypersensitivity reactions to tolnaftate are extremely unlikely. As with all topical medications, however, discontinuation is warranted if irritation, sensitization, or worsening of the skin condition occurs.

Tolnaftate (1% solution, cream, gel, powder, spray powder, or spray liquid) is applied sparingly twice daily after the affected area is cleaned thoroughly. Effective therapy usually takes 2–4 weeks although some individuals (patients with lesions between the toes or on pressure areas of the foot) may require treatment lasting 4–6 weeks. When medication is applied to pressure areas of the foot, where the horny skin layer is thicker than normal, concomitant use of a keratolytic agent (eg, Whitfield's ointment) may be advisable. Neither keratolytic agents nor wet compresses such as aluminum acetate solution (Burow's solution), which promote the healing of oozing lesions, interfere with the efficacy of tolnaftate. If weeping lesions are present, the inflammation should be treated before tolnaftate is applied.

As a cream, tolnaftate is formulated in a polyethylene glycol 400–propylene glycol vehicle. The 1% solution is formulated in polyethylene glycol 400 and may be more effective than the cream. The solution solidifies when exposed to cold, but if allowed to warm, it will liquefy with no loss in potency. These vehicles are particularly advantageous in superficial antifungal therapy because they are nonocclusive, nontoxic, nonsensitizing, water miscible, anhydrous, easy to apply, and efficient in delivering the drug to the affected area.

The topical powder formulation of tolnaftate uses cornstarch-talc as the vehicle. This vehicle not only is an effective drug delivery system but also offers a therapeutic advantage because the two agents retain water. The topical aerosol formulation of tolnaftate includes talc and the propellant vehicle.

Undecylenic Acid-Zinc Undecylenate

This combination is widely used and may be effective for various mild superficial fungal infections, excluding those involving nails or hairy parts of the body. It is fungistatic and effective in mild chronic cases of tinea pedis. Compound undecylenic acid ointment (USP XXI) contains 5% undecylenic acid and 20% zinc undecylenate in an ointment base. It is believed that zinc undecylenate liberates undecylenic acid (the active antifungal entity) on contact with perspiration. In addition, zinc undecylenate has astringent properties because of the presence of the zinc ion; this astringent activity decreases the irritation and inflammation of the infection. The FDA Advisory Review Panel on Over-the-Counter Antimicrobial Drug Products classified undecylenic acid and its derivatives (10–25% total undecylenate content) as Category I for the treatment of athlete's foot.[18]

Applied to the skin as an ointment, diluted solution, or dusting powder, the combination of undecylenic acid-zinc undecylenate is relatively nonirritating, and hypersensitivity reactions are rare. The undiluted solution, however, may cause transient stinging when applied to broken skin because of its isopropyl alcohol content. Caution must be exercised to ensure that these ingredients do not come into contact with the eye or that the powder is not inhaled.

The vehicle in compound undecylenic acid ointment has a water-miscible base, making it nonocclusive, removable with water, and easy to apply. The powder uses talc as its vehicle and absorbent. The aerosol contains menthol, which serves as a counterirritant and antipruritic. The solution contains 10% undecylenic acid in an isopropyl alcohol vehicle with either an applicator or a spray pump container.

The product is applied twice daily after the affected area is cleansed. When the solution is sprayed or applied to the affected area, the area should be allowed to air dry; otherwise, water may accumulate and further macerate the tissue. The relatively high alcohol concentration in these solutions could cause some burning, and the strong odor of undecylenic acid may be objectionable to some patients, possibly promoting patient noncompliance. The usual period required for therapeutic results depends on the severity of the infection. However, if improvement does not occur in 2–4 weeks, the condition should be reevaluated and an alternative medication used.

Salts of Aluminum

Because they do not have any direct antifungal activity, aluminum salts were not included in the final monograph for topical antifungal drug products. However, their effectiveness as astringents and their possible use in athlete's foot merit their inclusion in this chapter. Historically, aluminum acetate has been the foremost astringent used for both the acute, inflammatory type and the wet, soggy type of tinea pedis. Aluminum chloride is also used to treat the wet, soggy type of infection. However, each solution has potential for misuse (accidental childhood poisoning by ingesting the solutions or the solid tablets), and precautions must be taken to prevent this occurrence.

The action and efficacy of the aluminum salts appear to be two-pronged. First, these compounds act as astringents. Their drying ability probably involves the complexing of the astringent agent with proteins, thereby altering the proteins' ability to swell and hold water. Astringents decrease edema, exudation, and inflammation by reducing cell membrane permeability and hardening the cement substance of the capillary epithelium. Second, aluminum salts in concentrations greater than 20% possess antibacterial activity. Aluminum chloride (20%) may exhibit that activity in two ways: by directly killing bacteria and by drying the interspaces. Solutions of 20% aluminum acetate and 20% aluminum chloride demonstrate equal in vitro antibacterial efficacy.

Aluminum acetate for use in tinea pedis is generally diluted with about 10–40 parts of water. Depending on the situation, the patient may immerse the whole foot in the solution for 20 minutes up to three times a day (every 6–8 hours) or may apply the solution to the affected area in the form of a wet dressing.

For patient convenience, aluminum acetate solution (Burow's solution) or modified Burow's solution is available for immediate use in solution or in forms (powder packets, powder, and effervescent tablets) for dilution with water. These products are intended for external use only and should be kept away from contact with the eyes. Prolonged or continuous use of aluminum acetate solution may produce tissue necrosis. In the acute inflammatory state of tinea pedis, this solution should be used for less than 1 week. The pharmacist should instruct the patient to discontinue its use if inflammatory lesions appear or worsen.

Concentrations of 20–30% aluminum chloride have been the most beneficial for the wet, soggy type of athlete's foot.[12] Twice-daily applications are generally used until the signs and symptoms (odor, wetness, and whiteness) abate; after that, once-daily applications control the symptoms. In hot, humid weather, the original condition may return within 7–10 days after the application is stopped.

Aluminum salts do not entirely cure athlete's foot but are useful when combined with other topical antifungal drugs. Application of the aluminum salt merely shifts the disease process back to the simple dry type of athlete's foot, which can then be controlled with other agents such as tolnaftate.

Because aluminum salts penetrate skin poorly, their toxicity, like that of aluminum chloride, is low. However, a few cases of irritation have been reported in patients where deep fissures were present. Thus, the use of concentrated aluminum salt solutions is contraindicated on severely eroded or deeply fissured skin. In such a case, the salts must be diluted to a lower concentration (10% aluminum chloride) for initial treatment.

Other Drugs

Historically, some organic fatty acids (eg, caprylic acid), acetic acid (in the form of triacetin), some phenolic compounds (eg, salicylic acid), quaternary ammonium compounds (eg, benzethonium chloride), and quinoline derivatives (eg, 8-hydroxyquinoline) have been used to treat athlete's foot. However, in the final monograph for topical antifungal drug products, these were not included as safe and effective for self-care purposes. The reader is referred to the 10th edition of the *Handbook of Nonprescription Drugs* for a historical perspective and detailed descriptions of these agents.

Product Ingredients and Formulations

The primary drug delivery systems used in treating tinea pedis are creams, solutions, and powders. Powders, including those in aerosol product forms, generally are indicated for adjunctive use with solutions and creams. In very mild conditions, powders may suffice as the only therapy.

Solution and cream forms should be formulated in a vehicle that is:

- Nonocclusive because any moisture or sweat that is retained exacerbates the condition;
- Anhydrous because including water in the formulation introduces a variable that is one of the primary causes of the condition;
- Spreadable with minimal effort and without water;
- Water miscible or water washable (ie, removable with minimal cleansing efforts) because hard scrubbing of the affected area further abrades the skin;
- Nonsensitizing and nontoxic when applied to intact or denuded skin because it may be absorbed into the systemic circulation;
- Capable of efficient drug delivery (ie, it must not interact with the active ingredient but should allow that ingredient to penetrate to the seat of the fungal infection).

Most vehicles used to deliver topical solutions and creams are polyethylene glycol and alcohols, which meet these criteria. Polyethylene glycol bases deliver water-insoluble drugs topically and do it more efficiently than other water-soluble bases. This ability to deliver water-insoluble drugs is an added advantage because most topical antifungal drugs (eg, tolnaftate) are largely water insoluble.

Criteria for the powder form (shaker or aerosol) are basically the same as those for creams and solutions. Certain agents in powder forms (talc and cornstarch) are therapeutic and also serve as vehicles. Powders inhibit the propagation of fungi by adsorbing moisture and preventing skin maceration; thus, they actually alter the ecologic conditions of the fungi. The adsorbing material within the powder, rather than the intended active ingredient, may be responsible for much of the disease remission.

Many authorities consider cornstarch superior to talc for these formulations. This is because cornstarch is virtually free of chemical contamination and does not tend to produce granulomatous reactions in wounds as readily as talc. Moreover, cornstarch adsorbs 25 times more moisture from moisture-saturated air than talc.

Product Selection Guidelines

Patient compliance is influenced by product selection. Therefore, the pharmacist should recommend an appropriate drug and product form designed to cause the least interference with daily habits and activities without sacrificing efficacy. Product selection should be geared to the individual patient. For example, elderly patients may require a preparation that is easy to use; obese patients, in whom excessive sweating may contribute to the disease, should use topical talcum powders as adjunctive therapy.

Under certain patient circumstances, it may be necessary for the pharmacist to instruct the caregiver rather than the patient in the proper use of foot products.

Before recommending a nonprescription product, the pharmacist should review the patient's medical history. For example, persons with diabetes should have their blood glucose levels moderately controlled because increased glucose in perspiration may promote fungal growth. Patients with allergic dermatitides usually have a history of asthma, hay fever, or atopic dermatitis and thus are extremely sensitive to most oral and topical agents. By acquiring a good history, the pharmacist may be able to distinguish a tinea infection from atopic dermatitis and avoid recommending a product that may cause skin irritation.

The pharmacist should bear in mind that prescription drugs may sometimes be more beneficial than nonprescription products. In the soggy, macerated athlete's foot complicated by bacterial infection, the broad-spectrum antifungal agents (eg, econazole nitrate) are preferable to both tolnaftate and the prescription drug haloprogin.

The pharmacist should also bear in mind that product line extensions that have the same brand name do not necessarily have the same active ingredient(s). For example, the cream and solution formulations of Lotrimin AF contain clotrimazole, 1%, whereas the topical spray and powder formulations contain miconazole nitrate, 2%. In the case of the spray and powder formulations, it is prohibitively expensive for the manufacturer to pursue a new drug application that would be necessary to market these products with clotrimazole, 1%, as their active ingredient. It is more economically prudent to market them with an active ingredient that has already received FDA approval. Similarly, Desenex Maximum Strength Antifungal cream contains miconazole nitrate, 2%, whereas the traditional Desenex Cream contains undecylenic acid and zinc undecylenate in a 25% concentration.

Patient Education and Counseling

Pharmacists should advise patients not to expect dramatic remission of the condition. The onset of symptomatic relief may take several days. Patients should also be advised that, depending on certain factors (eg, the extent of the affected area and variable patient response to medication), medication should be used for a minimum of 2–4 weeks, as recommended by the FDA advisory panel.[18] If there is no improvement by then, the patient should consult a physician. Patients should also be told of the necessity to adhere strictly to the physician-prescribed dosage regimen or to the directions for use on the product label. Patient noncompliance contributes significantly to the failure of topical products in treating tinea pedis. Pharmacists may advise patients or caregivers to continue the medication for a few days beyond the recommended time to decrease the risk of relapse.

All topical antifungal products may induce various hypersensitivity reactions. Although the incidence of hypersensitivity is small, patients should be advised to discontinue the product if itching, swelling, or exacerbation of the disease occurs. In addition, patients should avoid contact of the product with the eyes. After applying the product, patients should thoroughly wash their hands with soap and water.

Pharmacists should inform patients of the need for adjunctive protective measures that assist the topical antifungal product in eradicating the fungal infection. They should emphasize the need for proper hygiene before effective drug therapy can begin. The feet should be cleansed with soap and water and thoroughly patted dry each day. However, patients should be cautioned against overzealous cleansing and drying between the toes so as not to further irritate the area. Patients should have their own washcloths and towels. After bathing, the feet should be dried last so the towel does not spread the infection to other sites, and they should be kept as dry as possible during the day.

General measures should be taken to eliminate the predisposing factors of heat and perspiration. Shoes and light cotton socks that allow ventilation should be worn. Wool and some synthetic fabrics interfere with foot moisture dissipation. Occlusive footwear, including canvas, leather, or rubber-soled athletic shoes, should not be worn for prolonged periods. Shoes should be alternated as often as possible so that the inside can adequately dry, and they should be dusted with medicated or unmedicated foot powders. Socks should be changed daily and washed thoroughly after use.

Contaminated clothing and towels should be laundered well in hot water. The feet, particularly the area between the toes, should be dusted with a medicated or unmedicated drying powder at every change of socks. Whenever possible, the feet should be aired to prevent moisture buildup. Cotton balls or Dr Scholl's Smooth Touch Pedi-spreads may be placed between the tips of the toes to keep the web spaces open and less moist. Pencil erasers have sometimes been recommended for this purpose, but they may contain sensitizing accelerators or antioxidants. Nonocclusive protective footwear (eg, rubber or wooden sandals) may be worn in areas of family or public use, such as home bathrooms or community showers.

Individuals whose feet perspire excessively may find odor-controlling insoles (eg, Odor Attackers and Sneaker Snuffers) useful for casual dress or sports activities. These insoles absorb moisture and prevent the growth of odor-causing bacteria. They also provide some support and cushioning for the feet. Patients must be advised, however, to change insoles routinely every 3–4 months or more often if the condition warrants.

More than 18 million adult Americans (70% women) suffer from nail fungus (tinea unguium). This condition can be very embarrassing because it can cause nails to become discolored, rough, and thick. For those patients who complain about unsightly finger- or toenails as a result of nail fungus, there is no approved nonprescription treatment. However, patients can use Fungal Nail Revitalizer, which is intended to reduce nail discoloration and smooth out the thick, rough nail. This product contains calcium carbonate and urea to debride nail tissue. The patient applies the cream over the entire surface of the infected nail, scrubs this for at least 1 minute with the provided nailbrush, and then washes and dries the nail completely. For optimum results, this procedure should be done daily for 3 weeks.

Tired, Aching Feet

It is estimated that two thirds of Americans suffer from tired, aching feet, the most common foot problem. People simply do not realize the daily abuse their feet must endure. With every step taken (repeated, on average, between 8 and 10,000 times each day), gravity-induced pressure of up to twice the body's weight bears down on each foot, releasing powerful shocks of energy that the foot's natural padding must struggle to absorb. In an unpadded shoe, the shock as the foot strikes the ground is absorbed throughout the foot, ankle, leg, and back. This shock can fatigue muscles, resulting in tired, aching feet and/or back pain.

The first way to avoid tired, aching feet is to use well-fitted footwear that has sufficient padding and cushioning. However, this might not be enough for active people or for those who must stand for prolonged periods during the day. Further, some active individuals prefer to wear shoes that look stylish rather than are orthopedic. Unfortunately, many stylish shoe models are not built to provide adequate support and cushioning; however, various shoe inserts are available to enhance the comfort of most well-fitting shoes.

Full shoe inserts, which can provide cushioning and absorb shock, are available in a variety of sizes and thicknesses to accommodate most individuals. Advanced shoe inserts are now available with enhanced shock-absorbing capability. For example, Back Guard is clinically proven to decrease the incidence of lower back pain associated with shock from walking. The person who is selecting an insert must realize that the insert should conform to the type of shoe worn. Thus, since a thick shoe insert may alter the fit of a woman's pump, a thin insole would be preferable.

Partial insoles are preferred when cushioning or support is desired in a certain portion of the shoe. For example, metatarsal arch supports, which fit into the ball-of-foot region of a woman's shoe, help lift the arch behind the toes to alleviate pain associated with the spreading of the foot, a condition that occurs with increasing age. For those women who wear high-heeled shoes, inserts (ie, Toe Squish Preventer cushions) are available to prevent the toes from becoming cramped in the pointed-toe box. A final example is the arch support insert intended to cushion and support painful longitudinal arches.

Twenty-one million adults are estimated to suffer from heel pain. The cause of heel pain is difficult to determine, which can make treatment prolonged and expensive. Depending on the location and extent of the pain, a heel cup or heel cushion may be indicated. For example, a heel cushion might be appropriate when the pain is confined to the bottom of the heel. The cushion can support the entire heel as it elevates the sensitive area to prevent further irritation. Alternatively, when the pain is widespread and diffuse, a heel cup might be more appropriate. Heel cups help relieve the pain caused by the breakdown of the heel's natural padding or intense athletic activity. Heel cups and cushions should be made of a lightweight, nonslip material that easily fits into any shoe, including athletic shoes.

Other Potentially Serious Conditions

It is important for the pharmacist to realize that selected chronic diseases predispose certain patients to foot problems. Most noteworthy is the diabetic patient in whom poor circulation and diminished limb sensitivity exist. These factors make this patient especially vulnerable to infectious foot problems. Other vulnerable patients include those with peripheral circulatory disease or arthritis. The pharmacist can identify these patients by asking appropriate questions about daily medication use or reviewing the patient's drug profile. Typical drug use patterns for high-risk patients include insulin, oral sulfonylureas, drugs for circulation (eg, cyclandelate, isoxsuprine, nylidrin, papaverine, and pentoxifylline), and drugs for arthritic conditions (eg, aspirin and nonsteroidal anti-inflammatory drugs [NSAIDs]).

Pharmacists are also in a position to advise patients with or without chronic conditions on self-treatment and prevention of ingrown toenails—a common foot problem. Frostbite—a less frequent but nonetheless potentially serious condition that often involves the feet—is another area in which pharmacists can educate patients and consumers about preventive measures.

Diabetes Mellitus

See Chapter 18, "Diabetes Care Products and Monitoring Devices," for a discussion of potentially serious foot disorders in persons with diabetes and of the proper way to care for the diabetic foot.

Poor Circulation

Patients with poor circulation of the feet and legs may complain of persistent and unusual feelings of cold, numbness, tingling, burning, or fatigue. Other symptoms may include discolored skin, dry skin, absence of hair on the feet or legs, or a cramping or tightness in the leg muscles. The most discriminating questions a pharmacist can ask this type of patient are (1) Do you experience aching in your calves when you walk? and (2) Do you have to hang your feet over the edge of the bed during sleep to relieve the soreness in your calves? A yes response to either question warrants referring the patient to a physician or podiatrist.

If a patient complains of coldness in only one foot, there may be a possible blockage (clot) of circulation to the foot. Sometimes the involved foot or lower leg will appear physically larger than the other, be red or waxy in appearance, have no hair growth on the toes, and exhibit thickened nails. If a review of the patient's medication history does not indicate the use of medications intended to relieve these symptoms, the patient with suspected circulatory problems should be advised to consult a physician or podiatrist for evaluation.

A daily footbath is a simple measure that will assist these patients. After the foot is patted dry, an emollient foot cream can be applied to aid in retaining moisture and pliability. The footbath also will soften brittle toenails for clipping and filing. The feet should be kept warm and moderately exercised every day.

Arthritis

Arthritic patients are also vulnerable to foot problems. Osteoarthritis is a noninflammatory, degenerative joint disease that occurs primarily in older people. Degeneration of the articular cartilage and changes in the bone result in a loss of resilience and a decrease in the skeleton's shock absorption capability. This condition, however, is also experienced by individuals in their late teens and early twenties as a secondary complication of a previous athletic injury. This might be evidenced by the development of hallux limitus or rigidus of the big toe (ie, a stiff toe or painful flexion of the big toe due to stiffness and spur formation in the metatarsophalangeal joint). Subsequently, these patients have a lot of difficulty with their shoes not fitting properly. They may also develop an osteoarthritic condition in the ankle joint. Referral to an orthopedic physician or podiatrist is appropriate.

Proper foot care is especially important for arthritic patients. These patients should wear properly fitted shoes, pad their shoes with insoles to protect their feet from the shock of hard surfaces, and undergo regular podiatric or medical examinations.

Ingrown Toenails

An ingrown toenail occurs when a section of nail presses into the soft tissue of the nail groove. The nail curves into the flesh of the toe corners and becomes embedded in the surrounding soft tissue of the toe, causing pain. Swelling, inflammation, and ulceration are secondary complications that can arise from this condition.

The frequent cause of ingrown toenails is incorrect trimming of the nails. The correct method is to cut the nail straight across without tapering the corners in any way. Nails that are left sharp or jagged-edged grow outward and eventually become embedded in the soft lip tissue of the nail bed. This results in microtears of the skin which, when coupled with invasion by opportunistic resident foot bacteria, can cause a superficial infection. Wearing pointed-toe or tight shoes, as well as hosiery that is too tight, has also been implicated. In these instances, direct pressure can force the lateral edge of the nail into the soft tissue, where the embedded nail may then continue to grow. Bedridden patients may develop ingrown toenails because tight bedcovers press the soft skin tissue against the nails. Nail curling, which can be hereditary or secondary to either incorrect nail trimming or a systemic, metabolic disease, can also result in ingrown toenails. Psoriatic arthritis is such a disease whose presence may be demonstrated in the nail.

Education is probably the best way to prevent the development of ingrown toenails. In the early stages of development, therapy is directed at providing adequate room for the nail to resume its normal position adjacent to soft tissue. This is accomplished by relieving the external source of pressure and applying medications that will harden the nail groove or help shrink the soft tissue. The patient should be referred to a podiatrist or physician if the condition is recurrent or gives rise to an oozing discharge, pain, or severe inflammation. Sometimes surgery is warranted, and even with subsequent systemic antibiotic therapy, the toe may take up to 3–4 weeks to heal.

Based on evidence currently available, the FDA in its final rule for ingrown toenail relief products did not propose any OTC active ingredient for ingrown toenail relief as safe and effective and not misbranded.[20] Thus, previously approved drugs, tannic acid and sodium sulfide,[21] were classified as Category III and withdrawn from the market.

The pharmacist, however, must be aware of brand name product reformulations to accommodate this rule. For example, Outgro Pain-Relieving Formula, which formerly contained tannic acid for the treatment of ingrown toenails, now contains benzocaine, 20%, for the relief of pain associated with ingrown toenails.

Patients with ingrown toenails often fail to realize that they may also be helped by oral medication intended to allay pain and inflammation. The pharmacist may recommend aspirin, ibuprofen, ketoprofen, or naproxen, four proven analgesics with anti-inflammatory activity, provided there are no contraindications to their use for a particular patient. (See Chapter 4, "Internal Analgesic and Antipyretic Products.")

Frostbite

Frostbite is defined as the actual freezing of tissues by excessive exposure to low temperatures. To maintain normal core temperature in cold weather, the body reflexly reduces the flow of blood to the skin surface and the extremities. Therefore, frostbite usually involves areas of the body (eg, feet, hands, earlobes, nose, and cheeks) that are the farthest from deep organs or large muscles. Minor frostbite may cause only blanching of the skin; severe frostbite may result in the loss of fingers and toes.

Predisposing factors to the development of frostbite include:

- Low temperatures (especially with high winds);
- Long periods of exposure to cold;
- Lack of proper clothing;
- Wet clothing;
- Poor nutrition, exhaustion, dehydration, and/or smoking;
- Circulatory disease;
- Immobility;
- Direct contact with metal or petroleum products at low temperatures;
- Individual susceptibility to cold.

Frostbite is not amenable to therapy with nonprescription drug products. The frostbitten part should be promptly and thoroughly rewarmed in water heated to 104–108°F (45.6–47.8°C). The water should *not* be hot to a normal hand at room temperature and should *not* be tested with the frozen part. The container of water should be large enough for the frozen part to move freely without bumping against the sides. Rewarming should be continued until a flush returns to the most distal tip of the thawed part. This usually takes about 20–30 minutes. Dry heat (eg, a heating pad) should be avoided because it is difficult to control the temperature and rewarm the frozen part evenly; overapplication of heat could actually burn the skin without the patient being aware. Once the injured part has been properly warmed, it should be soaked for about 20 minutes in a whirlpool bath once or twice daily until the healing process is complete.

The best treatment for frostbite is prevention; pharmacists should be able to provide a few simple rules to follow:

- Dress to maintain body warmth, taking into account the face, neck, and head as well as the extremities.
- Avoid exposure to cold during times of sickness or exhaustion.
- Do not exceed the body's tolerance to cold exposure.
- Avoid tight-fitting garments; dress with layered clothing.
- Wear clothing that allows ventilation and prevents perspiration buildup (water enhances heat loss).
- Wear insulated boots or shoes and socks (preferably wool) that fit snugly but are not tight in spots.
- Wear mittens instead of gloves in severe cold; the thumb should be with the rest of the fingers and not by itself.
- Never touch objects (especially cold metal or petroleum products) that facilitate heat loss.

When given the opportunity, the pharmacist should seek to correct a few misconceptions. It is dangerous to rub the affected area with ice or snow even though it seems to provide warmth; this can result in prolonged contact with the cold, and the ice crystals may lacerate cells. In addition, persons should refrain from drinking alcohol for "antifreeze" purposes, at least until they are in a warm place. Alcohol can induce a loss of body heat even though it may give the person a feeling of warmth when ingested. Finally, frostbite victims should avoid smoking. Nicotine can induce peripheral vasoconstriction and further reduce the blood supply to the frostbitten extremity. Thus, it would also seem prudent to forewarn individuals who want to stop smoking and are taking Nicorette (ie, nicotine polacrilex) or using one of the topical transdermal nicotine patches (Habitrol, Nicoderm, Nicotrol, or ProStep) that they should avoid excessive exposure to the cold. (See Chapter 36, "Smoking Cessation Products.")

Exercise-Induced Foot Problems

The pharmacist should be aware of the problem of exercise-induced foot injuries, particularly those caused by running, jogging, or other high-impact physical activities (Figure 4). Often, in their rush to recapture physical fitness, individuals fail to take certain precautions and dive headlong into a strenuous exercise program. Yet jogging, aerobic dance, and running are not without risk; one study documented that several exercise enthusiasts have died from heart attacks while jogging.[22] Some people, especially those over 35 years of age, should consult a physician before embarking on a fitness program. So, too, should patients with high blood pressure or a family history of heart disease or diabetes. Ultimately, a vigorous walking program may be a more prudent form of exercise for middle-aged, unconditioned individuals than jogging or running, and it may minimize potential orthopedic problems incurred from those more strenuous forms of exercise.

Specific Injuries

Shin Splints

The term *shin splint* is used generically by some to describe all the pain emanating from below the knee and above the ankle. Shin splints are an overuse phenomenon that occurs in runners or walkers who use hard surfaces. This condition may also occur from running on a banked track or on the sloped shoulder of a road, wearing improper footwear, or overstriding.

The typical complaint of a runner with shin splints is pain in the medial lower third of the shin that seems to increase gradually with exercise. The patient may admit that soreness begins after running; with a continual running program, the pain will eventually occur during and after running. Complaints of pain when walking or climbing stairs may also indicate a serious case of shin splints. If the discomfort is located on the anterior lateral aspect of the skin; is described as a cramping, burning tightness; and repeatedly occurs at the same distance or time during a run, self-treatment may be ill-advised and the runner should be referred to a physician, podiatrist, or physical therapist.

Rest and application of ice (eg, an ice bag or a cold compression wrap) to the painful area are good initial treatments. The cold anesthetizes the area and affects a decrease in pain. It is best to alternate compresses (10 minutes applied, 10 minutes off). To ensure greater contact with the injured part, the patient should be advised to use crushed or shaved ice. Aspirin or ibuprofen can also be used to relieve pain and reduce tissue inflammation. However, the use of analgesics to suppress pain or increase endurance during a workout is not recommended.

Stress Fracture

Stress fracture, also known as march, army, or fatigue fracture, may be encountered in runners, especially those who run repetitively on hard, inflexible surfaces. This injury usually involves the long bones of the foot or leg. It is not an overt break of the bone but rather an alteration in the architecture of the normal bone.

The onset of pain is associated with runners who drastically change aspects of their training routine (eg, running surface, speed, or distance). Although the pain begins insidiously, the person suffering from a stress fracture will often complain of deep pain in the lower leg with an area of extreme tenderness. A misconception among runners is that they can "work out" the problem by continuing to jog. Individuals must be instructed that pain is the body's communication mechanism to indicate that enough is enough and that something is abnormal.

Treatment for stress fractures is complete rest from running, sometimes for 4–6 weeks, or longer if the tibia is involved.

Achilles Tendinitis

Running on hills or the beach, wearing improper footwear (eg, running and jogging in shoes designed for racquet sports), and moving with excessive pronation (rolling in of the feet) are common causes of Achilles tendinitis. Yet this condition is not caused solely by running, and it may be an early sign of arthritis or rupture of a tendon; the exact cause of the problem is difficult to distinguish. Thus, Achilles tendinitis should be referred to a physician, podiatrist, or physical therapist.

By definition, Achilles tendinitis is a painful inflammation about the Achilles tendon. However, it may not show the classic signs of inflammation such as pain, erythema, increased skin temperature, or swelling. Typical symptoms are posterior heel pain, which is worse in the morning when getting out of bed, at the beginning of an exercise session, and when walking after prolonged sitting.

The best treatment is prevention with careful progression of training and replacement of worn footwear. Bony malalignments leading to excessive pronation should be accounted for with orthotic therapy. An orthotic device approximately positions the foot. The properties of shoe inserts (eg, flexible or rigid) vary; the choice of insert should be based on specific treatment objectives. Shoe inserts can be custom-made or purchased off the shelf. Arch supports are intended to provide buttressing for the foot.

Symptomatic self-treatment may consist of rest, new shoes, ice applications, appropriate NSAID use, physician-prescribed temporary heel lifts, and careful calf-stretching exercises.

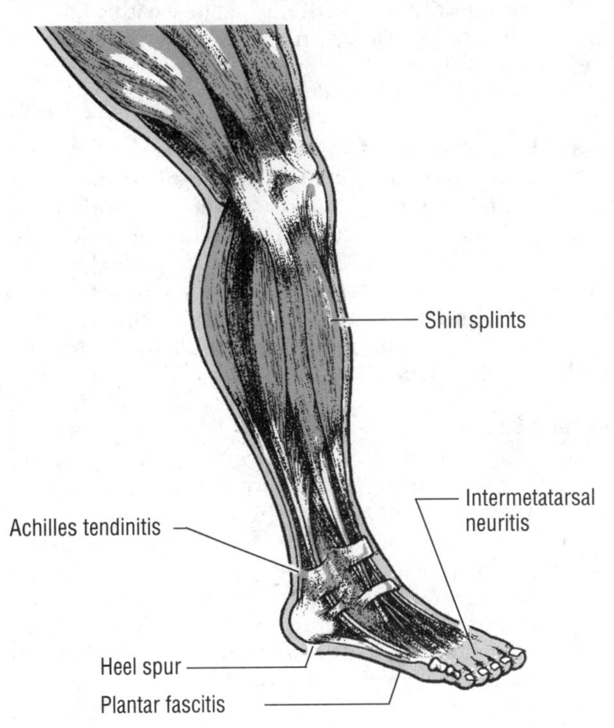

FIGURE 4 Selected foot and leg injuries associated with excessive impact shock.

Blisters

Ill-fitting footwear and inappropriate hosiery can often cause or contribute to the development of blisters. When shoes are worn while running, the shoe can place excessive pressure on a specific area of the skin between the stratum corneum and stratum lucidum. Fluid quickly accumulates at this site, often on the heel, the ball of the foot, and the ends or tops of the toes. Running barefoot can also cause blisters.

Again, prevention is the key to treating blisters. Cotton or woolen socks are preferred for running. The runner can wear two pairs of socks with ordinary talcum powder sprinkled between them. Some individuals with soft skin will continue to suffer from blisters until their skin toughens enough to withstand friction during running. Application of compound tincture of benzoin or of a flexible collodion product (eg, New Skin) will help toughen the skin.

Ankle Sprains

The typical mechanism of lateral ligament injury to the ankle is through rotation of the body over the fixed foot. This occurs most often in contact sports in which the foot remains stationary while the body is unintentionally rotated. The incidence of ankle sprains during jogging and running is low because runners usually do not take sharp diagonal cuts. However, stepping on an unnoticed stone or curb edge may also result in an ankle sprain.

The differential diagnosis of an ankle fracture from a sprained ankle is impossible without an x-ray. The immediate treatment of an ankle sprain involves applying a compressive bandage or wrap, elevating the ankle, and applying ice. If possible, the ankle should be bound with a wet elastic wrap while the cold is being applied; the wet wrap facilitates temperature transfer so that the ankle benefits most from the cold application. The recovery process can be made easier if the ankle is in a dorsiflexed position (foot toward the nose) when it is wrapped in the elastic bandage. Consistent with all sprains, including those of the neck and lower back, the use of alternating cold applications should continue for 24–72 hours, depending on injury severity.

Ice, compression, elevation (ICE) therapy is well accepted as the most appropriate immediate treatment for an ankle sprain. It remains controversial whether cold application without elevation is helpful or harmful. Regardless, treatment for a sprained ankle should be initiated as soon as possible. Sometimes an ankle sprain is perceived as a minor problem, even by trained professionals; however, the severity of the ligament damage can vary widely, and an extensive ligament rupture that has been given insufficient treatment may result in a permanently unstable ankle.

Intermetatarsal Neuritis

Intermetatarsal neuritis is characterized by pain and numbness between the toes, most often within the third interspace. The cause is linked to the foot jamming forward into the shoe without enough space to accommodate the foot. Nerves become inflamed when compressed or caught in the area between the metatarsal heads and digital bases.

The solution is correct-fitting shoes with the addition of a metatarsal pad or orthotic device. Lacing of the shoe can be modified by skipping the bottom two eyelets; this provides additional room for the ball of the foot.

Toenail Loss

Blisters under the toenail occur as a result of not keeping the toenails trimmed and of running in poorly fitted shoes. Long toenails catch on the sock or inside the shoe toe box, particularly when the individual is running downhill. This lifts the nail and separates it from the nail bed, and blood accumulates under the nail. This condition is very painful and can result in the temporary loss of the toenail.

Runner's Bunion

Bunion deformity and pain can increase in size. Management of the bunion should address the cause, such as tight-fitting or high-heeled shoes, excessive pronation, or a previous injury. Thus, self-treatment includes properly fitted shoes, a wide toe box, avoidance of high-heeled shoes, and protective padding, as well as appropriate anti-inflammatory drug therapy. If shoe adjustments fail to alleviate pain, referral to a properly trained health care professional is indicated.

Heel Pain

Heel pain in runners is a common and insidious injury. The common diagnosis is plantar fascitis and/or heel spur. The cause is excessive running or rapid gain in body weight. Like Achilles tendinitis, heel pain can be an early sign of systemic arthritis. The pain is worse when getting out of bed in the morning or when standing up after sitting.

Self-treatment includes replacing worn shoes or heel pads, using a night splint,[23] strapping or taping the arch, decreasing the amount of weight-bearing activity, and, if necessary, entering a weight reduction program. Anti-inflammatory treatment, including ice applications, is appropriate. When self-treatment fails, referral to an appropriate health care professional for evaluation of possible bony malalignments and possible orthotic therapy is indicated.

Treatment

The pharmacist may be called upon to play a triage role in treating an exercise-induced injury to the foot; that is, the pharmacist may have to decide whether to advise a self-treatment program or to refer the patient to a physician or podiatrist. The pharmacist must make this decision by asking the questions that are listed at the beginning of this chapter.

Responses to questions may indicate that the person has had a number of continuous days of high-intensity workouts. Because continual strenuous workouts cause accumulated fatigue and microtrauma, it is essential that the body be allowed to recuperate after vigorous exercise. Although some runners believe that the more mileage logged per week, the better their running ability, the incidence of acquired injuries among runners increases dramatically after 25–30 miles per week. An increased injury rate is also observed in runners who increase mileage too rapidly. A good training program entails "hard-easy" days, with extended mileage on 3 or 4 days per week and light, easy workouts on the remaining days.

If the runner or jogger has an injured leg or foot, that activity must occasionally be interrupted to allow the injured leg or foot to rest. Relative rest (ie, avoiding activities that produce the symptoms) is often indicated, but some runners resist this suggestion. The pharmacist should encourage alternative exercise modes, such as swimming or bicycling (stationary or outdoor), which would allow the serious runner to maintain aerobic conditioning despite missing regular exercise.

Preventive Measures

Prevention is the best way to treat foot problems. This entails the use of proper footwear, running surface, and running posture (ie, running erect). Most running injuries can be successfully treated with shoe modifications, in-shoe supports, correction for leg length discrepancies, modified training methods, ice applications, and stretching exercises.[24]

Proper Footwear

Shoes can be a powerful tool for manipulating human movement and can greatly influence the healing of injured tissues in both positive and negative ways.

The importance of appropriate footwear has been reported by McPoil et al.[25] These authors demonstrated that a well-designed shoe, even without an orthotic, can favorably alter the center-of-pressure recordings in individuals with foot deformities. Conversely, inappropriate shoes may be problematic, as observed by Frey et al,[26] who reported that a majority of the women surveyed indicated that they wore shoes too small for their feet and had foot pain with deformity.

A hallmark of the fitness shoe industry and the sports medicine community for decades has been that "good shoes can prevent injuries." Annually, shoe manufacturers modify their shoes with high-tech features purported to prevent injury. Unfortunately, there is little evidence to support these claims. It is interesting to note that there has been little or no change in the frequency and type of running injuries since 1977; a similar percentage of runners reported injuries in 1977 as in 1987,[27] and the types of injuries reported were also similar. This is despite the fact that running shoes have supposedly improved every year.

Shoe Store Selection There are several things an individual can do when selecting shoes. Simply stated, the first is to identify the right shoe store and the second is to find the right salesperson. There is probably a greater likelihood of finding a knowledgeable shoe salesperson in an independently owned and operated store than in a department store, discount store, or mail-order house. This usually means a higher price, but individuals with special needs should seek special service when searching for shoes. The owner or manager would be expected to be the most knowledgeable salesperson. The Prescription Footwear Association in Columbia, Md, has a certification process for shoe sales personnel (Pedorthist) and can provide a list of members.

Shoe Fit Two primary factors necessary to achieve proper shoe fit are shape and size. Proper fit is achieved when the shoe shape is matched to the foot shape. For example, an individual with a foot shaped inward like a pigeon's should use a shoe shaped inward, whereas an individual with a foot shaped like a duck's should select a shoe shaped outward.

A person's shoe size is determined by the person's foot length (based on longest foot, longest toe), arch length (the metatarsal head should be at the metatarsal break of the shoe), and foot width (comfortable at the first metatarsal joint and heel snug without lacing). The depth (vertical height) of the toe box is critical for individuals with abnormalities of toes or those requiring orthotics or padding. Extra-depth shoes, comfort shoes, and athletic shoes have similar depth.[28] Steel toe caps diminish the depth of the toe box and can be placed outside the shoe.

Related Issues Shoe manufacturers offer various types of shoes for different activities (eg, running, walking, racquetball sports). Injuries and problems often develop when sport-specific shoes are used for the inappropriate activity; for example, the heel on tennis shoes is too low for jogging. Cross-training shoes are an attempt to provide features generic to many athletic activities. Pharmacists should advise individuals to use proper equipment to prevent sport-related injuries.

Shoes are designed to provide stability and cushioning. Thus, as soon as a shoe becomes worn, it should be replaced. Studies on running shoes have demonstrated that the midsole of the shoe, which helps to reduce the impact on the foot by cushioning or absorbing shock, is the part of the shoe that fatigues first. Midsoles constructed of ethyl vinyl acetate or polyurethane lose 50% of their ability to attenuate force in as little as 250–500 miles of running.[29] Individuals with a history of stress fractures, osteoarthritis, or rigid high arches should not wait until the outer sole wears through before replacing shoes. It is wise to replace shoes early and often.

The Running Surface

The convenience, safety, and preferences of the runner often dictate the running surface (eg, concrete sidewalk, grassy surface, or dirt shoulder of roads). Because hard surfaces have no give and provide little shock-absorbing capacity, they cause intense shock to the legs, feet, and back; grassy surfaces, on the other hand, are often irregular, and the runner can easily incur a sprained ankle. Running on a sloping or banked surface may cause the foot to rotate excessively and may place additional stress on the tendons and ligaments of the leg and foot. Uphill running places a strain on the Achilles tendon and muscles of the lower back; downhill running places a lot of impact on the heel. The ideal running surface is relatively smooth, level, and resilient.

The ideal surface for a walker should also be relatively smooth, level, and resilient. Hard, inflexible surfaces should be avoided as much as possible. A walker who wants to increase energy expenditure may try walking on dirt or sand; these surfaces can boost energy expenditure by as much as one third. Similarly, walking on a mild, 14-degree slope requires more muscle power than walking on a straight, flat surface. However, walkers who become overzealous on these surfaces, can encounter the same problems (eg, sprained ankle) that runners encounter.

Patient Education and Consultation

A pharmacist can play an integral role in educating the exercise enthusiast, even if the pharmacist is not an enthusiast of that particular sport.

Hydration is crucial for joggers and runners, especially in summer when perspiration can effect a loss of body water. The runner is advised to drink 6–8 oz of water before a workout. If participating in runs of 5 km or greater, the runner should drink 6–8 oz of water every 20 minutes or about every 2.5 miles of running. In summer, joggers and runners should not overindulge in fluids but should attempt to keep the mouth moist. These athletes should avoid using salt (sodium chloride) tablets because they can induce an electrolyte imbalance by increasing potassium loss in perspiration.

When self-treatment is appropriate, the pharmacist can assist the patient in selecting nonprescription drugs (eg, aspirin, ibuprofen, or topical antibiotic ointments) and can make recommendations for their administration. Information and instructions about aspirin and nonprescription NSAID use are found elsewhere in this book (see Chapter 4, "Internal Analgesic and Antipyretic Products"), as is similar material about topical anti-infective ointments (see Chapter 26, "Dermatologic Products"). The pharmacist can also assist in selecting prescription accessories (eg, a compression ice wrap, ice bags, Ace bandages, arch supports, or heel cushions) that will alleviate injuries or problems. However, it is important to review some points about ice bags and cold wraps.

If an ice bag is used, the English type, which is identified by its commercial cloth material, is preferred because the patient does not have to wrap a towel around it to protect the skin. The ice should be broken into walnut-sized pieces with no jagged edges and should fill the bag to about one-half to two-thirds capacity. If the bag is overfilled, it will be difficult to apply because it will not rest on the contour of the body area. Once the bag has been filled, trapped air should be squeezed out, the outside dried, and the bag checked for leaks. The bag should then be applied to the specific body area. Usually, the ice should be replaced every 2–4 hours, depending on patient preference. Alternate applications (10 minutes applied, 10 minutes off) up to three to four times per day are suggested to avoid tissue damage. Because maximal swelling from an ankle sprain occurs within 48 hours of the injury, patients should continue applying ice for 2–3 days. Unfortunately, many people do not continue ice application for this long because it is inconvenient to do so and the ankle starts to feel a little better. After the ice bag is used, the patient should be encouraged to drain it and allow it to air dry. If possible, the bag should be turned inside out for more efficient drying. After this, the cap should be placed on the bag and the whole accessory stored in a cool, dry place.

Cold wraps are also useful for cold application. These can be either one-use products (eg, Faultless Instant Cold Pack) or those intended for multiple use. The patient activates the one-use product by squeezing the middle of the pack to burst the bubble, which initiates an endothermic reaction of ammonium nitrate, water, and special additives. Reusable products consist of a cold pack or gel pack that is stored in the freezer and a cloth cover that is kept at room temperature. Once placed in the freezer, the cold pack will reach optimal temperature within 2 hours. The patient removes the cold pack from the freezer, inserts it in the cloth cover, and applies it to the specific body area. The patient should be instructed that the cold pack should not be uncomfortable; if it is, it should be removed for a minute or two and then reapplied. After use, the cold pack is stored again in the freezer. Although some gel packs are nontoxic, all cold packs should be kept out of the reach of children.

Typically, an Ace bandage is used for an ankle sprain or knee sprain. However, the pharmacist must consider whether the patient will understand how to use the bandage in conjunction with an ice application so that additional damage is not incurred. If there is reason to believe the patient may cause further injury with a compression bandage through inappropriate use, the pharmacist should just recommend elevating the body part and applying an ice pack or, if warranted by the severity of the injury, consulting a physician.

If an Ace bandage is to be used, the width of bandage needed depends on the injury site. For example, a foot or an ankle requires a 2.5- to 3-in. bandage. At the time of purchase, the pharmacist should review with the patient the correct procedure for wrapping, which is also described on the bandage package. The patient should be advised to unwind about 12–18 in. of bandage at a time and to allow the bandage to relax. After the bandage is unwound, it can be soaked in water: when applied with ice, a wet elastic bandage facilitates the transfer of cold. The injured area should then be wrapped by overlapping the previous layer of bandage by about one third to one half its width. The point most distal from the ankle—that is, just above the toes—should be tightly wrapped, with decreasing tightness as the bandage is wrapped upward toward and past the ankle. Foot circulation should not be impaired (ie, cold toes). The patient should assess the degree of discomfort after wrapping the injury. If the bandage feels tight or uncomfortable, it should be removed and rewrapped. After use, it should be washed—not scrubbed—in lukewarm, soapy water; thoroughly rinsed; allowed to air dry on a flat surface; and then rolled to prevent wrinkles. It should not be ironed.

Case Studies

Case 34–1

Patient Complaint/History

AB, a 21-year-old college student, stops in to consult the pharmacist late one afternoon. He complains of a burning, itching sensation between the toes of his left foot. He says that these symptoms, which are becoming worse each day, are quite bothersome, particularly at bedtime when he is trying to fall asleep.

When questioned about the symptoms, AB reveals that the area between the toes is very red and seems to become worse after showering. He describes his toenails as normal in appearance; that is, the toenail beds show no apparent discoloration or brittleness. AB mentions that he showers every day in his residence hall and at the gymnasium after his varsity baseball team's workout. He also reports that his feet sweat a lot.

The patient admits to using Lotrimin AF cream intermittently for the past week in an attempt to resolve his problem. He says that the cream seems to help a little, but it just "doesn't get him over the hump." He also asks, "Why doesn't this stuff work? It used to be a prescription drug, didn't it?"

Except for the current foot problem, AB is in good general health, has no known diseases or allergies, and takes nonprescription medications only on rare occasions for relief of headaches or cold symptoms.

Clinical Considerations/Strategies

The following considerations/strategies are provided to aid the reader in (1) determining whether treatment of the patient's condition with nonprescription medications is warranted, (2) selecting the appropriate nonprescription medication, and (3) developing a patient counseling strategy to ensure optimal therapeutic outcomes:

- Assess the patient's symptoms to determine the most likely etiology and degree of severity.
- Formulate a realistic goal for treatment of the patient's problem (ie, relieve the symptoms and resolve the problem).
- Generate a list of therapeutic drug and nondrug interventions to address the patient's condition (eg, medical referral, nonprescription medication therapy, nondrug measures).
- Identify patient characteristics that either preclude or necessitate each therapeutic intervention.
- Create an optimal therapeutic intervention to resolve the patient's clinical condition.
- Create and agree upon a plan with the patient to monitor and document progress in resolving the problem.
- Develop a patient education/counseling strategy that will:
  - Support/justify the selected therapeutic strategy;
  - Aid patient adherence to the recommended therapeutic action plan;
  - Provide the patient with alternatives in the event of a less than optimal response to the recommended treatment.

Case 34–2

Patient Complaint/History

PJ, a 33-year-old obese female, presents to the pharmacy with a foot problem. Specifically, she complains of moderately severe pain in the fourth toe of each foot and of redness of the affected toes. She says that the pain makes walking to and from the bus stop each day difficult and interferes with her job as a retail sales clerk. She notes that a raised bump is apparent on the dorsal surface of each toe. Although the patient noticed the bumps several weeks ago, the affected toes have become painful only in the last few days.

Further questioning reveals that the pain is the most severe during the week when PJ wears high-heeled dress shoes. In an attempt to relieve the pain, she has been taking Advil 200 mg two tablets at least once a day for the past week. The analgesic helps until she walks more than a block in her high-heeled shoes. PJ is also currently taking Synthroid 0.075 mg one tablet QAM and Lo-Ovral one tablet hs for 21 days, 7 days off; she is allergic to penicillins and adhesive tape.

Clinical Considerations/Strategies

The following considerations/strategies are provided to aid the reader in (1) determining whether treatment of the patient's condition with nonprescription medications is warranted, (2) selecting the appropriate nonprescription medication, and (3) developing a patient counseling strategy to ensure optimal therapeutic outcomes:

- Assess the patient's symptoms to determine the most likely etiology and degree of severity.
- Formulate a realistic goal for treatment of the patient's problem (ie, relieve the symptoms and resolve the problem).
- Generate a list of all possible therapeutic interventions to address the patient's condition (eg, medical referral, nonprescription medication therapy, nondrug measures).
- Identify patient characteristics that either preclude or necessitate each therapeutic intervention.
- Create an optimal therapeutic regimen to relieve the patient's condition.
- Create a plan to monitor and document the patient's therapeutic response and progress in resolving the problem.
- Develop a patient education/counseling strategy that will:
  - Support/justify the selected therapeutic strategy;
  - Aid patient adherence to the recommended pharmacologic strategy;
  - Foster appropriate use of therapeutic agents as well as compliance with recommended nondrug and behavioral interventions;
  - Provide the patient with alternatives in the event of a less than optimal response to recommended treatment.

Summary

The nonprescription drug of choice in the treatment of corns, calluses, and warts is salicylic acid in a collodion-like vehicle or plaster product form, whichever is more convenient. Predisposing factors responsible for corns and calluses must be corrected. Plantar warts should be treated with a higher concentration of salicylic acid (20–40%); warts on thin epidermis require a lower concentration (10–20%). Because warts are usually self-limiting, treatment should be conservative; vigorous therapy with salicylic acid may scar tissue.

Historically, the nonprescription drug of choice to treat the dry, scaly type of athlete's foot has been tolnaftate. Other agents, such as clioquinol, clotrimazole, miconazole nitrate, and undecylenic acid and its derivatives, are also efficacious for this purpose. Their effectiveness will be limited, however, unless the patient eliminates other predisposing factors to tinea pedis. These drugs are effective in all their delivery systems, but the powder form should be reserved only for extremely mild conditions or as adjunctive therapy. Because the vehicle forms of solution and cream are spreadable, they should be used sparingly. When recommended for suspected or actual dermatophytosis of the foot, these drugs should be used twice daily, morning and night. Treatment should be continued for 2–4 weeks, depending on the symptoms. After this time, the patient and pharmacist should evaluate the effectiveness of the drug.

The value of any topical nonprescription product for treating the soggy, macerated type of athlete's foot is dubious. The complex nature of the topical flora (resident aerobic diphtheroids) superimposed on the fungal infection dictates rigorous therapy with broader-spectrum antifungals (eg, ciclopirox olamine or econazole nitrate). In addition, oral therapy with either griseofulvin or ketoconazole may be indicated. Soaks and compresses of astringent agents (eg, aluminum chloride) may be used as adjuvant therapy to dry the soggy, macerated tissue. Once this condition is converted to the dry form, appropriate use can be made of such agents as tolnaftate, clotrimazole, miconazole nitrate, and undecylenic acid derivatives.

To minimize noncompliance, patients should be advised that alleviation of the symptoms does not occur overnight. Patients should also be cautioned that frequent recurrence of any of these problems is an indication for consultation with a podiatrist or physician.

Patients with diabetes, circulatory problems, and/or arthritis pose special challenges to the pharmacist, who plays an important role in patient education. These patients should know not to self-medicate with any topical or oral nonprescription drug without first checking with their physician, podiatrist, or pharmacist. They should understand that there are certain ingredients in such products that may threaten the delicate balance that must be struck for their care. Misadventuring with nonprescription products could have devastating consequences and, at the least, may interfere with the attainment of intended patient outcomes.

Besides understanding concepts related to good foot care for patients with the above-mentioned chronic conditions, the pharmacist must be wary about drugs that can exacerbate these conditions or interact with other chronically used medications. Typically, persons with diabetes, for example, have other health problems (eg, hypertension, hyperlipidemia, or arthritis) and associated therapy regimens. Thus, the pharmacist must monitor patient progress carefully and be attuned to patient comments that might indicate the occurrence of drug-related problems.

In an era of physical fitness and health awareness, the pharmacist must be prepared to educate and assist patients who develop athletic injuries. With careful questioning, the pharmacist can help the patient determine whether the problem can be addressed through self-treatment or requires the assistance of a physician, podiatrist, or physical therapist. Most running injuries can be treated with shoe modifications, in-shoe supports, correction of leg length discrepancies, modified training methods, ice applications, and stretching exercises. It is important that the pharmacist be capable of providing informed recommendations to the sports enthusiast.

References

1. Brown JA, Scholl Inc. Personal communication. Memphis, Tenn: 1988.
2. Raskin J. Superficial fungal infections of the skin. In: Conn HF, ed. *Current Therapy 1976*. Philadelphia: WB Saunders; 1976: 611–4.
3. Gossel TA. The safe way to treat corns and calluses. *US Pharm*. 1987 Mar; 12: 41–2, 47–53.
4. Stewart WD, Danto JL, Maddin S. Callus. In: *Dermatologic Diagnosis and Treatment of Cutaneous Disorders*. 4th ed. St. Louis: CV Mosby; 1978: 129.
5. Reichman RC, Bonnez W. Papillomaviruses. In: Mandell GL, Douglas RG Jr, Bennett JE, eds. *Principles and Practice of Infectious Diseases*. 3rd ed. New York: Churchill Livingstone; 1990: 1191–7.
6. Vance JC et al. Intralesional recombinant alpha-2 interferon for the treatment of patients with condyloma acuminatum or verruca plantaris. *Arch Dermatol*. 1986 Mar; 122: 272–7.
7. Rock B, Shah KV, Farmer ER. A morphologic, pathologic and virologic study of anogenital warts in men. *Arch Dermatol*. 1992 Apr; 127: 495–500.
8. Melton JL, Rasmussen JE. Clinical manifestations of human papillomavirus infection in nongenital sites. *Dermatol Clin*. 1991 Apr; 9: 219–33.
9. Jarratt M. Viral infections of the skin: herpes simplex, herpes zoster, warts, and molluscum contagiosum. *Pediatr Clin North Am*. 1978 May; 25: 339–55.
10. Goldfarb MT et al. Office therapy for human papillomavirus infection in nongenital sites. *Dermatol Clin*. 1991 Apr; 9: 287–96.
11. *Federal Register*. 1990 Aug 14; 55(157): 33258–62.
12. Balkin SW. Treatment of corns by injectable silicone. *Arch Dermatol*. 1975 Sep; 111: 1143–5.
13. *Federal Register*. 1990 Aug 14; 55(157): 33246–56.
14. Smith EL. The occult removal of warts: a continuing practice. *Int J Dermatol*. 1979 Jan/Feb; 18: 89–91.
15. Hay RJ. Dermatophytosis and other special mycoses. In: Mandell GL, Douglas RG Jr, Bennett JE, eds. *Principles and Practice of Infectious Diseases*. 3rd ed. New York: Churchill Livingstone; 1990: 2017–28.
16. Goslen JB, Kobayashi GS. Dermatophytosis. In: Fitzpatrick TB et al, eds. *Dermatology in General Practice*. 3rd ed. New York: McGraw-Hill; 1987: 2193–248.
17. Jung JH et al. Isolation, via activity-directed fractionation, of mercaptobenzothiazole and dibenzothiazyl disulfide as 2 allergens responsible for tennis shoe dermatitis. *Contact Dermatitis*. 1988 Mar; 19: 254–9.
18. *Federal Register*. 1993 Sep 23; 58(183): 49890–9.
19. *Federal Register*. 1982 Mar 23; 47(56): 12480–566.
20. *Federal Register*. 1993 Sep 9; 58(173): 47602–6.
21. *Federal Register*. 1982 Sep 3; 47(172): 39120–5.
22. Thompson PD et al. Death during jogging or running. *JAMA*. 1979 Sep 21; 242: 1265–7.
23. Wapner KL, Sharkey PF. The use of night splints for treatment of recalcitrant plantar fasciitis. *Foot Ankle*. 1991; 12(3): 135–7.
24. Pinshaw R, Atlas V, Noakes TD. The nature and response to therapy of 196 consecutive injuries seen at a runner's clinic. *South Afr Med J*. 1984 Feb; 65: 291–8.
25. McPoil TG, Adrian M, Pidcoe P. Effects of foot orthotics on center of pressure patterns in women. *Phys Ther*. 1989; 69(2): 149.
26. Frey C et al. American Orthopaedic Foot and Ankle Society women's shoe survey. *Foot Ankle*. 1993; 14(2): 79–81.
27. Noakes TD. *Lore of Running*. Cape Town, South Africa: Oxford University Press; 1985.
28. Kay RA. The extra-depth toe box: a rational approach. *Foot Ankle*. 1994; 15(3): 146–50.
29. Cook SD, Kester MA, Brunet ME. Shock absorption characteristics of running shoe. *J Am Sports Med*. 1985; 13(4): 248–53.

CHAPTER 35

Herbs and Phytomedicinal Products

Varro E. Tyler and Steven Foster

Questions to ask in patient assessment and counseling

- *Have you used this product before?*
- *Are you allergic to any plant materials? If so, which specific materials or products?*
- *Is this product for personal use or for someone else (eg, a child)?*
- *Are you pregnant or breast-feeding?*
- *Are you aware of the importance of closely following label instructions for product dosages and duration of use?*
- *Are you taking prescription or nonprescription medications intended for the same purpose as this herb?*
- *Note: Because herbs and phytomedicinal products have a broad range of therapeutic use, many of the questions presented in other chapters are also applicable to these products.*

After an absence of nearly half a century, herbs and phytomedicinals have returned to the shelves of pharmacies—and with a vengeance. In 1992 they constituted the top growth category in American drugstores, up 57% from the previous year. However, annual sales in pharmacies amounted to only $53.1 million, a small fraction of the $1.5 billion estimated retail market.[1] Popularity of the products is increasing rapidly, with US sales predicted to top $5 billion annually by the year 2000. The present demand for certain products is truly amazing. Garlic sales in supermarkets increased 67% in 1993/94; sales of ginseng, the second best seller, advanced 247%. Drug company spokesmen no longer see herbal products as a "fad."[2]

Studies have shown that about one third of the US population now uses some form of unconventional medicine, if unconventional is defined in such broad terms as to include nutrition and other subjects not normally found in medical school curricula.[3] It is difficult to characterize the use of botanicals and phytomedicinals as unconventional when they are used so extensively by about three quarters of the world's population—in many cases, as their only medicines. No single factor accounts for the increasing popularity of herbal medicine. The reasons are probably something of an extension of the antiestablishment mentality of the sixties: increased appreciation of things "organic" and "natural" by members of the green movement; disenchantment with modern medicine (its inability to cure everything); reduced side effects caused by many gentle herbal remedies; and the low cost of herbal products, at least in comparison to patented single-chemical entities.

Herbs are defined in several ways, but for medical purposes they are simply botanicals used to treat disease states, often of a chronic nature, or to attain or maintain a condition of improved health. Phytomedicinals are galenicals—that is, preparations made by extracting herbs with various solvents, usually a hydroalcoholic menstruum, to produce tinctures, fluidextracts, extracts, and the like.

Obviously, it is imperative that pharmacists master the essentials of this complicated field in order to advise patients on the safe and effective use of these popular remedies. In view of the abundance of misinformation currently circulated and the educational deficiencies in many pharmacists, this is not an easy task. In the sections that follow, some of the more significant herbs are classified according to the disease syndromes or conditions they are intended to treat. The identity, chemical constituents, physiologic activity and therapeutic use, appropriate cautions concerning usage, and dosage of each are briefly discussed (see product table "Herbal and Phytomedicinal Products").

Safety and Effectiveness

Despite their intended use, most herbs and phytomedicinals are sold in the United States not as drugs but as dietary supplements. This reflects the fact that insufficient data concerning them have been submitted to the Food and Drug Administration (FDA) to permit that agency to classify them as safe and effective therapeutic agents. This does not necessarily mean that the herbs and phytomedicinals are unsafe and/or ineffective. It simply means that the FDA has not received sufficient data to permit these products to be placed in Category I. An understanding of this technicality is important; otherwise, one might think that peppermint is truly an unsafe and ineffective carminative and that prune concentrate (juice) is an unsafe and ineffective laxative. What these categorizations really mean is that the FDA has simply not properly evaluated these and many other products.

The reason for this situation is primarily economic. Having been used for hundreds—even thousands—of years, most classic herbs and their long-known constituents are not patentable. Therefore, no prospective marketer is willing to invest the hundreds of millions of dollars required to obtain sufficient clinical evidence to convince the FDA of their safety and utility. To do so would place that marketer at a distinct disadvantage compared with competitors who make no such investment.[4]

Although the FDA has been requested to adopt more reasonable standards of proof of efficacy for the long-used botanicals, it has not been willing to do so and, in 1993, even threatened to remove many of the products from the market. Lobbied intensively by an irate public, Congress passed the Dietary Supplement Health and Education Act of 1994, allowing herbs and phytomedicinals to be sold as "dietary supplements"—but without any labeled therapeutic or health claims. Under the act, a statement may appear on the label that describes the product's role in affecting structure or function in humans. However, this must be followed by a disclaimer noting that the statement has not been evaluated by the FDA and that the product is not intended to diagnose, treat, cure, or prevent any disease. In addition to this label information, accurate scientific information of a generic nature may be passed along to the consumer with the product.[5]

The situation is quite different in the advanced nations of Europe. There, following World Health Organization guidelines, relevant literature and research studies, as well as the experience of individual health care practitioners and patients, are additional parameters that are considered along with clinical evidence in evaluating the efficacy of herbs and phytomedicinals. The best system has been developed in Germany, where a special, broadly based Commission E, appointed by the Federal Health Agency, has been actively studying the safety and utility of botanicals since 1978. Using information derived from clinical trials, field studies, case collections, scientific literature, and the opinions of medical associations, that group has published about 300 monographs on herbs in the *Bundesanzeiger*, the German equivalent of our *Federal Register*. These monographs normally include nomenclature, part(s) used, constituents, range of application, contraindications, side effects, incompatibilities, dosage, use, and action of the herb.

Approximately two thirds of the monographs provide positive assessments of herbs found to be safe and effective. The remaining monographs are negative, usually because the drug—and these are considered to be drugs in Germany—presents an unsatisfactory risk-benefit ratio. Although not perfect, the Commission E monographs represent the most accurate summaries of information available anywhere on the safety and efficacy of herbs and phytomedicinals. Their conclusions will be cited extensively in the monographs that make up the bulk of this chapter.[6]

Ineffective Herbal Preparations

There are several types of preparations that will not be discussed in detail in this chapter. Herbal weight-loss preparations have become very popular; aside from their placebo effect, however, none of them is useful for this purpose. Most simply contain laxatives, such as senna, and diuretics, such as dandelion leaves, that produce a temporary illusion of weight loss. Another popular ingredient is ephedra (ma huang), which acts as a central nervous system (CNS) stimulant but is not an effective anorectic agent and may cause serious side effects in some consumers. Thus, herbal weight-loss preparations should not be recommended by pharmacists.[7] Other conditions for which no effective botanical remedy is currently available include arthritis, cancer, human immunodeficiency virus (HIV), and acquired immunodeficiency syndrome (AIDS).

Precautions

There are certain precautions that must be observed in the use of herbal dietary supplements. It is always necessary to remember that these are not approved drugs in the United States, so information pertaining to their proper use and especially necessary cautionary warnings do not always appear on the label. Consequently, prospective users should make every effort to obtain accurate information about the specific product prior to purchasing it. This is not always easy because of the prevalence of hyperbolic literature, written in many cases to promote the sale of the product rather than to inform the consumer accurately.

The FDA neither establishes nor regularly enforces any standards of quality for herbal products. This means that one must rely upon the reputation of the marketer for any quality assurance. Products are often misbranded, and often the quantities of the ingredients are not listed. In mixtures containing large numbers of herbal constituents, quantities sufficient to render a therapeutic effect are often lacking. The consumer is best advised to purchase a preparation containing a specified amount of a standardized extract marketed by a reputable firm. For example, Food and Drug Canada has recommended that feverfew products contain not less than 0.2% parthenolide. A 1993 study showed that some feverfew products purchased in Louisiana contained no parthenolide at all.[8] Now reputable companies are beginning to market in the United States feverfew preparations containing 125 mg of an extract standardized to contain 0.2% parthenolide. Such products are a distinct improvement over those of variable quality previously available.

Other concerns about herbal consumption must include a general prohibition of use by pregnant or nursing mothers and by young children, especially infants. This precaution applies particularly to stimulant laxatives and similar products that may lack adequate warning labels. Many botanicals lack the necessary long-term toxicity testing to ensure safety in cases of prolonged administration. Despite the deceptive legal classification as "dietary supplements," herbs used for therapeutic purposes are drugs, and proper dosage recommendations should be carefully observed.

Dosage Forms

A large variety of dosage forms of herbs and phytomedicinals is currently available. One of the most common is simply the coarsely comminuted botanical that is used to prepare an infusion (tea) or a decoction. This form is also used to prepare poultices for external application. More finely powdered herbs are either encapsulated or used to prepare compressed tablets. Some of these latter dosage forms may be enteric coated if their active constituents are inactivated by stomach acid. Herbs are also extracted with various solvents to produce liquid or solid phytomedicinals. Such extracts (galenicals) permit both concentration and standardization of the active principles—often a highly desirable feature. Because some herbal consumers are highly concerned about the nature of the products they ingest, special preparations, such as nongelatin capsules that are not prepared from animal by-products, and glycerites that do not use ethanol in their production, are occasionally encountered. Herbs derived from sources said to be "organic"—that is, grown without synthetic chemical fertilizers or pesticides—are often advertised.

Digestive System Disorders

Ginger

Ginger consists of the dried or fresh rhizome of *Zingiber officinale* Rosc., a member of the ginger family (Zingiberaceae), and preparations thereof.

Chemical Constituents

Ginger contains a volatile oil (1–3%) dominated by sesquiterpene hydrocarbons, including zingiberene, alpha-curcumene, beta-sesquiphellandrene, and beta-bisabolene. Also present is an oleoresin (4–7.5%) with nonvolatile pungent components, among which are gingerols and shogaols.[4,9]

Physiologic Activity and Therapeutic Use

Ginger is considered to be a carminative, an antiemetic, a cholagogue, and a positive inotropic. It promotes saliva and gastric juice secretion and is spasmolytic (in animals). Dried ginger root has been shown to stimulate the gastrointestinal (GI) tract, increasing both peristalsis and tone of the intestinal muscle. Use is primarily indicated for atonic dyspepsia, colic, and the prophylactic relief of symptoms of motion sickness.

Six human studies concerning ginger's effects on motion sickness have been conducted since 1982—four reporting positive results; two, negative results. Inappropriate low dose (<1 g per day) and inferior quality plant material could have contributed to the negative results. The German health authorities allow ginger products to be labeled as a remedy for dyspeptic complaints and a prophylactic for travel sickness.

Precautions

Given in amounts specified to prevent motion sickness, ginger has caused no reported side effects or toxic reactions. It has been suggested that the herb should be avoided for treatment of postoperative nausea; the rhizome is reported to inhibit thromboxane synthetase and to act as a prostacyclin agonist, possibly resulting in prolonged bleeding time and immunologic changes. Its use is also contraindicated in cases of gallstone pain and nausea associated with pregnancy.

Dosage

In the form of hard gelatin capsules, the dosage is two 500-mg capsules taken 30 minutes prior to travel departure, followed by 1 or 2 more 500-mg capsule(s) taken as needed every 4 hours. The daily dose is 2–4 g of the drug or equivalent preparations.[4,9]

Plantago Seed and Husk

Known as plantain or psyllium seed, the drug consists of the cleaned, dried, ripened seed of black psyllium (Spanish or French psyllium), *Plantago arenaria* Waldst. and Kit. (*Plantago psyllium* L. and *Plantago indica* L. are botanical names of invalid standing although official in *USP* XXII), and blonde psyllium, *Plantago ovata* Forssk., which primarily produces seed husk. These are members of the plantain family (Plantaginaceae). Major production areas include India and Pakistan, as well as southern France and Spain.[10,11]

Chemical Constituents

Seeds contain up to 80% insoluble fiber, and 10–30% of a hydrocolloid soluble fiber is concentrated in the epidermis. The hydrocolloid consists of acidic and neutral polysaccharide fractions which, upon hydrolysis, yield L-arabinose, D-galactose, D-galacturonic acid, L-rhamnose, and D-xylose.[10]

Physiologic Activity and Therapeutic Use

Plantago or psyllium seeds are bulk-forming laxatives. Their activity results from the swelling of the mucilaginous seed coats as they bind with fluid in the intestine; this increases intestinal content volume, causing a physical stimulation of the gut wall. At the same time, the bowels are lubricated by the seeds' mucilage, and accelerated transit through the colon is achieved.[11,12] Uses include treatment of chronic constipation and conditions necessitating soft stools, such as hemorrhoids, anal fissures, or rectal-anal surgery.[13]

The German health authorities allow plantago to be used in supportive therapy of irritable bowel syndrome (IBS). The drug's efficacy in producing a modest but significant lowering of total cholesterol and low-density lipoprotein levels is recognized.[13,14]

Precautions

Rare allergic reactions are reported in patients and in persons involved with industrial handling of the drug. Its use is contraindicated in the presence of bowel and GI tract obstructions as well as diabetes mellitus.[13]

Dosage

The dose is 7.5 g (average 4–20 g per day), taken with at least 150 mL of water for each 5 g of drug, 30–60 minutes after a meal or the administration of other drugs.[10,13]

Senna

The drug consists of the dried leaflet of Alexandria senna (*Cassia acutifolia* Del.) and Tinnevelly senna (*Cassia angustifolia* Vahl.), both of which are also referred to in recent botanical literature as *Senna alexandrina* Mill. Members of the Fabaceae (Leguminosae), these species are produced commercially in the Middle East, India, and elsewhere.[11]

Chemical Constituents

Dianthrone glycosides, particularly sennosides A, A_1, B, C, D, and G, are present along with various anthraquinone derivatives. Sennosides, a complex of total glycosides, is also official in the *USP*.[4,10]

Physiologic Activity and Therapeutic Use

Senna is cathartic; it is used for the treatment of constipation.[4,10]

Precautions

Patients may experience cramping discomfort in the GI tract. Use of stimulating laxatives should not continue beyond 1–2 weeks except under medical supervision. Chronic abuse or overdose can result in potassium loss, along with electrolyte and fluid imbalances. Such potassium loss may reduce the effectiveness of cardiac glycosides and antiarrhythmic drugs; it also increases the potential toxicity of the cardiac glycosides. Owing to the lack of sufficient toxicologic assessments, use of senna is not recommended during pregnancy or lactation.[15]

Dosage

The dose is 2 g or appropriate formulations as needed.[10,15]

Peppermint

The drug consists of the dried leaves and flowering tops of *Mentha × piperita* L., a member of the mint family (Lamiaceae, formerly Labiatae). Its essential oil is considered a separate but related drug. Peppermint is cultivated in Europe, Egypt, and the United States, especially in the states of Indiana, Michigan, Idaho, Oregon, and Washington.[16] The drug should contain not more than 2% of stems that measure 3 mm or greater in diameter.[16]

Chemical Constituents

The biologic activity of peppermint is attributed to its essential oil (0.5–4%, average 1.5%), which contains not less than 50% (50–78%) (−)-menthol and 5–20% menthol combined in esters, including the acetate or isovalerate. Menthol stereoisomers are also present; these include (+)-neomenthol (3%) as well as other monoterpenes such as menthone, menthofuran, eucalyptol, and limonene. The sesquiterpene viridoflorol provides a marker for oil identification.[4,10] Among other leaf constituents are flavonoids, rosmarinic acid, and tannin.[11]

Physiologic Activity and Therapeutic Use

Peppermint leaf and oil are currently in pharmaceutical use in the United States as flavoring agents. As a result of a decision by the FDA Advisory Review Panel on Over-the-Counter (OTC) Miscellaneous Internal Drug Products, the oil was dropped from nonprescription drug status in 1990. This decision does not necessarily reflect the oil's lack of safety or efficacy; it indicates only that no information on safety and efficacy was presented to the agency.[4]

Recent European interest has focused on the use of peppermint oil to treat IBS. The oil (enteric-coated capsules) has been reported to reduce symptoms of IBS characterized by recurrent colicky abdominal pain, a feeling of distention, and variations in bowel habits with minimal attendant side effects.[16] The German health authorities allow peppermint oil for the treatment of IBS, spastic discomfort of the upper GI tract, and other related conditions.[11]

Peppermint leaf is recognized as a carminative and choleretic, with a direct spasmolytic effect on smooth muscles of the digestive tract. The leaf is the subject of a positive German monograph indicating its use for spastic GI tract complaints.[17] Traditionally, peppermint leaf tea is used to treat dyspepsia, flatulence, and intestinal colic.[9]

Precautions

Peppermint tea is considered safe for normal individuals. Excessive use of the essential oil (0.3 g not enteric coated) may produce toxic reactions such as heartburn and relaxation of the lower esophageal sphincter.[16] Peppermint leaf tea should be used with caution in infants and small children because of possible laryngeal and bronchial spasms from volatilized menthol.[4] The oil may also irritate mucous membranes.

Dosage

The cut herb is used in hot infusions at an average daily dose of 1.5–3 g of the dried leaf.[17] For relief of stomach upset, an infusion is made by pouring 160 mL of boiling water on 1–1.5 g of the herb, steeping for up to 10 minutes, and ingesting it up to three or four times daily.[4] Each dose of enteric-coated peppermint oil is 0.2–0.4 mL, up to 0.6–1.2 mL per day.[18]

Chamomile

The drug consists of the dried flower head of German (also known as Hungarian) chamomile, *Matricaria recutita* L., which is referred to in older literature as *Matricaria chamomilla* or *Chamomilla recutita* (L.) Rauschert. It is the principal species available in world markets, including Europe and the United States. Primary production countries include Germany, Hungary, the Czech Republic, Egypt, and Argentina. Roman (also known as English) chamomile is obtained from *Chamaemelum nobile* (L.) All., which is referred to in older literature as *Anthemis nobilis* L. Its chemistry is different from that of German chamomile. Use of Roman chamomile is largely restricted to the United Kingdom, where most of the supply is grown. Both Roman and German chamomile are members of the Asteraceae (formerly Compositae).[11,19,20]

Chemical Constituents

German chamomile contains an essential oil (0.3–2%) with more than 120 components; the terpenoids (−)-alpha-bisabolol (up to 50% of the oil) and (−)-alpha-bisaboloxides A and B are important biologically active components. The characteristic blue color of the volatile oil results from the presence of chamazulene, which forms during steam distillation from the sesquiterpene lactone, matricin. Flavonoids, such as apigenin and apigenin-7-glucoside, in the dried flower heads contribute to the drug's antispasmodic activity.[4,9]

Physiologic Activity and Therapeutic Use

The dried flower heads and volatile oil have anti-inflammatory, spasmolytic, and antimicrobial activity. Thus, the German therapeutic monograph allows the flower preparations to be used for GI spasms and GI tract inflammatory diseases. The drug is also used for peptic ulcers. An infusion (as a mouthwash) is used to treat inflammatory conditions of the oral cavity and gums.[19,20]

Creams, ointments, and other topical products containing German chamomile flower extracts are widely available in Europe. The German Health Authorities allow topical products for the treatment of skin and mucous membrane inflammations and bacterial skin diseases.[4,9,21] Wound-healing effects include promotion of granulation and tissue regeneration. Flower extracts have also proven useful in the treatment of eczema.

Precautions

Numerous professional and popular references in the past decade have warned of possible anaphylactic shock from drinking chamomile tea. However, only five cases of allergy attributed to German chamomile have been identified between 1887 and 1982.[4] These figures would imply the drug's relative safety.

Dosage

For GI ailments, tea (150 mL hot water over 3 g dried flower heads, steeped for 10 minutes) is drunk three to four times daily between meals.

Milk Thistle

The drug consists of the seeds of *Silybum marianum* (L.) Gaertn., a member of the aster family (Asteraceae, formerly Compositae), and its standardized preparations. The seed is primarily produced in Germany, the Czech Republic, and other eastern European countries.[4]

Chemical Constituents

The main component of the seeds is a flavonolignan complex that was first designated silymarin (4–6% in ripe fruits) but was subsequently found to include several flavonolignans, including silybin, isosilybin, dehydrosilybin, silydianin, and silychristin. Products available in the United States generally consist of capsules containing varying amounts of a concentrated seed extract, standardized to 70–80% flavonolignans calculated as silybin.[4,22]

Physiologic Activity and Therapeutic Use

Milk thistle preparations are considered hepatoprotectants. Pharmacologic mechanisms for their hepatoprotective action include scavenging of free radicals, alteration of the outer liver membrane cell structure to protect liver cells from the entry of toxic substances, and stimulation of RNA polymerase A. The latter activity enhances ribosome protein synthesis, which activates the liver's regenerative capacity through cell development. Milk thistle seed preparations are widely used in Europe in the prophylaxis and treatment of chronic hepatotoxicity. They have been especially useful in inflammatory liver disorders and cirrhosis of the liver resulting from chronic hepatitis or fatty infiltration of the liver induced by alcohol and other chemicals.[4,22,23]

Precautions

Mild transient diarrhea has been reported in a small number of patients.[16]

Dosage

The average daily dose is 12–15 g of the seeds, corresponding to 200–420 mg per day of silymarin, or its equivalent in capsules or tablets, each containing 80–140 mg of silymarin in a concentrated extract.[4,22]

Licorice

The drug consists of the dried rhizome and roots of *Glycyrrhiza glabra* L. (European licorice), as well as *Glycyrrhiza uralensis* Fisch. (Chinese licorice) and other species and varieties of *Glycyrrhiza*, members of the pea family (Fabaceae, formerly Leguminosae).[4,8]

Chemical Constituents

Licorice contains a triterpene glycoside, glycyrrhizin (glycyrrhizic acid) at 2–14% of the dried root. A good-quality product contains at least 4% glycyrrhizin. This compound, 50 times sweeter than sugar, gives licorice its sweet taste. Upon hydrolysis, glycyrrhizin is converted to glycyrrhetinic acid (glycyrrhetic acid) and two molecules of glucuronic acid.[4]

Physiologic Activity and Therapeutic Use

The use of licorice in the treatment of peptic ulcers has been recognized since World War II. However, the dose must be carefully controlled to avoid side effects. Glycyrrhetinic acid has been found to inhibit two enzymes, 5-hydroxy-prostaglandin dehydrogenase and delta^{13}-prostaglandin reductase, which are important for the metabolism of prostaglandins E and F_{2a}. The resulting increase in prostaglandins in the stomach produces a protective effect on gastric mucosa, thereby promoting the healing of gastric ulcers. Other constituents in licorice, especially various flavonoids, add to the overall effect. Glycyrrhetinic acid also increases glucocorticoid concentrations in tissues responsive to mineralocorticoid, resulting in sodium retention, potassium excretion, and high blood pressure. The beneficial action and the side effects of glycyrrhetinic acid are inseparable, so the dose must be carefully controlled if the herb is to be used therapeutically.[4]

Licorice has also long been used as an ingredient in antitussive and expectorant formulations. Expectorant and secretolytic effects have been confirmed in laboratory animals (rabbits).[24]

Precautions

The German health authorities stipulate that use of licorice be limited to no longer than 4–6 weeks at a specified dose. An inappropriate dose or long-term use may result in mineralocorticoid effects, including sodium and water retention, potassium loss (with high blood pressure), and hypokalemia. Rare cases of myoglobinuria have also been reported.

Potassium loss may be increased by concurrent use of thiazide diuretics, resulting in an increased sensitivity to digitalis glycosides.

Use of licorice is contraindicated in liver cirrhosis, cholestatic liver disorders, hypertonia, and hypokalemia, as well as during pregnancy.

Dosage

An average daily dose of 5–15 g of the finely cut or powdered root (calculated to contain 200–600 mg of glycyrrhizin) in infusions is recommended for the treatment of gastric/duodenal ulcers. Duration of this regimen should not exceed 4–6 weeks.[24]

Kidney, Urinary Tract, and Prostate Disorders

Goldenrod

The drug consists of the dried flowering aerial (aboveground) parts of European goldenrod, *Solidago virgaurea* L. American species, including *Solidago serotina* Ait. (*Solidago gigantea* Ait.) and *Solidago canadensis* L., are used interchangeably. These species are members of the aster family (Asteraceae, formerly Compositae).

Chemical Constituents

The herb contains polygalic acid-based saponins, at least 12 clerodane diterpenes (solidagolactones I–VII, elongatolides C and E, and others), leiocarposide (a phenolic glycoside), miscellaneous flavonoids, phenolic acids, tannins, and other components.[9]

Physiologic Activity and Therapeutic Use

An aquaretic for use in irrigation therapy against lower urinary tract inflammation, the drug is also indicated for the prevention and treatment of urinary calculi and kidney stones.

Precautions

As with other members of the Asteraceae family, allergic cross-sensitivity to goldenrod can occur in certain individuals. Use of the drug should be avoided in cases of known allergies to aster family members. It is also contraindicated in the presence of edema due to impaired heart or kidney function.

Dosage

The herb is prepared as an infusion by pouring 240 mL boiling water over 3–5 g of the herb. Mean daily dose is 6–12 g.[4,25]

Bearberry

Bearberry, also known as uva-ursi, consists of the dried leaves of *Arctostaphylos uva-ursi* (L.) Spreng. (Ericaceae) and grows in cold temperate regions throughout the Northern Hemisphere.

Chemical Constituents

The phenolic glycosides arbutin and methylarbutin (6–10% of dried leaf) have an antiseptic action. Other constituents include flavonoids, tannins, and various organic acids. Arbutin is hydrolyzed in the intestinal tract, producing hydroquinone. After absorption, it is bound as glycuronides and sulfate esters and is excreted in the urine.

Physiologic Activity and Therapeutic Use

While bearberry is listed in most works as a diuretic, that activity is minimal; its primary activity is as an antibacterial for urinary tract infections (UTIs). Activation requires the urine pH to be alkaline, thereby releasing free hydroquinone from the conjugates. Administration should be in conjunction with a diet rich in milk, vegetables (such as tomatoes and potatoes), fruits and fruit juices, and other foods capable of inducing alkalinuria. Ingestion of 6–8 g of sodium bicarbonate a day will also produce alkalinity during treatment.[4]

Precautions

A small percentage of patients may experience nausea and vomiting.

Dosage

The dried cut or powdered herb is administered in a mean daily dose of 10 g (corresponding to 400–700 mg arbutin) macerated overnight in 150 mL of cold water (to reduce the tannin content extracted with hot water). Use should be limited to 1 week or less.[26]

Cranberry

Cranberry juice (sweetened diluted juice of the fruits) and extracts of the American cranberry *Vaccinium macrocarpon* Ait., a member of the Ericaceae family, are used to treat of UTIs.

Chemical Constituents

Cranberry juice contains fructose, carbohydrates, fiber, and various organic acids, including benzoic, citric, malic, and quinic acids. The constituents responsible for efficacy in the treatment of UTIs include fructose as well as a polymeric compound whose structure has not been elucidated.[4]

Physiologic Activity and Therapeutic Use

Cranberry juice has long been used by the public for self-treatment of UTIs. As early as the 1920s, it was postulated that the juice had a bacteriostatic effect owing to urinary acidification, but the scientific literature on the subject is conflicting. Any inherent benefits of cranberry juice or cranberry preparations in UTIs are no longer believed to be the result of direct antibacterial action. Instead, cranberry juice prevents the adhesion of *Escherichia coli* and other uropathogenic bacteria to the mucosal cells of the urinary tract.[4]

It has been suggested that cranberry juice can reduce the urinary odor of incontinent patients. This occurs because it lowers the pH enough to retard the degradation of urine by *Escherichia coli*, which produces the offensive ammoniacal odors.[27]

Precautions

No precautions are noted.

Dosage

As a UTI preventive, 90 mL of cranberry juice can be consumed daily; for UTI treatment, consumption should increase to 360–960 mL daily. Capsules containing dried cranberry and a dried, concentrated extract are available. Six capsules are reported to be equivalent to 90 mL of cranberry juice cocktail, about one third of which is cranberry juice.[4]

Saw Palmetto

The drug consists of the dried fruits of *Serenoa repens* (Bartr.) Small, a member of the palm family (Palmaceae) referenced in older literature as *Sabal serrulata* (Michx.) Hook. Fruits are harvested from wild populations in Georgia and Florida.

Chemical Constituents

Fruits contain 1–2% essential oil, as well as a fixed oil with 75% free fatty acids and 25% neutral substances, including free or esterified sterols or esters of fatty acids with alcohols. The antiandrogenic constituent(s) have not been specifically identified but are found in acidic lipophilic fractions of the fruits.[4,11]

Physiologic Activity and Therapeutic Use

Saw palmetto fruits and their preparations have antiandrogenic and anti-inflammatory activity and are widely used in Germany, France, and Italy for the treatment of symptoms associated with benign prostatic hyperplasia (BPH). Various studies have shown that liposterolic fruit extracts reduce testosterone and dihydrotestosterone in tissue samples by more than 40%. Anti-inflammatory and antiedematous activities have also been reported when using the fruit extracts. Antiedematous activity may be caused by inhibition of the arachidonic acid pathway.[4]

Placebo-controlled, double-blind studies of the use of saw palmetto extract carried out on more than 2,000 BPH patients in Germany confirmed its effectiveness. The German health authorities allow use of the fruit extract in the treatment of micturition difficulties associated with BPH stages 1 and 2.[4,28] According to the German monograph, the drug is used to relieve symptoms associated with enlarged prostate without reducing prostate enlargement. However, a recent study reports results of a 505-patient trial in which prostate size was reduced.[29]

Precautions

Stomach upset has been reported in rare instances.

Dosage

Average daily dose is 1–2 g of the ground, dried fruits or 320 mg of a lipophilic fruit extract.

Respiratory Tract Disorders

Ephedra

Commonly known by its Chinese name, *ma huang*, the drug consists of the aboveground aerial parts of three Asian species: *Ephedra sinica* Stapf. (most often cited as the source plant), *Ephedra intermedia* Schrank. and *Ephedra equisetina* Bunge. *Ephedra* is a genus in the primitive ephedra family (Ephedraceae), which consists of about 40 species native to warm, dry regions of the Americas, Asia, and Europe. Three species are found in the Mediterranean region, nine species and two hybrids are found in North American deserts; and the rest are found in South America and Asia.

The American species, *Ephedra nevadensis* S. Wats., known as Mormon or Brigham tea, is found in the southwestern deserts of the United States. It is traded on American dietary supplement markets. Ephedra alkaloids have been found to be absent from all North and Central American *Ephedra* species. Therefore, the inherent medicinal value of these species, if any, is owing to other, unidentified compounds.[11]

Chemical Constituents

The stem (herb) of ephedra contains a number of active compounds, including small amounts of an essential oil and, most important, 1–2% of an alkaloid mixture composed mainly of ephedrine and pseudoephedrine. The contained ephedrine ranges from 30 to 90% of the total, depending on the source. *Ephedra sinica* contains about 1.3% alkaloids with more than 60% ephedrine, *Ephedra intermedia* contains about 1.1% alkaloids with 30–40% ephedrine, and *Ephedra equisetina* contains about 1.7% alkaloids with 85–90% ephedrine. More than 50% of the alkaloids are concentrated in the stem internodes, with none in the root.[11]

Physiologic Activity and Therapeutic Use

Use of ephedra to treat bronchial asthma and related conditions has been known for at least 5,000 years. Alkaloid-containing Asian *Ephedra* species produce bronchodilation, vasoconstriction, and reductions in bronchial edema.[4]

Precautions

Ephedra should be avoided by patients suffering from heart conditions, hypertension, diabetes, or thyroid disease. Ephedrine and related alkaloids are CNS stimulants; overdose can result in nervousness, insomnia, and palpitation. Products containing ephedra herb, often spiked with ephedrine and/or pseudoephedrine, are commonly used in weight loss formulations although there is no evidence to suggest that ephedra or its alkaloids are safe and effective in reducing weight or appetite. Because of reports of toxicity, FDA regulatory action on such products is anticipated. Several states have restricted sales of ephedra herb because ephedrine is used as a precursor in the manufacture of the illicit drugs methamphetamine and methcathinone.[4]

Dosage

Two grams of the herb is steeped in 240 mL of boiling water for 10 minutes (equivalent to 15–30 mg of ephedrine) and drunk as a tea.[4]

Slippery Elm

The drug consists of the dried inner bark of *Ulmus rubra* Muhl. (referenced as *Ulmus fulva* Michx. in older literature), a member of the elm family (Ulmaceae) indigenous to the forests of eastern North America.

Chemical Constituents

The inner bark of slippery elm is high in mucilage (primarily consisting of a water-soluble polysaccharide), starch, and small amounts of tannins.

Physiologic Activity and Therapeutic Use

Slippery elm bark is a mucilaginous demulcent, emollient, and nutrient. It is used traditionally to soothe irritated mucous membranes or ulcerations of the digestive tract as well as to relieve gastritis, colitis, and gastric or duodenal ulcers.[9] The primary use in the United States is as a soothing demulcent for sore throat; it has received FDA approval for this purpose.

Precautions

No precautions are noted.

Dosage

Between 0.5 and 2 g of powdered bark steeped in 10 parts hot water (5–20 mL) is consumed as required. Commercially produced tablets and troches are also available.[9]

Horehound

The drug consists of the dried, aboveground parts of flowering *Marrubium vulgare* L., a member of the mint family (Lamiaceae, formerly Labiatae) native to Europe and widely naturalized in the United States.

Chemical Constituents

Minute amounts of a volatile oil (0.06%) as well as a bitter diterpenoid lactone, marrubiin (or its precursor premarrubiin), are found in the leaves.[4]

Physiologic Activity and Therapeutic Use

While horehound has been traditionally used as an expectorant and antitussive, its use as a cough suppressant has been recorded for at least 400 years.[4] Marrubiinic acid, a derivative of marrubiin, has strong choleretic activity. The herb is approved by the German health authorities for supportive treatment of coughs and colds, and as a digestive aid and an appetite stimulant.[30] Conversely, the FDA has declared it ineffective as a nonprescription cough suppressant and expectorant.

Precautions

No precautions are noted.

Dosage

Two grams of the dried cut herb is steeped in 240 mL of boiling water, with a daily consumption of 0.75–1 L of the infusion. Horehound-flavored candy is also widely used as a cough suppressant.[4]

Cardiovascular System Disorders

Hawthorn

The drug consists of the dried leaves with flower and/or fruits of *Crataegus laevigata* (Poir) DC. (referred to in older literature as *Crataegus oxyacantha* auct.) and *Crataegus monogyna* Jacq., both harvested from wild populations or cultivated supplies in Europe. *Crataegus pinnatifida* Bunge is used in China, and its dried fruits appear on the American market. Hawthorns are members of the rose family (Rosaceae).

Chemical Constituents

Biological activity of the drug is attributed to oligomeric procyanidins (catechin and epicatechin) as well as to flavonoids, including quercetin, hyperoside, vitexin, and vitexin rhamnoside.[4,12]

Physiologic Activity and Therapeutic Use

Hawthorn is widely used in European phytomedical practice for treatment of diminished cardiac performance (corresponding to stages I and II of the New York Heart Association classification), heart conditions not requiring digitalis, mild and stable forms of angina pectoris, and mild forms of dysrhythmia. Flowering tops are used in sleep-inducing preparations.[12]

Precautions

No toxicity has been noted; however, given the nature of indications, use of hawthorn should be considered only under medical supervision.[4]

Dosage

The German health authorities have established a minimum daily dose that is equivalent to 5 mg flavone (calculated as hyperoside), 10 mg total flavonoids, or 5 mg oligomeric procyanidins (calculated as epicatechin).[31] Products standardized to similar parameters have recently become available in the United States, where the crude herb is commonly sold.[1] The European Scientific Cooperative for Phytotherapy has proposed a daily dosage of 3–4 g of the dried drug administered in 1-g doses in the form of an infusion.[12]

Garlic

The drug consists of the dried or fresh bulbs of *Allium sativum* L. of the lily family (Liliaceae). A cultivar (not known from the wild) grown throughout the world, garlic has been cultivated for more than 5,000 years.

Chemical Constituents

The main components of garlic volatile oil are sulfur compounds, especially allicin, diallyl disulfide, and diallyl trisulfide (and more than 30 additional sulfur compounds). Ajoene (formed by the self-condensation of allicin) has also been shown to have antiplatelet aggregation and antibacterial activity. Allicin, generally considered the most important biologically active compound, is a derived product: when the bulb is crushed or bruised, alliin, an odorless, sulfur-containing amino acid, comes into contact with alliinase, an enzyme, and is converted to allicin. Commercial garlic products vary greatly in chemical composition.[32]

Physiologic Activity and Therapeutic Use

Garlic is considered antibacterial, antifungal, antithrombotic, and hypotensive; it activates fibrinolysis and is anti-inflammatory. Recent interest has focused on the potential use of garlic and its preparations for several purposes, including the treatment of high blood pressure, atherosclerosis, hypoglycemia, digestive ailments, colds, flu, and bronchitis, as well as for its blood cholesterol– and triglyceride-lowering activity.[32] Of all these activities, the best substantiated are those involving garlic's antihyperlipidemic properties.

Precautions

Garlic may cause GI discomfort; rare allergic reactions are also reported.

Dosage

The daily dosage is equivalent to 4–12 mg of alliin (2–5 mg of allicin) in appropriate formulations, 400–1,200 mg of dried powder, or 2–5 g of the fresh bulb.[9,33]

Ginkgo

The drug consists of the dried leaves of *Ginkgo biloba* L., the only surviving member of the ginkgo family (Ginkgoaceae), and appropriate formulations thereof.

Chemical Constituents

Active constituents include flavones; bioflavonoids such as the glycosides kaempferol, quercetin, and isorhamnetin; and organic acids. Novel diterpene lactones unique to ginkgo include ginkgolides (A, B, C, and M) and bilobalide, a sesquiterpene. Of the diterpenes, ginkgolide B is considered the most active. Most, if not all, of the more than 250 pharmacologic and clinical studies published in the last 20 years have involved a specific standardized ginkgo leaf extract. This extract is produced by a complex extraction process and standardized to 24% flavone glycosides as well as, in some cases, being further calibrated for ginkgolides and bilobalide. Potentially toxic ginkgoic acid is removed during the extraction process.[34]

Physiologic Activity and Therapeutic Use

The numerous pharmacologic and clinical studies of ginkgo leaf extract have demonstrated a positive effect in increasing vasodilation and the peripheral blood flow rate in capillary vessels and end arteries in various circulatory disorders. Among these are varicose conditions, post-thrombotic syndrome, chronic cerebral vascular insufficiency, short-term memory loss, cognitive disorders secondary to depression, dementia, tinnitus, vertigo, and obliterative arterial disease of the lower limbs. The drug also exerts a protective effect against hypoxia in normal healthy males and is thought to be useful in treating other conditions.[34]

A recent retrospective critical review analyzed the quality and methodology of 40 trials published since 1975 on the use of ginkgo extracts in cerebral insufficiency. The outcomes of the trials, all of which reported positive results, were interpreted in relation to their quality. Clinical trials reporting results in healthy volunteers were excluded. For most of the studies, the dosage was 120 mg per day of the ginkgo extract (given for at least 4–6 weeks). Of the 40 studies, 8 were deemed to be well performed. The two authors of this review note that, since no clear side effects were reported, they would both be willing to try ginkgo for symptoms for which the extracts are indicated. However, they stress the need for additional trials, carefully double-blinded and using a larger number of patients. Better descriptions of randomization procedures and patient characteristics are also needed, along with a more effective measurement of outcomes.[35]

Precautions

Ginkgo leaf extract has been reported to be generally free from side effects, except for minor reversible gastric disturbances (in 3.7 % of patients). Rare side effects include headache, dizziness, and vertigo.[36]

Dosage

The daily dose is 120–160 mg of standardized ginkgo leaf extract.[36]

Grapeseed and/or Pinebark

Grapeseed extract is derived from the seeds of *Vitis vinifera* L., a member of the grape family (Vitaceae). Pinebark extract is known in the trade as "pycnogenol," a chemical designation (as well as the trademark of a British company) for a mixture of water-soluble flavonoids derived from the bark of the European coastal pine *Pinus nigra* Arnold var *maritima* (also known as *Pinus maritima* Lam.).[37,38]

Chemical Constituents

Both pinebark and grapeseed extracts contain various proanthocyanidins (condensed tannins) that are polyphenol oligomers derived from the condensation of flavan–3–ols and flavan–3,4–diols.

Physiologic Activity and Therapeutic Use

Grapeseed and pinebark extracts are used as antioxidants. Grapeseed and pinebark extracts, available in the United States, are used in Europe as antioxidants and to treat circulatory disorders such as hypoxia from atherosclerosis, inflammation, and cardiac or cerebral infarction.[37,38] Much additional research is required to determine with certainty the effectiveness of oligomeric proanthocyanidins in preventing or treating these various conditions.

Precautions

No precautions are noted.

Dosage

Tablets or capsules of 75–300 mg are ingested daily for up to 3 weeks, followed by a maintenance dose of 40–80 mg daily.

Nervous System Disorders

Valerian

The drug consists of preparations of the dried or fresh root of *Valeriana officinalis* L., a member of the valerian family (Valerianaceae). Its natural range includes eastern, southeastern, and east-central Europe extending to south Sweden and the southern Alps. Locally naturalized westward in Europe, the plant is likewise naturalized in eastern North America. Major producers of common valerian root include Belgium, France, Russia, and China.[11]

Chemical Constituents

More than 120 chemical components have been identified from the root and its essential oil. A group of unstable iridoids known as valepotriates has been shown to possess sedative activity, as have some valepotriate degradation products. Other biologically active components may include valerenic acid and valerenone and/or an interaction of these constituents. Valerenic acid and the esters of eugenyl and isoeugenyl are spasmolytic. An as-yet unidentified water-soluble fraction has also been shown to possess sedative activity.[39]

Physiologic Activity and Therapeutic Use

Valerian is considered to be spasmolytic, mildly sedative, and a sleep aid. The German health authorities allow its use in sedative and sleep-inducing preparations to mediate states of excitation and difficulty in falling asleep due to nervousness.[40]

Precautions

Valeriana officinalis preparations are considered safe despite the known in-vitro cytotoxic activity of valepotriates.[12] However, because valerian's active constituents have not been specifically identified, additional controlled clinical trials are needed to establish its dose-response relationship and obtain other information required for its most effective use.

Dosage

Two to three grams of the drug are taken one to three times per day, or an equivalent dosage regimen is followed.

St John's Wort

The drug consists of the dried flowering tops of *Hypericum perforatum* L., a member of the St John's wort family (Hypericaceae). It is indigenous to Europe and naturalized in Asia, Africa, North America, and Australia.[11]

Chemical Constituents

The herb contains 0.05–0.3% of naphthodianthrone pigments, especially hypericin and pseudohypericin; flavonoids, including hyperoside (hyperin), quercetin, isoquercetin, quercetrin, isoquercetrin, rutin, and kaempferol; various flavanols; and small amounts of a volatile oil, among other components.[11]

Physiologic Activity and Therapeutic Use

While anxiolytic and anti-inflammatory activities have been ascribed to the herb, it is often described in the literature as a sedative; however, four clinical trials published since 1987 have concluded that St John's wort is best classified as an antidepressant. A recent clinical trial confirmed the results of previously reported studies. A psychiatrist, an internal specialist, and a general practitioner conducted a randomized, placebo-controlled, double-blind study with 105 outpatients diagnosed with mild to moderate depression or temporary depressive moods. Patients were given the equivalent of 300 mg of St John's wort extract (standardized to a hypericin content of 0.9 mg) or a placebo preparation daily for a period of 4 weeks. In the treatment group, 67% responded to treatment compared with only 28% in the placebo group. Treatment-group patients were assessed as having significant relief from depressive mood indicators (feelings of sadness, hopelessness, helplessness, and uselessness) as well as from emotional fear and difficult or disturbed sleep. No significant side effects were observed. These researchers concluded that, compared with synthetic antidepressants, the St John's wort extract produced side effects of minor significance and that the extract can be recommended for the treatment of mild and moderate depression.[41] It apparently functions as a monoamine oxidase inhibitor, but CNS-stimulating effects have also been reported.

Precautions

Hypericin is known to cause photodermatitis in light-skinned farm animals grazing on the plant. There are no reports of human photodermatitis from ingestion of hypericum products. However, cases of photodermatitis in humans have been reported in clinical trials involving synthetic hypericin. Light-skinned individuals are advised not to expose skin to direct sunlight after ingesting the herb.[11]

Dosage

In European phytomedicine, 2–4 g of herb (calculated to contain 0.2–1.0 mg hypericin) is used, usually in the form of capsules, for mild antidepressant action or nervous disturbances.[42]

Willow Bark

The drug consists of the dried bark of white willow, *Salix alba* L., as well as other species, including *Salix fragilis* L., *Salix purpurea* L., *Salix daphnoides* Villars, and *Salix pentandra* L. All of the above species are native to Europe but, with the exception of *Salix daphnoides*, have become naturalized in North America. They are members of the willow family (Salicaceae). The bark is collected from branches of the tree.[9]

Chemical Constituents

The bark contains phenolic glycosides (2.5–11%, depending upon species), predominately salicylates (not less than [NLT] 1% salicin in the form of its ester, salicortin) and tremulacin. Flavonoids are also present (1–4%), along with 8–20% tannins (generally of the catechin type), gallotannins, and various dimeric and trimeric procyanidins. Most literature notes that white willow (*Salix alba*) is the primary source of the drug; however, it is very low in salicin content (0.5–1%). Other species mentioned above have a much higher total phenolic glycoside content (calculated as salicin).[4,9]

Physiologic Activity and Therapeutic Use

Willow bark has been traditionally used as an anti-inflammatory and analgesic for rheumatic and arthritic conditions, as an antipyretic in cases of the common cold or influenza, and as an astringent. The root bark has also been used to treat mild headaches and gout.[9]

Phenolic glycoside esters in the bark, including salicortin, 2´-*O*-acetylsalicortin and tremulacin, are hydrolyzed to form salicin in alkaline intestinal fluid and then hydrolyzed to saligenin by intestinal flora. Once absorbed, this aglycone is oxidized in the blood and liver to produce salicylic acid, which has similar analgesic properties to acetylsalicylic acid but exerts no effect on platelet function. Pain is reduced by inhibiting prostaglandin synthesis in tissue and sensory nerves.[4,9]

Precautions

Because salicylates reported in the crude bark of various species are highly variable, it is estimated that 0.75–5 L of willow bark tea would have to be consumed to achieve a single average therapeutic dose. In light of the high tannin levels in the bark, such a dose is ill-advised.[4] In European phytomedicine, products standardized on the basis of salicin content are readily available, although they are not generally sold in the American market at this time.

Dosage

A decoction of 1–2 g of finely powdered dried bark, 1–2 mL of tincture (1:5 25% ethanol), or standardized forms corresponding to a total salicin content of 20–40 mg are taken three times a day, with the average daily dose calculated to 60–120 mg salicin.[9] These figures are apparently based on the low amount of salicin in commercially available bark samples and could not be expected to render an effective therapeutic dose (see Precautions). Consumers contemplating use of a crude willow bark preparation as an analgesic or anti-inflammatory are best advised to use aspirin or other appropriate nonsteroidal anti-inflammatory drugs.[4]

Feverfew

The drug consists of the dried leaves of *Tanacetum parthenium* (L.) Schulz Bip. (*Chrysanthemum parthenium* [L.] Bernh.), a member of the aster family (Asteraceae, formerly Compositae). Native to Europe, it is commonly grown as an ornamental flower in the United States.[43]

Chemical Constituents

The primary chemical constituents of feverfew are sesquiterpenes, especially parthenolide (0.1–1.27%). While parthenolide is the dominant sesquiterpene lactone in the species, several chemotypes have been found in which parthenolide is absent. Selection of parthenolide-containing germplasm is necessary for product development. Canadian regulatory authorities have proposed correctly identified whole dried leaf or leaf extract (with at least 0.2% parthenolide) as a minimum standard for reasonable certainty of efficacy in feverfew products; French authorities have proposed a level of 0.1%. The herb used in two published clinical trials on the effects of feverfew is comparable to the proposed Canadian standard. Parthenolide content of feverfew from various sources has been found to be highly variable.[44,45]

Physiologic Activity and Therapeutic Use

Traditionally, feverfew has been used to treat headaches, fevers, menstrual problems, and other painful maladies. Current primary use is as a prophylactic to reduce the frequency, severity, and duration of migraine headaches and to relieve associated symptoms such as nausea. Although the mechanism of action is not completely understood, migraine prophylaxis is attributed to inhibition of the release of 5-hydroxytryptamine (5-HT or serotonin) from blood platelets.[9,43–45]

Precautions

Some individuals may experience gastric discomfort following ingestion. Administration of fresh leaves has produced occasional mouth ulceration.

Dosage

The average daily dose of the dried leaves with a minimum content of 0.2% parthenolide is 125 mg; the herb is usually consumed in tablet or capsule form.[4]

Caffeine-Containing Plants

Caffeine-containing plants include coffee (dried ripe seed of *Coffea arabica* L., a member of the madder family [Rubiaceae]); tea (leaves and leaf buds of *Camellia sinensis* [L.] O. Kuntze, a member of the tea family [Theaceae]); kola (the dried cotyledon of *Cola nitida* [Vent.] Schott & Endl. and other *Cola* species, members of the cola family [Sterculiaceae]); cocoa, also known as cacao (the roasted seed of *Theobroma cacao* L. also a member of the cola family); guarana (crushed seeds of *Paullinia cupana* H.B.K., a member of the soapberry family [Sapindaceae]); and maté, also known as yerba maté (the dried leaves of *Ilex paraguariensis* St.-Hil., a member of the holly family [Aquifoliaceae]).[4]

Chemical Constituents

These herbs all contain caffeine (1,3,7-trimethylxanthine).[10]

Physiologic Activity and Therapeutic Use

All these herbs are CNS stimulants. They are used alone to overcome drowsiness and in combination with nonprescription analgesics, which they potentiate by as much as 40%. Combined with ergot alkaloids, caffeine has been used in preparations for the treatment of migraine headaches. Caffeine-containing beverages also have a weak diuretic activity of relatively short duration.[4]

Precautions

As CNS stimulants, caffeine-containing plants should be used with caution by persons with hypertension and related disorders.

Dosage

The daily dose is equivalent to 100–200 mg of caffeine.[4]

Metabolic and Endocrine Disorders

Black Cohosh

The drug consists of the dried rhizome and roots of *Cimicifuga racemosa* (L.) Nutt., a member of the buttercup family (Ranunculaceae), which is indigenous to the rich woods of the eastern deciduous forest of North America.

Chemical Constituents

The primary biologically active components of black cohosh are triterpene glycosides, including acetein and cimicifugoside (cimigoside). Isoflavones are also present, especially formononetin. Other constituents of minor importance include isoferulic and salicylic acids, tannins, resin, starch, sugars, and the like.

Physiologic Activity and Therapeutic Use

Black cohosh is primarily used in European phytomedicine (particularly in Germany) as an emmenagogue and for endocrine activity in the treatment of neurovisceral and psychic problems associated with menopause, premenstrual complaints, and dysmenorrhea. It is also used as a uterine antispasmodic. In a study involving 100 menopausal women, none of whom had received steroid replacement therapy for at least 6 months immediately preceding admission into the trial, an ethanolic extract of the rhizome was found to cause a selective reduction of serum concentrations of pituitary luteinizing hormone (LH). The extract has also been found to bind to estrogen receptors of rat uteri. LH reduction is attributed to three different chemical fractions, acting synergistically. Cimicifugoside is also believed to affect the hypothalamus–pituitary system, producing effects on the reproductive and nervous systems.[9] The German Commission E monograph allows use for premenstrual discomfort and dysmenorrhea.[46]

Precautions

GI disturbances have been reported from the use of black cohosh in some patients. Use is contraindicated during pregnancy and lactation.

Dosage

The dried rhizome is used in appropriate formulations, such as decoctions or tinctures (1:10, 60% ethanol), in amounts corresponding to a daily dosage of 40–200 mg. The German health authorities specify that duration of use should not exceed 6 months (presumably because information on long-term effects is lacking).[9]

Chaste Tree Berry

The drug consists of the fruits of *Vitex agnus-castus* L., a shrub or small tree native to West Asia and southwestern Europe that has become naturalized in much of the southeastern United States. It is a member of the verbena family (Verbenaceae).

Chemical Constituents

The fruits contain flavonoids, which are considered to be the primary active components. These include the major flavonoid casticin (quercetagetin-3,6,7,4′-tetramethyl ether), as well as orientin, 3,6,7,4′-tetramethyl ether of 6-hydroxykaempferol, and quercetagetin.[47] The dried fruits also contain an essential oil (up to 1.22%), as well as iridoid glycosides, including aucubin, eurostoside, and agnuside.[48]

Physiologic Activity and Therapeutic Use

Chaste tree has been used for at least 2,500 years to treat menstrual difficulties. A clinical survey of German gynecologists evaluated the effect of a chaste tree preparation (Agnolyt) on 1,542 women diagnosed with premenstrual syndrome (PMS). Administration of 40 drops daily continued for an average of 166 days. Both physicians and patients assessed efficacy, with 90% reporting complete relief of symptoms after an average treatment duration of 25.3 days. Two percent reported side effects, mostly GI in nature.[49] The German Commission E monograph on chaste tree fruits allows use of preparations for menstrual disorders due to primary or secondary corpus luteum insufficiency, PMS, mastalgia, menopausal symptoms, and inadequate lactation.[50]

Precautions

Chaste tree preparations are contraindicated during pregnancy. Noted side effects include early onset of menstruation following delivery (resulting from activation of the pituitary), as well as rare instances of itching, rashes, and GI discomfort. While no interactions with other drugs are reported, animal experiments indicate the possibility of interference with dopamine-receptor antagonists.[50]

Dosage

Preparations include alcoholic extracts (tinctures) of the pulverized fruits, formulated to provide an average daily dose equivalent to 20 mg of the crude fruit, or 30–40 mg of the fruits in decoction.[50]

Evening Primrose (Black Currant, Borage Seed) Oil

The drug consists of the oil expressed from the seeds of evening primrose (*Oenothera biennis* L.), native to eastern North America and widely naturalized elsewhere. It is a member of the primrose family (Onagraceae). The seed oils of black currant (*Ribes nigrum* L.) and borage (*Borago officinalis* L.) are also used for similar purposes.

Chemical Constituents

Evening primrose seed produces about 14% fixed oil consisting of *cis*-linoleic acid (50–70%) as the primary component, along with 7–10% *cis*-gamma-linolenic acid (GLA). The seed oil contains smaller amounts of palmitic, oleic, and stearic acids; steroids, including campesterol and beta-sitosterol, are also present.[11]

Physiologic Activity and Therapeutic Use

Studies suggest that the GLA found in dietary supplement sources, especially evening primrose oil (EPO), can be directly converted to the prostaglandin precursor dihomo-GLA and could be of benefit to individuals unable to metabolize *cis*-linoleic acid in addition to persons whose diets are low in that acid.[51]

GLA is present only in small amounts in normal dietary sources although it is a major component of human milk. Conversion of linoleic acid into GLA can be hampered by a number of factors such as aging, high cholesterol levels, high intake of saturated fats and *trans*-fatty acids, viral infections, stress, high alcohol intake, diabetes, eczema, and PMS.[51] Various studies have shown that supplementation with GLA is possibly beneficial in some of the above conditions. At specified doses, GLA may produce metabolites such as prostaglandin E_1 and 15-hydroxy-dihomo-GLA.[51,52]

A slow rate of 6-desaturation of essential fatty acids (EFAs) has been best documented in atopic eczema. A number of randomized, double-blind, placebo-controlled trials involving GLA-containing EPO have shown modest to insignificant improvement in symptoms associated with atopic eczema, especially relief from itching. In England, topical preparations of EPO are registered for use in the treatment of atopic eczema.[51,52]

Other plant oils, including those from the seeds of black currant and borage, also contain large amounts of GLA. However, the results of EPO research are difficult to apply to these species as the patterns of fatty acids present are different in these oils. Unlike the oils of the other plants, EPO contains no omega-3 EFAs and almost no saturated fatty acids, both of which are known to interfere with the biological activity and metabolism of omega-6 EFAs and may diminish the biological activity of the GLAs present in the oil. The triglyceride structures of the oils are also different and could produce different effects.[51]

Precautions

No precautions are noted.

Dosage

Relevant clinical conditions for GLA supplementation, such as alcoholism and inflammation, may require doses of 600–6,000 mg per day. For atopic eczema, the dosage is four 250-mg capsules taken twice daily.[51]

Arthritic and Musculoskeletal Disorders

All of the effective plant derivatives, mustard oil, methyl salicylate, etc, are covered in Chapter 5, "External Analgesic Products."

Disorders of the Skin, Mucous Membranes, and Gingiva

Witch Hazel

The botanical is derived from the twigs and leaves of *Hamamelis virginiana* L. (Hamamelidaceae), found in the eastern deciduous forest of North America. It is also commercially cultivated in Europe. Vernal witch hazel (*Hamamelis vernalis* Sarg.) may also be involved in the commercial supply. The witch hazel preparation commonly available in the United States is distilled witch hazel extract (also referred to as hamamelis water), which is prepared by steam distillation of the recently harvested, dormant twigs macerated in water, with 14% alcohol subsequently added. Conversely, hydroalcoholic extracts are commonly used in Europe.[4]

Chemical Constituents

Witch hazel leaves contain 8–10% tannin composed of hamamelitannin or digallyhamamelose, gallotannins, and proanthocyanidins. Tannins are considered responsible for the astringent activity of the herb; however, they are absent from the commonly available steam distillate, which relies on the added alcohol for its astringent effect.[4,11]

Physiologic Activity and Therapeutic Use

Witch hazel preparations are used to treat local inflammation of the skin and mucous membranes.[4] In Europe, hydroalcoholic extracts are also used as astringents, anti-inflammatories, and local hemostyptics for minor skin injuries, hemorrhoids, and varicose veins.[53]

Precautions

No precautions are noted.

Dosage

Witch hazel preparations are applied topically, as necessary.

Aloe Vera Gel

The drug consists of a mucilaginous gel obtained from the parenchymatous tissue in the center of the leaf of *Aloe vera* (L.) N. L. Burm., a member of the lily family (Liliaceae). It is also referred to in the literature as *Aloe barbadensis* Mill.; however, the *Aloe vera* binomial was published in 1768 and so has priority over the *Aloe barbadensis* binomial published subsequently. The gel should not be confused with the yellow latex or juice occurring in specialized cells just below the leaf epidermis, which is the source of the cathartic drug aloe.

Chemical Constituents

The gel primarily consists of several types of polysaccharides, including an acidic galactan, mannan, a glucomannan, an arabinan, and/or a glucogalactomannan. Polysaccharides constitute 0.2–0.3% of the fresh gel. The reported ratios of hexoses in each polysaccharide, as well as the molecular weights of the polysaccharides themselves, differ widely in various studies. Composition of the gel is still not clearly defined. A serine carboxypeptidase has been suggested as an antithermic agent in aloe gel.[11]

Physiologic Activity and Therapeutic Use

Fresh aloe gel, perhaps the most widely used folk medicine in the United States, is applied to first-degree burns and minor skin irritations. It has anti-inflammatory and emollient properties, and it also enhances wound healing. A recent review of the pharmacologic and clinical studies of aloe gel concluded that it also has possible therapeutic value in burns and a wide variety of soft tissue injuries: the authors found that it prevented progressive dermal ischemia following thermal injury, frostbite, and electrical trauma. Aloe gel penetrates injured tissue, relieves pain, and is anti-inflammatory; it acts to dilate capillaries, thus increasing the blood supply to the injury.[54]

Precautions

No precautions are noted.

Dosage
Fresh gel is applied topically as necessary.

Tea Tree Oil

Tea tree oil is the volatile oil that is steam distilled from the leaves of *Melaleuca alternifolia* (Maiden & Betche) Cheel (family Myrtaceae), a shrub or small tree growing up to 18 feet in height. The plant is found in swampy or wet ground on the northern coast of New South Wales (north of Port Macquarie) as well as in adjacent areas of southern Queensland in Australia. Production is generally limited to this region.

Chemical Constituents
Tea tree leaves contain about 2% of volatile oil, with terpene hydrocarbons including pinene, terpinene, cymene (about 30%), and 65% or more of oxygenated terpenes, particularly terpinen-4-ol (30–60%).[4] High-quality volatile oil (Australian Standard. "Oil of Melaleuca, Terpinen-4-ol type," AS 2782) contains 30–47% terpinen-4-ol and less than 15% cineole as major components. Cineole-rich oils are considered to be of inferior quality.[11]

Physiologic Activity and Therapeutic Use
Oil high in terpinen-4-ol is considered bacteriostatic and germicidal. The oil has been used for treating boils, abscesses, sores, cuts, and abrasions, as well as wounds with pus discharge. During World War II, the oil was mixed with machine-cutting oils in Australian ammunition factories to reduce infections from metal filing injuries.[4]

Other conditions for which use of the oil has been promoted include acne, arthritis, bruises, burns, cystitis, dermatitis, fungal infections, herpes, insect bites, muscular aches and pains, respiratory tract infections, sunburn, vaginal infections, varicose veins, and warts.[4] However, the oil's utility in many of these conditions requires verification.

A 1990 clinical trial involving 124 patients provided evidence that *Melaleuca alternifolia* oil is effective in the treatment of acne vulgaris. A 5% tea tree oil in a water-based gel was less effective (owing to slower onset of action) than a 5% benzoyl peroxide in water-based lotion; however, clinical assessment and self-reporting of side effects suggested that tea tree oil was better tolerated on facial skin with less skin scaling, dryness, pruritus, and irritation. The results of this study were less than conclusive.[55]

Tea tree oil products are widely marketed, often with hyperbolic claims.

Precautions
Tea tree oil may cause skin irritation or allergies in sensitive individuals. Generally, the oil has not been associated with toxicity.[4]

Dosage
The oil is applied topically in concentrations from 0.4 to 100%, depending upon the condition and area of treatment.[4]

Goldenseal

The drug consists of the dried rhizome and roots of *Hydrastis canadensis* L., a member of the buttercup family (Ranunculaceae) found in the rich, deciduous forests of the eastern United States.

Chemical Constituents
The rhizome and roots contain a number of isoquinoline alkaloids, including hydrastine (1.5–4%), berberine (1.7–4.5%), and canadine (0.5%).[9]

Physiologic Activity and Therapeutic Use
Root preparations have traditionally been used for their antimicrobial, astringent, and antihemorrhagic activities in the treatment of mucosal inflammation. Formerly, the hydrochlorides of hydrastine and berberine were used in ophthalmic products. The root is also used as a digestive tonic for the treatment of dyspepsia and gastritis. Hydrastine is considered to be vasoconstrictive, and hydrastine and berberine are thought to have choleretic, spasmolytic, and antibacterial properties. Unfortunately, despite its great popularity in the American herb market, there have been no recent pharmacologic or clinical studies of goldenseal.[9,56]

A modern folk use for goldenseal has been to mask illicit drugs in urinalysis tests. The herb's activity in this regard is a myth that has grown out of the fictional plot of the novel *Stringtown on the Pike*, published in 1900 by pharmacist John Uri Lloyd (1849–1936). There is no scientific evidence to support this use; in fact, it may instead promote false-positive readings. Some laboratories are now testing for the presence of hydrastine during urinalysis.[56,57]

Precautions
The use of goldenseal is contraindicated during pregnancy.

Dosage
The dosage is 0.5–1 g of the dried root or 2–4 mL of tincture (1:10, 60% ethanol) three times per day.[9]

Melissa

The drug consists of preparations of the leaves of Melissa, also commonly known as lemon balm (*Melissa officinalis* L.), a member of the mint family (Lamiaceae, formerly Labiatae).

Chemical Constituents
Melissa contains about 0.1–0.2% volatile oil composed mainly of oxygenated compounds such as citral (a and b), geraniol, caryophyllene oxide, and polyphenols (caffeic acid, protocatechuic acid, etc); a tannin composed of chlorogenic, caffeic, and rosmarinic acids; flavonoids; and other compounds.[11]

Physiologic Activity and Therapeutic Use
Historically, the leaves (primarily in tea form) have been used for their calmative, spasmolytic, and carminative activity. The German government allows the use of lemon balm preparations to alleviate difficulty in falling asleep

due to nervous conditions and to treat functional GI symptoms.[11]

More recently, antibacterial and antiviral activities have been confirmed. Oxidative products of caffeic acid and derivatives were found to have antiviral activity against herpes simplex virus type 1 (cold sores) and type 2 (genital herpes).[4] A European ointment corresponding to 0.7 g of leaf per gram has recently become available on the American market.

Two dermatologic centers carried out a randomized, placebo-controlled, double-blind study on the effect of a cream containing 1% dried extract of lemon balm leaves (drug extract 70:1) on herpes lesions. Case reports of 116 patients using lemon balm cream were evaluated for the study. The physicians and patients judged the lemon balm cream to be superior to the placebo. At the critical initial stage of treatment as well as during the second day, when the swelling began to decline, the treatment group showed significant improvement compared with those receiving a placebo. To achieve efficacy, it was found that treatment must be started at very early stages of the infection. Accelerated healing was most pronounced in the first 2 days of treatment.[58]

Precautions

No precautions are noted.

Dosage

Lemon balm preparations are applied topically as needed in appropriate formulations.

Performance and Endurance Enhancers

Ginseng

The drug consists of the dried root of Asian ginseng (*Panax ginseng* C.A. Meyer) and American ginseng (*Panax quinquefolius* L.), both members of the ginseng family (Araliaceae). The comments that follow focus primarily on Asian ginseng, the subject of the vast majority of scientific studies. Wild Asian ginseng is rare in its indigenous northeast Asian habitats, which include northeastern China, the Korean peninsula, and adjacent Russia. It is, however, extensively cultivated in China and Korea.[59]

Chemical Constituents

Asian ginseng contains as its primary active components at least 18 triterpenoid saponins, including ginsenosides R_0, R_{b-1}, R_{b-2}, R_{b-3}, R_c, R_d, R_e, R_f, $R_{20\text{-gluco-f}}$, R_{g-1}, and R_{g-2}. Traditionally, the root is harvested in the sixth year of growth. A recent 5-year study showed that the highest levels of ginsenosides were obtained at the end of summer of the fifth year. The root weight also doubles between the fourth and fifth years of growth. Other constituents include a trace of volatile oil, starch, polysaccharides (panaxans A–U in a concentration of 7–9%), pectin, free sugar, polyacetylenes, and the like.[11]

Physiologic Activity and Therapeutic Use

Traditionally characterized as an aphrodisiac and a tonic, ginseng has a documented use dating back well over 2,000 years. Numerous although conflicting pharmacologic and clinical benefits have been attributed to the root and its preparations, including radioprotective, antitumor, antiviral, and metabolic effects; CNS, reproductive performance, and lipid metabolism enhancement; and antioxidant, cholesterol-lowering, and endocrinologic activities.[60,61]

Ginseng is now designated as an adaptogen—an agent facilitating resistance to various kinds of stress. Extracts standardized to contain between 4 and 7% ginsenosides have been subjected to several clinical studies in Europe. Positive results reported include shortened reaction time to visual and auditory stimuli, elevated respiratory quotient, increased alertness, improved power of concentration, enhanced grasp of abstract concepts, and better visual and motor coordination. Conflicting results of various studies have been attributed to differences in the type of preparation, route of administration, dosage, and presence or absence of biologically active compounds, among other factors.[60,61] Additional randomized clinical trials with standardized ginseng preparations are needed to determine the degree of utility of this herb in the prevention and treatment of specific conditions in human beings. The German Commission E monograph allows ginseng's use as a tonic to treat fatigue, diminished work capacity, and loss of concentration, in addition to its use as a general aid during convalescence.[62]

Precautions

Ginseng is generally considered safe, given the relative infrequency of reports of significant side effects and its history of long-term use. Excessive consumption of ginseng of undefined origin (15 g per day) over a period of time has been reported to induce hypertension and nervousness.[4] These effects require verification.

Dosage

The daily dosage is 1–2 g of root in appropriate formulations.[62]

Eleuthero

The drug consists of the dried root of *Eleutherococcus senticosus* (Rupr. & Maxim.) Maxim., a shrubby member of the ginseng family (Araliaceae). The plant grows up to 9 feet tall and is found in eastern Siberia, northeastern China, adjacent Korea, and Hokkaido Island in Japan. In traditional Chinese medicine, the bark of the root was the plant part employed; today, the root, stems, and leaves enter commerce. The drug is widely marketed in the United States under the name "Siberian ginseng." Eleuthero was formerly said to be derived from *Acanthopanax senticosus* (Rupr.) Harms, a name still commonly seen in Chinese literature.[63]

Chemical Constituents

Numerous compounds have been identified from the root and are designated eleutherosides A–G. Their concentrations range from 0.6 to 0.9% in the roots and from 0.6 to 1.5% in the stems.[9] Although the common name *eleutheroside* would seem to imply similarity in chemical structure, such is not the case. Eleutheroside A is the sterol daucosterol; eleutheroside B is syringin, a phenylpropanoid; eleutheroside B_1 is isofraxidin-7-*O*-alpha-L-glucoside (beta-calycanthoside). Lignans include eleutheroside B_4 [(−)-sesamin], eleutheroside D [(−)-syringaresinol-di-*O*-beta-D-glucoside], and eleutheroside E (acanthoside D). Triterpenes include eleutherosides I–M. Senticosides A–F represent incompletely characterized oleanolic acid glycosides (possibly identical to other triterpenoid components).[11,64]

Physiologic Activity and Therapeutic Use

Numerous biologic activities have been described for eleuthero root ethanolic extracts, including adaptogenic activity in cases of hyperthermia, electroshock-induced convulsions, gastric ulcers, and x-ray irradiation. Among the positive effects demonstrated in vivo in animal studies are increased metabolic efficiency in swimming-induced stress, improved conditioned response to stimuli, inhibition of conditioned avoidance response, antioxidant (free-radical scavenging) activity, and a hypoglycemic effect along with antiedema, anti-inflammatory, diuretic, gonadotropic, estrogenic, and antihypertensive activities.[11] Eleuthero polysaccharides have also been reported to have immunostimulatory activity.[63,64]

Since the early 1960s, clinical studies involving more than 2,100 normal and stressed human subjects were conducted in Russia using an orally administered 33% ethanol root extract of *Eleutherococcus senticosus.* The root is the subject of a positive German Commission E monograph, which indicates its use as a tonic for invigoration during fatigue, debility, declining work capacity, and concentration as well as during convalescence. [9,63–65] Well-designed, randomized clinical trials with standardized preparations are required to determine which of the numerous claims of utility for eleuthero can be verified.

Precautions

Side effects have been rarely reported. Cautions against the use of eleuthero in cases of hypertension do appear in the literature.[65]

Dosage

The average daily dose is 2–3 g of the powdered or cut root in decoction. In Russian studies using a 33% ethanol extract of the root, dosages of 2–16 mL were taken one to three times a day for up to 60 consecutive days (with a 2- to 3-week resting interval between courses of administration). Up to five courses of the herb were administered within a period of 1 year.[64,65]

Echinacea

The drug consists of the aboveground parts and/or roots of *Echinacea purpurea* (L.) Moench., as well as the roots of *Echinacea angustifolia* DC and *Echinacea pallida* (Nutt.) Nutt., members of the aster family (Asteraceae, formerly Compositae). All of these species are indigenous to the midwestern United States. The entire supply of *Echinacea purpurea* is cultivated. While commercial cultivation of *Echinacea pallida* and *Echinacea angustifolia* has recently begun, most of the world's supply is harvested from indigenous habitats in the central United States.[66]

Chemical Constituents

Problems in identifying source plants used in chemical studies, with the exception of vouchered cultivated *Echinacea purpurea*, render chemical studies prior to 1988 unreliable.[67]

Echinacea purpurea, the best-studied species, contains cichoric acid, 1.2–3.1% in the flowering tops and 0.6–2.1% in the roots. It also contains other caffeic acid derivatives; an essential oil; alkylamides, including the isomeric dodeca-(2*E*,4*E*,8*Z*,10*E*/*Z*)-tetraenoic acid isobutylamides, along with 10 additional alkylamides possessing a 2,4-diene structure; and various polysaccharides.[67]

Echinacea angustifolia dried root contains cynarin; cichoric acid; an essential oil (less than 0.1%); alkylamides, including dodeca-(2*E*,6*Z*,8*E*,10*E*)-tetraenoic acid isobutylamide (echinacein, in a concentration of 0.01% in the dried roots); and 14 additional isobutylamides (0.009–0.151%). *Echinacea angustifolia* also contains polysaccharides. Echinacoside, once believed to be unique to *Echinacea angustifolia* (0.3–1.3% dry weight in the roots), has recently also been found in five additional *Echinacea* species.[67]

Physiologic Activity and Therapeutic Use

Echinacea products (oral dosage forms) are used as nonspecific immunostimulants, especially as prophylactics at the first sign of cold and flu symptoms, for treatment of *Candida albicans* infections, and for other related conditions.[66,67] A recent double-blind, placebo-controlled study indicates that a daily dose of 450 mg of *Echinacea purpurea* root extract (1:5 in 55% ethanol) significantly relieved the severity and duration of flu symptoms.[68] A double-blind, monocentric, placebo-controlled clinical trial examined the immunostimulating influence of an expressed fresh juice *Echinacea purpurea* preparation on the course and severity of colds and flulike symptoms in patients deemed to have greater than normal susceptibility to infections. At a dose of 2–4 mL per day, patients with diminished immune response (expressed by a low T4/T8 cell ratio) were found to benefit significantly from preventive treatment with the echinacea preparation.[69]

Topical preparations (ointment)—available in Germany but ordinarily not in the United States—of the fresh aboveground parts of *Echinacea purpurea* are used for the external treatment of hard-to-heal wounds, eczema, burns, psoriasis, herpes simplex, etc.[11,70]

Precautions

Echinacea, as well as nonspecific immunostimulants in general, are contraindicated in tuberculosis, leukosis, collagenosis, multiple sclerosis, HIV-infections, and other autoimmune diseases.[70] Historical confusion about plant identity in scientific studies (where vouchered specimens were lacking) and persistence of adulterated supplies of *Echinacea purpurea* root with *Parthenium integrifolium* L. have resulted in the publication of negative (not recommended) German therapeutic monographs on *Echinacea purpurea* root[71] as well as on *Echinacea angustifolia* root *and Echinacea angustifolia/Echinacea pallida* aerial parts.[72] Positive monographs have been published for preparations containing aerial parts of *Echinacea purpurea* and the roots of *Echinacea pallida.*[70,73]

Dosage

Of the expressed fresh juice of *Echinacea purpurea*, the dose is 6–9 mL per day for not longer than 8 weeks; after that period, the immunostimulatory effects decline.[70] For *Echinacea pallida* root preparations, the average daily dose corresponds to 900 mg per day, often administered in the form of a tincture (1:5) prepared with 50% ethanol.[73] Dosage of *Echinacea angustifolia* root in the form of capsules, tablets, or a tincture is 1 g, three times daily.[9]

Case Studies

Case 35-1

Patient Complaint/History

JS, a 16-year-old male student who participates actively in football, wrestling, and track and field events, asks the pharmacist about the availability of preparations that will enhance his physique and increase his performance/endurance in sports. He explains that body-building magazines regularly advertise dioscorea, sarsaparilla, and yohimbe as "natural testosterone sources." He then displays an advertisement that calls these products "steroid alternatives" and requests recommendations for suitable products containing the advertised or other related botanicals.

The patient is obviously a healthy teenager; his patient profile shows that he uses no prescription medications on a regular basis. His infrequent use of nonprescription products is limited to Advil 200 mg tablets prn for athletic aches/pains and Robitussin prn for symptoms related to occasional colds.

Clinical Considerations/Strategies

The following considerations/strategies are provided to aid the reader in (1) determining whether treatment of the patient's condition with nonprescription medications is warranted, (2) selecting the appropriate nonprescription medication, and (3) developing a patient counseling strategy to ensure optimal therapeutic outcomes:

- Assess this patient's actual versus perceived need for effective physique-enhancing drugs.
- Inform the patient of inaccuracies in herbal advertisements in a manner that will not "turn him off" to seeking professional advice or cause him to order useless products by mail.
- Advise the patient that certain steroidal compounds may be converted to active substances in the laboratory but not in the human body.
- Advise the patient that, in most instances, the safety and effectiveness of many products touted as wondrous cures or enhancers of mental and physical prowess—which are commonly sold by mail-order, telephone-order, health food stores, or nutrition centers—have not been clinically tested or proven in objective, controlled studies.
- Develop a patient/counseling strategy that will:
  - Reveal appropriate non–drug-assisted techniques for body building;
  - Help the patient understand that there are no shortcuts to the improvement of the mind and/or body and that all such "quick fixes" (promises) are irrational and without a basis in fact;
  - Further enlighten the patient as to the serious physical consequences that accompany the improper use of androgenic steroids to improve athletic performance;
  - Encourage the patient to seek professional advice on the safety and effectiveness of plant-derived products. Also, ask him to encourage his friends to seek professional advice if they have questions or concerns about these products.

Case 35–2

Patient Complaint/History

CP, an apparently healthy and obviously vigorous 64-year-old male, enters the consulting area and asks to speak privately with a pharmacist. The patient, who has patronized the pharmacy for several years, was diagnosed two years ago as having BPH for which his urologist prescribed Proscar 5 mg one tablet daily. His response to the medication has been excellent, but he now admits that the drug has greatly reduced his sexual potency. He also reveals that he plans to marry a 32-year-old woman; his first wife died 10 years ago.

CP has read the *Physician's Desk Reference*'s monograph on finasteride and is aware that the medication is probably the cause of his impotency. A friend who has no medical or pharmaceutical training advised him to quit taking finasteride and take saw palmetto standardized extract instead. CP asks whether this is a good idea. In addition to finasteride, he currently takes ascorbic acid (vitamin C) 250 mg one tablet daily and the standard nonprescription products for aches/pains and coughs/colds.

Clinical Considerations/Strategies

The following considerations/strategies are provided to aid the reader in (1) determining whether treatment of the patient's condition with nonprescription medications is warranted, (2) selecting the appropriate nonprescription medication, and (3) developing a patient counseling strategy to ensure optimal therapeutic outcomes:

- Assess the therapeutic use of saw palmetto as an alternative to finasteride.
- Assess the appropriateness of recommending a dietary supplement as a substitute for a prescription medication.
- Determine the best method for encouraging the patient's urologist to become involved, remembering that the therapeutic use of botanicals is not usually taught in US medical schools.
- Develop a patient education/counseling strategy that will:
  - Inform the patient of the need to consult his urologist before making any therapeutic decision;
  - Explain the effectiveness and limitations of saw palmetto standardized extract in treating BPH;
  - Aid the patient in selecting a specific botanical product and provide a suitable dosage regimen for the product (if the patient and his urologist collaborate and mutually approve a switch from Proscar to saw palmetto);
  - Explain the efficacy, side effect profile, and guidelines for proper use of Proscar (if the patient and his urologist decide the switch is not appropriate).

References

1. The right stuff: *Drug Store News* picks the categories taking off in '94. *Drug Store News*. 1994 Jan 17; 16(2): 15.
2. DeNitto E. Herbal remedies peal across US. *Advertising Age*. 1994 Apr 4; 65(14): 12.
3. Eisenberg D et al. Unconventional medicine in the United States. *N Engl J Med*. 1993 Jan 28; 328: 246–52.
4. Tyler VE. *Herbs of Choice: The Therapeutic Use of Phytomedicinals*. Binghamton, NY: Pharmaceutical Products Press; 1994.
5. Schepers A. Reading between the lines of the new "pill bill." *Environ Nutr*. 1994 Dec; 17(12): 2.
6. Schilcher H. The significance of phytotherapy in Europe. *Z Phytother*. 1993 Jun 15; 14: 132–9.
7. Tyler VE. *The Honest Herbal*. 3rd ed. Binghamton, NY. Pharmaceutical Products Press; 1993: 119–21.
8. Castañeda-Acosta J, Fischer NH, Vargas D. Biomimetic transformations of parthenolide. *J Nat Prod*. 1993 Jan; 56: 90–8.
9. Bradley PR, ed. *British Herbal Compendium*. Vol 1. Bournemouth, Dorset, England: British Herbal Medicine Association; 1992.
10. Tyler VE, Brady LR, Robbers JE. *Pharmacognosy*. 9th ed. Philadelphia, Pa: Lea & Febiger; 1988.
11. Leung AY, Foster S. *Encyclopedia of Common Natural Ingredients Used in Foods, Drugs, and Cosmetics*. 2nd ed. New York: John Wiley & Sons; 1995.
12. European Scientific Cooperative for Phytotherapy (ESCOP). *Proposal for European Monographs*. Vol 2. Bevrijdingslaan, The Netherlands: ESCOP Secretariat; 1992.
13. Monographie: Plantaginis ovatae testa (Indische Flohsamenschalen); Plantaginis ovatae semen (Indische Flohsamen). *Bundesanzeiger*. 1990 Feb 1.
14. Sprecher DL et al. Efficacy of psyllium in reducing serum cholesterol levels in hypercholesterolemic patients on high- or low-fat diets. *Ann Intern Med*. 1993 Oct 1; 119: 545–54.
15. Monographie: Sennae folium (Sennesblätter). *Bundesanzeiger*. 1993 Jul 21.
16. Foster S. *Peppermint*: Mentha x piperita. Botanical Series 306. Austin, Tex: American Botanical Council; 1991: 1–7.
17. Monographie: Menthae piperitae folium (Pfefferminzblätter). *Bundesanzeiger*. 1985 Nov 30; rev 1990 Mar 13.
18. Monographie: Menthae piperitae aetheroleum (Pfefferminzöl). *Bundesanzeiger*. 1990 Mar 13.
19. ESCOP. *Proposal for European Monographs*. Vol 1. Bevrijdingslaan, The Netherlands: ESCOP Secretariat; 1990.
20. Foster S. *Chamomile*: Matricaria recutita & Chamaemelum nobile. Botanical Series 307. Austin, Tex: American Botanical Council; 1991: 1–7.
21. Monographie: Matricariae flos (Kamillenblüten). *Bundesanzeiger*. 1984 Dec 5; rev 1990 Mar 13.
22. Foster S. *Milk Thistle*: Silybum marianum. Botanical Series 305. Austin, Tex: American Botanical Council; 1991: 1–7.
23. Monographie: Cardui mariae fructus (Mariendistelfrüchte). *Bundesanzeiger*. 1986 Mar 13.
24. Monographie: Liquiritiae radix (Süssholzwurzel). *Bundesanzeiger*. 1985 May 15; rev 1990 Mar 13.
25. Monographie: Solidaginis virgaureae herba (Echtes Goldrutenkraut). *Bundesanzeiger*. 1987 Oct 15; rev 1990 Mar 13.
26. Monographie: Uvae ursi folium (Bärentraubenblätter). *Bundesanzeiger*. 1984 Dec 5.
27. *Lawrence Rev Nat Prod*. 1994 Jul.
28. Monographie: Sabal fructus (Sägepalmenfrüchte). *Bundesanzeiger*. 1989 Mar 2; rev 1990 Feb 1; 1991 Jan 17.
29. Braeckman J. The extract of *Serenoa repens* in the treatment of benign prostatic hyperplasia: a multicenter open study. *Curr Ther Res*. 1994 Jul; 55: 776–85.
30. Monographie: Marrubii herba (Andornkraut). *Bundesanzeiger*. 1990 Feb 1.
31. Monographie: Cratageus (Weissdorn). *Bundesanzeiger*. 1984 Jan 3; rev 1988 May 5.
32. Foster S. *Garlic*: Allium sativum. Botanical Series 311. Austin, Tex: American Botanical Council; 1991: 1–7.
33. Monographie: Allii sativi bulbus (Knoblauchzwiebel). *Bundesanzeiger*. 1988 Jul 6.
34. Foster S. *Ginkgo*: Ginkgo biloba. Botanical Series 304. Austin, Tex: American Botanical Council; 1991: 1–7.
35. Kleijnen J, Knipschild P. *Ginkgo biloba* for cerebral insufficiency. *Br J Clin Pharmacol*. 1992 Oct; 34: 352–8.
36. Warburton DM. Clinical psychopharmacology of *Ginkgo biloba* extract. In: Fünfgeld EW, ed. *Rökan (Ginkgo biloba): Recent Results in Pharmacology and Clinic*. Berlin: Springer-Verlag; 1988: 327–45.
37. Liviero L et al. Antimutagenic activity of procyanidins from *Vitis vinifera*. *Fitoterapia*. 1994; 65: 203–9.
38. *Lawrence Rev Nat Prod*. 1991 Feb.
39. Foster S. *Valerian*: Valeriana officinalis. Botanical Series 312. Austin, Tex: American Botanical Council; 1991: 1–8.
40. Monographie: Valerianae radix (Baldrianwurzel). *Bundesanzeiger*. 1985 May 15.
41. Harrer G, Sommer H. Treatment of mild/moderate depressions with hypericum. *Phytomedicine*. 1994; 1: 3–8.
42. Monographie: Hyperici herba (Johanniskraut). *Bundesanzeiger*. 1984 Dec 5; rev 1989 Mar 2.
43. Foster S. *Feverfew*: Tanacetum parthenium. Botanical Series 310. Austin, Tex: American Botanical Council; 1991: 1–8.
44. Awang DVC et al. Parthenolide content of feverfew (*Tanacetum parthenium*) assessed by HPLC and ^{1}H-NMR spectroscopy. *J Nat Prod*. 1991 Nov–Dec; 54: 1516–21.
45. Heptinstall S et al. Parthenolide content and bioactivity of feverfew (*Tanacetum parthenium* (L.) Schultz-Bip.). Estimation of commercial and authenticated feverfew products. *J Pharm Pharmacol*. 1992 May; 44: 391–5.
46. Monographie: Cimicifugae racemosae rhizoma (Cimicifugawurzelstock). *Bundesanzeiger*. 1989 Mar 2.
47. Wollenweber E, Mann K. Flavonols from fruits of Vitex agnus castus. *Planta Med*. 1983 Jun; 48: 126–7.
48. Görler K, Oehlke D, Soicke H. Iridoidführung von *Vitex agnus-castus*. *Planta Med*. 1985 Dec; 51: 530–1.
49. Foster S. *Chaste tree*: Vitex agnus-castus. Botanical Series 315. Austin, Tex: American Botanical Council. In press.
50. Monographie: Agni casti fructus (Keuschlammfrüchte). *Bundesanzeiger*. 1985 May 15; replaced 1992 Dec 2.
51. Horrobin DF. Gamma linolenic acid, an intermediate in essential fatty acid metabolism with potential as an ethical pharmaceutical and as a food. *Rev Contemp Pharmacother*. 1990; 1(1): 1–41.
52. Briggs CJ. Evening primrose. *Can Pharm J*. 1986 May; 119: 248–54.
53. Monographie: Hamamelidis folium et cortex (Hamamelisblätter und -rinde). *Bundesanzeiger*. 1985 Aug 21; rev 1990 Mar 13.
54. Heggers JP, Pelley RP, Robson MC. Beneficial effects of *Aloe* in wound healing. *Phytother Res*. 1993 Spring special issue; 7: S48–S52.
55. Bassett IB, Pannowitz DL, Barnetson RStC. A comparative study of tea-tree oil versus benzoyl peroxide in the treatment of acne. *Med J Aust*. 1990; 153: 455–8.
56. Foster S. *Goldenseal*: Hydrastis canadensis. Botanical Series 309. Austin, Tex: American Botanical Council; 1991: 1–8.
57. Foster S. Goldenseal masking of drug tests. *HerbalGram*. 1989 Fall; (21): 7, 35.
58. Wöbling RH, Leonhardt K. Local therapy of herpes simplex with dried extract from *Melissa officinalis*. *Phytomedicine*. 1994; 1: 25–31.
59. Foster S. *Asian ginseng*: Panax ginseng. Botanical Series 303. Austin, Tex: American Botanical Council; 1991: 1–7.
60. Ng TB, Yeung HW. Scientific basis of the therapeutic effects of ginseng. In: Steiner RP, ed. *Folk Medicine, the Art and the*

Science. Washington, DC: American Chemical Society; 1986: 139–52.

61. Shibata S et al. Chemistry and pharmacology of *Panax*. In: Wagner H, Hikino H, Farnsworth NR, eds. *Economic and Medicinal Plant Research*. Vol 1. Orlando, Fla: Academic Press; 1985: 217–84.
62. Monographie: Ginseng radix (Ginsengwurzel). *Bundesanzeiger*. 1991 Jan 17.
63. Foster S. *Siberian ginseng*: Eleutherococcus senticosus. Botanical Series 302. Austin, Tex: American Botanical Council; 1991: 1–7.
64. Farnsworth NR et al. Siberian ginseng (*Eleutherococcus senticosus*): current status as an adaptogen. In: Wagner H, Hikino H, Farnsworth NR, eds. *Economic and Medicinal Plant Research*. Vol 1. Orlando, Fla: Academic Press; 1985: 155–215.
65. Monographie: Eleutherococci radix (Eleutherococcus-senticosus-Wurzel). *Bundesanzeiger*. 1991 Jan 17.
66. Foster S. Echinacea: The purple coneflowers. Botanical Series 301. Austin, Tex: American Botanical Council; 1991: 1–7.
67. Bauer R, Wagner H. Echinacea species as potential immunostimulatory drugs. In: Wagner H, Farnsworth NR, eds. *Economic and Medicinal Plant Research*. Vol 5. Orlando, Fla: Academic Press; 1991: 253–320.
68. Bräunig B, Dorn M, Knick E. Echinaceae purpureae radix: zur Stärkung der körpereigenen Abwehr bei grippalen Infekten. *Z Phytother*. 1992 Feb 15; 13: 7–13.
69. Schoneberger D. Einfluss der immunostimulierenden Wirkung von Preßsaft aus Herba Echinaceae purpureae auf Verlauf und Schweregrad von Erkältungskrankheiten. *Forum Immunologie*. 1992; 8: 2–11.
70. Monographie: Echinaceae purpureae herba (Purpursonnenhutkraut). *Bundesanzeiger*. 1989 Mar 2.
71. Monographie: Echinaceae purpureae radix (Purpursonnenhutwurzel). *Bundesanzeiger*. 1992 Aug 29.
72. Monographie: Echinaceae angustifoliae/ -pallidae herba (schmalblättriges Sonnenhutkraut/blassfarbenes Kegelblumenkraut); Echinacea angustifoliae radix (schmalblättrige Sonnenhutwurzel). *Bundesanzeiger*. 1992 Aug 29.
73. Monographie: Echinaceae pallidae radix (blassfarbene Kegelblumenwurzel). *Bundesanzeiger*. 1992 Aug 29.

CHAPTER 36

Smoking Cessation Products

Jack E. Fincham

Questions to ask in patient assessment and counseling

- *Are you currently a smoker? If so, how long have you smoked? How many cigarettes do you smoke per day?*
- *Have you tried to stop smoking before? If so, which smoking cessation methods did you try? If not, are you ready to stop smoking now? Have you talked with your physician about your desire to stop smoking?*
- *Are you interested in trying nicotine polacrilex therapy? If so, do you understand how to use the product? Are you aware that you cannot use nicotine polacrilex if you continue to smoke cigarettes, pipes, or cigars; use snuff; chew tobacco; or use nicotine prescription products (nicotine transdermal systems or nicotine nasal spray)?*
- *(If the patient is a woman) Are you pregnant or breast-feeding?*
- *Do you have heart disease or an irregular heart beat, or have you had a recent heart attack? Do you have high blood pressure not controlled with medication?*
- *Do you have, or have you had, esophagitis or peptic ulcer disease?*
- *Do you have diabetes? If so, do you use insulin to treat it?*
- *Do you have mouth or jaw problems such as active temporomandibular joint disease?*
- *Do you take prescription medications to treat asthma or depression?*
- *What other prescription or nonprescription medications are you currently taking?*

Despite more than 30 years of accumulative, substantial evidence describing the negative health effects of cigarette smoking on US society, smoking remains a highly promoted addiction. Although the percentage of adults who smoke has dropped to approximately 25% and the percentage of work sites that restrict or prohibit smoking has risen over 50%, many individuals still take up smoking and remain smokers for a long time.[1] Even though progress has been made in reducing smoking, much remains to be accomplished. For example, the estimated number of cigarettes sold in the United States in 1994 was equal to that of 1960: 480 billion.[2] These statistics are disturbing, especially considering that the percentage of smokers in the US population has decreased dramatically in 35 years. Based on the number of smokers in 1994, each smoker's per capita consumption of cigarettes was 2,493 cigarettes. Estimates place the number of smokers in 1996 at more than 55 million—more than at any other period.[3]

Pharmacokinetics of Nicotine

To become a nonsmoker, the individual must overcome the powerful addiction to nicotine. Tobacco use is a form of addiction that has effects comparable to opioid or narcotic addiction. These effects include euphoria during use and withdrawal symptoms after cessation of product use.[4] Traditionally, a reference to drugs of abuse implied substances such as heroin, morphine, cocaine, or alcohol. Nicotine, however, is also an addictive drug of abuse, and, as such, treatment should address nicotine-related withdrawal symptoms.[5] These symptoms have been referred to in terms normally reserved for the illicit drugs just mentioned: irritability, impatience, anxiety, confusion, impaired concentration, and/or restlessness.[6]

Nicotine acts as an agonist to nicotinic receptors in the peripheral and central nervous systems, producing both stimulant and depressant phases of action on all autonomic ganglia. The physiologic response to a nicotine dose delivered through a cigarette is almost immediate. Within seconds of inhaling the smoke, nicotine enters the pulmonary venous circulation and is taken to the heart where it subsequently is carried through internal carotid and anterior cerebral vessels to the brain. Tolerance to the effects of nicotine use may be caused by desensitization of nicotinic receptors at both the central and peripheral synapses.[7]

Addiction to nicotine is difficult to overcome even after a period of successful abstinence. Research has shown that relapse can occur years after cessation of use because of the complex character of nicotine addiction.[8] Maintaining cessation remains a difficult task for many individuals regardless of the smoking cessation method used.[9] Few individuals are successful in their first attempt; in fact, smoking cessation may be regarded as a cycle in which the individual smoker has to try several times to stop smoking before achieving that goal permanently.[10]

Consequences of Smoking

Financial Impact

Cigarette smoking is the most prevalent, modifiable risk factor for increased morbidity and mortality in the United States and perhaps the world.[11] In 1996 dollars, the direct and indirect costs associated with US cigarette consumption exceeded $100 billion. Smokers use the health care system at least 50% more often than do nonsmokers.[12–14] Health insurance coverage for the treatment of nicotine addiction remains sporadic; only seven states have third-party payers of medical care that offer reimbursement for such treatment.[15]

Social Impact

The issue of smoking is further compounded by a barrage of tobacco advertisements (eg, print, audio, video, billboards, clothing) that bombard the American public. Widespread advertisements entice nonsmokers to become smokers as well as encourage smokers to continue. Cigarette smoking remains a heavily promoted behavior; cigarette manufacturers spend more than $3 billion a year to promote nicotine addiction.[16] Many of the unwitting targets for this advertising blitz are the youth of our society. Studies have indicated that 25% of elementary school age children have smoked, and 12% have used smokeless tobacco. Children who use alcohol, cigarettes, and smokeless tobacco are also more likely to use other substances of abuse.[17]

Impact on Health and Existing Disease States

Cigarette smoking has a pervasive negative effect on countless health and disease states. It is the chief avoidable cause of death in the United States. Further, more adverse effects are being identified; discussion of some of the more common effects follows.

Active and Passive Smoking Mortality

The number of smokers dying each year from tobacco-related sequelae related to cardiovascular disease, pulmonary disease, and cancer is increasing. In the United States, smoking-related deaths are in excess of 500,000 each year, accounting for 16% of all deaths. The health risks of smoking are directly proportional to the number of cigarettes smoked per day, the number of years of cigarette smoking, and the amount of smoke inhaled. Smokers' risk for sudden cardiac death is two to four times greater than that of nonsmokers.[18] Unfortunately, these risks are not confined to only smokers: nonsmokers are affected by secondhand smoke (sidestream smoke); they, in effect, become passive smokers when exposed to cigarette smoke. Studies have indicated the association between cardiovascular mortality and passive smoking.[19] A recent report by the US Environmental Protection Agency estimated that second-hand cigarette smoke kills 53,000 nonsmokers per year and reported that cigarette smoke is a major cause of indoor air pollution.[20] The current public debate concerning passive smoking will only intensify in coming years as more links between passive smoking and various diseases are identified.

Cardiovascular Morbidity

Nicotine affects the cardiovascular system by increasing the blood pressure, stimulating the heart rate, inducing electrocardiographic changes (nonspecific ST and T wave changes, an increased conduction velocity, a propensity to arrhythmias), exacerbating angina in coronary patients, and diminishing left ventricular performance in coronary patients.[21]

Cancer

The US surgeon general's initial warning of the health risks of smoking, issued in 1994, was based on the correlation between cigarette smoking and lung cancer. Since that time many types of cancer have been linked to smoking, including bladder, breast, cervical, esophageal, kidney, laryngeal, lip, liver, lung, nasal, oral, pancreatic, pharyngeal, prostatic, skin, gastric, tongue, and tracheal.[22,23] These cancers have been shown to occur in active smokers. Several of the cancers (breast, cervical, lung) have been shown to occur also in passive smokers. In men the leading cause of smoking-related cancer mortality is lung cancer. For the past 40 years, the leading cause of smoking-related cancer mortality in women has been breast cancer; however, by the early 1990s, smoking-related lung cancer had overtaken breast cancer as the leading cause.

Respiratory Effects of Smoking

The respiratory effects of smoking were among the first to be quantified. As early as the 1870s, the negative effects of smoking upon chronic obstructive pulmonary disease (COPD) were reported. At present, cigarette smoking is the chief avoidable cause of COPD.[23] In fact, 80–90% of COPD is caused by cigarette smoking. Smokers have a higher prevalence of cough and greater production of phlegm in comparison with nonsmokers. Further, cigarette smoking is the major cause of COPD deaths in the United States. Rates of COPD mortality are greater in male smokers than in female smokers, reflecting the greater consumption of cigarettes by men.

Lung diseases resulting from smoking and/or conditions affected by smoking include allergies, asthma, bronchitis, emphysema, persistent cough, and pneumonia. In the large airways, smoking increases mucus secretion, cough, and sputum production, whereas it produces inflammation, ulceration, and squamous metaplasia in the smaller airways. These effects lead to fibrosis and airway narrowing.[24]

The most common symptoms related to passive smoking are eye irritation, headaches, cough, nasal irritation, wheezing, sore throat, and hoarseness.[25] Perhaps the most profound effect is on the lungs and respiratory system. In comparison with children of nonsmokers, children of smokers have higher rates of respiratory tract infections, pneumonia, wheezing, sore throats, asthma, and bronchitis.

Effects on Pregnancy

Smoking during pregnancy is harmful to the health of both mother and newborn. The adverse effects of smoking on pregnancy include miscarriages, full-term low birth-

TABLE 1 Selected disease states adversely affected by smoking

Disease state	Effect of smoking
Allergies[a]	Exacerbated allergic symptoms
Angina pectoris[a]	Increased angina symptomatology; more frequent attacks
Cataracts (posterior subcapsular)	Increased incidence of cataracts and lens opacities in moderate to heavy smoking
Chronic obstructive pulmonary disease[a]	Increased incidence of bronchitis, emphysema, asthma, and other respiratory disorders; limited daily activities; decreased tolerance for exercise; decreased quality of life
Depression	Common factors (stress, anxiety, etc) predispose individuals to both smoking and depressive symptomatology
Diabetes mellitus	Impaired glycemic control; increased gluconeogenesis
Graves' disease	Greatly increased risk for Graves' ophthalmopathy
Hypertension[a] (in smokers)	Elevated blood pressure
Gastrointestinal disease, infections, etc	Increased incidence of peptic ulcer disease; delayed ulcer healing; increased susceptibility to *Helicobacter pylori* infection
Periodontal disease	Negative impact on oral health
Peripheral vascular disease	Increased incidence of deep vein thromboses; intermittent claudication

[a]Active and passive (ie, those exposed to secondhand or sidestream smoke) smokers experience this effect.

weights, perinatal deaths, birth defects, and preterm births. The occurrence of sudden infant death syndrome (SIDS) has also been causally linked to parental smoking behavior.[26]

Other Diseases

Other disease states that are influenced by smoking[27–35] include allergies, Alzheimer's disease, cataracts, depression, diabetes, gastrointestinal disease (ulcers), Graves' ophthalmopathy, periodontal disease, and peripheral vascular disease (Table 1). Some of these relationships are presently tenuous; for example, the data linking Alzheimer's disease and smoking need further clarification and amplification. Other relationships, however, are firmly established (eg, allergies, angina, cardiovascular disease, congestive heart failure, hypertension, peripheral vascular disease). Still other relationships (eg, ulcers, other gastrointestinal disease) are influenced by factors such as alcohol consumption, eating habits, and duration of both the medical condition and smoking. Finally, diabetes is influenced by many factors: stress, diet, alcohol consumption, and smoking. Because nicotine can stimulate carbohydrate metabolism, diabetes is much harder to control in the smoker.

Effects on Drug Therapy

It may be difficult to distinguish the effect of smoking on disease states from its effect on the drugs used to treat the disease. Because of these dual effects, patients must be made aware of the influence of smoking on many physiologic, therapeutic, and disease state processes. Many interactions between smoking and medications have been identified. One interaction, the effect of smoking on drug metabolism, is well documented. The primary mechanism for interactions appears to be induction of hepatic microsomal enzymes by compounds present in tobacco smoke. The medications affected by smoking and the subsequent effects include[36–39]:

- *Analgesics*: decreased efficacy of acetaminophen and nonsteroidal anti-inflammatory drugs, resulting in the need for larger doses to achieve the desired effect;
- *Anticoagulants (heparin, sodium warfarin)*: increased platelet activity, resulting in diminished efficacy of the anticoagulants;
- *Cardiovascular agents (beta blockers, calcium channel blockers, furosemide and other loop-type diuretics, thiazide diuretics)*: decreased activity of the drugs, making the underlying conditions more difficult to treat;
- *Estrogens (estrogen replacements for postmenopausal women, oral contraceptives containing estrogens)*: increased risk in female smokers for thromboembolic disorders (eg, stroke, myocardial infarct, deep vein thromboses);
- *H_2-receptor antagonists (cimetidine, famotidine, nizatidine, ranitidine)*: increased acid production in the gut, resulting in decreased or negated effect of the H_2-receptor antagonists;
- *Insulin*: decreased subcutaneous insulin absorption, possibly requiring a decrease in insulin dosage;
- *Psychotropics (barbiturates, benzodiazepines, phenothiazines, and tricyclic antidepressants)*: decreased efficacy, delayed effects, or increased dose required;
- *Theophylline*: increased metabolism of theophylline, requiring increased doses because of the decreased half-life of theophylline and its derivatives;
- *Vitamins*: decreased levels of vitamin C.

Alternate therapy may be available for some patients who cannot stop smoking. For example, the ulcer patient could instead take sucralfate; it does not influence acid production but rather coats the site of ulceration with a spongy film, thus allowing the ulcerated lesion to heal. The continuance of smoking, however, will delay the healing. Patients with other conditions who stop smoking may need to decrease (eg, insulin) or increase (eg, theophylline) their medication dosages.

The precise mechanisms of these interactions remain unclear. It is not known whether the effect is caused by tobacco substrates (nicotine or others) or perhaps other byproducts of smoking (carbon monoxide). Nevertheless, it is important for patients to be aware of what is occurring and why. They may try to stop smoking if they can be convinced that it is futile to try to influence disease states and attendant drug therapies while continuing to smoke. Despite a drug's demonstrated efficacy in nonsmokers or appropriate compliance by the smoking patient, the negative health effects of smoking and the associated lack of response to the drug can eventually overcome and negate any drug therapy.

Treatment

Nicotine is similar to other addictive substances because of its psychoactive effect, compulsive use, and requirement to take more of the substance over time to obtain the same level of "high."[5] Henningfield and Nemeth-Coslett[5] have noted that in such addictions the chemical factor is in control of behavior, and treatment is helped by dealing with the drug-related factors. In the case of nicotine, the withdrawal symptoms that occur upon abstinence must be dealt with if smoking cessation is to be successful.

The response to withdrawal symptoms is highly variable among patients and depends on length of exposure (ie, how long a smoker), dose (ie, how much is smoked per day), and other unquantifiable effects. As with many other drugs, the individual physiologic response to nicotine varies from person to person. Thus, the addiction and response to nicotine are also patient specific. Some smokers can stop and suffer virtually no withdrawal symptoms; others are dramatically influenced by withdrawal symptoms. The recognition of this interindividual variation and subsequent occurrence of withdrawal symptoms is the key to pharmacists and others in helping patients successfully stop smoking. Successful programs address both the physical and psychologic aspects of nictotine addiction. None of the interventions will work optimally unless the smoker desires to stop smoking and maintain cessation.

Behavioral Interventions

Behavioral interventions used in smoking cessation therapies have included aversion therapy, educational programs, group therapy, hypnosis, and self-help literature. The success rate for each of these modalities has varied, and, as would be expected, is patient dependent.[40]

Some smokers can stop smoking through behavioral modification alone. Programs have been developed to help smokers learn to avoid certain stimuli to smoking. Patients are counseled to deal with the urge to smoke after a meal by taking a walk or doing exercise and to practice stress management as a method of controlling responses to stimuli, such as anxiety, that normally resulted in the patient smoking. Patients are also advised to avoid places or environments in which they usually smoked and to substitute alternate behaviors when the urge to smoke occurs. However, the more highly addicted smoker usually needs pharmacologic assistance.[40]

Self-Help Literature

This form of educational program has been used by various associations and societies (eg, American Cancer Society, American Heart Association, American Lung Association) to help smokers grapple with the periods before, during, and after smoking cessation. Literature and/or brochures are used to help smokers understand the reasons to stop smoking and how to do it. Again, success varies and is dependent upon individual motivations. Phone numbers for each of these organizations are listed in telephone directories in most communities.

Nicotine Replacement Therapy

Currently, three dosage forms of nicotine replacement are approved by the Food and Drug Administration (FDA): (1) nicotine transdermal systems (prescription only), (2) nicotine nasal spray (prescription only), and (3) nicotine polacrilex (available without a prescription). The initial intent of nicotine replacement therapy is to substitute pharmacologically dosed nicotine for "smoked" nicotine. Through a tapering of nicotine doses, the patient is gradually weaned from higher doses. Because the nicotine addiction is decreased, the smoker should have successfully modified behavior to the point that environmental and behavioral stimuli to smoke are no longer effective. Pharmacologic treatment with nicotine replacement therapy should always be accompanied by behavioral counseling and patient counseling.

Although replacing nicotine from smoking with a pharmacologic source and dose reduces the craving and withdrawal symptoms, the pharmacologic dose usually does not relieve these symptoms to the same degree as smoked nicotine. Thus, any smoker who expects the same "smoking effect" from nicotine replacement products may be disappointed.[41] Nicotine replacement therapy is designed to be used short term (6 months or less) to reduce the magnitude of the nicotine withdrawal syndrome experienced by smokers who stop smoking "cold turkey."

Currently, there is controversy about the use of nicotine replacement therapy during pregnancy. Cigarette smoking is a preventable cause of fetal morbidity and mortality; however, the pharmacologic adjuncts to smoking cessation currently available are contraindicated during pregnancy. Benowitz[42] has recommended examining in clinical settings the use of nicotine replacement in pregnant women who smoke, particularly in those who smoke 20 or more cigarettes per day and who have not been successful with behavioral smoking cessation therapies.

Nicotine Polacrilex

In 1996, the FDA approved nonprescription use of nicotine polacrilex resin[43] (see product table "Smoking Cessation Products"); this agent was first approved for prescription use in the United States in 1984. When used correctly, nicotine polacrilex (Nicorette) has been shown to reduce withdrawal symptoms and increase cessation rates when compared with the use of a placebo. Patients must understand how to use the resin dosage form (gum), how much to use per day, how long to use it, and how to stop use gradually. Strict patient compliance and cessation of product use are required if patients are to become free of nicotine use. Ensuring patient compliance with any therapy is difficult, let alone a therapy such as this that requires initial dosing of 12–24 units per day.

Dosage Nicotine polacrilex is available in two package sizes: a starter kit containing 108 units and a supplemental package containing 48 units. Each package size is available in either the 2-mg or 4-mg dose. The 4-mg dosage packages are targeted to those individuals who smoke more than 24 cigarettes per day.

Usage Guidelines The Nicorette package contains a cassette tape that provides instructions for use as well as a printed user's guide. The FDA considers these items to be part of the product labeling. Directions for use include the following[44]:

- Stop smoking completely when you begin using this product.
- Before using this product, read the enclosed user's guide and use the product according to the directions provided.
- Do not eat or drink for 15 minutes before using this product or while using it.
- Use this product according to the following 12-week schedule:
  - *Weeks 1–6*: Use one piece every 1–2 hours;
  - *Weeks 7–9*: Use one piece every 2–4 hours;
  - *Weeks 10–12*: Use one piece every 4–8 hours.
- Do not use more than 24 pieces a day.
- Stop using the product at the end of week 12. If you still feel the need for its use, talk with your physician.

Precautions Several of the warning statements that appear on the product labeling are as follows[44]:

- If you are pregnant or nursing a baby, seek the advice of a health professional before using this product.
- Do not use this product if you continue to smoke, chew tobacco, use snuff, or use a nicotine patch or other nicotine-containing product.
- Consult a physician before using this product if you:
  - Are under 18 years of age;
  - Have heart disease or an irregular heartbeat or have had a recent heart attack (Nicotine can increase your heart rate);
  - Have high blood pressure not controlled with medication (Nicotine can increase blood pressure);
  - Have a history of, or currently have, esophagitis or peptic ulcer disease;
  - Take insulin for diabetes;
  - Take prescription medications for depression or asthma. (Your prescription dose may need to be adjusted.)
- Stop using this product and see your physician if you have:
  - Mouth, teeth, or jaw problems;
  - Irregular heartbeat or palpitations;
  - Symptoms of nicotine overdose such as nausea, vomiting, dizziness, weakness, and rapid heartbeat.

Nicotine Transdermal Systems

During late 1991 and early 1992, four forms of prescription nicotine transdermal systems (NTS) were approved by the FDA for smoking cessation therapy. Only the United States still classifies nicotine transdermal products as prescription products. However, on April 19, 1996, an FDA advisory panel voted that two NTS products, Nicotrol and Nicoderm, should be available for nonprescription use. Although not bound by advisory panels' decisions, the FDA usually follows their advice. At the time this book went to press, NTS products were still available only by prescription.

If an NTS is used, the patient must understand the purpose of the patches, their proper application, and the appropriate time to stop using them.

Nicotine Nasal Spray

In March 1996, the FDA approved nicotine nasal spray for use as a prescription smoking cessation therapy. The patient using this therapy must understand the purpose of the spray, its proper use, and the appropriate method of stopping its use (ie, stopping use gradually at the appropriate time).

The Pharmacist's Role in Smoking Cessation

It is professionally important for pharmacists to encourage and counsel patients who smoke or use other forms of nicotine to become nicotine free. Pharmacists may be reluctant to counsel patients to stop smoking because they fear alienating them. However, as health professionals, pharmacists should not fear letting their patients understand that they care enough about them to encourage this important health promotion and disease prevention activity. Pharmacists can set a good example by not using nicotine and by discouraging colleagues from doing so as well. The sale of tobacco products in pharmacies has been much debated and remains an ethical and individual decision for pharmacists. Making the pharmacy area a smoke-free area also establishes a good example. Signs and reminders indicating that the area is smoke free can communicate the message without offending anyone. For patients who indicate that they do not want to stop smoking, pressing the issue can only lead to potential frustration. However, for the current smoker, even one who professes not to want to stop smoking, counseling on the benefits of smoking cessation should be performed tactfully at every pharmacist-patient encounter. This practice demonstrates a genuine concern for the patient.

Because of pharmacists' accessibility, patients view

them as trusted sources of information on any number of health concerns. Patients who smoke will not be surprised when a pharmacist asks questions about their nicotine use and counsels them to stop its use. Information about nicotine use should be noted on patient profiles. If a patient expresses a desire to stop nicotine use, pharmacists should advise them of available options.

Studies have shown that 60–70% of current smokers would like to stop smoking and that 70–90% would consider stopping.[45] Further, receiving advice on smoking cessation in lay terms from a health professional would increase the number of individuals who stop smoking by 5–10%.[45] Although numerous other studies have indicated the importance of health professionals as smoking cessation counselors, many patients have noted that no health professional counseled them to stop smoking.[46]

Patient Counseling

The success of any nicotine reduction therapy depends on a behavioral change in the patient. The patient must truly desire to stop smoking and must alter habits and behaviors to accommodate a nicotine-free existence. Support and encouragement (from family, friends, and health care providers) and proper patient counseling are also important in the patient achieving success with any of the smoking cessation therapies. When a patient begins to use these nicotine reduction therapies, use of other forms of nicotine must stop.

Pharmacists can significantly improve patients' cessation rates by providing consultation on behavioral modification and encouraging patients to join a class on smoking cessation behavioral modification. The effect of pharmacists' counseling on smoking cessation has been studied. One study of patients using nicotine transdermal therapy was conducted in more than 6,500 pharmacies with more than 40,000 patients participating. The data showed a 90% increase in cessation rates when compared with published cessation rates that did not involve counseling intervention.[47] Patients who were convinced by their pharmacist to attend a behavioral modification class showed a 175% increase in cessation rates when compared with the published rates that did not involve behavioral counseling.[48] A pharmacoeconomic analysis of several smoking cessation interventions, including pharmacists' consultation (at a rate of $75 for five interventions), showed that smoking cessation therapy consisting of nicotine transdermal systems, consultation with pharmacists, and participation in a behavioral modification class would be the most cost-beneficial.[48]

Specific counseling tips on the proper use of nicotine polacrilex include the following[49]:

- Do not start using nicotine polacrilex until you have stopped smoking.
- Do not smoke cigarettes or use other forms of nicotine (eg, nicotine patches, snuff, chewing tobacco, pipes, cigars, etc) while using nicotine polacrilex.
- Be aware that nicotine polacrilex is purposely made not to taste like ordinary chewing gum. It is a dose delivery device, not a chewing gum.
- Be aware that it may take several days to adjust to the product's taste and the special manner in which it should be used.
- If acidic drinks (eg, fruit juices, cola drinks, coffee) or foods (eg, catsup, soy sauce, or salsa or hot sauce) have been consumed, rinse the mouth with water before placing the gum in the mouth.
- To take advantage of the product's slow release formula, use the bite-park-bite rotation method:
  - Bite each piece slowly (10–15 times) until a peppery taste or tingling sensation occurs;
  - When this sensation begins, place the gum between the upper or lower cheek and gums for approximately 1 minute;
  - After the peppery taste fades, retrieve the dosing piece and repeat the process. (Keep the dosing piece in the mouth for approximately 30 minutes.)
- If biting the gum becomes tedious, push the gum from the outside of the cheek with a finger to expose a new surface of the gum to the saliva.
- Be aware that chewing the gum too quickly will result in an unpleasant taste caused by too much nicotine in the saliva and, if the nicotine is swallowed, may cause effects similar to those produced by excess smoking (eg, nausea [especially if the stomach is empty], irritation of the throat, hiccups, light-headedness.)
- If jaw ache or belching occurs, combine the nicotine polacrilex gum with a small amount of sugar-free gum to soften the nicotine-containing gum and reduce the swallowing of air. Use the bite-park-bite rotation method with the gum mixture.
- Take the product on a scheduled rather than an as-needed basis.
- Follow the dosage regimen carefully and reduce the dosage at the recommended intervals.
- If a problem or severe symptoms develop, report them to a pharmacist or physician.
- Carry at least one full sleeve of nicotine polacrilex (12 doses per sleeve) at all times. Keep it in the same place where cigarettes were normally kept (eg, shirt pocket or purse).
- Do not expose the product to extreme temperatures (ie, place in a glove box, next to a source of heat, etc).
- Remember to keep an extra sleeve of the product in the car, at work, and/or by the telephone.
- Keep this product out of the reach of children or pets.

Parking the gum between the cheek and gum permits nicotine in the saliva to be absorbed into the bloodstream through the buccal mucosa. If the nicotine is swallowed with saliva or washed down when drinking a hot or cold liquid, it will not be effective and may cause side effects such as heartburn, upset stomach, or hiccups. A basic pH is required for the nicotine to be properly released from the dosing piece into the saliva and then through the buccal mucosa. Thus, the consumption of acidic liquids must be avoided while the dosing piece is in the mouth.

Nicotine polacrilex is sugar free and, although somewhat sticky, suitable for use by many denture wearers. If additional gum is mixed with the nicotine polacrilex, a sugar-free gum should be used because sugar also produces acidity in the mouth and would hinder absorption of the nicotine.

If the patient complains of hiccups, nausea, an upset stomach, or a sore throat, the product is probably not being used properly. The patient needs to be counseled not to chew the dosing piece like regular chewing gum but to park and retrieve the dose of nicotine polacrilex sporadically. After a few days, the patient will automatically adjust the rate of dosing through the park and retrieval process.

After a patient completes a course of nicotine replacement therapy, the pharmacist must be prepared to support the patient through discontinuance of the therapy. The true measure of success lies in examining the cessation rate after the patient is weaned from the product. The cessation rate can be improved through appropriate behavioral counseling of the former smoker. Pharmacists should help the patient to understand the following:

- Behaviors to avoid that traditionally reinforced the urge to smoke;
- Places or activities to avoid in which the individual previously would smoke;
- Social and psychologic stimulators to avoid that previously influenced smoking.

Case Studies

Case 36–1

Patient Complaint/History

IJ, a 35-year-old female, presents to the pharmacist holding a carton of cigarettes and a 108-unit 4-mg package of Nicorette. Numerous prior attempts to help the patient stop smoking were unsuccessful. When questioned about the Nicorette, the patient indicates that she wishes to try to stop smoking "a little at a time" using this product. On separate occasions she previously tried a 24-hour and a 16-hour NTS without success. The patient admits that she just could not stop smoking, even when using the NTS.

A review of IJ's patient profile reveals the following current prescriptions: propranolol 40 mg one tablet bid for hypertension (#60 filled monthly) and Nordette one tablet daily (#28 filled monthly). While filling the oral contraceptive prescription, the pharmacist notes the presence of tobacco flakes behind the tape covering the label on the container.

Clinical Considerations/Strategies

The following considerations/strategies are provided to aid the reader in (1) determining whether treatment of the patient's condition with nonprescription drugs is warranted, (2) selecting the appropriate nonprescription medication, and (3) developing a patient counseling strategy to ensure optimal therapeutic outcomes:

- Counsel the patient on potential interactions between smoking and her current medications.
- Assess the willingness of the patient to stop smoking.
- Determine why the NTS therapies might have failed.
- Develop a pharmaceutical care plan for the patient's smoking cessation efforts and continue to educate and counsel the patient on smoking cessation options.
- Contact the patient's physicians and explain the pharmaceutical care plan.

Case 36–2

Patient Complaint/History

SL, a 55-year-old male, calls the pharmacy to complain of a "racing heart beat." He reports that this effect first occurred when he began using nicotine polacrilex (40 4-mg dosing pieces a day) 10 days earlier and has continued throughout the therapy. He also complains of a sore throat that occurs after he drinks his customary six cups of coffee in the morning. When questioned about the presence of other symptoms, the patient reports that he has not suffered any withdrawal symptoms to date. He wants to stay off the cigarettes; however, the racing heart beat is frightening to him.

A review of SL's patient profile reveals the following prescription medications: Theo-Dur 450 mg one tablet tid for asthma (#90 filled monthly); amoxicillin 500 mg one capsule tid for 10 days (filled 3 days earlier); Beconase AQ nasal spray 25 g two sprays in each nostril bid (filled monthly); and Claritin-D one tablet bid for 10 days (#20 filled 3 days earlier).

Clinical Considerations/Strategies

The following considerations/strategies are provided to aid the reader in (1) determining whether treatment of the patient's condition with nonprescription drugs is warranted, (2) selecting the appropriate nonprescription medication, and (3) developing a patient counseling strategy to ensure optimal therapeutic outcomes:

- Assess the probable cause of the patient's symptoms.
- Contact the patient's primary physician to explain the symptoms as described by the patient.
- Encourage the patient to come to the pharmacy for counseling.
- Review with the patient the proper dosing technique for administration of the nicotine polacrilex therapy.
- Suggest a dosage regimen and caution the patient about concurrent consumption of acidic beverages.
- Develop a pharmaceutical care plan for the patient's smoking cessation program.
- Work with the physician and the patient to determine a potential revision in the theophylline dosage.

Summary

An estimated 3 million tobacco-related deaths will occur in the world during the 1990s alone.[50] There has never been a better time for pharmacists to become involved as smoking cessation and patient advocates. Pharmacists must first identify which patients are smokers and then counsel those who wish to stop about the various options available and the success potential of each option. After a treatment plan (whatever the make-up) is started, the pharmacist should be prepared to deliver pharmaceutical care by helping the patient follow through on the therapeutic plan. Helping the smoking patient stop smoking is one of the most needed and rewarding activities for pharmacists. Encouraging smoking cessation, monitoring patients who are using pharmacologic treatment for smoking cessation, and supporting the patients throughout the withdrawal symptom stage can provide therapeutic benefits for patients, savings on health care costs, economic benefits for pharmacists, and long-term enhancement of the patients' quality of life.

References

1. Marwick C. Advocates say smoke free society eventually may result from more curbs, taxes on tobacco use. *JAMA*. 1993; 269: 724.
2. Giovino GA, Schooley MW, Zhu BP, et al. Surveillance of selected tobacco-use behaviors—United States, 1900–1994. *MMWR*. 1994; 43(SS–3): 1–43.
3. Fiore MC, Novotny TE, Pierce JP, et al. Trends in cigarette smoking in the United States: projections to the year 2000. *JAMA*. 1989; 261: 61–5.
4. Cohen C, Pickworth WB, Henningfield JE. Cigarette smoking and addiction. *Clin Chest Med*. 1991; 12(4): 701–10.
5. Henningfield JE, Nemeth-Coslett R. Nicotine dependence: interface between tobacco and tobacco-related disease. *Chest*. 1988; 93(suppl): 37S–55S.
6. Brunton SA, Henningfield JE. *Nicotine Addiction and Smoking Cessation*. New York: Medical Information Services; 1991.
7. Volle RL. Nicotine and ganglion blocking drugs. In: Smith CM, Reynard AM, eds. *Textbook of Pharmacology*. Philadelphia: WB Saunders; 1992: 119–26.
8. Cohen S, Lichtenstein E, Prochaska JO, et al. Debunking myths about self-quitting: evidence from 10 prospective studies of persons who attempted to quit smoking by themselves. *Am Psychol*. 1989; 44: 1355–65.
9. McIlvain HE, McKinney ME, Thompson AV, et al. Application of the MRFIT smoking cessation program to a healthy, mixed sex sample. *Am J Prevent Med*. 1992; 8(3): 165–70.
10. Fisher EB, Bishop DB, Goldmuntz J, et al. *Chest*. 1988; 93(2): 69S–78S.
11. Lee EW, Dalonzo GE. Cigarette smoking, nicotine addiction, and its pharmacologic treatment. *Arch Intern Med*. 1993; 153: 34–48.
12. Nixon JC, West JF. Cost reductions from a smoking policy. *Employee Benefits J*. 1989; 14(1): 26–30.
13. Weis WL. Can you afford to hire a smokers? *Personnel Administrator*. 1981; 71–8.
14. Kristein MM. Economic issues in prevention. *Prevent Med*. 1977; 6: 252–64.
15. Centers for Disease Control, State Tobacco Prevention and Control Activities. Results of the 1989–1990 association of state and territorial health officials survey final report. *MMWR*. 1991; 40(RR–11): 32.
16. Federal Trade Commission. *1988 FTC Report to Congress*. Washington, DC: US Government Printing Office; 1989.
17. Gottlieb A, Pope SK, Rickert VI, et al. Patterns of smokeless tobacco use by young adolescents. *Pediatrics*. 1993; 91(1): 75–8.
18. Public Health Service, Office on Smoking and Health. *The Health Consequences of Smoking: Cardiovascular Disease*. DHHS (PHS) Pub No 84–50204. Washington, DC: US Department of Health and Human Services; 1983.
19. Glantz SA, Parmley WW. Passive smoking and heart disease: Epidemiology, physiology, and biochemistry. *Circulation*. 1991; 83(1): 1–12.
20. Lesmes GR, Donofrio KH. Passive smoking: the medical and economic issues. *Am J Med*. 1992; 93(1A): 38S–42S.
21. Stimmel B. Cardiovascular effects of mood-altering drugs. New York: Raven Press; 1979: 200.
22. Doll R. Tobacco: an overview of health effects. In: Zaridze D, Peto R, eds. *Tobacco—A Major Health Hazard*. Lyon, France: International Agency for Research on Cancer; 1986: 11–22.
23. Public Health Service, Office on Smoking and Health. *The Health Consequences of Smoking, Cancer: A Report of the Surgeon General*. DHHS (PHS) Pub No 83–50203: Washington, DC: US Department of Health and Human Services; 1982.
24. Brunton SA. *Nicotine Addiction and Smoking Cessation*. New York: Medical Information Services; 1991: 7.
25. Eriksen MP, LeMaistre CA, Newell GR. Health hazards of passive smoking. *Ann Rev Pub Health*. 1988; 9: 47–70.
26. Haglund B, Cnattingius S. Cigarette smoking as a risk factor for sudden infant death syndrome: a population-based study. *Am J Pub Health*. 1990; 80: 29–32.
27. McGill HC. The cardiovascular pathology of smoking. *Am Heart J*. 1988; 115: 250–7.
28. Alderon MR, Lee PN, Wang R. Risks of lung cancer, chronic bronchitis, ischemic heart disease, and stroke in relation to type of cigarette smoked. *J Epidemiol Commun Health*. 1985; 39: 286–93.
29. Amler RW, Eddins DL. Cross-sectional analysis: precursors of premature death in the United States. In: Amler RW, Dull HB, eds. *Closing the Gap: The Burden of Unnecessary Illness*. New York: Oxford University Press; 1987: 181–7.
30. Lane MR, Lee SP. Recurrence of duodenal ulcer after medical treatment. *Lancet*. 1988; 1(8595): 1147–9.
31. Hankinson SE, Willett WC, Colditz GA, et al. A prospective study of cigarette smoking and risk of cataract surgery in women. *JAMA*. 1992; 268(8): 994–8.
32. Breslau N, Kilbey MM, Andreski P. Nicotine dependence and major depression—new evidence from a prospective investigation. *Arch Gen Psychiatr*. 1993; 50: 31–5.
33. Locker D, Leake JL. Risk indicators and risk markers for periodontal disease experience in older adults living independently in Ontario, Canada. *J Dent Res*. 1993; 72(1): 9–17.
34. Prummel MF, Wiersinga WM. Smoking and the risk of Graves' disease. *JAMA*. 1993; 269(4): 479–82.
35. Bateson MC. Cigarette smoking and Helicobacter pylori infection. *Postgrad Med J*. 1993; 69: 41–4.
36. Lipman A. How smoking interferes with drug therapy. *Modern Med*. 1985; 53(8): 141–2.
37. Ferguson T. *The Smoker's Book of Health: How to Keep Yourself Healthier and Reduce Your Smoking Risks*. New York: The Putnam & Grosset Group; 1987.
38. Piepho RW, Culbertson VL, Rhodes RS. Drug interactions with the calcium entry blockers. *Circulation*. 1987; 75: 191–4.
39. Deanfield J, Wright C, Krikler S, et al. Cigarette smoking and the treatment of angina with propranolol, atenolol, and nifedipene. *N Engl J Med*. 1984; 310(15): 951–4.
40. Schwartz JL. *Review and Evaluation of Smoking Cessation Methods: The United States and Canada, 1978–85*. Bethesda, Md: US Department of Health and Human Services, Public Health Service, Division of Cancer Prevention and Control, National Cancer Institute. NIH Pub No (NCI) 87–2940; 1987.
41. Kumar R, Cooke EC, Lader MH, et al. Is nicotine important in tobacco smoking? *Clin Pharm Therapeut*. 1977; 21: 520–9.
42. Benowitz NL. Nicotine replacement therapy during pregnancy. *JAMA*. 1991; 262(22): 3174–7.
43. OTC Nicorette will be available in retail stores by late spring following Feb 9 approval. *F-D-C Reports—The Tan Sheet*. Chevy Chase, Md: F-D-C Reports: 1996; 4(7): 4–5.
44. Nicorette® product and packaging information. Pittsburgh, Pa: SmithKline Beecham Consumer Healthcare, LP; 1996.

45. Coultas DB. The physician's role in smoking cessation. *Clin Chest Med.* 1991; 12(4): 755–68.

46. Haire-Joshu D, Morgan G, Fisher EB. Determinants of cigarette smoking. *Clin Chest Med.* 1991; 12(4): 711–25.

47. Smith MD, McGhan WF, Lauger GL. Pharmacist counseling and outcomes of smoking cessation. *Am Pharm.* 1995; NS35(8): 20–32.

48. McGhan WF, Smith MD. Pharmacoeconomic analysis of smoking-cessation interventions. *Am J Health-Syst Pharm.* 1996; 53: 45–52.

49. Fincham JE, Smith MC. The role of the pharmacist in smoking cessation counseling. *Drug Topics.* 1989 Jun 19: 133(suppl): 1S–24S.

50. World Health Organization, Consultative Group on Statistical Aspects of Tobacco-Related Mortality. The future worldwide health effects of current smoking patterns. Paper presented at Perth, Western Australia: Seventh World Conference on Tobacco and Health; 1990 Apr 3.

Index

Boldface entries designate either a chapter title, medical condition, therapeutic drug class, nonprescription agent, dosage form, patient population, or other major chapter topic.

Entries in regular lightface type designate subordinate chapter topics or subheads of major topics.

Italic entries in which all major words are capitalized designate product trade names.

Other italic entries designate the genus and species of plants or organisms.

The italic designations *a*, *f*, and *t* that follow a page number indicate an appendix, figure, or table, respectively.

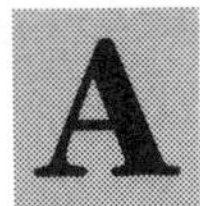

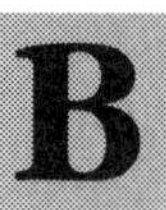

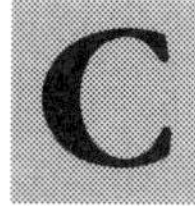

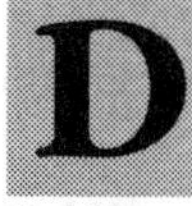

E

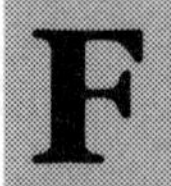

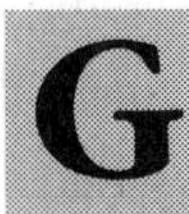

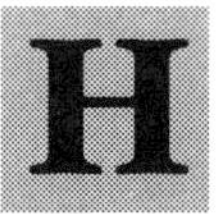

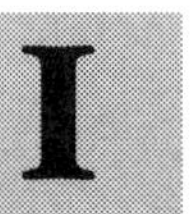

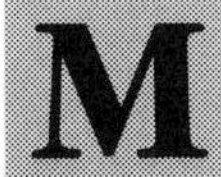

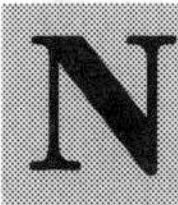

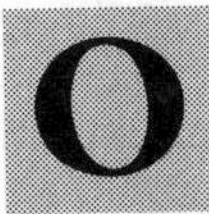

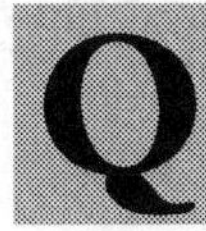

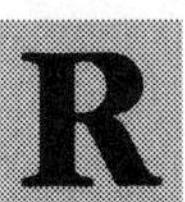

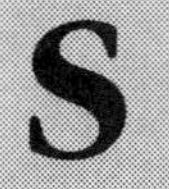

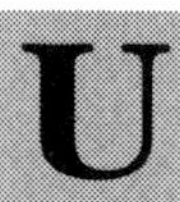

V

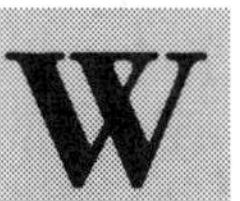

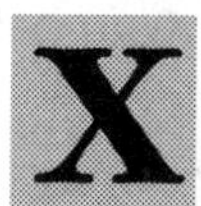

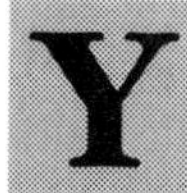

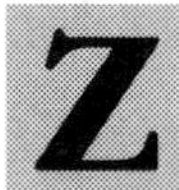